Gynecologic and Obstetric Surgery

Challenges and Management Options

The Editors donate the royalties of this book to Ammalife (UK Registered Charity 1120236: www.ammalife.org) for the advancement of non-physician clinicians (clinical officers) in Africa.

This book is dedicated to my inspirational teachers in Valalai, Idaikkadu, Paththamani, Paruthithurai, Chennai and Forest Gate, for opening the doors of curiosity, knowledge and discernment.

Arri Coomarasamy

I would like to dedicate this book to my family: Naseem, Imran, Omar and Mohsin Shafi.

Mahmood I. Shafi

My contributions to this book are dedicated to the many clinical fellows, residents, researchers and observers who have given me the impetus to continue to acquire and, more importantly, share knowledge. Otherwise, life would be rather boring.

G. Willy Davila

Gynecologic and Obstetric Surgery

Challenges and Management Options

Edited by

Arri Coomarasamy, MBChB, MD, FRCOG

Professor of Gynecology and Reproductive Medicine, College of Medical and Dental Sciences, University of Birmingham; Consultant Gynecologist and Subspecialist in Reproductive Medicine and Surgery, Birmingham Women's NHS Foundation Trust, Birmingham, UK

Mahmood I. Shafi, MB BCh, MD, DA, FRCOG

Consultant Gynecologic Surgeon and Oncologist, Cambridge University Hospitals NHS Foundation Trust, Addenbrooke's Hospital, Cambridge, UK

G. Willy Davila, MD, FACOG

Center Director, Women's Health Institute (Florida); Chairman, Department of Gynecology and Head of Section of Urogynecology and Reconstructive Pelvic Surgery, Cleveland Clinic Florida, Weston/Fort Lauderdale, Florida, USA

Kiong K. Chan, MBBS, FRCS, FRCOG

Emeritus Consultant Gynecologic Oncologist, Pan-Birmingham Gynecologic Cancer Center, City Hospital, Sandwell and West Birmingham Hospitals NHS Trust, Birmingham, UK

Section Editors

T. Justin Clark, MBChB, MD (Hons), MRCOG
Birmingham Women's NHS Foundation Trust; University of Birmingham, Birmingham, UK
Janesh Gupta, MSc, MD, FRCOG
University of Birmingham; Birmingham Women's NHS Foundation Trust, Birmingham, UK
Pallavi Latthe, MD, MRCOG
Birmingham Women's NHS Foundation Trust; University of Birmingham, Birmingham, UK
Phil Moore, MD, FRCA, FFPMRCA
Birmingham Women's NHS Foundation Trust, Birmingham, UK
Kavita Singh, MBBS, MD, FRCOG
City Hospital, Sandwell and West Birmingham Hospitals NHS Trust, Birmingham, UK

Editorial Coordinator

Helen Marie Williams, BSc (Hons)
Research Associate, College of Medical and Dental Sciences, University of Birmingham, Birmingham, UK

WILEY Blackwell

Contents

Section 7: Gynecologic Oncology
Editors: Kavita Singh, Mahmood I. Shafi, and Kiong K. Chan

Contributors

Hany Abdel-Aleem, MBBCh, MD
Faculty of Medicine, Assiut University, Assiut, Egypt

Parveen Abedin, MRCOG, DFFP, MSc
Birmingham Women's NHS Foundation Trust, Birmingham, UK

Basim Abu-Rafea, MD, FRCSC, FACOG
Dalhousie University, Halifax, Nova Scotia, Canada

Yousri Afifi, PhD, MD, MRCOG
Birmingham Women's NHS Foundation Trust, Birmingham, UK

Masoud Afnan, MBBS, FRCOG
Beijing United Family Hospital, Beijing, China

Tariq Ahmad, MA, MBBChir, FRCS, FRCS (Ed), FRCS (Plast)
Addenbrooke's Hospital, Cambridge University Hospitals NHS Foundation Trust, Cambridge, UK

Catherine Aiken, MBBChir, PhD, MRCOG
University of Cambridge, Cambridge, UK

Djavid Alleemudder, MRCOG, MRCS (Ed)
Salisbury NHS Foundation Trust, Salisbury, UK

Y. Zaki Almallah, MD, FRCS (Urol)
University Hospitals Birmingham NHS Foundation Trust, Birmingham, UK

Firas Al-Rshoud, MBBS, MD
Medical School, Hashemite University; Prince Hamza Hospital, Zarqua, Jordan

Bassel H. Al Wattar, MD, PGD
Women's Health Research Unit, Blizard Institute, Queen Mary University of London, London, UK

Margarita M. Aponte, MD
New York University Langone Medical Center, New York, USA

Sherif Awad, PhD, FRCS
School of Clinical Sciences, University of Nottingham; East Midlands Bariatric and Metabolic Institute (EMBMI), Royal Derby Hospital, Nottingham, UK

Gubby Ayida, MA, FRCOG, DM
Chelsea and Westminster Hospital NHS Foundation Trust, London, UK

John Ayuk, MD, FRCP
University Hospitals Birmingham NHS Foundation Trust; University of Birmingham, Birmingham, UK

Janos Balega, MD, MRCOG
City Hospital, Sandwell and West Birmingham Hospitals NHS Trust, Birmingham, UK

Elizabeth Ball, MD, PhD, MRCOG
Barts Health NHS Trust; Blizard Institute, Queen Mary University of London, London, UK

Moji Balogun, MBChB, MRCP, FRCR
Birmingham Women's NHS Foundation Trust, Birmingham, UK

Mohammed Belal, MA, MBBChir, FRCS (Urol)
University Hospitals Birmingham NHS Foundation Trust, Birmingham, UK

Helen Bolton, DLM, MRCOG, PhD
Hinchingbrooke Hospital, Hinchingbrooke Health Care NHS Trust, Huntingdon, UK

Jeremy Brockelsby, PhD, MRCOG
Rosie Maternity Hospital, Cambridge, UK

Claire Burton, BMedSci, BMBS, MRCOG
Portsmouth Hospitals NHS Trust, Portsmouth, UK

Jennifer Byrom, MD, BSc, MBBS, MRCOG
Birmingham Women's NHS Foundation Trust, Birmingham, UK

Sanoj Chacko, MBBS, MRCP
University Hospitals Birmingham NHS Foundation Trust, Birmingham, UK

Manas Chakrabarti, MBBS, MRCOG
Apollo Gleneagles Cancer Hospital, Kolkata, India

Kiong K. Chan, MBBS, FRCS, FRCOG
Pan-Birmingham Gynecologic Cancer Center, City Hospital, Sandwell and West Birmingham Hospitals NHS Trust, Birmingham, UK

Shiao-yng Chan, MBBChir, PhD, FRCOG
Yong Loo Lin School of Medicine, National University of Singapore; National University Hospital, Singapore

Rohan Chodankar, MBBS, MD, MRCOG
Frimley Health NHS Foundation Trust, Frimley, Surrey, UK

Anneke Chu, MBChB, BMedSci
City Hospital, Sandwell and West Birmingham Hospitals NHS Trust, Birmingham, UK

Justin Chu, MBChB, MRCOG
Birmingham Women's NHS Foundation Trust, Birmingham, UK

T. Justin Clark, MBChB, MD (Hons), MRCOG
Consultant Obstetrician and Gynecologist, Birmingham Women's NHS Foundation Trust; Honorary Professor of Obstetrics and Gynecology, University of Birmingham, Birmingham, UK

Alessandro Conforti, MD
Minimally Invasive Therapy Unit and Endoscopy Training Center, The Royal Free Hospital, London, UK

Arri Coomarasamy, MBChB, MD, FRCOG
College of Medical and Dental Sciences, University of Birmingham; Birmingham Women's NHS Foundation Trust, Birmingham, UK

Naomi S. Crouch, MBBS, MD, MRCOG
St Michael's Hospital, Bristol, UK

Justin Davies, MA, MBMChir, FRCS (Gen Surg), EBSQ (Coloproctology)
Addenbrooke's Hospital, Cambridge University Hospitals NHS Foundation Trust; University of Cambridge, Cambridge, UK

G. Willy Davila, MD, FACOG
Women's Health Institute (Florida); Cleveland Clinic Florida, Weston/Fort Lauderdale, Florida, USA

Amelia Davison, MBChB, MRCOG
Homerton University Hospital, London, UK

Joseph de Bono, BMBCh, MA, FRCP, DPhil
University Hospitals Birmingham NHS Foundation Trust, Birmingham, UK

Joanna K. Dowman, MBChB
University of Birmingham; City Hospital, Sandwell and West Birmingham Hospitals NHS Trust, Birmingham, UK

Karolynn T. Echols, MD, FACOG, FPMRS
Cooper Medical School of Rowan University and Cooper University Hospital, Camden, New Jersey, USA

Sohier Elneil, MBChB, PhD (Cantab), FRCOG
National Hospital for Neurology and Neurosurgery, University College London Hospitals NHS Foundation Trust; University College London, London, UK

Ahmed M. El-Sharkawy, MBBS, MRCS
School of Clinical Sciences, University of Nottingham, Nottingham, UK

Yaso Emmanuel, MBChB, MRCP, DPhil
Adult Congenital Heart Disease Unit, University Hospitals Birmingham NHS Foundation Trust, Birmingham, UK

Luis Manuel Espaillat-Rijo, MD
Cleveland Clinic Florida, Weston/Fort Lauderdale, Florida, USA

Rami Fares, MSc, MRCS
Pan-Birmingham Gynecologic Cancer Center, City Hospital, Sandwell and Birmingham Hospitals NHS Trust, Birmingham, UK

Alan Farthing, MD, FRCOG
Imperial College Healthcare NHS Trust, London, UK

Robert Freeman, MD, FRCOG
Plymouth Hospitals NHS Trust, Plymouth, UK

Chieh Lin Fu, MD
Cleveland Clinic Florida, Weston/Fort Lauderdale, Florida, USA

Ketan Gajjar, MBBS, MD, MRCOG
Addenbrooke's Hospital, Cambridge University Hospitals NHS Foundation Trust, Cambridge, UK

Ioannis Gallos, DMS, MD, MRCOG
University of Birmingham; Birmingham Women's NHS Foundation Trust, Birmingham, UK

Gamal M. Ghoniem, MD, FACS
University of California, Irvine; Long Beach Memorial Medical Center, Long Beach, California, USA

Vibha Giri, MBBS, MD, MRCOG
Good Hope Hospital, Heart of England NHS Foundation Trust, Sutton Coldfield, West Midlands, UK

James Gray, MBChB, MRCP, FRCPath
Birmingham Women's NHS Foundation Trust, Birmingham, UK

Ian A. Greer, MBChB, MD, MRCP, FRCP (Glas), MFFP, FRCP (Edin), FRCOG, FRCP (London)
University of Manchester; Manchester Academic Health Science Center (MAHSC), Manchester, UK

Samuel Grimsley, FRCS (Urol), MSc (Cancer Sciences), MBChB
Doncaster and Bassetlaw Hospitals NHS Foundation Trust, Doncaster, UK

Janesh Gupta, MSc, MD, FRCOG
Professor of Obstetrics and Gynecology, University of Birmingham; Consultant Obstetrician and Gynecologist, Birmingham Women's NHS Foundation Trust, Birmingham, UK

Khalid Hasan, MBBS, FRCA, PGCME
University Hospitals Birmingham NHS Foundation Trust, Birmingham, UK

Nir Haya, MD, DU, RANZCOG
Royal Brisbane and Women's Hospital, Brisbane, Queensland, Australia

Lynsey Hayward, BSc (Hons), MBChB (Hons), MRCOG, FRANZCOG
Middlemore Hospital, Auckland, New Zealand

Khaled M.K. Ismail, MBBCh, MSc, MD, PhD, FRCOG
College of Medical and Dental Sciences, University of Birmingham; Birmingham Women's NHS Foundation Trust, Birmingham, UK

Fidan Israfil-Bayli, MBChB, PhD
Birmingham Women's NHS Foundation Trust, Birmingham, UK

Simon Jackson, MD, FRCOG
John Radcliffe Hospital, Oxford University Hospitals NHS Trust, Oxford, UK

Ariella Jakobsen-Setton, MD
Sheba Medical Center and Tel Aviv University, Tel Hashomer, Israel

Swati Jha, MD, FRCOG
Sheffield Teaching Hospitals NHS Foundation Trust; University of Sheffield, Sheffield, UK

Alfredo Jijon, MD
Cleveland Clinic Florida, Weston/Fort Lauderdale, Florida, USA

Danita Jones, DO, MPH
Cleveland Clinic Florida, Weston/Fort Lauderdale, Florida, USA

Howard Joy, MBBS, BSc, FRCS (General Surgery)
City Hospital, Sandwell and West Birmingham Hospitals NHS Trust, Birmingham, UK

Deborah R. Karp, MD
School of Medicine, Emory University, Atlanta, Georgia, USA

Amie Kawasaki, MD
Cleveland Clinic Florida, Weston/Fort Lauderdale, Florida, USA

Rohna Kearney, MD, MRCOG, MRCPI
St Mary's Hospital, Central Manchester University Hospitals NHS Foundation Trust, Manchester, UK

Chris Keh, MD, FRCS (Gen Surg)
University Hospitals Birmingham NHS Foundation Trust, Birmingham, UK

Jennie Kerr, MBChB, FRCA
University Hospitals Birmingham NHS Foundation Trust and Birmingham Women's NHS Foundation Trust, Birmingham, UK

Mohammed Khairy, MBBCh, MSc
Birmingham Women's NHS Foundation Trust, Birmingham, UK

Sohail Q. Khan, BSc (Hons), MBChB, MD, MRCP
University Hospitals Birmingham NHS Foundation Trust, Birmingham, UK

Su-Yen Khong, MBChB, MRCOG, FRANZCOG
University of Malaya; University of Malaya Medical Center, Kuala Lumpur, Malaysia

Cara R. King, DO, MS
University of Pittsburgh Medical Center, Pittsburgh, Pennsylvania, USA

Kathleen C. Kobashi, MD, FACS
Virginia Mason Medical Center, Seattle, Washington, USA

Mohan Kumar, MBBS, MRCOG
Good Hope Hospital, Heart of England NHS Foundation Trust, Sutton Coldfield, West Midlands, UK

Heinke Kunst, MD, FRCP, MSc
Queen Mary University of London; Barts Health NHS Trust, London, UK

Ramy Labib, MBBCh, FRCA
Worcestershire Acute Hospitals NHS Trust, Worcestershire, UK

Alan Lam, MBBS (Hons), FRANZCOG, FRCOG
Center for Advanced Reproductive Endosurgery, University of Sydney, Royal North Shore, St Leonards, Australia

Thomas G. Lang, MD, MSc
Bethesda Memorial Hospital, Boynton Beach; Charles E. Schmidt College of Medicine, Florida Atlantic University, Boca Raton, Florida, USA

Pallavi Latthe, MD, MRCOG
Consultant in Obstetrics and Gynecology and Subspecialist in Urogynecology, Birmingham Women's NHS Foundation Trust; Honorary Senior Lecturer, University of Birmingham, Birmingham, UK

Sophie Lee, MBChB, FRCP, FRCPath
University Hospitals Birmingham NHS Foundation Trust, Birmingham, UK

Tim Lees, MBChB, FRCS, MD
Freeman Hospital, Newcastle upon Tyne Hospitals NHS Foundation Trust, Newcastle upon Tyne, UK

Will Lester, MBChB, BSc, FRCP, FRCPath, PhD
University Hospitals Birmingham NHS Foundation Trust and Birmingham Women's NHS Foundation Trust, Birmingham, UK

Rebekah Ley, LLB (Hons), MSc
Cambridge University Hospitals NHS Foundation Trust, Cambridge, UK

Naomi Low-Beer, MBBS, MD, MRCOG, MEd
Chelsea and Westminster Hospital NHS Foundation Trust, London, UK

David M. Luesley, MA, MD, FRCOG
University of Birmingham; City Hospital, Sandwell and West Birmingham Hospitals NHS Trust, Birmingham, UK

Jane MacDougall, MBBChir, MD, FRCOG, MEd
Addenbrooke's Hospital, Cambridge University Hospitals NHS Foundation Trust, Cambridge, UK

Adam Magos, BSc, MBBS, MD, FRCOG
The Royal Free Hospital, London, UK

Amita Mahendru, MD, MRCOG
Nottingham University Hospitals NHS Trust, Nottingham, UK

Christopher FRANZCOG, CU, PhD
University of Queensland; Royal Brisbane and Women's Hospitals; Wesley Hospital, Brisbane, Australia

Ayesha Mahmud, MBBS, DRCOG, MRCOG
Birmingham Women's NHS Foundation Trust; University of Birmingham, Birmingham, UK

Suketu Mansuria, MD, FACOG
University of Pittsburgh Medical Center, Pittsburgh, Pennsylvania, USA

Howard Marshall, MBChB, FRCP, MD
University Hospitals Birmingham NHS Foundation Trust, Birmingham, UK

Syeda Batool Mazhar, MBBS, FCPS (Pak), FRCOG (UK)
Shaheed Zulfiqar Ali Bhutto Medical University; Mother and Child Health Center, Pakistan Institute of Medical Sciences, Islamabad, Pakistan

G. Rodney Meeks, MD
University of Mississippi School of Medicine, Jackson, Mississippi, USA

Mohamed Mehasseb, MBBCh, MSc, MD, MRCOG, PhD
Glasgow Royal Infirmary, Glasgow, UK

Emanuele Lo Menzo, MD, PhD
Digestive Disease Institute, Cleveland Clinic Florida, Weston/Fort Lauderdale, Florida, USA

Rachel J. Miller, MD, FACOG
Children's Hospitals and Clinics of Minnesota; University of Minnesota, Minneapolis, Minnesota, USA

Aarthi R. Mohan, BSc, PhD, MRCOG, MRCP
St Michael's Hospital, Bristol, UK

Ash Monga, BMBS, MRCOG
Southampton University Hospital Trust, Southampton, UK

Phil Moore, MD, FRCA, FFPMRCA
Consultant Anesthetist, Birmingham Women's NHS Foundation Trust, Birmingham, UK

Karen Louise Moores, MRCOG, DFSRH, MBChB
Shrewsbury and Telford Hospitals NHS Trust, Telford, Shropshire, UK

Alfred Murage, MBChB, MMed, MRCOG, PMETB
Aga Khan University Hospital, Nairobi, Kenya

David Muthuveloe, MBBS, BSc, MRCS
University Hospitals Birmingham NHS Foundation Trust, Birmingham, UK

Anjana Nair, MBBS, MD
Advanced Surgical Specialties for Women, Carolinas Healthcare System, Charlotte, North Carolina, USA

Saloney Nazeer, MBBS, MD
International Network for Control of Gynecologic Cancers (INCGC), Geneva Foundation for Medical Education and Research (GFMER), World Health Organization (WHO) Collaborating Center in Education and Research in Human Reproduction, Geneva, Switzerland

Asia Nazir, MBBS
Pakistan Institute of Medical Sciences, Islamabad, Pakistan

Shaista Nazir, MBBS, FCPS
Alexandra Hospital, Worcestershire Acute Hospitals NHS Trust, Redditch, Worcestershire, UK

Catherine Nelson-Piercy, MBBS, FRCP, FRCOG
Women's Health Academic Center, King's Health Partners, St Thomas' Hospital; Guy's and St Thomas' Hospitals NHS Foundation Trust, London, UK

Philip N. Newsome, MBChB, PhD, FRCPE
College of Medical and Dental Sciences, University of Birmingham; University Hospitals Birmingham NHS Foundation Trust, Birmingham, UK

Aaron Ndhluni, MBChB (Hons), FCS (SA)
Groote Schuur Hospital, Cape Town, South Africa

Victor W. Nitti, MD
New York University Langone Medical Center, New York, USA

Natalie P. Nunes, MBBS, MRCOG, PGD (Med Ed)
West Middlesex University Hospital, London, UK

Barry A. O'Reilly, MBBCh, MD, FRCPI, FRCOG, FRANZCOG
Cork University Maternity Hospital, Cork, Ireland

Orfhlaith E. O'Sullivan, MRCSI, MCh, MRCPI, MRCOG
Cork University Maternity Hospital, Cork, Ireland

Mohamed Otify, MRCOG
King's College Hospital, London, UK

Spyros Papaioannou, MD, FRCOG
Heartlands Hospital, Heart of England NHS Foundation Trust, Birmingham, UK

John Parkin, BSc, MBBS, FRCS (Urol)
Pan-Birmingham Gynecologic Cancer Center, City Hospital, Sandwell and Birmingham Hospitals NHS Trust, Birmingham, UK

William Parry-Smith, MBBS, BSc (Hons)
Shropshire Women and Children's Center, Princess Royal Hospital, Telford, Shropshire, UK

Matthew Parsons, MBChB, DFSRH, MD, FRCOG
Birmingham Women's NHS Foundation Trust; University of Birmingham, Birmingham, UK

Resad Pasic, MD, PhD
University of Louisville, Louisville, Kentucky, USA

Bhavin Patel, MD
Virginia Mason Medical Center, Seattle, Washington, USA

Richard Popert, MS, FRCS (Urol)
Guy's and St Thomas' Hospitals NHS Foundation Trust, London, UK

Neelam Potdar, MBBS, MD, MSc, MRCOG
University Hospitals of Leicester NHS Trust, and University of Leicester, Leicester, UK

Andrew Prentice, BSc, MA, MD, FRCOG, FHEA
University of Cambridge; Addenbrooke's Hospital, Cambridge University Hospitals NHS Foundation Trust, Cambridge, UK

Natalia Price, MD, MRCOG
John Radcliffe Hospital, Oxford University Hospitals NHS Trust, Oxford, UK

Najum Qureshi, MBBS, FRCOG, MA
Birmingham Women's NHS Foundation Trust, Birmingham, UK

Zahida Qureshi, MBChB, MMed (Obs/Gyn)
University of Nairobi, Nairobi, Kenya

Suneetha Rachaneni, MBBS, MRCOG
University of Birmingham, Birmingham, UK

Simon Radley, MBChB, MD, FRCS
Birmingham Bowel Clinic, Birmingham, UK

Anuradha Radotra, MD, FRCOG, DFFP
Shrewsbury and Telford Hospitals NHS Trust, Shropshire, UK

Smita Rajshekhar, MBBS, MS, MRCOG
Addenbrooke's Hospital, Cambridge University Hospitals NHS Trust, Cambridge, UK

Kalaivani Ramalingam, MBBS, DGO, MRCOG
Apollo Hospitals, Chennai, India

Edward Rawstorne, MBBCh, BSc, MRCS
Heart of England NHS Foundation Trust, Birmingham, UK

Joanne Kathleen Ritchie, MBChB
Shrewsbury and Telford Hospitals NHS Trust, Shropshire, UK

Lynne Robinson, MBChB, MD, MRCOG
Birmingham Women's NHS Foundation Trust, Birmingham, UK

Peter L. Rosenblatt, MD
Mount Auburn Hospital, Cambridge, Massachusetts, USA

Raul J. Rosenthal, MD
Cleveland Clinic Florida, Weston/Fort Lauderdale, Florida, USA

Jackie A. Ross, BSc (Hons), MBBS, FRCOG
King's College Hospital, London, UK

Ted M. Roth, MD, FPMRS
Central Maine Medical Center, Lewiston, Maine, USA

Virgilio Salanga, MD, MS, FAAN
Cleveland Clinic Florida, Weston/Fort Lauderdale, Florida, USA

Ertan Saridogan, MD, PhD, FRCOG
University College London Hospitals NHS Foundation Trust; University College London, London, UK

Kris Ann P. Schultz, MD
Children's Hospitals and Clinics of Minnesota, Minneapolis, Minnesota, USA

Indrani Sen, MCh
Christian Medical College, Vellore, Tamil Nadu, India

Mahmood I. Shafi, MBBCh, MD, DA, FRCOG
Addenbrooke's Hospital, Cambridge University Hospitals NHS Foundation Trust, Cambridge, UK

Khaldoun Sharif, MD, FRCOG, MFFP
Istishari Fertility Center, Amman, Jordan

Manjeet Shehmar, MMedEd, MRCOG, MBBS, BSc
Birmingham Women's NHS Foundation Trust, Birmingham, UK

Emanuela Silva, MD
Cleveland Clinic Florida, Weston/Fort Lauderdale, Florida, USA

Kavita Singh, MBBS, MD, FRCOG
Consultant Gynecologist and Gynecologic Oncologist, City Hospital, Sandwell and West Birmingham Hospitals NHS Trust, Birmingham, UK

Mark Slack, MMed, FCOG (SA), FRCOG
Addenbrooke's Hospital, Cambridge University Hospitals NHS Foundation Trust, Cambridge, UK

Christopher Smart, MBBS, FRCS
East Lancashire Hospitals NHS Trust, Blackburn, UK

Robbert Soeters, MD, PhD
University of Cape Town, Groote Schuur Hospital; Vincent Pallotti Hospital, Cape Town, South Africa

Michael L. Sprague, MD
Cleveland Clinic Florida, Weston/Fort Lauderdale, Florida, USA

Edward Stanford, MD, MS, MHA, FACOG, FACS, CDIP
Oasis International Hospital, Beijing, China

Phil Steer, BSc, MD, FRCOG
Imperial College London, London, UK

Edwin Stephen, MS
Northern Vascular Center, Freeman Hospital, Newcastle upon Tyne Hospitals NHS Foundation Trust, Newcastle upon Tyne, UK

Kevin J.E. Stepp, MD, FACOG, FPMRS
Advanced Surgical Specialties for Women, Carolinas Healthcare System, Charlotte, North Carolina, USA

Helen Stevenson, MBChB
Birmingham Women's NHS Foundation Trust, Birmingham, UK

Sudha Sundar, MBBS, MPhil, MRCOG
College of Medical and Dental Sciences, University of Birmingham; Pan-Birmingham Gynecologic Cancer Center, City Hospital, Sandwell and West Birmingham Hospitals NHS Trust, Birmingham, UK

Samuel Szomstein, MD
Cleveland Clinic Florida, Weston/Fort Lauderdale, Florida, USA

Nirmala Rai Talapadi, MBBS, MRCOG
College of Medical and Dental Sciences, University of Birmingham, Birmingham, UK

Toh Lick Tan, MBBS (London), MRCOG
KK Women's and Children's Hospital, Singapore

Ranee Thakar, MBBS, MD, FRCOG
Mayday University Hospital; St George's University, London, UK

Sara A. Thorne, MBBS, MD, FRCP
University Hospitals Birmingham NHS Foundation Trust, Birmingham, UK

Tamara V. Toidze, MD, FACOG
Cooper Medical School of Rowan University, Camden, New Jersey, USA

Philip Toozs-Hobson, MBBS, MD, FRCOG
Birmingham Women's NHS Foundation Trust, Birmingham, UK

Jonathan N. Townend, BSc, MBChB, MD, FRCP
University Hospitals Birmingham NHS Foundation Trust; University of Birmingham, Birmingham, UK

Martyn Underwood, MBChB, MRCOG
Shrewsbury and Telford Hospitals NHS Trust, Telford, Shropshire, UK

Hemant N. Vakharia, MBBS, BSC (Hons), MRCOG
Birmingham Women's NHS Foundation Trust, Birmingham, UK

Dukaydah van der Berg, MBChB, DRCOG
Frankly Health Practice, Birmingham, UK

Rajesh Varma, MA (Cantab), PhD, MRCOG
Guy's and St Thomas' Hospitals NHS Foundation Trust, London, UK

Monika Vij, MBBS, MS, MRCOG
Derriford Hospital, Plymouth Hospitals NHS Trust, Plymouth, UK

Sara S. Webb, MPhil, BSc, Dip HE (Midwifery), RM
Birmingham Women's NHS Foundation Trust, Birmingham, UK

Steven D. Wexner, MD, PhD (Hon), FACS, FRCS, FRCS (Ed)
Cleveland Clinic Florida, Weston/Fort Lauderdale, Florida, USA; Florida International University, Florida, USA

Olivia Will, MBChB, MRCS, PhD
Addenbrooke's Hospital, Cambridge University Hospitals NHS Foundation Trust, Cambridge, UK

Sarah Winfield, BSc (Hons), MBBS, MRCOG
Leeds General Infirmary, Leeds Teaching Hospitals NHS Trust, Leeds, UK

Idnan Yunas, MBBChir, MA (Cantab), DCH, DRCOG, DFSRH, MRCGP
University Medical Practice Edgbaston; Health Education West Midlands, Birmingham, UK

Stephen E. Zimberg, MD, MSHA
Cleveland Clinic Florida, Weston/Fort Lauderdale, Florida, USA

Preface

Our book has the aim of stimulating resourceful thinking and offering insightful management options to many challenges a gynecologic or obstetric surgeon may face before, during and after an operation. This book addresses two primary issues of concern at the coalface of practice: how to avoid getting into trouble, and if you are already in trouble, how to get out of it. It is thus a highly practical manual, with very little in the way of fine print.

We, the editors, are under no delusion that a book alone will make one an effective and safe surgeon. Competence in surgery is acquired by diligent and intelligent training under expert guidance. This book is designed to complement that process.

The book is divided into two parts, the first covering general preoperative, intraoperative, and postoperative challenges, and the second covering challenges specific to various gynecologic and obstetric operations within the subspecialty areas. Chapters are brief, starting with (i) a case history that presents the challenge, then (ii) a discussion about the challenge, and finally (iii) the management options that are available, with reasoning and available evidence. A summary Key points box is provided with each chapter, and is ideal for "elevator reading," i.e., speedy checking up of facts on the way to facing a challenge in an operating room or elsewhere.

How will you get the most out of this book? We suggest you read the case history, and work out some management solutions yourself before reading the rest of the chapter. Compare and contrast your solutions with the options in the book. Discuss with your seniors and juniors. And if you have a better option than that outlined in the book, please let us know; if we agree with you, we will acknowledge your contribution in the next edition.

A.C., M.I.S., G.W.D., K.K.C.

List of Abbreviations

AAE	arterial air embolism
AAGL	American Association of Gynecologic Laparoscopists
ABC	airway, breathing, circulation
ABCDE	airway, breathing, circulation, disability, exposure/examination
ABG	arterial blood gases
ABPI	ankle-brachial pressure index
ACC/AHA	American College of Cardiology/American Heart Association
ACCP	American College of Chest Physicians
ACE	angiotensin-converting enzyme
ACHD	adult congenital heart disease
ACOG	American College of Obstetricians and Gynecologists
ACTH	adrenocorticotropic hormone
AED	antiepileptic drug
AF	atrial fibrillation
AFP	α-fetoprotein
AIS	anti-incontinence surgery
AKI	acute kidney injury
ALP	alkaline phophatase
ALS	advanced life support
ALSO	advanced life support in obstetrics
ALT	alanine aminotransferase
anti-HBs	hepatitis B surface antibody
anti-HBc	total hepatitis B core antibody
anti-HBe	hepatitis B e antibody
AOC	advanced ovarian cancer
AP	anteroposterior
APS	antiphospholipid syndrome
aPTT	activated partial thromboplastin time
ARDS	acute respiratory distress syndrome
ART	assisted reproductive technology
ASA	American Society of Anesthesiologists
AST	aspartate aminotransferase
ATP	anti-tachycardia pacing
BCSH	British Committee for Standards in Haematology
b.d.	twice daily
bHCG	β-human chorionic gonadotropin
BM	Boehringer Mannheim (test to measure blood glucose levels)
BMI	body mass index
BMS	bare metal stent
BP	blood pressure
bpm	beats per minute
BPI	brachial plexus injury
BSO	bilateral salpingo-oophorectomy
BSUG	British Society of Urogynecology
CABG	coronary artery bypass grafting
CAD	coronary artery disease
CAIS	congenital androgen insensitivity syndrome
CARP	Coronary Artery Revascularization Prophylaxis
CDC	Centers for Disease Control and Prevention
CE	Conformité Européenne
CEA	carcinoembryonic antigen
CEMACH	Confidential Enquiry into Maternal and Child Health
CHA$_2$DS$_2$-VASc	congestive heart failure, hypertension, age, diabetes mellitus, stroke, vascular disease, age, sex category
CI	confidence interval
CIC	clean intermittent catheterization
CIN	cervical intraepithelial neoplasia
CISC	clean intermittent self-catheterization
CIWA-Ar	Clinical Institute Withdrawal Assessment of Alcohol Scale, Revised
CKC	cold-knife cone
CKD	chronic kidney disease
CME	continuing medical education
COPD	chronic obstructive pulmonary disease
CPAP	continuous positive airway pressure
CPR	cardiopulmonary resuscitation
CRH	corticotropin releasing hormone
CRP	C-reactive protein
CRT	cardiac resynchronization therapy
CS	cesarean section
CSF	cerebrospinal fluid
CSP	cesarean scar pregnancy
CT	computed tomography
CTG	cardiotocography
CTP	Child-Turcotte-Pugh (scoring system)
CTS	category, time, site
Cu-IUD	copper intrauterine device
CVP	central venous pressure
D&C	dilatation and curettage
DAP	dose-area product
DDAVP	desmopressin acetate (1-desamino-8-D-arginine vasopressin, a synthetic analog of the pituitary hormone 8-arginine vasopressin)
DDD	dual chamber (dual pacing, dual activity sensing, dual response)
DES	drug-eluting stent
DIC	disseminated intravascular coagulation
DIEP	deep inferior epigastric perforator
DKA	diabetic ketoacidosis
DMARDs	disease-modifying antirheumatic drugs
DNAR	do not attempt resuscitation
DO	detrusor overactivity
DSD	disorders of sex development
DSM	Diagnostic and Statistical Manual of Mental Disorders
DVT	deep vein thrombosis
EAS	external anal sphincter
EAU	endoanal ultrasound
ECF	extracellular fluid
ECG	electrocardiography, electrocardiogram
EHRA	European Heart Rhythm Association
ELISA	enzyme-linked immunosorbent assay
EMG	electromyography

EmOC	emergency obstetric care
ENT	ear, nose and throat
EPO	erythropoietin
ER	enhanced recovery
ERAS	enhanced recovery after surgery
ERPC	evacuation of retained products of conception
ESA	erythropoiesis-stimulating agent
ESBL	extended spectrum β-lactamase
ESC	European Society of Cardiology
ESR	erythrocyte sedimentation rate
ESTReP	Enhanced Surgical Treatment and Recovery Programme
ETCO$_2$	end-tidal carbon dioxide
EUA	examination under anesthesia
EWS	early warning score
FBC	full blood count
FDA	Food and Drug Administration
FDG	fluorodeoxyglucose
FFP	fresh frozen plasma
FEV$_1$	forced expiratory volume in 1 s
FGM	female genital mutilation
FIGO	International Federation of Gynecology and Obstetrics
FNA	fine needle aspiration
FRC	functional residual capacity
FSH	follicle-stimulating hormone
FVC	functional vital capacity
G&S	group and save
GABA	γ-aminobutyric acid
GDC	Gartner's duct cyst
GECS	graduated elastic compression stockings
GFR	glomerular filtration rate
GIFTASUP	Guideline on Intravenous Fluid Therapy for Adult Surgical Patients
GIST	gastrointestinal stromal tumor
GMC	General Medical Council
GnRH	gonadotropin-releasing hormone
GP	general practitioner
GTN	glyceryl trinitrate
HAART	highly active antiretroviral therapy
HAS-BLED	**h**ypertension, **a**bnormal renal or liver function, **s**troke, **b**leeding, **l**abile INRs, **e**lderly, **d**rugs and/or alcohol
Hb	hemoglobin
HBeAg	hepatitis B e antigen
HBIG	hepatitis B immunoglobulin
HBsAg	hepatitis B surface antigen
HBV	hepatitis B virus
HCAI	healthcare-associated infection
HCG	human chorionic gonadotropin
HCV	hepatitis C virus
HCW	healthcare worker
HDU	high-dependency unit
HGCIN	high-grade cervical intraepithelial neoplasia
HIV/AIDS	human immunodeficiency virus/acquired immunodeficiency syndrome
HMB	heavy menstrual bleeding
HNPCC	hereditary non-polyposis colorectal cancer
HPA	hypothalamic-pituitary-adrenal
HPV	human papillomavirus
HrHPV	high-risk human papillomavirus
HRT	hormone replacement therapy
HSG	hysterosalpingography
IAP	intra-abdominal pressure

IAS	internal anal sphincter
ICD	implantable cardioverter defibrillator
ICF	intracellular fluid
ICI	International Consultation on Incontinence
ICIQ-VS	International Consultation on Incontinence Questionnaire on Vaginal Symptoms
ICS	International Continence Society
ICSI	intracytoplasmic sperm injection
IDDM	insulin-dependent diabetes mellitus
IEA	inferior epigastric artery
IgM anti-HBc	IgM antibody to hepatitis B core antigen
i.m.	intramuscular (injection)
IMCA	independent mental capacity advocate
INR	International Normalized Ratio
IOTA	International Ovarian Tumor Analysis
IPC	intermittent pneumatic compression
IPL	infundibulopelvic ligament
ISD	intrinsic urethral sphincter deficiency
ITA-IEA	internal thoracic artery/inferior epigastric artery
ITC	isolated tumor cell
ITP	immune-mediated thrombocytopenic purpura
ITU	intensive therapy unit
IU	international unit(s)
IU(C)D	intrauterine (contraceptive) device
IUGA	International Urogynecology Association
IUS	intrauterine system
i.v.	intravenous (injection)
IVC	inferior vena cava
IVF	*in vitro* fertilization
IVIG	intravenous immunoglobulin
IVP	intravenous pyelography
IVU	intravenous urography
KCl	potassium chloride
LAVH	laparoscopic-assisted vaginal hysterectomy
LDH	lactate dehydrogenase
LDUH	low-dose unfractionated heparin
LEEP	loop electrosurgical excision procedure
LEER	laterally extended endopelvic resection
LFT	liver function test
LH	luteinizing hormone
LLETZ	large loop excision of the transformation zone
LM	laparoscopic myomectomy
LMA	laryngeal mask airway
LMWH	low-molecular-weight heparin
LNG-IUS	levonorgestrel intrauterine system
LRH	laparoscopic radical hysterectomy
LRINEC	laboratory risk indicator for necrotizing fasciitis
LUTS	lower urinary tract symptoms
LVH	left ventricular hypertrophy
LVSI	lymphovascular space invasion
MAOIs	monoamine oxidase inhibitors
MAP	mean arterial pressure
MCA	Mental Capacity Act
MCV	mean cell volume
MDCT	multirow detector helical computed tomography
MELD	Model for End-stage Liver Disease (score)
MEWS	Modified Early Warning Score
MHRA	Medicines and Healthcare products Regulatory Agency
MI	myocardial infarction
micro-TESE	microdissection testicular sperm extraction

MMSE	Mini Mental State Examination
MR	magnetic resonance
MRgFUS	magnetic resonance-guided focused ultrasound
MRI	magnetic resonance imaging
MRKH	Mayer-Rokitansky-Kuster-Hauser (syndrome)
MROP	manual removal of placenta
MRSA	methicillin-resistant *Staphylococcus aureus*
MSU	midstream specimen of urine
MUCP	maximal urethral closure pressure
MUS	mid-urethral sling
MVA	manual vacuum aspiration
NACT	neoadjuvant chemotherapy
NGT	nasogastric tube
NHS	National Health Service
NHSLA	NHS Litigation Authority
NICE	National Institute for Health and Care Excellence
NIDDM	non-insulin-dependent diabetes mellitus
NOAC	novel anticoagulant
NPO/NBM	nothing by mouth
NPSA	National Patient Safety Agency
NPWT	negative pressure wound therapy
NSAIDs	non-steroidal anti-inflammatory drugs
OAB	overactive bladder
OASIS	obstetric anal sphincter injuries
OR	odds ratio
ORS	ovarian remnant syndrome
OT	operating theater
PA	posteroanterior
PAE	paradoxical air embolism
PAF	paroxysmal atrial fibrillation
PALS	Patient Advice and Liaison Service
PCA	patient-controlled analgesia
PCI	percutaneous coronary intervention
PDS	poly(p-dioxanone)
PE	pulmonary embolism
PEA	pulseless electrical activity
PEEP	positive end-expiratory pressure
PEP	post-exposure prophylaxis
PESA	percutaneous epididymal sperm aspiration
PET	positron emission tomography
PFMT	pelvic floor muscle training
PID	pelvic inflammatory disease
POD	pouch of Douglas
PONV	postoperative nausea and vomiting
POP	pelvic organ prolapse
POP-Q	pelvic organ prolapse quantification
PPH	postpartum hemorrhage
PRBC	packed red blood cells
PSH	port-site herniation
PT	prothrombin time
PTFE	polytetrafluoroethylene
PVR	post-void residual
q.d.s.	four times daily
RA	rheumatoid arthritis
RBC	red blood cell
RCOG	Royal College of Obstetricians and Gynaecologists
RCT	randomized controlled clinical trial
RLS	reporting and learning system
RMI	risk of malignancy index
RR	relative risk
RVE	rectovaginal endometriosis

RVF	rectovaginal fistula
RVT	radical vaginal trachelectomy
SCJ	squamocolumnar junction
SCr	serum creatinine
SFT	solitary fibrous tumor
SIADH	syndrome of inappropriate antidiuretic hormone secretion
SIRS	systemic inflammatory response syndrome
SLE	systemic lupus erythematosus
SLN	sentinel lymph node
SLNB	sentinel lymph node biopsy
SN	sentinel node
SNAPP	**s**epsis, **n**utrition, **a**ssess anatomy, **p**rotect skin, **p**lanned surgery
SOCRATES	**s**ite, **o**nset, **c**haracter, **r**adiation, **a**ssociations, **t**iming, **e**xacerbating factors, **s**everity
SPRM	selective progesterone receptor modulator
SSF	sacrospinous fixation
SSI	surgical site infection
SSL	sacrospinous ligament
SSLF	sacrospinous ligament fixation
SSRI	selective serotonin reuptake inhibitor
SST	short Synacthen test
STARR	stapled transanal rectal resection
STI	sexually transmitted infection
SUI	stress urinary incontinence
T_4	thyroxine
T_3	triiodothyronine
TAH	total abdominal hysterectomy
TAP	transversus abdominis plane
TCAs	tricyclic antidepressants
TCRE	transcervical resection of the endometrium
t.d.s.	three times daily
TEE	transesophageal echocardiography
TESA	testicular sperm aspiration
TESE	testicular sperm extraction
TFT	thyroid function test
TH	thyroid hormone
TIA	transient ischemic attack
TIBC	total iron-binding capacity
TIVA	total intravenous anesthesia
TLH	total laparoscopic hysterectomy
TME	total mesorectal excision
TMET	transmyometrial transfer
TNF	tumor necrosis factor
TOT	transobturator tape
TPN	total parenteral nutrition
TPP	tubal perfusion pressure
TPU	transperineal ultrasound
TRALI	transfusion-related acute lung injury
TRAM	transversus rectus abdominis muscle
TSH	thyroid-stimulating hormone
TTE	transthoracic echocardiography
TVH	total vaginal hysterectomy
TVS	transvaginal ultrasonography
TVT	tension-free vaginal tape
TVTO	tension-free vaginal tape obturator
TWOC	trial without catheter
U&E	urea and electrolytes
UC	ulcerative colitis
UFE	uterine fibroid embolization

UFH	unfractionated heparin	**VCUG**	voiding cystourethrography
UNFPA	United Nations Population Fund	**VF**	ventricular fibrillation
UNICEF	United Nations Children's Fund	**VLPP**	Valsalva leak point pressure
US-FNAC	ultrasound-guided fine needle aspiration cytology	**VT**	ventricular tachycardia
USI	urodynamic stress incontinence	**VTE**	venous thromboembolism
USS	ultrasound scan	**VVF**	vesicovaginal fistula
UTI	urinary tract infection	**VVP**	vaginal vault prolapse
UVF	urethrovaginal fistula	**vWF**	von Willebrand factor
VAC	vacuum-assisted closure	**WBC**	white blood cell
VAE	venous air embolism	**WHO**	World Health Organization
VAIN	vaginal intraepithelial neoplasia		

PART I

General Preoperative, Intraoperative, and Postoperative Challenges

Section 1
Preoperative Care
Editors: Phil Moore and Arri Coomarasamy

CHAPTER 1

Patient with Poor ASA Score

Phil Moore

Birmingham Women's NHS Foundation Trust, Birmingham, UK

Case history: An obese 79-year-old woman with chronic obstructive pulmonary disease, angina, hypertension and insulin-dependent diabetes requires abdominal hysterectomy for endometrial cancer.

Background

The idea of a physical status classification system was originally suggested by the American Society of Anesthetists in 1940, and three physicians – Saklad, Rovenstine and Taylor – produced a six-point scale. In 1963 this was published with two modifications by Dripps *et al.* as the current five-point scale, which was subsequently amended to become the American Society of Anesthesiologists physical status system for assessing the fitness of patients before surgery. This eponymous system consists of five grades (Table 1.1). The system was later modified to include a sixth grade for brain-dead patients whose organs are being removed for donation. In cases of emergency surgery, the grade is modified by the addition of an 'E' (e.g., 5E).

Table 1.1 American Society of Anesthesiologists (ASA) physical status system.

ASA grade	Physical status
1	A normal healthy patient
2	A patient with mild systemic disease
3	A patient with severe systemic disease
4	A patient with severe systemic disease that is a constant threat to life
5	A moribund patient who is not expected to survive without the operation

The score has been criticized for being subjective and prone to inter-observer variability. Additionally, it takes no account of the nature of the surgical procedure being carried out. Nevertheless, it is simple and quick to administer, rapidly communicated, and has been shown to be broadly correlated with adverse outcomes from surgery (Table 1.2).

Table 1.2 Percentage perioperative mortality categorized by ASA status.

ASA physical status class	Vacanti *et al.* [1]	Marx *et al.* [2]
1	0.08%	0.06%
2	0.27%	0.47%
3	1.8%	4.4%
4	7.8%	23.5%
5	9.4%	50.8%

In view of the increased morbidity and mortality rate, patients with high ASA scores undergoing major surgery need appropriate preoperative investigations and preparation and, in order to optimize their outcome, require the involvement of senior surgical and anesthetic staff at all stages of their management.

Management

The management of patients with a poor ASA score is based on three important principles.

1 A multidisciplinary assessment of the risks and benefits of the proposed procedure, and a frank discussion of these issues with the patient, and her relatives if appropriate.

In the case described, surgery may be necessary to save the woman's life; nevertheless, the severity of the underlying diseases must be taken into account, to ensure that surgery will result in not only prolonged life, but also a return to a quality of life deemed acceptable to the patient. However, it can be very difficult to quantify the risks and benefits associated with the proposed surgical procedure, and the decision to proceed is often based on a consensus opinion of the specialists involved. It is sometimes appropriate, especially in cases of disagreement among the healthcare professionals, to obtain opinions from clinicians not directly involved in the case. Discussions with the patient should include provision of published risk data if available, although this may be difficult to apply to an individual patient's clinical situation. The General Medical Council (UK) has stressed the importance of providing adequate information to enable patients to make a decision about their care. The patient may ask for the clinician's opinion about whether to proceed, and while it is appropriate to provide this, it should be made clear that this decision ultimately lies with the patient. It is almost always mandatory to seek the consent of patients before involving their relatives in discussions about their care. All discussions should be documented, in addition to obtaining signed written consent.

Sometimes the risks of surgery and anesthesia may dictate that a decision not to operate is the most appropriate course of action, with symptomatic, supportive or palliative care provided instead, with the patient's consent.

2 Preoperative optimization of physiology and pre-existing morbidity, including the involvement of other medical specialists as appropriate.

Gynecologic and Obstetric Surgery: Challenges and Management Options, First Edition. Edited by Arri Coomarasamy, Mahmood I. Shafi, G. Willy Davila and Kiong K. Chan.
© 2016 John Wiley & Sons, Ltd. Published 2016 by John Wiley & Sons, Ltd.

In the case described, the woman should be reviewed by the cardiologists, diabetologists, respiratory or general physicians, and geriatricians as necessary. The aim of preoperative preparation is to optimize management of the patient's pre-existing comorbidities, and it may be appropriate to perform this either in the outpatient department or after hospital admission. This process may involve changing the patient's medication, or optimizing the dose and frequency of the drugs already in use. In the case described, review will include the patient's inhaled bronchodilators (Chapter 8), insulin (Chapter 9), and antihypertensive drug therapy (Chapter 7). It might be necessary to carry out further investigations or even interventional procedures, for example coronary angiography and stenting if her angina is inadequately controlled (Chapter 3). Arrangements should also be made for the postoperative management of these conditions. Although other specialists will likely make a valuable contribution to the patient's management, the final decision to proceed with anesthesia and surgery lies with the consultant surgeon and anesthetist caring for the patient. After listing for surgery, the patient should be reviewed by an anesthetist at the earliest possible opportunity, to allow planning of the perioperative management of her comorbidities. Physiological variables such as intravascular volume and plasma electrolyte levels should be optimized as far as possible. Some patients will benefit from preoperative admission to a critical care area where oxygen delivery to body tissues can be optimized with goal-directed therapy utilizing intravenous fluids and inotropes, and with invasive cardiovascular monitoring. Arrangements should also be made for higher-level care postoperatively, if required, and good communication with the nursing staff who will care for the patient will allow any special equipment or arrangements to be organized; for example, in this case, the patient is obese and may require specialist equipment for manual handling. It is important that discharge planning also commences at this stage, as non-standard care or equipment may also be needed in the community, and early assessment of these will avoid a prolonged and inappropriate stay in hospital.

3 The involvement of consultant-level surgical and anesthetic personnel and senior nursing staff in the planning and implementation of intraoperative and postoperative care. It may be important to also involve other healthcare and allied professionals, such as physiotherapists, dietitians, and social workers. It may be appropriate for very senior surgical and anesthetic trainees to manage high-risk cases; however, close supervision and involvement of consultant staff is mandatory for high-risk patients at all stages of their hospital stay. This is particularly true intraoperatively, as minimizing time under anesthesia may reduce complications and enhance recovery. The World Health Organization (WHO) surgical checklist provides an opportunity for all the staff involved with the procedure to highlight issues or potential problems, and to ensure everyone understands the procedure being undertaken, and the particular risks associated with the patient's pre-existing conditions.

Although avoidance of general anesthesia by using spinal or epidural anesthesia may be advantageous from the point of view of this patient's lung disease, it may be associated with increased cardiovascular risk, requiring careful risk–benefit consideration by an experienced anesthetist. Depending on the planned incision, regional techniques may not provide adequate anesthesia.

Arrangements for recovery and high-level postoperative care (in a high-dependency or intensive therapy unit) should be in place in advance of surgery, and these should be confirmed on the day. It is sometimes necessary to review and clarify the patient's

resuscitation status before surgery. High-risk patients may have 'Do not attempt resuscitation' (DNAR) orders in place, and as a number of the activities involved in general anesthesia may be interpreted as being resuscitative in nature (e.g., lung ventilation), DNAR orders may have to be withdrawn or suspended intraoperatively, dependent on local policy. Alternatively, it may be appropriate to agree limits on the interventions which may be used, for example stipulating that cardiac compressions in the event of cardiac arrest would be inappropriate. These issues should be fully discussed with the patient and/or relatives as appropriate.

Prevention of complications

All discussions and plans should be carefully documented in the medical records, and good lines of communication should be established to ensure that all staff involved in the patient's care are aware of these.

Most medication should be continued up to the time of surgery, although this may require discussion with the anesthetist and appropriate medical specialists (Chapter 2). It may be necessary to repeat investigations such as blood tests after admission to hospital, to provide up-to-date baseline data in advance of surgery. The patient should be closely monitored postoperatively to allow early identification and treatment of complications arising from anesthesia or surgery. Regular review by senior medical staff is mandatory during the early postoperative period.

Scheduling the patient for surgery early in the day allows early postoperative complications to be detected and dealt with during daylight hours. It may be inadvisable to operate on these patients just before a weekend, as weekend medical cover is often reduced.

KEY POINTS

Challenge: Surgery for the patient with a poor ASA score.

Background
- The ASA physical status scale correlates with perioperative morbidity and mortality.
- Patients' physical condition should be optimized before surgery.
- Senior surgical and anesthetic staff must be involved in all stages of patient management.

Prevention
- Careful planning of all stages of perioperative care.
- Multidisciplinary involvement.
- Scheduling of operation early in the day.

Management
Preoperative
- Multidisciplinary assessment of risks and benefits of surgery, and discussion of these with the patient and her relatives.
- Optimization of pre-existing medical conditions by medical specialists.
- Optimization of physiological variables: goal-directed therapy.
- Multidisciplinary advance planning of perioperative management.

Intraoperative
- Direct involvement of consultant surgical and anesthetic staff.
- Minimization of operative time.

Postoperative
- Close monitoring to identify complications early.
- Consideration for transfer to HDU or ITU for postoperative care.
- Regular senior surgical and anesthetic or critical care review of patient during postoperative period.

References

1 Vacanti CJ, VanHouten RJ, Hill RC. A statistical analysis of the relationship of physical status to postoperative mortality in 68,388 cases. *Anesth Analg* 1970; 49:564–566.
2 Marx GF, Mateo CV, Orkin LR. Computer analysis of postanesthetic deaths. *Anesthesiology* 1973; 39:54–58.

Further reading

Cecconi M, Corredor C, Arulkumaran N *et al.* Clinical review: Goal-directed therapy: what is the evidence in surgical patients? The effect on different risk groups. *Crit Care* 2013; 17:209.
Cooper N, Forrest K, Cramp P. Optimising patient before surgery. In: *Essential Guide to Acute Care*, 2nd edn. Blackwell Publishing, Oxford, 2006.
General Medical Council (UK). *Consent: patients and doctors making decisions together*. GMC, London, 2008. Available at http://www.gmc-uk.org/GMC_Consent_0513_Revised.pdf_52115235.pdf
Keats A. The ASA classification of physical status: a recapitulation. *Anesthesiology* 1978; 49: 233–236 .
Roizen ME, Fleisher LA. Anesthetic implications of concurrent diseases. In: Miller RD (ed.) *Miller's Anesthesia*, 7th edn, pp. 1067–1150. Churchill Livingstone Elsevier, Philadelphia, 2010.

CHAPTER 2

Patient on Medication

Arri Coomarasamy

College of Medical and Dental Sciences, University of Birmingham, Birmingham, UK

Case history: An elderly woman taking phenytoin for epilepsy and prednisolone 20 mg daily for COPD is scheduled to have laparotomy for ovarian cancer.

Background

Medications may affect, or be affected by, surgery. For instance, drugs can interact with anesthetic agents, impair clotting, or affect wound healing; conversely, surgery can wreak havoc on established treatment regimens, for example insulin or steroid therapy. A common preoperative challenge is deciding whether a drug should be stopped, continued as normal, or continued with a modified regimen. Another challenge is what should be done with oral medications during the preoperative fasting period and the postoperative period until oral feeding is re-established. This chapter focuses on medications and surgery; however, medications are often prescribed for specific chronic illnesses, and the management of patients with common chronic illnesses is addressed elsewhere in the book.

Medication and anesthesia interactions

Several drugs can result in a hazardous interaction [1,2]. Some key drugs that may interact with anesthetic agents include aminoglycosides, beta-blockers, ACE inhibitors, clindamycin, cyclophosphamide, erythromycin, monoamine oxidase inhibitors, droperidol, haloperidol, magnesium, ritonavir, procainamide, quinidine, lithium, and tricyclic antidepressants. To reduce the risk of interactions, a full history of drugs and allergies should be taken during preoperative assessment and drug interactions should be carefully considered.

Stress hormones

Operations associated with minimal stress (many minor operations) do not result in the release of stress hormones; however, operations associated with moderate or severe stress result in the release of cortisol and catecholamines [3]. The stress hormone response is of importance in women with adrenocortical suppression or diabetes.

Poor gastrointestinal function

After major abdominal surgery, the patient may suffer with nausea, vomiting and ileus, preventing oral intake of medicines or resulting in poor absorption. Alternative routes of administration (e.g. intravenous, rectal or transdermal) will need to be considered.

Clotting complications

Venous thromboembolism may occur following major surgery, particularly if the surgery is prolonged and associated with immobility and other risk factors. Oral contraceptives and hormone replacement therapy will increase the risk of venous thromboembolism (VTE). Women on anticoagulant or antiplatelet therapy are at risk of intraoperative and postoperative bleeding.

Management

Medications on the day of the operation

To avoid the risk of aspiration of stomach contents, food needs to be avoided for at least 6 hours before general anesthesia. However, water can be taken in small quantities for up to 2 hours before surgery. This will allow patients to take oral medications with sips of water until a few hours before an operation.

Drugs that need to be continued and discontinued

Unless there is a contraindication, medicines should be continued through the perioperative period to avoid relapse of the condition being treated and to prevent the effects of drug withdrawal. Continuation may require administration via a route other than oral; however, a change of route may alter the bioavailability of a drug and thus may also necessitate a change of dose. Involvement of pharmacy information services and drug level monitoring may be necessary to ensure an effective therapeutic regimen is achieved. Categories of common drugs and whether they should be continued or discontinued is provided in Table 2.1. For detailed discussion of management of patients on anticoagulant/antiplatelet therapy and steroid therapy, see Chapters 16 and 17, respectively.

Gynecologic and Obstetric Surgery: Challenges and Management Options, First Edition. Edited by Arri Coomarasamy, Mahmood I. Shafi, G. Willy Davila and Kiong K. Chan.
© 2016 John Wiley & Sons, Ltd. Published 2016 by John Wiley & Sons, Ltd.

Table 2.1 Perioperative use of medications.

Medication class	Perioperative recommendation	Alternatives for prolonged "nil by mouth"
Cardiovascular medications (Chapters 3–7)		
Antihypertensives	Continue most antihypertensives, including a dose on the morning of surgery *Withhold diuretics on the morning of surgery to reduce the risk of volume depletion and hypokalemia* *Withhold ACE inhibitors on the night before and the morning of surgery* Consider prophylactic beta-blockers in patients at high risk of perioperative cardiac morbidity (controversial)	Consider transdermal alternatives to α_2-agonists Consider intravenous alternatives to beta-blockers (e.g., esmolol) Nitropaste is an alternative to oral nitrates
Antiarrhythmics (digoxin, sotalol, amiodarone)	Continue; consider serum levels	Amiodarone i.v.
Lipid-lowering drugs	Continue statins, including on the morning of surgery *Discontinue bile acid sequestrants (cholestyramine, colestipol) and fibric acid derivatives (gemfibrozil) and other agents*	
Pulmonary medications (Chapters 8 and 53)	Continue inhaled agents (beta-agonists, ipratropium and steroids) Continue chronic corticosteroids and increase dosage to account for surgical stress Continue leukotriene inhibitors Theophylline: no clear advice	Consider nebulized therapy Consider intravenous steroids
Medications affecting hemostasis (Chapters 14–16)	Antiplatelet agents can be continued in patients having minor surgery	Consider bridging anticoagulation with LMWH for patients at high risk of thrombosis
Aspirin, clopidogrel (irreversible platelet function)	*Stop 5 days before surgery*	
Dipyridamole	No clear advice	
NSAIDs (reversible platelet dysfunction)	*Stop 3 days before surgery*	
Cox-2 inhibitors (little or no platelet effect)	Continue	
Warfarin	*Stop 4 days before surgery, and check INR the night before surgery. Most operations are safe when INR <1.5.* For emergency surgery, warfarin effect can be reversed by 2 units of FFP over 30 min (recheck INR after 1 hour) or 10 mg of intramuscular vitamin K (recheck INR after 6 hours)	
Unfractionated heparin (UFH)	*Discontinue full-dose anticoagulation 4–6 hours before surgery*	
Low-molecular-weight heparin (LMWH)	*Discontinue full-dose anticoagulation 24 hours before surgery*	
Endocrine medications (Chapters 9, 10 and 17)		
Diabetic agents	*Withhold oral hypoglycemics on the day of surgery and resume when patient starts eating. If the half-life of the agent is >24 hours, stop 2 days before surgery* *Discontinue metformin for 2 days before surgery* Insulin: individualized regimens are required. For intermediate and long-acting insulin, half the usual dose is normally given on the night before and the morning of the operation, with dextrose infusion and sliding scale insulin	Use intermediate and long-acting insulin for "basal coverage" with sliding scale insulin
Thyroid agents	Continue thyroxine Continue antithyroid medications	
Steroid therapy	If the patient is on >10 mg of prednisolone (or equivalent) per day, use the following: • For minor surgery: hydrocortisone 25 mg i.v. at induction • For moderate surgery: hydrocortisone 50 mg i.v. at induction, and 25 mg every 8 hours for 48 hours, and then resume usual oral dose • For major surgery: hydrocortisone 100 mg i.v. at induction and 50 mg every 8 hours for 48–72 hours and resume usual oral dose	Use intravenous hydrocortisone therapy Discuss with endocrinologist
Oral contraceptives and hormone replacement therapy	*Stop combined estrogen/progesterone preparations 4 weeks before major surgery* Continue progesterone-only preparations	
Gastrointestinal medications	Continue H_2 blockers Continue proton pump inhibitors	Consider intravenous therapy
Neurologic and psychotropic medications (Chapters 18 and 19)	Continue anti-seizure medications Hold anti-Parkinsonian agents briefly Continue agents for myasthenia gravis Continue SSRIs Continue tricyclic antidepressants, benzodiazepines, lithium, and antipsychotics *Discontinue MAOIs 10–14 days before surgery*	Benzodiazepines can be used parenterally The antipsychotic agents haloperidol and olanzapine can be given parenterally
Herbal medications	Discontinue 1 week before surgery	

Restarting medications

Most drugs that are discontinued preoperatively can be restarted as soon as the patient is able to tolerate oral intake. For anticoagulants and for drugs that predispose to VTE, the time of recommencement will need to be individualized. If a patient is unable to take oral medications for more than 1 or 2 days, then alternative routes should be considered, in consultation with the medical and pharmacy teams as appropriate.

Resolution of the case

The patient will need to be reviewed by an anesthetist and medical specialists to optimize her condition preoperatively. Necessary tests, including blood count, biochemistry, chest X-ray, ECG, lung function, and possibly cardiac function, will need to be performed. Phenytoin will need to be continued perioperatively, including on the morning of surgery. This can be taken with a small sip of water up to 2 hours before surgery.

It is very likely that this woman's adrenal axis will have been suppressed and normal steroid response to stress will have been blunted with 20 mg/day of regular prednisolone. As this is major surgery, hydrocortisone 100 mg i.v. should be given at induction, followed by 50 mg i.v. every 8 hours for 48–72 hours; after this period, the usual oral dose of steroid can be resumed.

Prevention

A full drug and allergy history is essential to identify and avoid potentially serious drug and anesthetic interaction. When reviewing the medications, consider the indication for the medication, the effects of stopping the drug, absorption, half-life, metabolism, and elimination. Involvement of anesthetists, physicians, and pharmacists may be necessary for patients on complex medical regimens. Even if patients are "nil by mouth," they may still take oral medications with a sip of water until 2 hours before the operation; postoperatively, the aim should be to restart the medicine on day 1.

KEY POINTS

Challenge: Patient on medication.

Background
- Medications may affect or be affected by surgery.
- For each drug, a decision needs to be made to stop, continue as normal, or modify the regimen.
- Major surgery is associated with release of the stress hormones cortisol and catecholamines; this has implications for patients with adrenocortical suppression and diabetes.
- Abdominal surgery can be associated with nausea, vomiting, and ileus; this may necessitate a non-oral route of drug administration.

Prevention
- A full drug and allergy history should be taken preoperatively.
- When reviewing medications, consider indication, effect of withdrawal, absorption, half-life, metabolism, and elimination.
- Involve physicians, anesthetists, and pharmacists for women with complex medical regimens.

Management
- Patients may take oral medications with a sip of water until 2 hours before surgery.
- Postoperatively, aim to start oral medications on day 1. If oral medication is not tolerated, consider alternative routes temporarily.
- For specific recommendations about perioperative use of commonly used medicines, see Table 2.1.

References

1 Drugs in the peri-operative period. 1. Stopping or continuing drugs around surgery. *Drug Ther Bull* 1999; 37:62–64.
2 Dawson J, Karalliedde L. Drug interactions and the clinical anaesthetist. *Eur J Anaesthesiol* 1998; 15:172–189.
3 Chernow B, Alexander HR, Smallridge RC *et al.* Hormone responses to graded surgical stress. *Arch Intern Med* 1987; 147:1273–1278.

Further reading

Cohn SL (ed.) *Perioperative Medicine*. Springer Verlag, London, 2011.

CHAPTER 3
Patient with Ischemic Heart Disease

Sohail Q. Khan and Jonathan N. Townend

University Hospitals Birmingham NHS Foundation Trust, Birmingham, UK

Case history: A 75-year-old woman with an ovarian mass is scheduled to have surgery under general anesthesia. During the course of history-taking, it became apparent that she had symptoms of chest pain on minimal exertion and on two occasions had been woken at night with typical ischemic chest pain necessitating the use of her GTN spray. Her cardiac biomarkers were within the normal range.

Background

Coronary artery disease (CAD) is common and affects around 12% of the female population over 70. In patients with stable or asymptomatic CAD undergoing non-cardiac surgery, trials have shown no benefit from prophylactic coronary revascularization at reducing subsequent operative risk [1]. However, chest pain *at rest* is a symptom of unstable angina, a form of acute coronary syndrome which if untreated carries a high risk of adverse events including myocardial infarction (MI) and mortality. Thus, further investigation with coronary angiography is warranted as there is a significantly increased risk of postoperative MI, cardiac arrest and death to the patient. Even if treated by percutaneous coronary intervention (PCI) with coronary stents, a delay in performing surgery is mandated. It has been shown that patients undergoing non-cardiac surgery within 6 weeks of a PCI procedure have a higher risk of mortality when compared with patients undergoing surgery after 6 weeks [2]. Published guidelines are available for risk assessment and management of patients with CAD who need to undergo non-cardiac surgery [3].

If coronary revascularization is undertaken by PCI, there are concerns related to the need for dual antiplatelet therapy and operative bleeding. This, on the other hand, has to be balanced with the risk of stent thrombosis associated with early discontinuation of dual antiplatelet drugs in patients who have had recent deployment of a stent.

Coronary revascularization prior to non-cardiac surgery

The Coronary Artery Revascularization Prophylaxis (CARP) trial [1] investigated the value of medical therapy versus revascularization in stable patients undergoing non-cardiac surgery. The revascularization strategy included both PCI and coronary artery bypass grafting (CABG). There was no difference in perioperative MI or long-term mortality when medical therapy was compared with coronary revascularization. Outside the perioperative setting, when non-invasive ischemia testing is employed, patients with evidence of moderate to severe ischemia (defined as >10% myocardium at risk) seem to benefit prognostically from PCI compared with medical therapy alone [4]. This strategy reduces the risk of death or MI especially if the ischemic burden is reduced to less than 5%. No trial, however, has specifically addressed the role of prophylactic coronary revascularization in patients with unstable angina symptoms requiring non-cardiac surgery.

PCI with BMS versus DES

Coronary artery stents broadly comprise two categories: the bare metal stent (BMS) and the drug-eluting stent (DES). The latter were introduced in the early 1990s as a result of the high rate of restenosis seen with the deployment of BMS in the early (3–6 months) postoperative phase. Minor restenosis caused by neointimal hyperplasia (also called late luminal loss) is universal and occurs as part of the normal healing process within the vascular wall, and leads to scar tissue formation within the lumen of the stent. In about 30% of cases when a BMS is used, the degree of restenosis is severe leading to recurrent flow limitation. This can cause symptoms of recurrent angina and on occasion result in occlusion of the vessel and subsequent MI [5]. Risk factors for the development of restenosis with implantation of a BMS have been identified and include the presence of diabetes, current smoking, a reference vessel diameter of less than 3.25 mm, and lesion length of more than 30 mm [6].

A DES differs from a BMS in that it has an antiproliferative drug coating that inhibits smooth muscle proliferation and neointimal hyperplasia. The use of drug-eluting compared with bare metal stents results in a significant reduction in the subsequent need for target vessel revascularization, with no difference in rates of death or MI [7]. The use of DES modulates vascular inflammation preventing restenosis but also leads to delayed re-endothelialization and impairment of endothelial function, which increases the requirements for duration of dual antiplatelet therapy.

Coronary stents and antiplatelet therapy

Stent thrombosis is a feared outcome, with reported mortality rates up to 45% [8]. Stent thrombosis can be categorized as early (0–30 days), late (>30 days), and very late (>12 months). The presence of metal within the coronary tree creates a thrombogenic area; fortunately

Gynecologic and Obstetric Surgery: Challenges and Management Options, First Edition. Edited by Arri Coomarasamy, Mahmood I. Shafi, G. Willy Davila and Kiong K. Chan.
© 2016 John Wiley & Sons, Ltd. Published 2016 by John Wiley & Sons, Ltd.

there are antiplatelet drugs available which reduce the risk of stent thrombosis to less than 1%. Aspirin and clopidogrel have long been considered mandatory. Recently, however, there have been newer antiplatelet drugs (ticagrelor, prasugrel) which further reduce the risk of stent thrombosis but with an increased risk of bleeding [9,10].

After implantation of a BMS it is recommended that the patient remains on a dual antiplatelet regimen for 4 weeks. For a DES, the recommendation is 6–12 months to allow adequate endothelialization of the stent [11]. Early discontinuation of antiplatelet drugs is considered the most potent risk factor for stent thrombosis [8]. Surgery also induces a state of hypercoagulability with reduced fibrinolysis and increased platelet reactivity, thus conferring an increased risk of stent thrombosis [12].

There were initial concerns that the presence of a DES may confer an increased risk of stent thrombosis, but recent studies do not suggest this [13]. It is also becoming evident that although early discontinuation of dual antiplatelet therapy carries a substantially increased relative risk of stent thrombosis, absolute risks are low and shorter durations of treatment (as little as 3 months) may be adequate when necessary [14].

Bleeding risk with dual antiplatelet therapy

Some types of surgery increase the risk of bleeding and ideally should be undertaken with single or no antiplatelet therapy (e.g., prostatectomy, intracranial surgery, and myomectomy). However, patients who have had recent stent implantation should continue on aspirin when undergoing surgery. The decision to continue with clopidogrel will depend on the type of surgery and the type of coronary stent inserted. In certain surgical procedures, continuing with clopidogrel has been shown to increase the risk of bleeding, the need for blood transfusion, and hospital stay. The risk of bleeding will therefore need to be carefully balanced against the risk of developing stent thrombosis if clopidogrel is discontinued.

Management

A cardiologist and an anesthetist will need to be involved in the management of a patient with CAD. The first step is to assess the extent and stability of CAD as well as the presence of any comorbidities (e.g., hypertension, diabetes, renal disease). Appropriate investigations may include ECG, echocardiography, exercise stress test, and coronary angiography.

Preoperative optimization of medical conditions should include cessation of smoking, good control of hypertension and cholesterol, and management of comorbidities such as diabetes.

The key decisions are best made in a multidisciplinary setting, and should include consideration of whether warfarin, aspirin or clopidogrel need to be stopped, and whether preoperative revascularization (e.g., with PCI) is needed.

A systematic review of randomized trials found that regional (spinal or epidural) anesthesia is safer than general anesthesia, with a reduction in overall mortality with regional anesthesia (OR 0.7; 95% CI 0.5–0.9) [15]. Although research evidence supports a more widespread use of regional anesthesia, it is recognized that an individualized approach will need to be taken with each patient.

Postoperatively, vigilance is required; if myocardial ischemia is suspected, an ECG and measurement of cardiac troponins, as well as review by a cardiologist, should be arranged.

Resolution of the case

The management involved close discussion with surgeons and cardiologists. In view of the history of chest pain, the patient in the case history underwent a cardiac perfusion scan which confirmed significant ischemia in the left anterior descending artery territory (>10%). In light of this finding, she underwent urgent coronary angiography. There were concerns about the possible malignant nature of the ovarian mass and the indication for urgent surgery was clear. However, the high risks of dangerous cardiac complications when performing surgery on patients with unstable angina are well known and prominent in all relevant guidelines, so surgery was delayed. Angiography revealed a critical stenosis in the proximal left anterior descending artery (Figure 3.1). In view of this and the large amount of myocardium in jeopardy, she proceeded to PCI (Figures 3.2 and 3.3). It was clear that the patient would need

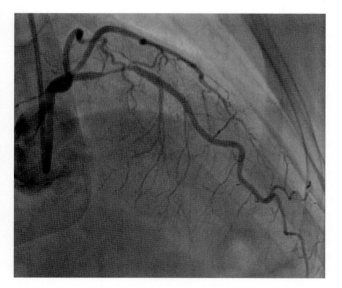

Figure 3.1 Coronary angiogram showing significant proximal left anterior descending (LAD) artery stenosis.

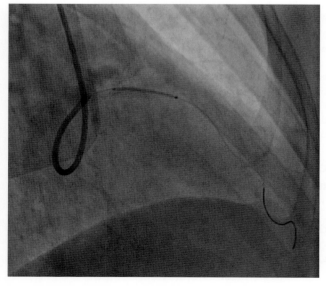

Figure 3.2 Successful positioning of 3.0 × 18 mm bare metal stent in proximal LAD.

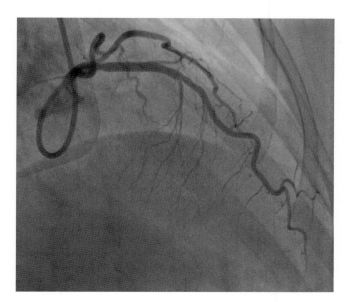

Figure 3.3 Successful stent deployment and final angiographic result after expansion of stent with a 3.5 mm non-compliant balloon.

to go to surgery in the near future and so a bare metal stent was successfully deployed. Dual antiplatelet therapy was given for only 4 weeks post PCI. At 6 weeks the patient remained on aspirin therapy together with statins and underwent a successful general anesthetic procedure and surgical exploration.

In patients with stable angina there is no clear role for prophylactic revascularization prior to non-cardiac surgery but it is believed that optimal medical therapy including aspirin and statins reduces the risk of adverse cardiac events. However, in this patient, because of the unstable nature of symptoms and large burden of myocardium at risk, it was important for her to undergo undertake coronary angiography and revascularization by PCI.

Prevention

A key goal of preoperative assessment is to identify hitherto undiagnosed heart disease. A cardiovascular condition may be suspected if the patient has unexplained chest pain, shortness of breath, claudication, lower extremity edema, erectile dysfunction, or past history of cerebrovascular events. All patients over the age of 60 years should have routine preoperative ECG.

If screening suggests a cardiovascular condition, appropriate investigations (e.g., ECG, exercise treadmill ECG, 24-hour ECG, and echocardiogram) should be arranged, and management planned with the help of a cardiologist and consultant anesthetist.

Preoperatively, the patient's condition should be optimized, with cessation of smoking and good control of blood pressure, cholesterol and body weight. There is conflicting evidence on the use of preoperative beta-blocker therapy, although it is suggested that it can be considered in patients who have known ischemic heart disease or myocardial ischemia [16]. The use of preoperative statins also has a IIa recommendation. Meta-analysis has shown that statins can reduce postoperative MI [17]; this is most likely a class effect and if statin treatment is considered, it should be initiated 4 weeks before non-cardiac surgical procedures.

KEY POINTS

Challenge: Patient with ischemic heart disease.

Background
- CAD is common in those over 70 years of age.
- In stable or asymptomatic CAD, it is believed that optimal medical therapy including aspirin and statins reduces the risk of adverse cardiac events.
- Unstable angina carries a high risk of adverse events including MI and death, warranting further investigation with coronary angiography.
- If PCI is indicated, surgery should be delayed for 6 weeks if possible.
- Elective surgery should be delayed for 3–6 months after MI.

Prevention (of complications)
- Perform a thorough preoperative assessment to identify undiagnosed heart disease.
- Perform ECG on all patients over 60 years of age.
- Optimize preoperative condition: cessation of smoking, good control of hypertension and cholesterol, and management of comorbidities such as diabetes.
- Refer patients with unstable cardiac symptoms to a cardiologist for evaluation of symptoms as they are at increased risk of cardiac complications.
- Patients with unstable cardiac symptoms and/or substantial myocardium at risk should undergo revascularization and deployment of a BMS.
- There are conflicting data on the use of preoperative beta-blocker therapy, and routine use is not recommended for the purpose of postoperative risk reduction.
- There are promising data on the use of preoperative statins to reduce postoperative cardiovascular complications.

Management
- Involve a cardiologist and an anesthetist.
- Assess the extent and stability of CAD.
- Assess the presence of comorbidities, particularly hypertension, high cholesterol, diabetes, and renal disease.
- Arrange necessary investigations (e.g., ECG, echocardiography, exercise stress test, and coronary angiography).
- Take key decisions in a multidisciplinary setting:
  - When to stop and restart warfarin.
  - Whether and when to stop and restart aspirin and clopidogrel.
  - Whether to organize preoperative revascularization (e.g., stent) and delay the operation.
  - Whether to use regional (spinal or epidural) or general anesthesia.
- Postoperatively, if myocardial ischemia is suspected, arrange an ECG and measurement of cardiac troponins, as well as review by a cardiologist.

References

1 McFalls EO, Ward HB, Moritz TE et al. Coronary-artery revascularization before elective major vascular surgery. N Engl J Med 2004; 351:2795–2804.
2 Nuttall GA, Brown MJ, Stombaugh JW et al. Time and cardiac risk of surgery after bare-metal stent percutaneous coronary intervention. Anesthesiology 2008; 109:588–595.
3 Poldermans D, Bax JJ, Boersma E et al. Guidelines for pre-operative cardiac risk assessment and perioperative cardiac management in non-cardiac surgery. Eur Heart J 2009; 30:2769–2812.
4 Shaw LJ, Berman DS, Maron DJ et al. Optimal medical therapy with or without percutaneous coronary intervention to reduce ischemic burden. Circulation 2008; 117:1283–1291.
5 Rathore S, Kinoshita Y, Terashima M et al. Comparison of clinical presentations, angiographic patterns and outcomes of in-stent restenosis between bare metal stents and drug eluting stents. EuroIntervention 2010; 5:841–846.
6 Park CB, Park HK. Identification of independent risk factors for restenosis following bare-metal stent implantation: role of bare-metal stents in the era of drug-eluting stents. Exp Ther Med 2013; 6:840–846.
7 Kaiser C, Galatius S, Erne P et al. Drug-eluting versus bare-metal stents in large coronary arteries. N Engl J Med 2010; 363:2310–2319.
8 Iakovou I, Schmidt T, Bonizzoni E et al. Incidence, predictors, and outcome of thrombosis after successful implantation of drug-eluting stents. JAMA 2005; 293:2126–2130.

9 Wiviott SD, Braunwald E, McCabe CH *et al.* Prasugrel versus clopidogrel in patients with acute coronary syndromes. *N Engl J Med* 2007; 357:2001–2015.

10 Steg PG, Harrington RA, Emanuelsson H *et al.* Stent thrombosis with ticagrelor versus clopidogrel in patients with acute coronary syndromes: an analysis from the prospective randomized PLATO trial. *Circulation* 2013; 128:1055–1065.

11 Wijns W, Kolh P, Danchin N *et al.* Guidelines on myocardial revascularization: the Task Force on myocardial revascularization of the European Society of Cardiology (ESC) and the European Association for Cardio-Thoracic Surgery (EACTS). *Eur Heart J* 2010; 31:2501–2555.

12 Blake GJ, Ridker PM. Inflammatory bio-markers and cardiovascular risk prediction. *J Intern Med* 2002; 252:283–294.

13 Mauri L, Hsieh WH, Massaro JM *et al.* Stent thrombosis in randomized clinical trials of drug-eluting stents. *N Engl J Med* 2007; 356:1020–1029.

14 Kim BK, Hong MK, Shin DH *et al.* A new strategy for discontinuation of dual antiplatelet therapy: the RESET Trial (REal Safety and Efficacy of 3-month dual antiplatelet Therapy following Endeavor zotarolimus-eluting stent implantation). *J Am Coll Cardiol* 2012; 60:1340–1348.

15 Rodgers A, Walker N, Schug S *et al.* Reduction of postoperative mortality and morbidity with epidural or spinal anaesthesia: results from overview of randomised trials. *BMJ* 2000; 321:1493.

16 Kristensen SD, Knuuti J, Saraste A *et al.* 2014 ESC/ESA Guidelines on non-cardiac surgery: cardiovascular assessment and management. *Eur Heart J* 2014; 35:2383–2431.

17 Winchester DE, Wen X, Xie L, Bavry AA. Evidence of pre-procedural statin therapy: a meta-analysis of randomized trials. *J Am Coll Cardiol* 2010; 56:1099–1109.

CHAPTER 4

Patient with Arrhythmias

Sanoj Chacko and Joseph de Bono

University Hospitals Birmingham NHS Foundation Trust, Birmingham, UK

Case history: *A 76-year-old woman attended for preoperative assessment, as she was awaiting hysterectomy. She was known to have had hypertension for 10 years and was diagnosed to be in atrial fibrillation (AF) 1 month previously on ECG. She had a DDD pacemaker implanted 3 years ago for an episode of collapse and asystole and had remained stable since then with satisfactory pacemaker check annually. Her medications included warfarin, amlodipine 10 mg once daily, and digoxin 125 μg once daily. On assessment she was asymptomatic, BP 130/80 mmHg, pulse 80–90/min irregularly irregular, but physical examination was otherwise unremarkable. Her 12-lead ECG confirmed rate-controlled AF, and echocardiography showed mild concentric LVH, good left ventricular systolic function, normal cardiac dimensions, and no significant valvular lesion; 24-hour tape showed rate-controlled AF.*

Background

Atrial fibrillation (AF) is the most common cardiac arrhythmia, occurring in 1–2% of the general population. The prevalence of AF increases with advancing age, from less than 0.5% at 40–50 years to 5–15% at 80 years. About one-third of the patients with AF are asymptomatic, which aggravates the problem of timely detection and early management. The Framingham Heart Study showed that AF was associated with increased morbidity and mortality in both men and women. The adverse consequences of AF are related to reduced cardiac output and to thromboembolic manifestations. The arrhythmia is associated with a fivefold increase in stroke, and anticoagulation has been shown to reduce mortality by approximately two-thirds.

Definition and classifications

AF is a cardiac arrhythmia characterized by surface ECG showing irregular RR intervals with no distinct P waves. The hemodynamic consequence is a result of loss of coordinated atrial contraction, irregular ventricular response, and decrease in myocardial blood flow.

AF is broadly divided into valvular and non-valvular AF and the term "valvular AF" is used to imply that AF is associated with rheumatic valvular disease or prosthetic heart valves. Depending on the nature of the arrhythmia, AF can be characterized as follows.
- New-onset AF: first diagnosed AF, regardless of the duration, presence or absence of symptoms.

- Paroxysmal AF (PAF): PAF is intermittent and self-terminating AF, with two or more episodes in less than 7 days.
- Persistent AF: this is when AF fails to terminate spontaneously within 7 days and continues until reverted chemically or electrically.
- Permanent AF: this term is used to identify patients with persistent AF in whom the chances of restoring sinus rhythm are unlikely; therefore a rate control strategy is adopted.
- Lone AF: no underlying structural heart disease.

Management

Management of AF is aimed not only at reducing the risks of death, stroke and other thromboembolic consequences, but also at reducing hospitalization and improving quality of life.

When a patient presents with new-onset AF, a rapid assessment of her symptoms (palpitations, breathlessness, fatigue, dizziness), hemodynamic status (ventricular rate, hypotension, hypoxia), and underlying causes (structural heart disease, heart failure, ischemia, electrolyte abnormalities, thyroid dysfunction, pulmonary disease, chronic renal disease) is important. A focused assessment and relevant investigations are crucial for an initial work-up. Initial investigations include full blood count, renal profile, thyroid function, inflammatory markers, chest X-ray, ECG, and echocardiography.

Risk stratification

All patients need to be assessed for anticoagulation therapy. Unless a patient is under 65 with no risk factors or has a major contraindication, she should be anticoagulated with warfarin or a novel anticoagulant (NOAC). The thromboembolic risk is similar in individuals with paroxysmal, persistent, or permanent AF and the risk stratification can be performed using clinical and echocardiographic variables. All patients with valvular AF need anticoagulation. In non-valvular AF, the modified CHA_2DS_2-VASc score (Table 4.1) can be used to assess for thromboembolic risk. The risk of major bleeding, in particular intracranial bleed, is the most feared complication of anticoagulation therapy. Hence the decision to consider anticoagulation must be carefully balanced against the risk of bleeding. While there are several bleeding risk assessment tools, the widely recommended HAS-BLED tool (Table 4.2) offers simple and reliable bleeding risk prediction. For patients with

Gynecologic and Obstetric Surgery: Challenges and Management Options, First Edition. Edited by Arri Coomarasamy, Mahmood I. Shafi, G. Willy Davila and Kiong K. Chan.
© 2016 John Wiley & Sons, Ltd. Published 2016 by John Wiley & Sons, Ltd.

Table 4.1 CHA$_2$DS$_2$-VASc scoring, adapted with permission from MDCalc.com©.

C	Congestive heart failure	1
H	Hypertension	1
A$_2$	Age >75 years	2
D	Diabetes mellitus	1
S$_2$	Stroke/TIA/thromboembolism	2
V	Vascular disease (previous MI, peripheral arterial disease or aortic plaque)	1
A	Age between 65 and 74 years	1
Sc	Female	1

Source: Lip *et al.*, 2010 [2]. www.mdcalc.com. Reproduced with permission of the American College of Chest Physicians.

Table 4.2 HAS-BLED scoring, adapted with permission from MDCalc.com©

H	Hypertension	1
A	Abnormal renal function	1
A	Abnormal liver function	1
S	Stroke	1
B	Bleeding	1
L	Labile INRs	1
E	Elderly (age >65 years)	1
D	Drugs	1
D	Alcohol	1

Source: Pisters *et al.*, 2010 [3]. www.mdcalc.com. Reproduced with permission of the American College of Chest Physicians.

a HAS-BLED score of 3 or above, anticoagulation should be considered with caution and close monitoring is recommended while modifying the risk factors. Warfarin has been the choice for anticoagulation therapy for more than 50 years; however, more recently, NOACs such as direct thrombin inhibitor (dabigatran) and factor Xa inhibitors (rivaroxaban and apixaban) have also been used in selected patients with non-valvular AF. The indication for anticoagulation in patients with AF is shown in Figure 4.1.

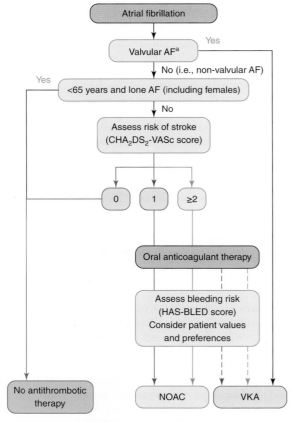

Figure 4.1 Antithrombotic therapy. AF, atrial fibrillation; NOAC, novel oral anticoagulant; OAC, oral anticoagulant; VKA, vitamin K antagonist. CHA$_2$DS$_2$-VASc score: green = 0; blue = 1; red ≥2. Solid line represents best option; dashed line represents alternative option. ^{a} Includes rheumatic valvular disease and prosthetic valves. From Camm *et al.*, 2012 [1] with permission of Oxford University Press (UK). © European Society of Cardiology, www.escardio.org/guidelines.

Antiarrhythmic therapy

The general principles of management of AF are to determine the urgency of therapy and the choice between a rate control and a rhythm control strategy. A rate control strategy is generally adopted for patients with permanent AF, and this is achieved with drugs that slow conduction through the atrioventricular node. While an optimum rate goal has not been determined, achieving a heart rate of 80 bpm or less at rest and 110 bpm or less during moderate exercise would be ideal. The efficacy of rate control can be assessed by various methods, such as resting 12-lead ECG, 6-min walk test, and 24-hour ambulatory monitor. A rhythm control strategy is adopted for patients with symptomatic paroxysmal or persistent AF, and consists of antiarrhythmic drugs, cardioversion, and radiofrequency ablation.

The most commonly used drugs for rate and rhythm control are shown in Table 4.3. The choice of antiarrhythmic drug generally depends on underlying pathology. In patients with significant structural heart disease and associated heart failure, in whom rhythm control is required, the choice of drug therapy is limited to amiodarone. However, in patients with minimal or no structural heart disease, therapy with sotalol, flecainide, propafenone, and dronedarone is effective.

Table 4.3 Pharmacotherapy for arrhythmia.

Rate control
Beta-blockers (atenolol, metoprolol, bisoprolol)
Calcium antagonists (diltiazem, verapamil)
Digoxin
Amiodarone

Rhythm control
Sotalol
Flecainide
Amiodarone
Dronedarone
Propafenone

Indications for urgent cardioversion

The American College of Cardiology/American Heart Association/European Society of Cardiology (ACC/AHA/ESC) guidelines recommend direct current cardioversion in four circumstances.
1 Myocardial ischemia.
2 Hypotension and organ hypoperfusion.
3 Heart failure.
4 Pre-excited AF with fast ventricular response.

Perioperative management

Antiarrhythmic drugs should ideally not be discontinued perioperatively. The risk of bleeding during surgery in patients taking anticoagulant therapy depends on several factors, such as the patient's age, type of surgery, coexisting disease, and anticoagulation regimen. Continuation of anticoagulation increases the risk of bleeding, and interruption of such therapy may increase the risk of thromboembolism. Timely interruption and resumption of anticoagulant therapy and appropriate use of alternative bridging anticoagulation therapy, using subcutaneous low-molecular-weight heparin or intravenous heparin, has been used to minimize the perioperative complications.

Elective surgery

Most patients with AF can discontinue oral anticoagulation for up to 7 days around elective surgery. However, in patients who are at very high risk of embolic events (e.g., CHADS-VASc >3), treatment-dose low-molecular-weight heparin may be given perioperatively. Warfarin has a long half-life of 36–48 hours, and it takes 2–3 days for the INR to fall below 2 and 4–6 days for it to normalize. Once warfarin is restarted it takes up to 5 days for the INR to rise above 2. In general, warfarin is discontinued 5 days before surgery and recommenced as soon after possible afterwards. It is therefore estimated that in the perioperative period patients will have a subtherapeutic INR for 8–10 days.

NOACs have a rapid onset of action, achieving peak anticoagulant activity 2–3 hours after ingestion, with an elimination half-life of 12–14 hours. Unlike rivaroxaban and apixaban, dabigatran excretion is dependent on renal clearance, and therefore in patients with severe renal impairment the elimination half-life of dabigatran is significantly prolonged. In general, NOACs should be discontinued 1–2 days before surgery depending on the risk of perioperative bleeding. For those patients with renal failure with a creatinine clearance of less than 50 mL/min, dabigatran should be discontinued 3–5 days before surgery. Postoperatively, even when hemostasis has been achieved, caution should be taken when resuming NOACs due to their rapid onset of action. Following surgery associated with a high risk of hemorrhage, it is sensible to delay resuming NOACs for 2–3 days.

Emergency surgery

In emergency surgery, urgent reversal of anticoagulation is required. In patients on warfarin, the drug should be withheld, and 2.5–5 mg of intravenous vitamin K needs to be administered. If more immediate reversal is required, for example within minutes to hours, fresh frozen plasma or prothrombin complex concentrate should be given in addition to vitamin K. In patients on NOACs, the anticoagulation effect can be assessed by checking aPTT for dabigatran and PT or factor Xa assay for rivaroxaban and apixaban; however, there is a poor correlation between these measures and actual anticoagulation effect. NOACs do not have specific antidotes; however, in an emergency setting reversal of anticoagulation can be achieved by administering prothrombin complex concentrate or activated recombinant factor VII and by replacing blood products. Close collaboration with a hematologist is essential.

New-onset perioperative AF

It is not uncommon for patients to develop new-onset AF following surgery, usually due to electrolyte imbalance or infection. It may also be a manifestation of pulmonary embolism or acute coronary syndrome. Careful clinical assessment is crucial to look for an underlying cause, and prompt management is essential. Rate control should be achieved using a beta-blocker, calcium channel antagonist, or digoxin. Digoxin is particularly useful in patients with low blood pressure or cardiac failure. In the high-dependency setting, sinus rhythm

can often be achieved with intravenous amiodarone but this must be given into a central vein. In patients who become acutely hemodynamically compromised with sudden-onset AF, sinus rhythm should be restored with DC cardioversion. If AF persists or recurs, then the patient should be risk stratified for anticoagulation and referred to a cardiologist for consideration of outpatient DC cardioversion.

Resolution of the case

The patient should be referred to a cardiologist for assessment prior to listing her for elective surgery.

The patient had persistent asymptomatic AF with a CHA$_2$DS$_2$-VASc score of 3, giving her an estimated annual stroke risk of 3.2%. She had a low HAS-BLED score and hence had a low bleeding risk. She remained asymptomatic with no clinical evidence of cardiac decompensation and her AF seemed very well rate-controlled on resting 12-lead ECG and 24-hour ambulatory monitor. Echocardiography found evidence of mild concentric left ventricular hypertrophy consistent with long-standing hypertension but was otherwise unremarkable with no significant valvular lesion. In her case, a rate-control strategy with long-term anticoagulation with either warfarin or NOACs would be appropriate.

She could stop her anticoagulation preoperatively and this should be started again as soon as possible postoperatively. Her current antiarrhythmic drug should be continued during surgery and if she needs any additional rate-limiting drug postoperatively, then a beta-blocker could be added to achieve optimum heart rate control.

She had a dual chamber pacemaker implanted for asystole in the past and therefore there is a potential risk of asystole during surgery in the current pacing mode. Hence a cardiac physiologist should be asked to reprogram her pacemaker to asynchronous pacing mode should electrocautery be used during surgery or care should be taken to use short bursts of electrocautery with arterial pressure monitoring.

KEY POINTS

Challenge: Patient in atrial fibrillation.

Background
- AF is the commonest arrhythmia, and becomes more common with advancing age.
- It may be asymptomatic, but is associated with increased morbidity and mortality.
- The adverse effects are related to decreased cardiac output and thromboembolic manifestations.
- Anticoagulation reduces mortality.

Prevention (of complications)
- In patients with AF, risk stratification is essential to determine appropriate therapy to reduce the risk of stroke.
- Appropriate knowledge of perioperative management of anticoagulation is crucial for a favorable surgical outcome.
- Balance the risk of stopping anticoagulation and causing thromboembolic complications against the increased risk of surgical hemorrhage if it is continued.

Management
- Involve a cardiologist.
- Continue rate-control drugs perioperatively.
- New-onset AF identified during perioperative period needs careful evaluation.
- Evaluate symptoms, hemodynamic status, and underlying causes.
- Anticoagulate if indicated, considering type of surgery.
- Institute rate or rhythm control as appropriate.

- The timing of discontinuation and recommencement of anticoagulation is dependent on the type of surgery and the risk of adverse cardiovascular events.
  - In general, warfarin is stopped 5 days before surgery, and recommenced as soon after possible afterwards.
  - In general, NOACs are stopped 1 or 2 days before surgery, and recommenced only when risk of serious bleeding has passed (usually 2 or 3 days after surgery).
- Reverse anticoagulation in an emergency situation if necessary.
  - Stop warfarin and give vitamin K 2.5–5 mg i.v.
  - If immediate reversal is required, give fresh frozen plasma or prothrombin complex concentrate, in addition to vitamin K.
  - For patients on NOACs, discuss with a hematologist, and give prothrombin complex concentrate or activated recombinant factor VII, and replace blood products.

References

1 Camm AJ, Lip GY, De Caterina R *et al*. 2012 focused update of the ESC Guidelines for the management of atrial fibrillation: an update of the 2010 ESC Guidelines for the management of atrial fibrillation. Developed with the special contribution of the European Heart Rhythm Association. *Eur Heart J* 2012; 33:2719–2747.

2 Lip GY, Nieuwlaat R, Pisters R, Lane DA, Crijns HJ. Refining clinical risk stratification for predicting stroke and thromboembolism in atrial fibrillation using a novel risk factor-based approach: the Euro Heart Survey on atrial fibrillation. *Chest* 2010; 137:263–272.

3 Pisters R, Lane DA, Nieuwlaat R, de Vos CB, Crijns HJ, Lip GY. A novel user-friendly score (HAS-BLED) to assess 1-year risk of major bleeding in atrial fibrillation patients: The Euro Heart Survey. *Chest* 2010; 138:1093–1100.

Further reading

Ahrens I, Lip GY, Peter K. New oral anticoagulant drugs in cardiovascular disease. *Thromb Haemost* 2010; 104:49–60.

Camm AJ, Kirchhof P, Lip GY *et al*. Guidelines for the management of atrial fibrillation: the Task Force for the Management of Atrial Fibrillation of the European Society of Cardiology (ESC). *Europace* 2010; 12:1360–1420.

Gallagher AM, Setakis E, Plumb JM *et al*. Risks of stroke and mortality associated with suboptimal anticoagulation in atrial fibrillation patients. *Thromb Haemost* 2011; 106:968–977.

Healey JS, Connolly SJ, Gold MR *et al*. Subclinical atrial fibrillation and the risk of stroke. *N Engl J Med* 2012; 366:120–129.

Lane DA, Lip GYH. Use of the CHA2DS2-VASc and HAS-BLED scores to aid decision making for thromboprophylaxis in non-valvular atrial fibrillation. *Circulation* 2012; 126:860–865.

MDCalc. CHA2DS2-VASc Score for Atrial Fibrillation Stroke Risk. MDCalc© 2015. Available at http://www.mdcalc.com/cha2ds2-vasc-score-for-atrial-fibrillation-stroke-risk/ (accessed May 2015).

MDCalc. HAS-BLED Score for Major Bleeding Risk. MDCalc© 2015. Available at http://www.mdcalc.com/has-bled-score-for-major-bleeding-risk/ (accessed May 2015).

Patel MR, Mahaffey KW, Garg J *et al*. Rivaroxaban vs warfarin in nonvalvular atrial fibrillation. *N Engl J Med* 2011; 365:883–891.

Sie P, Samama CM, Godier A *et al*. Surgery and invasive procedures in patients on long-term treatment with direct oral anticoagulants: thrombin or factor-Xa inhibitors. Recommendations of the Working Group on Perioperative Haemostasis and the French Study Group on Thrombosis and Haemostasis. *Arch Cardiovasc Dis* 2011; 104:669–676.

CHAPTER 5

Patient with a Pacemaker or Implantable Defibrillator

Howard Marshall

University Hospitals Birmingham NHS Foundation Trust, Birmingham, UK

Case history: A 26-year-old girl with an ectopic pregnancy requires emergency surgery. Her previous medical history included a diagnosis of long QT3 which presented with an out-of-hospital VF arrest. She had an implantable dual chamber defibrillator in situ which had last been checked 6 months ago at her local hospital (not yours).

Background

The prevalence of patients with pacemakers and implantable cardioverter defibrillators (ICDs) is increasing worldwide. The latest figures across Europe [1] demonstrate a new implant rate of 697 per million for pacemakers, 146 per million for ICDs, and 142 per million for cardiac resynchronization therapy (CRT) devices for heart failure; figures are similar across the USA [2]. While it is clear that these devices are largely implanted in an older population, there are increasing numbers of younger patients, either with a primary bradycardia indication or more often with accompanying complex cardiac disease. In addition to the management of the pacemaker, many of these patients will need close anesthetic assessment of their other medical problems.

Management

Identifying the type of device

Patients with a pacemaker or ICD should be under regular follow-up and carry a device registration card. Information regarding the device will be available from the patient's follow-up clinic. If these sources of information are unavailable, a chest X-ray should help determine what sort of device a patient has [3]. The size of the generator will help determine whether a device is a pacemaker or ICD, as ICDs are generally bigger than pacemakers, approximately 6–7 × 4–5 cm versus 4–5 × 2–3 cm. Individual manufacturers can be identified by radiographic markers within the header cap of the device. In addition, the leads connecting the generator to the heart have different appearances: an ICD lead has one or two coils along its length that allow delivery of a high-energy shock in the event of a life-threatening ventricular arrhythmia. In contrast, a pacemaker tends to have thinner leads and none will have the shocking coils required by a defibrillator (Figures 5.1, 5.2 and 5.3). A biventricular

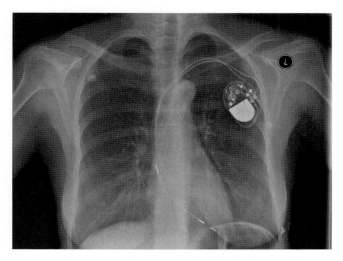

Figure 5.1 PA chest X-ray of a woman with a dual chamber pacemaker. Note the small generator with thin leads without shocking coils.

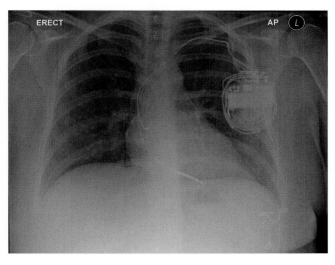

Figure 5.2 PA chest X-ray of a woman with a dual chamber implantable defibrillator. Note the larger generator and shocking coil on ventricular lead.

Gynecologic and Obstetric Surgery: Challenges and Management Options, First Edition. Edited by Arri Coomarasamy, Mahmood I. Shafi, G. Willy Davila and Kiong K. Chan.

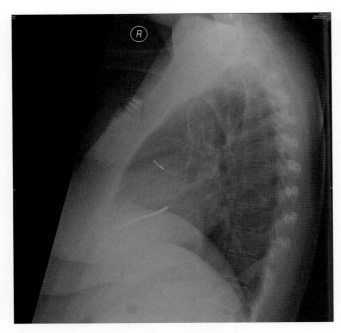

Figure 5.3 Lateral chest X-ray of a woman with a dual chamber implantable defibrillator. Note the shocking coil on ventricular lead.

device (used to treat heart failure) will have two leads overlying the ventricular part of the cardiac shadow and may be either a pacemaker or a defibrillator.

The primary device management issues for pacemaker or defibrillator patients undergoing surgery (gynecologic or otherwise) are:

1 ensuring the pacemaker is functioning normally to provide heart rate support perioperatively;
2 disabling defibrillator function during surgery to avoid inappropriate activation with the use of diathermy (appropriate safety and resuscitation facilities need to be in place);
3 planning of diathermy to avoid suppression of pacing.

Assessing pacemaker function

Pacemaker patients should routinely attend their pacemaker clinic on at least an annual basis. It may be possible to conduct follow-up and device testing remotely using wireless technology. If there is evidence that the pacemaker has had a satisfactory check within 3–6 months before surgery, then no additional check is required. It is prudent, however, to document the pacemaker model and programming and to determine how dependent the patient is on the pacemaker (as this may influence the use of diathermy). Patients should carry a device identity card, which will give details of the device, programming, and the hospital providing follow-up.

If there has not been a recent check, or there is doubt about pacing function, the device should be checked at the patient's usual clinic (for elective surgery) or by the local cardiology department in the case of an acute admission. Where emergency surgery is unavoidable, it may not be possible to obtain a pacemaker check preoperatively; an ECG is the minimum requirement in this circumstance.

Disabling implantable defibrillator function

It is imperative that the defibrillator and anti-tachycardia pacing (ATP) function of an ICD is disabled before surgery. This is because the electrical signals produced by diathermy may be misinterpreted by the ICD, resulting in inappropriate (and possibly proarrhythmic) delivery of a shock or ATP. In the elective or urgent setting, this should be arranged through the local cardiology department. The device should be disabled as close to the scheduled surgery as possible (ideally in the anesthetic room) and re-enabled before the patient returns to the ward. The cardiology team will need to know at least the manufacturer of the device to enable selection of the correct programmer. This information should be available on the patient's device identity card or from the patient's normal follow-up hospital.

In the emergency setting, it may not be possible to disable the ICD using a programmer. Under these circumstances, it is possible to disable the device temporarily with the use of a magnet, which should be available from the local cardiology department, the emergency department, or the coronary care unit. A magnet applied directly over the device will disable defibrillator and ATP function as long as it is kept in place. In this situation, it is advisable to tape the magnet in place firmly for the duration of the surgery. The device should be checked as soon as possible postoperatively.

Planning of diathermy

Diathermy generates an electrical signal which may be misinterpreted by a pacemaker. Even if the defibrillator function of a device has been disabled, its pacing function may be suppressed by the use of diathermy. This is particularly important when patients are pacemaker dependent (i.e., when the pacemaker is working all the time to support the heart rate). To minimize the risk of inhibiting the pacemaker, diathermy use should be optimized.

Where possible, bipolar diathermy should be used; this restricts the electrical output to the surgical field. The vast majority of cardiac devices are implanted on the anterior chest wall but occasionally one may be positioned in the rectus sheath; this will incur additional risk from even bipolar diathermy and there will be surgical implications if a midline or paramedian incision is used for a laparotomy. Specialist advice should be sought under such circumstances.

Where bipolar diathermy is not feasible, monopolar diathermy can be used with caution. The indifferent electrode should be placed as far from the pacemaker as possible (e.g., the thigh) and with cardiac monitoring, diathermy can be used in short pulses. If extensive prolonged diathermy is required, the pacemaker can be reprogrammed to an "asynchronous" mode, which will provide fixed-rate pacing even during electrical interference. However, this may be proarrhythmic and is rarely required.

Prevention

The key to avoiding problems with pacemakers and defibrillators is planning. Identification of patients at pre-admission clinic is essential so that appropriate liaison with the patient's follow-up hospital can take place in advance of surgery. In the emergency setting this can be more difficult, but out-of-hours contact with the cardiology team is usually possible. In any event, full resuscitation facilities need to be available in the operating room.

KEY POINTS

Challenge: Safe management of a patient with a pacemaker or implantable defibrillator during gynecologic surgery.

Background
- Pacemakers and defibrillators are increasingly common in cardiological practice and require special precautions to ensure patient safety during surgery.
- They can stimulate atria, ventricles, or both, and be on-demand (if heart rate is too slow) or asynchronous (function regardless of heart rate).

Management
- Identification of the device is essential and this can be accomplished via the patient's device identity card, local cardiology center, or chest X-ray.
- If no recent pacemaker check has taken place (3–6 months before surgery), it should be sought preoperatively if possible.

- An implantable defibrillator needs to be disabled preoperatively (ideally in the anesthetic room) and reactivated after surgery. A magnet placed directly over the device can perform this function in the emergency setting.
- Diathermy use:
  - Use bipolar diathermy where possible.
  - Can use monopolar diathermy, but with caution and only if absolutely necessary.
  - If prolonged diathermy is anticipated, the pacemaker can be programmed to "asynchronous" mode, which will provide fixed-rate pacing even during electrical interference.

Prevention
- Liaison with the patient's cardiology center in advance of all elective surgery will prevent last minute issues.
- MRI is an absolute contraindication in patients with pacemakers.

References

1 Auricchio A, Kuck K-H, Hatala R, Arribas F. *The EHRA White Book 2012. The Current Status of Cardiac Electrophysiology in ESC Member Countries.* European Heart Rhythm Association, Sophia Antipolis, France, 2012. Available at http://www.escardio.org/static_file/Escardio/Press-media/press-releases/2012/ehra-white-book-2012.pdf

2 Greenspon AJ, Patel JD, Lau E *et al.* Trends in permanent pacemaker implantation in the United States from 1993 to 2009: increasing complexity of patients and procedures. *J Am Coll Cardiol* 2012; 60:1540–1545.

3 Jacob S, Shahzad MA, Maheshwari R, Panaich SS, Aravindhakshan R. Cardiac rhythm device identification algorithm using X-rays: CaRDIA-X. *Heart Rhythm* 2011; 8:915–922.

Further reading

Medicines and Healthcare Products Regulatory Agency. *Guidelines for the perioperative management of patients with implantable pacemakers or implantable cardioverter defibrillators, where the use of surgical diathermy/electrocautery is anticipated.* MHRA, London, 2006. Available at http://heartrhythmuk.org.uk/files/file/Docs/Guidelines/MHRA%20guidelines%20surgery%20and%20ICDs.pdf

CHAPTER 6

Patient with Complex Congenital Heart Disease (Fontan Circulation)

Yaso Emmanuel and Sara A. Thorne
University Hospitals Birmingham NHS Foundation Trust, Birmingham, UK

Case history: A 30-year-old woman with tricuspid atresia had been surgically palliated with a Fontan circulation (extracardiac total cavopulmonary connection). Prior to pregnancy she was well with good ventricular function. During her first pregnancy she developed life-threatening atrial arrhythmia requiring cardioversion in the first trimester. Delivery at 32 weeks of gestation by cesarean section became necessary for obstetric reasons.

Background

The Fontan circulation was first reported in 1971 as a surgical strategy to manage tricuspid atresia. It has since been applied to palliate a variety of different forms of congenital heart disease in which there is a single functioning ventricle and two-ventricular repair is not possible. This approach has transformed the outlook for many patients with complex forms of congenital heart disease.

The basic principle of the Fontan circulation is to use the single ventricle to support the systemic circulation, leaving the systemic venous return to flow passively into the pulmonary arteries without the support of a ventricle. This is achieved by redirecting the systemic venous return straight to the pulmonary arteries without passing through a subpulmonary ventricle. There have been various modifications to the surgical technique over the years and the most common current approach is to connect the inferior vena cava directly to the pulmonary artery using an extracardiac conduit.

The Fontan circulation relies on high systemic venous filling pressures to help drive transpulmonary blood flow and maintain left ventricular preload. The absence of a subpulmonary ventricle also means that transpulmonary blood flow also relies on minimal resistance across the pulmonary bed. The high systemic venous pressures can also promote the development of venovenous collaterals, resulting in right-to-left shunting of blood flow and therefore a degree of cyanosis. Congestion of the abdominal organs, particularly the liver, may also develop. Sometimes a small fenestration is required to allow controlled right-to-left shunting in order to decompress the venous system.

In the long term, patients develop problems related to impaired pulmonary blood flow, ventricular dysfunction, arrhythmias, and thrombosis. Although the pulmonary and systemic circulations have been separated, they remain in series and the single ventricle

provides the sole pump for the circulation. The ventricle may also be congenitally abnormal and over time the increased afterload faced by the single ventricle often results in impaired ventricular function.

Atrial arrhythmias are common as a result of both increased atrial stretch and multiple previous atrial surgical scars. These arrhythmias are poorly tolerated and potentially fatal for patients with a Fontan circulation because of the consequent hemodynamic changes. During the arrhythmia, the atria become congested and ventricular dysfunction may also ensue as a result of both tachycardia and loss of atrial contribution to ventricular filling. The atrial congestion leads to a rise in atrial pressure and a reduction in the transpulmonary gradient. Pulmonary blood flow and therefore cardiac output may fall with potentially catastrophic consequences. Therefore atrial arrhythmias require urgent assessment and sinus rhythm should be restored as soon as safely possible.

The physiologic changes associated with pregnancy pose significant risks for these patients. The heart rate and circulating volume progressively increase from the beginning of pregnancy. However, the Fontan circulation is limited in its ability to increase cardiac output to cope with the demands of pregnancy or major surgery and heart failure may develop. The increased circulating volume also results in increased atrial stretch, which increases the risk of developing atrial arrhythmias.

Intracardiac thrombus may form as a result of atrial arrhythmias and slow flow within dilated atria. Patients are therefore routinely anticoagulated with warfarin. Pregnancy is also a hypercoagulable state and patients with a Fontan circulation are already at risk of developing intracardiac thrombus. Anticoagulation must therefore be continued throughout pregnancy. As warfarin is teratogenic, patients should be converted to low-molecular-weight heparin with close monitoring of anti-factor Xa levels to ensure therapeutic levels between 0.7 and 1.2 IU/mL.

Management

The specialist congenital heart disease team should be informed of these cases prior to surgery to ensure that an appropriate management plan is made.

Presurgical management should ensure that systemic venous filling is maintained. Patients should therefore be kept well hydrated with

Gynecologic and Obstetric Surgery: Challenges and Management Options, First Edition. Edited by Arri Coomarasamy, Mahmood I. Shafi, G. Willy Davila and Kiong K. Chan.
© 2016 John Wiley & Sons, Ltd. Published 2016 by John Wiley & Sons, Ltd.

intravenous fluids while fasting. In patients who have a right-to-left shunt, such as a fenestration or venovenous collaterals, any air bubbles that enter the venous system may pass directly to the systemic circulation. Therefore filters should be used on all intravenous lines to prevent paradoxical emboli. Patients with a Fontan circulation should be on long-term anticoagulation with warfarin or low-molecular-weight heparin with regular hematologic monitoring of anti-factor Xa levels during pregnancy. Patients who are still on oral anticoagulation should have this stopped 3 days prior to surgery and be commenced on a therapeutic dose of low-molecular-weight heparin or intravenous unfractionated heparin, when the INR falls below 2.0.

During surgery the physiologic aims are to maintain ventricular preload, minimize increases in intrathoracic pressures, and keep the systemic vascular resistance low. The case should involve a cardiac anesthetist familiar with the Fontan circulation. Intraoperative monitoring of the ECG, oxygen saturations, and hemodynamic status using an arterial line and central venous line should be performed. It is important to be aware that the superior vena cava is anastomosed to the pulmonary artery and not the right atrium so care should be taken when inserting the line and the position of the tip of the line should be confirmed. If regional anesthesia is used then this should be with a slow epidural technique to minimize reduction in systemic venous filling pressures. Atrial arrhythmias should be treated promptly.

Postoperatively, patients should be monitored in a high-dependency setting. Patients who have had general anesthesia should be extubated as early as possible to encourage a normal negative intrathoracic pressure ventilatory pattern. Anticoagulation should be restarted as soon as surgically appropriate. Early mobilization should be encouraged to help promote venous return and maintain systemic venous filling.

KEY POINTS

Challenge: Surgery in a patient with Fontan circulation.

Background
- The Fontan circulation is used to palliate a variety of different forms of congenital heart disease in which there is a single functioning ventricle and two-ventricular repair is not possible.
- The systemic venous return to the pulmonary arteries is passive and relies on high systemic venous filling pressures.
- In the long term, patients can develop problems related to impaired pulmonary blood flow, ventricular dysfunction, arrhythmias, and thrombosis.
- Atrial arrhythmias are poorly tolerated and potentially fatal because of the consequent hemodynamic changes, and require urgent assessment and restoration of sinus rhythm.
- The physiologic changes associated with pregnancy cause significant additional risks of heart failure, atrial arrhythmias, and intracardiac thrombus formation.
- Anticoagulation is continued throughout pregnancy.

Management
- Patients with a Fontan circulation are complex and the specialist ACHD team should be involved in planning the perioperative management.
- Patients should be kept well hydrated with intravenous fluids while fasting to maintain systemic venous filling.

- In patients who have a right-to-left shunt, filters should be used on all intravenous lines to prevent paradoxical air emboli.
- Patients who are still on oral anticoagulation should have this stopped 3 days prior to surgery and be commenced on a therapeutic dose of low-molecular-weight heparin or intravenous unfractionated heparin, when the INR falls below 2.0.
- Specialist advice from a cardiac anesthetist should be requested.
- During surgery the physiologic aims are to:
  - Maintain ventricular preload.
  - Minimize increases in intrathoracic pressures.
  - Keep the systemic vascular resistance low.
- Intraoperative monitoring should include arterial line and central venous line.
- Particular care is needed when positioning the central line.
- Regional anesthesia is possible using a slow epidural top-up technique to minimize reduction in systemic venous filling pressures.
- Atrial arrhythmias should be treated promptly.
- After general anesthesia, patients should be extubated as early as possible.
- Patients should be monitored in a high-dependency setting postoperatively.
- Early mobilization should be encouraged.
- Anticoagulation should be restarted as soon as surgically appropriate.

Further reading

Baum VC, de Souza DG. Anesthetic considerations for the pregnant patient with Fontan circulation. Available at http://www2.pedsanesthesia.org/meetings/2010winter/syllabus/pdfs/pblds/Table%20-%2012.pdf

Chugh R. Management of pregnancy in women with repaired CHD or after the Fontan procedure. *Curr Treat Options Cardiovasc Med* 2013; 15:646–662.

Fontan F, Baudet E. Surgical repair of tricuspid atresia. *Thorax* 1971; 26:240–248.

Fredenburg TB, Johnson TR, Cohen MD. The Fontan procedure: anatomy, complications and manifestations of failure. *Radiographics* 2011; 31:453–463.

Nayak S, Booker PD. The Fontan circulation. *Contin Educ Anaesth Crit Care Pain* 2008; 8:26–30.

CHAPTER 7

Hypertensive Patient

Aarthi R. Mohan[1] and Catherine Nelson-Piercy[2]

[1] St Michael's Hospital, Bristol, UK

[2] Guy's and St Thomas' Hospitals NHS Foundation Trust, London, UK

Case history: You are asked to see a 60-year-old woman who is scheduled to have a total abdominal hysterectomy later in the morning. She has a past medical history of hypertension for which she takes atenolol 50 mg once daily and hydrochlorothiazide 25 mg once daily. She has not been taking her medications for 2 days including the morning of her operation, as she thought her doctor told her not to take them preoperatively. Her BP is 179/101 mmHg. What do you do now?

Background

Hypertension affects one-quarter of the UK adult population, with more than half of those over 60 years of age having a blood pressure greater than or equal to 140/90 mmHg [1]. This is thought to be due to the change in demographics of the population towards an older, more obese and sedentary population.

Poorly controlled hypertension is one of the most common medical indications for deferring elective surgery [2]. Patients with chronic uncontrolled hypertension undergoing surgery have an increased risk of morbidity and mortality perioperatively, and a meta-analysis of 30 studies including 12,995 patients suggests an association between hypertension and increased cardiovascular risk [3]. The concerns include increased myocardial oxygen consumption, subendocardial hypoperfusion, and myocardial ischemia. Non-cardiac complications include increased risks of stroke, renal dysfunction, and surgical bleeding.

Normotensive patients may develop elevated blood pressure and tachycardia due to sympathetic activation during the induction of the anesthesia [4]. This response is increased in patients with untreated hypertension, where the systolic blood pressure may increase by as much as 90 mmHg and heart rate by 40 bpm.

Intraoperative hypertension is associated with acute pain-induced sympathetic stimulation leading to vasoconstriction, and in the early post-anesthesia period, hypertension is associated with sympathetic stimulation, hypothermia, hypoxia, or intravascular volume overload from excessive intraoperative fluid therapy.

Management

Assess risk

When booking a hypertensive patient for an elective operation, a careful history regarding their disease and medications should be taken. A search for end-organ damage should be carried out by checking urea and electrolytes, urine dipstick for hematuria and proteinuria for evidence of renal dysfunction, an ECG, and possibly a recent echocardiogram for evidence of LVH, and by taking a history for myocardial infarction, stroke or transient ischemic attack. Secondary causes of hypertension, especially in the younger patient, should also be excluded. The etiology of the hypertension should be sought and severity calculated (stages 1–3, Table 7.1) [5].

Table 7.1 Definition and classification of blood pressure levels.

Category	Systolic arterial pressure (mmHg)	Diastolic arterial pressure (mmHg)
Optimal	<120	<80
Normal	120–129	80–84
High normal	130–139	85–89
Hypertension		
Stage 1	140–159	90–99
Stage 2	160–179	100–109
Stage 3	≥180	≥110

Source: Mancia *et al.,* 2007 [5]. Reproduced with permission from Oxford University Press.

Mild to moderate hypertension (stage 1 or stage 2 hypertension) affects patients with a systolic BP below 180 mmHg and a diastolic BP below 110 mmHg. The American College of Cardiology and American Heart Association (ACC/AHA) Guidelines on Perioperative Cardiovascular Evaluation and Care for Non-cardiac Surgery considers uncontrolled stage 1–2 hypertension a "minor risk factor" for perioperative cardiovascular events and these patients do not appear to be at increased risk of adverse cardiovascular outcomes [6].

Gynecologic and Obstetric Surgery: Challenges and Management Options, First Edition. Edited by Arri Coomarasamy, Mahmood I. Shafi, G. Willy Davila and Kiong K. Chan.
© 2016 John Wiley & Sons, Ltd. Published 2016 by John Wiley & Sons, Ltd.

Look for cause

Although a cause is not identified in 95% of those with hypertension, it necessary to rule out potentially serious causes of hypertension, especially in young patients. The key causes to consider include renal disease, pheochromocytoma, hyperaldosteronism, Cushing's syndrome, obstructive sleep apnea, drugs (e.g., TCAs, cocaine), and uncommon conditions such as coarctation of the aorta. Some of the underlying conditions will have specific perioperative risks (e.g., sleep apnea and airway problems, Cushing's syndrome and metabolic abnormalities). These risks will need to be managed with the involvement of appropriate specialists.

Optimize antihypertensive treatment

The patient's antihypertensive medication should be optimized well in advance and ideally the patient should be normotensive (i.e., BP <140/90 mmHg) for several months prior to elective surgery. It is important to rule out hypokalemia and hypomagnesemia in patients on diuretics, and to bear in mind that the normal response of tachycardia may be missing in patients on beta-blockers.

It is recommended not to delay surgery if the initial evaluation establishes stage 1–2 hypertension with no associated metabolic abnormalities, and intraoperative and postoperative blood pressures should be carefully monitored to prevent hypertensive or hypotensive episodes. However, when hypertension has caused end-organ disease such as congestive heart failure and renal insufficiency, the probability of adverse cardiac outcome in the perioperative period increases significantly [7]. It is important to weigh the benefits of delaying surgery to optimize blood pressure control with the risk of delaying surgery for stage 3 hypertension (i.e., systolic BP ≥180 mmHg and diastolic BP ≥110 mmHg).

Continue antihypertensive treatment

Antihypertensive medications should be continued preoperatively until the time of the surgery [8]. The patient in the case history should have been advised to continue her atenolol on the morning of her surgery. Her current blood pressure (179/101 mmHg) is not a contraindication to the surgery; however, she could be given a beta-blocker prior to the operation.

Care should be taken not to abruptly discontinue some medications, for example beta-blockers and clonidine (a centrally acting α2-adrenergic agonist), as this is associated with significant rebound hypertension. If necessary, intravenous propranolol or labetalol can be administered to patients taking beta-blockers, and transdermal clonidine can be given to patients taking clonidine. For a hypertensive patient taking ACE inhibitors preoperatively, it is recommended that the ACE inhibitors be discontinued 24 hours before surgery and resumed after the patient's intravascular volume has been stabilized [8].

Laparoscopic surgery in the hypertensive patient

Laparoscopic procedures incur a cardiac stress similar to that of open procedures. The pneumoperitoneum used in these procedures results in elevated intra-abdominal pressure, leading to a reduction in venous return and a decrease in cardiac output [8]. It is important to bear this in mind when seeing patients with chronic hypertension who are having relatively minor "day-case" laparoscopic procedures.

Emergency surgery in the hypertensive patient

When patients undergo emergency gynecologic surgery, the risks and benefits of proceeding with the surgery immediately need to be weighed against delaying surgery in order to optimize blood pressure control. If surgery cannot be delayed, a parenteral antihypertensive drug can be used to lower the blood pressure in the perioperative period.

Postoperative care

Careful management to minimize hemodynamic instability is important. If there is postoperative hypertension, it is important to exclude other causes of hypertension such as pain, hypercarbia, hypoxia, hypervolemia, and bladder distension. Once this is done, antihypertensive medication can be used to treat a persistent blood pressure above 180 mmHg or a diastolic blood pressure above 110 mmHg. Once the patient is able to take medications orally, she can resume her preoperative antihypertensive medications.

KEY POINTS

Challenge: Perioperative management of the hypertensive patient.

Background
- Hypertension affects one-quarter of the UK adult population and half of those above 60 years of age.
- Patients with chronic hypertension are at increased risk of cardiovascular complications, stroke, renal dysfunction, and surgical bleeding.
- Hypertension does not have a cause in most patients; however, consider renal disease, pheochromocytoma, hyperaldosteronism, Cushing's syndrome, obstructive sleep apnea, drugs (e.g., TCAs, cocaine), and uncommon conditions such as coarctation of the aorta.
- Postoperative hypertension can result from pain, hypothermia, hypoxia, or fluid overload.

Management
- Assess risks: history and examination to rule out end-organ disease (check U&E, urine for hematuria and proteinuria, perform an ECG, and consider an echocardiogram).
- Grade the hypertension:
  - Stage 1: 140–159/90–99 mmHg.
  - Stage 2: 160–179/100–109 mmHg.
  - Stage 3: ≥180/≥110 mmHg.
- Decide whether to proceed with or postpone the operation:
  - Stage 1 and 2 pose minor risks of complications, and therefore an operation does not need to be postponed.
  - In stage 3 hypertension, it is thought to be safer to postpone the operation until the BP is gradually corrected.
- Optimize antihypertensive treatment: aim for BP <140/90 mmHg for several months prior to elective surgery.
- Continue antihypertensive treatment in the perioperative period: antihypertensive drugs should be continued until the day of surgery, and restarted as soon as the patient tolerates oral intake.
- If the patient is undergoing emergency surgery which cannot be postponed, a parenteral antihypertensive agent may be used to lower BP.
- Postoperative care: minimize hemodynamic instability and avoid triggers of hypertension (pain, hypercarbia, hypoxia, hypervolemia, bladder distension).

References

1 National Clinical Guideline Centre. *Hypertension: The Clinical Management of Primary Hypertension in Adults: Update of Clinical Guidelines 18 and 34.* NICE Clinical Guidelines, No. 127. Royal College of Physicians, London, 2011.
2 Dix P, Howell S. Survey of cancellation rate of hypertensive patients undergoing anaesthesia and elective surgery. *Br J Anaesth* 2001; 86:789–793.
3 Howell SJ, Sear JW, Foëx P. Hypertension, hypertensive heart disease and perioperative cardiac risk. *Br J Anaesth* 2004; 92:570–583.
4 Erstad BL, Barletta JF. Treatment of hypertension in the perioperative patient. *Ann Pharmacother* 2000; 34:66–79.

5 Mancia G, De Backer G, Dominiczak A *et al.* 2007 Guidelines for the management of arterial hypertension: The Task Force for the Management of Arterial Hypertension of the European Society of Hypertension (ESH) and of the European Society of Cardiology (ESC). *Eur Heart J* 2007; 28:1462–1536.

6 Fleisher LA, Beckman JA, Brown KA *et al.* ACC/AHA 2007 guidelines on perioperative cardiovascular evaluation and care for noncardiac surgery: a report of the American College of Cardiology/American Heart Association Task Force on Practice Guidelines. *Circulation* 2007; 116:418–499.

7 Goldman L, Caldera DL, Nussbaum SR *et al.* Multifactorial index of cardiac risk in noncardiac surgical procedures. *N Engl J Med* 1977; 297:845–850.

8 Poldermans D, Bax JJ, Boersma E *et al.* Guidelines for pre-operative cardiac risk assessment and perioperative cardiac management in non-cardiac surgery. *Eur Heart J* 2009; 30:2769–2812.

Further reading

Nelson-Piercy C. *Handbook of Obstetric Medicine*, 4th edn. Informa Healthcare, London, 2010.

CHAPTER 8
Patient with Respiratory Disease

Heinke Kunst

Queen Mary University of London, London, UK

Case history: A 67-year-old female with known bronchiectasis and an exercise tolerance of less than 182 m (200 yards) is advised to have a total abdominal hysterectomy. She requires a general anesthetic as she is unable to have spinal anesthesia due to previous spinal surgery. She has a history of recurrent chest infections in the last 6 months and there is concern that she is not fit for surgery.

Background

Patients with underlying respiratory disease undergoing pelvic surgery may be at risk of postoperative pulmonary complications. Asthma is characterized by mostly *reversible* airway obstruction, and is generally not a risk factor for postoperative pulmonary complications; on the other hand, chronic obstructive pulmonary disease (COPD) is characterized by mostly *irreversible* airway obstruction, and is associated with a threefold increase in pulmonary complications.

Risk factors for pulmonary complications in patients with COPD include age over 70 years, ASA class above 2, poor exercise capacity, cigarette smoking, obstructive sleep apnea, general anesthesia (when compared with regional anesthesia), and prolonged or emergency surgery.

Atelectasis

Atelectasis is a common perioperative complication; it is observed in more than 80% of all anesthetized patients and is consistent with an area of collapsed lung leading to ventilation–perfusion mismatch [1]. The main mechanisms underlying the formation of atelectasis are compression, loss of surfactant or impaired surfactant, leading to a decrease in functional vital capacity (FVC), forced expiratory volume (FEV_1), and partial pressure of oxygen in blood (PaO_2) [1]. Laparotomy, supine position, and general anesthesia inevitably lead to lung atelectasis and decrease in functional residual capacity (FRC) resulting in ventilation–perfusion mismatch.

In order to minimize complications, patients with chronic respiratory diseases such as COPD, bronchiectasis, interstitial lung disease or neuromuscular respiratory disorders should have a clear perioperative plan.

Management

Assess the extent and stability of the respiratory disorder

Patients will need an assessment of exercise tolerance (e.g., inability to climb at least two flights of stairs, breathless on dressing, unable to complete a sentence). Preoperative 6-min walk test is thought to be a poor predictor of postoperative pulmonary complications in abdominal surgery but may be of benefit in patients with more severe pulmonary disease.

Patients with underlying lung disease should undergo chest radiography before surgery. There is insufficient evidence to support routine lung functions tests such as spirometry for patients with underlying pulmonary disease; however, in patients with more severe disease and poor exercise tolerance it may be advisable to perform lung function tests including spirometry.

In patients with evidence of underlying right heart failure, echocardiography may be helpful to estimate the postoperative risk of complications.

Optimize the management of the respiratory disorder

Elective surgery should be delayed to optimize management, and treat any acute exacerbations and respiratory tract infections.

Although asthma is not a significant risk factor for pulmonary complications, patients with severe asthma may benefit from a course of preoperative steroids (e.g., 1-week course of oral prednisone 20–40 mg/day, or an intravenous steroid). Patients with mild asthma symptoms may only require doubling of the dose of inhaled steroids for a week before the surgery. In patients with COPD, nebulized salbutamol 2.5–5 mg q.d.s. and ipratropium 0.5 mg q.d.s. should be considered.

Patients with underlying bronchiectasis and a history of recurrent exacerbations may benefit from a preoperative course of intravenous antibiotics and physiotherapy including postural drainage.

In restrictive diseases such as neuromuscular disorders or chest wall deformities (e.g., kyphoscoliosis), mucociliary clearance can be impaired due to decreased cough. Physiotherapy with regard to lung expansion maneuvers and sputum clearance should be offered

Gynecologic and Obstetric Surgery: Challenges and Management Options, First Edition. Edited by Arri Coomarasamy, Mahmood I. Shafi, G. Willy Davila and Kiong K. Chan.
© 2016 John Wiley & Sons, Ltd. Published 2016 by John Wiley & Sons, Ltd.

Table 8.1 Prevention of postoperative complications in patients undergoing pelvic surgery.

Underlying respiratory disease	Preoperative investigations	Preoperative and postoperative interventions
Chronic obstructive pulmonary disease	Full pulmonary function tests Echocardiogram if clinical evidence of pulmonary hypertension Chest X-ray	Smoking cessation Optimization of inhaled bronchodilators Pulmonary rehabilitation/physiotherapy
Severe asthma	Full pulmonary function test Chest X-ray	Consider preoperative steroids
Bronchiectasis	Full pulmonary function tests Chest X-ray	Consider preoperative course of intravenous antibiotics Pulmonary rehabilitation/physiotherapy
Obstructive sleep apnoea Obesity/hypoventilation	Full pulmonary function tests Chest X-ray	Consider postoperative CPAP or non-invasive ventilation
Interstitial lung disease	Full pulmonary function tests Chest X-ray	Pulmonary rehabilitation/physiotherapy
Chronic restrictive lung disease (kyphoscoliosis and neuromuscular disease)	Full pulmonary function tests Chest X-ray	Pulmonary rehabilitation/physiotherapy

to these patients perioperatively and non-invasive ventilation may need to be considered in the postoperative period to avoid atelectasis and lung collapse.

Cessation of smoking

Smoking is an independent risk factor for pulmonary complications in those with and without COPD [2]. Smoking increases airway secretions and reactivity. Cessation of smoking more than 2 months before surgery is recommended to reduce the risk of pulmonary complications.

Consider intraoperative steps to reduce risk

The first key decision is whether regional anesthesia could be performed instead of general anesthesia, as regional anesthesia is associated with a reduction in pneumonia and respiratory failure [3]. Regional anesthesia is not suitable for every patient, but this should be the preferred option. The operative time should be limited to the shortest possible period. Laparoscopic surgery, compared with laparotomy, is known to reduce postoperative pain and pulmonary complications [4] and is therefore the preferred surgical approach in patients with underlying pulmonary disease, especially those undergoing minor pelvic surgery [5].

Arrange lung expansion interventions

There is good evidence that lung expansion interventions including deep breathing exercises, chest physiotherapy, incentive spirometry, and continuous positive airway pressure (CPAP) reduce pulmonary complications. Elderly patients undergoing pelvic surgery have a greater risk of postoperative pulmonary complications and mortality. Therefore elderly patients with underlying lung disease may benefit from pulmonary rehabilitation before surgery [6].

One example of a deep breathing exercise is taking eight to ten breaths, with a 3–5 s inspiratory hold, every 1–2 hours; the inspiratory hold should be followed by forced expiration and coughing [3].

Postoperative care

Patients should be mobilized early. Effective analgesia is important to facilitate deep breathing; however, opiates can blunt respiratory drive and thus attention should be paid to dosing. Postoperative epidural analgesia may be suitable for some patients. Regular physiotherapy is important to prevent atelectasis. Routine antibiotics are not needed, but if symptoms or signs of chest infection develop, sputum culture and chest X-ray should be arranged, and antibiotics commenced. Use of nebulized bronchodilators is recommended until the patient is fully mobile.

A summary of preoperative and postoperative approaches to minimize pulmonary complications in patients with respiratory disease is given in Table 8.1.

Resolution of the case

The patient was referred for full lung function tests, which showed an obstructive defect and a reduced transfer factor of 50% of predicted. Chest radiography was consistent with signs of moderate bronchiectasis. The patient was referred for pulmonary rehabilitation including physiotherapy and admitted preoperatively for a course of intravenous antibiotics. Postoperatively she was seen daily by the physiotherapist to ensure sputum clearance. The patient had an uneventful recovery.

KEY POINTS

Challenge: Patient with respiratory disease needing surgery.

Background
- Patients with underlying chronic respiratory disease undergoing pelvic surgery are at risk of postoperative pulmonary complications, increased length of hospital stay, and mortality.
- Risk factors for pulmonary complications include age over 70 years, ASA class above 2, poor exercise capacity, cigarette smoking, obstructive sleep apnea, general anesthesia (when compared with regional anesthesia), and prolonged or emergency surgery.
- Atelectasis is very common, causes ventilation–perfusion mismatch and is exacerbated by laparotomy, supine position, Trendelenburg position, and general anesthesia.
- The incidence of complications may be reduced by pulmonary rehabilitation, including physiotherapy.

Management
- Careful clinical evaluation of the patient. Ask if she can climb at least two flights of stairs.
- Arrange investigations to assess the severity of the disease, including chest radiography and lung function tests (spirometry) in patients with severe chronic lung disease.
- Perform echocardiography if pulmonary hypertension is suspected.
- Optimize inhaled and other medication preoperatively. Consider a course of preoperative steroids for patients with severe asthma.
- Get the patient to stop smoking, ideally at least 2 months before the operation.
- Arrange preoperative pulmonary rehabilitation (deep breathing exercises and physiotherapy).

- Use regional anesthesia to avoid general anesthesia if possible.
- Use a laparoscopic approach if possible.
- Arrange postoperative deep breathing exercises, incentive spirometry, physiotherapy, and CPAP to reduce pulmonary complications.
- If mucociliary clearance is decreased because of impaired cough, consider non-invasive ventilation in the postoperative period to avoid atelectasis and lung collapse.

References

1   Lindberg P, Gunnarsson L, Tokics L *et al.* Atelectasis and lung function in the postoperative period. *Acta Anaesthesiol Scand* 1992; 36:546–553.
2   Arozullah AM, Lawrence VA. Asthma and COPD. In: Cohn SL, Smetana GW, Weed HG (eds) *Perioperative Medicine: Just The Facts*, pp. 141–147. McGraw-Hill Medical, New York, 2006.
3   Smetana GW, Conde MV. Pulmonary evaluation. In: Cohn SL, Smetana GW, Weed HG (eds) *Perioperative Medicine: Just The Facts*, pp. 135–141. McGraw-Hill Medical, New York, 2006.
4   Solomon ER, Muffly TM, Barber MD. Common postoperative pulmonary complications after hysterectomy for benign indications. *Am J Obstet Gynecol* 2013; 208:54.e1–5.
5   Joris J, Kaba A, Lamy M. Postoperative spirometry after laparoscopy for lower abdominal or upper abdominal surgical procedures. *Br J Anaesth* 1997; 79: 422–426.
6   Manku K, Bacchetti P, Leung JM. Prognostic significance of postoperative in-hospital complications in elderly patients. I. Long-term survival. *Anesth Analg* 2003; 96:583–589.

CHAPTER 9
Patient with Diabetes

Arri Coomarasamy[1] and Dukaydah van der Berg[2]
[1] College of Medical and Dental Sciences, University of Birmingham, Birmingham, UK
[2] Frankly Health Practice, Birmingham, UK

Case history 1: A 44-year-old woman with insulin-dependent diabetes presented with heavy and irregular menstrual bleeding, and was found to have complex hyperplasia with atypia on endometrial biopsy. She elected to have an abdominal hysterectomy. On the day before surgery, she was admitted to the ward, and was found to have a BM of 19 mmol/L. However, there was no evidence of ketoacidosis.

Case history 2: A 32-year-old woman with non-insulin-dependent diabetes was booked to have laparoscopic sterilization on a day-case list. On the morning of operation, she was found to have a BM of 2 mmol/L.

Background

Diabetes affects 3% of the UK population. The primary perioperative concern is the control of blood glucose. Diabetic patients are at increased risk of nausea and vomiting, aspiration due to gastroparesis, pulmonary complications, wound infection, pressure sores and, rarely, renal failure, myocardial infarction or stroke. Autonomic neuropathy, associated with symptoms such as postural hypotension and urinary retention, may result in abnormal responses to local and general anesthesia.

Overly tight control of perioperative glucose levels is unnecessary: the aim should be to maintain blood glucose between 6 and 10 mmol/L. For most patients with non-insulin-dependent diabetes mellitus (NIDDM) having minor surgery (as in Case history 2), this can be achieved with diet, oral hypoglycemic drugs, and occasionally subcutaneous insulin. A variable-rate insulin infusion pump is recommended for all women with diabetes having major surgery, whether they have NIDDM or insulin-dependent diabetes mellitus (IDDM), and all women with IDDM (whether they are having minor or major surgery). Invasive investigative procedures (e.g., barium enema) should be treated as minor surgery.

Management

Hyperglycemia

Hyperglycemia up to 25 mmol/L is not a medical emergency, as long as there is no ketoacidosis (Case history 1). Non-emergency surgery can be deferred to allow time to achieve glycemic control. The management aim is to reduce the sugar level in a controlled fashion, and this can usually be achieved with a small starting dose of 4–8 units of subcutaneous insulin. The patient is likely to know a great deal about her illness and management, and thus ask her about previous episodes of uncontrolled hyperglycemia and what insulin regimen was employed to control it; the answers should not be taken as confirmed facts, but may still be useful in tailoring her management. Avoid the temptation to start an insulin pump unless control cannot be achieved with subcutaneous insulin or the patient is acutely ill: insulin pump will require 1–2 hourly monitoring of blood sugar levels, with the undesirable result of giving the woman a sleepless night before major surgery. Investigations for the woman in Case history 1 include checking urea and electrolytes, testing urine for ketones, and if ketones are present, checking blood gases and bicarbonate to rule out ketoacidosis.

Ketoacidosis is a condition in which the patient has an elevated glucose concentration, ketosis (at least ++ ketones in urine), and acidosis (pH <7.2 or HCO_3^- <15 mmol/L). This is a medical emergency: seek help from the medical team. Emergency resuscitation in diabetic ketoacidosis (DKA) will include protecting the airway, facial oxygen, intravenous fluids (1 L normal saline bolus, with addition of K+ if potassium <3.0 mmol/L), administration of 4–8 units of Actrapid if glucose above 20 mmol/L, and institution of an insulin sliding scale (Table 9.1). Glucose, K+ and arterial blood gases (to assess acidosis) will need to be checked hourly until the patient is stable.

Hypoglycemia

Hypoglycemia (blood glucose <3.5 mmol/L; Case history 2) can lead to convulsions, unconsciousness, and permanent cerebral dysfunction unless it is rapidly and effectively managed. If the patient in Case history 2 is conscious, give her a sweet drink, followed by biscuits or a sandwich. If she is unable to eat, give 50 mL of 50% dextrose intravenously. If venous access is not possible, give glucagon 1 unit intramuscularly or rub glucose gel (e.g., Hypostop) on the gums. If the operation was deferred, once stable glycemic control is achieved, the operation can be rebooked.

Prevention

In working up diabetic patients, particularly those with IDDM scheduled to undergo major surgery, it is important to liaise closely with the diabetic team and the anesthetist. In complex cases, obtain a written plan for preoperative, intraoperative, and postoperative management from the diabetic team.

Preoperative history should elicit previous problems with glycemic control as well as any existing complications, including retinopathy, nephropathy, ischemic heart disease, peripheral vascular disease, cerebrovascular disease, and neuropathy. Blood pressure

Gynecologic and Obstetric Surgery: Challenges and Management Options, First Edition. Edited by Arri Coomarasamy, Mahmood I. Shafi, G. Willy Davila and Kiong K. Chan.
© 2016 John Wiley & Sons, Ltd. Published 2016 by John Wiley & Sons, Ltd.

Table 9.1 An example intravenous insulin infusion regimen for perioperative care.

10% glucose + 10 mmol KCL at 50 mL/hour
Plus 50 units of insulin (Actrapid) in 50 mL of 0.9% saline as prescribed below:

Insulin sliding scale

Blood sugar (mmol/L)	Gentle regimen (units insulin/hour)	Standard regimen (units insulin/hour)	Aggressive regimen (units insulin/hour)
<3.5 or signs of hypoglycemia: give 50 mL of 50% dextrose i.v. and call doctor			
<4	0.25	0.5	1
4.0–9	0.5	1	2
9.1–11	1	2	4
11.1–17	2	3	8
17.1–28	4	4	10
>28	6 and call doctor	6 and call doctor	12 and call doctor
Monitor glucose hourly for 6 hours, then 2-hourly if stable.			

Source: Cooper *et al.*, 2006 [1]. Reproduced with permission from Wiley.

should be checked and the aim is to have a BP below 160/90 mmHg preoperatively. Check urine for ketones and protein, take blood for HbA$_{1c}$, urea and electrolytes, and if over the age of 30 arrange an ECG. Schedule the patient first on the operating list to minimize the risk of unscheduled prolongation of fasting.

A patient with diet-controlled diabetes often requires no special preparation, if the glucose and urea and electrolytes are normal. Oral hypoglycemic drugs will need to be omitted on the day of surgery; however, if the patient is taking long-acting hypoglycemics (e.g., chlorpropamide and glibenclamide), these should be discontinued 24–48 hours before surgery. If long-acting drugs are continued, watch for hypoglycemia in the perioperative period

(Case history 2). If the patient undergoes minor surgery, she will be eating and drinking soon after the procedure, so no further special management is required.

For patients with IDDM, omit the usual dose of insulin on the day of surgery, and start an intravenous insulin regimen early on the morning of surgery. If the patient is on long-acting insulin, this should be stopped the night before surgery and an intravenous insulin regimen started. A typical intravenous insulin regimen is given in Table 9.1; however, local hospitals may have their own regimens that most staff are familiar with, and these should be used if available. The infusion is continued until the patient starts to drink and eat normally.

KEY POINTS

Challenge: Poor preoperative glycemic control in diabetic patients.

Background
- 3% of UK population have diabetes.
- Surgery-related risks include poor glycemic control, aspiration, pulmonary complications, wound infection, pressure sores, renal failure, myocardial infarction, and stroke.
- Aim of perioperative care is to maintain blood glucose level between 6 and 10 mmol/L.

Prevention (of complications)
- Liaise with the diabetic team and the anesthetist.
- Preoperative assessment:
  - Obtain history about usual glycemic control and pre-existing diabetic complications.
  - Check BP and urine (for ketones and protein).
  - Take blood for HbA$_{1c}$, urea and electrolytes, and FBC.
  - If patient >30 years of age, arrange ECG.
- Schedule first on the operating list.
- Patients with diet-controlled diabetes and normal U&E and glycemic control often require no special preparation.

NIDDM
- Omit the usual oral hypoglycemic drug on the day of surgery; however, if the patient is taking long-acting hypoglycemics (e.g., chlorpropamide and glibenclamide), these should be discontinued 24–48 hours before surgery.
- For major surgery, an insulin infusion regimen is required.

IDDM
- Omit the usual dose of subcutaneous insulin on the day of surgery, and commence insulin infusion.
- If the patient is on long-acting insulin, this should be stopped the night before surgery and an intravenous insulin regimen started.
- Continue insulin infusion until patient resumes oral intake.

Management (of poor perioperative glycemic control)
Hyperglycemia
- Defer non-urgent surgery until glycemic control is achieved.
- If glucose <25 mmol/L and there is no ketoacidosis, use 4–8 units of subcutaneous insulin to gradually reduce the sugar level.
- If ketoacidosis is present, seek immediate medical help. For emergency management of diabetic ketoacidosis:
  - Protect the airway and give facial oxygen.
  - Give intravenous fluids (1 L normal saline bolus, with addition of K+ if potassium <3.0 mmol/L).
  - Administer 4–8 units of Actrapid if glucose >20 mmol/L and start an insulin sliding scale.
  - Check glucose, K+ and ABG (to assess acidosis) hourly until the patient is stable.

Hypoglycemia
- If patient is conscious, give sweet drink followed by biscuits or a sandwich.
- If patient is unconscious, give 50 mL of 50% dextrose intravenously.
- If intravenous access is not possible, give glucagon 1 unit intramuscularly or rub glucose gel on to the gum.

Reference

1 Cooper N, Forrest K, Cramp P. Optimising patient before surgery. In: *Essential Guide to Acute Care*, 2nd edn. Blackwell Publishing, Oxford, 2006.

Further reading

Cooper N, Forrest K, Cramp P. Optimising patient before surgery. In: *Essential Guide to Acute Care*, 2nd edn. Blackwell Publishing, Oxford, 2006.

French G. Clinical management of diabetes mellitus during anaesthesia and surgery. *Update in Anaesthesia* 2000; 11:66–73.

Hattersley A, Saddler J. Endocrine and metabolic disorders. In: Nicholls A, Wilson I (eds) *Perioperative Medicine*, pp. 161–172. Oxford University Press, Oxford, 2000.

Marks JB. Perioperative management of diabetes. *Am Fam Physician* 2003; 67:93–100.

CHAPTER 10
Patient with Thyroid Disease

Ramy Labib[1] and Shiao-yng Chan[2]
[1] Worcestershire Acute Hospitals NHS Trust, Worcestershire, UK
[2] Yong Loo Lin School of Medicine, National University of Singapore, Singapore

Case history 1: *A 32-year-old woman presented with heavy vaginal bleeding secondary to a miscarriage of a molar pregnancy. Clinical examination found sinus tachycardia, excessive sweating, and a fine tremor. Thyroid function tests confirmed thyrotoxicosis with a fully suppressed TSH (<0.03 mU/L; normal range in first trimester 0.1–2.5 mU/L) and markedly elevated free T_4 and T_3 serum concentrations. The patient needed an urgent evacuation of the uterus.*

Case history 2: *A 49-year-old woman presented for an ovarian cystectomy. She was known to have hypothyroidism treated with levothyroxine but admitted to non-compliance with treatment. Clinical examination found a large goiter causing difficulty in swallowing and hoarseness of voice. Thyroid function tests showed a markedly elevated serum TSH of 56 mU/L accompanied by low serum concentrations of free T_4 and T_3.*

Background

Thyroid disorders are more prevalent in women than in men [1], mainly as a result of estrogen effects on thyroid cell growth and function [2]. Thyroid disorders have been associated with many gynecologic conditions such as menstrual irregularities, infertility, abnormal uterine bleeding, and premature menopause [3]. The epidemiology of common thyroid disorders in iodine-replete areas is summarized in Table 10.1, but a higher prevalence for all thyroid disorders is reported in iodine deficient areas [1].

Table 10.1 The epidemiology of common thyroid disorders in iodine-replete areas.

Thyroid disorder	Prevalence (F:M ratio)	Prevalence in women*	Annual incidence in women	Effect of age on prevalence
Hyperthyroidism	10:1	0.3–0.5%	0.4–1 per 1000	Rises with age
Hypothyroidism	10:1	0.3–2%	3.5–5 per 1000	Higher in elderly
Goiter	4:1	6.4%	—	Peaks in premenopause

* Prevalence of previously undiagnosed cases.
Source: Vanderpump, 2011 [1]. Reproduced with permission from Oxford University Press.

In pregnancy, normal physiologic changes result in alterations to thyroid function. Biochemical hyperthyroidism (gestational transient thyrotoxicosis) is found in about 3% of normal pregnancies in the first and early second trimester, usually associated with hyperemesis gravidarum. The transient changes spontaneously normalize to a euthyroid state by late second trimester. This is attributed to the thyrotrophic effect of human chorionic gonadotropin (HCG); thus conditions with higher levels of HCG, such as molar pregnancies and multiple pregnancies, may be particularly associated with transient thyrotoxicosis [4].

Patients with previously undiagnosed thyroid disorders often have non-specific symptoms or are asymptomatic and clinical detection of new cases can be promoted by having a high index of suspicion.

Hyperthyroidism

Hyperthyroidism is the excessive production of thyroid hormone (TH), most commonly due to an autoimmune disorder known as Graves' disease or to a multinodular goiter. Thyrotoxicosis describes the presence of excessive circulatory TH and is diagnosed by a suppressed thyroid-stimulating hormone (TSH) associated with elevated free thyroxine (FT_4) and free triiodothyronine (FT_3) serum concentrations. It is characterized by sympathetic overactivity and increased metabolic rate despite normal levels of catecholamines [5].

Clinical features of thyrotoxicosis include tremor, palpitations, weight loss, sweating, anxiety, and heat intolerance. Cardiac arrhythmias are common, typically sinus tachycardia but can also take the form of atrial fibrillation.

Surgical stress puts patients with uncontrolled thyrotoxicosis at high risk of developing a thyroid crisis. This is an acute hypermetabolic state known as "thyroid storm" with mortality rates as high as 90% if untreated, but dropping to less than 20% with early recognition and optimal management [6]. It is characterized by hyperthermia, tachycardia, sweating, and dyspnea [6]. If not managed promptly it can lead to heart failure or cardiac arrest. Therefore, thyrotoxic patients should have surgery delayed until they are clinically and biochemically euthyroid.

Hypothyroidism

Hypothyroidism is diagnosed by an elevated serum TSH concentration accompanied by a low serum FT_4 concentration. While iodine deficiency is the most common cause worldwide, autoimmune Hashimoto thyroiditis is the most common cause in iodine-replete areas [7]. The clinical picture can range from being asymptomatic to a life-threatening "myxedema coma."

Gynecologic and Obstetric Surgery: Challenges and Management Options, First Edition. Edited by Arri Coomarasamy, Mahmood I. Shafi, G. Willy Davila and Kiong K. Chan.
© 2016 John Wiley & Sons, Ltd. Published 2016 by John Wiley & Sons, Ltd.

Common features of hypothyroidism include fatigue, weight gain, cold intolerance, hair loss, dry skin, water retention, and depression. Cardiovascular effects include bradycardia, reduced cardiac contractility, and increased systemic vascular resistance resulting in hypertension [7]. Chronic hypothyroidism can lead to congestive heart failure with impaired systolic and diastolic function [8].

During the perioperative period, patients with uncontrolled hypothyroidism are at greater risk of cardiovascular depression, hypothermia, and aspiration due to delayed gastric emptying. Airway management can also be difficult because of generalized edema, particularly in pregnant patients. There is also controversial evidence that wound healing could be compromised [9].

Goiter

Goiter is a non-specific term for enlargement of the thyroid gland, which can present with or without thyroid dysfunction. Thyroid dysfunction, if present, should be treated before surgery. The enlargement may be secondary to a single nodule or to a multinodular or diffuse goiter. External compression on the trachea could cause airway obstruction in about 33% of adult patients presenting with goiter [10]. History of dysphagia, dysphonia, snoring, breathing difficulty, and retrosternal goiter should raise the suspicion of a difficult airway [11].

Management

Patients should be rendered euthyroid before elective surgery to reduce perioperative mortality and morbidity.

Hyperthyroidism

Euthyroidism is usually achieved by the use of antithyroid medications such as propylthiouracil, methimazole, or carbimazole. The most serious side effect of these drugs is agranulocytosis, which occurs in 0.2–0.5% of patients treated [12]. Antithyroid drugs have a slow onset of action, taking 6–8 weeks to render a patient euthyroid. Propranolol is a commonly used beta-blocker to ameliorate most thyrotoxic symptoms [6,12].

Patients with uncontrolled thyrotoxicosis presenting for emergency surgical interventions (e.g., Case history 1) require early involvement of anesthesiologists, endocrinologists, and intensivists to reduce the risk of thyroid storm [7]. The choice of treatment will depend on the time available for preoperative preparation. All patients should be started on beta-blockers, unless contraindicated,

with intravenous preparations such as esmolol infusion [12]. Antithyroid drugs should still be started with a view to controlling TH production in the postoperative period [12]. In addition to propylthiouracil, intravenous hydrocortisone helps to reduce peripheral conversion of T_4 to T_3 [12]. Plasmapheresis has been used successfully for rapid clearance of circulating TH for both preoperative preparation and in the event of thyroid crisis [13]. Regional anesthesia should be considered because of its additional benefit of sympathetic blockade [14]. With general anesthesia, great care should be taken to attenuate the autonomic responses to surgical stimuli as well as intubation and extubation.

Hypothyroidism

In an emergency, treatment with T_3 as well as T_4 is recommended in the management of myxedema coma [11], as T_3 has a half-life of 1.5 days (compared with 7 days for T_4) and is available in an intravenous preparation. Again, the involvement of a multidisciplinary team is required with early referral to anesthesiologists and endocrinologists. Corticosteroid cover should be considered because of the risk of unmasking adrenal insufficiency [11]. Regional anesthesia is preferred in patients with uncontrolled hypothyroidism because of the increased risk of respiratory depression following general anesthesia [8,11].

Goiter

A respiratory flow–volume loop can help detect airway obstruction even in asymptomatic patients [10,11]. Anesthesiologists and ENT surgeons should be involved in preoperative assessment. Indirect laryngoscopy provides useful information with regard to the view and movement of vocal cords [11]. Radiography, CT and MRI may be helpful in assessing the degree of tracheal deviation and narrowing [11]. Regional anesthesia should be considered.

Prevention

Gynecologists should consider the possibility of thyroid dysfunction while investigating patients. The majority of patients with thyroid dysfunction presenting for gynecologic surgery are well controlled on treatment. Patients with uncontrolled thyroid dysfunction are at higher risk of perioperative morbidity and mortality. If possible, elective surgery should be delayed until patients are euthyroid. If urgent surgery is required, prompt assessment and preparation in conjunction with endocrinologists and anesthesiologists are needed.

KEY POINTS

Challenge: Patient with uncontrolled thyroid disorder presenting for surgery.

Background
- Thyroid disorders and goiter are more prevalent in women than in men.
- Thyroid dysfunction is associated with many gynecologic conditions.
- Surgical stress in uncontrolled or undiagnosed thyrotoxicosis can lead to life-threatening "thyroid storm," characterized by hyperthermia, tachycardia, sweating, and dyspnea. If not managed promptly it can lead to heart failure or cardiac arrest.
- Chronic hypothyroidism can be associated with cardiac failure, a difficult airway, hypothermia, and aspiration due to delayed gastric emptying.
- Goiter is associated with airway obstruction in a significant proportion of cases.

Prevention
- Previously undiagnosed patients often have non-specific symptoms or are asymptomatic and there should be a low threshold for preoperative thyroid function testing.
- Surgery should be postponed, if possible, until the patient is rendered euthyroid.

Management (if urgent surgery is required)
- Early involvement of endocrinologists and anesthesiologists.
- Regional anesthesia should be considered for all patients.
- Thyrotoxic patients should be started on beta-blockers (unless contraindicated) and antithyroid medication (propylthiouracil, methimazole or carbimazole). Plasmapheresis may be useful. Aim to reduce resting heart rate to <90 bpm.

- Management of thyroid storm includes [15]:
  - Oxygen by face mask.
  - Cooling with ice bags.
  - Hydrocortisone 100–300 mg i.v.
  - Propranolol 1 mg i.v. boluses (up to 10 mg).
  - Digoxin if fast AF.
  - Correction of electrolyte imbalance and dehydration.
- Hypothyroid patients should receive T_3 treatment in addition to T_4, and steroid cover should be considered because of the risk of unmasking adrenal insufficiency.

- Emergency management of myxedema coma includes [15]:
  - Oxygen by face mask.
  - Warm air blankets.
  - Hydrocortisone 100 mg i.v. every 8 hours.
  - T_3 5–20 μg by slow intravenous injection.
- Patients with a goiter should undergo radiologic imaging and a respiratory flow–volume loop to help detect airway obstruction.

References

1 Vanderpump MPJ. The epidemiology of thyroid disease. *Br Med Bull* 2011; 99:39–51.

2 Santin AP, Furlanetto TW. Role of estrogen in thyroid function and growth regulation. *J Thyroid Res* 2011;Article ID 875125. http://dx.doi.org/10.4061/2011/875125 (accessed 19 June 2013).

3 Poppe K, Velkeniers B, Glioer D. Thyroid disease and female reproduction. *Clin Endocrinol* 2007; 66:309–321.

4 Glineor D. The regulation of thyroid function in pregnancy: pathways of endocrine adaptation from physiology to pathology. *Endocr Rev* 1997; 18:404–433.

5 Coulombe P, Dussault JH, Walker P. Plasma catecholamine concentration in hyperthyroidism and hypothyroidism. *Metabolism* 1976; 25:973–978.

6 Singhal A, Campell D. Thyroid storm. Available at http://emedicine.medscape.com/article/925147-overview (accessed 19 June 2013).

7 Chakera AJ, Pearce SHS, Vaidya B. Treatment for primary hypothyroidism: current approaches and future possibilities. *Drug Des Devel Ther* 2012; 6:1–11.

8 Bennett-Guerro E, Kramer DC, Schwinn DA. Effect of chronic and acute thyroid hormone reduction on perioperative outcome. *Anesth Analg* 1997; 85:30–36.

9 Safer JD, Crawford TD, Hollick MF. A role for thyroid hormone in wound healing through keratin gene expression. *Endocrinology* 2004; 145:2357–2361.

10 Gittoes NJL, Miller MR, Daykin J, Sheppard MC, Franklyn JA. Upper airways obstruction in 153 consecutive patients presenting with thyroid enlargement. *BMJ* 1996; 312:484.

11 Farling PA. Thyroid disease. *Br J Anaesth* 2000; 85:15–28.

12 Langley RW, Burch HB. Perioperative management of the thyrotoxic patient. *Endocrinol Metab Clin North Am* 2003;32:519–534.

13 Ezer A, Caliskan A, Parlakgumus A, Belli S, Kozanoglu I, Yildirim S. Preoperative therapeutic plasma exchange in patients with thyrotoxicosis. *J Clin Apher* 2009; 24:111–114.

14 Varela A, Yuste A, Villazala A, Garrido J, Lorenzo A, Lopez E. Spinal anaesthesia for emergency abdominal surgery in uncontrolled hyperthyroidism. *Acta Anaesthiol Scand* 2004; 49:100–103.

15 Chikwe J, Walther A, Jones P. Thyroid disease. In: *Perioperative Medicine: Managing Surgical Patients with Medical Problems*, 2nd edn. Oxford University Press, Oxford, 2009.

CHAPTER 11
Patient with Renal Disease

Khalid Hasan

University Hospitals Birmingham NHS Foundation Trust, Birmingham, UK

Case history: A 51-year-old woman with long-standing hypertension and diabetes and consequent renal impairment presents for laparoscopic-assisted vaginal hysterectomy. Her serum creatinine is 120 mg/L and the estimated GFR is 46 mL/min per 1.73 m².

Background

The prevalence of renal disease in the UK is estimated at 8.5%; females are over-represented with a prevalence of about 10.8%. As people age, there is a physiologic reduction in glomerular filtration rate (GFR), which can be rapidly accelerated by additional comorbidity. Renal disease may be completely silent, with no symptoms or signs to alert the clinician to its status and etiology.

It is important to be aware of the patient with renal disease; they have a twofold to fivefold increase in the risks of death and cardiovascular complications, and a higher risk of postoperative sepsis, fluid overload, acid–base disturbance, acute kidney injury, bleeding, and thromboembolism. Within the context of renal disease, emergency surgery has a significantly greater detrimental effect. Renal insults can be divided into prerenal, renal, and obstructive in origin; organ function preservation is the goal of therapy.

The current NICE classification of chronic kidney disease (CKD) can aid identification of at-risk patients (Table 11.1).

Table 11.1 Chronic kidney disease staging.

Stage	Renal dysfunction
1	Kidney damage with normal or increased GFR ≥90 mL/min per 1.73 m²
2	Kidney damage with mild reduction in GFR 60–89 mL/min per 1.73 m²
3*	Moderate reduction in GFR 30–59 mL/min per 1.73 m²
4	Severe reduction in GFR 15–29 mL/min per 1.73 m²
5	Kidney failure <15 mL/min per 1.73 m² (or dialysis)

* Some authors recommend splitting stage 3 into stages 3a and 3b, 3a with GFR 45–59 mL/min per 1.73 m² and 3b GFR 30–44 mL/min per 1.73 m².

Management

The key principle of management is to identify the at-risk patient and avoid or minimize the factors that will damage renal function any further. Any further acute kidney injury in this context is associated with increased risks of serious morbidity and mortality. Many specific renal protective therapies have been evaluated, including the use of dopamine infusion, mannitol, and furosemide. Currently, the data to support such strategies are lacking. Attention to hydration status and euvolemia remain the main aims at present.

Identify important risk factors

Renal disease may be related to underlying risk factors such as hypertension, diabetes, heart disease, pulmonary disease, liver disease (especially ascites), advanced age and, less commonly, autoimmune and connective tissue disorders, tumors, and sepsis. Drugs and toxins may also precipitate and exacerbate renal disease and dysfunction.

Patients with CKD stage 3 or above require careful perioperative care, ensuring full assessment and management of comorbidities. If surgery is not urgent, consider deferring elective surgery if hypertension or diabetic control requires optimization.

Check blood pressure

It is important to check the patient's BP. If there is a known history of hypertension, is it well controlled? If the BP is above 150 mmHg systolic, involve the primary care physician so that the BP can be rechecked and treated if appropriate. Poorly controlled hypertension leads to poor renal outcomes. In the presence of hypertensive disease, the renal system will not tolerate significant hypotension, and optimal management should aim to keep the BP within 20% of the preoperative value.

Perform baseline investigations

Investigations should include a recent blood urea and electrolytes, together with FBC (anemia is common) and ECG. If the patient has diabetes, HBA_{1c} should be checked (Chapter 9). Poor diabetic control can increase the risk of surgical complications such as postoperative infections and delayed wound healing.

Avoid nephrotoxic drugs

It is necessary to check if the patient is taking nephrotoxic drugs such as NSAIDs, disease-modifying drugs, diuretics, or lithium. These drugs can precipitate or exacerbate renal disease. Check if ACE inhibitors or aspirin can be withheld before surgery. In the postoperative period, avoid NSAIDs, as they increase the risk of acute-on-chronic renal failure. Consider PCA morphine or

Gynecologic and Obstetric Surgery: Challenges and Management Options, First Edition. Edited by Arri Coomarasamy, Mahmood I. Shafi, G. Willy Davila and Kiong K. Chan.
© 2016 John Wiley & Sons, Ltd. Published 2016 by John Wiley & Sons, Ltd.

regional anesthesia as an alternative. Other drugs used perioperatively will also require due consideration. Antimicrobial prophylaxis may need dose adjustment dependent on renal function. There is a risk that drugs (or active metabolites) that are renally excreted may accumulate; morphine is one such drug that should be used with care.

Monitor fluid and electrolyte balance

The use of frequent electrolyte (potassium) and acid–base analysis may be necessary to help guide renal support, together with careful charting of fluid balance. Adequate preoperative hydration and avoidance of intraoperative hypotension are vital, with additional appropriate circulatory support if bleeding intervenes. Consider blood transfusion if the hemoglobin is less than 9 g/dL. Careful attention should be paid to avoid fluid overload when transfusing a euvolemic patient in whom diuresis cannot be satisfactorily achieved. At the renal level, avoidance of nephrotoxic drugs (e.g., NSAIDs) and careful use of drugs that interfere with renal arterial autoregulation (e.g., prostaglandins and vasoactive drugs) is advisable.

When CKD stage 3 or above is present, a perioperative indwelling urinary catheter should be considered. A degree of intraoperative oliguria is normal. Postoperative oliguria should be managed carefully with limited fluid challenges and invasive central venous pressure monitoring. A level 2 critical care bed may be needed to offer the appropriate level of nursing care.

Discuss with anesthetist

Preoperative insertion of central line and invasive arterial line may be necessary to guide appropriate fluid resuscitation and inotropic support. Some patients may require postoperative HDU or ITU admission. In particular, patients undergoing biliary surgery, aortic surgery, and emergency surgery are at increased risk of postoperative renal failure.

Care must be taken with regard to pneumoperitoneum; pressure above 15 mmHg for prolonged periods is an independent risk factor contributing to oliguria.

Prevention

Avoidance of prolonged preoperative starvation, and omission of any ACE inhibitors, should be considered; it is best to liaise with the anesthetist involved as individual practice may vary. ACE inhibitors, if administered on day of surgery, can produce hypotension that is refractory to usual measures (intravenous fluids and sympathomimetic drugs), exacerbating the risk of acute kidney injury.

Care should be exercised if contrast imaging is required. The dyes used can have a detrimental effect on renal function, especially if there is any element of dehydration or if there is a prerenal cause for the renal failure.

Stage 1 and 2 kidney disease are not associated with increased mortality, or major complications in the perioperative phase, provided pathologic albuminuria is not present. However, the patient will still require high-quality care to prevent any element of acute kidney injury occurring.

While there is little RCT evidence about the use of cell salvage perioperatively, it is prudent to reduce reliance on autologous blood transfusion. DDAVP is useful for treating uremia-induced bleeding.

KEY POINTS

Challenge: Patient with renal disease.

Background
- 10.8% of women have chronic renal disease.
- CKD stage 3 and above is associated with increased risk of morbidity, mortality, and hospital stay.
- Renal disease may be silent.
- Measures to maintain organ perfusion and avoid nephrotoxic drugs are key.

Prevention
- Identify the at-risk patient.
- Establish current renal function and etiology of impairment.
- Liaise with physicians and anesthetist preoperatively.
- Limit pneumoperitoneum duration and intra-abdominal pressure.
- Plan location of postoperative care.

Management
- Minimize starvation time.
- Omit ACE inhibitors on day of surgery.
- Maintain normal BP preoperatively and intraoperatively.
- Monitor fluid balance. Do not allow patient to become dehydrated.
- Consider transfusion if Hb<9 g/dL.
- Use an indwelling catheter.
- Check serial K+ and H+ levels to guide fluid replacement therapy.
- Modify doses of drugs that are renally excreted.
- Avoid NSAIDs and be cautious with opiates postoperatively.

Further reading

Foëx P, Sear JW. The surgical hypertensive patient. *Contin Educ Anaesth Crit Care Pain* 2004; 4: 139–143.

National Institute for Health and Care Excellence. *Early identification and management of chronic kidney disease in adults in primary and secondary care.* NICE Clinical Guidance 73. NICE, London, 2008. Available at https://www.nice.org.uk/guidance/cg73

Schaffer AC, Stefan MS. Chronic kidney disease. In: Cohn SL (ed.) *Perioperative Medicine*, pp. 493–501. Springer, London, 2011.

Yentis S, Hirch N, Smith G. *Anaesthesia and Intensive Care A–Z*, 4th edn. Churchill Livingstone, London, 2009.

CHAPTER 12
Patient with Liver Disease

Joanna K. Dowman[1] and Philip N. Newsome[2]
[1] City Hospital, Sandwell and West Birmingham Hospitals NHS Trust, Birmingham, UK
[2] College of Medical and Dental Sciences, University of Birmingham, Birmingham, UK

Case history: A 55-year-old woman with a 15-year history of excessive alcohol intake presented with abdominal pain and distension. Blood tests revealed Hb 10.5 g/dL, albumin 32 g/L, bilirubin 36 μmol/L, ALT 60 IU/L, INR 1.4, platelets 105 × 10⁹/L, and creatinine 105 μmol/L. Ultrasound scan of the abdomen and pelvis showed a small irregular liver, splenomegaly and small amount of ascites, with note also made of large intramural fibroids, for which she was due to have an elective hysterectomy the following week. After exclusion of other causes of liver disease she was diagnosed with alcohol-related cirrhosis.

Background

Several factors contribute to an increased risk of surgery in patients with liver disease. In stable chronic liver disease, surgery can precipitate hepatic decompensation, especially if synthetic function is compromised [1]. Operative risk depends on severity of the underlying liver disease and nature of the surgical procedure, in addition to age and any additional comorbidities. Open abdominal and emergency surgery are considered higher-risk procedures [1].

The severity of liver disease can be assessed using the Child–Turcotte–Pugh (CTP) score (Table 12.1) or the Model for End-stage Liver Disease (MELD) score, both of which have been demonstrated to correlate with perioperative risks [1].

Table 12.1 Child–Turcotte–Pugh scoring system.

Parameter	Points		
	1	2	3
Albumin	>35	28–35	<28
Bilirubin	<34	34–50	>50
INR	<1.7	1.71–2.3	>2.3
Ascites	None	Mild	Moderate to severe
Encephalopathy	None	Grade I–II	Grade III–IV
Total points			
Class A: 5–6			
Class B: 7–9			
Class C: 10–15			

Source: Pugh *et al.*, 1973 [4]. Reproduced with permission of Wiley.

Studies have reported mortality rates for patients undergoing surgery of 10%, 30% and 76–82% for patients with Child's A, Child's B, and Child's C cirrhosis, respectively [1–3]. Child's class was also associated with the frequency of postoperative complications, including liver failure, bleeding, infection, renal failure, and encephalopathy [1]. The general consensus is that elective surgery is usually well tolerated in Child's class A cirrhosis, permissible in Child's class B, with the exception of high-risk procedures, and contraindicated in Child's class C cirrhosis [1].

The MELD score is a linear regression model based on serum bilirubin and creatinine levels and the INR, calculated as follows:

$$MELD = 9.57 \times \ln(creatinine) + 3.78 \times \ln(bilirubin) + 11.2 \times \ln(INR) + 6.43$$

MELD is a useful tool for predicting perioperative mortality, with increased precision over the CTP score [1,5,6]. A large study of 772 patients with cirrhosis undergoing abdominal, orthopedic, and cardiovascular surgery demonstrated 30-day mortality rates of 5.7% in those with MELD score of 7 or less, 10.3% in those with MELD score 8–11, 25.4% in those with MELD score 12–15, and more than 53% with MELD score over 20 [5]. Age and ASA status were the other major contributors to mortality risk, with ASA class V the strongest predictor of 7-day mortality and MELD score the strongest predictor of mortality after 7 days and in the longer term [5].

The following liver-related conditions are associated with high operative risk, and are generally recognized to be contraindications to elective surgery: acute liver failure and/or acute renal failure, alcoholic hepatitis, acute viral hepatitis, alcoholic cardiomyopathy, hypoxemia (e.g., due to hepatopulmonary syndrome or portopulmonary hypertension), and severe coagulopathy (prolonged INR > 1.5 that does not correct with vitamin K) [1].

Management

Management should involve a liver specialist and an experienced anesthetist, as well as other specialists depending on the comorbidities.

Preoperative management

Assess and optimize patient's condition
Elective surgery in patients with liver disease should only be undertaken after detailed assessment of the perioperative risk, and should not be performed in the presence of known contraindications, including acute liver failure, acute hepatitis, and severe coagulopathy. The patient should receive supportive treatment including vitamins

Gynecologic and Obstetric Surgery: Challenges and Management Options, First Edition. Edited by Arri Coomarasamy, Mahmood I. Shafi, G. Willy Davila and Kiong K. Chan.
© 2016 John Wiley & Sons, Ltd. Published 2016 by John Wiley & Sons, Ltd.

and nutritional optimization, and should abstain from alcohol. Diuretics should be prescribed to reduce ascites, if present, with careful monitoring of renal function. When the patient's condition is stable, surgical risk should be assessed using the MELD score to assess the severity of liver disease, with additional assessment of important risk factors including presence of portal hypertension, ascites, anemia, coagulopathy, malnutrition, and hypoalbuminemia.

In the absence of contraindications, elective surgery can be undertaken in stable patients with low MELD scores or Child's class A or B cirrhosis after optimization of liver function, clotting, renal function, anemia, and nutritional status.

Entry of the ASA status, age, and INR, serum bilirubin and creatinine into an online calculator, available at http://www.mayoclinic.org/meld/mayomodel9.html, allows calculation of mortality risk at specific time points after surgery, and can be used to counsel patients regarding the risk of mortality from surgery [5].

Admit
Patients should be admitted 2–3 days before the operation. Adjust medications for hepatic impairment and start on intravenous vitamins. Portal hypertension increases blood loss from all abdominal surgery. Correct coagulopathy with vitamin K, and consider FFP to optimize hemostasis. In patients who are potential liver transplant candidates, consideration should be given to performing surgery at liver transplant centers [5].

Drain ascites
Ascites and hepatic pneumothorax should be drained preoperatively. Massive ascites may need paracentesis. FBC and clotting screen should be performed prior to draining.

Correct fluid and electrolyte imbalance
A strict fluid balance should be maintained. Look for signs of hyponatremia, which is common in hepatic failure. Serum Na^+ should be monitored twice daily and careful attention paid to preventing fluid overload and worsening hyponatremia. Also check for hyperkalemia, which may result from use of spironolactone or from renal failure. Consider switching to loop diuretics if K^+ is greater than 5.0 mmol/L.

Intraoperative management
In the operating theater, careful attention is required to optimize perfusion and oxygenation, and surgeons should be aware of the risk of mechanical decrease in hepatic blood flow induced by intermittent positive pressure ventilation and pneumoperitoneum during laparoscopic surgery [1]. It is important to aim to reduce surgical time to the minimum necessary, and to pay attention to hemostasis.

Postoperative management
Postoperative admission to HDU or ITU for patients with Child's class B or C cirrhosis or a high MELD score should be considered.

Look for signs of decompensation
In the postoperative period, patients with cirrhosis should be monitored closely for signs of hepatic decompensation, including encephalopathy, jaundice, renal dysfunction, coagulopathy, and ascites. Nephrotoxic or hepatotoxic drugs should be avoided, and morphine doses should be reduced because of increased half-life and consequent sedative effects.

Optimize fluid management
Particular attention should be paid to optimizing fluid management. This can be a challenge in cirrhosis, as reduced circulating volume can precipitate renal dysfunction and hepatic underperfusion,

while infusion of excessive fluid, particularly crystalloid, can exacerbate extravascular volume overload with worsening ascites, and peripheral and pulmonary edema [1]. Monitor urinary output hourly and perform daily weight measurements. Blood glucose levels should also be monitored regularly, particularly if there are signs of liver failure with consequent risk of hypoglycemia.

Perform daily coagulation screen
After major surgery, a daily coagulation screen should be carried out, including the measurement of prothrombin time which is a sensitive marker of reduced liver function.

Resolution of the case

Despite only moderate elevations in bilirubin, creatinine and INR, this patient has a MELD score of 15, with Child's class B cirrhosis, which would indicate a significantly increased risk of perioperative mortality and decompensation. This patient's ultrasound scan and laboratory results indicate cirrhosis with early liver dysfunction. This incurs a risk of decompensation during any surgical intervention, and therefore elective surgery should be delayed until her condition has been optimized.

She should receive supportive treatment including vitamins and nutritional optimization, and most importantly abstinence from alcohol. Diuretics should be prescribed to reduce her ascites, with careful monitoring of renal function. Deficiencies of iron, folate or vitamin B_{12} contributing to her anemia should be addressed with replacement therapy. When her condition is stable, surgical risk should be assessed using the MELD score to assess the severity of her liver disease, with additional assessment of important risk factors including presence of portal hypertension, ascites, anemia, coagulopathy, malnutrition, and hypoalbuminemia.

Prevention

Malnutrition is common in patients with cirrhosis, with those presenting with alcoholism at particular risk. Consideration should therefore be given to preoperative enteral or parenteral nutritional supplementation prior to surgery to optimize recovery [7]. Patients with alcoholic liver disease who are still actively drinking are at risk of withdrawal on admission to hospital, and should receive specific monitoring and treatment using tools such as the Clinical Institute Withdrawal Assessment for Alcohol (CIWA-Ar) scoring system and appropriate benzodiazepine treatment. Specific consideration should also be given to the choice of drugs used in the perioperative period because of the reduced capacity of the liver to metabolize many commonly used agents.

Minor elevations of a single liver function test, such as AST or ALP, are very common and unlikely to indicate liver disease that would increase operative risk. However, in the elective situation it is sensible to investigate any liver function test abnormalities detected preoperatively with full history and examination, ultrasound imaging, and blood tests to exclude significant causes such as viral hepatitis, autoimmune liver disease, and metabolic disorders. After exclusion of such diseases, and in the absence of excess alcohol intake, the most common cause of minor elevation in transaminases is non-alcoholic fatty liver disease, which should be suspected in the presence of metabolic risk factors such as obesity, glucose intolerance, hypertension, and dyslipidemia. The presence of such abnormalities should also alert clinicians to the likelihood of increased cardiovascular risk.

KEY POINTS

Challenge: Patient with liver disease.

Background

- Operative risk is increased in patients with liver disease and related to the nature of the operation, severity of liver disease, age, and ASA status.
- Operative risks can be quantified using the CTP score and the MELD score.
- Elective surgery is contraindicated in acute liver failure, acute hepatitis, severe coagulopathy, and advanced decompensated chronic liver disease.

Prevention

- Encourage abstinence from alcohol.
- Consider nutritional supplementation prior to surgery.
- If the patient is a candidate for transplantation, consider performing surgery at a liver transplant center.
- Incidental minor liver test abnormalities detected preoperatively should be investigated prior to surgery, but are unlikely to indicate liver disease that would significantly increase operative risk.

Management

- Elective surgery should only be undertaken after detailed preoperative assessment including evaluation of liver disease severity using MELD score, ASA status and other risk factors including portal hypertension, coagulopathy, sepsis, malnutrition, hypoalbuminemia, anemia, and hypoxemia.
- Liver function, clotting, renal function, anemia, and nutritional status should be optimized preoperatively.
- Careful attention should be paid to fluid balance and oxygenation in the perioperative period.
- Pharmacologic agents should be chosen carefully to minimize adverse effects on liver function.
- Patients should be monitored closely postoperatively for signs of hepatic decompensation.
- Daily bloods, including a coagulation screen, should be performed postoperatively.

References

1 Friedman LS. Surgery in the patient with liver disease. *Trans Am Clin Climatol Assoc* 2010; 121: 192–204.

2 Garrison RN, Cryer HM, Howard DA, Polk HC Jr. Clarification of risk factors for abdominal operations in patients with hepatic cirrhosis. *Ann Surg* 1984; 199: 648–655.

3 Mansour A, Watson W, Shayani V, Pickleman J. Abdominal operations in patients with cirrhosis: still a major surgical challenge. *Surgery* 1997; 122: 730–735.

4 Pugh RN, Murray-Lyon IM, Dawson JL, Pietroni MC, Williams R. Transection of the oesophagus for bleeding oesophageal varices. *Br J Surg* 1973; 60:646–649.

5 Teh SH, Nagorney DM, Stevens SR *et al*. Risk factors for mortality after surgery in patients with cirrhosis. *Gastroenterology* 2007; 132: 1261–1269.

6 Kamath PS, Wiesner RH, Malinchoc M *et al*. A model to predict survival in patients with end-stage liver disease. *Hepatology* 2001; 33: 464–470.

7 Keegan MT, Plevak DJ. Preoperative assessment of the patient with liver disease. *Am J Gastroenterol* 2005; 100: 2116–2127.

CHAPTER 13

Patient with Rheumatologic Diseases

Amita A. Mahendru[1] and Justin Chu[2]
[1] Nottingham University Hospitals NHS Trust, Nottingham, UK
[2] Birmingham Women's NHS Foundation Trust, Birmingham, UK

Case history: *A 50-year-old woman with long-standing rheumatoid arthritis is due to undergo an abdominal hysterectomy. She is on regular diclofenac 75 mg twice daily for analgesia. She takes methotrexate 7.5 mg weekly, oral prednisolone 25 mg daily, and infliximab 3 mg/kg i.v. every 8 weeks to manage the symptoms of arthritis. She also has a painful and stiff neck.*

Background

Rheumatologic diseases affect women more than men and cause damage to bones, joints, and connective tissues. While some autoimmune disorders are organ-specific (Graves' disease, Hashimoto's thyroiditis, insulin-dependent type 1 diabetes, and inflammatory bowel disease), rheumatologic disorders may involve multiple organ systems; examples include systemic lupus erythematosus (SLE), psoriatic arthritis, rheumatoid arthritis (RA), and Wegener's granulomatosus [1]. Women with these conditions are usually on long-term immunosuppressant and anti-inflammatory medications, such as steroids, methotrexate and biologic agents to maintain disease remission.

Rheumatologic diseases may be associated with deranged function of one or more organs either as a result of the disease process or secondary to the effects of long-term medications. Women with rheumatologic conditions are at increased risk of postoperative morbidity and mortality from cardiovascular complications, pneumonia, septicemia, stroke, pulmonary embolism, and wound complications [2,3]. The perioperative risks depend on the specific organs affected by the disease (e.g., cardiovascular, respiratory, metabolic or hematologic), type and duration of surgery, as well as type and duration of immunosuppressant medications taken by the patient.

The aim of perioperative care is to reduce organ-specific risks, manage the immunosuppressant medications, reduce the risk of disease relapse, prevent wound complications and infections, and minimize the risk of thrombosis.

Management of patients with rheumatoid arthritis

Patients with long-standing RA are likely to have joint involvement and mobility problems, and increased cardiovascular risk. The first step is to conduct a thorough preoperative history and examination to diagnose medical comorbidities and assess cardiovascular and thrombotic risks and overall health.

Drug management

A detailed history of medications, including immunosuppressant and anti-inflammatory drugs, is required. Long-term use of drugs such as methotrexate may lead to bone marrow suppression, and derangement of liver and renal function. Therefore, a preoperative full blood count to check for anemia, leukopenia, thrombocytopenia or bone marrow suppression, as well as renal and liver enzyme assays, should be performed.

Patients with RA often use non-steroidal anti-inflammatory agents (NSAIDs). NSAIDs confer an increased risk of perioperative bleeding and therefore diclofenac should be withheld for 7–10 days before surgery to reverse the antiplatelet effects. If discontinuation is not acceptable, her management should be discussed with the hematologist and anesthetist. Long-term NSAID use can also cause renal impairment and therefore renal function should be checked.

Long-term high-dose prednisolone leads to suppression of the stress-induced response of the hypothalamic–pituitary–adrenal axis. Patients using long-term steroids are at risk of having intraoperative Addisonian crisis, manifested by circulatory collapse and hypotension. Perioperative exogenous steroid cover with intravenous hydrocortisone 100 mg every 12 hours is required to avoid this problem. The dose can then be tapered quickly over 1–2 days to the usual preoperative prednisolone dose.

Many patients with RA use disease-modifying antirheumatic drugs (DMARDs) such as methotrexate or biologic agents such as infliximab to ensure that the disease is maintained in remission. Stopping these medications can precipitate an exacerbation of autoimmune inflammatory activity. Based on the existing literature, there is no increased risk of postoperative infection or other complications with DMARDs and it is generally safe to continue methotrexate and other DMARDs such as hydroxychloroquine, azathioprine, and sulfasalazine [4]. Intraoperative antibiotics should be given and postoperative antibiotics considered in view of an increased risk of wound infection.

Infliximab, an inhibitor of tumor necrosis factor (or anti-TNF), is a biologic agent used for immunosuppression. It is administered intravenously as it is destroyed by the gastrointestinal tract, and is given every 8 weeks as a maintenance dose. It should be stopped 1 week before surgery and restarted at least 1 week after the surgery. It would be ideal

Gynecologic and Obstetric Surgery: Challenges and Management Options, First Edition. Edited by Arri Coomarasamy, Mahmood I. Shafi, G. Willy Davila and Kiong K. Chan.
© 2016 John Wiley & Sons, Ltd. Published 2016 by John Wiley & Sons, Ltd.

to plan surgery in the middle of the 8-week interval to minimize the risk of infection and to enable satisfactory wound healing.

Musculoskeletal risks

Surgery requiring general anesthesia in patients with RA places them at risk of spinal cord injuries during intubation due to inflammatory arthropathy affecting the cervical spine. Particular attention should be paid to radicular symptoms (where paresthesia travels down the arms). Therefore, preoperative anesthetic review to assess the airway and to discuss the various anesthetic options should be arranged. Thoracic and lumbar spine involvement may make use of regional anesthesia such as epidural or spinal anesthesia difficult or impossible.

Details of any previous joint replacement surgery (especially of the lower limbs) should also be ascertained so that due care can be exercised when maneuvering patients in the operating room.

Cardiorespiratory risks

RA can affect both the heart and lungs and therefore a detailed history of exercise tolerance, breathing difficulties, and wheeze is required. Patients can have reduced exercise tolerance and aerobic function because of their immobility. In addition, RA can cause valvular heart disease as well as pericarditis and pulmonary fibrosis, rheumatoid pulmonary nodules, and pleural effusion. Therefore, preoperative investigations should include 12-lead ECG and chest radiography. Pulmonary function tests as well as an echocardiogram may also be needed.

Venous thromboembolism risks

As a result of their restricted mobility, patients with RA are at increased risk of venous thromboembolism. Intermittent pneumatic compression of the legs should be used in the intraoperative and postoperative periods. Prophylactic subcutaneous low-molecular-weight heparin (LMWH) should also be implemented.

Wound care

Diligent wound care and patient education regarding medications are important to reduce wound-related complications. It may be necessary to stop some immunosuppressive treatments such as azathioprine or biologic agents such as infliximab to reduce the risk of wound complications. This issue must be carefully balanced with the risks of exacerbation if these medications are stopped.

Resolution of the case

The patient in the case history should have a detailed preoperative history and examination; this would ideally be done by the anesthetist who will be present at the time of her hysterectomy. At the same time the anesthetic options and potential airway difficulties should be identified and discussed. A full blood count and renal and liver function tests should be carried out to identify any organ impairment secondary to the medications that this patient is taking. The patient should discontinue her diclofenac 7–10 days prior to surgery and also be given intraoperative hydrocortisone due to the long-term use of prednisolone. Her methotrexate and infliximab should be managed with the input of her rheumatologist. Appropriate thromboprophylaxis should be implemented and meticulous wound care undertaken.

Other rheumatologic disorders

Similar considerations to those discussed are needed for all patients with other rheumatic disorders, such as SLE, systemic sclerosis, Wegener's granulomatosis, and spondyloarthropathies (Table 13.1).

Table 13.1 Perioperative management of specific risks in patients with rheumatologic diseases.

Category	Management
Cardiac (Chapters 3–7)	Preoperative investigations: ECG, chest X-ray. Continue medications: antihypertensives, diuretics, nitrates, calcium channel blockers. Stop antiplatelet agents: aspirin and clopidogrel 5–7 days before surgery, to be resumed 24–48 hours postoperatively
Immunosuppressants	Assess renal function, risk of infections and wound complications. Glucocorticoids: continue, administer stress dose. Methotrexate: continue unless renal compromise or high risk of respiratory or wound healing complications. 5-Aminosalicylates, azathioprine, 6-mercaptopurine: discontinue on the day of surgery and resume 3 days after surgery if normal renal function. Cyclosporine: continue and carefully monitor for opportunistic infections. Biologics (anti-TNF agents): stop for a week before surgery and recommence once reduced risk of wound complications. May need to continue in cases of inflammatory bowel disease
Hematologic (Chapters 14–16)	Check FBC. Balance risk of thrombosis against risk of bleeding: for anticoagulation, replace warfarin with LMWH or UFH 5 days prior to surgery
Gastrointestinal	Hepatic function: may be affected by medications such as methotrexate. Inflammatory bowel disease: risk of adhesions and increased intraoperative surgical time, malabsorption, malnutrition, and delayed wound healing
Renal (Chapter 11)	Preoperative renal function assessment. Avoid nephrotoxic drugs. Consider risk of acute kidney injury due to surgical trauma and perioperative hemodynamic instability

Key issues in the perioperative management of patients with these rare rheumatologic diseases also center around minimizing cardiovascular risks, modification of immunosuppressive medications (in order to balance the risk of relapse of disease against the risk of surgical site infections and wound healing complications), and consideration of risks of thrombosis [3,4]. Multidisciplinary management involving the anesthetist, physician, immunologist, and rheumatologist is necessary to minimize intraoperative and postoperative complications.

Patients with SLE may have hematologic complications such as thrombocytopenia and antiphospholipid syndrome (APS). These cases should be managed in liaison with a hematologist. Women with thrombocytopenia may require preoperative steroids to increase their platelet count, and elective procedures should be deferred until the platelet count is deemed adequate for the surgery. These women may require perioperative steroid cover.

Women with APS have an increased risk of arterial and venous thrombosis. The general consensus is for bridging anticoagulation with LMWH or unfractionated heparin (UFH) in the preoperative period, after stopping warfarin 5 days preoperatively. Anticoagulation should be recommended postoperatively as soon as possible, once hemostasis is achieved.

KEY POINTS

Challenge: Perioperative management of patients with rheumatologic diseases.

Background
- Rheumatic diseases are chronic diseases, often with other comorbidities.
- Women are usually on long-term immunosuppressant and anti-inflammatory medications to maintain disease remission.
- Increased perioperative risks can be a result of cardiovascular compromise, wound complications, postoperative infections, septicemia, and thrombotic complications.
- Aim of perioperative care is to identify the various organs involved and manage immunosuppressive medications.

Prevention of complications
- Liaise with immunologist, hematologist, anesthetist, and physician depending on comorbidities.
- Obtain detailed history, examination, and appropriate preoperative investigations to assess the organ systems affected.
- Consider reducing the dose of steroids if possible and provide perioperative cover with intravenous hydrocortisone.

- Continue DMARDs unless the planned surgery is complicated with increased risk of pulmonary infection or there is pre-existing renal compromise. If so, stop them a week before surgery and restart when reduced risk of wound complications.
- Weigh risk of thrombosis versus risk of bleeding and consider bridging anticoagulation with all other appropriate measures of thromboprophylaxis.
- Anti-inflammatory and antiplatelet drugs should be stopped 7–10 days before surgery if high risk of bleeding. Seek advice from hematologist, cardiologist, and anesthetist.

Management
Major surgery
- Modify immunosuppressants and disease-modifying medications, as appropriate.
- Give intraoperative steroids.
- Give intraoperative antibiotic prophylaxis.
- Monitor for postoperative infection.
- Arrange mechanical and pharmacologic thromboprophylaxis.
- Encourage early mobilization.

References

1 Davidson A, Diamond B. Autoimmune diseases. *N Engl J Med* 2001; 345: 340–350.
2 Lin JA, Liao CC, Lee YJ, Wu CH, Huang WQ, Chen TL. Adverse outcomes after major surgery in patients with systemic lupus erythematosus: a nationwide population-based study. *Ann Rheum Dis* 2014; **73**:1646–1651.
3 Akkara Veetil BM, Bongartz T. Perioperative care for patients with rheumatic diseases. *Nat Rev Rheumatol* 2011; 8:32–41.
4 Bissar L, Almoallim H, Albazli K, Alotaibi M, Alwafi S. Perioperative management of patients with rheumatic diseases. *Open Rheumatol J* 2013; 7:42–50.

Further reading

Goh L, Jewell T, Laversuch C, Samata A. Should anti-TNF therapy be discontinued in rheumatoid arthritis patients undergoing elective orthopaedic surgery? A systematic review of the evidence. *Rheumatol Int* 2012; 32:5–13.
Grennan DM, Gray J, Loudon J, Fear S. Methotrexate and early postoperative complications in patients with rheumatoid arthritis undergoing elective orthopaedic surgery. *Ann Rheum Dis* 2001;60:214–217.

CHAPTER 14
Patient with Hematologic Disorders

Chieh Lin Fu

Cleveland Clinic Florida, Weston/Fort Lauderdale, Florida, USA

Case history: A 35-year-old woman with a fibroid uterus elected to have a total abdominal hysterectomy for menorrhagia. Investigations found red blood cell count 4.0 × 10⁶/μL, hemoglobin 7.1 g/dL, mean cell volume (MCV) 70 fL, white blood cell count 4.3 × 10³/μL, platelet count 10 × 10³/μL, iron saturation 10% (serum iron/TIBC), and ferritin 10 ng/mL. She has petechiae and easy bruising. She had a deep vein thrombosis (DVT) on oral contraceptive in the past. Her mother has menorrhagia and had a DVT in the past too.

Anemia

Background and management
Anemia, consistent with iron deficiency, is frequently noted with menorrhagia. A low ferritin is consistent with iron deficiency and is supported by a low mean cell volume (MCV) and a low iron saturation (iron/TIBC) below 20%. Elemental iron 150 mg daily should be considered for oral supplementation. For acute intervention, transfusion of 1 unit of packed red blood cells will raise the hemoglobin by 1 g/dL. Iron supplementation should continue until a normal ferritin level is reached. Oral supplementation can raise the hemoglobin by more than 1 g/dL within a month. Intravenous iron infusion is an alternative option for those who cannot tolerate oral iron therapy [1].

If the ferritin is not low, other etiologies for anemia should be sought. For a microcytic anemia, if the MCV to RBC ratio is less than 13, a hereditary anemia such as thalassemia is a possibility.

An evaluation of anemia should include the complete blood cell count with differential, a reticulocyte count, and review of the peripheral smear. A macrocytic anemia can suggest vitamin B₁₂ or folate deficiency or a hematologic disorder. An elevated reticulocyte count with an elevated indirect bilirubin can suggest a hemolytic anemia. A low reticulocyte count would suggest decreased erythropoiesis from bone marrow suppression. A pancytopenia or an abnormal differential can suggest a hematologic disorder or an inflammatory state, and will need further evaluation.

Thrombocytopenia

Background and management
An isolated thrombocytopenia in the context of a normal hemoglobin and white cell count can suggest immune-mediated thrombocytopenic purpura (ITP). ITP is more common in women and can be associated with viral and autoimmune disorders, but is more often idiopathic. The acute intervention for ITP is intravenous immunoglobulin (IVIG) 1–2 g/kg given in divided doses over 2–4 days to improve the platelet count. Oral corticosteroids such as prednisone 1 mg/kg daily can also improve the platelet count in ITP. Alternate managements for ITP include anti-D antibody, rituximab (a CD20 monoclonal antibody directed to the B-cell lymphocytes) to suppress the immune system, thrombopoietin receptor agonist (romiplostim or eltrombopag) to increase platelet production, or splenectomy [2].

The diagnosis of ITP is by exclusion; therefore if an alternative diagnosis such as disseminated intravascular coagulation, heparin-induced thrombocytopenia, thrombotic thrombocytopenic purpura, or primary bone marrow suppression is suspected, additional clinical evaluation and further laboratory tests need to be performed. Thrombocytopenia from splenic sequestration would manifest as splenomegaly, and will need investigation.

A platelet count above 50 × 10³/μL is needed before surgery. Other than ITP, for which management is primarily with immunosuppressants, other causes of thrombocytopenia can be supported with platelet transfusion if there is evidence of bleeding. A transfusion of 4–6 units of pooled platelets or 1 unit of apheresed platelets around the time of surgery can increase the platelet count to 30–50 × 10³/μL [3].

Bleeding disorders

Background and management
Von Willebrand factor (vWF) deficiency is the most common bleeding disorder, with a prevalence of 5–20% in women with menorrhagia. The vWF antigen is necessary for platelet adhesion to the endothelial cell surface to achieve hemostasis. The activity is measured by the ristocetin cofactor. Additionally, the vWF antigen is a carrier of clotting factor VIII in circulation. Therefore initial testing for the vWF deficiency includes the von Willebrand factor antigen, ristocetin cofactor activity, factor VIII levels, and the activated partial thromboplastin time (aPTT). The subtypes of vWF deficiency include evaluation for the vWF multimer pattern. Because the vWF studies can be below normal in blood type O and can be normal in mild vWF deficiency in inflammatory states, the diagnosis requires clinical correlation. In mild vWF deficiency, one dose of desmopressin (DDAVP) 0.3 μg/kg given intravenously perioperatively can be adequate. Nasal DDAVP (Stimate) can be given for menorrhagia with vWF deficiency [4].

Gynecologic and Obstetric Surgery: Challenges and Management Options, First Edition. Edited by Arri Coomarasamy, Mahmood I. Shafi, G. Willy Davila and Kiong K. Chan.
© 2016 John Wiley & Sons, Ltd. Published 2016 by John Wiley & Sons, Ltd.

Platelet dysfunction can increase the risk of bleeding intraoperatively and is primarily acquired from the use of inhibitors of platelet aggregation, including aspirin, NSAIDs, and thienopyridines such as clopidogrel. Platelet dysfunction can also be seen in uremia. The bleeding time evaluated by various instruments has not been definitively correlated with surgical bleeding risk [5].

A prolonged prothrombin time (PT) or aPTT can suggest a bleeding disorder. A mixing study on the PT or the aPTT is first performed to evaluate for correction of the PT or aPTT. If there is correction with addition of normal plasma to the patient's plasma, a clotting factor deficiency is suggested, and needs to be identified. A prolonged aPTT suggests factor VIII, IX, or XI deficiency. A prolonged PT suggests factor VII deficiency. A prolonged PT and aPTT suggests an acquired factor II or factor X deficiency, such as from warfarin. There are other rare bleeding disorders that are not detected by the PT or aPTT and would need further evaluation if a bleeding disorder is suspected (e.g., a fibrinogen defect or factor XIII deficiency). If there is no correction on the mixing study, an inhibitor known as a lupus anticoagulant or other clotting factors need to be identified.

For most emergency procedures, fresh frozen plasma (FFP) can be given to correct the coagulopathy (~10 mL/kg; about 4 units of FFP) to achieve hemostasis. If factor VIII or factor IX deficiency is identified, a recombinant factor is given. If factor XI deficiency is identified, FFP is given. Activated factor VII (Novoseven) is given for factor VII deficiency and in cases of uncontrolled bleeding. For rare cases of dysfibrinogenemia or hypofibrinogenemia, cryoprecipitate derived from FFP would be given [6].

Tranexamic acid (Lysteda) is approved for the transient management of menorrhagia. Tranexamic acid is an antifibrinolytic agent that inhibits the lysis of a clot. It is considered a non-hormonal alternative to control menorrhagia.

Venous thrombosis

Background and management

Oral contraceptives can increase the risk of venous thromboembolism (VTE) to three times the normal risk. The estrogen content increases the risk [7]. A thrombophilia is considered if there is no provoking event or an atypical presentation. Factor V Leiden and prothrombin gene mutation are the two common thrombophilias in the white population. Protein C, protein S, and antithrombin deficiency are less common. Antiphospholipid antibody syndrome is an acquired cause for venous and arterial thrombosis [8].

Because the risk for VTE in gynecologic surgery is considered moderate at 3%, prophylactic anticoagulation with medical and mechanical prophylaxis should be contemplated [9]. Therapeutic anticoagulation should be undertaken for at least 3 months for a provoked event. Elective surgery should be delayed for at least a month with an acute VTE in order to minimize risk of propagation. The duration of anticoagulation in thrombophilia patients will depend on clinical evaluation [10].

Resolution of the case

The patient in the case history has iron-deficiency anemia. Oral elemental iron 150 mg daily is recommended until an adequate hemoglobin is achieved before surgery. Alternatively, transfusion of packed red blood cells would be provided as needed for acute intervention.

Because the RBC count is normal for the degree of hemoglobin, there is likely a hemoglobinopathy for which hemoglobin electrophoresis can be helpful, along with review of the peripheral smear.

In addition, clinically the patient has immune-mediated thrombocytopenic purpura. Prednisone 1 mg/kg would be initiated until the platelet count is above $50 \times 10^3/\mu L$ before surgery. IVIG 1–2 g/kg in divided doses over 2–4 days can be given if surgery is planned within 1–2 weeks.

DVT prophylaxis would be considered if the platelet count was adequate postoperatively. Because of the family history of DVT and the personal history of DVT (while on oral contraceptives), thrombophilia work-up would be discussed.

Because of the menorrhagia and family history of bleeding, vWF deficiency should be considered. Nasal desmopressin (Stimate) can be given for vWF deficiency during the time of menses. Intravenous desmopressin 0.3 µg/kg would be given perioperatively for mild vWF deficiency.

KEY POINTS

Challenge: Hematologic issues in gynecologic surgery.

Anemia
- Iron-deficiency anemia is associated with low hemoglobin, ferritin, MCV, and iron saturation (iron/TIBC).
- Full evaluation of anemia should include complete blood cell count with differential, a reticulocyte count, and review of the peripheral smear.
  - Microcytic anemia with normal ferritin suggests a hereditary anemia such as thalassemia.
  - A macrocytic anemia suggests vitamin B_{12} or folate deficiency or a hematologic disorder.
  - An elevated reticulocyte count with elevated indirect bilirubin suggests a hemolytic anemia.
  - A low reticulocyte count suggests decreased erythropoiesis from bone marrow suppression.
  - A pancytopenia or abnormal differential suggests a hematologic disorder or an inflammatory state.
- Treatment of iron-deficiency anemia:
  - Oral iron 150 mg daily can raise hemoglobin by more than 1 g/dL within a month.
  - For acute intervention, blood transfusion: 1 unit of packed cells can raise the hemoglobin by 1 g/dL.
  - For those who cannot tolerate oral iron, intravenous iron infusion can be used.

Thrombocytopenia
- An isolated thrombocytopenia with normal hemoglobin and white cell count suggests ITP.
- The diagnosis of ITP is by exclusion, so consider (and exclude by additional investigations if necessary):
  - Disseminated intravascular coagulation.
  - Heparin-induced thrombocytopenia.
  - Thrombotic thrombocytopenic purpura.
  - Primary bone marrow suppression.
- A platelet count $>50 \times 10^3/\mu L$ is needed before surgery.
- Treatment of ITP:
  - IVIG 1–2 g/kg in divided doses over 2–4 days or prednisone 1 mg/kg daily.
  - Other management options include anti-D antibody, rituximab, thrombopoietin receptor agonist (romiplostim or eltrombopag), or splenectomy.
- For other thrombocytopenic conditions, consider transfusion of 4–6 units of pooled platelets or 1 unit of apheresed platelets around the time of surgery.

Bleeding disorders
- Von Willebrand factor deficiency:
  - Is the most common bleeding disorder, with a prevalence of 5–20% in women with menorrhagia.

- Order vWF antigen, ristocetin cofactor activity, factor VIII levels, aPTT for evaluation.
- DDAVP 0.3 µg/kg can be given over 30 min perioperatively for mild vWF deficiency to achieve adequate hemostasis for surgery (with peak 30–90 min after infusion).
- Bleeding disorders need full evaluation as replacement depends on the identified deficiency. However, FFP (~10 mL/kg; about 4 units of FFP) can be given for an undiagnosed coagulopathy.
- Tranexamic acid can be considered for menorrhagia as a non-hormonal treatment if thrombotic risk is low.

References

1 Centers for Disease Control and Prevention (CDC). Recommendations to prevent and control iron deficiency in the United States. *MMWR* 1998; 47(RR-3): 1–36. Available at http://www.cdc.gov/mmwr/pdf/rr/rr4703.pdf

2 Neunert C, Lim W, Crowther M, Cohen A, Solberg L Jr, Crowther MA. The American Society of Hematology 2011 evidence-based practice guideline for immune thrombocytopenia. *Blood* 2011; 117: 4190–4207.

3 Slichter SJ. Evidence-based platelet transfusion guidelines. *Hematology Am Soc Hematol Educ Program* 2007:172–178.

4 Nichols WL, Hultin MB, James AH *et al.* von Willebrand disease (VWD): evidence-based diagnosis and management guidelines, the National Heart, Lung, and Blood Institute (NHLBI) Expert Panel report (USA). *Haemophilia* 2008; 14:171–232.

5 Konkle BA. Acquired disorders of platelet function. *Hematology Am Soc Hematol Educ Program* 2011:391–396.

6 O'Shaughnessy DF, Atterbury C, Bolton Maggs P *et al.* Guidelines for the use of fresh-frozen plasma, cryoprecipitate and cryosupernatant. *Br J Haematol* 2004; 126: 11–28.

7 Vandenbroucke JP, Rosing J, Bloemenkamp KW *et al.* Oral contraceptives and the risk of venous thrombosis. *N Engl J Med* 2001; 344:1527–1535.

8 Wu O, Robertson L, Twaddle S *et al.* Screening for thrombophilia in high-risk situations: systematic review and cost-effectiveness analysis. The Thrombosis: Risk and Economic Assessment of Thrombophilia Screening (TREATS) study. *Health Technol Assess* 2006; 10(11): 1–110.

9 Gould MK, Garcia DA, Wren SM *et al.* Prevention of VTE in nonorthopedic surgical patients: Antithrombotic Therapy and Prevention of Thrombosis, 9th edn. American College of Chest Physicians Evidence-Based Clinical Practice Guidelines. *Chest* 2012; 141(2 Suppl): e227S–e277S.

10 Kearon C, Akl EA, Comerota AJ *et al.* Antithrombotic therapy for VTE disease: Antithrombotic Therapy and Prevention of Thrombosis, 9th edn. American College of Chest Physicians Evidence-Based Clinical Practice Guidelines. *Chest* 2012; 141(2 Suppl): e419S–e494S.

CHAPTER 15

Patient at High Risk of Venous Thrombosis

Ian A. Greer

Faculty of Medical and Human Sciences, University of Manchester, UK

Case history: A 38-year-old woman with a BMI of 36 kg/m² is admitted at 36 weeks of gestation with pre-eclampsia. She has a cesarean section complicated by a major postpartum hemorrhage of 2.3 L, requiring blood transfusion. In the course of this, she develops a coagulopathy. Seven days following delivery she is found to have wound infection requiring antibiotics and drainage. Her mobility has been poor since delivery.

Background

The mechanisms of venous thromboembolism (VTE) risk in surgical patients are described by Virchow's triad: venous stasis, endothelial injury, and hypercoagulability. These three factors can influence both procedure-related risks and patient-related risks.

Procedure-specific factors include open abdominal or pelvic procedures, which are associated with a higher risk of VTE than laparoscopic procedures, and the extent and duration of the procedure. Patient-specific factors have been established from large studies of VTE risk in mixed surgical populations. Key risk factors include age over 60 years, previous VTE, cancer, bed rest for more than 4 days, sepsis, pregnancy, and central venous access.

Gynecologic surgery

Overall, the risk of VTE associated with gynecologic surgery is similar to the risk of VTE in general surgical patients. Pulmonary embolism (PE) is associated with a substantial proportion of the deaths associated with gynecologic surgery, particularly in patients with cancer [1]. Routine thromboprophylaxis is now well established for gynecologic surgery.

Obstetric surgery

The risk of VTE after cesarean section is around 5 in 1000. Pregnancy itself is a risk factor for VTE, and surgical procedures in pregnant patients result in the interaction of risk factors. The increased risks are explained by hormonal changes, mechanical compression by the uterus, and reduced mobility of the patient. VTE during pregnancy (often presenting as DVT in the lower limbs or PE) accounts for 10% of all maternal deaths. The major and minor risk factors for postpartum VTE are summarised in Table 15.1.

Table 15.1 Risk factors for postpartum VTE.

Major risk factors
Massive postpartum hemorrhage (loss of ≥1 L) with surgery
Antepartum immobility (strict bed rest for ≥1 week)
Previous history of VTE
Pre-eclampsia with fetal growth restriction
Thrombophilia
Antithrombin deficiency
Factor V Leiden (homozygous or heterozygous)
Prothrombin G20210A (homozygous or heterozygous)
Medical conditions
Active SLE
Heart disease (e.g., heart failure)
Sickle cell disease
Blood transfusion
Postpartum infection
Minor risk factors
BMI >30 kg/m²
Multiple pregnancy
Cesarean section
Postpartum hemorrhage >1 L
Smoking >10 cigarettes/day
Fetal growth restriction
Thrombophilia
Protein C deficiency
Protein S deficiency
Pre-eclampsia
Family history of VTE

Source: adapted from Bates *et al.*, 2013 [6].

Management

The benefits of thromboprophylaxis should be balanced against the risks of complications from perioperative bleeding [2,3]: therefore it is important to conduct a careful presurgical risk assessment. Risk scoring systems (e.g., Roger's or Caprini scores) have been used, although these have not been validated specifically in gynecologic or obstetric surgery [4–6].

The overall rate of bleeding associated with pharmacologic thromboprophylaxis is low; however, most studies have excluded patients at high risk of bleeding complications [6]. Previous major bleeding, an untreated bleeding disorder, renal or liver failure, thrombocytopenia, acute stroke, uncontrolled hypertension, and sepsis are associated with increased bleeding risk.

For a patient at high risk of VTE but not at high risk of bleeding complications, there is substantial evidence from high-quality trials

---

Gynecologic and Obstetric Surgery: Challenges and Management Options, First Edition. Edited by Arri Coomarasamy, Mahmood I. Shafi, G. Willy Davila and Kiong K. Chan.
© 2016 John Wiley & Sons, Ltd. Published 2016 by John Wiley & Sons, Ltd.

that thromboprophylaxis with either low-dose unfractionated heparin (LDUH) or low-molecular-weight heparin (LMWH) will reduce the risk of mortality from PE by more than 40% [6]. There is also evidence of a substantial reduction in non-fatal VTE. Further, this substantially outweighs the risk from non-fatal bleeding [6]. Many authorities now prefer LMWH over LDUH because of once-daily dosing and ease of administration.

There are fewer data to evaluate mechanical techniques such as intermittent pneumatic compression (IPC). These interventions may be valuable in women at high risk of VTE who are also at high risk of bleeding complications, but pharmacologic prophylaxis with LMWH is still generally considered preferable unless the baseline risk of major bleeding exceeds 4%. In this situation mechanical techniques are best used, at least until the risk of bleeding has subsided [6]. When the risk of bleeding diminishes, pharmacologic prophylaxis can be initiated.

For the patient at high risk of thrombosis, there may be benefit from combining pharmacologic thromboprophylaxis with IPC or graduated elastic compression stockings (GECS).

For a patient undergoing extensive surgery for gynecologic cancer, extended thromboprophylaxis for 4 weeks may be valuable; it appears to offer additional protection from non-fatal VTE without a significant increase in bleeding risk [6].

Cesarean section in women at high risk of VTE is a major perioperative challenge for thromboprophylaxis [7,8]. Thromboprophylaxis with LMWH is recommended and may be combined with GECS or IPC. Modeling has estimated a greater than 50% reduction in VTE in high-risk patients receiving LMWH following cesarean section [8]. Mechanical techniques alone may be used if there is a significant risk of bleeding. Extended thromboprophylaxis for up to 6 weeks needs to be considered in patients at high risk of thromboembolism [8].

Specific high-risk gynecologic situations
Specific high-risk situations, such as a patient on long-term oral anticoagulants, may be encountered in practice. For a woman with a mechanical heart valve, or a problem such as atrial fibrillation requiring long-term anticoagulation, it is usual to provide bridging anticoagulation with heparin during the interruption of oral anticoagulant therapy. Expert hematologic input is usually appropriate for these women.

In a woman with a recent coronary stent who is receiving dual antiplatelet therapy, with clopidogrel and aspirin for example, the bleeding risk is substantial and it is best to defer surgery for at least 6 weeks after the placement of a bare metal stent, and for at least 6 months after placement of a drug-eluting stent, rather than operate during these periods [9].

Specific high-risk obstetric situations
A specific high-risk situation for cesarean section is the patient with a recent thrombosis. These women will be on therapeutic treatment. This will require to be interrupted for the operation to take place. It is important to consider whether or not a temporary inferior vena cava (IVC) filter should be used. In general these should be restricted to women with proven DVT who have recurrent PE despite adequate anticoagulation, complications of anticoagulation preventing its use, and VTE complications where anticoagulation is contraindicated. This is because experience with these devices during pregnancy is limited and there is significant risk of filter migration and IVC perforation [10]. The use of an IVC filter for primary prevention of PE even when LMWH or mechanical methods are not possible is not recommended.

Note that temporary filters are not always retrieved and one large systematic review found a non-retrievable rate of more than 30% [10]. The complications associated with filters include DVT, filter migration, vena cava thrombosis or stenosis, and fracture of the filter.

Resolution of the case

At the time of delivery, this woman had multiple risk factors: age over 35, high BMI, pre-eclampsia, pregnancy, cesarean section, coagulopathy, and blood transfusion. Risk factors interact and so the level of risk of VTE in this case was exceptionally high and thus she required thromboprophylaxis. However, immediately postpartum she had a coagulopathy and potential bleeding problem.

Given the features present prior to cesarean section, combined mechanical and pharmacologic prophylaxis would have been appropriate, and IPC or GECS could have been used during surgery. After the operation, LMWH should have been delayed until the coagulopathy resolved, and the patient would therefore have required continued mechanical techniques at least until LMWH could be prescribed. A wound infection, reduced mobility, and high BMI created significant ongoing risk of VTE for weeks after delivery, and she would have benefited from extended prophylaxis for 6 weeks following delivery with both GECS and LMWH.

KEY POINTS

Challenge: Managing patients at high risk of venous thrombosis.

Background
- VTE is associated with substantial morbidity and mortality and varies depending on patient and procedural risk factors.
- Mechanisms are described by Virchow's triad: venous stasis, endothelial injury, and hypercoagulability.

Management
- The benefits of thromboprophylaxis always have to be balanced against the risks of complications from perioperative bleeding; therefore conduct a careful presurgical risk assessment.
- Use pharmacologic and non-pharmacologic prophylaxis/treatment options:
  - Pharmacologic: LMWH, fondaparinux, and new oral agents such as rivaroxaban, apixaban and dabigatran.
  - Non-pharmacologic: early ambulation, GECS, and IPC.
- LMWH is usually indicated for women at high VTE risk.
- Where heparin has to be avoided, e.g., because of a high risk of bleeding, mechanical techniques such as IPC should be used alone until LMWH can be prescribed.
- IVC filters are rarely indicated.
- Maintain adequate hydration.
- Recognize early warning signs.
- Make a further risk assessment prior to discharge as many high-risk patients will require extended thromboprophylaxis for 4–6 weeks.
- Obtain expert hematologic assistance when managing patients on long-term anticoagulation or with a history of a recent thrombotic event.

References
1 Nicolaides A, Fareed J, Kakkar AK *et al.* Prevention and treatment of venous thromboembolism. International Consensus Statement. *Int Angiol* 2013; 32:132–139.
2 Nelson-Piercy C, Powrie R, Borg JY *et al.* Tinzaparin use in pregnancy: an international, retrospective study of the safety and efficacy profile. *Eur J Obstet Gynecol Reprod Biol* 2011;159:293–299.

3 Nicolaides A, Fareed J, Kakkar AK *et al.* Prevention and treatment of venous thromboembolism. International Consensus Statement. *Int Angiol* 2013; 32:223–224.

4 Bahl V, Hu HM, Henke PK, Wakefield TW, Campbell DA Jr, Caprini JA. A validation study of a retrospective venous thromboembolism risk scoring method. *Ann Surg* 2010; 251:344–350.

5 Rogers SO Jr, Kilaru RK, Hosokawa P, Henderson WG, Zinner MJ, Khuri SF. Multivariable predictors of postoperative venous thromboembolic events after general and vascular surgery: results from the patient safety in surgery study. *J Am Coll Surg* 2007 ;204:1211–1221.

6 Gould MK, Garcia DA, Wren SM *et al.* Prevention of VTE in nonorthopedic surgical patients: Antithrombotic Therapy and Prevention of Thrombosis, 9th edn. American College of Chest Physicians Evidence-Based Clinical Practice Guidelines. *Chest* 2012; 141(2 Suppl): e227S–e277S.

7 Nelson-Piercy C, MacCallum P, Mackillop L. *Reducing the Risk of Thrombosis and Embolism During Pregnancy and the Puerperium.* RCOG Green-top Guideline No.

37a. Royal College of Obstetricians and Gynaecologists, London, 2015. https://www.rcog.org.uk/globalassets/documents/guidelines/gtg-37a.pdf (accessed August 2011).

8 Bates SM, Greer IA, Middeldorp S, Veenstra DL, Prabulos AM, Vandvik PO. VTE, thrombophilia, antithrombotic therapy, and pregnancy: Antithrombotic Therapy and Prevention of Thrombosis, 9th edn. American College of Chest Physicians Evidence-Based Clinical Practice Guidelines. *Chest* 2013; 141(2 Suppl): e691S–e736S.

9 Douketis JD, Spyropoulos AC, Spencer FA *et al.* Perioperative management of antithrombotic therapy: Antithrombotic Therapy and Prevention of Thrombosis, 9th edn. American College of Chest Physicians Evidence-Based Clinical Practice Guidelines. *Chest* 2012; 141 (2 Suppl): e326S–e350S.

10 Greer IA, Nelson-Piercy C. Low-molecular-weight heparins for thromboprophylaxis and treatment of venous thrombo-embolism in pregnancy: a systematic review of safety and efficacy. *Blood* 2005; 106:401–407

CHAPTER 16
Patient on Anticoagulant Therapy

Sophie Lee and Will Lester

University Hospitals Birmingham NHS Foundation Trust, Birmingham, UK

Case history 1: A 65-year-old woman with a mechanical mitral valve who is on warfarin (INR target 3.0) requires a hysterectomy with bilateral salpingo-oophorectomy for endometrial cancer. A perioperative plan of anticoagulation is required for the patient.

Case history 2: A 30-year-old pregnant woman with an otherwise unremarkable pregnancy presents with sudden pain and swelling in the left leg at 35 weeks of gestation. A therapeutic dose of LMWH was commenced pending further investigations. A Doppler ultrasound scan of the leg did not identify a thrombus; however, based on clinical suspicion, an MRI scan of the pelvis was requested which confirmed occlusive thrombosis of the common iliac vein. She continued enoxaparin 1 mg/kg b.d. and was fitted with a class 2 below-knee graduated compression sock. She is now 38 weeks pregnant. She wishes to have an elective cesarean section. She requires a birth plan for anticoagulant management.

Background

Patients requiring gynecologic surgery may be on oral anticoagulants for a variety of reasons. The American College of Chest Physicians (ACCP) recommends an individualized approach to determine the need for bridging anticoagulation based on the patient's estimated thromboembolic risk and periprocedural bleeding risk (Table 16.1).

Table 16.1 Bridging anticoagulation therapy according to risk of thrombosis.

Low risk (no bridging therapy required)
Patients with low-risk AF (no prior stroke or TIA)
Patients with a bileaflet aortic mechanical heart valve with no other risk factors

Intermediate risk (prophylactic LMWH bridging therapy required)
Patients with VTE more than 3 months earlier

Higher risk (high-dose LMWH bridging therapy usually required)
INR target range 3–4
Less than 3 months after a deep venous thrombosis
Recurrent thrombosis on anticoagulants or with active cancer
AF with previous stroke or TIA or other multiple risk factors
Mechanical prosthetic heart valves (unless low risk)
Antiphospholipid syndrome on long-term anticoagulation

Management

Preoperative care
A detailed history should be obtained regarding the indication for anticoagulant therapy. In the case of a patient with a prosthetic valve,

the type and age of the prosthetic heart valve should be ascertained. Other risk factors for thromboembolism should also be identified (e.g., atrial fibrillation, previous valve thrombosis). The patient's INR target and usual warfarin dose should be established.

In patients having major surgery, warfarin should be stopped 5 days before surgery. Low-molecular-weight heparin (LMWH) is the most commonly used agent for bridging as it is far more convenient and predictable than unfractionated heparin.

After stopping warfarin, therapeutic LMWH such as enoxaparin 1 mg/kg every 12 hours should be started 3 days before surgery with the last dose being more than 24 hours before surgery. Dosing must take into account the renal function of the patient. Some experts recommend that the last preoperative dose is halved for high-risk surgery.

Postoperative care
Following surgery, the timing and dose of bridging LMWH remain controversial. Bridging therapy can clearly increase the risk of perioperative bleeding (conferring a more than threefold overall risk of major bleeding). The British Committee for Standards in Haematology (BCSH) guidelines recommend that therapeutic postoperative bridging should not be started until at least 48 hours after surgery with high bleeding risk.

There is some evidence from meta-analysis that postoperative prophylactic or intermediate-dose LMWH is associated with less bleeding without increasing thromboembolic event rates. For most elective procedures, warfarin can be started at the usual preoperative dose in the evening or on the day after surgery if there is adequate hemostasis, as the onset of an anticoagulant effect will be delayed for a number of days.

Prophylactic-dose LMWH is given until at least day 2 after surgery when the dose can then be increased to a therapeutic dose. LMWH should then be continued until the INR is above 2.5.

Special circumstances

Emergency surgery for patients on warfarin
For surgery that requires reversal of warfarin and that can be delayed for 8–24 hours, the INR can be corrected by giving intravenous vitamin K.

For emergency surgery that requires urgent reversal of warfarin, the INR can be corrected by giving a four-factor prothrombin complex concentrate (25–50 units/kg depending on INR) and 5–10 mg intravenous vitamin K.

Gynecologic and Obstetric Surgery: Challenges and Management Options, First Edition. Edited by Arri Coomarasamy, Mahmood I. Shafi, G. Willy Davila and Kiong K. Chan.
© 2016 John Wiley & Sons, Ltd. Published 2016 by John Wiley & Sons, Ltd.

Table 16.2 Recommendations on how long to withhold anticoagulant therapy before surgery.

	Dabigatran		Apixaban		Rivaroxaban	
	Low risk	High risk	Low risk	High risk	Low risk	High risk
CrCl ≥80 mL/min	≥24 hours	≥48 hours	≥24 hours	≥48 hours	≥24 hours	≥48 hours
CrCl 50–80 mL/min	≥36 hours	≥72 hours	≥24 hours	≥48 hours	≥24 hours	≥48 hours
CrCl 30–50 mL/min	≥48 hours s	≥96 hours	≥24 hours	≥48 hours	≥24 hours	≥48 hours
CrCl 15–30 mL/min	Not indicated	Not indicated	≥36 hours	≥48 hours	≥36 hours	≥48 hours

CrCl, creatinine clearance.

Source: adapted from Heidbuchel *et al.*, 2013 [1]. Reproduced with permission from Oxford University Press.

New oral anticoagulants (oral direct inhibitors): perioperative management

Several newer oral anticoagulants are now in routine clinical use. The aPTT and PT may provide a semi-quantitative assessment of the presence of dabigatran and rivaroxaban; however, more specialist laboratory assays are required to actually quantify drug levels of oral direct inhibitors and these may not be available in an emergency situation. Based on drug half-life, recommendations on how long to withhold oral direct inhibitors prior to surgery are given in Table 16.2.

Post-procedure prophylactic LMWH can be initiated 6–8 hours after surgery if hemostasis has been achieved. New anticoagulants should ideally be deferred for 48–72 hours before recommencing.

Antiplatelet agents: perioperative management

Aspirin and clopidogrel are irreversible inhibitors of platelet function. If used for primary cardiovascular prophylaxis only and the surgery has a significant bleeding risk, they should be stopped for 7 days to allow platelet recovery. Clopidogrel is generally associated with a higher bleeding risk than aspirin. If surgery cannot be delayed and there is a very high bleeding risk, platelet transfusions may be effective as the drug half-life is approximately 8 hours.

NSAIDs and dipyridamole cause milder reversible inhibition of platelet function so they can be stopped 24–48 hours and on the day of surgery, respectively.

Appropriate LMWH prophylaxis should still be given postoperatively as antiplatelet agents are not considered adequate for prophylaxis against venous embolism. There is likely to be an increased bleeding risk when using a combination of LMWH and antiplatelet agent. Antiplatelet agents can be restarted on the day after surgery unless high bleeding risk or thrombocytopenia is present.

For high-risk patients (e.g., with recent insertion of a drug-eluting stent) seek specialist advice and delay surgery if possible. It is preferable to avoid stopping clopidogrel whenever possible and aspirin should not be stopped unless absolutely necessary.

Anticoagulation in an obstetric patient

LMWH should be stopped as soon as a woman is in established labor or thinks she is in labor. For elective cesarean section, LMWH should be stopped for at least 24 hours. The same recommendation could be used for induction of labor; however, one may need to consider additional doses of LMWH for high-risk women who are not in active labor during the induction period.

Regional anesthesia should not be used until at least 12 hours after a prophylactic dose of LMWH and for at least 24 hours after the last dose of therapeutic LMWH. LMWH should be delayed for 4 hours after an epidural catheter has been removed or for 6 hours if there are concerns about local trauma. Removing the catheter before restarting LMWH may be safer in terms of minimizing the risk of spinal hematoma. Otherwise, it should not be removed

within 12 hours of a prophylactic dose. It is often recommended that LMWH should not be given for 4 hours after spinal anesthesia, although the risks of bleeding are much lower than with an epidural.

In women receiving therapeutic doses of LMWH, wound drains (abdominal and rectus sheath) should be considered at cesarean section and the skin incision should be closed with staples or interrupted sutures to allow drainage of any hematoma.

Resolution of the cases

Case history 1

Warfarin should be stopped 5 days before the surgery date. LMWH 1 mg/kg b.d. should be started 3 days prior to her operation and then stopped before 24 hours prior to the surgery.

Postoperatively, the warfarin is restarted at the patient's usual dose on the day after surgery. A prophylactic dose of LMWH is given for 48 hours after surgery, and then the treatment dose is recommended at 1 mg/kg b.d. This LMWH should continue until the INR is above 2.5.

Case history 2

The last dose of LMWH should be given at 7 AM the day before admission for elective cesarean section at 39 weeks. Spinal anesthesia can be used for the cesarean section. Taking into account the early pregnancy weight of 78 kg, enoxaparin 40 mg is given 4 hours after the operation. Enoxaparin 40 mg b.d. is then given on the first postoperative day. The dose is increased to 80 mg b.d. on day 2 after cesarean section, if no abnormal bleeding is identified by the obstetric team.

If the patient is not keen on attending clinic for the regular INR monitoring required for warfarin, she can be discharged on enoxaparin 120 mg once daily to complete a total of 3 months of anticoagulation. She can continue to breast-feed throughout the treatment period. The patient should be advised to have prophylactic LMWH in any future pregnancy both antenatally and for 6 weeks postpartum.

KEY POINTS

Challenge: Perioperative care of patient on anticoagulant therapy.

Background
- Patients on oral or parenteral anticoagulants who need surgery require a perioperative plan that takes into account the risks of bleeding and thromboembolism.
- There is a paucity of clinical trials to give evidence-based guidance.

Managing anticoagulants and antiplatelet agents for major surgery and delivery
- Perioperative management of patient on warfarin:
  - Warfarin should be stopped for 5 days before surgery.
  - The need for LMWH bridging and dose required depends on the underlying risk of thrombosis. A typical regimen for bridging

therapy is enoxaparin 1 mg/kg every 12 hours started 3 days before surgery, with the last dose being more than 24 hours before surgery.
- For most elective procedures, warfarin can be started at the usual preoperative dose on the day after surgery if there is adequate hemostasis, as the onset of an anticoagulant effect will be delayed for a number of days.
- Prophylactic-dose LMWH is given until at least day 2 after surgery when the dose can then be increased to a therapeutic dose. LMWH should then be continued until the INR is above 2.5.
- Emergency surgery for patients on warfarin:
  - If the operation can be delayed for 8–24 hours, the INR can be corrected by giving intravenous vitamin K.
  - For emergency surgery that requires urgent reversal of warfarin, the INR can be corrected by giving a four-factor prothrombin complex concentrate (25–50 units/kg depending on INR) and intravenous vitamin K 5–10 mg.
- If deemed necessary after risk assessment, antiplatelet drugs clopidogrel and/or aspirin should be stopped for 7 days before surgery.
- New oral anticoagulants (oral direct inhibitors) should be stopped with reference to renal function (usually up to 48 hours before surgery).
- Therapeutic doses of LMWH should be stopped at least 24 hours before and prophylactic LMWH 12 hours before surgery or planned cesarean section or regional anesthesia.
- Therapeutic anticoagulation should be delayed for at least 48 hours after major surgery.

Further reading

Douketis JD, Spyropoulos AC, Spencer FA *et al.* Perioperative management of antithrombotic therapy: Antithrombotic Therapy and Prevention of Thrombosis, 9th edn. American College of Chest Physicians Evidence-based Clinical Practice Guidelines. *Chest* 2012;141(2 Suppl):e326S–e350S.

Heidbuchel H, Verhamme P, Alings M *et al.* European Heart Rhythm Association Practical Guide on the use of new oral anticoagulants in patients with non-valvular atrial fibrillation. *Europace* 2013;15:625–651.

Horlocker TT, Wedel DJ, Benzon H *et al.* Regional anesthesia in the anticoagulated patient: defining the risks (the second ASRA Consensus Conference on Neuraxial Anesthesia and Anticoagulation). *Reg Anesth Pain Med* 2003;28:172–197.

Keeling D, Baglin T, Tait C *et al.* British Committee for Standards in Haematology Guidelines on oral anticoagulation with warfarin, 4th edn. *Br J Haematol* 2011;154:311–324.

Nelson-Piercy C, MacCallum P, Mackillop L. *Reducing the Risk of Thrombosis and Embolism During Pregnancy and the Puerperium*. RCOG Green-top Guideline No. 37a. Royal College of Obstetricians and Gynaecologists, London, 2015. https://www.rcog.org.uk/globalassets/documents/guidelines/gtg-37a.pdf

Thomson AJ, Greer IA. *Thromboembolic Disease in Pregnancy and the Puerperium: Acute Management*. RCOG Green-top Guideline No. 37b. Royal College of Obstetricians and Gynaecologists, London, 2015. https://www.rcog.org.uk/globalassets/documents/guidelines/gtg-37b.pdf

Siegal D, Yudin J, Kaatz S, Douketis JD, Lim W, Spyropoulos AC. Periprocedural heparin bridging in patients receiving vitamin K antagonists: systematic review and meta-analysis of bleeding and thromboembolic rates. *Circulation* 2012;126:1630–1639.

Reference

1 Heidbuchel H, Verhamme P, Alings M *et al.* EHRA practical guide on the use of new oral anticoagulants in patients with non-valvular atrial fibrillation: executive summary. *Eur Heart J* 2013; 34:2094–2106.

CHAPTER 17
Patient on Steroid Therapy

Shaista Nazir¹ and John Ayuk²
¹ Alexandra Hospital, Redditch, Worcestershire, UK
² University Hospital Birmingham, Birmingham, UK

Case history: A 45-year-old woman with a history of uterine fibroids and menorrhagia was admitted for elective abdominal hysterectomy. Her past medical history included systemic lupus erythematosus (SLE), and she had been prescribed prednisolone 60 mg/day for a flare-up 3 months ago. The dose was subsequently tapered down and she was currently on prednisolone 10 mg daily. Her baseline blood tests were normal apart from long-standing iron-deficiency anemia. Her pulse rate was 80 bpm and regular, with blood pressure of 120/70 mmHg. During her preoperative assessment, the issue of how to manage her steroids perioperatively was raised.

Background

The primary role of the endocrine system is maintenance of the normal physiologic functioning of many organ systems of the body. The adrenal cortex plays a crucial role in the endocrine response to major stress. Cortisol has long been recognized as a requirement for survival in critical illness [1].

Cortisol promotes protein catabolism and liver gluconeogenesis and, by antagonizing insulin, ensures normal blood glucose concentrations during fasting. Glucocorticoids are essential for the normal cardiovascular response to stress; without them, the cardiovascular system becomes unresponsive to catecholamines [2].

Normal physiology of hypothalamic–pituitary–adrenal axis

The production of glucocorticoids by the adrenal cortex is regulated by adrenocorticotropic hormone (ACTH), secreted by the anterior pituitary under the influence of hypothalamic corticotropin-releasing hormone (CRH). ACTH and CRH are under direct negative feedback from cortisol [1].

Effect of surgery and stress on HPA axis

Glucocorticoids are responsible for maintaining blood pressure, blood glucose, and energy levels during times of physiologic stress, such as illness, surgery or injury [3]. Stress activates the hypothalamic–pituitary–adrenal (HPA) axis, resulting in increased plasma ACTH and cortisol concentrations [4]. Stress can be physical (surgery, anesthesia, trauma, burns), psychologic (pain, anxiety) or physiologic (hypoglycemia, fever, hypotension, exercise, cold exposure) [4].

Surgery is one of the most potent activators of the HPA axis. During a major surgical procedure, CRH, ACTH, and cortisol levels rise significantly. Plasma ACTH levels rise at the time of incision and during surgery. The maximum ACTH and cortisol levels are reached in the early postoperative period, especially during reversal of anesthesia, extubation, and the immediate postoperative recovery period. During stress, from a normal daily secretion of 15–20 mg, cortisol production increases to 75–150 mg/day [1].

The increased cortisol level enhances survival by increasing cardiac contractility, cardiac output, and sensitivity to catecholamines, and also maintains vascular tone, work capacity of skeletal muscles and blood glucose levels by mobilizing energy sources [1].

While ACTH levels return to the normal range within 24 hours, cortisol levels decline more slowly, reaching high normal values about 48–72 hours after surgical procedures [4].

HPA axis suppression

Glucocorticoids, when given in supraphysiologic doses, may cause suppression of the HPA axis and lead to adrenal gland atrophy and adrenal insufficiency [5]. The resulting reduced cortisol response in stressful conditions like surgery and anesthesia can result in a variety of hemodynamic abnormalities, such as hypovolemic or circulatory shock, and inadequate host defense against infections, resulting in significant morbidity and mortality [6,7].

"Stress-dose" steroids are administered during the perioperative period to prevent complications of secondary hypoadrenalism due to HPA axis suppression, which can occur after long-term steroid treatment [8,9].

Management

Perioperative management: to replace or not to replace?

Preoperative assessment is of crucial importance in identifying patients with HPA axis suppression and the severity of its effects (Figure 17.1). The important questions to be considered include the following.
- Is the patient at risk of developing adrenal crisis (is the HPA axis suppressed)?
- What is the dose of steroids required to cover the perioperative period?
- What is the duration of stress-dose steroid cover?

Gynecologic and Obstetric Surgery: Challenges and Management Options, First Edition. Edited by Arri Coomarasamy, Mahmood I. Shafi, G. Willy Davila and Kiong K. Chan.
© 2016 John Wiley & Sons, Ltd. Published 2016 by John Wiley & Sons, Ltd.

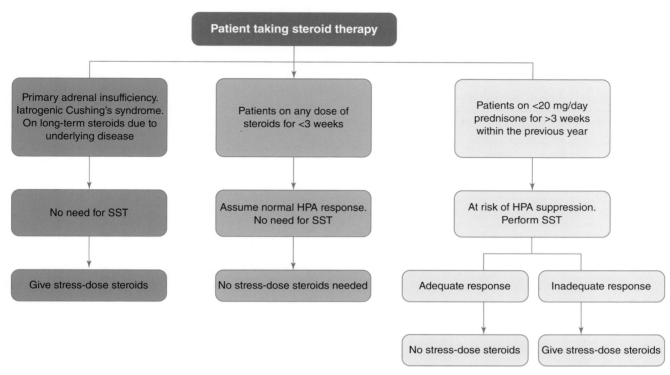

Figure 17.1 Algorithm for perioperative management of a patient on steroids [1,10,11].

The short Synacthen test (SST) or ACTH stimulation test is a reliable means of assessing adrenocortical function (Box 17.1). It is also a reliable guide to the integrity of the entire HPA axis. Because hypothalamic–pituitary function recovers before adrenocortical function, a normal response to ACTH stimulation indicates normal hypothalamic–pituitary function as well [10]. Testing can be performed at any time of the day [1].

BOX 17.1. ACTH STIMULATION (SHORT SYNACTHEN TEST)

Method
Withhold exogenous glucocorticoids for 24 hours
Give cosyntropin 250 μg as i.v. bolus or i.m. injection
Measure plasma cortisol at 30 or 60 min after injections

Interpretation
Plasma cortisol >18 μg/dL (>580 nmol/L) at 30 or 60 min indicates adequate response
Source: Axelrod, 2003 [10] with permission.

It is generally reported that there is no risk of HPA axis suppression in patients who are taking doses equivalent to replacement doses (no more than 25 mg hydrocortisone, 5 mg prednisone, 4 mg triamcinolone or 0.75 mg dexamethasone) unless it is administered later in the day, in which case it may inhibit the diurnal surge of ACTH release [10]. However, most patients on these doses are either on

replacement for adrenal insufficiency, or have been weaned down from higher initial doses, and so may well have suppressed HPA axis. Recovery from HPA axis suppression can take up to 12 months, so steroid use within the previous year must be considered [10].

Individuals with known adrenal insufficiency due to hypothalamic, pituitary or adrenal disease will require perioperative supplemental glucocorticoids [11].

Patients who have been on more than 20 mg prednisone per day for more than 3 weeks, or patients with clinical features of iatrogenic Cushing's syndrome, are assumed to have functional suppression of the HPA axis. Such patients do not require assessment of the HPA axis, and should be prescribed stress-dose steroids to cover surgery [1]. Preoperative assessment of the HPA axis would also not be necessary in a patient for whom interruption of steroid therapy could not be tolerated (e.g., due to the underlying disease process or need for immune suppression therapy in an organ transplant recipient), as they require continuation of steroids during the perioperative period [10].

Patients taking less than 20 mg/day of prednisolone for more than 3 weeks within the previous year may have suppressed HPA axis function depending on the dose and duration of steroid therapy, and the individual patient. These patients need to be assessed for HPA axis function before surgery if time allows, or should be given stress-dose steroids empirically [1].

Steroid replacement regimens
Over the past decade, there has been a shift in clinical practice in favor of giving lower doses and shorter duration of stress-dose glucocorticoids, according to the severity and duration of illness

or surgery [4]. Typical regimens for steroid cover are given in Table 17.1. Current recommendations suggest replacing the amount equivalent to normal physiologic response to surgical stress. The dose and duration of steroid supplementation should be based on the magnitude of surgical stress [12].

Table 17.1 Examples for perioperative glucocorticoid therapy [4,11].

Degree of surgical stress	Examples	Glucocorticoid dose
Minimal	<1 hour under local anesthesia (e.g., routine dental work, skin biopsy)	Usual replacement dose, hydrocortisone 15–30 mg/day
Minor	Cesarean section Inguinal hernia repair Colonoscopy Dental procedures requiring >1 hour under local anesthesia (e.g., multiple extractions, periodontal surgery)	Intravenous hydrocortisone 25 mg or equivalent at start of procedure. Usual replacement dose after procedure Double the daily dose of glucocorticoid on day of procedure (e.g., 40 mg oral hydrocortisone). Usual replacement dose the next day
Moderate	Abdominal hysterectomy Open cholecystectomy Segmental colon resection Lower limb revascularization Total joint replacement	Intravenous hydrocortisone 75 mg/day on day of procedure (e.g., 25 mg 8-hourly). Taper down over next 1–2 days to usual replacement dose in uncomplicated cases
Severe	Labor Cardiothoracic surgery Whipple's procedure Oesophagogastrectomy Total proctocolectomy Dental procedures under general anesthesia	Intravenous hydrocortisone 150 mg/day (e.g., 50 mg 8-hourly). Taper down over next 2–3 days to usual replacement dose in uncomplicated cases
Critical illness, intensive care	Major trauma Life-threatening complication	Maximum 200 mg/day intravenous hydrocortisone (e.g., 50 mg 6-hourly, or by continuous infusion)

Once the major stress of surgery is resolved and the patient is stable and free of complications (e.g., fever, vomiting, hemorrhage, wound infection, reoperation, sepsis, thrombosis, pulmonary embolism, acute renal failure, need for intensive care, ARDS [13]), hydrocortisone can be tapered down over a few days (halve the dose daily) to the usual maintenance dose (Box 17.2) [1]. Postoperatively, steroid doses should not be tapered excessively to a level below that known to control the underlying disease for which the steroids are required [1]. Studies of the normal cortisol response to surgery support the recommendation that increased glucocorticoid cover is not required beyond 3 days in uncomplicated surgical cases. Potential side effects of prolonged or excessive steroid use include hyperglycemia, impaired wound healing, and increased susceptibility to infection caused by immune suppression [4].

BOX 17.2. EXAMPLE OF POSTOPERATIVE STEROID TAPERING

Day 1 Hydrocortisone 100 mg i.v. every 8 hours, starting from induction of anesthesia
Day 2 If patient stable and major postoperative stress resolved, lower dose of steroids to 50 mg i.v. every 8 hours
Day 3 Hydrocortisone 25 mg every 8 hours
Day 4 Hydrocortisone 25 mg b.d.
Day 5 Maintenance dose (hydrocortisone 12–15 mg/m² daily): 15–20 mg AM; 5–10 mg PM

Source: Jabour, 2001 [1] with permission.

Prevention (of complications)

There is no alternative to a thorough history and clinical examination in identifying patients at risk of HPA axis suppression. Steroid use in the previous year must be considered. Adrenal insufficiency should be considered if there is unexplained or refractory hypotension.

Patient education and identification with a medical alert bracelet are important. Patients may also benefit from having an ampoule of hydrocortisone at home or when traveling (together with appropriate syringe, needles, and instructions) for use in an emergency. Hospital stickers can be developed for use on drug charts to draw attention to a patient's steroid dependency. Ideally, a red flag system on the electronic patient record should be developed for those with steroid dependency [14].

KEY POINTS

Challenge: Patients on steroid therapy.

Background
- Glucocorticoids are essential for the normal cardiovascular response to stress.
- Surgery is one of the most potent activators of the HPA axis.
- Plasma ACTH levels rise at time of incision and during surgery; maximum levels are reached in the early postoperative period.

Management
- It is important to identify patients at risk of developing perioperative adrenal crisis.
- The following require stress-dose steroids during the perioperative period without the need to test HPA axis function:
  - Patients with known adrenal insufficiency due to hypothalamic, pituitary, or adrenal disease.
  - Patients taking more than 20 mg prednisone daily for more than 3 weeks.
  - Patients with clinical features of iatrogenic Cushing's syndrome.
- Test for HPA axis suppression before surgery in patients taking more than replacement dose equivalent, but less than 20 mg daily.
- Once the stress is over, taper down steroids (by 50% daily) over a few days to maintenance dose.

Prevention (of complications)
- Take a careful history to detect steroid use within the previous year.
- Alert staff to steroid use with medical alert bracelets and medical note flagging.

References

1 Jabour AS. Steroids and the surgical patient. *Med Clin North Am* 2001; 85:1311–1317.
2 Davies M, Hardman J. Anaesthesia and adrenocortical disease. *Contin Educ Anaesth Crit Care Pain* 2005; 5:122–126.
3 Ahmet A, Kim H, Spier S. Adrenal suppression: a practical guide to the screening and management of this under-recognized complication of inhaled corticosteroid therapy. *Allergy Asthma Clin Immunol* 2011; 7:13.
4 Jung C, Inder WJ. Management of adrenal insufficiency during the stress of medical illness and surgery. *Med J Aust* 2008; 188:409–413.
5 Krasner AS. Glucocorticoid-induced adrenal insufficiency. *JAMA* 1999; 282:671–676.
6 Gordijn MS, Gemke RJ, van Dalen EC, Rotteveel J, Kaspers GJ. Hypothalamic–pituitary–adrenal (HPA) axis suppression after treatment with glucocorticoid therapy for childhood acute lymphoblastic leukaemia. *Cochrane Database Syst Rev* 2012; (5): CD008727.
7 Wakim JH, Sledge KC. Anesthetic implications for patients receiving exogenous corticosteroids. *AANA J* 2006; 74:133–139.
8 Yong SL, Coulthard P, Wrzosek A. Supplemental perioperative steroids for surgical patients with adrenal insufficiency. *Cochrane Database Syst Rev* 2013; (10):CD005367.

9 Aytac E, Londono JM, Erem HH, Vogel JD, Costedio MM. Impact of stress dose steroids on the outcomes of restorative proctocolectomy in patients with ulcerative colitis. *Dis Colon Rectum* 2013; 56:1253–1258.

10 Axelrod L. Perioperative management of patients treated with glucocorticoids. *Endocrinol Metab Clin North Am* 2003; 32:367–383.

11 Coursin DB, Wood KE. Corticosteroid supplementation for adrenal insufficiency. *JAMA* 2002; 287:236–240.

12 Shaikh S, Verma H, Yadav N, Jauhari M, Bullangowda J. Applications of steroid in clinical practice: a review. *ISRN Anesthesiology* 2012, Article ID 985495.

13 Dindo D, Demartines N, Clavien PA. Classification of surgical complications. A new proposal with evaluation in a cohort of 6336 patients and results of a survey. *Ann Surg* 2004; 240: 205–213.

14 Wass JA, Arit W. How to avoid precipitating an acute adrenal crisis. *BMJ* 2012; 345:e6333.

CHAPTER 18
Patient with Epilepsy

Danita Jones and Virgilio Salanga
Cleveland Clinic Florida, Weston/Fort Lauderdale, Florida, USA

Case history: *A 28-year-old woman with well-controlled epilepsy is scheduled for total abdominal hysterectomy under general anesthesia. She is on a single antiepileptic medication (levetiracetam 750 mg every 12 hours) with no seizure activity for several years. Her gynecologist notifies her neurologist of her impending surgery and requests collaboration in her perioperative management.*

Background

Epilepsy is defined as two or more unprovoked seizures. Seizures may present at various ages and have numerous clinical manifestations. A patient may retain consciousness but manifest sensory or motor symptoms, as seen in simple partial seizures. In complex partial or generalized seizures, a patient can become unresponsive, with varying degrees of generalized muscle contractions. The choice of antiepileptic medication is based on the type of seizure as well as the patient's medical comorbidities.

Well-controlled epilepsy is not associated with increased perioperative risks. Risks during the perioperative period can be from non-compliance with antiepileptic medications or from other medications decreasing the seizure threshold. Approaches to reduce risks include ensuring compliance with medications, encouraging early mobilization after surgery, maintaining a low threshold to check for electrolyte imbalance, and providing effective hydration and analgesia.

Management

Preoperative management
The type and frequency of seizure should be assessed with special emphasis on the last known or documented seizure episode. Disease control and medication review are important to ensure the highest degree of neurologic stability. Patient counseling and reassurance by the surgeon and neurologist prior to surgery are essential.

The patient should continue to take her oral antiepileptic drug (AED) until the time for no oral intake (NPO). Inadvertent delay or withdrawal of AEDs may trigger breakthrough seizures. If necessary, intravenous doses of AEDs may be given while the patient remains NPO (postoperatively also, in case of an ileus) in order to ensure adequate drug levels. Certain types of antiepileptic medications are available in parenteral preparations.

Intraoperative management
Most general anesthetic drugs pose no additional risk of triggering seizures, and many in fact have anticonvulsant properties. If the surgery takes longer than expected, the patient's AED can be administered intravenously by the anesthesiologist (e.g., levetiracetam 750 mg i.v.).

The total plasma volume of the patient should be a focus of the anesthesiologist's attention. Although renally excreted, antiepileptic medications such as levetiracetam have significantly fewer drug–drug interactions; other AEDs whose metabolism involves hepatic enzyme pharmacokinetics (cytochrome P450 induction or inhibition) have potential interactions with a multitude of additional medications and anesthetics. Interactions within the cytochrome P450 system may lead to either an increase or decrease in the medication's metabolism, thereby grossly affecting the duration and efficacy of the specific drug.

A patient's fluid volume can play a correlative effect on an antiepileptic medication's drug level. As with any surgical procedure, women undergoing surgery are given additional fluids intravenously to compensate for any loss of bodily fluids during the procedure. If the change in plasma volume becomes extreme, either positive or negative, the concentration of an antiepileptic medication may be significantly altered. This could result in either subtherapeutic dosing or toxicity.

It is important to be vigilant and avoid seizure triggers, such as reduced PaO_2, hyponatremia, hypocalcemia, and hypoglycemia.

Postoperative management
When oral medications are allowed, the patient's AED should be resumed. If resumption of oral intake needs to be delayed, parenteral AED should be instituted. If the patient is on an oral AED without comparable parenteral formulation, the neurologist may temporarily employ another parenteral AED with comparable mechanism of action.

Pain management and choice of sedative medications should also be reviewed when caring for an epileptic patient. Certain medications, such as ketorolac and meperidine, have been shown to lower the seizure threshold, thereby making any patient more susceptible to breakthrough seizures. An epileptic patient would be at an even greater risk, and therefore alternate medications should be considered.

Gynecologic and Obstetric Surgery: Challenges and Management Options, First Edition. Edited by Arri Coomarasamy, Mahmood I. Shafi, G. Willy Davila and Kiong K. Chan.
© 2016 John Wiley & Sons, Ltd. Published 2016 by John Wiley & Sons, Ltd.

After surgery, AED serum concentrations should be closely monitored with an expected prompt return to the patient's antiepileptic dose prior to surgery.

If a patient's underlying disease is stable (as is the case for the patient in the case history), there should be no further risk.

If a patient's epilepsy is less stable, requiring multiple AEDs, the perioperative care will require close collaboration with a neurologist.

KEY POINTS

Challenge: Patient with epilepsy undergoing surgery.

Background
- Epilepsy is defined as two or more unprovoked seizures.
- Seizures are of various types and may be partial or generalized, have sensory or motor symptoms, and may or may not be associated with loss of consciousness.
- The choice of antiepileptic medication depends on the type of seizure and other comorbidities.
- Most patients with epilepsy are stable on one AED with well-understood pharmacokinetics, while others are less stable requiring multiple AEDs with varied pharmacokinetics that lead to therapeutic complexity.

Prevention (of complications)
- Close collaboration of the surgeon and neurologist is important, especially in a patient with unstable epilepsy, to ensure drug therapy is optimized.
- Attention to potential drug–drug interactions is necessary.
- Avoid medications that potentially lower seizure threshold.

- Inadvertent "withdrawal" or delay of AEDs must be avoided.
- Extreme changes in plasma volume may affect AED plasma concentration, requiring adjustments to dose and/or frequency of administration.

Management
- The main focus of perioperative care for a patient with epilepsy is maintaining the baseline level of medical control of seizures, and avoidance of triggering breakthrough seizures.
- Continue normal oral medication until commencement of preoperative starvation.
- Maintain drug levels by using intravenous (parenteral) preparations of the medication(s) as necessary until oral intake resumes postoperatively.
- If an intravenous preparation is not available, a drug with a similar mechanism of action may be used under supervision of the neurologist.
- Be vigilant to avoid seizure triggers, such as reduced PaO_2, hyponatremia, hypocalcemia, and hypoglycemia.
- Monitor AED plasma levels if appropriate.
- Allow for the effect of anesthetic and perioperative medications which may increase or decrease the seizure threshold.

Further reading

Harden CL, Hopp J, Ting TY *et al.* Practice parameter update: management issues for women with epilepsy – focus on pregnancy: obstetrical complications and change in seizure frequency: report of the Quality Standards Subcommittee and Therapeutics and Technology Assessment Subcommittee of the American Academy of Neurology and American Epilepsy Society. *Neurology* 2009; 73:126–141.

CHAPTER 19
Patient with a Psychiatric Condition

Idnan Yunas

University Medical Practice Edgbaston, Birmingham, UK

Case history 1: A patient with a past medical history of severe depression and currently taking an antidepressant medication was admitted for an elective hysterectomy.

Case history 2: A young patient with a diagnosis of schizophrenia, controlled by antipsychotic medication, was admitted for a myomectomy.

Background

It is estimated that one in four people experience some form of mental health problem in the course of a year [1]. Psychiatric disorders can complicate surgical outcomes. Conversely, surgery can exacerbate pre-existing psychiatric illness [2,3]. Psychiatric illness affecting surgical patients may include depression, bipolar disorder, schizophrenia, and psychoses.

Many of the difficulties faced by patients with a history of psychiatric illness undergoing surgery are related to their medication. However, other factors can also be relevant; for example, poor diet and nutritional status may influence recovery, and lack of motivation may influence engagement with follow-up after surgery. Patients with poor insight may often find it difficult to report their concerns, making them difficult to monitor for complications. They are also more likely to suffer with postoperative delirium and confusion [2,4]. Patients with psychiatric problems also tend to be more socially isolated and vulnerable. Careful management is required in the preoperative, intraoperative, and postoperative periods.

Management

Assessment
The preoperative assessment must include a full history and examination. Thorough assessment of the preoperative mental and functional state of the patient is crucial to establish a baseline in case of future deterioration. The medication history and the patient's compliance with psychiatric medications should be determined. This will allow consideration of the choice of anesthetic agents used and continuation of current therapy in light of interactions and risks [5]. These decisions will need to be made with input from the psychiatric and anesthetic teams managing the patient. Medication

history should also include the presence of allergies and any drug or alcohol dependence. Drug dependence often requires medical treatment of its own to avoid withdrawal.

Preoperative investigations often include blood tests to determine electrolyte levels and drug levels to elucidate potential toxicity. A baseline ECG is required when psychiatric medication such as antipsychotics are used as they are associated with arrhythmia [6,7].

Each patient is unique and so their perioperative plan must be treated as such. An individualized plan should be formulated with input from a multidisciplinary team.

Capacity and consent
It is assumed that all adult patients have the capacity to make decisions about their care. A patient is deemed to lack capacity only if he or she is unable to understand and retain information to make a decision despite all practical efforts being made to help the patient make that decision. Capacity may be transiently affected by factors such as delirium, pain, and medication side effects. In patients who lack capacity to make an informed decision, the care-providing team may make decisions in their "best interest." It is good practice to involve the next of kin in such best interest decisions. There will be instances in which a court of law has to make these decisions, as capacity and consent are legal as well as ethical considerations for surgery [8].

Medical management

Selective serotonin reuptake inhibitors
SSRIs are the most frequently used class of antidepressants for mild to moderate depression. They have very few side effects and a relatively short half-life, so are continued throughout the perioperative period. This is to avoid discontinuation syndrome [3,5,9].

Discontinuation syndrome
Discontinuation syndrome is a withdrawal phenomenon due to the abrupt cessation of antidepressants. It is more likely with antidepressants with a short half-life, such as SSRIs. It is characterized by low mood, anxiety, abdominal pain, and nausea which can commence within a few days of stopping antidepressant treatment. The syndrome can be treated by reintroducing the antidepressant [9,10].

Gynecologic and Obstetric Surgery: Challenges and Management Options, First Edition. Edited by Arri Coomarasamy, Mahmood I. Shafi, G. Willy Davila and Kiong K. Chan.
© 2016 John Wiley & Sons, Ltd. Published 2016 by John Wiley & Sons, Ltd.

Serotonin syndrome

A severe risk associated with the use of SSRIs is the development of serotonin syndrome. It is a potentially fatal adverse drug reaction resulting from increased serotonin levels in the brain and spinal cord. It is usually precipitated by the use of more than one serotonergic drug concurrently.

Tricyclic antidepressants

TCA treatment is continued throughout the perioperative period. The few indications for cessation of therapy include the presence of significant cardiac disease [5]. TCAs have α-adrenergic blocking activity. Potential interactions with anesthetic agents include cardiac arrhythmias and hypotension. Hypotension in such cases should be corrected with care to avoid hypertensive crisis.

Monoamine oxidase inhibitors

MAOIs are rarely used in current practice due to their adverse side effects. They are usually stopped 2 weeks prior to surgery following discussion with the psychiatry team to ensure the risk of discontinuation syndrome is minimized. If the risks of stopping treatment for 2 weeks are too high, a careful and tailored anesthetic regimen should be used [5]. Concurrent serotonergic medication should be avoided. Pethidine and indirect acting sympathomimetics are absolutely contraindicated.

Atypical antidepressants such as venlafaxine and mirtazapine should generally be continued through the perioperative period.

Antipsychotics

Antipsychotics are the mainstay of treatment for patients with schizophrenia. Discontinuation of therapy can cause acute withdrawal resulting in psychosis. Therefore, typical and atypical antipsychotic drugs are continued throughout the perioperative period. The use of antipsychotics is associated with hypotension, neuroleptic malignant syndrome, sudden cardiac death and arrhythmia due to prolongation of the QT interval. A preoperative ECG is a necessity, with careful perioperative monitoring [2,3,5,11,12].

Patients taking clozapine should also continue it perioperatively. They need to be monitored for agranulocytosis [5].

Neuroleptic malignant syndrome

This is an adverse reaction to neuroleptic (antipsychotic) medication characterized by hyperthermia, autonomic dysfunction, and acute confusion [12]. Its management requires prompt recognition, and treatment is usually in the intensive care setting.

Lithium

Lithium is used as a mood stabilizer in bipolar disorder. Subtle electrolyte and fluid shifts can result in toxicity when using it. Lithium also has direct effects which can be dangerous perioperatively. There is no withdrawal syndrome on cessation of treatment, so it is discontinued 72 hours prior to surgery [5]. Treatment is reinstituted postoperatively when the patient is hemodynamically stable and electrolytes are within their normal ranges. Lithium blood levels should be closely monitored in the first week.

Other mood stabilizers such as valproate should be continued perioperatively.

Postoperative considerations

- If patients are nil by mouth for a prolonged period, parenteral forms of psychiatric medication should be considered to avoid relapse and withdrawal.

- Patients should be provided with a stable and familiar environment to allow them to "normalize" and orientate themselves.
- In patients with an altered mental state compared with their baseline, non-psychiatric causes of delirium should also be considered.
- Effective analgesia is important: depressed patients may perceive a greater intensity of pain, and thus have greater requirements for analgesia. Schizophrenic patients, on the other hand, tend to under-report pain and may have decreased perception of it [12]. Antipsychotics themselves have analgesic properties [13].

Prevention

Careful multidisciplinary and holistic management of patients with psychiatric problems is necessary to minimize adverse drug interactions, withdrawal symptoms, and relapse. Identifying potential problems is achieved through careful and thorough history-taking, which includes a comprehensive drug history; clinical examination with baseline mental state examination and relevant investigations are also needed. The multidisciplinary team includes the surgical, anesthetic, and psychiatry teams.

KEY POINTS

Challenge: Patient with a psychiatric condition.

Background
- A significant proportion of patients undergoing surgery suffer with psychiatric problems.
- Psychiatric conditions range from depression and bipolar disorder to schizophrenia and other psychoses.

Prevention
- A multidisciplinary approach with surgical, anesthetic, and psychiatric colleagues is crucial.
- Thorough history and clinical examination with comprehensive baseline mental state examination are necessary.
- Investigations should include bloods and baseline ECG.

Management
- Assessment includes full history and clinical examination with appropriate investigations.
- Consent and capacity issues must be considered in all cases.
- SSRIs: continue perioperatively. *Caution:* discontinuation and serotonin syndrome.
- TCAs: continue perioperatively. *Caution:* hypotension and cardiac arrhythmias.
- MAOIs: discontinue 2 weeks prior to surgery. *Caution:* significant adverse effects.
- Antipsychotics: continue perioperatively. *Caution:* prolongation of QT interval, sudden cardiac complications, hypotension, and neuroleptic malignant syndrome.
- Lithium: discontinue 72 hours prior to surgery. *Caution:* toxicity.
- Postoperatively: provide a supportive and stable environment, effective analgesia, and also consider non-psychiatric causes in cases of delirium.

References

1 Singleton N, Bumpstead R, O'Brien M, Lee A, Meltzer H. *Psychiatric Morbidity Among Adults Living in Private Households, 2000*. The Stationery Office, London, 2001.

2 Copeland L, Zeber J, Pugh M, Mortensen E, Restrepo M, Lawrence V. Postoperative complications in the seriously mentally ill: a systematic review of the literature. *Ann Surg* 2008; 248: 31–38.

3 Desan P, Powsner S. Assessment and management of patients with psychiatric disorders. *Crit Care Med* 2004; 32(4 Suppl):S166–S173.

4   Daumit G, Pronovost P, Anthony C, Guallar E, Steinwachs DM, Ford DE. Adverse events during medical and surgical hospitalizations for persons with schizophrenia. *Arch Gen Psychiatry* 2006; 63:267–272.

5   Huyse F, Touw D, van Schijndel R, de Lange J, Slaets J. Psychotropic drugs and the perioperative period: a proposal for a guideline in elective surgery. *Psychosomatics* 2006; 47:8–22.

6   Buckley N, Sanders P. Cardiovascular adverse effects of antipsychotic drugs. *Drug Saf* 2000; 23:215–228.

7   Glassman A, Bigger J. Antipsychotic drugs: prolonged QTc interval, torsade de pointes, and sudden death. *Am J Psychiatry* 2001; 158:1774–1782.

8   Department of Health. Mental Capacity Act. HMSO, London, 2005.

9   Kudoh A, Katagai H, Takazawa T. Antidepressant treatment for chronic depressed patients should not be discontinued prior to anesthesia. *Can J Anaesth* 2002; 49:132–136.

10 Haddad P. Antidepressant discontinuation syndromes. *Drug Saf* 2001; 24:183–197.

11 Kudoh A, Katagai H, Takazawa T. Effect of preoperative discontinuation of antipsychotics in schizophrenic patients on outcome during and after anesthesia. *Eur J Anaesth* 2004; 21:414–416.

12 Kudoh A. Perioperative management for chronic schizophrenic patients. *Anesth Analg* 2005; 101:1867–1872.

13 Patt R, Proper G, Reddy S. The neuroleptics as adjuvant analgesics. *J Pain Sympt Manage* 1994; 9:446–453.

CHAPTER 20
Patient with Organ Transplant

Sarah Winfield
Leeds General Infirmary, Leeds Teaching Hospitals NHS Trust, Leeds, UK

Case history: A 25-year-old woman with a live-donor renal transplant 2 years ago is in a planned first pregnancy. She is stable on tacrolimus 1 mg twice daily and azathioprine 125 mg once daily, and her blood pressure has been, until now, well controlled with labetalol 100 mg twice daily. Her renal function is stable with a serum creatinine (SCr) of 120 μmol/L. At 34 weeks of gestation she develops pre-eclampsia and a semi-elective cesarean section is arranged.

Background

With advances in transplantation surgery and immunosuppressive regimens there is improved prognosis for patient and graft alike. Furthermore, the success of transplantation has also meant that children who received organ transplants are now reaching child-bearing age [1], and may wish to become pregnant.

Transplant patients are usually admitted and managed under specialist teams. However, they may require non-transplant surgery under the care of a gynecologist or obstetrician, and thus a clinician should be aware of the key issues relating to transplant patients. The key issues include risk of rejection and organ failure, risks related to chronic immunosuppression (cancer and infections), side effects of immunosuppressive drugs, and comorbidities.

Management

Preoperative management

Comorbid conditions after transplantation are common [2–4] and include hypertension, diabetes, anemia, and an increased risk of osteopenia, osteoporosis and fractures. The assessment of the patient should include at least the following issues.

- Is the patient in good general health?
- Is there adequate and stable graft function (determined using organ-specific criteria)? (Note that non-renal as well as renal recipients should have SCr ≤160 μmol/L, and preferably ≤125 μmol/L.)
- Is there evidence of graft rejection?

- Is there adequate immunosuppression with suitable drug(s) and stable dosing?
- Are comorbidities optimally managed?
- Is there evidence of any infection? Chronic immunosuppression puts patients at risk of infection.

If the preoperative assessment elicits any concerns, it is important to obtain specialist help from appropriate experts or team, and delay elective surgery to allow optimization of the patient's condition.

The surgeon should, if possible, view the transplant surgery operation notes in order to be aware of the site of the graft and thus avoid injury during surgery. A review of the transplant or any previous surgery anesthetic records can provide the anesthetist with valuable information.

Postoperative care

Postoperative care should ideally be provided in a high dependency unit. Postoperatively there is still the risk of graft rejection and clinical deterioration, so careful monitoring of fluid balance and immunosuppression levels is important. Graft rejection may be indicated by non-specific features (e.g., low-grade fever and malaise), organ-specific features (e.g., for renal transplant rejection, oliguria, rising U&E, and fluid retention), and lymphocytosis. Graft assessment for rejection may necessitate a biopsy (which will show cellular necrosis and lymphocyte infiltration if there is rejection).

Postoperatively, immunosuppressive drugs may need to be adjusted, but this should be in consultation with the relevant experts. NSAIDs need to be avoided due to the risk of nephrotoxicity, particularly in patients taking cyclosporine or tacrolimus. Thromboprophylaxis should be provided.

Cesarean section in a renal transplant patient

Transplant patients can achieve vaginal delivery as kidney grafts rarely cause obstructive problems [4–6]. There is one report of kidney injury at cesarean section when the lower pole of the graft was accidentally transected [7], but fortunately injury at cesarean section is rare. An appropriately constituted multidisciplinary team should provide pregnancy and operative care.

Gynecologic and Obstetric Surgery: Challenges and Management Options, First Edition. Edited by Arri Coomarasamy, Mahmood I. Shafi, G. Willy Davila and Kiong K. Chan.
© 2016 John Wiley & Sons, Ltd. Published 2016 by John Wiley & Sons, Ltd.

KEY POINTS

Challenge: Perioperative care of an organ transplant patient.

Background
- Patients with solid organ transplants (e.g., renal, heart, or liver) may need to have non-transplant operations, including gynecologic procedures and cesarean section.
- Risks related to transplant include:
  - Risks of rejection and organ failure.
  - Risks related to chronic immunosuppression (cancer and infections).
  - Side effects of immunosuppression.
  - Comorbidities (anemia, hypertension, osteoporosis, and fractures).
- Care should be provided with the involvement of appropriate specialists. Immunosuppressive drugs should not be altered or stopped without specialist advice.

Management
- Assess the patient:
  - Is the patient in good general health?
  - Is there adequate and stable graft function?
  - Is there evidence of graft rejection?
  - Is there adequate immunosuppression with suitable drug(s) and stable dosing?
  - Are comorbidities optimally managed?
  - Is there evidence of any infection?
- Get specialist advice from transplant team:
  - Optimize immunosuppressive regimens.
  - Optimize medical comorbidities.
- Review past surgery and anesthetic records.
- Postoperative care:
  - Provide care in HDU.
  - Close monitoring, particularly fluid balance and immunosuppression levels.
  - Look for any evidence of graft rejection: non-specific features (low-grade fever and malaise); organ-specific features (e.g., for renal transplant rejection, oliguria, rising U&E, and fluid retention), and lymphocytosis. Patient may need a biopsy if graft rejection is suspected.
  - Avoid NSAIDs, especially in patients taking cyclosporine or tacrolimus.
  - Provide thromboprophylaxis.

References

1 Armenti VT, Moritz MJ, Davison JM. Pregnancy in female pediatric solid organ transplant recipients. *Pediatr Clin North Am* 2003; 50:1543–1560.
2 Mastrobattista JM, Gomez-Lobo V. Pregnancy after solid organ transplantation. *Obstet Gynecol* 2008; 112:919–932.
3 McKay DB, Josephson MA. Pregnancy in recipients of solid organs: effects on mother and child. *N Engl J Med* 2006; 352:1281–1293.
4 Armenti VT, Moritz MJ, Davison, JM. Pregnancy after transplantation. In: James DK, Steer PJ, Weiner CP, Gonik B (eds) *High Risk Pregnancy: Management Options*, 4th edn, pp. 961–971. Elsevier Saunders, St Louis, 2011.
5 National Transplantation Pregnancy Registry. NTPR Annual Report 2012. Available at www.NTPR.giftoflifeinstitute.org
6 Winfield S, Davison JM. The patient with organ transplantation. In: Macklon NS, Greer IA, Steegers EAP (eds) *Textbook of Periconceptional Medicine*, pp. 57–68. Informa Healthcare, London, 2008.
7 Shrestha BM, Throssell D, McKane W, Raftery AT. Injury to a transplanted kidney during caesarean section: a case report. *Exp Clin Transplant* 2007; 1:618–620.

CHAPTER 21

Patient with Hepatitis B or C

Firas Al-Rshoud[1] and Arri Coomarasamy[2]
[1] Medical School, Hashemite University, Zarqua, Jordan
[2] College of Medical and Dental Sciences, University of Birmingham, Birmingham, UK

Case history: A 35-year-old woman requires an urgent laparotomy for ruptured ectopic pregnancy. She is known to be a carrier for hepatitis B.

Background

Hepatitis B
Hepatitis B virus (HBV) is one of the commonest infections in the world, affecting more than one-third of world's population. About 5–10% fail to clear the virus, resulting in a worldwide chronic carrier rate of approximately 5%. About 25% of HBV carriers develop serious complications such as cirrhosis and liver cancer.

Interpretation of hepatitis B serology often causes much confusion, but an understanding of the serologic response to HBV (Figure 21.1) will aid interpretation (Table 21.1).

Hepatitis C
Hepatitis C virus (HCV) infection is generally asymptomatic, and thus its true prevalence is unknown; however, many European countries report a prevalence between 0.5 and 2%. The World Health Organization (WHO) estimates that about 3% of world's population are infected with HCV, and there are more than 170 million carriers worldwide. The carriers are at risk of cirrhosis and liver cancer.

Table 21.1 Interpretation of HBV serology.

Test	Result	Interpretation
HBsAg	Negative	Susceptible
anti-HBc	Negative	
anti-HBs	Negative	
HBsAg	Negative	Immune due to natural infection
anti-HBc	Positive	
anti-HBs	Positive	
HBsAg	Negative	Immune due to hepatitis B vaccination
anti-HBc	Negative	
anti-HBs	Positive	
HBsAg	Positive	Acutely infected
anti-HBc	Positive	
IgM anti-HBc	Positive	
anti-HBs	Negative	
HBsAg	Positive	Chronically infected
anti-HBc	Positive	
IgM anti-HBc	Negative	
anti-HBs	Negative	
HBsAg	Negative	Interpretation unclear, with four possibilities:
anti-HBc	Positive	1 Resolved infection (most common)
anti-HBs	Negative	2 False-positive anti-HBc, thus susceptible
		3 "Low-level" chronic infection
		4 Resolving acute infection

Source: US Centers for Disease Control and Prevention [1]. http://www.cdc.gov/vaccines/

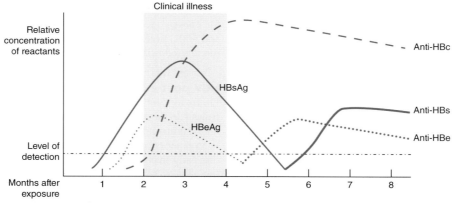

Figure 21.1 Serologic responses to HBV infection.

Gynecologic and Obstetric Surgery: Challenges and Management Options, First Edition. Edited by Arri Coomarasamy, Mahmood I. Shafi, G. Willy Davila and Kiong K. Chan.

Transmission risk from needlestick injury

HBV and HCV (and HIV) transmission risk following sharp needle injury is summarized in Table 21.2.

Table 21.2 Transmission risk with sharp needle injury.

Source	Transmission risk
HBV	up to 1 in 3
HCV	1 in 30
HIV	1 in 300

Source: Health Protection Agency [2].

Management

Management of patients with HBV or HCV infection

Assessing the risk of surgery in patients with liver disease is an important preoperative step (Chapter 12). Patients with liver disease often have abnormalities in plasma protein binding and detoxification and excretion processes, with implications for the pharmacokinetic behavior of anesthetics, muscle relaxants, analgesics, and sedatives. Coagulopathy increases bleeding risk, while changes in the hepatic reticuloendothelial cells and other changes to the immune system heighten the likelihood of infection. Perhaps most importantly, a diseased liver is particularly susceptible to the hemodynamic changes that accompany surgery. However, operative risk is probably not increased in the vast majority of patients with liver disease in whom liver function is preserved.

Patients infected with HBV and HCV at substantial risks of complications include those with:
- acute hepatitis;
- hepatic failure;
- severe coagulopathy (prolongation of PT >3 s despite vitamin K administration; platelet count <50,000/μL);
- cardiac complication such as heart failure and/or cardiomyopathy;
- acute renal failure;
- extrahepatic complications.

Patients in an acute phase of hepatitis should avoid elective surgery until the acute phase resolves. If emergency surgery is required, consultation with a liver specialist is needed. Patients will need to have their liver function and clotting (particularly PT and platelets) tested before surgery. It will be necessary to correct clotting defects in consultation with a hepatologist and hematologist before any surgery.

It is generally recommended to avoid hepatically metabolized anesthetic and other drugs, or to reduce the dose or frequency of administration if appropriate. Fluid balance (intake/output) should be managed and it is often necessary to limit sodium intake.

In the postoperative period, patients with liver disease should be monitored closely for any sign of hepatic failure, such as worsening of jaundice, coagulopathy, encephalopathy, and ascites, and if necessary liver function and clotting studies can be arranged. It is also important to monitor (i) renal function in case of hepatorenal syndrome, and (ii) serum glucose levels in case of hypoglycemia.

Prevention of transmission of HBV and HCV from the patient to healthcare workers

There are greater risks of HBV and HCV transmission than HIV transmission through occupational exposure during surgical work.

Sharp needlestick injuries are recorded in 1–15% of surgical procedures, and around 60% of all such injuries occur while suturing fascia. It is therefore important to utilize the highest standards of infection control, involving (i) the most effective known protective barriers to prevent contact with patient body fluids and (ii) universal precautions.

Steps to reduce the risk of HBV or HCV infection to healthcare workers (HCWs) during surgical procedures include:
- double-gloving and/or regular changes of gloves during long procedures;
- blunt-tipped needles and stapling devices;
- face and/or eye protection (goggles) to prevent mucocutaneous transmission;
- instruments for retraction (rather than hand or fingers);
- instruments to handle sharps;
- instruments to remove scalpels.

HBV post-exposure management

If a surgeon sustains a needlestick injury, he or she should stop the operation; if it is unsafe to pause the surgery, another surgeon should continue the surgery. The first and immediate step is to squeeze around (*not on*) the puncture site to express as much blood as possible. The puncture site should be washed with soap or antiseptic solution. The subsequent management will depend on local policies, but key principles are given below and in Table 21.3.
- Post-exposure prophylaxis (PEP) involves vaccination against HBV and (if necessary) immunoglobulin.
- Immunoglobulin is given at a different site and does not reduce any immune response to the vaccine.
- PEP may be indicated even if the exposed individual has previously been vaccinated against HBV.
- PEP should be initiated within 24 hours and no more than 7 days after exposure.

Studies suggest it may be possible to prevent infection in 70–90% of cases by either (i) initiating the HBV vaccine series within 12–24 hours of exposure to the virus or (ii) combining both vaccination and hepatitis B immunoglobulin (HBIG). Among known non-responders to vaccination, one dose of HBIG has been shown to be 70–90% effective in preventing HBV when administered within 7 days of percutaneous HBV exposure, and multiple doses have been shown to be 75–95% effective.

Any sharps injury or contamination incident from a (possible) source of hepatitis B must be followed by a risk assessment for booster vaccination and HBIG. Non-response to vaccination and HBIG necessitates precautionary testing for HBsAg at 3 and 6 months following the incident.

HCV post-exposure management

Efforts to identify effective prophylaxis to HCV have not yet been fruitful. In the meanwhile, immunoglobulin and antiviral agents are not recommended, but acutely infected patients should be referred to an experienced specialist for early treatment. Recent data suggest that early treatment of acute hepatitis C with interferon is highly (perhaps 98%) effective. The optimum regimen of therapy and duration of treatment are still uncertain but it is reasonable to monitor for any spontaneous and acute recurrence throughout a period of 8–12 weeks after exposure.

HCWs exposed to hepatitis C-infected patients should have regular monitoring for HCV RNA in addition to HCV antibodies, because HCV RNA testing has been shown to identify acute infection

Table 21.3 Recommended PEP for HBV.

Vaccination and/or antibody response status of exposed individual[a]	Treatment when source patient is:		
	HBsAg positive	HBsAg negative	Source unknown or unavailable for testing
Unvaccinated Non-immune	HBIG[b] ×1 Initiate HBV vaccine series	Initiate HBV vaccine series	Initiate HBV vaccine series
Previously vaccinated Known responder[c]	No treatment	No treatment	No treatment
Previously vaccinated Known non-responder[d]	HBIG ×1 Initiate revaccination or HBIG ×2[e]	No treatment	No treatment unless known high-risk source necessitates treatment as if HBsAg positive
Previously vaccinated Response unknown	Single vaccine booster dose	No treatment	No treatment unless known high-risk source necessitates treatment as if HBsAg positive
Still undergoing vaccination	HBIG ×1 Complete series	Complete series	Complete series

[a] Persons who have previously been infected with HBV are immune to reinfection and do not require postexposure prophylaxis.

[b] Hepatitis B immune globulin; dose is 0.06 mL/kg i.m.

[c] A responder is a person with adequate levels of serum antibody to HBsAg (i.e., anti-HBs ≥10 mIU/mL).

[d] A non-responder is a person with inadequate response to vaccination (i.e., serum anti-HBs <10 mIU/mL).

[e] The option of giving one dose of HBIG and reinitiating the vaccine series is preferred for non-responders who have not completed a second three-dose vaccine series. For persons who previously completed a second vaccine series but failed to respond, two doses of HBIG are preferred.

Source: US Centers for Disease Control and Prevention [3]. http://www.cdc.gov/mmwr/preview/mmwrhtml/rr5011a1.htm

within 2 weeks of exposure, whereas antibody tests take longer to become positive. Seroconversion with the ELISA antibody test occurs in 50% of patients within 9 weeks of exposure, in 80% of patients within 15 weeks of exposure, and in at least 97% of patients within 6 months of exposure. The ELISA test is highly sensitive but relatively non-specific, resulting in a low positive predictive value in low-prevalence populations. A positive HCV ELISA antibody test result should be verified with a quantitative viral load assay such as HCV PCR.

KEY POINTS

Challenge: Management of a patient infected with HBV or HCV, to reduce the risks resulting from surgical procedures for both the patient and HCWs.

Background
- HBV: one of the commonest infections, affecting one-third of world's population; chronic carrier rate is 5%.
- HCV: prevalence is 0.5–2% in Europe, and 3% worldwide.
- Patients with HBV or HCV may have abnormal liver function, clotting defects, high risk of infection, and abnormal drug metabolism.
- Transmission risk from needlestick injury:
  - HBV: up to 1 in 3.
  - HCV: 1 in 30.
- HCWs exposed to HBV or HCV should receive post-exposure HBV vaccination, counseling, testing, and medical evaluation.

Management
Management of patients with HBV or HCV infection
- Review history and seek opinion from hepatologist.
- Defer surgery in patients with acute hepatitis if it is safe to do so.
- Check liver function tests and clotting.
- Correct clotting defects and platelets in consultation with hepatologist and hematologist.

- Avoid or adjust dose or frequency of hepatically metabolized anesthetic and other drugs.
- Manage fluid balance and limit sodium intake.
- Postoperatively, monitor for worsening liver function, coagulopathy, renal function (to assess for hepatorenal syndrome), and serum glucose levels.

Management of HCWs exposed to HBV or HCV needlestick injury
- Stop operating; find an alternative surgeon to continue if necessary.
- Squeeze around (*not on*) the puncture site to express blood.
- Wash thoroughly with soap or antiseptic solution.
- Follow local policies for post-exposure prophylaxis: HBV vaccine should ideally be given within 24 hours.

Prevention of transmission of HBV and HCV to HCWs
- Use two pairs of gloves; change gloves regularly for long procedures.
- Use blunt-tipped needles and stapling devices.
- Wear face and eye protection (goggles) to prevent mucocutaneous transmission.
- Use instruments for retraction (rather than hand or fingers).
- Use instruments to handle sharps.
- Use instruments to remove scalpels.

References

1 US Centers for Disease Control and Prevention, Division of Viral Hepatitis. http://www.cdc.gov/hepatitis/HBV/PDFs/SerologicChartv8.pdf (accessed August 5, 2014).
2 Health Protection Agency. *Eye of the Needle. United Kingdom Surveillance of Significant Occupational Exposure to Bloodborne Viruses in Healthcare Workers.* HPA, London, 2012. Available at https://www.gov.uk/government/uploads/system/uploads/attachment_data/file/337065/Eye_of_the_needle_2012_accessible.pdf
3 US Centers for Disease Control and Prevention. Updated U.S. Public Health Service Guidelines for the Management of Occupational Exposures to HBV, HCV, and HIV and Recommendations for Postexposure Prophylaxis. http://www.cdc.gov/mmwr/preview/mmwrhtml/rr5011a1.htm (accessed August 6, 2014).

CHAPTER 22
Patient with HIV

Firas Al-Rshoud¹ and Arri Coomarasamy²
¹ Medical School, Hashemite University, Zarqua, Jordan
² College of Medical and Dental Sciences, University of Birmingham, Birmingham, UK

Case history: A 55-year-old woman requires a hysterectomy for stage 1a endometrial carcinoma. She is known to be infected with human immunodeficiency virus (HIV), with a CD4 cell count of 300/µL and a viral load of 1000 copies/mL. She is currently undergoing highly active antiretroviral therapy (HAART).

Background

The number of people now living with HIV or AIDS worldwide is estimated to be more than 34 million. Over two-thirds of the patients are located in sub-Saharan Africa, but the condition is not confined to low-income countries. Estimates of the number of cases in the UK increased to 100,000 (0.15% of the population) in 2012. As many as one in four (24%) of those infected may be undiagnosed and unaware of their infection. The incidence among men (0.2%) is greater than among women (0.09%).

Perioperative risks in HIV patients
HIV-infected patients tolerate surgery well, particularly when they have good CD4 cell counts (>200/µL) and low viral loads (<10,000 copies/mL), and have no comorbidities. However, there are a number of potential risks in HIV patients [1], including:
- cytopenias (thrombocytopenia, anemia, and leukopenia), which can predispose patients to infections (particularly pneumonia) and bleeding;
- coagulopathy;
- drug-induced hepatotoxicity and nephrotoxicity;
- HIV-associated nephropathy;
- adrenal insufficiency;
- metabolic disorders (e.g., insulin resistance);
- malnutrition;
- increased risk of allergic reactions.

Preoperative assessment will need to consider the possibility of all these potential risk factors.

Risk of transmission to healthcare workers
The risk of transmission to healthcare workers (HCWs) from needlestick injury is approximately 0.3%, while the risk of transmission from splashes to mucous membrane is lower at 0.1%. The risk of infection is higher from (i) patients with high viral loads, (ii) hollow needles, (iii) deeper tissue injury, and (iv) injuries during phlebotomy. Precautions are needed not only with blood but also when handling other biofluids such as semen and vaginal secretions.

Management

Preoperative assessment
Review of the patient and notes should elicit the duration of disease, most recent CD4 count and viral load, history of opportunistic infections, and medical comorbidities. Medication history should include antiretroviral regimen and any infection prophylaxis. A clinical examination is needed to assess for oropharyngeal thrush, lymphadenopathy, and signs of infection (particularly chest infection). A recent (<6 months) CD4 count, viral load, and blood count are essential; other blood tests (e.g., clotting, renal and liver function tests) can be performed if clinically indicated. If test results for tuberculosis, syphilis, HBV, and HCV are not documented, testing for these should be considered.

Preoperative management
As complications are mostly related to uncontrolled HIV, non-urgent operations in a patient with high viral loads should be delayed to give antiretroviral regimens a chance to lower the viral load. Prophylactic antibiotic treatment should be commenced, based on disease status and past history of opportunistic infections. Comorbid conditions should be optimized, and nutrition improved in malnourished patients.

It is important to minimize breaks in antiretroviral medications, and preferably continue them even when the patient is NPO, in consultation with anesthetist, pharmacist, and HIV specialist.

Postoperative management
In the postoperative period, patients infected with HIV may be at risk of complications including thromboembolic disease, pneumothorax, pneumonia, and severe pain that requires high doses of pain medication.

HIV-infected patients are particularly vulnerable to postoperative thromboembolic complications as a result of hypercoagulability [2]. Patients should receive prophylactic heparin and mobilization as soon as feasible. Pneumothorax may be the cause of acute postoperative chest pain and shortness of breath, and should also be managed appropriately.

Gynecologic and Obstetric Surgery: Challenges and Management Options, First Edition. Edited by Arri Coomarasamy, Mahmood I. Shafi, G. Willy Davila and Kiong K. Chan.
© 2016 John Wiley & Sons, Ltd. Published 2016 by John Wiley & Sons, Ltd.

Methadone replacement therapy and/or chronic exposure to opiates may necessitate the treatment of HIV-infected patients with higher than usual doses of analgesics during the postoperative period.

Data collected in studies to date are insufficient to determine any effect of HIV infection on postoperative wound healing. Standard perioperative prophylactic antibiotic therapy is recommended.

Resolution of the case

The patient in this case history has a good CD4 count and low viral load, and is on potent antiretroviral therapy. Following appropriate preoperative assessment and management, she is suitable to have the scheduled operation.

Prevention of transmission of HIV from the patient to HCWs

Sharp needlestick injuries are recorded in 1–15% of surgical procedures [3], and there are estimates that more than half of needlestick injuries involving suture needles occur during the suturing of fascia or muscle [4,5]. It is important to use the highest standards of infection control, involving the most effective known protective barriers to prevent contact with the patient's body fluids and universal precautions [6].

Steps to reduce the risk of HCWs acquiring HIV infection during surgical procedures include:
- double-gloving and/or regular changes of gloves during long procedures;
- blunt-tipped needles and stapling devices;
- face and/or eye protection (goggles) to prevent mucocutaneous transmission;
- instruments for retraction (rather than hand or fingers);
- instruments to handle sharps;
- instruments to remove scalpels.

Post-exposure management
If a surgeon sustains a needlestick injury, he or she should stop the operation; if it is unsafe to pause the surgery, another surgeon should continue the surgery. The first and immediate step is to squeeze around (not on) the puncture site to express as much blood as possible. The puncture site should be washed with soap or antiseptic solution.

The US Centers for Disease Control and Prevention (CDC) recommend antiretroviral chemoprophylaxis for HCWs exposed through surgical procedures to HIV in blood or body fluids. Local guidelines for post-exposure prophylaxis (PEP) regimens can be followed, but the first dose should ideally be given within 1 hour [7]. HCWs should be followed up in an occupational health or HIV clinic; they should be offered counseling, post-exposure testing, and medical evaluation regardless of whether they receive PEP. HIV antibody testing by enzyme immunoassay is appropriate to check for seroconversion for at least 6 months. After baseline testing at the time of exposure, follow-up testing could be performed at 6, 12, and 26 weeks. Extended follow-up (for 12 months) is recommended for those coinfected with both HIV and HCV.

KEY POINTS

Challenge: Perioperative management of a patient infected with HIV, to reduce the risks resulting from surgical procedures for both the patient and HCWs.

Background
- There are 34 million people with HIV or AIDS worldwide.
- One in four of those infected with HIV may not know that they have the infection.
- HIV patients generally tolerate surgery well, particularly when they have:
  - Good CD4 cell counts (>200/µL).
  - Low viral loads (<10,000 copies/ml).
  - No comorbidities.
- Potential risks in HIV-infected patients having surgery include:
  - Cytopenias (thrombocytopenia, anemia, and leukopenia) which can predispose patient to infections (particularly pneumonia) and bleeding.
  - Coagulopathy.
  - Drug-induced hepatotoxicity and nephrotoxicity.
  - HIV-associated nephropathy.
  - Adrenal insufficiency.
  - Metabolic disorders (e.g., insulin resistance).
  - Malnutrition.
  - Increased risk of allergic reactions.
- The risk of transmission to HCWs from needlestick injury is approximately 3%; the risk of infection is higher from (i) patients with high viral loads, (ii) hollow needles, (iii) deeper tissue injury, and (iv) injuries during phlebotomy.

Management
Preoperative assessment
- Elicit the duration of disease, most recent CD4 count and viral load, history of opportunistic infections, and medical comorbidities.
- Obtain history of antiretroviral regimen and any infection prophylaxis.
- Perform clinical examination to assess for oropharyngeal thrush, lymphadenopathy, and signs of infection (particularly chest infection).
- Arrange CD4 count, viral load, and blood count if these have not been performed within 6 months before the operation.
- Consider other tests: clotting, renal and liver function tests.

Preoperative management
- Delay non-urgent operations in a patient with high viral loads to administer antiretroviral regimens to lower the viral load.
- Commence prophylactic antibiotic treatment, based on disease status and past history of opportunistic infections.
- Optimize comorbid medical conditions.
- Improve nutrition in malnourished patients (high calorie and protein diet).
- Minimize breaks in antiretroviral medications, and preferably continue them even when the patient is NPO.

Postoperative management
- Be vigilant for thromboembolic disease, pneumothorax, pneumonia, and worsening medical comorbidities.

Management of HCWs exposed to HIV needlestick injury
- Stop operating; find an alternative surgeon to continue if necessary.
- Squeeze around (not on) the puncture site to express blood.
- Wash thoroughly with soap or antiseptic solution.
- Follow local policies for PEP, which should ideally be given within 1 hour.
- Arrange follow-up for HCW in an occupational health or HIV clinic.

Prevention of transmission of HIV to HCWs
- Use two pairs of gloves; change gloves regularly for long procedures.
- Use blunt-tipped needles and stapling devices.
- Wear face and eye protection (goggles) to prevent mucocutaneous transmission.
- Use instruments for retraction (rather than hand or fingers).
- Use instruments to handle sharps.
- Use instruments to remove scalpels.

References

1   Brooks R. HIV. In: Cohn SL (ed.) *Perioperative Medicine*. Springer-Verlag, London, 2011.
2   New York State Department of Health. *Perioperative management of HIV-infected patients*. New York State Department of Health, New York, 2012.
3   American College of Surgeons. Statement on sharps safety. *Bull Am Coll Surg* 2007; 92(10).
4   Jagger J, Bentley M, Tereskerz P. A study of patterns and prevention of blood exposures in OR personnel. *AORN J* 1998; 67:979–981, 983–984, 986–987.
5   American College of Surgeons. Statement on blunt suture needles. *Bull Am Coll Surg* 2005; 90(11).
6   American College of Surgeons. Statement on the surgeon and HIV infection. *Bull Am Coll Surg* 2004; 89(5).
7   Chikwe J, Walther A, Jones P. *Perioperative Medicine*, 2nd edn. Oxford University Press, Oxford, 2009.

CHAPTER 23
Obese Patient

Phil Moore

Birmingham Women's NHS Foundation Trust, Birmingham, UK

Case history 1: A 35-year-old woman with a BMI of 55 presented with urinary incontinence and was listed for TVT insertion.

Case history 2: A 28-year-old woman with a BMI of 61 was listed for elective cesarean section at 37 weeks of gestation.

Background

Obesity has reached epidemic proportions in many Western countries; in the UK, 25% of men and 26% of women are classed as obese. The consequences of obesity involve every major organ system and it is associated with many pathologic conditions including hypertension, diabetes, hyperlipidemia, cholelithiasis, gastroesophageal reflux disease, cirrhosis, degenerative joint and disk disease, venous stasis and thromboembolic disease, sleep disorders, and body image and psychological disorders. Additionally, carrying out surgery involves physical challenges for the operating surgeon because of the increased weight and body fat thickness, while changes to the cardiorespiratory system provide particular challenges for the anesthetist. Consequently, obesity has been highlighted as a risk factor for increased perioperative morbidity and mortality in a number of national reports. The UK Confidential Enquiry into Maternal Deaths for the 2003–2005 triennium found that half of the women who died from direct or indirect causes were overweight or obese and that 15% were morbidly or supermorbidly obese. It is therefore mandatory that special attention is paid to the preoperative preparation and perioperative and peripartum management of this group of patients.

Management

Preoperative preparation

Both the cases described should be identified as high risk before admission to hospital, either in the outpatient or preoperative clinic, or in the antenatal clinic. The BMI should be routinely calculated for all patients undergoing surgery or booking for delivery. Local protocols should dictate which patients are referred for further review, according to type and urgency of surgery and BMI, with particular attention being paid to pre-existing morbidity which further increases risk (e.g., respiratory or cardiovascular disease and type 2 diabetes); under these circumstances the patient should be referred to appropriate specialties for preoperative optimization of the underlying conditions (Chapter 1).

Although surgeons are usually aware of obese patients when they list them for surgery, it is important that a care pathway is in place to alert other healthcare professionals who will be involved in their care at the earliest opportunity, to ensure that adequate assessment and planning can occur in advance of admission. This includes preoperative clinic nursing staff, anesthetists, ward nursing staff, operating room staff, and allied professionals such as physiotherapists and dietitians. Often these patients are reviewed in a dedicated anesthetic pre-assessment clinic by the anesthetist who will care for them. It is important for a senior surgeon and anesthetist to outline the intended benefits of surgery, along with the risks of anesthesia and surgery, both to ensure that the patient is certain that the benefits she hopes to accrue are worth the risks involved, and also to provide an incentive for weight loss. This applies particularly to Case history 1 as surgery could be delayed pending weight loss. The need to provide prompt delivery of the baby in Case history 2 means there is little alternative but to proceed with the surgery; these patients would normally be flagged up earlier in pregnancy to allow more time for preparations to be made.

Intraoperative management

Obese patients should ideally be operated on early in the day to allow adequate immediate postoperative time during daylight hours to detect and treat any complications which arise. Most obese patients will require an overnight stay, especially if systemic opioid drugs have been used. However, it may be possible to perform minor or intermediate surgery as an outpatient, if sufficient time is allowed for full recovery from the sedative anesthetic drugs and opioids, reducing the chance of obstructive apnea and desaturation which could cause cardiovascular complications during the first postoperative night.

Senior surgical and anesthetic staff should perform or supervise the procedure and extra time should be factored in for all stages of the operation and recovery. The anesthetic management may be complicated by difficult venous access and airway management, and back-up plans and equipment should be available for both these eventualities; it may be necessary to insert a central venous catheter and perform awake fiber-optic intubation. Invasive arterial blood

Gynecologic and Obstetric Surgery: Challenges and Management Options, First Edition. Edited by Arri Coomarasamy, Mahmood I. Shafi, G. Willy Davila and Kiong K. Chan.
© 2016 John Wiley & Sons, Ltd. Published 2016 by John Wiley & Sons, Ltd.

pressure monitoring may be desirable or necessary if non-invasive measurement is difficult or impossible due to the size of the upper arm. Obese patients are prone to hypertension and cardiomegaly, which may lead to left ventricular failure perioperatively; invasive monitoring also allows cardiovascular parameters to be monitored more closely intraoperatively to allow abnormalities to be detected and treated more promptly.

Depending on the patient's weight, specialist transfer equipment may be needed for moving between operating table and bed or trolley, and it is important to check that all equipment is rated to support the necessary mass. Safe positioning of the patient can be challenging, and adequate padding must be applied to avoid putting undue pressure on pressure points, and especially nerves and nerve plexuses. Depending on the surgery, additional surgical assistance may be needed to provide adequate retraction of the tissues, and this is especially the case with abdominal surgery.

Mechanical ventilation can be challenging in these patients because of both the weight of the chest wall and the additional abdominal fat pushing up on the diaphragm. This is exacerbated if the patient requires head-down tilt intraoperatively. Surgery should be expedited as far as possible. Avoidance of opioid analgesia by using other analgesic drugs and regional or local anesthetic techniques is desirable to reduce the chances of postoperative hypoventilation and obstructive sleep apnea.

Postoperative management

Patients should be nursed in a semi-recumbent position as far as possible in order to aid respiratory excursion and minimize the chance of hypoxemia. Obese patients are at risk of obstructive sleep apnea after anesthesia, even if this was not a pre-existing problem, and they should be closely monitored for this, especially if they have received opioids for analgesia. It is important that they receive supplemental oxygen therapy, particularly overnight, and continuous positive airway pressure (CPAP) may be necessary even in those who did not require it previously.

Obese patients are at high risk of postoperative venous embolic disease, and pulmonary embolus is the commonest cause of mortality within 30 days of surgery in this group; a clear plan for thromboprophylaxis should be in place, comprising both physical and pharmacologic interventions, as well as encouragement of early ambulation.

In emergency situations, morbidly obese patients requiring surgery should have the senior surgical and anesthetic clinicians responsible for their care informed of their admission at the earliest opportunity, so that they may attend the hospital to plan and manage the procedure.

Prevention

If time allows, obese patients should be encouraged to lose weight before surgery. Sometimes, surgery may be declined unless the patient loses weight, for example patients needing assisted conception. A dietitian or GP referral may be useful. Even small amounts of weight loss may reduce the risk of perioperative complications. Although it is desirable that obese patients should lose weight in advance of their surgery, it is often difficult for them to achieve this; nonetheless, dietary advice and support should be offered. Hospitals should have an agreed pathway to ensure that obese patients are appropriately prepared for surgery, and all

relevant staff are informed. Special equipment may be needed in theater and on the wards to ensure that the patient can be handled and moved safely.

KEY POINTS

Challenge: Surgery for the obese patient.

Background
- 25% of the UK population are overweight or obese.
- Obesity is associated with many comorbidities, including hypertension, diabetes, hyperlipidemia, gastroesophageal reflux disease, cirrhosis, degenerative joint and disk disease, thromboembolic disease, and sleep disorders.
- Obese patients are at increased risk of perioperative complications.
- National guidelines recommend local protocols and senior involvement in their perioperative care.

Prevention
- Few patients will be able to lose significant amounts of weight before surgery; nonetheless this should be advised.
- Defined care pathways should be in place to ensure that all necessary preparations are made.
- Morbid obesity (BMI >40) is a contraindication to day-case surgery.

Management
- Identify and optimize any comorbidities (e.g., hypertension and diabetes).
- Operate early in the day.
- Involve senior staff at all stages.
- Allow for increased anesthetic and surgical time.
- Ensure appropriate equipment is arranged in advance.

Anesthetic
- Consider regional technique if appropriate, although insertion may not be easy.
- Avoid or minimize the use of opioid drugs if possible.
- Make contingency plans for difficult venous access and airway management (e.g., central venous catheter, awake fiber-optic intubation).
- Position with particular regard to pressure areas.

Surgical
- Engage extra surgical assistance for adequate tissue retraction.
- Consider suturing techniques to avoid wound breakdown.

Postoperative care
- May need an ITU or HDU bed.
- Nurse patients in a semi-recumbent position.
- Monitor patients for sleep apnea, especially if they received opioids; consider supplemental oxygen, particularly overnight, and CPAP therapy.
- Arrange thromboprophylaxis: heparin, compression stockings, and pneumatic compression boots.
- Consider chest physiotherapy.
- Encourage early ambulation.

Further reading

Lewis G (ed.). *Saving Mothers' Lives: Reviewing Maternal Deaths to Make Motherhood Safer, 2003–2005*. The Seventh Report on Confidential Enquiries into Maternal Deaths in the United Kingdom. Confidential Enquiry into Maternal and Child Health (CEMACH), London, 2007.

Public Health England. About obesity. Available at http://www.noo.org.uk/NOO_about_obesity (accessed 1 September 2013).

Roizen M, Fleisher L. Anesthetic implications of concurrent diseases. In: Miller RD (ed.) *Miller's Anesthesia*, 7th edn, pp. 1067–1150. Churchill Livingstone Elsevier, Philadelphia, 2010.

CHAPTER 24
Patient with Poor Nutritional Status

Phil Moore

Birmingham Women's NHS Foundation Trust, Birmingham, UK

Case history 1: A 65-year-old cachectic woman with dementia and known ovarian carcinoma was admitted as an emergency with abdominal pain and distension.

Case history 2: A thin 45-year-old woman is admitted for TAH. She has a history of Crohn's disease with previous small bowel resection and is currently on home total parenteral nutrition (TPN).

Background

Poor nutrition may be a result of inadequate calorific intake or an inability to absorb nutrition from the gut. In either case, poor nutrition may lead to perioperative complications and impaired wound healing or infection and so, if time allows, attempts should be made to improve nutrition preoperatively. Well-nourished patients undergoing uncomplicated surgery can reasonably tolerate up to 4 days of fasting. However, if malnourishment is pre-existing, it is important to re-establish feeding or supplementation as soon as possible postoperatively, as the normal metabolic stress response to surgery includes catabolism, hypermetabolism, hyperglycemia, and lipolysis.

Severe starvation, from any cause, can lead to acidosis, hypokalemia, hypomagnesemia, diabetes insipidus, and severe endocrine abnormalities; it is important these are corrected before surgery. Severe protein deficiency may lead to ECG changes, including prolonged QT interval, atrioventricular block and other arrhythmias.

Management

In Case history 1, emergency surgery may be necessary, with little time to address the patient's nutritional state. However, the patient should have any electrolyte imbalance corrected preoperatively, with measurement of serum sodium, potassium, magnesium, and phosphate levels (Chapter 56). If time allows, the patient should be referred to a dietitian, who can provide a plan for enhanced nutrition postoperatively with high calorific supplements; these can usually be given orally, although if the patient's condition is likely to delay this, gastric or jejunal tube feeding can be considered. Failure of enteral routes should trigger a prompt switch to parenteral feeding, despite the increased complications associated with this route.

In Case history 2, the cause of the poor nutrition is malabsorption, and parenteral feeding via a central venous catheter is already in progress, under the supervision of specialist dietitians. Arrangements should be made for this to be continued throughout the perioperative period, with close monitoring to allow the TPN solution to be appropriately tailored to the patient's needs around the time of surgery. The solution is constituted with careful reference to serial measurements of blood electrolyte levels, as well as including appropriate calories in the form of glucose and fat, and nitrogen in the form of protein. Vitamins, minerals, and trace elements are also included, as well as appropriate amounts of water. Liver and renal functions are monitored frequently. Box 24.1 shows the process followed when preparing TPN for a patient.

> **BOX 24.1 STEPS IN THE PREPARATION OF TPN SOLUTION FOR A PATIENT**
>
> - What is the patient's energy need in kcal/day?
> - How much protein/nitrogen is needed per day?
> - How much fluid does the patient need and can tolerate?
> - How much fat is needed?
> - How much carbohydrate is needed?
> - Which electrolytes are required? In what amounts?
> - Which vitamins and minerals are needed and how much?
> - What route of feeding is being used?
> - What is the osmolality of the solution?

Meticulous asepsis is required in the care of the central venous catheter used for TPN feeding to avoid iatrogenic line infections, and it should not be used for other purposes such as drug administration.

Complications of supplemental feeding include refeeding syndrome, overfeeding, and hyperglycemia. Refeeding syndrome may occur in severely malnourished patients during the first few days of nutritional support. Clinical features include weakness, respiratory and cardiac failure, arrhythmias, and seizures, and it can be fatal. In these patients, feeding should be introduced slowly, and gradually increased after 4 days at 25–50% of energy requirements. Supplemental thiamine and B vitamins should be given, along with appropriate electrolyte supplementation.

Gynecologic and Obstetric Surgery: Challenges and Management Options, First Edition. Edited by Arri Coomarasamy, Mahmood I. Shafi, G. Willy Davila and Kiong K. Chan.
© 2016 John Wiley & Sons, Ltd. Published 2016 by John Wiley & Sons, Ltd.

In view of the cardiovascular complications of malnutrition, intraoperative invasive monitoring with an arterial line and central venous catheter is indicated in both these cases. These will also allow blood electrolytes to be easily checked and corrected if surgery is prolonged.

Prevention

Outpatient detection of poor nutrition may allow community-based intervention to improve matters in advance of admission, if the surgery is elective. The general practitioner should be alerted as the main coordinator of care and can involve community dietitians and community services as appropriate. It may be necessary for district nurses to visit regularly, especially if the patient is elderly or suffering with dementia, to ensure adequate calorific intake. Poor nutrition in young women can be due to psychiatric conditions such as anorexia nervosa and bulimia; under these circumstances psychiatric services should be involved and, depending on the urgency of the surgery, in some cases use of sectioning under the Mental Health Act may be needed to protect the woman's own best interests.

KEY POINTS

Challenge: Patient with poor nutritional status.

Background
- Poor nutrition may be due to inadequate calorific intake or malabsorption.
- Poor nutrition increases the risk of perioperative infections, delayed healing, and wound dehiscence.
- Starvation may lead to severe metabolic and cardiovascular effects.
- Well-nourished patients undergoing uncomplicated surgery can generally tolerate a maximum of 4 days of fasting.

Prevention
- In elective patients, calculation of the BMI in outpatients may allow detection of poor nutrition and corrective intervention in the community.

- Refer to dietitian and gastroenterologist as necessary.
- Monitor calorific intake and weight gain.
- Reinstate feeding as soon as possible postoperatively.

Management
- If time allows, calorific supplementation should be instigated in advance of hospital admission.
- For emergency surgery, at least electrolyte (serum sodium, potassium, magnesium, and phosphate levels) and fluid imbalances should be corrected before surgery.
- Feeding should be started promptly postoperatively, by enteral route if possible but parenterally if this is not possible or delayed.
- For patients needing TPN, meticulous asepsis is required in the care of the central venous catheter used for TPN feeding to avoid iatrogenic line infections.

Further reading

Stroud M, Duncan H, Nightingale J. Guidelines for enteral feeding in adult hospital patients. *Gut* 2003; 52(Suppl 7):vii1–vii12.

Weissman C. Nutrition and metabolic control. In: MillerRD (ed.) *Miller's Anesthesia*, 7th edn, pp. 2923–2956. Churchill Livingstone Elsevier, Philadelphia, 2010.

CHAPTER 25

Pregnant Patient Requiring Non-obstetric Surgery

Arri Coomarasamy

College of Medical and Dental Sciences, University of Birmingham, Birmingham, UK

Case history: A woman who is 20 weeks pregnant has been diagnosed with appendicitis requiring an appendectomy.

Background

Incidental non-obstetric surgery is required in 0.2–1.0% of pregnant women. Appendectomy and cholecystectomy are the two common non-obstetric operations in pregnancy; other operations include surgery for adnexal masses and ovarian torsion. Although it is often recommended to defer operations to the second trimester, if a patient is unwell the benefits of surgery may outweigh any harm; therefore surgery may need to be performed at any gestation.

Physiologic changes in pregnancy

There are key changes in cardiovascular, respiratory, renal, and hematologic physiology that the anesthetist and surgeon need to take into consideration [1,2].

Cardiovascular changes
* Heart rate increases by 10%.
* Blood pressure decreases by 20 mmHg systolic and 10 mmHg diastolic by 20 weeks.
* Cardiac output and stroke volume increase by 50%, peaking at 16 weeks.
* Plasma volume increases by 50%, peaking by 30 weeks.
* Soft systolic murmur and non-sustained S3 gallop may be present.

Respiratory changes
* Minute ventilation increases.
* Tidal volume increases by 50%.
* As a result of normal hyperventilation of pregnancy, PaO_2 increases slightly and $PaCO_2$ decreases to 28–32 mmHg.
* Mild respiratory alkalosis (pH ~7.44) may be present.
* Functional residual capacity can decrease by up to 70% when the woman is supine.

Renal changes
* Glomerular filtration rate increases by 50%.
* Creatinine clearance increases by 50% to about 150 mL/min.
* 24-hour protein excretion increases up to 300 mg.

Hematologic changes
* Hemodilution results in low hemoglobin (10–11 g/dL).
* CRP and ESR are elevated, and not useful tests in pregnancy.
* Slight increase in white cell count, but no changes in platelets.

Testing in pregnancy

Appropriate preoperative testing should be arranged depending on history, symptoms, and signs. For instance, a patient with a loud murmur should have an echocardiogram and cardiology review before an operation. Chest X-ray can be performed with abdominal shielding to reduce the risk of radiation exposure to the fetus. MRI, CT, and ventilation–perfusion (*V/Q*) scans can be performed in pregnancy; however, CT of the abdomen should generally be limited to no more than two scans [1,2].

Management

Loss of maternal airway is the most common cause of anesthesia-related maternal deaths, and thus regional anesthesia should be considered to avoid the risks associated with intubation and airway management [2]. A multidisciplinary approach should be the aim, with the involvement of gynecologists, obstetricians, anesthetists, and medical specialists as appropriate.

Patient positioning and fetal monitoring

A pregnant patient should be positioned in the left lateral decubitus position with a pelvic wedge or pillow under the right hip to reduce the effects of aortic and vena caval compression from the pregnant uterus. An alternative to the use of a wedge is to tilt the operating table to the left by 20–30° [3]. Fetal heart rate monitoring may be considered after 24 weeks of gestation, although depending on the operation and the operative approach, this may not be possible intraoperatively. A minimum standard is to perform fetal monitoring before and after the procedure.

Surgical approach

The decision on whether the approach should be via laparoscopy or laparotomy should be individualized. Historically, pregnancy was considered a relative contraindication for laparoscopy, but now it

Gynecologic and Obstetric Surgery: Challenges and Management Options, First Edition. Edited by Arri Coomarasamy, Mahmood I. Shafi, G. Willy Davila and Kiong K. Chan.
© 2016 John Wiley & Sons, Ltd. Published 2016 by John Wiley & Sons, Ltd.

is recognized to have a role, possibly up to 28 weeks of gestation [4]. Laparoscopy is associated with limited handling of the pregnant uterus, optimal exposure, rapid resumption of mobility (and thus reduced risk of VTE), early resumption of bowel function, less pain and analgesic requirement, and reduced risk of scar dehiscence or herniation during labor [4,5].

The three major concerns with laparoscopy are (i) penetration injury to the uterus, (ii) potential harmful effects of CO_2 pneumoperitoneum on fetal well-being, and (iii) risk of fetal loss.

Although many studies have documented the use of Veress needle to create pneumoperitoneum in pregnant patients, particularly in early gestations, it is safer (and thus recommended) to use an open (Hasson) technique to minimize the risk of penetration injury to the pregnant uterus. A Palmer's point entry would be another option to minimize the risk of penetration injury.

Fetal hypercapnia and acidosis are possible from CO_2 absorption. High CO_2 pressure can also decrease maternal venous return and cardiac output [4]. The pneumoperitoneum pressure should ideally be maintained between 10 and 12 mmHg [5], and should certainly be no more than 15 mmHg [4]. End-tidal CO_2 monitoring to ensure $PaCO_2$ remains within a safe range (30–40 mmHg) is recommended [3]. Operative time should generally be restricted to less than 60 min [6].

A systematic review of 11 low-grade observational studies suggested a doubling in the risk of fetal loss with laparoscopy compared with laparotomy for appendectomy [7]. However, this finding was dominated by one large retrospective registry-based study [8], and removal of this study from the meta-analysis negated the association between laparoscopy and fetal loss. The evidence on the risk of fetal loss with laparoscopy is equivocal, and better data are needed.

Postoperative care

Tocolysis (e.g., indomethacin 100 mg suppository or oxytocin antagonist infusion) may be useful if there is evidence of uterine contractions, but should only be given in consultation with obstetricians and with fetal heart rate monitoring.

Resolution of the case

The diagnosis of appendicitis can be made from a combination of clinical features, blood results, and ultrasound scan. The site of pain often moves up on the right side of the abdomen with advancing gestation. If there is diagnostic uncertainty, MRI is the next useful test, and if there is still some uncertainty then CT can be useful. If appendicitis is diagnosed, it is important to proceed to operative treatment in a timely manner to avoid the risk of appendiceal perforation and sepsis, which are associated with poor maternal and fetal outcomes.

The first port should be at least 3–4 cm above the pregnant uterus, and can be in the midline between the umbilicus and the xiphoid process (Figure 25.1) [3]. Two lateral ports can then be placed under direct vision and the appendectomy operation can be completed taking into account the various precautions addressed in this chapter.

Prevention

Although there is often an understandable reluctance to perform operations in pregnant women, those with surgical emergencies should have the necessary operation without undue delay, regardless of gestation. The harms of non-action are likely to outweigh the

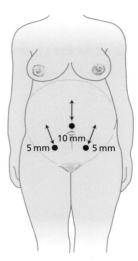

Figure 25.1 Trocar placement for laparoscopic appendectomy in different stages of pregnancy. Adapted from Chung *et al.*, 2013 [3] with permission from the Canadian Medical Association.

benefits for both mother and baby. The risk of appendiceal perforation is, for example, known to be higher in pregnant women [9], and this may be related to delayed diagnosis or surgery, or both. Prevention of complications requires rapid diagnostic work-up (including MRI and CT as necessary), multidisciplinary care, and timely surgical management.

KEY POINTS

Challenge: Pregnant patient requiring non-obstetric surgery.

Background
- Incidental non-obstetric surgery is required in 0.2–1.0% pregnant women.
- Appendectomy and cholecystectomy are the two common non-obstetric operations in pregnancy.
- There are significant cardiovascular, respiratory, renal, and hematologic changes in pregnancy.

Prevention
- Rapid diagnostic work-up, multidisciplinary care, and timely surgery are needed to avoid complications associated with surgical emergencies such as appendicitis.

Management
- Consider regional anesthesia.
- Avoid aortocaval compression by positioning the patient in the left lateral decubitus position with the aid of a wedge or pillow, or by tilting the operating table by 20–30°.
- Monitor fetal heart rate before and after the procedure.
- Individualize decision about laparoscopy or laparotomy. Laparoscopy is an option until 28 weeks of gestation, and in some cases even beyond 28 weeks.
- Laparoscopy:
  - Do not use Veress needle due to the risk of uterine puncture. Use open (Hasson) technique. Consider Palmer's point entry.
  - The first port should be at least 3–4 cm above the pregnant uterus.
  - Maintain pneumoperitoneum pressure below 15 mmHg, and ideally 10–12 mmHg. This is to minimize the risk of CO_2 absorption and fetal acidemia and improve maternal venous return and cardiac output.
  - Consider end-tidal CO_2 monitoring; ensure $PaCO_2$ remains between 30 and 40 mmHg.
  - The evidence on the association between laparoscopy and fetal loss is equivocal, although the available evidence suggests a doubling in the risk of fetal loss compared with open operations.
- Tocolysis should be considered if there are uterine contractions.

References

1 Lewis BG, Carson MP. The pregnant surgical patient. In: Cohn SL (ed.) *Perioperative Medicine*. Springer-Verlag, London, 2011.

2 Carson MP. The pregnant surgical patient. In: Jaffer AK, Grant PJ (eds) *Perioperative Medicine: Medical Consultation and Co-Management*. Wiley-Blackwell, Hoboken, NJ, 2012.

3 Chung JC, Cho GS, Shin EJ, Kim HC, Song OP. Clinical outcomes compared between laparoscopic and open appendectomy in pregnant women. *Can J Surg* 2013; 56: 341–346.

4 Fatum M, Rojansky N. Laparoscopic surgery during pregnancy. *Obstet Gynecol Surv* 2001; 56:50–59.

5 Machado NO, Grant CS. Laparoscopic appendicectomy in all trimesters of pregnancy. *JSLS* 2009; 13:384–390.

6 Jackson H, Granger S, Price R *et al.* Diagnosis and laparoscopic treatment of surgical diseases during pregnancy: an evidence-based review. *Surg Endosc* 2008; 22:1917–1927.

7 Wilasrusmee C, Sukrat B, McEvoy M, Attia J, Thakkinstian A. Systematic review and meta-analysis of safety of laparoscopic versus open appendicectomy for suspected appendicitis in pregnancy. *Br J Surg* 2012; 99:1470–1478.

8 McGory ML, Zingmond DS, Tillou A, Hiatt JR, Ko CY, Cryer HM. Negative appendectomy in pregnant women is associated with a substantial risk of fetal loss. *J Am Coll Surg* 2007; 205:534–540.

9 Corneille MG, Gallup TM, Bening T *et al.* The use of laparoscopic surgery in pregnancy: evaluation of safety and efficacy. *Am J Surg* 2010; 200:363–367.

Section 2
Intraoperative Care
Editors: Arri Coomarasamy and Mahmood I. Shafi

CHAPTER 26

Transverse Incision on the Abdomen Inadequate for Surgery

Arri Coomarasamy

College of Medical and Dental Sciences, University of Birmingham, Birmingham, UK

Case history: *A woman with a fibroid uterus elected to have a total abdominal hysterectomy. The surgeon opened the abdomen through a Pfannenstiel incision, and found the uterus to be larger than expected and to have restricted mobility. It was not possible for him to exteriorize the uterus or access the pedicles to carry out the hysterectomy.*

Background

Adequate exposure and access are fundamental requirements for successful surgery. While some women prefer a below bikini-line cut, this should not be at the expense of adequate exposure. A surgeon needs to consider the pathology being treated, the proposed surgery, patient's body habitus, and previous abdominal scars while planning the incision.

Reported advantages of transverse incisions include better cosmetic appearance, less pain, and low incidence of hernia formation. However, transverse incisions can result in poor access, and are associated with greater blood loss, higher risk of hematoma formation and local nerve injury (which can result in paresthesia of the overlying skin) when compared with a midline incision.

The midline incision is versatile and allows a quick and almost bloodless entry into the abdominal cavity, and is easily extendable in length if necessary. The presumed disadvantages of a midline incision, compared with a transverse incision, include an increased risk of wound dehiscence and hernia formation. However, recent studies find little difference in dehiscence rates between properly closed midline and transverse incisions [1,2,3]. A gynecologist does not, therefore, have any excuse for compromising safety by evading a midline incision when it is indicated.

Management

The options for this woman are either modifying the Pfannenstiel incision to make more room or reducing the size of the uterus by performing a myomectomy.

Making more room by modifying the incision

Because of the effect of rectus muscles, a simple increase in the length of the Pfannenstiel skin incision will not improve exposure or access. The options for improving access are (i) converting the Pfannenstiel into a Cherney incision; (ii) if the original incision was over the body of the rectus, then converting it into a muscle-cutting Mayland incision; or (iii) adding a vertical midline incision to the existing incision to give an inverted-T incision.

Cherney incision

In a Pfannenstiel incision, the rectus muscles are not cut. In a Cherney incision [4], the rectus muscles are transected at their tendinous insertion to the pubic symphysis. The first step is the sharp dissection of the pyramidalis muscle. Then a plane is developed between the fibrous tendons of the rectus muscle and the underlying tranversalis fascia. Using diathermy, the rectus tendons are then cut from the pubic bone (Figure 26.1). The rectus muscles can then be retracted upwards, which results in improvement in access and particularly good exposure of the pelvic sidewall.

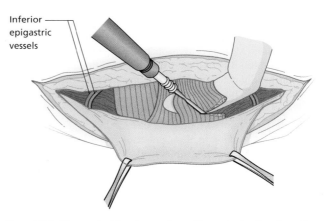

Inferior epigastric vessels

Figure 26.1 Cherney incision: transection of the rectus tendons from the pubic symphysis.

During closure, the cut end of the rectus tendons are approximated to the lower flap of the rectus sheath with five or six interrupted mattress non-absorbable sutures.

Gynecologic and Obstetric Surgery: Challenges and Management Options, First Edition. Edited by Arri Coomarasamy, Mahmood I. Shafi, G. Willy Davila and Kiong K. Chan.
© 2016 John Wiley & Sons, Ltd. Published 2016 by John Wiley & Sons, Ltd.

Maylard incision

If the original Pfannenstiel incision was higher on the abdomen such that the incision lay over the body of the rectus muscle, the muscle-cutting Maylard incision may be appropriate [5]. Through the transverse incision on the anterior rectus sheath, the inferior epigastric vessels (which lie on the posterior lateral border of each rectus muscle) should first be identified, teased away from their attachments by gentle figure dissection, clamped, cut and ligated. The rectus muscle is then completely transected with diathermy (Figure 26.2).

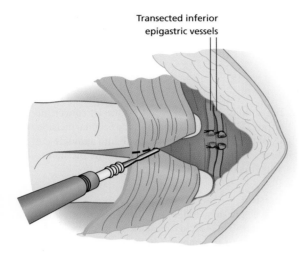

Transected inferior
epigastric vessels

Figure 26.2 Maylard incision: transection of the rectus muscle after ligation of the inferior epigastric vessels.

During closure of a standard Maylard incision, the rectus muscles need not be brought together. However, when a Pfannenstiel is converted to Maylard incision, muscle approximation with mattress sutures is required. It is the adherence of the rectus muscles to the anterior rectus sheath with several transverse inscriptions that normally prevents the rectus muscles from retracting after a Maylard incision; in a Pfannenstiel to Maylard conversion, the anterior rectus sheath would already have been dissected away from the rectus muscles (as part of the Pfannenstiel incision) and thus reapproximation of the cut ends of the rectus muscles is necessary to prevent muscle retraction.

Inverted-T incision

If Cherney or Maylard incision does not give adequate exposure and access, or if the pathology requires it, a vertical midline incision can be added to the Pfannenstiel incision, producing an inverted-T scar. The vertical incision is generally closed before closure of the transverse incision. Where the two incisions meet is a weak point in the closure and prone to ischemia and dehiscence.

Reducing the size of the uterus by performing a myomectomy

The uterine incision(s) for myomectomy would depend on the location and size of fibroids. Removal of a few large fibroids may be sufficient to allow exteriorization of the uterus, which may then allow hysterectomy to be performed. In an effort to reduce the blood loss during myomectomy, if access permits, the infundibulopelvic ligaments can be ligated and cut and a tourniquet can be placed around the neck of the uterus. A Foley catheter tied tightly around the uterus acts as an excellent tourniquet, and the uterine or internal iliac artery can be clipped or sutured.

Prevention

All steps should be taken to minimize the chances of encountering unexpected pathology during surgery. This requires examination of the abdomen and pelvis and, where appropriate, imaging with ultrasound, CT, or MRI. MRI scan is particularly useful in the three-dimensional assessment of a fibroid uterus.

Women waiting to have surgery for fibroids can be given GnRH analogs or ulipristal acetate to reduce the size of the fibroids and thus the overall size of the uterus. Monthly injections of GnRH analog or daily ulipristal acetate 5 mg orally for 3 months will reduce the fibroid volume by about half.

Examination under anesthesia before starting the surgery presents the final opportunity to prevent the situation described in this case history. A thorough pelvic examination assessing the size and mobility of the uterus and the adnexae may have prompted the surgeon to choose a vertical midline incision. In this context, appropriate consenting is important: a woman scheduled to have a hysterectomy through a transverse incision should be warned that a final assessment on the appropriateness of this incision will be made in the operating theater, and that there is a possibility that she may require a vertical incision.

KEY POINTS

Challenge: Transverse incision on the abdomen inadequate for surgery.

Background
- The choice of abdominal incision should depend on the pathology, proposed surgery, body habitus, abdominal scars, and the findings of examination under anesthesia.
- Transverse incisions may offer better cosmetic appearance, less pain, and low incidence of hernia formation. However, they are associated with poor exposure and access, greater blood loss, higher risk of hematoma formation and local nerve injury.

Prevention
- Comprehensive preoperative assessment, including ultrasound, CT or MRI, can help decide on the appropriate incision.
- Women waiting to have surgery for fibroids are likely to benefit from GnRH or ulipristal acetate therapy to reduce fibroid size.
- Thorough examination under anesthesia before commencing surgery is necessary to determine the optimal incision.

Management
- Improve access and exposure by modifying the Pfannenstiel incision to:
  - Cherney incision: transection of the rectus tendons from the pubic symphysis.
  - Maylard incision: transection of the rectus muscle after ligating the inferior epigastric vessels.
  - Inverted-T incision: addition of a vertical incision to the Pfannenstiel incision.
- Reduce the size of the uterus by first performing a myomectomy.

References

1 Makela JT, Kiviniemi H, Juvonen T, Laitinen S. Factors influencing wound dehiscence after midline laparotomy. *Am J Surg* 1995; 170:387–390.

2 Weiland DE, Bay RC, Del Sordi S. Choosing the best abdominal closure by meta-analysis. *Am J Surg* 1998; 176:666–670.

3 Cliby WA. Abdominal incision wound breakdown. *Clin Obstet Gynecol* 2002; 45:507–517.

4 Brand E. The Cherney incision for gynaecological cancer. *Am J Obstet Gynecol* 1991; 165; 235.

5 Rock JA, Jones HW (eds) *Te Linde's Operative Gynecology*, 10th edn. Lippincott Williams & Wilkins, Philadelphia, 2008.

CHAPTER 27
Previous Multiple Abdominal Scars

Mohammed Khairy¹ and Arri Coomarasamy²
¹Birmingham Women's NHS Foundation Trust, Birmingham, UK
²College of Medical and Dental Sciences, University of Birmingham, Birmingham, UK

Case history: A patient who had three previous abdominal surgeries via midline incision is scheduled to have a hysterectomy for menorrhagia, secondary to fibroids.

Background

Management of patients with previous multiple abdominal or pelvic surgeries represents a high-risk and surgically challenging situation. The risks and potential complications of pelvic surgery are increased because of the possibility of adhesions and distorted anatomy. There can be challenges in access and exposure, with subsequent increased risks of bleeding and bowel, ureteric and visceral injury. Other potential complications include development of severe sepsis, wound infection and dehiscence and, less commonly, adhesive bowel obstruction or enterocutaneous fistula. A particular risk of laparoscopic surgery in these women is "through-and-through" bowel injury at insertion of the primary trocar which may escape notice by an unwary surgeon [1].

The extent of the risk is mainly related to the indication and type of previous surgery and the type of incisions. The risk of bowel involvement is worse after midline incisions, especially those extending above the umbilicus, after surgery for peritonitis, oncologic procedures, radiation, or where bowel resection was performed [2].

Management

Pre-admission care

Consider alternative options
Given the risks associated with surgery, alternatives should be actively considered. For instance, the patient in the case history may benefit from levonorgestrel IUS, endometrial ablation, uterine fibroid embolization (UFE), or magnetic resonance-guided focused ultrasound (MRgFUS) treatment.

Discuss risks of surgery
Proper counseling should include the risks or potential complications of the intended surgery and how these can be minimized, as well as the consequences of these complications.

Arrange investigations
In addition to routine investigations to assess fitness for surgery, the patient should have specific investigations to assess the risks from previous multiple operations.

MRI of the abdomen and pelvis can be useful to assess the presence of any bowel loops attached to the anterior abdominal wall or the uterus. MRI will delineate the urinary tract and can detect hydroureter or hydronephrosis. CT with contrast or MRI with intravenous urography (IVU) in combination (CT urography or MR urography) can evaluate the proximity of the ureters to any pelvic pathology (e.g., endometrioma, adnexal mass, or fibroid uterus) and help in the decision-making on whether ureteric stenting is required [3].

Liaise with other relevant specialists
With complex operations, it is necessary to discuss in advance with gastroenterology or colorectal surgeon and urologist to seek advice regarding the approach to surgery and to be available to participate in surgery if need arises.

Preoperative care
The following general measures should be used for patients with previous multiple abdominal surgeries.

Bowel preparation
The aim of bowel preparation is to reduce enteric volume and bacterial load, which can help with handling and packing of the bowel.

One method of bowel preparation is mechanical cleansing with either isotonic lavage solutions or enemas. Examples include use of sodium phosphate and a clear fluid-only diet from noon the day before surgery. This can be combined with chemical (antibiotic) preparations using minimally absorbable oral antibiotics such as neomycin or erythromycin and metronidazole [4,5]. The following regimen is an example of mechanical cleansing and antibiotic preparation.
- From 06:00 onwards on the day before surgery, only clear liquids allowed (e.g., broth, tea, fruit juices). This should continue for the rest of the day. No milk or dairy products allowed.
- At 07:00 on the day before surgery, a half bottle of Fleet Phospho-Soda (22 mL) diluted with 120 mL of water is taken.

Gynecologic and Obstetric Surgery: Challenges and Management Options, First Edition. Edited by Arri Coomarasamy, Mahmood I. Shafi, G. Willy Davila and Kiong K. Chan.
© 2016 John Wiley & Sons, Ltd. Published 2016 by John Wiley & Sons, Ltd.

- At 10:00 on the day before surgery, 1 g of oral neomycin and 400 mg of oral metronidazole are taken. Further doses of neomycin and metronidazole are taken at 14:00 and 18:00 on the day before surgery.
- Fleet Phospho-Soda is also given at 19:00 on the night before surgery. Clear fluids can be taken up to 2 hours prior to surgery.

Although literature from RCTs is still inconclusive on the effects of preoperative bowel preparations, some surgeons still recommend bowel preparations if bowel injury or involvement is likely [4,5].

Antibiotic prophylaxis

Administration of a single dose of broad-spectrum antibiotic parenterally 30–60 min before the start of surgery is recommended. If the surgery is prolonged over 3 hours, antibiotic administration may need to be repeated [4].

Intraoperative care

Positioning of the patient

When involvement of ureter, rectosigmoid or bowel is suspected and adequate exposure of these organs is required, it may be advantageous to place the patient in the low dorsal lithotomy (Lloyd Davies) position. This allows intraoperative pelvic examination and exposure of the bladder and rectum. An assistant can stand between the stirrups and help by elevation of vaginal apex if necessary. This position also allows assessment of bladder and rectosigmoid integrity, ureteric stenting, and rectal anastomosis if needed [4].

Abdominal entry and incisions

Despite all efforts at careful mapping of intra-abdominal structures, there will remain uncertainty about the position of viscera especially bowel when entering the abdomen. Virginal areas of the abdomen and non-classical incisions may be used to decrease risk of visceral injury (Figure 27.1). The left upper quadrant of the abdomen is often a virginal area, and a Palmer's point entry with a 5-mm laparoscope can be used to map adhesions and the position of bowel and other viscera before a planned laparotomy [2].

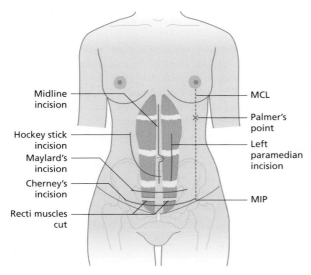

Figure 27.1 Abdominal incisions.

Open laparoscopic entry (e.g., Hasson technique) does not reduce risk of bowel injury. If conventional umbilical entry is used without prior Palmer's point entry, it is imperative to inspect the entry site perpendicularly and to withdraw the optics within the trocar to see if any bowel wall is seen, indicating transfixation injury of bowel loop under the umbilicus.

Other possible incisions that may be of use in these situations are the paramedian incisions and Maylard muscle-cutting suprapubic transverse incisions that can be transformed if needed into hockey stick (J-shaped) incisions for adequate exposure.

Adhesiolysis and restoration of anatomy

Once a safe abdominal entry is achieved, performing the intended surgery may be challenged by the presence of extensive adhesions with distorted anatomy and bowel involvement, impeding access to pelvic structures. The principles of dealing with adhesions include the following.

- Start with areas of recognizable anatomy.
- Follow the natural plane parallel to the recognizable viscera (e.g., a loop of bowel).
- Controlled traction and counter-traction will allow the visualization of anatomic planes: usually a thin white line is seen between the adhesions and their peritoneal attachment.
- Start with the translucent adhesions, which can be lysed sharply without difficulty.
- Use sharp dissection and avoid excessive tearing force.
- In case of dense adhesions, gentle blunt dissection and palpation with the index finger and thumb often allows identification of any involved bowel and can usually help to identify a translucent adhesive band that can then be dissected [5].

Use of extraperitoneal approach

This approach is invaluable in cases of large uteri or dense pelvic adhesions with high risk of injury to ureters (e.g., pelvic endometriosis) or in cases of malignancy. It involves opening the round ligament and extending the incision to the retroperitoneal space parallel to infundibulopelvic ligament above its crossing to the iliac vessels. The ureter will consistently be identified in the medial leaf of the broad ligament which can be mobilized medially and visualized throughout its course. This approach allows safe mobilization of the ureter, and the ligation of the uterine artery at its origin from the internal iliac vessel, in case of a hysterectomy. It also helps displacement of the bowel medially along the medial leaf of broad ligament and mobilization of bowel in case of bowel adhesions or injury [6,7].

Tests to check visceral integrity

Cystoscopy and confirmation of ureteric efflux with or without the use of intravenous methylene blue or indigo carmine dye should be used to confirm ureteric integrity in cases where an injury is suspected (Chapter 36). If this situation is foreseen, it might be prudent to insert a ureteric stent before starting the procedure. This will not reduce risk of injury but it allows easy identification of the site of injury.

To check for small bladder injuries, methylene blue dye diluted in sterile water can be instilled through an indwelling urinary catheter to identify watertight integrity [8].

Gas inflation of rectosigmoid with a Foley catheter and observation of its integrity under water (absence of gas bubbles) should be used whenever the rectosigmoid has been dissected off adnexae and uterus, or when an injury is otherwise suspected.

Small bowel loops can be checked by manual and visual inspection, starting from the ileocecal valve using hand-to-hand technique with milking movement to check for any minor cuts. Injuries are usually easily identified, with leak of bowel contents or evidence of thermal injury [5]. If an injury is suspected, management will need to be planned and implemented with the involvement of the relevant specialists (Chapter 37).

Prevention of adhesions

Because the risk of adhesion formation and its late consequences (abdominopelvic pain and intestinal obstruction) are high in these patients, it is important to take all possible measures to reduce the risk of reformation of adhesions or *de novo* adhesions. These measures include gentle handling of tissues, constant irrigation, meticulous hemostasis, minimal use of energy with preference for bipolar over unipolar energy, and avoidance of excessive suturing and use of less antigenic sutures on serosal surfaces. Use of agents that prevent adhesion (e.g., peritoneal instillates such as icodextrin 4%) has been shown to be effective in reducing the risk of adhesions following surgery.

A technique called "full conditioning" of the peritoneal cavity has been shown in an RCT to be effective in preventing adhesion formation. This technique comprises 86% CO_2, 10% N_2O, and 4% O_2, cooling of the peritoneal cavity, humidification, and use of heparinized rinsing solution and dexamethasone 5 mg [9,10].

Postoperative care

Postoperative feeding

Although early postoperative feeding is widely practiced in modern gynecologic surgery, it is prudent in cases with extensive bowel dissection and adhesiolysis to await evidence of bowel function and to gradually reintroduce normal diet.

Postoperative monitoring

Early recognition and management of the following symptoms and signs of postoperative complications are essential to reduce morbidity and mortality.

- Ileus: abdominal distension, vomiting, absent or hypoactive bowel sounds, tympanic note on abdominal percussion.
- Small bowel obstruction: abdominal pain, worsening bilious vomiting, hyperactive high-pitched bowel sounds and, in later stages, tenderness, rebound tenderness, and rigidity indicative of ischemic necrosis of bowel segments and peritonitis.
- Enterocutaneous fistula: similar to obstruction, followed by persistent or intermittent high-volume wound discharge with wound breakdown.
- Urinary obstruction: loin pain, fever, rigors, nausea and vomiting, hematuria, ascites, and peritonitis may develop in cases of undiagnosed ureteric or bladder injury.

These postoperative symptoms or signs should prompt appropriate diagnostic investigations (erect abdominal X-ray, water-soluble contrast CT with small bowel follow-through, or MR urography) and appropriate corrective measures.

Delayed bowel perforation and evidence of peritonitis may develop 72–96 hours after electrodiathermy injury of the bowel.

Postoperative thromboprophylaxis

Adequate thromboprophylaxis should be instituted with combined use of hydration, early ambulation, use of thromboembolic deterrent stockings, and low-molecular-weight heparin.

KEY POINTS

Challenge: Patient with previous multiple abdominal scars.

Background
- Surgery in patient with previous multiple abdominal scars can be challenging due to distorted anatomy and adhesions.
- Patients with multiple abdominal scars are at increased risk of bowel injury, ureteric injury, sepsis, wound dehiscence and, less commonly, enterocutaneous fistula.

Management
Preoperative care
- Consider alternatives to surgery.
- Discuss potential risks and benefits of surgery.
- Arrange appropriate imaging to assess risks of bowel and other visceral involvement (e.g., MRI of the abdomen and pelvis, CT urography).
- Bowel preparation with isotonic lavage solution is advisable in high-risk patients.
- Give prophylactic intravenous antibiotics 30–60 min before start of surgery.

Intraoperative management
- Careful choice of entry method and site of entry; a Palmer's point entry with a 5-mm laparoscope may be invaluable in these cases even before intended laparotomy to assess and minimize risk of bowel injury.

- Adhesiolysis and restoration of anatomy using principles of adhesiolysis outlined in this chapter.
- Use of extraperitoneal approach in cases of extensive bowel adhesions or large pelvic mass.
- Tests to check visceral (bowel, urinary bladder, ureteric) integrity as appropriate.
- Measures to prevent formation of adhesions (gentle handling of tissues, meticulous hemostasis, avoidance of desiccation, avoidance of use of antigenic materials, and use of adhesion prevention agents).

Postoperative care
- Vigilance for early symptoms and signs of visceral injury or dysfunction (e.g., ileus, bowel obstruction) is important.
- Appropriate investigations should be arranged to confirm or refute any suspected complication.
- Thromboprophylaxis is essential after complex surgery.

Prevention
- Careful planning can minimize the additional risks from previous surgery.
- Use of appropriate imaging will help plan the surgical approach.

References

1   Ahmad G, Duffy JM, Farquhar C *et al.* Barrier agents for adhesion prevention after gynaecological surgery. *Cochrane Database Syst Rev* 2008; (2); CD000475.

2   Nezhat C, Nezhat C, Nezhat F, Ferland R. Principles of laparoscopy. In: Nezhat C, Nezhat F, Nezhat C (eds) *Nezhat's Operative Gynecologic Laparoscopy and Hysteroscopy*, 3rd edn, pp. 40–56. Cambridge University Press, New York, 2008.

3   Silverman SG, Leyendecker JR, Amis ES Jr. What is the current role of CT urography and MR urography in the evaluation of the urinary tract? *Radiology* 2009; 250: 309–323.

4   Markham SM, Rock JA. Preoperative care. In: Rock JA, Jones HW III (eds) *Te Linde's Operative Gynecology*, 10th edn, pp. 113–132. Lippincott Williams and Wilkins, Philadelphia, 2008.

5 Molpus KL. Intestinal tract in gynecologic surgery. In: RockJA, Jones HW III (eds) *Te Linde's Operative Gynecology*, 10th edn, pp. 1097–1130. Lippincott Williams and Wilkins, Philadelphia, 2008.

6 Dubisson JB, De Dycker Y, Yaron M. The retroperitoneal approach in minimally invasive pelvic surgery. *Ann NY Acad Sci* 2006; 1092:187–198.

7 Hsu WC, Chang WC, Huang SC, Sheu BC, Torng PL, Chang DY. Laparoscopic-assisted vaginal hysterectomy for patients with extensive pelvic adhesions: a strategy to minimise conversion to laparotomy. *Aust NZ J Obstet Gynaecol* 2007; 47:230–234.

8 Nezhat C, Fisher D. Additional procedures for the pelvic surgeon: cystoscopy. In: Nezhat C, Nezhat F, Nezhat C (eds) *Nezhat's Operative Gynecologic Laparoscopy and Hysteroscopy*, 3rd edn, pp. 537–540. Cambridge University Press, New York, 2008.

9 Ten Broek RP, Stommel MW, Strik C, Van Laarhoven CJ, Keus F, Van Goor H. Benefits and harms of adhesion barriers for abdominal surgery: a systematic review and meta-analysis. *Lancet* 2014; 383:48–59.

10 Koninckx PR, Corona R, Timmerman D, Verguts J, Adamyan L. Peritoneal full conditioning reduces postoperative adhesions and pain: a randomised controlled trial in deep endometriosis surgery. *J Ovarian Res* 2013; 6:90.

CHAPTER 28

Patient with Previous Mesh Incisional Hernia Repair Requiring a Laparotomy

Christopher Smart[1] and Chris Keh[2]
[1] East Lancashire Hospitals NHS Trust, Blackburn, UK
[2] University Hospitals Birmingham NHS Foundation Trust, Birmingham, UK

Case history: A 44-year-old woman requires laparotomy for a large pelvic mass. Aged 27 she underwent lower midline laparotomy for perforated appendicitis. She developed an incisional hernia, which was repaired laparoscopically 7 years ago. She says "I think the surgeon put some mesh in."

Background

Laparotomy remains the mainstay for removal of large pelvic masses or pelvic cancer surgery. It is not uncommon that the operating surgeon will have to see, assess, and subsequently operate on a variety of patients that have had previous abdominal surgery.

The incidence of incisional hernia after major laparotomy is up to 20% but at least 10% of wounds will have a defect that is symptomatic [1]. Most present within the first year and the rates are doubled in the presence of infection at the index operation. Over 100,000 ventral incisional and primary hernia repairs are performed each year in the USA alone [2].

The modern management of incisional hernia is very varied and many techniques and meshes have been popularized over the last 20 years to try to surgically ameliorate this common problem. High rates of recurrence with suture repair (up to 54%) [3] have promoted the routine use of mesh to reduce recurrence rates [4]. Laparoscopic repair may have benefits in primary ventral or incisional hernia repair and the technique has been shown to be safe when compared with open surgery [5,6].

It is important to have a basic understanding of the different approaches to incisional hernia repair and the different meshes that are used, to enable a safe approach to managing patients who require a subsequent laparotomy. The large number of defects created, subsequent repairs, routine use of mesh, and vogue for laparoscopic surgery makes this a challenge for the operating surgeon. As patients live longer and more repairs are performed, we conclude this will become an increasingly common challenge.

Many patients requiring laparotomy may have had intra-abdominal meshes placed laparoscopically for the treatment of primary ventral hernia. Scars from this procedure may be difficult to see as there is no primary incision. However, these will generate the same issues of concern for the operating surgeon on entry to, and closure of, the abdomen. It is important to look for evidence of this repair, both clinically and in the past surgical history assessment. Most scars will be found laterally toward the mid-axillary line, as a lateral approach to port placement is required to facilitate mesh placement.

Similarly, some mesh techniques use a small incision in the skin and the rectus sheath but are used to place large meshes (up to 30 cm) caudally and cephalad undermining the respective layers (e.g., Stoppa repair).

Types of mesh and surgical approach

The combination of different types of mesh, surgical approach, and the layer in which the mesh is placed generates a large number of possible outcomes. They are all treated similarly at repeat laparotomy but knowledge of what might be found and in what layer may help the surgeon, especially if a mesh is unexpectedly encountered.

Mesh types

There are two types of mesh: synthetic meshes (e.g., polypropylene or polyester) and biological collagen-based meshes. Both are used as a material to reinforce or facilitate a hernia repair.

Synthetic meshes are subdivided into two broad types: simple or component meshes. Simple meshes are inert polymers that form a matrix for intense fibrosis to strengthen a repair. They cause a local reaction that changes the nature of the underlying and overlying tissues, and the subsequent fibrosis (characterized by an intense white reaction) reinforces what would otherwise be a weak repair. They are commonly used as they are cheap and readily available. They are generally used for repairs where the mesh is placed *outside the peritoneum* because of concerns of mesh enterocutaneous fistulation or adhesive small bowel obstruction.

Component meshes were conceived to combat this problem and allow intraperitoneal placement to facilitate repairs where mesh could not be placed outside the peritoneal cavity. These usually comprise one of the simple polymers but have a specialist layer that is hydrophilic in nature and safer in contact with bowel (e.g., Physiomesh™, Ethicon; Parietex™, Covidien). It is important to remember that these meshes are designed to facilitate regeneration of the peritoneum, with a full covering within 2 weeks. Subsequently, they can be difficult to see if the abdomen is opened away from the hernia site repair.

Gynecologic and Obstetric Surgery: Challenges and Management Options, First Edition. Edited by Arri Coomarasamy, Mahmood I. Shafi, G. Willy Davila and Kiong K. Chan.
© 2016 John Wiley & Sons, Ltd. Published 2016 by John Wiley & Sons, Ltd.

Biological meshes are normally porcine collagen-based matrices that are designed to be incorporated into the patient's tissues rather than rejected with the subsequent fibrous reaction. Their use is increasing as they offer a solution to incisional hernia repairs in cases where the risk of infection is very high (e.g., recurrent hernia due to infected mesh).

Surgical techniques

It is not necessary to know the intimate details of all types of repairs but some fundamental knowledge will help the operating gynecologist react to, and manage, patients with a previous mesh insertion.

Whether the mesh is placed laparoscopically or via open surgery is largely irrelevant, but all laparoscopic meshes are placed *within the abdomen* and normally fixed with a combination of sutures and tacking devices. In general, large meshes are used to obtain a greater than 5-cm overlap of the defects to reduce recurrence.

At open surgery there are three main layers where the mesh can be placed.

1 Intraperitoneal, using a specialist mesh as described (similar to laparoscopic repair).
2 Intramuscular layers, called "inlay" or "sublay" techniques: the mesh is placed in one of the potential layers in the musculature of the abdominal wall. A common eponymous description is the Stoppa repair, which puts mesh over a closed posterior sheath.
3 Onlay repair: the mesh is placed on top of a closed repair to reinforce it.

The layer in which the mesh is placed determines when it will be met on entry to the abdomen. If biological meshes are used, these can be difficult to determine as most are incorporated into existing tissues after remodeling.

Management

Surgical technique for entry to the abdomen

It is important that the operating surgeon should make every effort to establish the nature of the previous repair(s) before surgery is undertaken. As illustrated, previous mesh repairs can be a surgical challenge and help from a general surgeon or an experienced colleague is advisable. Adhesions are common and mobilizing small bowel can be time-consuming and demanding.

The basic principles of entry apply to previous mesh repairs or any previous laparotomy incision.

1 Try to enter in a virgin section of abdomen, either open or laparoscopically (Figure 28.1).
2 If entering through the old incision, expect the unexpected. The mesh will normally appear as a normal layer and can be cut with a knife or diathermy. Carefully dissect off any adherent bowel or omentum in the midline, working down the wound in section to allow all layers to be opened fully.

Closure of the abdominal wall

There is a paucity of evidence to direct an evidence-based approach to closure of the abdominal wall. The incision in the case history was closed routinely with mass closure using a non-absorbable suture to facilitate a lasting repair to hold the mesh together. In our experience, mass closure in clean or clean contaminated surgery is safe. In patients with gross contamination, an assessment of mesh

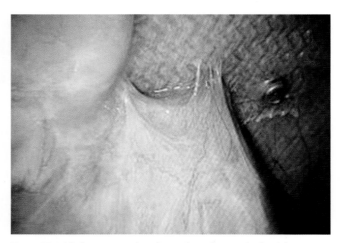

Figure 28.1 Mesh at reoperation: the mesh can be seen in the right upper section with peritoneum covering it, giving a chevron appearance. The small bowel is widely adherent and a metal tack is seen.

removal versus routine closure should be made. Mesh can be difficult to remove and adding extensive dissection to an already long operation may confer little benefit and create more problems than it solves. If there is concern over closing the abdominal wall after mesh removal, a biological mesh can be inserted.

The general surgeon may be of help in these scenarios, not only surgically but also in the decision-making process and the governance issues. A commitment to understanding previous surgical intervention and assessment of the potential pitfalls preoperatively is essential. This will enable a general surgeon to be involved if the clinician feels this is indicated.

The impact of a mesh can be very variable, ranging from cases where the operating surgeon is unaware when mesh has been dissected through, to the cases discussed here where careful dissection is required for a safe outcome.

KEY POINTS

Challenge: Patient with previous mesh incisional hernia repair requiring a laparotomy.

Background
- Primary abdominal and incisional hernias are common.
- Repair is normally augmented with a mesh in the modern management of hernia.

Prevention
- Aim to determine what type of repair has been undertaken and what mesh was used.
- Involve a general surgeon early in learning curve or with difficult cases.
- Look for the scars of hernia repair, particularly laparoscopic scars.

Management
- Keep to the basic surgical principles of entry into an abdomen with previous surgery (Chapter 27):
  - If possible, enter in a virginal section of the abdomen, either open or laparoscopically.
  - Layer by layer dissection.
  - Expect the mesh and adhesions to it and seek help where necessary.
- Mass closure of the abdomen should be safe with a non-absorbable suture to facilitate a lasting repair. In grossly contaminated cases, consider mesh removal but assess benefits with general surgeon before committing the patient to extensive dissection to remove the mesh.
- If mesh removal is performed, consider insertion of a biological mesh.

References

1 Israelsson LA, Jonsson T. Incisional hernia after midline laparotomy: a prospective study. *Eur J Surg* 1996; 162:125–129.
2 Rutkow IM. Demographic and socioeconomic aspects of hernia repair in the United States in 2003. *Surg Clin North Am* 2003; 83:1045–1051, v–vi.
3 Paul A, Korenkov M, Peters S, Köhler L, Fischer S, Troidl H. Unacceptable results of the Mayo procedure for repair of abdominal incisional hernias. *Eur J Surg* 1998; 164:361–367.
4 den Hartog D, Dur AHM, Tuinebreijer WE, Kreis RW. Open surgical procedures for incisional hernias. *Cochrane Database Syst Rev* 2008; (3):CD006438.
5 Salvilla SA, Thusu S, Panesar SS. Analysing the benefits of laparoscopic hernia repair compared to open repair: a meta-analysis of observational studies. *J Minim Access Surg* 2012; 8:111–117.
6 Sauerland S, Walgenbach M, Habermalz B, Seiler CM, Miserez M. Laparoscopic versus open surgical techniques for ventral or incisional hernia repair. *Cochrane Database Syst Rev* 2011;(3):CD007781.

CHAPTER 29

Patient with Previous Mesh Incisional Hernia Repair Requiring a Laparoscopy

Emanuele Lo Menzo, Samuel Szomstein, and Raul J. Rosenthal

Bariatric and Metabolic Institute, Cleveland Clinic Florida, Weston/Fort Lauderdale, Florida, USA

Case history: A 54-year-old woman with a history of morbid obesity and open abdominal hysterectomy developed a suprapubic incisional hernia. She underwent laparoscopic incisional hernia repair with a polyester-based mesh. She now presents with recurrent episodes of small bowel obstruction resolving with non-operative treatment. A CT scan shows a transition point in the right lower quadrant. Because of the multiple and close recurrent episodes, the patient was offered a diagnostic laparoscopy.

Background

Incisional hernias are a frequent complication of abdominal surgery and they occur in up to 20% of laparotomies [1,2]. Since up to 65% of ventral hernias repaired primarily will recur, tension-free repair with the use of mesh is now considered the standard of care for defects greater than 3–4 cm [3]. It is thus obvious that abdominal explorations in patients with previous mesh have become more prevalent.

For the safe laparoscopic approach of abdomens with previous mesh, a knowledge of the size, location and, if possible, the type of mesh (Chapter 28) would be beneficial.

Management

Patient positioning

The patient is positioned supine with all the pressure points adequately padded. Preoperative antibiotics are administered within 30 min of the incision and usually consist of a first- or second-generation cephalosporin. If both the operator and the assistant are expected to be working from the same side of the patient, the ipsilateral arm should be tucked along the body. The monitor is aligned with the targeted area and triangulation of the trocars and optics should be maintained whenever possible. Usually at least two monitors, one on each side of the patient, are required. Working against the camera should be avoided to ensure optimal dexterity, and angle laparoscopes (30 or 45°) are used to allow different views of the adhesions, in order to minimize bleeding and enterotomies.

Essential laparoscopic instruments include atraumatic graspers, scissors, and energy sources (diathermy and ultrasonic energy). It

is paramount to remember that different energy sources dissipate lateral energy in different amounts.

Abdominal access

Whenever possible, the laparoscopic access to the abdominal cavity should be gained outside the perimeter of the mesh itself, in order to avoid dense adhesions, viscus injury, and potential mesh infection. The outside perimeter of the mesh can be established by CT scan, if available, or by identifying the small scars of transfascial fixation sutures, if the previous hernia repair was done laparoscopically (Figure 29.1). Access can be gained by either open approach (Hasson technique), blind Veress needle insufflation, or by direct visualization of the abdominal wall layers via optical trocars. In general the subcostal areas are safer choices for access, as adhesions are less common in these areas. Although access with the Veress techniques has been proven to be safe, our preference is to utilize either the open Hasson technique or the optical trocar method, especially in obese individuals [4,5]. If access through the mesh is required, then an open technique with division of the mesh is the only option. Careful digital exploration would follow prior

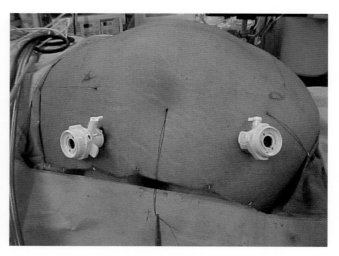

Figure 29.1 Transfascial sutures delineating the outside perimeter of the intra-abdominal mesh during laparoscopic ventral hernia repair.

Gynecologic and Obstetric Surgery: Challenges and Management Options, First Edition. Edited by Arri Coomarasamy, Mahmood I. Shafi, G. Willy Davila and Kiong K. Chan.
© 2016 John Wiley & Sons, Ltd. Published 2016 by John Wiley & Sons, Ltd.

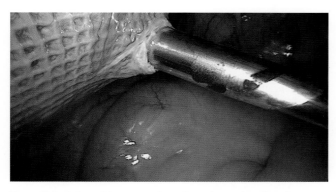

Figure 29.2 A 5-mm blunt trocar through a polyester-based mesh.

to insertion of the Hasson cannula in order to assure presence of adequate space. Whenever good mesh incorporation is found, and in the setting of lack of contamination, the old mesh can be simply reapproximated at the end of the procedure.

Insertion of the additional trocars should always be done under direct visualization, and in order to facilitate identification of the trajectory of the trocar a 14-gauge needle can be introduced through the abdominal wall. If necessary trocars can be inserted through the mesh, especially if not e-PTFE based (Figure 29.2).

Lysis of adhesions

Laparoscopic lysis of adhesions is feasible even in the presence of a small bowel obstruction as long as there is no massive abdominal distension limiting access to the abdominal cavity or limiting adequate working space. The laparoscopic approach is also indicated provided that there is no frank peritonitis, hemodynamic instability, or cardiopulmonary morbidity precluding the use of pneumoperitoneum [4].

The technique of the adhesiolysis should be tailored to the type of adhesions encountered. Fine filmy adhesions are easily approached with both blunt and sharp dissection, whereas the densely vascularized ones might require an energy source to limit bleeding obscuring the tissue planes; great care should be taken when applying thermal energy in proximity to bowel. In general the use of sharp dissection is preferred whenever the close presence of bowel cannot be ruled out, and some additional bleeding is tolerated more than a missed or delayed enterotomy (Figure 29.3). In fact, electrical injury to the bowel can manifest itself several days after the procedure. The entire tip of the instruments should be in view at all times in order to

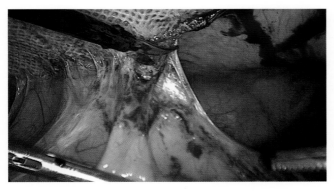

Figure 29.3 Gentle traction allows for visualization of a filmier dissection plane. Note the use of sharp dissection in the presence of bowel.

avoid unwanted injuries, and if the tips of the scissors can be visualized through the adhesions, these can be safely cut. Whenever the anatomy is unclear, changing the angle of view of the camera can help in better visualizing the loops of bowels. If visualization remains suboptimal, additional trocars should be inserted. The challenges of laparoscopic adhesiolysis are determined by the lack of free space to place working trocars, limited visualization, and presence of dense adhesions [4]. If the mesh–bowel interface is too densely adherent and separation might result in enterotomy, portions of the mesh can be detached from the abdominal wall and left on the bowel serosa, provided no evidence of erosion or obstruction is present.

Serosal tears should be promptly addressed and repaired with interrupted serosal apposition including the submucosal layer (Lembert sutures). Whenever a bowel loop is severely damaged or the repair might lead to a stricture, resection and re-anastomosis should be carried out. The latter can be delayed until the entire lysis of adhesions is completed, in order to address all the questionable area at the same time. It is recommended to mark the questionable areas as encountered, in order to avoid missing some of them and to expedite the evaluation at the end of the adhesiolysis. Depending on the skills of the surgeon, bowel repairs and resections can be accomplished laparoscopically or by limited laparotomies.

A totally laparoscopic approach offers a multitude of advantages. First, the incidence of additional ventral hernias is reduced from the 12.9% of standard laparotomy to 2.4% using laparoscopy [6]. Secondly, laparoscopy has also been well established in decreasing the incidence of wound infection and postoperative pulmonary complications and shortening hospital stay because of a more rapid return of bowel function and decreased postoperative pain [7].

Postoperative management

Early patient mobilization is a key aspect for expediting postoperative recovery and decreasing pulmonary complications. Mechanical and pharmacologic prophylaxis of deep vein thrombosis is routinely used in the perioperative period, and is continued based on the individual risk factors of the patient.

If extensive adhesiolysis or small bowel resection has been performed, nasogastric decompression is warranted until signs of bowel function recovery. Any delays in the normal postoperative recovery, unexplained elevation of the white cell count, or fever should be promptly worked up. Besides the common potential etiology of atelectasis and urinary and wound infections, early evaluation with CT is indicated to diagnose potentially missed enterotomies or anastomotic leaks. In the setting of clinical deterioration, with or without pertinent physical signs, early diagnostic exploration might be warranted. In fact, the sooner the enterotomy or anastomotic leak is diagnosed, the more favorable the outcome.

In the presence of small bowel enterotomy or small bowel anastomotic leak, resection with primary anastomosis is usually possible. Only in cases of hemodynamic instability and extensive fecal contamination should diverting ostomies be considered. In the latter scenario, meshes well incorporated to the abdominal wall can be left *in situ*, whereas if fecal contamination exists near exposed meshes, removal of the mesh is imperative. The subsequent abdominal wall closure becomes challenging and should be accomplished by primary technique (with or without fascial release) or by using biologic materials. As a last resort, temporary abdominal wall closure techniques can be performed with the intent of returning to the operating room for washouts and definitive closure in the following 24–48 hours.

Prevention

Laparoscopic re-exploration after placement of intra-abdominal mesh is feasible. Care must be taken during the initial abdominal wall entry, with preference for the bilateral subcostal areas or a non-meshed site. The laparoscopic lysis of adhesions has to proceed in a standardized fashion, maximizing traction and counter-traction to expose planes of dissection. In the majority of cases sharp and blunt dissection is used, and energy sources should be used sparingly and away from bowel. Any derangement from the standard postoperative recovery necessitates prompt work-up and even re-exploration if clinically warranted.

KEY POINTS

Challenge: Laparoscopy in a patient with previous mesh hernia repair.

Background
- Incisional hernias are a frequent complication of abdominal surgery and occur in up to 20% of laparotomies.
- Since up to 65% of the ventral hernias repaired primarily will recur, tension-free repair with the use of mesh is now considered the standard of care.

Management
- An abdominal CT scan can establish the outside perimeter of a mesh.
- Whenever possible, the laparoscopic access should be outside the perimeter of the mesh itself. The left (Palmer's point) or right upper quadrants are usually chosen.
- An open Hasson technique or direct visualization with optical trocar is usually preferred. If access through the mesh is required, then an open technique with division of the mesh is the only option.

- Lysis of adhesions should be done bluntly or sharply to avoid energy injury.
- If the mesh–bowel interface is too densely adherent and separation might result in enterotomy, portions of the mesh can be detached from the abdominal wall and left on the bowel serosa, provided no evidence of erosion or obstruction is present.
- Inadvertent enterotomies can be repaired laparoscopically or via a mini laparotomy.
- Any incision on the old mesh can be simply reapproximated at the end of the procedure.
- Any delays in postoperative recovery, unexplained elevation of the white cell count, or fever should be promptly worked up, and occult enterotomy should be high in the differential diagnosis.

Prevention
- Care is needed during initial abdominal entry, preference being given to the bilateral subcostal areas or a non-meshed site.

References

1 Burger JW, Luijendijk RW, Hop WC, Halm JA, Verdaasdonk EG, Jeekel J. Long-term follow-up of a randomized controlled trial of suture versus mesh repair of incisional hernia. *Ann Surg* 2004; 240:578–583; discussion 583–585.

2 Mudge M, Hughes LE. Incisional hernia: a 10 year prospective study of incidence and attitudes. *Br J Surg* 1985; 72:70–71.

3 Pierce RA, Perrone JM, Nimeri A *et al.* 120-day comparative analysis of adhesion grade and quantity, mesh contraction, and tissue response to a novel omega-3 fatty acid bioabsorbable barrier macroporous mesh after intraperitoneal placement. *Surg Innov* 2009; 16:46–54.

4 Szomstein S, Lo Menzo E, Simpfendorfer C, Zundel N, Rosenthal RJ. Laparoscopic lysis of adhesions. *World J Surg* 2006; 30:535–540.

5 Sato Y, Ido K, Kumagai M *et al.* Laparoscopic adhesiolysis for recurrent small bowel obstruction: long-term follow-up. *Gastrointest Endosc* 2001; 54:476–479.

6 Duepree HJ, Senagore AJ, Delaney CP, Fazio VW. Does means of access affect the incidence of small bowel obstruction and ventral hernia after bowel resection? Laparoscopy versus laparotomy. *J Am Coll Surg* 2003; 197:177–181.

7 Chopra R, McVay C, Phillips E, Khalili TM. Laparoscopic lysis of adhesions. *Am Surg* 2003; 69:966–968.

CHAPTER 30

Unexpected Pathology: Ovarian Cyst

Mohan Kumar

Good Hope Hospital, Heart of England NHS Trust, Sutton Coldfield, West Midlands, UK

Case history 1: A 30-year-old woman is undergoing a laparoscopy for suspected appendicitis; the appendix appears normal, but the surgeon notices a 6 × 6 cm cyst on the right ovary.

Case history 2: A 50-year-old woman presents with abdominal pain and constipation for over 1 week. Ultrasound scan shows small bilateral ovarian cysts and large bowel loaded with feces. During laparotomy for suspected bowel obstruction, surgeon notices bilateral ovarian cysts with metastasis to bowel and omentum and disseminated peritoneal deposition.

Background

Unexpected ovarian cysts are common, but the vast majority of cysts in premenopausal women are benign. Up to 10% of women will have some form of surgery during their lifetime for the presence of an ovarian mass. Most often women with ovarian cysts are asymptomatic and are diagnosed incidentally by imaging. Many cysts are simple and unilocular, and resolve spontaneously within three menstrual cycles. Up to 0.3% of symptomatic cysts are malignant in premenopausal women.

The unexpected finding of an ovarian cyst is a relatively common discovery during surgery, especially in emergency circumstances. Appropriate management at that time is often a challenge and will depend on the nature of the cyst. Gynecologists may be called to theater intraoperatively by the surgeons to given an opinion on an unexpected ovarian cyst. The gynecologist will need to make very careful assessment before deciding on management of the cyst, particularly in the context of lack of patient consent for any procedure on the ovary.

Adnexal cysts can be benign or malignant ovarian cysts, or indeed non-ovarian in origin (Table 30.1).

Management

To biopsy or not?

If the cyst is fluid-filled, a biopsy should not be attempted because of the risk of fluid leak that can upstage a cancer, if cancer is the diagnosis. If the cyst is solid, then biopsy may be taken along with peritoneal washings. If there are any depositions in other areas, then multiple biopsies may be taken to aid accurate diagnosis.

Table 30.1 Types of adnexal cysts.

Benign ovarian cysts

Functional cysts: follicular or corpus luteal
Endometriomas
Serous cystadenoma
Mucinous cystadenoma
Mature teratoma (dermoid cyst)

Malignant ovarian cysts

Epithelial carcinoma
Sex-cord stromal tumors
Germ-cell tumors
Secondary ovarian tumors

Non-ovarian cysts

Tubo-ovarian abscess
Fimbrial cysts
Hydrosalpinx
Appendicular abscess
Diverticular disease
Peritoneal inclusion cysts

When to operate on the ovary without consent

Management of unexpected finding of an ovarian cyst intraoperatively depends on the type and nature of the cyst. Careful assessment needs to be made to attempt to differentiate between benign and malignant cysts, and healthy and necrosed ovaries. A second opinion may have to be sought from another gynecologist, especially if the plan is to proceed with surgery on the ovary. If the cyst appears benign and the ovary is healthy, then no attempt should be made to remove the cyst or the ovary; management can be conservative, as most of the cysts will resolve spontaneously. If the cyst has undergone torsion and necrosed, then performing oophorectomy without consent may be justified as this would prevent another operation and associated risks.

Investigations for cysts diagnosed before an operation

If a cyst is identified before surgery, serum CA125 levels should be measured. If the woman is under 40 years, germ cell tumor markers including human chorionic gonadotropin (HCG), α-fetoprotein (AFP), and lactate dehydrogenase (LDH) should be measured. If cancer is suspected, CT scan of the pelvis, abdomen, and thorax is

Gynecologic and Obstetric Surgery: Challenges and Management Options, First Edition. Edited by Arri Coomarasamy, Mahmood I. Shafi, G. Willy Davila and Kiong K. Chan.
© 2016 John Wiley & Sons, Ltd. Published 2016 by John Wiley & Sons, Ltd.

recommended to determine the extent of the disease. Management plan should be discussed at an oncology multidisciplinary team meeting and the patient should be managed at a cancer center.

Common cysts and their management

Functional (simple) cysts
These are unilocular cysts that are benign and can be managed conservatively or surgically. If the cyst is more than 5–7 cm in size and persists over 6 months, laparoscopic cystectomy may be considered, if tumor markers (AFP, CEA, HCG and LDH in premenopausal women) are normal. In postmenopausal women, the risk of malignancy needs to be ascertained before planning surgery by calculating a risk of malignancy index (RMI). Aspiration of simple cysts either under ultrasound guidance or laparoscopically is less effective as it is associated with a high incidence of cyst recurrence.

Endometrioma
When performing surgery in women with an ovarian endometrioma, gynecologists should perform cystectomy instead of drainage as cystectomy reduces endometriosis-associated pain [1]. Many gynecologists will consider operating on cysts that are symptomatic or 4 or 5 cm or larger in size.

Dermoid cyst
Dermoid cysts are the commonest ovarian germ cell tumors. These are usually benign, but are a common cause of torsion. Laparoscopic cystectomy is the standard operation. All precautions should be taken to avoid spillage of the cyst as it may lead to chemical peritonitis. If the cyst is ruptured accidentally, thorough washing of the peritoneal cavity should be performed using warm saline.

Borderline ovarian cyst
About 15% of ovarian cysts are borderline tumors. They usually occur in young women. They have low malignant potential and have a very good prognosis. Surgical resection is the primary treatment. Referral to a gynecologic oncologist and a multidisciplinary approach should be considered as a borderline tumor can be difficult to differentiate from stage 1 ovarian cancer. They may be treated by cystectomy or unilateral oophorectomy in women who wish to preserve fertility. Pelvic clearance with hysterectomy and bilateral salpingo-oophorectomy is recommended in women who have completed the family.

Ovarian cancer
If a malignant ovarian cyst is suspected intraoperatively, care must be taken not to damage the cyst as this can potentially disseminate the disease. Multiple biopsies from the peritoneal surface, omentum, diaphragmatic surface, and any other lesions should be obtained along with peritoneal cytology. Small biopsy from the ovarian mass itself can be taken only in the solid areas; this can help in the accurate histologic diagnosis and aid decisions on neoadjuvant chemotherapy if the patient is deemed not suitable for primary debulking surgery.

Resolution of the cases

Case history 1
The surgeon needs to make a thorough assessment of the cyst; as the laparoscopy was performed for abdominal pain, there is a high possibility of torted ovarian cyst. If the ovary is torted, the surgeon can untwist the ovary to check whether it has retained its perfusion. In this age group it is very unlikely the cyst is malignant; therefore, an ovarian cystectomy can be performed if ovarian torsion is thought to be the case and the cyst does not appear to be malignant. If there is any doubt about the nature of the cyst, cystectomy should not be attempted. If the ovarian cyst is torted and necrosed, an oophorectomy may be carried out as this would be in the patient's best interest. After the operation the patient needs to be debriefed appropriately by the operating surgeon.

Case history 2
In this case, the patient was taken to theater by the colorectal surgeons for suspected bowel obstruction and the intraoperative findings were unexpected. When called for help, the gynecologist has to make a complete assessment of the pathology including the extent of disease to all intra-abdominal structures. This is most likely advanced ovarian carcinoma and if there is no bowel obstruction found, it is best not to proceed with the operation. Multiple biopsies from the different metastatic areas should be taken from peritoneal, omental, and diaphragmatic areas. Postoperatively, CT scan of the pelvis, abdomen, and thorax should be organized along with blood tests for tumor marker levels. Once all the reports are available, multidisciplinary management has to be considered. Once the type of ovarian carcinoma is confirmed, the patient may require neoadjuvant chemotherapy followed by delayed debulking surgery in a multidisciplinary setting at a cancer center.

Prevention

A complete preoperative evaluation of the patient can reduce the risk of surprises during surgery. A detailed clinical assessment, appropriate investigations, and imaging would lead to accurate diagnosis. As clinical examination is poor at identifying pelvic masses, and pelvic ultrasound is a ubiquitously available investigation, a case can be made for all patients to have a pelvic scan before abdominopelvic surgery.

KEY POINTS

Challenge: Patient with unexpected ovarian cyst.

Background
- Ovarian cysts are common in both premenopausal and postmenopausal women.
- Most ovarian cysts are benign. Only 0.3% of symptomatic cysts are malignant in premenopausal women.
- Adnexal masses:
  - Benign ovarian cysts: functional cyst, endometrioma, serous cystadenoma, mucinous cystadenoma, and mature teratoma (dermoid cyst).
  - Malignant ovarian cysts: epithelial carcinoma, sex-cord stromal tumors, germ-cell tumors, and secondary ovarian tumors.
  - Non-ovarian cysts: tubo-ovarian abscess, fimbrial cysts, hydrosalpinx, appendicular abscess, diverticular disease, and peritoneal inclusion cysts.

Prevention
- A full preoperative assessment including history, clinical examination (abdominal and pelvic), and ultrasound scan can reduce the risk of finding unexpected pathology at surgery.

Management
- When an ovarian cyst is seen unexpectedly at surgery, should it be biopsied?
  - If the cyst is fluid-filled, a biopsy should not be attempted due to the risk of upstaging possible cancer.
  - If the cyst is solid, then biopsy may be taken along with peritoneal washings.
  - If there are depositions in other areas, then multiple biopsies should be taken from the peritoneal surface, omentum, and diaphragmatic surface, along with peritoneal washings.
- Management of an unexpected ovarian cyst depends on the type and nature of the cyst. Careful assessment needs to be made to differentiate between:
  - benign and malignant cysts, and
  - healthy and necrosed ovaries.
- If surgery is proposed for unexpected ovarian cyst, and without prior patient consent, seek a second opinion from another gynecologist.
- If there is evidence of ovarian torsion or necrosis, it can be reasonable to operate on an ovary without prior patient consent.
- If a cyst is identified before surgery, assess the risk of malignancy and perform tumor marker tests: serum CA125, and in women under 40 years of age HCG, AFP, and LDH. If cancer is suspected, arrange CT scan of pelvis, abdomen, and thorax.
- Where malignancy is considered possible, prompt referral to a gynecologic oncologist should be made; a multidisciplinary approach in a cancer center is the standard of care.

Reference

1 Hart RJ, Hickey M, Maouris P, Buckett W. Excisional surgery versus ablative surgery for ovarian endometriomata. *Cochrane Database Syst Rev* 2008; (2):CD004992.

CHAPTER 31

Unexpected Pathology: Abnormal Appearance of the Uterus

Arri Coomarasamy

College of Medical and Dental Sciences, University of Birmingham, Birmingham, UK

Case history 1: During a diagnostic laparoscopy, the surgeon notes a uniformly enlarged "boggy" uterus.

Case history 2: During a diagnostic laparoscopy, the surgeon is concerned that an irregular and "lumpy" uterus could be a sarcoma. The serosa appears normal.

Background

Unexpected large uteri are common; they are often due to fibroids, the incidence of which is up to 25% of all women [1]. Although fibroids or other uterine masses are often diagnosed before an operation, occasionally the surgeon encounters a uterine mass intraoperatively. Diagnosis of some masses is straightforward (e.g., fibroids), while some can present a diagnostic challenge (e.g., adenomyosis or uterine sarcoma).

Management

Enlarged uterus

The key differential diagnosis, associated diagnostic features, and possible intraoperative actions are given in Table 31.1. Some women will have simple myometrial hypertrophy [2], which is regarded as a diagnosis of exclusion, after definite pathologies have been excluded.

Pregnancy

All patients should have a menstrual history taken and a pregnancy test performed (if pregnancy could be possible) *before* any operation, particularly if intrauterine instrumentation is planned. If a pregnancy test has been omitted, and an enlarged uterus is encountered, a small sample of urine can be obtained with a catheter and a pregnancy test can be carried out. If the pregnancy test is positive, intrauterine instrumentation should be strictly avoided, and uterine handling should be reduced to the minimum necessary. Other causes of a raised bHCG should be considered, particularly ectopic pregnancy and ovarian germ cell tumor (thus the ovaries should be examined). Occasionally, intraoperative transvaginal ultrasonography may be necessary and is straightforward to perform; however, this is only necessary if it is considered the

Table 31.1 Differential diagnosis for a uterine mass.

Differential diagnosis	Diagnostic features	Possible intraoperative actions
Pregnancy	Uniformly enlarged and "boggy" uterus. One ovary may be slightly enlarged with a corpus luteum	Unless the operation is urgent (e.g., cancer, ovarian accident), consider abandoning the procedure. Strictly no intrauterine instrumentation
Adenomyosis	Smooth enlargement of the uterus; possibility of coexisting endometriosis	None. Postoperative ultrasound or MRI
Endometrial cancer	Smooth or irregular enlargement of the uterus. Mass visible on speculum or easy bleeding on uterine instrumentation	Endometrial biopsy is indicated. An addition of hysteroscopy (even without prior consent) may be justifiable in the interest of patient
Uterine sarcoma	Smooth or irregular enlargement of the uterus; fibroid uterus	None. Postoperative MRI. No reliable tests, but rapid growth and indistinct borders should raise the possibility
Congenital uterine abnormalities	Typical appearance of various congenital abnormalities, including rudimentary horn, uterus didelphys or bicornuate uterus	EUA to assess for vaginal or cervical abnormalities (e.g., vaginal septum or double cervix). Postoperative three-dimensional ultrasound or MRI, and renal tract ultrasonography
Rare conditions to consider	Abnormal pregnancies (e.g., interstitial pregnancy, causing uterine cornual end enlargement; cesarean scar pregnancy, bulging under the bladder), uterine tuberculosis, pyometra, hematometra, and bladder or bowel tumor invading into the uterus	

diagnosis will influence management, which most often is not the case, and thus the ultrasonography can often be safely deferred to the postoperative period.

To biopsy or not?

When an abnormal mass is encountered, it is tempting to perform a biopsy. A biopsy can certainly be useful for diagnosing conditions such as adenomyosis [2], uterine sarcoma, or endometrial

Gynecologic and Obstetric Surgery: Challenges and Management Options, First Edition. Edited by Arri Coomarasamy, Mahmood I. Shafi, G. Willy Davila and Kiong K. Chan.
© 2016 John Wiley & Sons, Ltd. Published 2016 by John Wiley & Sons, Ltd.

cancer. However, if the serosa appears normal and has no breaches, a transmyometrial biopsy should not be performed. If the diagnosis does turn out to be cancer, the breach of the serosa from the biopsy instrument can upstage the cancer. If the serosa itself looks abnormal, a biopsy can be appropriate as there is no risk of upstaging a cancer. In all cases with abnormal and unidentified abdominopelvic masses, peritoneal washings should be taken and sent for cytology.

Transcervical biopsy

A Pipelle biopsy or curettage of the endometrium is a straightforward procedure with minimal risks, and can therefore be performed if necessary. As this may be regarded as an extended part of examination, many clinicians consider it reasonable to perform this even when prior consent was not specifically obtained for such a procedure. An early diagnosis of cancer can be to the patient's advantage.

Transmyometrial biopsy

If cancer risk is low and histologic diagnosis is considered to be useful for management, transmyometrial biopsies can be performed to confirm or refute the diagnosis of adenomyosis. Under laparoscopic guidance, a 14-gauge Tru-cut needle through the abdominal wall has been used for taking biopsies, and has been shown to have excellent accuracy for diagnosing adenomyosis [2]. It is necessary to take multiple biopsies (as many as 10) and to take the biopsies from the thickest myometrial areas and as close to the serosa as possible to avoid taking endometrial biopsies [2]. Pitressin (e.g., 20 units in 10 mL of normal saline) can be infiltrated into the myometrium to reduce the risk of uterine bleeding. An alternative to laparoscopically guided biopsies is the use of transvaginal ultrasound-guided myometrial biopsy [3]. Alternatively, performing an MRI scan after surgery would give a good indication as to the possibility of adenomyosis.

Abnormal serosal surface

An abnormal serosal or indeed any peritoneal surface could be due to primary peritoneal cancer (very rare), secondary peritoneal cancer (particularly from the ovary), borderline tumors of the ovary, pseudomyxoma peritonei, peritoneal mesothelioma, tuberculosis, pelvic inflammatory disease, endometriosis, and other causes. If any peritoneal abnormality is observed, the first step is to collect peritoneal washings for cytology; the surgeon will then need to perform a thorough examination of the peritoneal surfaces and obtain multiple peritoneal biopsies.

Resolution of the cases

Case history 1

The surgeon needs to exclude pregnancy with a urine pregnancy test. If the patient is pregnant, intrauterine instrumentation should be avoided, uterine handling should be minimized, and the operation may need to be abandoned unless it is considered urgent. If the patient is not pregnant, then the operation can continue as planned.

Case history 2

It is not possible to make a diagnosis of uterine sarcoma on laparoscopy. However, if the surgeon is concerned, postoperative investigations, particularly MRI of the pelvis, can be arranged. Transmyometrial biopsy should not be performed as it may upstage cancer.

Prevention

The key to avoiding surprises is to undertake a full preoperative assessment. In addition to a full clinical history, all patients should have either an abdominopelvic examination or pelvic ultrasound scan. Every female patient of reproductive age should have menstrual history taken and a pregnancy test performed on the day of or the day before the operation.

KEY POINTS

Challenge: Patient with abnormal appearance of the uterus.

Background
- Uterine masses are common, particularly fibroids, adenomyosis, and pregnancy.

Prevention
- A full preoperative assessment should include an abdominopelvic examination or, ideally, a pelvic ultrasound scan.
- All women of reproductive age should have a urine pregnancy test on the day of or the day before the operation.

Management
- When an enlarged uterine mass of uncertain nature is encountered, do *not* perform a transmyometrial biopsy as this may upstage a cancer; take peritoneal washings and fully examine the abdomen and the pelvis.
- Enlarged uterus: differential diagnosis and management:
  - Pregnancy: obtain urine with a catheter and check for pregnancy; do not instrument uterus; minimize handling of the uterus; abandon operation if non-urgent; consider other causes of raised bHCG (ectopic pregnancy and ovarian germ cell tumors); arrange postoperative ultrasonography.
  - Adenomyosis: continue with the scheduled operation; arrange postoperative ultrasound or MRI; laparoscopic-guided multiple Tru-cut biopsies are reported to have very high accuracy for diagnosing adenomyosis, but may not be necessary for clinical management.
  - Endometrial cancer: endometrial biopsy (Pipelle or curette) and consider hysteroscopy.
  - Uterine sarcoma: difficult to diagnose; arrange postoperative MRI.
  - Congenital uterine abnormalities: assess also for vaginal or cervical abnormalities; arrange postoperative three-dimensional ultrasound scan or MRI and renal tract ultrasonography.
  - Myometrial hypertrophy: diagnosis of exclusion, after significant pathologies have been excluded.
  - Rare conditions: abnormal pregnancies (e.g., interstitial pregnancy, cesarean scar pregnancy, trophoblastic disease), uterine tuberculosis, pyometra, hematometra, and bladder or bowel tumor invading into the uterus.
- Abnormal serosal (or peritoneal) surface:
  - Take peritoneal washings.
  - Examine abdominal and pelvic peritoneum and obtain multiple peritoneal biopsies.
  - An abnormal serosal or peritoneal surface could be due to primary peritoneal cancer, secondary peritoneal cancer (particularly from the ovary), borderline tumors of the ovary, pseudomyxoma peritonei, peritoneal mesothelioma, tuberculosis, pelvic inflammatory disease, endometriosis, and other causes.

References

1 Buttram VC Jr, Reiter RC. Uterine leiomyomata: etiology, symptomatology, and management. *Fertil Steril* 1981; 36:433–445.

2 Jeng CJ, Huang SH, Shen J, Chou CS, Tzeng CR. Laparoscopy-guided myometrial biopsy in the definite diagnosis of diffuse adenomyosis. *Hum Reprod* 2007; 22:2016–2019.

3 Walker WJ, Jones K. Transvaginal ultrasound guided biopsies in the diagnosis of pelvic lesions. *Minim Invasive Ther Allied Technol* 2003; 12:241–244.

CHAPTER 32

Unexpected Pathology: Severe Pelvic Adhesions

Stephen E. Zimberg and Michael L. Sprague
Cleveland Clinic Florida, Weston/Fort Lauderdale, Florida, USA

Case history: A 40-year-old female presents with complaints of pelvic pressure, menorrhagia, severe dysmenorrhea, dyspareunia, abdominal bloating, and anemia. Physical examination revealed a 14-week uterus that was tender to manipulation. Ultrasound showed an enlarged uterus with multiple small fibroids and heterogeneity consistent with adenomyosis. She has finished her childbearing and wishes definitive procedure. Of note, her past medical history is significant for a ruptured ectopic pregnancy at age 24 which required a laparotomy. The patient was scheduled for a laparoscopic hysterectomy. At the time of surgery, severe pelvic adhesive disease was encountered with small bowel adherent to the anterior abdominal wall completely obscuring the uterus. The uterus was firmly adherent to the anterior abdominal wall and bladder.

Background

One of the more vexing problems facing the laparoscopic surgeon, and indeed the general gynecologic surgeon, is the unexpected finding of severe pelvic adhesive disease at the time of surgery.

Adhesion formation

The problem is usually the result of previous surgery but can occur from endometriosis or pelvic and abdominal inflammatory processes, such as pelvic inflammatory disease or bowel disease. The pathogenesis is the result of damage to peritoneal surfaces resulting in the deposition of fibrin at the site of injury. Normally, fibrinolysis occurs as the tissues heal, but connective tissue scars occur and adhesions develop if the process is disrupted [1].

Similarly, the uterus is often adherent to the anterior abdominal wall after procedures such as cesarean delivery and myomectomy, and less commonly after tubal and ovarian surgery. The practice of non-closure of the peritoneum after cesarean delivery has contributed to the increased adherence of the uterus to the anterior abdominal wall and bladder, whereas closure of the peritoneum can result in markedly fewer adhesions [2].

Risks of adhesions

The clinical implications of adhesions include chronic pelvic pain, infertility, and intestinal obstruction. Indeed, the most common cause of small bowel obstruction is intra-abdominal adhesions. Long-term morbidity occurs in approximately 5% of all women who undergo open gynecologic surgery, risking adhesion-related

readmission up to 10 years from the original surgery [3]. The incidence of pelvic adhesions reported during second-look laparoscopy after surgery has been reported to be 50–100% [4].

Management

Entry into abdomen through a virginal area

When operating for pelvic pain, endometriosis, or adhesions, placement of a 3-mm or 5-mm trocar above the umbilicus for the laparoscopic telescope is preferable to the umbilical approach. This gives a greater panoramic view and is less likely to involve midline adhesions if they are already present. Similarly, the left upper quadrant approach (Palmer's point) will yield similar benefits with minimal risk. However, one caveat in using the left upper quadrant approach is in patients with previous bariatric sleeve surgery, as the port used to narrow the stomach is usually placed in the area that would normally be used for insertion. Remaining accessory trocars are then placed under direct visualization once the patient has been placed in the Trendelenburg position. Trocar placement will vary depending on the location of the adhesions and the best operative angle to achieve adhesiolysis.

Adhesiolysis

Traditional traction and counter-traction techniques are utilized to divide the adhesions using atraumatic graspers such as Debakey graspers. Scissors are optimal to lyse bowel adhesions as there is less danger of unintended thermal injury to sensitive structures. Most bowel adhesions can be divided with meticulous dissection as would be performed in open surgery. In the event of serosal damage to the bowel, oversewing the area with interrupted 3-0 Vicryl or PDS sutures is optimal, taking care not to narrow the lumen. For more involved injuries, consultation with a general surgeon is advised (Chapter 37).

For uterine adherence to the anterior abdominal wall, a harmonic energy device may be used. This allows division of the densely adherent tissue from the anterior fascia or musculature with minimal bleeding and minimal thermal spread. Moving the uterus away from the abdominal wall with traction and filling the bladder with dilute indigo carmine or methylene blue solution is helpful in delineating planes and identifying incidental cystotomy. In the event of injury, the bladder is repaired using a two-layer closure

Gynecologic and Obstetric Surgery: Challenges and Management Options, First Edition. Edited by Arri Coomarasamy, Mahmood I. Shafi, G. Willy Davila and Kiong K. Chan.
© 2016 John Wiley & Sons, Ltd. Published 2016 by John Wiley & Sons, Ltd.

with 3-0 Vicryl or PDS suture. The inner layer suture includes the bladder mucosa and muscularis and the outer includes the serosa. Retrograde filling of the bladder after repair will confirm closure and cystoscopy is warranted to evaluate the integrity of the closure and patency of the ureters (Chapters 35 and 36).

Lighted ureteral stent

An instrument that can be helpful in extensive adhesiolysis is the lighted ureteral stent (Figure 32.1). These can be obtained from Cook Medical (Bloomington, IN, USA) and are solid stents that are connected to traditional light sources. Lighting of the ureters along the pelvic sidewalls can be of significant value when planes are not apparent. The stents are easily removed at the end of the procedure [5].

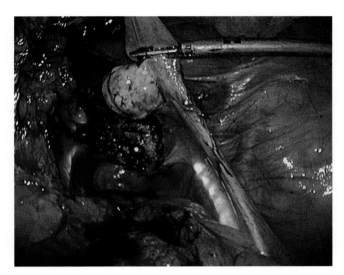

Figure 32.1 Lighted stents illuminating both ureters in a supracervical hysterectomy with adhesions.

While minimally invasive surgery is the ideal approach for adhesions, it is important to realize that occasionally this cannot be done safely via a laparoscopic route and a laparotomy will be necessary to complete the surgery. The criteria for conversion to laparotomy will vary depending on the skill set and experience of the surgeon, but the welfare of the patient should be paramount.

Prevention of adhesions

Obviously, prevention of abdominal and pelvic adhesions is preferable to having to deal with the immediate and long-term complications as well as reoperations. Prevention can be subdivided into surgical methods, barrier, and chemical substances.

Meticulous surgical technique includes minimizing tissue trauma, achieving optimal hemostasis, minimizing the risk of infection, and avoiding contaminants such as glove powder, urine, or fecal material. The Canadian Adhesion Prevention Task-force recommendations include performing surgical procedures using the least invasive method, preferentially a laparoscopic surgical approach, limiting packing, crushing and manipulation of tissues [6].

Barrier agents are devised to create a synthetic barrier between opposing pelvic structures and thus reduce adhesion formation. Oxidized regenerated cellulose (Interceed®) is a woven sheet that transforms into a gel membrane that lasts 2 weeks and has been

shown to reduce adhesions in open and laparoscopic cases. Interceed can actually induce adhesion formation by creating a stable fibrin matrix if blood is present. The barrier is placed over the injured area and is moistened with saline to keep it in place.

Sodium hyaluronate and carboxymethylcellulose (Seprafilm®) is a sheet placed over the injured areas and becomes a gelatin which is absorbed within 7 days and excreted within 28 days. It is approved for use in laparotomy but can be used laparoscopically by making a slurry of chopped sheets and saline to coat the desired areas [7]. Gore-Tex® polytetrafluoroethylene surgical membrane has also been shown to prevent adhesions but has the disadvantage of being non-absorbable and requiring suture fixation. A Cochrane review of barrier agents concluded that these reduce the incidence of postoperative adhesions but are not a substitute for good surgical technique [8].

Icodextrin 4% solution (Adept®) is the only approved solution for broad coverage in pelvic gynecologic surgery. It has been confirmed as safe but its efficacy is in question in preventing adhesion formation after surgery [9].

Conclusion

The discovery of severe pelvic adhesions at the time of pelvic surgery is a challenge requiring patience and sound surgical technique. Use of microsurgical and bowel surgical skills will help, and use of adhesion barriers will likely be of value in preventing further adhesion formation. No single technique or substance has been shown to work in all settings and the ability to shift to alternatives is important. Laparoscopy is the preferred approach but laparotomy may be necessary depending on the skill set of the surgeon and condition of the patient.

KEY POINTS

Challenge: Unexpected severe pelvic adhesive disease encountered during planned gynecologic surgery.

Background
- Pelvic adhesive disease is common after previous surgery, endometriosis, pelvic inflammatory disease, or inflammatory bowel disease.
- Pathogenesis results from damage to peritoneal surfaces, resulting in deposition of fibrin at the site of injury and inadequate fibrinolysis.
- Risks of adhesions include chronic pelvic pain, infertility, and intestinal obstruction.
- Long-term morbidity occurs in approximately 5% of all women who undergo gynecologic surgery, risking adhesion-related readmission up to 10 years or more from original surgery.

Management
- Initial abdominal entry in a virginal area: make a small (3 or 5 mm) initial incision above the umbilicus or in Palmer's point in left upper quadrant to allow for panoramic visualization and decreased risk of initial trocar injury. For upper abdominal or Palmer's point entry, first deflate the stomach with a nasogastric tube.
- Use conventional traction and counter-traction techniques to separate bowel loops and adhesions, with minimal use of energy devices.
- For uterine adhesions to the anterior abdominal wall:
  - Instrument the uterus and move it away from the abdominal wall in order to place adhesions under tension.
  - Fill the bladder with indigo carmine or methylene blue to delineate planes and identify incidental cystotomy.
  - Use harmonic energy device to dissect the dense adhesions.

- Place remaining ports under direct vision required by the pathology encountered. Do not be wed to the umbilicus or extremely low entry points.
- Use of lighted ureteral stents may be helpful in delineating anatomy in difficult cases.
- Conversion depends on skill set and experience of surgeon; safety and well-being of the patient are paramount.

Prevention
- Can be subdivided into surgical methods, barriers, and chemical substances.
- Meticulous surgical technique minimizing tissue trauma, achieving hemostasis, minimizing risk of infection, and avoiding contaminants is key.
- Closure of the peritoneal layers may reduce adhesions.
- Barrier agents create a synthetic barrier between opposing structures to reduce adhesion formation. Chemical substances such as 4% icodextrin solution are approved to minimize adhesion formation but challenges remain.
- Laparoscopy is the preferred approach for gynecologic surgery.

References

1 Imudia AN, Kumar S, Saed GM, Diamond MP. Pathogenesis of intra-abdominal and pelvic adhesion development. *Semin Reprod Med* 2008; 26:289–297.
2 Lyell DJ, Caughey AB, Hu E, Daniels K. Peritoneal closure at primary cesarean delivery and adhesions. *Obstet Gynecol* 2005; 106:275–280.
3 Al-Jabri S, Tulandi T. Management and prevention of pelvic adhesions. *Semin Reprod Med* 2011; 29: 130–137.
4 di Zerega GS. Contemporary adhesion prevention. *Fertil Steril* 1994; 61: 219–235.
5 Redan JA, McCarus SD. Protect the ureters. *JSLS* 2009; 13:139–141.
6 Robertson D, Lefebvre G, Leyland N *et al.* Adhesion prevention in gynaecological surgery. *J Obstet Gynaecol Can* 2010; 32:598–608.
7 Lipetskaia L, Silver DF. Laparoscopic use of a hyaluronic acid carboycellulose membrane slurry in gynecologic oncology. *JSLS* 2010; 14:91–94.
8 Ahmad G, Duffy JM, Farquhar C *et al.* Barrier agents for adhesion prevention after gynaecological surgery. *Cochrane Database Syst Rev* 2010; (2):CD000475.
9 Trew G, Pistofidis G, Pados G *et al.* Gynaecological endoscopic evaluation of 4% icodextrin solution: a European, multicentre, double-blind, randomized study of the efficacy and safety in the reduction of de novo adhesions after laparoscopic gynaecological surgery. *Hum Reprod* 2011; 25:2015–2027.

CHAPTER 33

Unexpected Pathology: Abnormal Appearance of Bowel

Olivia Will and Justin Davies
Addenbrooke's Hospital, Cambridge University Hospitals NHS Foundation Trust, Cambridge, UK

Case history: A 45-year-old woman with previous pelvic inflammatory disease presented with fever, offensive vaginal discharge, and pelvic pain. An ultrasound scan showed a left tubo-ovarian abscess. At laparoscopy, the sigmoid colon was found to have extensive diverticular disease causing a colo-vaginal fistula and pelvic abscess.

Background

Gynecologists not infrequently encounter intestinal pathology such as diverticular disease intraoperatively. Partly this is because symptoms such as lower abdominal pain, episodic pelvic discomfort, bloating, palpable lower abdominal masses, weight loss, and even vaginal discharge may have an intestinal or gynecologic etiology. Occasionally the preoperative history or imaging may be misleading and suggest gynecologic pathology as causative, but frequently the excellent intra-abdominal view afforded by laparoscopy leads to incidental diagnosis of intestinal conditions. Therefore, this chapter reviews both the common intestinal conditions that mimic gynecologic complaints, and those that are encountered unexpectedly during laparoscopy.

Management

At laparoscopy, a general surgeon can be consulted if unexpected bowel pathology is encountered. It would be impossible to totally avoid diagnosis of unexpected bowel pathology intraoperatively. However, focused questions in history-taking may help to identify patients with long-standing bowel symptoms who might benefit from preoperative CT scan, and preoperative planned referral to general surgery.

Appendicitis

Appendicitis and pelvic inflammatory disease (PID) can be difficult to distinguish at presentation. Both conditions are frequent in young women. Suggestive clinical history for appendicitis may include initiation of pain in the periumbilical area, anorexia, and diarrhea, whereas PID may be recurrent, associated with cervical or vaginal discharge, and have fewer signs of generalized sepsis [1]. Cervical motion tenderness will be present in appendicitis if there is

significant peritoneal irritation. Both conditions can often improve rapidly with antibiotics, and appendicitis may recur if non-operative management is employed. A CT scan can be helpful to visualize the appendix to confirm appendicitis, but entails radiation exposure, whereas pelvic ultrasound scans are frequently inconclusive, even when performed transvaginally. When an abscess has formed in the right iliac fossa, it may be difficult to identify its source with any imaging technique, and occasionally the tip of the appendix may become involved in a tubo-ovarian abscess. Therefore, the young female with pain in the right iliac fossa may pose a diagnostic dilemma for both general surgeons and gynecologists.

However, since a ruptured appendix may cause life-threatening sepsis, and further long-term complications of adhesional bowel obstruction and reduced fertility, laparoscopy is a safe diagnostic procedure where there is diagnostic doubt. If appendicitis is confirmed, the appendix should be removed. A laparoscopic approach also allows copious lavage of the abdominal cavity to be performed if there is an abscess or purulent peritonitis. Occasionally there is significant involvement of the cecal base, and general surgeons will often use a laparoscopic stapling device to deal with this situation.

Diverticular disease and diverticulitis

Diverticular disease is a common benign condition that is now increasingly seen in younger patients. Often noted incidentally as small pockets on the colonic surface, diverticular disease is frequently localized to the sigmoid colon, but is sometimes more widespread.

The term "diverticulitis" is used when there is acute inflammation associated with a segment of diverticular disease. Patients may present with lower abdominal or pelvic pain, often a constant ache that is made worse with movement or coughing. There is typically an associated fever and raised inflammatory markers. Diverticular abscess, like appendix abscess, may involve the fallopian tubes [2]. Sometimes, particularly in those who have had a hysterectomy, a diverticular fistula may connect bowel (most commonly the sigmoid colon) to the vaginal vault, causing fecal discharge and gas per vagina.

When encountered unexpectedly at laparoscopy, mild diverticulitis requires antibiotics only. If there is an associated abscess or purulent peritonitis with no clear site of colonic perforation, laparoscopic

Gynecologic and Obstetric Surgery: Challenges and Management Options, First Edition. Edited by Arri Coomarasamy, Mahmood I. Shafi, G. Willy Davila and Kiong K. Chan.
© 2016 John Wiley & Sons, Ltd. Published 2016 by John Wiley & Sons, Ltd.

lavage may be performed with abdominal drainage and continuation of antibiotics (in consultation with a colorectal or general surgeon). However, a perforation with fecal peritonitis requires immediate general surgical consultation and intervention as this is managed with a colonic resection and either end colostomy (Hartmann's procedure) or primary anastomosis with or without diverting loop ileostomy. In the case of less acute presentations, such as abscess or vaginal fistula, preoperative imaging (including CT with rectal contrast or pelvic MRI) is helpful to establish the diagnosis.

Meckel's diverticulum

A Meckel's diverticulum is a remnant of the embryologic vitello-intestinal duct and occurs in 1–2% of people. Usually this remnant is broad-based and 2–5 cm in length, seen on the antimesenteric surface of the small intestine approximately 60 cm from the ileocecal valve. Commonly, Meckel's diverticula are benign incidental findings, but some may contain ectopic pancreatic or gastric mucosal tissue which can bleed, cause pain, or lead to perforation and peritonitis. Diagnostic laparoscopy for abdominal pain should therefore always exclude the presence of a Meckel's diverticulum [3]. Sometimes they may remain attached to the undersurface of the umbilicus, usually by a fibrotic band, causing possible small bowel obstruction/torsion or intraoperative tethering of the bowel. If thought to be symptomatic they may be removed by a wedge excision and closure of the resultant enterotomy.

Inflammatory bowel disease

Inflammatory bowel disease – Crohn's disease or ulcerative colitis (UC) – may cause abdominal pain, diarrhea, and weight loss. Since UC usually causes more florid colonic symptoms like diarrhea and rectal bleeding, it is more usually Crohn's disease that presents unexpectedly to gynecologists. Sometimes abdominal pain may be the sole presenting feature of Crohn's disease, resulting in laparoscopy being performed for pathology such as ovarian cysts that were, in retrospect, incidental. At laparoscopy, the small bowel (usually the terminal ileum) looks reddened and dilated, with wrapping of the mesenteric fat around the bowel (a change pathognomonic for Crohn's disease [4]). Crohn's disease can lead to fistulation and possible resultant pelvic abscess or enteric fistula to the ovary, fallopian tube, uterus, or vagina.

Since resection is not curative in Crohn's disease, the surgical aim is to remove only bowel that cannot be rescued with medical therapy. Unsalvageable bowel may include fibrotic strictures and severely diseased bowel causing abscesses or fistulae. When encountered incidentally at laparoscopy, it is helpful for future management to "run the small bowel," documenting the number of sites involved; however, resection is often best avoided in this setting.

Bowel adhesions and strictures

Bowel obstruction secondary to adhesions usually presents to general surgeons with symptoms of acute bowel obstruction: cramping abdominal pain, distension, vomiting, and failure to open bowels. However, most adhesions seen at laparotomy or laparoscopy by gynecologists are usually long-standing. Adhesiolysis risks serosal tears and enterotomies, and may cause prolonged ileus postoperatively. Thus asymptomatic adhesions ought to be left undisturbed where possible.

Strictures of the small bowel may similarly present with acute bowel obstruction, but sometimes the obstruction may be of gradual onset. Therefore, loops of dilated small bowel may be found as an incidental finding, with collapsed loops seen distal to the obstruction. Radiation damage and Crohn's disease can cause multilevel narrowings, and intraoperative decision-making involves addressing only those areas which are causing symptoms [5]. Usually a short segment of obstructed bowel is resected, or a strictureplasty to widen the narrowed area may be considered in Crohn's disease. Since bypass of small bowel segments may cause bacterial overgrowth in excluded small intestinal loops, resection is performed where possible; however, bypass may be necessary in the palliative setting where it may not be possible to mobilize small bowel away from a tumor in the pelvis, for example. A third option is to perform a diverting stoma, which avoids anastomosis of thickened edematous bowel.

Bowel tumors

Colorectal malignancy is often asymptomatic, particularly when occurring in the proximal colon. Tumors may be noted incidentally if they have breached the serosal surface of the bowel, or if there is evidence of bowel obstruction. Colonic tumors may also be an underlying cause of fistulae and abscesses. Importantly, Lynch syndrome (HNPCC, hereditary non-polyposis colorectal cancer), a highly penetrant inherited predisposition for bowel cancer, may cause endometrial, ovarian, and colonic cancer, and cancers of the small bowel [6]. In addition, colorectal cancer may metastasize to the ovary(s), a condition known as Krukenberg tumor. Therefore bowel cancer is not infrequently seen in patients with malignancy of the gynecologic tract.

When encountered incidentally, immediate surgical management is not indicated. The diagnosis is usually confirmed by colonoscopic biopsy (unless there are obvious peritoneal nodules which can be sampled at the initial laparoscopy) and imaging undertaken for staging purposes. Further management is then decided by the multidisciplinary team, and may include options such as bowel resection with or without stoma, colonic stenting, and the possibility of neoadjuvant therapy.

Hernias

Incisional hernias often complicate entry into the abdomen. In the case of umbilical hernias, entry into the abdomen by entering the hernia sac is often straightforward, and careful closure of the port site will often suffice to coincidentally repair the hernia. Pneumoperitoneum may make inguinal hernias evident externally, and at laparoscopy bowel may be noted to enter the inguinal canal. Inguinal hernias and larger incisional hernias require a mesh repair; to reduce the risks of infection, hernia repair is best done as a stand-alone procedure where possible.

Incisional hernias arising from scars in the lower abdomen can be challenging to repair laparoscopically via a transabdominal approach. Since the bladder is an extraperitoneal organ, bladder expansion will tend to strip the mesh off the undersurface of the abdominal wall. For this reason, some surgeons repair this hernia by creating an extraperitoneal pocket for the inferior edge of the mesh.

Resolution of the case

Diverticular disease is increasingly common in younger patients, and is often asymptomatic. Spasmodic abdominal pain or changes in bowel habit due to diverticulitis may be ascribed to irritable bowel syndrome; and pelvic pain, fever, tubo-ovarian masses, and vaginal discharge may be thought to result from PID.

Immediate definitive operative management of the diverticular disease is usually not indicated, but the opportunity afforded by laparoscopy can help in two ways. Firstly, collections of pus can be drained, and laparoscopic lavage may also help to control infection. However, in cases of life-threatening sepsis and gross fecal contamination, an emergency Hartmann's procedure may be required.

Secondly, laparoscopy can allow a general surgeon an opportunity for planning future operative intervention in patients less acutely unwell. For example, he or she may want to ascertain the extent of the diverticular disease and the potential involvement of adjacent and retroperitoneal structures.

Prevention

A good clinical history and examination may allow some differentiation between gynecologic and intestinal causes; if bowel pathology is likely, appropriate investigations (e.g.,

CT with contrast) and a surgical opinion can help to reduce the risk of finding unexpected bowel pathology during laparoscopy by a gynecologist. Patients with pelvic pain or other symptoms may have coexisting bowel pathology; thus a diagnostic laparoscopy should examine the bowel, particularly the appendix and exclude Meckel's diverticulum. In cases at high risk of bowel pathology, having a general or colorectal surgeon on standby is prudent. If unexpected bowel pathology is identified and a surgeon is not available for an intraoperative opinion, a video recording of systematic examination of the bowel can help later review by the surgeon.

Conclusion

Intestinal disease may mimic, underlie, or coexist with gynecologic pathology. Close team-working between general surgeons and gynecologists will ensure the best outcomes for women with intestinal problems presenting to gynecologic surgeons.

KEY POINTS

Challenge: Bowel pathology encountered in gynecologic operations.

Background
- Bowel pathology is encountered frequently by operative gynecologists because of disease coincidence, misleading preoperative imaging, and incidental findings at laparoscopy.
- There is significant overlap in signs and symptoms of common gynecologic and bowel conditions.

Common bowel pathologies that mimic gynecologic conditions and which are often diagnosed on laparoscopy
- Infection and abscess:
  - Appendicitis
  - Diverticulitis
  - Inflammatory bowel disease
- Pain or mass:
  - Inflammatory bowel disease
  - Colonic tumors
  - Strictures

- Operative/postoperative complications: adhesions, hernias.
- Incidental oddities: Meckel's diverticulum.

Prevention
- Clinical history and examination to identify women at risk of bowel disease; if bowel pathology is suspected, appropriate investigations (e.g., CT with contrast) and preoperative surgical opinion.
- Given the risk of coexistence of gynecologic and bowel pathology, always examine bowel systematically, and rule out appendicitis and Meckel's diverticulum.
- In cases at high risk of bowel pathology, either operate with a surgeon or have a surgeon on standby.

Management
- Management depends on the pathology.
- Involve general or colorectal surgeons.
- Intraoperative consultation if required to aid postoperative decision-making.
- If unexpected bowel pathology is encountered and an intraoperative surgical opinion cannot be obtained, take a full video recording with systematic examination of bowel for later surgical review.

References

1 Rock JA, Jones HW (eds) *Te Linde's Operative Gynecology*, 9th edn. Lippincott Williams & Wilkins, Philadelphia, 2003.
2 Nichols DH, Anderson GW. *Clinical Problems, Injuries, and Complications of Gynecologic Surgery*. Williams & Wilkins, Baltimore, 1988.
3 Méndez-García CC, Suárez-Grau JM, Rubio-Chaves C, Martín-Cartes JA, Docobo-Durántez F, Padillo-Ruiz J. Surgical pathology associated with Meckel's diverticulum in a tertiary hospital: 12 year review. *Rev Esp Enferm Dig* 2011; 103: 50–254.

4 Sheehan AL, Warren BF, Gear MW, Shepherd NA. Fat-wrapping in Crohn's disease: pathological basis and relevance to surgical practice. *Br J Surg* 1992; 79:955–958.
5 Gershenson DM, DeCherney AH, Curry SL (eds) *Operative Gynecology*. WB Saunders, Philadelphia, 1993.
6 Win AK, Lindor NM, Young JP *et al.* Risks of primary extracolonic cancers following colorectal cancer in Lynch syndrome. *J Natl Cancer Inst* 2012; 104:1363–1372.

CHAPTER 34

Unexpected Pathology: Retroperitoneal Mass

Mohamed Mehasseb

Glasgow Royal Infirmary, Glasgow, Scotland, UK

Case history 1: A 37-year-old woman with chronic left lower abdominal pain is undergoing laparoscopic surgery for a suspected left ovarian endometrioma, suggested on ultrasound scan. Intraoperatively, the cyst is found to lie behind the sigmoid colon, in the retroperitoneum, and sitting closely or infiltrating the wall of the iliac vessels and the inferior vena cava/aorta. The left ovary is normal.

Case history 2: A 45-year-old woman presented with abdominal discomfort and bloatedness and a right lower quadrant abdominal mass. CT scan suggested an 8-cm heterogeneous mass in the right adnexal region, with right hydroureter and hydronephrosis. CA125 was normal. The general gynecologist proceeded with a planned hysterectomy and bilateral salpingo-oophorectomy through a Pfannenstiel incision to face normal ovaries and a retroperitoneal mass.

Background

Preoperative diagnosis of retroperitoneal masses can be deceptive. As ovarian and uterine masses are common, a gynecologic cause is typically suspected when a pelvic mass is discovered clinically or radiologically. Retroperitoneal masses can therefore be mistaken for gynecologic pathology, and can be seen as an unanticipated finding at the time of planned gynecologic surgery. Adult primary retroperitoneal tumors represent an uncommon but diverse group of neoplasms (0.2–0.5% of all malignant tumors). The retroperitoneal masses may be cystic or solid, and benign or malignant (Tables 34.1 and 34.2). The majority of solid retroperitoneal tumors are malignant (80%). Abdominopelvic pain or pressure is the commonest presentation, although symptoms could be non-specific or absent [1,2].

Retroperitoneal masses present the clinician with a diagnostic and management dilemma. Because of the clinical implications of and therapeutic strategies for retroperitoneal masses, the ability to differentiate between both entities using imaging criteria is desirable. However, a final diagnosis can sometimes only be made at the time of surgery or following surgical biopsy [2].

Anatomy of the retroperitoneum

The retroperitoneum extends from the diaphragm superiorly to the pelvis inferiorly and is situated between the posterior parietal peritoneum anteriorly and the transversalis fascia posteriorly

Table 34.1 Key features of cystic primary pelvic retroperitoneal masses [4,5,6].

	Clinically	Imaging
Cystic neoplasms		
Lymphangioma	In isolation or part of Klippel–Trenaunay–Weber syndrome	Unilocular or multilocular mass, crossing different compartments
Myxoma or pseudomyxoma	Fifth decade	High T2 MRI signal, mild or no enhancement, non-cystic appearance on USS, internal septa
Presacral teratoma	Children or adults, recurrent pilonidal infections	Fat/fluid level, cystic component, and calcification
Cystic mesothelioma	Abdominal pain	Multilocular
Mullerian cyst	Obese, on hormonal therapy	Unilocular or multilocular
Epidermoid cyst	Middle-aged, constipation	Unilocular, presacral area
Tailgut cyst	Any age, infection/malignant degeneration	Multilocular, presacral space
Degenerated paraganglioma or neurogenic tumor	Elderly, indolent, hypertension	Well-defined, complex mass, variable enhancement
Cystic non-neoplastic pathology		
Lymphocele	Surgery (lymphadenectomy)	Long-standing, thin irregular wall, extending between structures without luminal invasion
Urinoma	Trauma	Hydronephrosis
Hematoma	Trauma	Hyper-attenuating lesion with fluid
Congenital pelvic arteriovenous malformation	Chronic pelvic pain, vaginal bleeding, hematuria, and a pulsatile mass	Multiple feeding vessels, with early opacification of the draining vein
Klippel–Trenaunay–Weber syndrome	Sporadic, present at birth	Multiple venous varicosities, multiple phleboliths, coexistent lymphatic malformation

Gynecologic and Obstetric Surgery: Challenges and Management Options, First Edition. Edited by Arri Coomarasamy, Mahmood I. Shafi, G. Willy Davila and Kiong K. Chan.
© 2016 John Wiley & Sons, Ltd. Published 2016 by John Wiley & Sons, Ltd.

Table 34.2 Key features of solid primary pelvic retroperitoneal masses [4,5,6].

	Clinically	Imaging
Solid neoplasms		
Lipoma or liposarcoma	Elderly	Purely fat-containing mass (lipoma); solid components, local invasion, or distant metastases (liposarcoma)
Myelolipoma	Elderly	Presacral mass, containing fat and soft tissue
Retoperitoneal sarcoma	Non-specific	Heterogeneous, calcification, local invasion (possibly IVC) or metastases
Solitary fibrous tumor (SFT)	Fifth decade, 5% present with hypoglycemia	Hypervascular mass with a fibrous component, intense persistent arterial enhancement
Schwannoma	Asymptomatic, large	High T2 signal with moderate enhancement, along expected course of nerves
Plexiform neurofibroma	Neurofibromatosis type 1	Target-like pattern on MRI, bilateral symmetric pelvic masses, widening of neural foramina
Extraintestinal gastrointestinal stromal tumors	Extremely rare	Hypervascular mass with hypointense areas (fibrous component) on T2 MRI
Extra-adrenal pheochromocytoma	Excess catecholamines, urinary levels of vanillylmandelic acid and serum norepinephrine	Below aortic bifurcation, T2 MRI hyperintense, hypervascular mass
Solid non-neoplastic pathology (rare)		
Rejected transplant kidney	Prior surgery	Cortical calcification, evidence of vascular anastomosis to iliac vessels

(Figure 34.1). The retroperitoneum is broadly divided into the anterior and posterior pararenal, perirenal, and great vessels spaces. The anterior pararenal space is subdivided into the pancreatico-duodenal and the pericolonic spaces. The great vessels space is the fat-containing region that surrounds the aorta and the inferior vena cava (IVC) and lies anterior to the vertebral bodies and psoas muscles. Below the level of the kidneys, the anterior and posterior pararenal spaces merge to form the infrarenal retroperitoneal space, which communicates inferiorly with the prevesical space and extraperitoneal compartments of the pelvis. The pelvic retroperitoneum forms a part of the pelvic extraperitoneal space but is less well understood than the abdominal retroperitoneum, and includes: (i) the region within the pelvis posterior to the parietal peritoneal reflection, and (ii) the presacral and retrorectal spaces.

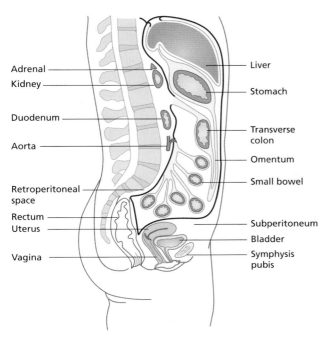

Figure 34.1 Anatomy of the retroperitoneum.

Management

Faced with an unanticipated retroperitoneal mass, the surgeon has to consider several issues: deciding on the most appropriate action, the absence of consent for additional procedures, any existing comorbidities of the patient, and the additional morbidity of any extra procedure. Surgical resection is technically challenging because of the large size often attained before the establishment of a diagnosis, the uninhibited growth, and the lack of fascial boundaries [3]. Their relative rarity, the lack of familiarity with the anatomy and pathologic processes of the pelvic retroperitoneum, and the proximity to vital vascular and neural structures as well as intra-abdominal organs add to the dilemma.

A multidisciplinary skill-mix, often not within the remit of the general gynecologic surgeon, is required for the optimal resection/management of these cases. Additional operations and/or procedures are often required to diagnose and plan the management of retroperitoneal masses, and the surgeon must consider his or her own limitations, the operating room and hospital facilities, and the immediate availability of additional surgical expertise and other services that might be required (e.g., vascular or urologic surgery).

The retroperitoneal space is deep, with rich vascularity. Thus, an adequate surgical incision and approach to allow exposure and easy hemostasis are important. As such, a midline laparotomy is advantageous. The surgeon faced with the situation might want to consider modifying the Pfannenstiel incision or converting to a midline incision (Chapter 26). Laparoscopic surgery can have its limitations in this context.

If resection is deemed feasible and the expertise is available, the "pseudomembrane" of the mass should be identified and dissection should be carried along this plane (less bleeding and prevents inadvertent injury of surrounding structures). The surgeon should control proximal blood flow before separating the tumor, and should have the techniques to handle and reconstruct injured vessels.

However, accurate and complete diagnostic and staging evaluation, before ultimate surgical intervention, provides the best option for the management of these retroperitoneal masses, particularly in case of solid masses. This may mean abandoning the current procedure without attempting removal of the retroperitoneal mass, obtaining a surgical biopsy, and deferring the ultimate treatment and further work-up until a definite diagnosis is established.

Prevention

All steps should be taken to minimize the chances of encountering an unexpected pathology during surgery. Although there is substantial overlap of imaging findings in various retroperitoneal masses (Figure 34.2), some specific features, along with clinical characteristics, may favor a specific diagnosis. Histologic examination is often required for definitive diagnosis. CT and MRI play an important role in characterization and in assessment of the extent of the disease and involvement of adjacent and distant structures [4]. Although CT is best for assessing calcification, MRI has superior soft-tissue contrast, which is useful for staging and the assessment of vascular invasion, as well as for evaluating the fat content of lesions. Ultrasonography plays a relatively limited role in the evaluation of retroperitoneal masses [4,5,6].

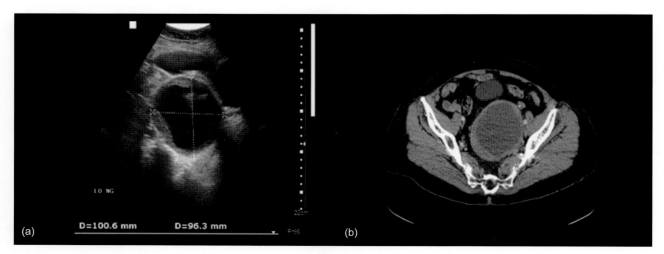

(a)   D=100.6 mm   D=96.3 mm   (b)

Figure 34.2 (a) Ultrasound scan and (b) CT scan of a schwannoma, mistakenly thought to be a left ovarian mass on preoperative diagnosis.

KEY POINTS

Challenge: Incidental finding of retroperitoneal mass during gynecologic surgery.

Background

- Primary retroperitoneal masses are rare (0.2–0.5% of all malignant tumors).
- Retroperitoneal masses can be mistaken for gynecologic conditions on clinical examination and imaging.
- The masses can be cystic or solid, and benign or malignant.
  - Cystic neoplasms: lymphangioma, myxoma or pseudomyxoma, presacral teratoma, cystic mesothelioma, Mullerian cyst, epidermoid cyst, tailgut cyst, degenerated paraganglioma, neurogenic tumor.
  - Cystic non-neoplastic pathology: lymphocele, urinoma, hematoma, congenital pelvic arteriovenous malformation, Klippel–Trenaunay–Weber syndrome.
  - Solid neoplasms: lipoma or liposarcoma, myelolipoma, retoperitoneal sarcoma, solitary fibrous tumor (SFT), schwannoma, plexiform neurofibroma, extraintestinal GIST, extra-adrenal pheochromocytoma.
  - Solid non-neoplastic pathology: rejected transplant kidney.

Management

- Surgical management of a retroperitoneal mass requires a diagnosis first, and therefore the appropriate course of action is generally to defer treatment until definitive diagnosis is established.
- If the mass is solid (i.e., not cystic or vascular) and the peritoneum has been breached, a biopsy can be taken to help with the diagnosis. If the peritoneum has not been breached, it is advisable to avoid an incisional biopsy because of the risk of seeding and peritoneal cavity contamination. This substantially decreases the cure rate and increases the risk of recurrent disease and death from retroperitoneal malignancies. A Tru-Cut needle core biopsy may be acceptable if hemostasis can be assured and contamination of the peritoneal cavity avoided.
- Surgical removal of retroperitoneal masses is often technically challenging due to the proximity of the mass to major vascular and neural structures, and should only be undertaken by an appropriately skilled team.

Prevention

- An important step that may reduce the risk of finding unexpected retroperitoneal pathology is careful examination of imaging results. CT and MRI can be useful in cases where uncertainty remains after abdominal or pelvic ultrasound imaging.

References

1 Cuschieri A. Disorders of the abdominal wall and peritoneal cavity. In: Cuschieri A, Steele RJC, Moossa AR (eds) *Essential Surgical Practice: Higher Surgical Training in General Surgery*, 4th edn, pp. 165–167. Arnold Publishers, London, 2002.
2 Murtaza B, Saeed S, Khan NA *et al.* Retroperitoneal masses: different clinical scenarios. *Journal of Ayub Medical College, Abbottabad: JAMC* 2008; 20:161–164.
3 Tseng WW, Wang SC, Eichler CM, Warren RS, Nakakura EK. Complete and safe resection of challenging retroperitoneal tumors: anticipation of multi-organ and major vascular resection and use of adjunct procedures. *World J Surg Oncol* 2011; 9:143.
4 Yang DM, Jung DH, Kim H *et al.* Retroperitoneal cystic masses: CT, clinical, and pathologic findings and literature review. *Radiographics* 2004; 24:1353–1365.
5 Rajiah P, Sinha R, Cuevas C, Dubinsky TJ, Bush WH Jr, Kolokythas O. Imaging of uncommon retroperitoneal masses. *Radiographics* 2011; 31:949–976.
6 Shanbhogue AK, Fasih N, Macdonald DB, Sheikh AM, Menias CO, Prasad SR. Uncommon primary pelvic retroperitoneal masses in adults: a pattern-based imaging approach. *Radiographics* 2012; 32:795–817.

CHAPTER 35
Bladder Injury

Arri Coomarasamy[1] and Richard Popert[2]

[1] College of Medical and Dental Sciences, University of Birmingham, Birmingham, UK
[2] Guy's and St Thomas' Hospitals NHS Foundation Trust, London, UK

Case history 1: During a cesarean section, an unintentional 2-cm hole is created on the anterior bladder wall.

Case history 2: During mobilization of the bladder from the cervix in a hysterectomy, a 2-cm ragged hole is found to have been created in the posterior bladder wall.

Case history 3: A posterior wall bladder injury during a hysterectomy was repaired appropriately. The bladder was drained with a urethral and suprapubic Foley catheter, and the pelvis was drained with a Robinson drain. On the third postoperative day, copious amounts of clear fluid were noted in the Robinson drain, raising the probability of bladder leak.

Background

We address the management of bladder injuries in open surgery in this chapter. Laparoscopic management of bladder injury is addressed in Chapter 72, and the management of bladder injury during various urogynecologic procedures is addressed in Section 6.

The reported incidence of bladder injury varies between 0.5 and 2% of major gynecologic operations, with over 90% recognized and corrected intraoperatively [1,2]. Bladder injuries recognized and treated intraoperatively result in virtually no complications, whereas those that are unrecognized and therefore untreated can result in ileus, urinary ascites, intra-abdominal abscess, peritonitis, sepsis, and eventually vesicovaginal fistulae [3].

Risk factors for bladder injury include obesity, inadequate incision, large pelvic masses, congenital abnormalities, endometriosis, extensive pelvic dissection, bleeding from bladder base, previous pelvic surgery or cesarean section, malignancy, and radiotherapy [3].

Site and mechanism of injury

The typical site of injury is on the posterior bladder wall or between the ureteric orifices on the trigone, and injury often occurs while mobilizing the base of the bladder off the cervix and upper vagina. Another mechanism of injury is catching the posterior wall of the bladder with a suture while closing the vaginal vault. Injuries associated with cesarean section are often on the anterior wall or base of the bladder.

Direct mechanisms for injury are cutting, tearing, diathermizing, or including bladder in a suture; direct injuries are often immediately recognized and repaired, resulting in good outcomes. Indirect injuries result from devascularization, often due to injudicious dissection or

use of diathermy, or abscess formation around stitches; such injuries are often not diagnosed intraoperatively and can result in fistulae.

If the damage to bladder is not full thickness and only involves the muscularis and not the mucosa, then a "bubble" of mucosa can be seen bulging through the injury in the muscularis; in such a situation, the muscularis can simply be brought together with continuous or interrupted sutures, and the bladder drained for 7 days with a urethral catheter.

Management

If an injury is diagnosed, inform the anesthetist and the operating room staff, and seek the input of a urologist, particularly if the injury is suspected to involve the ureters. It is also important to give prophylactic antibiotics, for example intravenous gentamicin 3 mg/kg body weight.

Diagnosis of bladder injury

Straw-colored fluid (urine) in the operative field, blood in the catheter bag, or a difficult bladder dissection should initiate a meticulous examination of the bladder for injury. Water or dilute methylene blue can be introduced into the bladder via a urethral catheter to assess for a bladder hole. To define the extent of the bladder injury a cystoscopy or an intentional cystotomy (opening of the anterior wall of the bladder) may be necessary. If cystotomy is needed, first distend the bladder with 200 mL of water (and not saline because of the need for diathermy), then place stay sutures above and below the edges of the intended line of incision on the anterior bladder wall, and finally make a transverse incision with a diathermy knife.

Instruments and sutures

While a repair can be made with generally available instruments and sutures, the following are of particular value [4]: DeBakey vascular forceps (atraumatic and ideal for handling bladder mucosa and periureteric tissues); Lahey forceps (the right-angled forceps is ideal for going under the ureters for example); Babcock or Allis forceps (ideal for elevating edges); nylon tape or vascular slings; ureteric catheters (6–10 Fr); suprapubic catheter; Robinson drain; and fine absorbable sutures (e.g., 2-0, 3-0 and 4-0 Monocryl or Vicryl).

Gynecologic and Obstetric Surgery: Challenges and Management Options, First Edition. Edited by Arri Coomarasamy, Mahmood I. Shafi, G. Willy Davila and Kiong K. Chan.
© 2016 John Wiley & Sons, Ltd. Published 2016 by John Wiley & Sons, Ltd.

Bladder repair

The principles of bladder repair are tension-free approximation of bladder mucosa and muscularis, and continuous unobstructed bladder drainage. It is often necessary to extend the bladder incision or injury to better define the extent of the damage and to assess the base of the bladder and the ureters.

Closure technique

Although the bladder can often be closed with a single layer as a continuous suture, it is best repaired in two layers with 2-0 or 3-0 absorbable sutures. The mucosa is closed as a continuous layer (Figure 35.1). The muscularis can also be closed as a continuous layer (Figure 35.2); however, interrupted sutures to reduce tension are better when the bladder wall is thin or when the injury is on the posterior wall or the trigone (Figure 35.3).

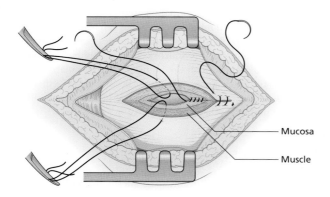

Figure 35.1 Closure of the mucosa of the bladder. From Popert, 2004 [4] with permission from Elsevier.

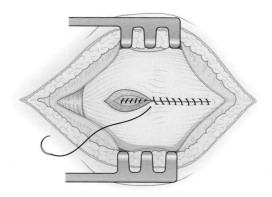

Figure 35.2 Closure of the muscle layer of the bladder. From Popert, 2004 [4] with permission from Elsevier.

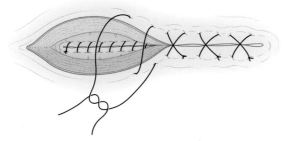

Figure 35.3 Interrupted suturing of the muscle layer of the bladder. From Popert, 2004 [4] with permission from Elsevier.

Posterior wall injuries

If there is injury to the posterior wall or the trigone, it is essential to assess the integrity of the ureters. This may require an intentional cystotomy on the anterior bladder wall (see Diagnosis of bladder injury above) and catheterization of the ureters, before the bladder injury is repaired. Ureteric catheterization can be performed with double-J stents, and fluoroscopy (or at least a plain radiograph) should be performed intraoperatively to ascertain correct insertion of the stents [5]; the stents can be removed 6 weeks postoperatively. With posterior bladder wall or trigone repairs, omentum can be mobilized and interposed between suture lines of bladder repair and vaginal vault closure to minimize the risk of fistulation [4].

Testing the closure

Once bladder injury has been repaired, the adequacy of the repair should be checked by bladder distension. If any leaks are identified, these can be closed with interrupted figure-of-eight sutures.

Bladder drainage

With difficult repairs, bladder drainage with both suprapubic and urethral catheter is advisable as this will avoid the risk of a solitary catheter blocking and causing vesical leak [4]. A suprapubic Foley catheter can be brought out through the bladder closure, although it may be safer to bring it out through a separate stab on the bladder (before the bladder is closed). The urethral catheter can be removed after 48 hours as the risk of blocking with a clot is negligible beyond that point. The suprapubic catheter should remain in place for 7–10 days, and can be clamped and removed if there are no significant residuals. If the patient has only the urethral catheter, this will need to be maintained for 7–10 days. If the repair is uncomplicated, then a cystogram is unnecessary but should be done if there is any concern about a possible urinary leak beyond 10 days. Most repairs heal with rest and time.

Pelvic drainage

With significant bladder injuries, a Robinson drain in the pelvis is mandatory to remove inflammatory exudate and any temporary urinary leak (not uncommon). This drain can be removed when the drainage is less than 25 mL in 24 hours.

Management of urinary leak

Postoperatively, if excessive clear fluid is observed in the pelvic drain, a leaking bladder or an unrecognized ureteric injury needs to be considered. A sample of drainage fluid should be sent for urea and electrolytes; if the urea and creatinine levels are equivalent to serum levels, then the drainage fluid is not urine, and both the surgeon and the patient can be reassured. If, however, the urea and creatinine levels are very high, then urine leakage is the diagnosis, and urgent investigations should be arranged to investigate and identify the location of the leak.

Relevant investigations include urinary tract ultrasound, cystogram (to assess for bladder leak), IVU (to assess for ureteric leak), abdominal CT cystography and, if appropriate, cystoscopy with retrograde study and stenting.

If the cystogram shows a leak from the bladder, the first step is to ensure that the suprapubic and urethral catheters are not blocked, by flushing them gently with 25 mL of saline. The urethral catheter can be changed for a larger one. Expectant management for a few days for the leak to dry up is then appropriate. Bilateral nephrostomies may be considered to encourage the leak to dry up. If the patient is unwell, a more aggressive approach is needed, and may include intensive management with antibiotics for Gram-negative bacteria, percutaneous nephrostomy, repeat laparotomy and repair, and bilateral intubated ureterostomies [4].

If intravenous pyelography shows a ureteric injury, this will require specialist management (Chapter 36).

Resolution of the cases

Case history 1
A standard two-layer closure with continuous suturing with a fine absorbable suture (2-0 or 3-0 Vicryl) is appropriate. The bladder should be drained for 7–10 days.

Case history 2
The integrity of the ureters should be assessed before repair is carried out; this is simply done by gently passing ureteric catheters or 6 Fr infant feeding tubes up the ureter. This may require an intentional cystotomy on the anterior bladder wall. The posterior defect should be carefully defined and can then be repaired with interrupted sutures in two layers. The initial closure should be intravesical and the muscular component may be more easily closed posteriorly on the outside across the site of the injury. Once the repair is completed and if the surgeon is happy there is no ureteric injury, then the ureteric catheters can be removed. The bladder and pelvis should have drainage, as discussed.

Case history 3
The drainage fluid should be sent for urea and creatinine to assess if the fluid is urine. If it is urine, ensure the bladder catheters are not blocked, and arrange a cystogram (to look for any bladder leak) and IVU (to look for any ureteric leak), and plan further management according to the investigation results.

Prevention

A high index of suspicion for bladder injury, deliberate check of the anatomy, and early recourse to necessary investigations are the keys to minimize complications. There should be a low threshold to involve a urologist if injury is suspected.

An empty bladder has a low likelihood of sustaining damage, and thus bladder catheterization is necessary for all significant pelvic operations. In patients at high risk of bladder injury, it may sometimes be better to open the bladder anteriorly or at the dome to aid dissection, rather than risk a large uncontrolled accidental damage. Meticulous sharp dissection with counter-traction on the bladder is the key to preventing a bladder injury.

KEY POINTS

(See also Chapter 72 and Section 6)

Challenge: Bladder injury in open surgery.

Background
- Incidence of bladder injury varies between 0.5 and 2% of major gynecologic operations.
- Bladder injuries recognized and treated intraoperatively result in virtually no complications.
- Unrecognized and untreated bladder injuries can result in ileus, urinary ascites, intra-abdominal abscess, peritonitis, sepsis, and vesicovaginal fistulae.
- Risk factors for bladder injury include obesity, inadequate incision, large pelvic masses, congenital abnormalities, endometriosis, extensive pelvic dissection, bleeding from bladder base, previous pelvic surgery or cesarean section, malignancy, and radiotherapy.
- Typical site of injury is posterior bladder wall or between the ureteric orifices on the trigone; injury occurs while mobilizing the bladder off the cervix.

Prevention
- Maintain a high index of suspicion in difficult cases.
- Keep bladder empty during all significant pelvic operations.
- Consider an intentional cystotomy if difficult bladder dissection is anticipated.
- Meticulous sharp dissection with appropriate counter-traction.

Management
- Involve urologist if the injury is near the ureters.
- Give intravenous antibiotics to cover Gram-negative bacteria.
- Diagnosis of injury and assessment of extent of injury may require instillation of dilute methylene blue in the bladder, cystoscopy, or intentional anterior bladder wall cystotomy.
- Ureteric stenting with double-J stents may be required if ureteric injury is suspected (likely with posterior bladder wall or trigone injury) before the bladder injury is repaired.
- Bladder repair:
  - Use 2-0 or 3-0 Vicryl.
  - Close mucosa with continuous suturing.
  - Close muscularis with continuous suturing; however, if the bladder wall is thin use interrupted figure-of-eight stitches.
- Posterior wall injury: interpose omentum between the bladder and the vaginal vault to minimize the risk of fistulation.
- Test the repair by distending the bladder with water.
- Drain the bladder with urethral and/or suprapubic catheter for 7–10 days. Dual catheterization will minimize the risk of bladder leak from the injury repair site from a blocked catheter.
- Drain the pelvis with a Robinson drain. Remove drain when drainage <25 mL in 24 hours.

References

1 Wharton LR. Methods of preventing injury to the ureters and bladder during gynecological operations. *Ann Surg* 1956; 143:752–763.
2 Graber EA, O'Rourke JJ, McElrath T. Iatrogenic bladder injury during hysterectomy. *Obstet Gynecol* 1964; 23:267–273.
3 Gomez RG, Ceballos L, Coburn M et al. Consensus statement on bladder injuries. *BJU Int* 2004; 94:27–32.
4 Popert R. Techniques from the urologists. In: MaxwellDJ (ed.) *Surgical Techniques in Obstetrics and Gynaecology*. Elsevier, London, 2004.
5 Monaghan J, Lopes T, Naik R. The management of injuries to the urinary tract. In: *Bonney's Gynaecological Surgery*, 10th edn. Blackwell Science Ltd, Oxford, 2004.

CHAPTER 36
Ureteric Injury

Arri Coomarasamy¹ and Richard Popert²
¹College of Medical and Dental Sciences, University of Birmingham, Birmingham, UK
²Guy's and St Thomas' Hospitals NHS Foundation Trust, London, UK

Case history 1: During a hysterectomy for a fibroid uterus, a ureteric injury is thought to have been caused in the vicinity of the uterine artery and the cervix.

Case history 2: During para-aortic lymph node dissection, a complete transection injury to the ureter is sustained at approximately 4 cm above the pelvic brim.

Case history 3: Five days after a hysterectomy, a pelvic drain is found to discharge large amounts of clear fluid; urea and electrolytes from the drain fluid showed very high levels of urea and creatinine, suggesting intra-abdominal urine leak. A CT scan with contrast found a leaking right ureter, approximately at the level of the pelvic brim.

Background

We address ureteric injury in open surgery in this chapter; the management of ureteric injury in laparoscopic surgery is addressed in Chapter 73.

The incidence of ureteric injury varies between 0.2 and 1% for most obstetric and gynecologic operations [1]. Many ureteric injuries are not recognized or reported, and thus the true incidence is likely to be higher than the reported rates.

Risk factors for ureteric injury include an enlarged uterus (particularly by cervical or broad ligament fibroids), previous pelvic surgery, ovarian neoplasms, endometriosis, pelvic adhesions, distorted pelvic anatomy, coexistent bladder injury (Chapter 35), massive intraoperative hemorrhage, radical hysterectomy, and history of pelvic irradiation.

Sites and mechanism of injury
The two common sites of injury are where the distal ureter lies close to the uterine artery, uterosacral ligaments or the vaginal cuff, and where the ureter crosses the pelvic brim at the base of the infundibulopelvic ligament. During laparoscopy the ureter is injured most frequently adjacent to the uterosacral ligaments [2].

The ureter may be injured in several ways. Intraoperatively, there may be ligation, crushing by a clamp, complete or partial transection, devascularization, or diathermy-related injury. In the postoperative period, avascular necrosis may occur following extensive dissection of periureteric tissue, crushing or diathermy injury, or compression from hematoma or other masses.

Management

As the ureter is the sole conduit from the kidney, renal deterioration is inevitable unless urine flow is restored. The key variables guiding a surgeon's approach to management include time of diagnosis, etiology, length and location of the injury, and the condition of the woman. The precise nature of the injury should be defined before deciding on the best method of repair. The management should be by a urologist. Prophylactic antibiotics should be given, and urea and electrolytes should be checked.

Diagnosis
Approximately half of the ureteric injuries are diagnosed intraoperatively and the other half postoperatively. Intraoperative diagnosis can allow prompt repair, resulting in better outcomes compared with postoperative diagnosis and repair.

Intraoperative diagnosis
A good method for diagnosing intraoperative ureteric injury is by entering the retroperitoneum and fully exposing the ureter. If this is not feasible, intravenous methylene blue or indigo carmine (5 mL) can be given to assess the integrity of the ureters. A cystoscopy will need be performed 10–15 min after the dye injection to visualize the two ureteric orifices; if blue urine jets are ejected from both ureteric orifices, then patency of the ureters is confirmed; if bubbles or blood-stained urine is seen and blue jets of urine are absent, the likely diagnosis is ureteric injury. Retrograde ureterography (Figure 36.1) can help to identify the nature and location of the injury.

Postoperative diagnosis
Clinical features are often non-specific and include fever, hematuria, flank pain, abdominal distension, peritonitis, ileus, sepsis, oliguria or anuria, and urine leakage from the vagina, abdominal wound or pelvic drain. Useful tests include urine culture, drain culture, renal ultrasonography, IVU and CT with intravenous contrast [1].

Gynecologic and Obstetric Surgery: Challenges and Management Options, First Edition. Edited by Arri Coomarasamy, Mahmood I. Shafi, G. Willy Davila and Kiong K. Chan.
© 2016 John Wiley & Sons, Ltd. Published 2016 by John Wiley & Sons, Ltd.

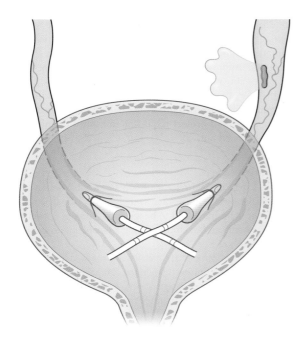

Figure 36.1 Retrograde ureterography to identify the nature and location of ureteric injury. From Popert, 2004 [3] with permission from Elsevier.

Management of intraoperatively diagnosed ureteric injury

Expose the ureter and identify the site of injury

The standard approach is to enter the retroperitoneum by opening the round ligament, advance through the loose areolar tissue on the lateral pelvic wall between the peritoneum and the iliac vessels, and identify the ureter attached to the pelvic peritoneum. Alternatively, the retroperitoneum can be entered at the pelvic brim and the ureter first identified at that level. The ureter can be slung to aid further dissection. The dissection can be advanced into the pelvis by dividing the adventitia overlying the division of the common iliac artery and the origin of the internal and external iliac vessels, and following it until its division into obliterated umbilical, superior vesical, and uterine arteries. The uterine artery can be ligated and divided, demonstrating the entire course of the ureter in the pelvis as well as the nature, length, and location of any ureteric injury.

Plan the repair

The surgical approach will depend on the nature and location of the injury. While the approach should be individualized for each patient, some guiding principles are provided in Table 36.1.

Injury to upper or middle third of the ureter: perform a spatulated end-to-end anastomosis (ureteroureterostomy) over a stent

The two transected ends of the ureter are cleanly divided (Figure 36.2a), spatulated (Figure 36.2b), and sutured using 4-0 Vicryl (Figure 36.2c). Spatulation refers to incising the cut ends of the ureter and splaying it open to create an elliptical anastomosis of wide circumference. The anastomosis needs to be tension free, and this may require mobilization of the ureter, or occasionally mobilization of the kidney. A watertight closure needs to be achieved, but the surgeon should be mindful not to use more stitches than necessary

Table 36.1 General principles for management of ureteric injury.

Injury	Management
Needle injury	No action needed unless bleeding or urine leakage
Partial transection	Repair over a ureteral stent
Transection away from the bladder (upper and middle third of the ureter)	Ureteroureterostomy (spatulated anastomosis) over a ureteral stent. If complicated injury, may require ileal conduit
Transection close to the bladder (lower third of the ureter)	Ureteroneocystostomy (ureteric implantation into bladder) over stent; with or without psoas hitch; with or without Boari flap
Ligation injury	Removal of the stitch, assessment of viability of the ureter and stent placement. If not viable, resection of the injured segment, mobilization of the ureter, and spatulated anastomosis over a stent
Thermal or crushing injury	Resection of injured area, and management as per transection

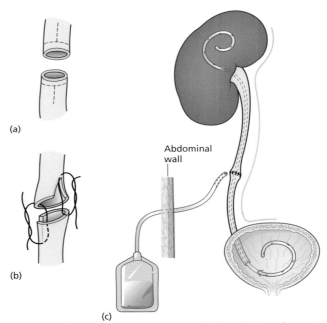

Figure 36.2 End-to-end ureteric anastomosis: (a) clean division of ureteric ends; (b) spatulated repair; (c) completed anastomosis. Adapted from Underwood, 2008 [4].

to avoid the risk of ureteric end necrosis and infection. An omental "wrap" can be used to cover the anastomosis to aid healing through neovascularization and to avoid the development of fibrosis.

Injury to lower third of the ureter: implant the ureter into the bladder (ureteroneocystostomy)

As the blood supply to the lower third of the ureter is more tenuous and can often be compromised after an injury, it is considered safer to implant the ureter directly into the bladder. It is also more difficult to mobilize the two ends of the ureter in the pelvis. The damaged distal part of the ureter, still attached to the bladder, can be simply ligated as it is no longer required. The damaged end of the proximal ureter is cleanly divided and implanted into a new point of entry into the bladder, over a ureteric stent (Figure 36.3). To achieve a

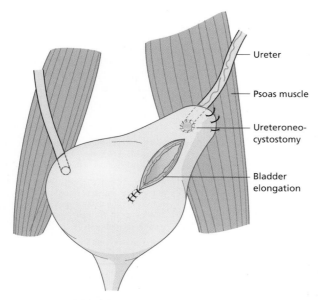

Figure 36.3 Psoas hitch. Adapted from Underwood, 2008 [4].

tension-free anastomosis, the bladder is mobilized from symphysis pubis, and if necessary elevated toward the ureter by a psoas hitch (Figure 36.3). The psoas hitch is a versatile procedure to bridge the gap between the bladder and the ureter, and is achieved by lifting the bladder up and suturing it to the surface of the psoas muscle. The Boari flap is another approach to bridge the gap between the ureter and bladder, and is achieved by fashioning a flap of bladder wall (Figure 36.4).

Complex ureteric injuries

If it is not possible to bridge the gap between the ureter and bladder, more complex operations such as a trans-ureteroureterostomy

(Figure 36.5) or an ileal conduit (Figure 36.6) may be necessary. A temporary measure is intubated ureterostomy in which an 8 or 10 Fr infant feeding tube is passed into the renal pelvis through a 0.5–1 cm ureterotomy or transected ureteric end at the level of the pelvic brim or above and well away from the pelvic injury; the distal end of the tube is exteriorized through an abdominal stab incision and sutured to the skin. This procedure will allow drainage of urine from the kidney, and protect renal function until definitive treatment can be carried out.

Postoperative care

The double-J stent in the ureter is usually left for 2–6 weeks to allow tissues to heal; however, in women with a history of pelvic radiation or fibrosis, the stent may need to be left for as long as 3 months [3]. The double-J stent can be removed using a flexible cystoscope in the outpatient clinic.

The pelvic or abdominal drain is left for a few days to assess for urine leak, and can be removed when the drainage is less than 25 mL in 24 hours. The bladder drainage is achieved by urethral or suprapubic catheters and needs to be retained for 7–10 days (Chapter 35).

An IVU or CT with contrast should be performed postoperatively to test the integrity of any anastomosis.

Management of postoperatively diagnosed ureteric injury

The principles of management are aggressive treatment of any infection, prompt (same day) drainage of the obstructed renal tract, and planning of definitive surgery for the ureteric injury. The drainage of obstructed renal tract can be achieved with a radiologically guided percutaneous nephrostomy, and it is essential to do this promptly to preserve renal function. When the ureteric blockage is due to compression from a mass (e.g., hematoma) or nearby surgical suture, it may be possible to pass a ureteric catheter to relieve the blockage.

There is debate over when definitive surgery for ureteric injury is best carried out, but generally this should not be

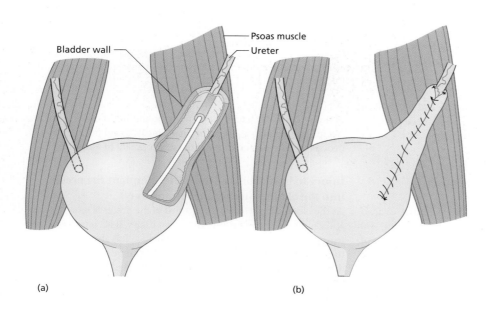

(a)   (b)

Figure 36.4 Boari flap: (a) development of the flap from the bladder wall; (b) suturing of the flap to form a tube. Adapted from Underwood, 2008 [4].

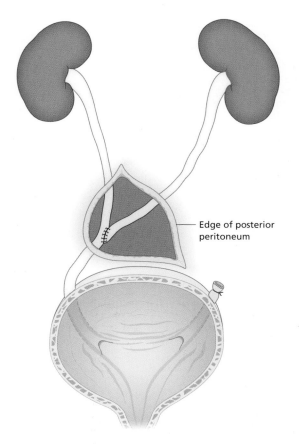

Figure 36.5 Trans-ureteroureterostomy. From Popert, 2004 [3] with permission from Elsevier.

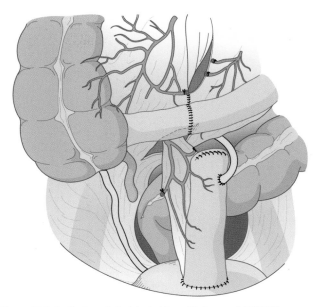

Figure 36.6 An ileal conduit. Adapted from Underwood, 2008 [4].

delayed, unless there is sepsis, abscess, hematoma, or the patient is unstable [1].

Resolution of the cases

Case history 1
Operating room staff need to be informed and intravenous antibiotics need to be given. Intraoperative diagnosis of ureteric injury can be made by exposing the ureter, and antegrade methylene blue injection combined with a cystoscopy. If ureteric injury is diagnosed within the lower third of the ureter, appropriate management can be ureteric reimplantation into the bladder (ureteroneocystostomy) over a stent with or without a psoas hitch or Boari flap. See previous text for postoperative management.

Case history 2
An end-to-end spatulated anastomosis (ureteroureterostomy) over a ureteric stent is appropriate management.

Case history 3
The patient's clinical condition needs to be assessed and any infection should be aggressively treated. An IVU or CT with contrast can be used to demonstrate the likely level of a ureteric injury. The obstructed renal tract needs to be relieved with a radiologically guided percutaneous nephrostomy. Once the patient is stable, definitive surgery for the ureteric injury can be carried out laparoscopically or via a laparotomy.

Prevention

Intraoperative measures to prevent injury include an appropriate operative approach, adequate exposure, full examination of the disease in the pelvis, and seeking early urologic assistance where appropriate. The key approach to prevent injury is constant awareness of the location of the ureter, and mobilization and direct visualization of the ureter when in any doubt. It is important to preserve the adventitia on the ureter during any dissection.

There is no evidence that preoperative IVU, CT, or stenting has any role in preventing ureteric injuries in routine gynecologic surgery; however, in complex cases, they may have a role. The complex cases where a preoperative IVU needs to be considered include women with procidentia, large adnexal masses, large cervical or broad ligament fibroids, or endometriosis [3].

If there is bleeding from around the cervix, it is important to resist the temptation to blindly underrun the bleeding area; with such an approach, it is easy to catch the ureter, which runs under the uterine vessels ("water under the bridge"). The safe approach is to define the anatomy, in particular trace the ureter (from the pelvic brim if necessary), dissect and sling the ureter, isolate and tie off superior vesical and uterine vessels, and once the ureter has been identified clearly the bleeding can be controlled safely.

Laparoscopic injury to the ureter is often diathermy-related; the surgeon needs to be mindful of the depth of penetration of diathermy effect, and minimize this by using short applications of diathermy.

Edge of posterior peritoneum

KEY POINTS

Challenge: Ureteric injury during gynecologic surgery.

Background
- Incidence of ureteric injury is 0.2–1% of obstetric and gynecologic operations.
- Risk factors include an enlarged uterus (particularly by cervical or broad ligament fibroids), previous pelvic surgery, ovarian neoplasms, endometriosis, pelvic adhesions, distorted pelvic anatomy, coexistent bladder injury, intraoperative hemorrhage, radical hysterectomy, and history of pelvic irradiation.
- The two common sites of injury are near the cervix and near the infundibulopelvic ligament.
- Ureteric injury mechanisms: ligation, crushing by a clamp, complete or partial transection, devascularization, or diathermy-related injury.

Prevention
- Appropriate operative approach and adequate exposure.
- Seek early urologic assistance where appropriate.
- Maintain constant awareness of the location of the ureter, and mobilize and visualize the ureter when in any doubt.
- Preserve the adventitia on the ureter during any dissection.
- Consider preoperative IVU, CT with contrast, and ureteric stenting in selected complex cases.
- Avoid blind underrunning of bleeding areas.
- Aim for short applications of diathermy near the ureter.
- Cool instruments which generate heat before touching the ureter.

Management
- Involve urologist.
- Give prophylactic intravenous antibiotics.

Diagnosis
- Confirm diagnosis intraoperatively by full retroperitoneal exposure of the ureter, and antegrade intravenous methylene blue, combined with a cystoscopy.

- Postoperative diagnosis of ureteric injury can be made by renal tract ultrasound, IVU and CT with contrast.

Ureteric injury management
- Needle injury: no action.
- Partial transection: repair over a ureteric stent.
- Ureteric injury in the upper or middle third of the ureter: ureteroureterostomy (end-to-end anastomosis) over a ureteral stent. If complicated injury, consider ileal conduit.
- Ureteric injury in the lower third of the ureter: ureteroneocystostomy (ureteric implantation into bladder) over stent; with or without psoas hitch; with or without Boari flap.
- Ligation injury: remove the stitch, assess viability of the ureter and consider stent placement.
- Thermal or crushing injury: resect injured area, and manage as above depending on the location of the injury.

Postoperative care
- Remove ureteric stent after 2–6 weeks; leave in for longer for those with pelvic irradiation or fibrosis.
- Remove abdominal drain when drainage <25 mL in 24 hours.
- Remove bladder catheter after 7–10 days.
- Perform IVU or CT with contrast postoperatively to test the ureteric repair.

Management of postoperatively diagnosed ureteric injury
- Treat infection and stabilize patient.
- Same-day drainage of obstructed renal tract with percutaneous nephrostomy.
- When the patient is stable, definitive management for the injury can be planned.

References

1 Jha S, Coomarasamy A, Chan KK. Ureteric injury in obstetric and gynaecological surgery. *Obstetrician and Gynaecologist* 2004; 6:203–208.
2 Grainger DA, DeCherney AH. Hysteroscopic management of uterine bleeding. *Bailliere's Clin Obstet Gynaecol* 1989; 3:403–414.
3 Popert R. Techniques from the urologists. In: Maxwell DJ (ed.) *Surgical Techniques in Obstetrics and Gynaecology*. Elsevier, London, 2004.
4 Underwood P. Operative injuries to the ureter. In: Rock J, Jones HW (eds) *Te Linde's Operative Gynecology*, updated 10th edn. Lippincott Williams & Wilkins, Philadelphia, 2008.

CHAPTER 37
Small and Large Bowel Injury

Howard Joy
City Hospital, Sandwell and West Birmingham Hospitals NHS Trust, Birmingham, UK

Case history 1: Small bowel enterotomy occurs during adhesiolysis of a patient with a previous laparotomy for appendicitis. No contamination resulted and injury was immediately recognized.

Case history 2: Two days after a radical hysterectomy for recurrent cervical cancer, a patient is noted to be systemically unwell, pyrexial and tachycardic, with an ileus and lower abdominal peritonism.

Case history 3: A patient who has undergone a hysterectomy for a large fibroid uterus 6 days previously presents with a wound infection. She is systemically well. Upon removing the skin staples, pus and small bowel contents are noted to discharge.

Background

Bowel injury is a well-recognized complication during both laparoscopy and laparotomy for gastrointestinal disorders and other pathologies not related to the bowel. Injury caused by laparoscopic instruments may occur out of view so may not be recognized promptly.

The principal risk factor is extensive adhesions due to prior surgery, particularly in the pelvis, where bowel may become densely adherent to the pelvic sidewalls and floor. Obstructed bowel is distended, delicate, and easily damaged by sharp or blunt dissection. Irradiated bowel, while no more prone to injury, is less likely to heal, thus favoring resection over repair of injuries.

Site and mechanism of injury

The stomach and the duodenum are rarely injured. Both are in the upper abdomen away from the pelvic organs. The duodenum is relatively protected as it is largely retroperitoneal.

The small bowel and sigmoid colon and rectum are the most commonly injured segments of the bowel during gynecologic surgery. The small bowel is most likely to be injured during adhesiolysis. The sigmoid is at risk during mobilization to identify the left ovarian vessels and ureter. The rectum is prone to injury during cervical mobilization and the development of the rectovaginal plane.

Injury may also occur to the large or small bowel mesentery. This is particularly likely during excision of visceral peritoneal nodules, typically during surgery for ovarian cancer and granulosa cell tumor.

Diathermy injury to the bowel can occur when using diathermy injudiciously close to the bowel. This is often a small-diameter burn of 1–3 mm, but full thickness. This does not usually cause

an enterotomy, and the white burn mark is often transitory, so this injury may easily be missed. A later postoperative perforation can develop, if the injury is not noted and repaired at the time.

Injury on entry into the peritoneal cavity may also occur due to adhesions to the anterior abdominal wall. This can occur during open and laparoscopic surgery. The incidence of bowel injury is said to be higher with Veress needle insertion compared with open Hasson entry, but there is no risk-free entry technique.

Management (see also Chapters 74 and 75)

Bowel injury is a potentially lethal complication. The time of diagnosis is the principal factor determining the outcome. An immediate intraoperative finding allows for minimal contamination and often a simple repair with minimal risks of complications. Delayed recognition, often several days later, may lead to profound physiologic compromise and peritonitis, with a prolonged complicated recovery requiring multiple procedures and critical care, or even death.

The risk of sepsis must also be considered in all patients. With any enterotomy, even without spillage of enteric contents, the procedure is clean-contaminated at best. Prophylactic antibiotics to cover Gram-negative bacilli and anaerobes (co-amoxiclav or gentamicin plus metronidazole) should be given if not administered on induction of anesthesia. If enteric or fecal contamination occurs, local control with aspiration and extensive lavage to clean the peritoneal cavity is essential. This should be augmented with a therapeutic course of antibiotics to cover the expected microorganisms.

Choice of operative approach for repair

The site and magnitude of the bowel injury, whether the damage is via a clean cut or with crushing of the edges, and the degree of devitalization are the main factors in determining the mechanism of repair (i.e., primary repair, resection or stoma formation). A clean cut, with no evidence of blood supply compromise, can be amenable to primary repair. If there has been substantial crushing or tearing of the edges, or if there is evidence of devitalization (e.g., darkening of the bowel), resection needs to be considered.

The physiologic status of the patient must be considered. Peritonitic patients are best served by defunctioning stomas, and lavage and drainage of sepsis. Furthermore, intraoperatively noted injuries may not be suitable for primary repair if the patient is hypotensive and hypothermic after prolonged operations with significant hemorrhage.

Gynecologic and Obstetric Surgery: Challenges and Management Options, First Edition. Edited by Arri Coomarasamy, Mahmood I. Shafi, G. Willy Davila and Kiong K. Chan.
© 2016 John Wiley & Sons, Ltd. Published 2016 by John Wiley & Sons, Ltd.

In such circumstances, compromised healing processes may lead to failure of technically adequate primary repairs.

Management of intraoperatively diagnosed small bowel injury

Small bowel serosal or seromuscular injury

Small (<1 cm) serosal or seromuscular injuries are most common with adhesiolysis. There is no associated contamination. Repair should be undertaken immediately because small injuries are often difficult to identify later. This is even more applicable to diathermy injuries because the obvious white mark of the burn fades rapidly, and the site of this potential full-thickness injury is usually impossible to locate later. Repair with interrupted, absorbable, seromuscular sutures (3-0 Vicryl or PDS on an atraumatic round-bodied needle) is sufficient.

Small bowel full-thickness injury

A full-thickness enterotomy may be suitable for a similar technique. It is usually sensible to request gastrointestinal instruments, as bowel clamps may be necessary to control ongoing contamination during the repair. Soft bowel clamps (Doynes) applied to the "first click" are usually sufficient to curtail gastrointestinal content without compromising bowel vascularity. After aspirating any enteric spillage, an assessment of the vascularity should be made. The small bowel has a rich blood supply, and so is usually very forgiving of injury repaired competently. Interrupted, absorbable, seromuscular sutures which invert the mucosa are needed. The repair must be performed transversely not longitudinally to avoid narrowing the bowel (Figure 37.1).

Ischemic bowel should be resected and a primary anastomosis performed, bringing together well-vascularized proximal and distal ends of bowel (Figure 37.2). This may be achieved with sutures or a stapling technique. Both techniques are equivalent in terms of patency and leakage. The differing opinions of surgeons are largely due to esthetic concerns, personal experience, and habit. A surgeon should perform a repair that he or she is most confident in performing.

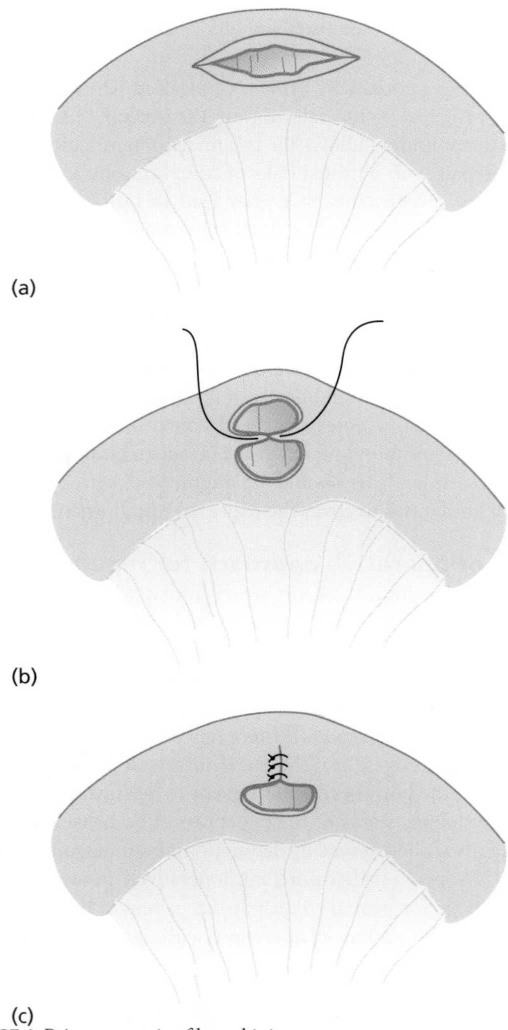

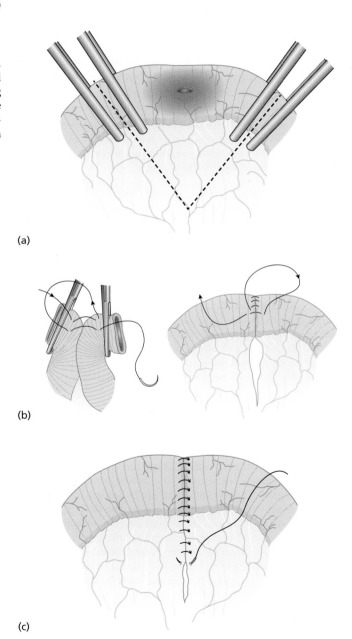

(a)

(b)

(c)

Figure 37.2 Resection and repair of small bowel: (a) resection of damaged small bowel; (b) suturing of small bowel; (c) closing of the mesenteric edges. From Monaghan et al., 2004 [1] with permission from Wiley.

(a)

(b)

(c)
Figure 37.1 Primary repair of bowel injury.

Bowel repairs and anastomoses can be covered by omentum. This may improve vascularity and seal tiny leaks. However, this may be merely calming the surgeon's nerves, akin to tucking one's children in at night, in other words a step that is not necessarily a bad move.

Mesenteric injury

A mesenteric injury requires careful assessment and management due to potential bowel ischemia. Simple visceral peritoneal defects do not require any repair. A full-thickness mesenteric defect should be closed to prevent a site of internal herniation. However, care should be taken to avoid large "bites" with the suture, as doing so will compromise the mesenteric vasculature and can result in bowel ischemia. Mesenteric bleeding can be controlled with judicious diathermy to tiny vessels or clip and ligature or underrunning suture of larger vessels. Good hemostasis is essential, not least because a subsequent mesenteric hematoma can cause ischemia of the overlying bowel.

After hemostasis or defect closure is achieved, a thorough assessment of the overlying bowel vascularity needs to be made. Ischemia may be evident immediately with a dusky appearance of the bowel. However, it is always prudent to check again at the end of the procedure, prior to closure, as ischemia may become apparent later.

Management of intraoperatively diagnosed large bowel injury

The principles detailed in the previous section also apply to the management of large bowel injury. However, the relatively poorer blood supply makes the colon less forgiving of injury, and more prone to leak from repair and anastomoses than small bowel; it is worth remembering the adage that the integrity of colorectal anastomoses is due to three factors: blood supply, blood supply, and blood supply.

Serosal and seromuscular tears may be primarily repaired if not too large (<1 cm). Full-thickness injuries need to be managed with much more caution. A primary repair can be performed safely if the vascularity is good, in other words a healthy bowel, small defect, young patient (no atherosclerosis), no mesenteric injury, no significant hemorrhage, and physiologically stable. If, however, there is any doubt about the vascularity, a formal resection should be performed. Indications for a resection include large defect, older patient with atherosclerosis, watershed area (splenic flexure), mesenteric injury, irradiated bowel, hemorrhage over 1500 mL, and physiologically unstable patient.

Despite the better vascularity of the proximal portion of ileocolic anastomoses, these concerns are still valid with right colon resections. Leakage rates from right hemicolectomies are similar to those from left hemicolectomies. However, the consequences are usually worse, with fecal peritonitis a typical presentation of an ileocolic anastomotic leak, compared with partially contained sepsis in the pelvis with a colorectal anastomotic leak.

Stoma

Following a resection, a decision needs to be made about anastomosis or stoma formation. Again, this is largely a question related to vascularity. If both proximal and distal ends of the colon or rectum are well vascularized and can be brought together without tension, an anastomosis is usually reasonable. Again, sutured or stapled anastomoses are equally valid. Exceptions need to be made where hemorrhage has been significant (>1500 mL), or when the patient is malnourished, physiologically unstable, or has residual

intraperitoneal cancer. With residual intraperitoneal cancer, a local recurrence at the anastomosis is highly likely, and can lead to obstruction. Care must also be given to the likely functional outcome of a low colorectal anastomosis in elderly women with poor anal sphincter function. Quality of life may be much better with a stoma than following a low anastomosis, with the attendant risks of significant urgency and fecal incontinence.

Any significant concerns over vascularity should prompt the surgeon to exteriorize the proximal end of the resection as an end colostomy or end ileostomy via a separate left or right iliac fossa trephine. It may be necessary to mobilize further the proximal bowel, such as by taking down the splenic flexure, to ensure adequate mobility and thus no tension. It is essential that the stoma, like an anastomosis, has a good blood supply. Poor blood supply is a particular challenge in obese patients where the subcutaneous fat may be more than 10 cm thick; in such patients, it may be safer to site the stoma higher than the umbilicus where the subcutaneous fat is considerably thinner. Ischemic stomas do not function, can necrose, and may retract into the peritoneal cavity. Significant necrosis and retraction often occurs 1 week postoperatively, which is about the worst time to re-enter the abdomen due to adhesions and friable bowel. This situation is sure to cause dread to colorectal colleagues, and all efforts should be made to prevent it.

It is also possible to defunction an anastomosis with a proximal stoma. Loop ileostomies are preferred to loop colostomies because a loop ileostomy is easier to manage and reversal is technically easier and less prone to leak. Low colorectal anastomoses are commonly defunctioned with a loop ileostomy. This does not reduce the leak rate, but it does reduce the consequences to local pelvic contamination rather than possible fecal peritonitis, as the fecal stream is diverted. However, this only applies if the colon is empty. Defunctioning an anastomosis with a colon full of feces makes no sense. Consequently, if a gynecologist suspects that the gynecologic procedure may require a left-sided bowel resection, preoperative bowel preparation (Kleen Prep, Picolax) should be prescribed. However, in the context of bowel injury, no such bowel preparation is likely to have taken place. This makes it more likely to need a resection with an end colostomy, rather than risk an anastomosis. It may be feasible to perform an on-table colonic lavage to allow an anastomosis and defunctioning ileostomy.

Reversing a loop ileostomy is a much more minor procedure than a Hartmann's reversal, with much less morbidity and fewer complications. Many patients with a "temporary" Hartmann's procedure never have it reversed because of lack of enthusiasm to undergo a further major operation by either the patient or the surgeon.

Management of postoperatively diagnosed bowel injury

An unnoticed bowel injury will leak gastrointestinal contents either immediately or after a few days when necrosis occurs from a full-thickness diathermy burn. Free leakage into the peritoneal cavity will result in fecal peritonitis. The patient will have significant pain, an ileus, and a rigid and tender abdomen, and be systemically unwell with systemic inflammatory response syndrome (SIRS). If inadequately treated, septic shock and death will occur. These, hopefully few, patients require prompt diagnosis and urgent resuscitation preferably in critical care with invasive monitoring, intravenous antibiotics and emergency surgery. Do not wait for confirmatory imaging in unstable patients. Fecal peritonitis is a clinical not a radiologic diagnosis. The cause of the sepsis is controlled by surgery with aspiration and lavage, resection of the injured segment of bowel, and proximal stoma formation. A colorectal injury or leak should not be managed by a local repair because of the very high risk of failure in a critically ill patient. Even small bowel injuries in this context require a cautious approach. Lavage and formation of a proximal stoma is always safer.

If the leakage is small and contained (e.g., in the pelvis), it may present insidiously with an ileus, fever, and a leukocytosis, without pain. CT with oral and intravenous contrast may demonstrate a pelvic or abdominal collection. This may be amenable to percutaneous drainage, intravenous antibiotics, total parenteral nutrition, and bowel rest. Diet can be restarted once drainage ceases and inflammatory markers normalize. Failure to respond or clinical deterioration should prompt urgent surgery.

A minor small bowel leak may also present as an enterocutaneous or enterovaginal fistula. Enterovaginal fistulae always require surgical repair. Enterocutaneous fistulae commonly present as a wound infection about 5 days postoperatively, with an associated ileus. On removing the skin sutures or staples to drain the expected pus, the enteric leak becomes evident. If the injury is small and the underlying bowel is healthy with no distal obstruction, an enterocutaneous fistula may be managed conservatively. This is most appropriately done in the hands of colorectal colleagues according to the principles of SNAPP (sepsis, nutrition, assess anatomy, protect skin, planned surgery). Again, failure to respond or deterioration should prompt urgent surgery.

Postoperative management

After repair or resection of bowel, postoperative management is largely the same as following major gynecologic surgery. If there was no contamination, only prophylactic antibiotics are required. If there was contamination, a full 5-day therapeutic antibiotic course is required.

There is no advantage in resting the bowel after successful repair or resection. The gut obtains its nutrition principally from the lumen, and not intravascularly as other organs. It requires luminal nutrition to maintain mucosal integrity and the gut mucosal barrier to bacterial translocation. Normal diet should be instituted as soon as it can be tolerated. Early oral nutrition is a key feature of enhanced recovery. Clearly this does not apply to a patient with ileus or suspected ongoing bowel leak.

Patients can be discharged once comfortable with oral analgesia, independently mobile, tolerating a normal diet, and have their bowel open or are managing their stoma.

Resolution of the cases

Case history 1

Intravenous antibiotics should be administered if not previously given on induction of anesthesia. Soft bowel clamps are applied to prevent enteric spillage. A primary transverse repair is performed with interrupted, absorbable, seromuscular sutures. A thorough washout is performed at the end of the procedure.

Case history 2

Fecal peritonitis is diagnosed. Prompt resuscitation is performed while the patient is transferred to critical care for invasive monitoring. Intravenous antibiotics should be given. Once resuscitation is adequate, an emergency laparotomy should be performed. The contamination should be cleared and the site of leak identified, mobilized, resected, and an end stoma fashioned.

Case history 3

An enterocutaneous fistula is diagnosed and the patient should be referred to colorectal surgeons for SNAPP management:

- Sepsis: intravenous antibiotics and percutaneous drainage of intra-abdominal collection.
- Nutrition: NBM, TPN, bowel rest with loperamide, codeine, octreotide and proton pump inhibitors.
- Assess anatomy: CT with oral and intravenous contrast, small bowel meal, and fistulogram.
- Protect skin: stoma bag to collect and measure fistula output, and barrier ointments to protect the skin.
- Planned surgery: if spontaneous closure does not occur.

Prevention

Careful entry into the abdomen, ideally in a virginal area, will reduce the risk of bowel injuries that occur due to adhesions of bowel to parietal peritoneum, or injuries from bowel protruding through incisional hernias. Palpation of previous scars with the patient upright might demonstrate incisional hernias.

During gynecologic procedures, the bowel should be mobilized as necessary and packed away from the pelvis. This should avoid bowel injury and improve the view of the operative field.

The prolonged morbidity and potential mortality of bowel injury during laparotomy or laparoscopy requires the surgeon to be careful and vigilant in the peritoneal cavity. The bowel is all too easily injured, particularly if dissecting too close to it with diathermy. Laparoscopic instruments should always be used under direct vision, particularly during insertion and withdrawal, and kept within the rather narrow field of view. Bowel should only be manipulated with laparoscopic instruments when it is within the field of view of the laparoscope.

Bowel should be handled with care and unnecessarily forceful retraction should be avoided, particularly in patients who have cancer or have had irradiation.

KEY POINTS

Challenge: Small or large bowel injury during gynecologic surgery.

Background
- Key risk factors for bowel injury are adhesions from prior surgery, pelvic infection, endometriosis, or cancer.
- In gynecologic surgery, small bowel, sigmoid colon and rectum are the most commonly injured bowel segments.
- Injury to mesentery can occur during excision of peritoneal nodules. Mesenteric injury can result in delayed bowel ischemia and injury.
- Diathermy injury can be small (1–3 mm) and therefore easily missed; but it is often full thickness and can result in delayed bowel perforation.
- Risks of bowel injury include sepsis, abscess, fistula formation, multiple organ failure, and death.

Prevention
- Bowel preparation if the patient is at high risk for bowel injury.
- Forewarn gastrointestinal or general surgeon if complex surgery is anticipated.
- Careful entry into the abdomen, preferably in a virginal area of the abdomen.
- Correct packing of the bowel away from the pelvis before starting a gynecologic procedure.
- Laparoscopic instruments should always be used under direct vision, particularly during insertion and withdrawal.

Management

- Management depends on the time of diagnosis, site and magnitude of the bowel injury, whether the damage is via a clean cut or with crushing of the edges, and the degree of devitalization.
- An immediate intraoperative diagnosis and management is associated with good outcome. Delayed diagnosis is associated with critical complications.
- Give prophylactic antibiotics in all cases of bowel injury; include cover for Gram-negative bacilli and anaerobes.
- If enteric contamination occurs, perform extensive lavage of the peritoneal cavity.
- Injuries should be repaired immediately as small (particularly diathermy) injuries can be difficult to identify later.
- Repair is usually with interrupted, absorbable, seromuscular sutures (3-0 Vicryl or PDS on an atraumatic round-bodied needle).
- Surgical approach:
  - Clean cut with no compromise of blood supply: primary repair.
  - Substantial crushing or tearing of the edges or vascular supply compromised: resection and anastomosis. Anastomosis can be performed with sutures or stapling devices.
  - Complex injuries, or peritonitic or unwell patients: defunctioning stomas.
- Bowel repairs can be covered with omentum to improve vascularity and seal tiny leaks.
- Mesenteric injury: needs careful assessment due to risk of bowel ischemia; full-thickness mesenteric injuries should be repaired but without compromising mesenteric vasculature in the sutures.
- Management of postoperatively diagnosed bowel injury:
  - Prompt diagnosis and urgent resuscitation preferably in critical care with invasive monitoring, intravenous antibiotics and emergency surgery.
  - Lavage of the abdomen.
  - Resection of the injured segment of bowel and proximal stoma formation.
- Postoperative management:
  - If there was contamination, a 5-day therapeutic antibiotic course is needed.
  - Normal diet should be instituted as soon as tolerated. There is no advantage in prolonged bowel resting.
  - Vigilance for peritonitis and sepsis.
  - White cell count, CRP, and CT scan may be needed if clinically indicated.
  - Involvement of stoma therapist.

Reference

1 Monaghan J, Lopes T, Naik R. The management of injuries to the urinary tract. In: *Bonney's Gynaecological Surgery*, 10th edn. Blackwell Science Ltd, Oxford, 2004.

CHAPTER 38
Inferior Epigastric Vessel Injury

Manas Chakrabarti[1] and Sudha Sundar[2]

[1] Apollo Gleneagles Cancer Hospital, Kolkata, India
[2] City Hospital, Sandwell and West Birmingham Hospitals NHS Trust, Birmingham, UK

Case history: *During a laparoscopic sterilization in an obese woman, the initial pneumoperitoneum is uneventful; however, bleeding from the left-sided port is noted after insertion of accessory 5-mm trocar. Bipolar diathermy stopped the bleeding initially but soon after a hematoma is seen to form.*

Background

Trauma to abdominal wall blood vessels occurs in 0.2–2% of laparoscopic procedures [1]. The majority are due to trauma to inferior epigastric artery (IEA) during trocar insertion.

Anatomy

The IEA arises from the external iliac artery just above the inguinal ligament. The initial ascending course is subperitoneal, running along the medial border of the internal inguinal ring, which can be identified by following the round ligament as it exits the pelvis via this ring before being inserted onto labia majus. IEA becomes more superficial as it ascends, perforating transversalis fascia to lie between rectus muscle and posterior lamella of rectus sheath. IEA divides into few branches below the navel to anastomose with the superior epigastric artery. Average thickness of the IEA is significant at 3.4 mm; hence, when injured it can cause extensive bleeding [2].

Management (see Chapters 40 and 76)

Various methods have been used for hemostasis when there is bleeding from IEA.

Bipolar diathermy

Bipolar diathermy (Figure 38.1) via opposite accessory port is tempting but in cases of complete transectional injury of IEA, the ends of the vessel can retract preventing adequate hemostasis. It can also cause damage to the abdominal wall. Hence this method should be used with caution.

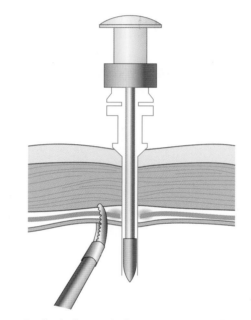

Figure 38.1 Bipolar diathermy of inferior epigastric artery (©Maher/Francis).

Foley balloon tamponade

Perhaps the quickest way to stop bleeding is to introduce a large-diameter Foley catheter through the bleeding port, inflate the balloon with an adequate amount of fluid, pull it against the abdominal wall, and secure the tamponade by externally clamping it with hemostatic forceps (Figure 38.2). A 5-mm port should be able to accommodate a 14 Fr Foley catheter. Larger-diameter Foley catheters have been used in various published reports. A number of studies have reported control of bleeding using this technique with removal of the catheter after 24 hours, by which time hemostasis had been achieved. Aharoni *et al.* [3] found no cases of repeat bleeding when a Foley catheter was removed after 24 hours in their 12-patient case series. However, there is a risk of delayed hematoma formation and artery forceps can permanently crush the fluid channel of a Foley catheter.

Gynecologic and Obstetric Surgery: Challenges and Management Options, First Edition. Edited by Arri Coomarasamy, Mahmood I. Shafi, G. Willy Davila and Kiong K. Chan.
© 2016 John Wiley & Sons, Ltd. Published 2016 by John Wiley & Sons, Ltd.

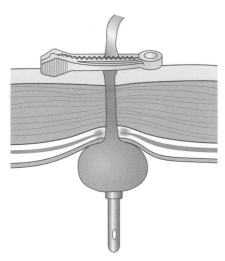

Figure 38.2 Foley balloon tamponade of inferior epigastric artery (©Maher/Francis).

Laparoscopic sutures

If bleeding persists or if definitive treatment is desired, the ideal technique is to place intramural sutures to proximal and distal ends of inferior epigastric vessels to secure both arterial and venous bleeding. Laparoscopic port closure needle or suture passers could aid in placing such sutures. Obviously, it requires some dexterity to place laparoscopic sutures and Foley tamponade should be used if there is a delay in getting help. Transmural non-absorbable sutures have also been used but they should be removed after approximately 24 hours postoperatively, given that these sutures have been reported to cause abdominal wall necrosis when left in place for 72–96 hours [4].

Laparotomy

In a minority of cases bleeding may continue despite trying all these measures. In such cases, and where the patient is becoming hemodynamically unstable, prompt conversion to laparotomy and ligation of the vessel should be undertaken. During intra-abdominal entry a hemoperitoneum may be encountered. Early communication with the anesthetist is important as these patients require appropriate fluid resuscitation.

Postoperative care

It is important to remain vigilant during the postoperative period. Despite apparent intraoperative hemostasis, significant bleeding can still occur leading to blood transfusion requiring reoperation to control bleeding. Although the majority of hematomas resolve, some may form abscesses and require drainage [5]. Attempts to aspirate a hematoma are not recommended as it can transmit infection and cause further vascular injuries. An enlarging hematoma causing hemodynamic instability must be corrected by surgery and adequate antibiotic cover should be provided [4].

It is worth noting that the IEA can play an important role in creating transversus rectus abdominis muscle (TRAM) or deep inferior epigastric perforator (DIEP) flap for breast reconstruction. In addition, the internal thoracic artery/inferior epigastric artery (ITA/IEA) pathway maintains a limb-saving collateral in aortoiliac occlusive disease (Leriche's syndrome) [6]. Hence, occlusion of the IEA should be clearly documented in operative notes and the patient should be adequately informed.

Prevention

Knowledge of the course of the IEA and its branches is invaluable for a laparoscopic surgeon. Traditionally, the surface marking of IEA has been the straight line from mid-inguinal point (midpoint between anterior superior iliac spine and symphysis pubis) to umbilicus [7]. However, the anatomic path of IEA and its branches are highly variable, being further complicated by obesity and previous laparotomy. Cadaveric studies have shown that if trocars are inserted more than two-thirds of the distance along a horizontal line between the midline and the anterior superior iliac spine, injury to the main stem of IEA can be mostly avoided [8]. Furthermore, IEA branches are least frequently found in the lowest part of the abdomen lateral to the artery.

Instead of relying solely on surface marking, direct visualization of the artery is recommended. The lower subperitoneal part of the IEA (before it pierces transversalis fascia) is easier to visualize through a laparoscope prior to insertion of lateral ports. Use of a transillumination technique by placing a 30° laparoscope against the abdominal wall in a dark operating room is not helpful in detecting deep vessels such as the IEA [9]. In thinner and light-skinned women, a transillumination technique can be helpful in detecting superficial epigastric vessels, which are branches of femoral vessels.

Every attempt should be made to identify any vessel injury after removal of the port at the end of an operation. Surgeons must remember that often the pneumoperitoneum and trocar can produce an artificial temporary tamponade, which stops the bleeding temporarily. This results in vascular injury being missed at surgery and can result in significant postoperative hemoperitoneum and a critically ill patient.

Insertion of accessory ports must be performed under continuous direct visualization. The direction of insertion of accessory ports is also important to prevent injuries. The direction should be perpendicular through the abdominal wall and any tilt to avoid visceral injury can be done just before puncturing the peritoneum. This is important in obese patients where the distance from the skin to abdominal cavity can be considerable, increasing the risk of error. Surgeons may want to request assistants to hold the laparoscope while utilizing both hands for trocar insertion to ensure controlled perpendicular entry through the abdominal wall. It is recommended to maintain an intra-abdominal pressure of 20–25 mmHg until all the accessory ports are inserted safely. Following port insertion, the pressure should be reduced to 12–15 mmHg for the operative procedure.

KEY POINTS

Challenge: Inferior epigastric injury and bleeding.

Background
- Trauma to abdominal wall blood vessels occurs in 0.2–2% of laparoscopic procedures, and the majority are due to trauma to IEA.
- Average thickness of the IEA is significant at 3.4 mm; hence, when injured it can cause extensive bleeding.

Prevention
- Knowledge of the course of the IEA and its branches is important:
  - Surface marking of IEA is a straight line from mid-inguinal point (midpoint between anterior superior iliac spine and symphysis pubis) to umbilicus; however, the course of the IEA is highly variable, particularly in obese women.
  - If trocars are inserted more than two-thirds of the distance along a horizontal line between the midline and the anterior superior iliac spine, injury to the main stem of the IEA can be mostly avoided.
- Laparoscopic visualization of the artery prior to port insertion and removal of port under direct vision is recommended.
- Pneumoperitoneum and trocar can produce an artificial temporary tamponade which can stop the bleeding temporarily from an injured IEA.

- After removal of trocars, a careful laparoscopic assessment of lateral port sites is recommended.

Management
- Inform all relevant staff, gain large-bore intravenous access, and arrange blood count and bloods (Chapter 40).
- Bipolar diathermy via opposite accessory port might control the bleeding in some women, but is unlikely to be helpful with transectional injury of IEA as the ends of the vessel often retract and therefore are not accessible to diathermy.
- Foley balloon tamponade:
  - Introduce a 14 Fr Foley catheter through the bleeding port.
  - Inflate the balloon with adequate amount of fluid.
  - Secure tamponade by externally clamping the Foley catheter with a hemostatic forceps.
  - Remove the Foley catheter 24 hours postoperatively.
- If the expertise is available, intramural sutures to proximal and distal ends of the inferior epigastric vessels can be placed through a laparoscopic approach. If transmural sutures are placed, they will need to be released 24 hours later to avoid abdominal wall necrosis.
- If all other measures fail, or if the patient is hemodynamically unstable, laparotomy to ligate the vessels should be undertaken without delay.

References

1 Saber AA, Meslemani AM, Davis R, Pimentel R. Safety zones for anterior abdominal wall entry during laparoscopy: a CT scan mapping of epigastric vessels. *Ann Surg* 2004;239:182–185.
2 Nezhat C, Nezhat F, Nezhat C (eds) *Nezhat's Video-assisted and Robotic-assisted Laparoscopy and Hysteroscopy*, 4th edn. Cambridge University Press, New York, 2013.
3 Aharoni A, Condea A, Leibovitz Z, Paz B, Levitan Z. A comparative study of Foley catheter and suturing to control trocar-induced abdominal wall haemorrhage. *Gynaecol Endosc* 1997; 6:31–32.
4 Vazquez-Frias JA, Huete-Echandi F, Cueto-Garcia J, Padilla-Paz LA. Prevention and treatment of abdominal wall bleeding complications at trocar sites: review of the literature. *Surg Laparosc Endosc Percutan Tech* 2009; 19:195–197.
5 Hurd WW, Pearl ML, DeLancey JO *et al*. Laparoscopic injury of abdominal wall vessels: a report of three cases. *Obstet Gynecol* 1993; 82(4 Pt 2 Suppl):673–676.
6 Yurdakul M, Tola M, Ozdemir E, Bayazit M, Cumhur T. Internal thoracic artery-inferior epigastric artery as a collateral pathway in aortoiliac occlusive disease. *J Vasc Surg* 2006; 43:707–713.
7 Lewis WH (ed.) *Gray's Anatomy of the Human Body*, 20th edn. Bartleby.com, New York, 2000.
8 Epstein J, Arora A, Ellis H. Surface anatomy of the inferior epigastric artery in relation to laparoscopic injury. *Clin Anat* 2004; 17:400–408.
9 Quint EH, Wang FL, Hurd WW. Laparoscopic transillumination for the location of anterior abdominal wall blood vessels. *J Laparoendosc Surg* 1996; 6:167–169.

CHAPTER 39

Bleeding from Retracted Pedicular (Pelvic Sidewall) Vessels

Michael L. Sprague and Stephen E. Zimberg

Cleveland Clinic Florida, Weston/Fort Lauderdale, Florida, USA

Case history: During hysterectomy for a large fibroid uterus through a midline incision, the surgeon encountered a 6-cm ligamentous myoma lateral to the cervix. During mobilization of the ligamentous myoma, the right uterine artery was transected. The vessel retracted laterally toward the pelvic sidewall and hemorrhage ensued.

Background

Distorted anatomy, poor dissection technique, and inadequately secured vessels may lead to hemorrhage from retracted vascular pedicles within the pelvis. Lack of plan, poor visualization, and surgeon panic may lead to increased bleeding because of further vascular trauma or injury to bowel, bladder, or ureter. Hemorrhage from retracted pelvic sidewall vessels is life-threatening and pelvic surgeons must be prepared to manage this surgical emergency.

Management (see Chapter 40)

A pelvic surgeon must maintain composure and employ a systematic approach when managing bleeding from retracted pelvic sidewall vessels. Steps that should be taken immediately after encountering bleeding from retracted pelvic vessels include:

1 alerting operating room team of bleeding and ensuring sufficient ancillary staff are available for assistance;
2 obtaining adequate exposure of the pelvis through methods such as conversion to laparotomy for vaginal or laparoscopic procedures, extending the incision, or placement of a self-retaining retractor;
3 controlling bleeding by direct tamponade or by occluding the aorta;
4 obtaining necessary blood products;
5 obtaining necessary supplies, such as suture, energy device, or hemostasis clips.

Autologous transfusion with blood rescued using cell salvage devices is appropriate, when available. Although useful for diffuse bleeding, topical hemostatic agents are rarely sufficient for retracted arterial pedicles. Bleeding from all operative and vascular access sites is suggestive of disseminated intravascular coagulation, which needs be swiftly corrected.

Identify and secure the retracted pedicle and vessel

In certain cases, the bleeding vessel can be readily identified near the site of transection, secured with a fine clamp, and the bleeding controlled with a suture ligature. Oftentimes, however, the pelvic sidewall must be explored to adequately secure a retracted pedicle.

The uterine arteries arise from the anterior division of the internal iliac vessels. Firstly, the round ligament remnant is placed on traction and an incision is made in the peritoneum overlying the psoas muscle to expose the structures at the pelvic brim. The ureter is observed as it courses over the iliac bifurcation and is retracted medially. The anterior division of the internal iliac artery is identified, and the branches of the vessel are carefully exposed and mobilized. The uterine artery arises proximal to the origin of the superior vesical artery and courses laterally and in close proximity to the pelvic ureter. At the level of the cervical isthmus, the uterine artery courses medially over the ureter. Once the course of the vessel is confirmed, the uterine artery may be secured using suture-ligature or a vascular clip under direct visualization of the ureter. Temporary vascular clips to the internal iliac artery or pressure on the aorta (or vascular clamp) can be used to diminish blood flow to the operative area to allow visualization if this is impeded by significant hemorrhage. Depending on the degree of hemorrhage, a vascular surgeon and a hematologist should be consulted.

Ligation of anterior division of the internal iliac artery

If persistent bleeding or distorted anatomy precludes safe dissection of the pelvic sidewall, the anterior division of the internal iliac artery may be ligated. Unilateral ligation of the anterior division of the internal iliac artery yields a 77% reduction in pulse pressure ipsilaterally, and 85% if ligation is undertaken bilaterally [1]. The structures of the pelvic brim are exposed, the common iliac artery is identified at the pelvic brim and the ureter is retracted medially. A right-angle clamp is placed from lateral to medial beneath the anterior division of the internal iliac artery distal to the posterior division. Two large-gauge suture ligatures are fed into the clamp and the knots secured. An assistant should check that femoral or dorsal pedal pulses are palpable in order to confirm that the external iliac artery has not been occluded.

Gynecologic and Obstetric Surgery: Challenges and Management Options, First Edition. Edited by Arri Coomarasamy, Mahmood I. Shafi, G. Willy Davila and Kiong K. Chan.
© 2016 John Wiley & Sons, Ltd. Published 2016 by John Wiley & Sons, Ltd.

Arterial embolization

For those instances when bleeding cannot be controlled surgically, it is reasonable to perform arterial embolization to control bleeding. Angiographic insertion of vaso-occlusive spheres or gelatin pledgets can be performed intraoperatively and is effective at controlling bleeding from pelvic vessels. Direct tamponade can be performed to optimize resuscitation and minimize blood loss while waiting for the staff and the necessary interventional radiology equipment to arrive.

Pelvic packing

Pelvic packing is a salvage procedure employed to manage intractable pelvic bleeding. Sterile sponges are employed to apply direct pressure to the sites of ongoing bleeding and the skin is closed. The patient remains sedated while the patient's anemia, coagulopathy, hypothermia, and metabolic disorders are corrected. Intravenous antibiotics are administered. The packing remains in place for 24–72 hours, after which time it is removed in the operating room. For cases in which a colpotomy has been made, a pelvic pressure pack can be placed intraoperatively and the packing removed through the vagina 48 hours later [2].

Prevention

Hemorrhage from retracted pedicular vessels is a common but preventable complication of abdominal surgery. Sound surgical technique including proper placement of surgical clamps, careful division of pedicles, and precise securing of suture knots minimizes, but does not eliminate, the risk of bleeding from "slipped" or retracted pedicles. A pelvic surgeon must be alert, observant, and prepared to manage life-threatening intraoperative bleeding.

KEY POINTS

Challenge: Bleeding from retracted pedicular (pelvic sidewall) vessels.

Background
- Distorted anatomy, poor dissection technique, and inadequately secured pedicles may lead to catastrophic bleeding from retracted pelvic sidewall vessels.

Prevention
- Good knowledge of surgical anatomy and reliable surgical techniques such as sound dissection technique, proper clamp placement, careful division of pedicles, and careful securing of surgical knots may reduce the incidence of bleeding from retracted sidewall vessels.

Management
- The immediate steps to managing acute bleeding from retracted sidewall pedicles include:
  - Alert operating room team of acute bleeding and request additional assistance, resources and blood products.
  - Obtain adequate exposure (e.g., conversion of laparoscopy to laparotomy, or extension of existing abdominal incision).
  - Apply direct tamponade to the bleeding vessel.
- Expose and secure the bleeding vessel with care not to injure nearby structures:
  - Place round ligament on traction and incise the peritoneum to expose the retroperitoneal structures all the way to the pelvic brim.
  - Identify and retract the ureter medially.
  - Identify the anterior division of the internal iliac artery, and expose the branches.
  - Ligate the bleeding vessel while keeping the ureter out of the way.
- If basic interventions are unsuccessful, advanced interventions include:
  - Ligation of anterior division of internal iliac artery: identify common iliac artery at the pelvic brim, and retract ureter medially; place a right-angle clamp from lateral to medial beneath the anterior division of the internal iliac artery, distal to the posterior division; use large-gauge suture to ligate the vessel.
  - Angiography and arterial embolization.
  - Pelvic packing for 24–72 hours.
- Consultation with a vascular surgeon and a hematologist may be indicated.

References

1 Burchell RC. Physiology of internal iliac ligation. *J Obstet Gynaecol Br Commonw* 1968; 75:642–651.

2 Logothetopulos K. An absolutely certain method of stopping bleeding during abdominal and vaginal operations. *Zentralbl Gynakol* 1926; 50:3202–3204.

CHAPTER 40
Massive Hemorrhage

Karen Louise Moores, William Parry-Smith, and Martyn Underwood
Shrewsbury and Telford Hospitals NHS Trust, Telford, Shropshire, UK

Case history 1: A woman at 37 weeks of gestation with a history of abdominal pain and contractions had an ultrasound scan that confirmed intrauterine fetal death and suspected abruption. She collapsed and was taken to theater for an urgent laparotomy.

Case history 2: A woman with heavy menstrual bleeding and a large fibroid uterus opted to have a hysterectomy, but bled heavily during the procedure.

Background

Massive hemorrhage can be defined as a loss of 50% of circulating blood volume within 3 hours or blood loss of at least 150 mL/min. Massive obstetric hemorrhage is often defined as a total blood loss of over 1500 mL or a loss of over 25% of circulating blood volume [1]. Hemorrhage is an important cause of morbidity and mortality; while it is a decreasing cause of direct maternal deaths, the rate remains significant at 5 per 100,000 maternities for 2006–2008 in the UK [2]. Half of these cases are due to postpartum hemorrhage, one-quarter to placenta praevia, and one-quarter to placental abruption. Mortality risk increases if postoperative hemoglobin levels fall below 7 g/dL [3].

In this chapter, we address principles and management of massive hemorrhage; for specific management of bleeding, refer to Chapters 38, 39 and 76, as well as Section 8 (Obstetric surgery).

Classification of hemorrhagic shock

Hemorrhagic shock can be classified into four groups (Table 40.1) [4]. Tachycardia is an early sign of significant blood loss, followed by a drop in blood pressure and oliguria. In a normal adult, a tachycardia indicates at least a 15% loss in blood volume (>750 mL) [5].

Management

Immediate steps

Early recognition of massive hemorrhage can be life-saving. Immediate management involves summoning appropriate help; in Case history 1, a senior anesthetist and obstetrician. Prior to transfer to operating room, urgent measures must be instigated, namely administration of facial oxygen, insertion of two large-bore cannulae (16 gauge or larger), urgent 6 units of blood cross-match and 4 units of FFP, plus FBC, coagulation studies, and renal and liver function studies. The senior anesthetist should consider invasive monitoring for arterial blood pressure or central venous pressure. Fluid replacement should be initiated with crystalloids (Hartmann's) and a Foley urinary catheter inserted. Consideration should be given to transfusion of group O rhesus-negative blood.

Transfusion of blood and blood products

In a case of massive hemorrhage, a major transfusion protocol must be instigated with involvement from the consultant hematologist

Table 40.1 Classification of hemorrhagic shock based on initial presentation.

	Class I	Class II	Class III	Class IV
Blood loss (mL)	Up to 750	750–1500	1500–2000	>2000
Blood loss (% blood volume)	Up to 15%	15–30%	30–40%	>40%
Pulse rate (bpm)	<100	100–120	120–140	>140
Systolic blood pressure	Normal	Normal	Decreased	Decreased
Pulse pressure	Normal or increased	Decreased	Decreased	Decreased
Respiratory rate	14–20	20–30	30–40	>35
Urine output (mL/hour)	>30	20–30	5–15	Negligible
CNS/mental status	Slightly anxious	Mildly anxious	Anxious, confused	Confused, lethargic
Initial fluid replacement	Crystalloid	Crystalloid	Crystalloid and blood	Crystalloid and blood

Source: American College of Surgeons, 2012 [4]. Reproduced with permission from the American College of Surgeons.

Gynecologic and Obstetric Surgery: Challenges and Management Options, First Edition. Edited by Arri Coomarasamy, Mahmood I. Shafi, G. Willy Davila and Kiong K. Chan.
© 2016 John Wiley & Sons, Ltd. Published 2016 by John Wiley & Sons, Ltd.

and anesthetist. Early communication with the transfusion laboratory is essential to provide warning that a patient has major bleeding, or is anticipated to require a lot of blood products. Hypothermia increases the risk of disseminated intravascular coagulation (DIC) and other complications, and therefore it is important to pre-warm resuscitation fluids and obtain a temperature-controlled blood warmer if possible.

Group compatible blood can be available within 15 min from receipt of the patient's blood sample in most UK National Health Service hospitals. If needed more urgently, emergency blood (group O rhesus D negative) can be transfused.

FFP 1 unit can be given with each unit of packed red cells, but this should be in accordance with advice from the consultant hematologist. Large volumes of FFP may be required to improve fibrinogen and other coagulation factor deficiencies. However, if fibrinogen levels remain low (<1.0 g/L), cryoprecipitate therapy should be considered. One adult dose (2 pools) of cryoprecipitate and one adult dose (1 unit) of platelets can be transfused for every 6–8 units of red cells. Platelets should not be allowed to fall below 50×10^9/L in acutely bleeding patients. Again, this must be with advice from the consultant hematologist. Coagulation studies should be monitored frequently in these patients to evaluate the need for, and efficacy of, component therapy; a minimum guide of 4-hourly and after each therapy is suggested [6].

Transfusion of blood products can pose serious risks to patients, for example transfusion-related acute lung injury (TRALI) and hemolysis [6]. Therefore, products must be used appropriately, following local guidelines and in consultation with a hematologist; if feasible, the patient should be counseled on the risks and benefits of blood products.

Medical drug interventions

Consider use of intravenous tranexamic acid 1–2 g to prevent acidosis and hypothermia [6]. Furthermore, in patients with known von Willebrand disease, intravenous desmopressin 0.15–0.3 µg/kg infused over 30 min can be used [7]. Additionally, intravenous antifibrinolytics such as aprotinin can help preserve platelet adhesion during hemorrhage, given as an initial bolus dose of 2,000,000 KIU followed by an intravenous infusion of 500,000 KIU/hour [7].

If there is continuing hemorrhage despite surgical or radiologic intervention, or these techniques are not available, consider use of a recombinant form of activated factor VII (rVIIa, NovoSeven, Novo Nordisk, Copenhagen, Denmark). Evidence exists to support use of rVIIa to enhance hemostasis at the site of bleeding without systemically activating the coagulation cascade (and the associated risk of distant thrombosis). Vials of rVIIa can be requested by the consultant hematologist and are administered by intravenous bolus at a dose of 60 µg/kg [8]. Acidosis and thrombocytopenia must be corrected prior to use of rVIIa. rVIIa should be used cautiously in patients with a history of venous or arterial thrombosis, cerebrovascular disease and DIC because of the risk of thrombotic complications [8].

Massive obstetric hemorrhage

The management of massive obstetric hemorrhage is addressed in detail in Section 8. Surgical techniques to reduce ongoing hemorrhage include under-suturing of the placental bed, an intrauterine balloon, a B-Lynch compression suture, uterine artery or internal iliac artery ligation, and hysterectomy as a last resort. Interventional radiologic techniques such as arterial embolization or balloon catheters are available in some hospitals. In addition, cell salvage can be considered if facilities and expertise exist; this technique avoids risks associated with blood transfusion.

Massive gynecologic hemorrhage

Meticulous surgical technique and appropriate application of hemostatic sutures with or without Surgicel®, an absorbable hemostat, is essential. However, if these techniques are unsuccessful in controlling the hemorrhage, consideration should be given to the use of other hemostatic agents, such as FloSeal® (gelatin–thrombin matrix), which can be beneficial in achieving hemostasis and which are applied immediately and directly to bleeding tissue [9]. Furthermore, coagulation agents such as tranexamic acid, vitamin K and NovoSeven can be contemplated [6,8]. Embolization techniques or hysterectomy need to be considered in cases of ongoing hemorrhage. Consideration should be given to the insertion of a pelvic drain to alert the medical team to postoperative intra-abdominal bleeding.

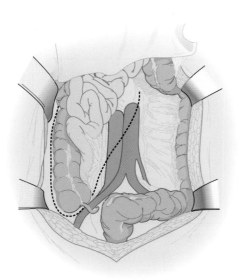 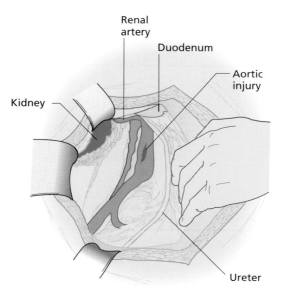

Figure 40.1 Laparotomy incision for exposure of aorta and inferior vena cava. Adapted from Lopes et al., 2011 [9] with permission from Wiley.

Aortic or inferior vena cava injury

An immediate midline laparotomy should be performed (Figure 40.1) while requesting the urgent presence of a vascular surgeon. Direct pressure should be applied to the bleeding vessel to allow time for the anesthetist to obtain appropriate central venous access and blood products to be requested. Manual compression can be replaced with mechanical compression using Satinsky or Fogerty vascular non-crushing clamps proximal and distal to the site of injury. Prior to mechanical clamping, a bolus dose of 100 units/kg of heparin should be administered. The defect can then be repaired using a small-calibre Prolene suture (4-0 or 5-0) [9].

Iliac artery injury

Principles similar to those above are used to apply non-crushing clamps proximally and distally to the injury site. Internal iliac artery injury can be repaired or alleviated by clipping or ligating the vessel and its branches [9].

Presacral bleeding

The most effective measure to control bleeding is to apply direct pressure over the presacral plexus for 20–30 min, while blood products are obtained and appropriate monitoring commenced. Fibrin sealants can then be used to ensure hemostasis [9].

Postoperative care

Postoperatively, repeat testing at least every 4 hours to monitor hematology and coagulation is essential until results have begun at least to normalize; microsampling, arterial blood gas sampling and near-patient testing are techniques that can be used to optimize rapid intervention as required [10]. Recovery may need to take place in the high-dependency unit or intensive treatment unit depending on the severity of the hemorrhage and the availability of local facilities.

It is important to ensure that appropriate thromboprophylactic measures are in place to reduce the risk of venous thromboembolism; this may include early hydration, patient mobilization, and subcutaneous low-molecular-weight heparin. In addition, a senior member of the healthcare team or the operating surgeon should debrief the patient and next of kin with regard to the events of the patient's admission, surgery, future care plans, and prognosis. Iron therapy or erythropoietin, alone or in combination, can be commenced after discussion with a hematologist.

Resolution of the cases

Case history 1

The obstetrician evacuated a macerated fetus and over 3 L of blood from the uterine cavity. The major transfusion protocol was instigated with involvement from the hematologist. A B-Lynch compression suture was unsuccessful at controlling the hemorrhage; after cardiac arrest on the operating table and in consultation with the family, a decision was made to proceed with hysterectomy with conservation of ovaries. The patient made a satisfactory recovery in HDU.

Case history 2

The gynecologist encountered massive bleeding of over 2 L from the uterine arteries and vaginal vault intraoperatively despite meticulous surgical technique. After successfully securing the uterine vessels, FloSeal was used successfully to control the remaining small bleeding points.

Prevention

Preoperatively, it is important to identify at-risk patients for massive hemorrhage, namely those who are obese, have had previous surgery, have a known thrombophilia or clotting disorder, and those in whom complex surgery is anticipated. Hemoglobin levels should be optimized prior to surgery; options include preoperative ferrous sulfate, parenteral iron or, in Case history 2, therapies to reduce ongoing heavy menstrual loss, such as oral tranexamic acid. Furthermore, GnRH agonists or ulipristal acetate (Esmya) 5 mg orally once daily for up to 3 months can also be used to reduce the size of fibroids, which may help with the surgical procedure [11]. A recent hemoglobin level and group and save should be available, and cross-matched blood if there is a high anticipated risk of hemorrhage. Furthermore, cell salvage can be considered if facilities and expertise exist. Again, if massive hemorrhage is anticipated, consideration should be given to invasive monitoring by the anesthetist.

How to avoid massive hemorrhage and vessel injury

It may not always be possible to avoid major hemorrhage, particularly in the emergency obstetric setting. By recognizing the emergency situation early, seeking senior support early, and working as a multidisciplinary team, we can aim to reduce blood loss, minimize complications, and expedite the patient's care.

In Case history 2, this is an elective situation so there is more time to plan and ensure a senior gynecologist is available to perform the surgery with an appropriate assistant. Blood products can be requested prior to starting, and additional equipment which may be needed (i.e., cell salvage and vascular clamps) can be made available. By following the basic surgical principles of adequate exposure, lighting, and knowledge of the anatomy, injury to vessels and important structures such as the ureters can be minimized. When tying off important vessels, such as ovarian pedicles, ensure that they are secured with a free tie first and then secured with a suture to avoid vessel hematomas and slippage of knots.

KEY POINTS
(See also Chapters 38, 39 and 76, and Section 8)

Challenge: Intraoperative care of major hemorrhage.

Background
- Massive hemorrhage is a loss of 50% of circulating blood volume within 3 hours or blood loss of 150 mL/min.
- Massive obstetric hemorrhage is a total blood loss of over 1500 mL or a loss of more than 25% of circulating blood volume.
- Hemorrhage is an important cause of morbidity and mortality.

- Mortality risk increases if postoperative hemoglobin levels fall below 7 g/dL.
- Tachycardia >120 bpm, hypotension, oliguria <15 mL/hour, and confused mental status are all late signs of massive hemorrhage of more than 30% of circulating volume.

Management
- Early recognition and management can be life-saving; summon appropriate help including senior gynecologist or obstetrician, anesthetist, and hematologist.
- Immediate steps: two large-bore cannulae (16 gauge or larger); 6 units cross-match; 4 units FFP; FBC and coagulation studies; fluid replacement

with warmed crystalloids; Foley urinary catheter. Transfusion with group O rhesus-negative blood for pregnant women if cross-match not immediately available.

- Follow local major transfusion protocol with senior hematologist input:
  - Transfuse blood.
  - Consider giving 1 unit FFP with each unit of packed red cells. Large volumes of FFP may be required if coagulation defects have developed.
  - If fibrinogen levels are low (<1.0 g/L), consider cryoprecipitate therapy: one adult dose (2 pools) of cryoprecipitate and one adult dose (1 unit) of platelets can be transfused for every 6–8 units of red cells.
  - Keep platelets above 50×10^9/L in acutely bleeding patients.
  - Be aware of serious transfusion risks such as TRALI and hemolysis.
- Consider intravenous tranexamic acid, desmopressin, aprotinin, rVIIa, cell salvage, Surgicel, FloSeal, and arterial embolization.
- Massive obstetric hemorrhage: surgical techniques include under-suturing of placental bed, intrauterine balloon, B-Lynch suture, uterine or internal iliac artery ligation, and hysterectomy.
- In elective gynecologic surgery, consider preoperative ferrous sulfate or parenteral iron to optimize hemoglobin; consider tranexamic acid to reduce ongoing heavy menstrual loss; use GnRH agonists or Esmya to reduce fibroid size before surgery.
- Aortic or IVC injury:
  - Perform an immediate midline laparotomy, while requesting the urgent presence from a vascular surgeon.
  - Apply direct pressure to the bleeding vessel to allow time for the anesthetist to obtain appropriate central venous access and blood products.

- Manual compression can be replaced with mechanical compression using Satinsky or Fogarty vascular non-crushing clamps proximal and distal to the site of injury.
- Prior to mechanical clamping, a bolus dose of 100 units/kg of heparin should be administered.
- The vascular surgeon can repair the defect using a small-calibre Prolene suture (4-0 or 5-0).
- Iliac artery injury: similar principles to management of aortic or IVC injury. Internal iliac artery injury can be repaired or the vessel and its branches can be ligated.
- Presacral bleeding: apply direct pressure over the presacral plexus for 20–30 min, while blood products are obtained and appropriate monitoring commenced. Fibrin sealants can then be used to ensure hemostasis.
- Postoperative care:
  - Manage in HDU or ITU.
  - Repeat testing to check hematology and coagulation, at least every 4 hours.
  - Ensure appropriate thromboprophylaxis.

Prevention
- Identify at-risk patients. Arrange FBC and G&S or cross-match. Organize cell salvage. Involve anesthetist, hematologist, and interventional radiologist.
- Optimize preoperative hemoglobin.
- Follow good surgical principles, including adequate exposure, lighting, good appreciation of anatomy, and meticulous dissection techniques.

References

1 Santoso JT, Saunders BA, Grosshart K. Massive blood loss and transfusion in obstetrics and gynecology. *Obstet Gynecol Surv* 2005; 60:827–837.

2 Lewis G. The women who died 2006–2008. In: Cantwell R (ed.) *Saving Mothers Lives: Reviewing Maternal Deaths to Make Motherhood Safer, 2006–2008.* The Eighth Report of the Confidential Enquiries into Maternal Deaths in the United Kingdom (CEMACE). *BJOG* 2011;118(Suppl 1):30–56.

3 Carson JL, Noveck H, Berlin JA, Gould SA. Mortality and morbidity in patients with very low postoperative Hb levels who decline blood transfusion. *Transfusion* 2002; 42:812–818.

4 American College of Surgeons. *Advanced Trauma Life Support Student Source Manual,* 9th edn. American College of Surgeons, Chicago, 2012.

5 American College of Surgeons. *Advanced Trauma Life Support for Doctors,* 8th edn. American College of Surgeons, Chicago, 2008.

6 Stainsby D, MacLennan S, Thomas D, Isaac J, Hamilton PJ. British Committee for Standards in Haematology: Guidelines on the management of massive blood loss. *Br J Haematol* 2006; 135:634–641.

7 Wali A. Novel techniques in treatment of intractable obstetric hemorrhage. *Rev Mex Anestesiol* 2008; 31:S48–S50.

8 Lavigne-Lissalde G, Aya G, Mercier F et al. Recombinant human FVIIa for reducing the need for invasive second-line therapies in severe refractory postpartum hemorrhage: a multicenter, randomized, open controlled trial. *J Thromb Haemost* 2015; 13:520–529.

9 Lopes T, Spirtos NM, Naik R, Monaghan JM. *Bonney's Gynaecological Surgery,* 11th edn, p. 245. Wiley-Blackwell, Oxford, 2011.

10 Price CP. Clinical review: point of care testing. *BMJ* 2001; 322:1285–1288.

11 Esmya (ulipristal acetate). http://www.esmya.co.uk/home/ (accessed April 2014).

CHAPTER 41

Broken Needle

Joanne Kathleen Ritchie, Anuradha Radotra, and Martyn Underwood
Shrewsbury and Telford Hospitals NHS Trust, Telford, Shropshire, UK

Case history 1: During suturing of the vaginal vault in a total laparoscopic hysterectomy, the needle breaks off and falls into the pelvis.

Case history 2: During the closure of the deep myometrial layers in an abdominal myomectomy, it becomes evident that the tip of the needle had been broken.

Background

Surgical needles can be lost during both open and minimal-access endoscopic procedures. Manipulation of instruments in restricted and deep areas in the pelvis is a risk factor for broken needles.

A broken needle can become lodged between bowel and omentum and so can easily be lost from view. The implications of a broken needle include additional surgical time, pain, infection, damage to internal structures (including fistula formation), nerve irritation, and medicolegal repercussions. Even when there is no physical harm, patient with a broken needle in the body can have psychological effects including fears about harm to the sexual partner or a fetus. These all suggest a swift and safe retrieval should be sought.

Management

Intraoperative

Perform a visual examination

Once a needle is recognized to have broken off, the surgeon should not withdraw the needle holder or avert his or her gaze from the surgical field. All available light should be directed to the surgical field. A thorough visual search for the needle should then be performed without moving anything as this may cause the needle to become buried further. At laparoscopy, it may be possible to increase the light to see if the needle can be detected from the glare created, and then consider reducing the light, which may reduce glare from other background structures and enable visualization of the needle.

Move tissues carefully to look for the needle

If looking alone fails to uncover the needle, a further search involving careful hand and instrument movements should be performed.

Care should be taken to not cause any damage to the internal structures during the search and to try to prevent causing the needle to become further misplaced. When searching during an open procedure the surgeon should be cautious to not sustain a needle injury and if this happens to follow the local guidelines for needle injuries. If the needle has broken off while removing the needle from the abdomen, it may be helpful to check the port sites.

Use X-ray or fluoroscopy

If a visual search fails to identify the missing item, then X-ray should be used, preferably with AP or PA with or without lateral views, to maximize the chance of locating the lost needle. The surgeon can use X-ray detectable items such as surgical instruments (e.g., the needle holder) to act as a reference point for locating the position of the needle on the X-ray. If a needle under 15 mm in size is lost, this is unlikely to be seen on X-ray, unlikely to be found, and unlikely to cause any damage if left behind, but the patient should nevertheless be informed [1] and an incident form should be completed, not least in case of later discovery during any other future treatments (such as unrelated CT scans). Real-time video fluoroscopy may be helpful in the operating room to allow retrieval of the needle under direct vision.

Use strong magnet

Magnetic-tipped devices can be used to attract the metallic needle and avoid laparotomy for a broken/missing needle [2]. In open surgery, a strong magnet can be placed inside a sterile glove or sterile medical condom before being introduced into the surgical field. A magnet may also be used if the missing/broken needle has been misplaced outside of the abdominal cavity by sweeping the floor and immediate operating table area with a larger magnet.

Postoperative

In the case of a post-surgery presentation, a CT scan may be useful. Serial CT scans can be performed to evaluate any migration of the needle toward any vital structures.

Finally, it is important to be open and honest with the patient, explain the implications and apologize for the issue. An incident form should be completed so that the event can be fully investigated.

Gynecologic and Obstetric Surgery: Challenges and Management Options, First Edition. Edited by Arri Coomarasamy, Mahmood I. Shafi, G. Willy Davila and Kiong K. Chan.
© 2016 John Wiley & Sons, Ltd. Published 2016 by John Wiley & Sons, Ltd.

Prevention

A broken needle is the result of a combination of undue or wrongly applied force by the surgeon, inappropriate needle, injudicious needle handling, and often resistance from tough tissues. The properties of the tissues for suturing should be considered, and an appropriate needle for the task should be carefully selected. When grasping the needle with the needle holder, the location and angle of grasping is important: generally a perpendicular grasp at midpoint of the needle is appropriate. Occasionally, an obtuse or acute angle hold is necessary, and in such instances getting the needle as close to a perpendicular position as feasible will make the driving of the needle easier to accomplish. In tough or fibrosed tissues, the needle should be grasped between the tip and the midpoint; as the needle is advanced, the needle holder is repositioned to the midpoint, and the needle is driven further into the tissue in what is called the "ratchet technique."

Needles generally bend before they break; if a needle begins to bend, the surgeon will need to change the approach and/or choose a stronger needle. Once a needle has bent, it should not be reused.

The *WHO Guidelines for Safe Surgery 2009* includes a list of recommendations to ensure the retention of needles is prevented [3]. These include completing the WHO checklist [4] to ensure the correct number of needles at the start and end of the procedure. Furthermore, the WHO guideline states that needles should not be left free on the table and instead should have an appropriate container, often an adhesive pad, to reduce the chance of them going missing.

KEY POINTS

Challenge: Broken or lost needle.

Background
- Needles can be broken off or lost during open or laparoscopic surgery.
- A broken needle is the result of a combination of undue or wrongly applied force by the surgeon, inappropriate needle, injudicious needle handling, and often resistance from tough tissues.
- Risks of a broken needle include infection, damage to internal structures (including fistula formation), nerve irritation, and psychological effects including fear of harm to a sexual partner or fetus.
- A needle less than 15 mm in size is unlikely to cause any damage; however, with any broken or lost needle, the ideal is to identify and remove it.

Management
- First perform a thorough visual search:
  - Do not withdraw the needle holder, avert your gaze from the surgical field, or move any tissues.
  - Direct all available light to the surgical field.
- At laparoscopy, consider increasing the light to produce a needle glare, or reducing the light to reduce tissue glare.

- During a physical search, care should be taken to not displace the needle, cause any damage to tissues, or sustain a needlestick injury.
- If a visual search fails to identify the missing item, X-ray or fluoroscopy should be used.
- Consider magnetic devices both intra-abdominally and in surrounding area; strong magnets can be placed inside a sterile glove or sterile medical condom before being introduced to the surgical field.
- Complete an incident form, so a full investigation can be carried out.
- If a needlestick injury is sustained, follow local hospital protocol.
- Postoperatively, serial CT scans can be useful to track a migrating needle.

Prevention
- Choose the correct needle for the task.
- As far as possible, grasp the needle perpendicularly at midpoint of the needle. For tough tissues, use the "ratchet technique."
- If any needle is bent, discard it. Do not even straighten bent needles.
- Always conduct a pre-procedure needle count, by two people and spoken aloud.
- Have an appropriate container (adhesive pad) to reduce the chance of needles going missing.

References

1 NoThing Left Behind: A national surgical patient-safety project to prevent retained surgical items. Available at http://www.nothingleftbehind.org/Resources.html (accessed 9 April 2014).
2 Kandioler-Eckersberger D, Niederle B, Herbst F *et al*. A magnetic probe to retrieve broken metallic parts of instruments during laparoscopic procedures. *Surg Endosc* 2002; 16:208–209.

3 World Health Organization. *WHO Guidelines for Safe Surgery 2009: Safe Surgery Saves Lives*. WHO, Geneva, 2009.
4 WHO Surgical Safety Checklist, January 2009, World Health Organization. Available at http://www.nrls.npsa.nhs.uk/resources/?entryid45=59860 (accessed 9 April 2014).

CHAPTER 42

Lost Swab, Needle or Instrument

Joanne Kathleen Ritchie, Martyn Underwood, and William Parry-Smith
Shrewsbury and Telford Hospitals NHS Trust, Telford, Shropshire, UK

Case history 1: A 24-year-old woman is readmitted 4 days after a Neville Barnes forceps delivery and repair of a 3b tear. She is pyrexial, tachycardic, and has offensive vaginal discharge. On speculum a retained swab is found.

Case history 2: A 46-year-old woman is undergoing a total abdominal hysterectomy for menorrhagia and a large fibroid uterus. While performing the WHO checklist for safe surgery 2009, it is discovered that the instrument count is incorrect: one non-tooth dissecting forceps is missing.

Background

The occurrence of an unintentionally retained swab (sponge) or instrument post procedure is on the NHS Core List of Never Events [1]. The incidence of retained instruments and swabs has been estimated to be as high as 1 in 1000 procedures [2]. Dependent on the type and size, these lost items may be discovered shortly after the procedure or, on rare occasions, up to several months or years later.

Retained swabs can be a focus for infection and lead to sepsis, whereas surgical instruments can cause life-threatening damage to bodily organs and internal bleeding. Both can result in the need for additional surgery to remove the lost item(s) and to treat any subsequent complications.

Incidents of missing or retained swabs and instruments that were reported to the Reporting and Learning System (RLS) demonstrated that obstetrics and gynecology as a specialty is ranked as second highest for the number of cases identified (second only to surgery), with 145 cases reported between April 2007 and March 2008 [3].

Swabs

The incident of a lost swab most commonly occurs during abdominal or pelvic surgery and at operative vaginal deliveries. In obstetrics, retained swabs can be lost during operative vaginal deliveries, particularly during suturing or if tampons and vaginal packs are needed. Between April 1, 2000 and March 31, 2010 there were 186 claims to the NHS litigation authority (NHSLA) for retained swabs, which amounted to a cost of £3,021,910 [4].

Patients may notice the swab themselves or they may present symptomatically days later. The retained swabs can lead to pain, infection, and secondary postpartum hemorrhage as well as possible psychological sequelae. In gynecology, swabs can be lost during laparotomies when they are placed intra-abdominally and then missed at the subsequent swab count. If missed, the retained swab may not be noticed until the patient presents with pain, infection, and a swinging temperature. Occasionally a lost swab may be incidentally detected on a scan, and may be misdiagnosed as an abscess or tumor.

The risk of having retained swab, needle or instrument is highest during emergency procedures, when there is an unexpected change of surgical procedure, and in the obese patient. Extra care is needed under these circumstances.

A gossypiboma [5] is the official term for a lost swab after surgery, derived from the Latin *gossypium* (cotton) and the Swahili word *boma* (place of concealment).

Instruments and needles

Surgical instruments and needles can be lost during both open and minimally invasive endoscopic procedures. While it would be difficult to lose a surgical instrument in a patient during a vaginal delivery, stress and confusion can still be caused while trying to locate the missing equipment. Missing instruments can potentially cause bowel perforation, fistula, infection, and internal bleeding.

Management

Intraoperative

Should any item be missing from a delivery repair pack or swab count, a thorough search of the patient, any pathology specimen, the suturing trolley, bins, bags and surrounding areas should be conducted. All staff involved in the care of the patient should be informed.

On searching, swabs may be easily identified and should be removed from the vagina. The tray used to receive the placenta should be checked along with the placenta. The clinical and domestic waste bags and laundry should remain in the room (and be included in the search) until the missing item is found.

If a visual search fails to identify the missing item, then X-ray should be used, preferably with AP or PA with or without lateral views, to maximize the chance of locating the lost item. If a needle

Gynecologic and Obstetric Surgery: Challenges and Management Options, First Edition. Edited by Arri Coomarasamy, Mahmood I. Shafi, G. Willy Davila and Kiong K. Chan.
© 2016 John Wiley & Sons, Ltd. Published 2016 by John Wiley & Sons, Ltd.

under 15 mm in size is lost this is unlikely to be seen on X-ray, unlikely to be found, and unlikely to cause any damage if left behind, but the patient should nevertheless be informed [6] and an incident form should be completed, not least in case of later discovery during any future tests or treatments (such as unrelated CT scans). Real-time video fluoroscopy may be helpful in theater to allow retrieval of the instrument or needle under direct vision.

In Case history 1, the swab count went wrong or was omitted and the missing swab was not identified. In such cases, a patient presenting with pyrexia and pain after delivery will require a speculum to look for and remove any retained swab, and broad-spectrum antibiotics.

Postoperative

In the case of a post-surgery presentation, a CT scan may be useful. It is important to be open and honest with the patient and apologize for the issue. An incident form should also be completed so that the event can be fully investigated.

Prevention

Preoperative

It is essential that a pre-procedure swab count is completed prior to vaginal delivery or an operation. Everyone involved in the procedure should be aware of (and trained in) the importance of counting swabs, although the surgeon must ultimately take the responsibility of ensuring the count occurs correctly.

It may be helpful to ensure that all sterile delivery and suture packs contain X-ray detectable swabs to facilitate identification of a lost swab. By standardizing all kits such as suture repair packs to contain the same number of swabs and instruments, it is possible to minimize the chance of an error occurring.

Intraoperative

In addition to the initial count (swab, needle, and instrument), a count should occur before every closure of a cavity and additionally at skin closure. A repeat count should occur at any time that care is handed over to another practitioner (e.g., if the case is handed over to a more senior colleague). It may be helpful to use a standardized form or whiteboard on which to write the swab and instrument count in all operating rooms. The count should be completed aloud by two people undisturbed (at least one a registered practitioner) and all swabs should be separated during counting. Providing an appropriate receptacle to collect the used swabs will reduce the chances of error, and no equipment should be removed from the room until all counts are correct.

If a tampon or large swab in the vagina is used to aid suturing or packing, then it can be attached with a clip to the drapes, so that it is less likely to be forgotten. The surgeon can also minimize the risk of retained items by not inserting loose swabs in body cavities, and instead using the tape already attached to the swab to fix the swab to the surgical drapes outside the body. If a small swab needs to be used in the pelvis, a suture can be placed through the swab and attached to the outside drape.

Preventive WHO guidelines

The *WHO Guidelines for Safe Surgery 2009* includes a list of recommendations to ensure the retention of instruments and sponges in surgical wounds is prevented [2]. These recommendations mention that each department should have a standardized protocol for counting swabs and instruments. By completing the WHO checklist, all members of the team may be confident that the instrument and swab count is correct and the instruments are sterile at the start of the operation.

The guideline states that needles should not be left free on the table and instead should be placed in an appropriate container to reduce the chance of them going missing. The loss of part of an instrument is more likely than the loss of the whole and so each instrument should be counted with its component parts. Most of these procedures will be carried out by the scrub nurse, but the surgeon should be aware that the checks are taking place and ensure they are completed properly.

Moreover, WHO endorses that the surgeon should perform a "methodical wound exploration" before closing any body cavity.

KEY POINTS

Challenge: Lost swab, needle or instrument.

Background
- Unintentionally retained swab or instrument is classified as a "never event" (i.e., it should never happen).
- Despite the "never event" status, the incidence of retained swabs or instruments is estimated to be as high as 1 in 1000 procedures.
- Retained swabs can be a focus of infection; retained instruments can cause life-threatening organ damage, including bowel perforation, fistula, and bleeding.

Management
- If any item is missing, halt the procedure if safe to do so and keep the patient anesthetized until the issue is resolved.
- If anything is lost, conduct a full search of body cavities, pathology specimens, trolleys, bins, bags, and the floor.
- Intraoperative imaging:
  - Use X-ray with all views: PA or AP with or without lateral views.
  - Real-time video fluoroscopy can be particularly useful.
- X-ray, CT, and ultrasound may all have a role in postoperative diagnosis of missing swab or instrument.
- Complete an incident form, so a full investigation can be carried out.

Prevention
- Always conduct a pre-procedure swab, instrument and needle count, by two people and spoken aloud.
- If any swabs or instruments are missing preoperatively, ensure the team are all aware and it is clearly documented.
- Use X-ray detectable swabs and instruments/devices.
- Use whiteboards to document the counts.
- Use the tape on the swab to attach the swab to the drapes.
- Perform swab, instruments and needle counts at all relevant parts of the procedure: follow the WHO safe surgery guideline.
- Ensure the abdomen is empty of swabs and instruments before closure of the wound and that the count is confirmed by the operating room staff.
- Ensure the final count is complete.

References

1. NHS Core List of Never Events. Available at http://www.nrls.npsa.nhs.uk/resources/collections/never-events/core-list/
2. World Health Organization. *WHO Guidelines for Safe Surgery 2009: Safe Surgery Saves Lives*. WHO, Geneva, 2009.
3. WHO Surgical Safety Checklist, January 2009, World Health Organization. Available at http://www.nrls.npsa.nhs.uk/resources/?entryid45=59860 (accessed 9 April 2014).
4. NHS Litigation Authority. *Tens Years of Maternity Claims: An Analysis of NHS Litigation Authority Data*. Available at http://www.nhsla.com/safety/Documents/Ten%20Years%20of%20Maternity%20Claims%20-%20An%20Analysis%20of%20the%20NHS%20LA%20Data%20-%20October%202012.pdf
5. Morgan MA, Rusinov VB *et al*. Gossypiboma. Available at http://radiopaedia.org/articles/gossypiboma
6. NoThing Left Behind: A national surgical patient-safety project to prevent retained surgical items. Available at http://www.nothingleftbehind.org/Resources.html

Section 3
Postoperative Care
Editors: Arri Coomarasamy and Janesh Gupta

CHAPTER 43
Postoperative Care

Janesh Gupta[1], Robbert Soeters[2], and Aaron Ndhluni[2]
[1] College of Medical and Dental Sciences, University of Birmingham, Birmingham, UK
[2] Groote Schuur Hospital, Cape Town, South Africa

Case history: A 40-year-old woman had a hysterectomy through a midline laparotomy for significant size fibroids, but is progressively getting worse with dehydration and abdominal distension at 3 days after the operation.

Background

Because of the physiologic stress caused by surgery, catecholamines including adrenaline (epinephrine) and noradrenaline (norepinephrine) are released as a result of the activation of the hypothalamic–pituitary–adrenal axis. Emotional stress has also been shown to increase the production and release of cortisol. This additional cortisol can affect the postoperative patient, for example by increasing metabolism, water excretion, cardiovascular tone, temperature, and blood glucose levels. Cortisol also diminishes inflammation by suppressing the body's immune response, thereby hindering wound healing [1].

As a result of the body's physiologic response to stress and the inherent surgical risk of hemorrhage and shock, regular postoperative observations are essential in maintaining patient care. The nature of the operation, the patient's condition, and the method of pain control will determine how regularly such observations need to be performed. A reduction in systolic blood pressure can indicate hypovolemic shock, which can ultimately lead to multiple organ failure (Chapter 52). However, it is important to note that blood pressure measurements can be variable due to the body's compensatory mechanisms. Therefore, it is useful to consider the early signs of reduced tissue perfusion when detecting signs of shock [2]. These include increased respiratory rate and tachycardia as a precursor to hypotension, low urine output (<0.5 mL/kg per hour), restlessness or confusion, and cold peripheries.

Infection is one of the main causes of postoperative morbidity in abdominal surgery [3], with wound infections being one of the most common presentations (Chapter 47). Such infections present with localized pain, redness, and slight discharge usually caused by skin staphylococci. The microorganisms causing surgical site infection are usually endogenous, related to skin. Exogenous infection occurs when microorganisms from instruments or other sources contaminate during the operation or before the skin is sealed. It

is rare for microorganisms to cause a surgical site infection from hematogenous spread.

Wound cellulitis and abscesses usually occur after bowel-related surgery and most commonly present within the first week. In terms of treatment, cellulitis is treated with antibiotics whereas abscesses require surgical exploration. The wound may sometimes have to be left open to heal by secondary intention (Chapter 47). Further complications of postoperative infection include failure of the surgical procedure, sepsis, organ failure, and even death. Other postoperative complications include thrombosis (Chapters 15 and 57), which is increased in patients with comorbidities such as diabetes, obesity, older age, emergency operations and those who develop infection [4].

There are important principles that should not be ignored in the first 14 days after surgery (Figure 43.1). Postoperative care should involve observation for signs of visceral damage that can occur as a result of direct injury (within 3 days) or delayed (up to 14 days) which can occur due to avascular necrosis. Common viscera that can be damaged are bowel (Chapter 37), bladder (Chapter 35), and ureters (Chapter 36).

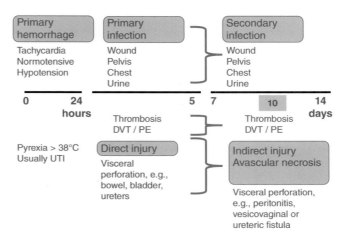

Figure 43.1 Principles of postoperative care: timelines for indicating possible causes.

Gynecologic and Obstetric Surgery: Challenges and Management Options, First Edition. Edited by Arri Coomarasamy, Mahmood I. Shafi, G. Willy Davila and Kiong K. Chan.
© 2016 John Wiley & Sons, Ltd. Published 2016 by John Wiley & Sons, Ltd.

Prevention and management

In order to combat the effects of increased cortisol, nutrition plays an important role in postoperative care. Cortisol can deplete protein stores, therefore reducing muscle mass. It has been suggested that patients can be fed orally, even in the early stages following major abdominal surgery, without increasing their risk of paralytic ileus or dehiscence of a gut anastomosis [5].

Surgical drain output can be an unreliable method of determining blood loss since they can become blocked with clots. Some patients may benefit from central venous pressure (CVP) monitoring to determine circulatory volume. Chest X-rays are useful in detecting pulmonary edema.

If hypovolemic shock is observed, the primary aim of treatment it to restore adequate tissue perfusion to prevent organ failure. This is usually achieved through fluid resuscitation with crystalloid or colloid and increased oxygenation to maintain hemoglobin saturation above 95% (Chapter 52). Excessive blood loss may require a blood transfusion or even further surgical intervention to control the bleeding (Chapter 40).

Postoperative infection can be reduced with good surgical technique (Chapter 47). This includes not shaving the skin before skin incision, administering antibiotic prophylaxis to patients before surgery, preparing the skin with antiseptic immediately before incision, avoiding surgical drains, and covering the wound for at least 48 hours with a waterproof dressing postoperatively [4].

Thrombosis can be prevented with prophylactic anticoagulation with low-molecular-weight heparin (LMWH) for the duration of hospital stay and the use of anti-thromboembolic stockings (to be used until mobilization is no longer significantly reduced or for at least 6 weeks postoperatively). Patients have an increased risk of developing venous thromboembolism if their mobility is expected to be significantly reduced for 3 days or more, or if the operation lasts more than 90 min or more than 60 min if the surgery is in the pelvis or leg(s). Early mobilization and early resumption of normal diet can reduce these risks. Early discharge from hospital also results in lower risks of postoperative complications and hospital-acquired infections such as MRSA [6]. These approaches form part of the principles of the Enhanced Recovery Partnership currently being implemented in the NHS in the UK [7].

Resolution of the case

This patient has signs of intra-abdominal visceral injury, likely to be bowel. She has progressively worsened over the 3 days after midline abdominal hysterectomy. It is likely that she has sustained a bowel perforation, which has gone unnoticed at the time of surgery as she is presenting within 3 days with peritonitis. The timeline for presentation of symptoms is usually a good indicator for what type of postoperative complication has taken place (Figure 43.1). In general, patients should progressively get better, even after major surgery, and not worse. If there is any doubt, an aggressive management policy to identify a potential cause should be followed. For management of bowel injury, see Chapter 37.

KEY POINTS

Challenge: Postoperative care complications.

Background
- Key postoperative complications include hemorrhage, infection, visceral damage, and thrombosis.
- Visceral injury can occur as a result of direct injury (within 3 days) or delayed (up to 14 days) which can occur due to avascular necrosis.
- The timeline for presentation of symptoms is usually a good indicator for what type of postoperative complication has taken place.
- Common viscera that can be damaged are bowel, bladder or ureters, especially in abdominal surgery.

Prevention and management
- See postoperative patients at least once a day, and if there are any concerns twice or thrice a day. There should be low threshold for getting a second, senior or specialist review.
- Ask the patient if she is drinking, eating, moving about the ward, passing urine, and opening bowels.
- Review pulse, temperature, blood pressure, oxygen saturation, drainage, fluid balance, wound, blood results, and drug chart.
- Early mobilization and resumption of fluids and diet within 24 hours after major surgery will enhance recovery.
- In general, patients should progressively get better, even after major surgery, and not worse. If there is any doubt, an aggressive management policy to identify a potential cause should be followed.
- Thromboprophylaxis includes compression stockings and LMWH.
- Postoperative infection can be reduced with good surgical technique. This includes not shaving the skin before skin incision, administering antibiotic prophylaxis to patients before surgery, preparing the skin with antiseptic immediately before incision, avoiding surgical drains, and covering the wound for at least 48 hours with a waterproof dressing postoperatively.

References

1 Hughes E. Principles of post-operative patient care. *Nursing Standard* 2004; 19(5): 43–51.
2 Anderson ID (ed.) *Care of the Critically Ill Surgical Patient*, 2nd edn. Hodder Arnold, London, 2003.
3 Pessaux P, Msika S, Atalla D, Hay JM, Flamant Y. Risk factors for postoperative infectious complications in noncolorectal abdominal surgery: a multivariate analysis based on a prospective multicenter study of 4718 patients. *Arch Surg* 2003; 138:314–324.
4 Torpy JM, Burke AE. Postoperative infections. *JAMA* 2010; 303:2544.
5 Bisgaard T, Kehlet H. Early oral feeding after elective abdominal surgery: what are the issues? *Nutrition* 2002; 18: 944–948.
6 Collins AS. Preventing health care-associated infections. In: Hughes RG (ed.) *Patient Safety and Quality: An Evidence-based Handbook for Nurses*, chapter 41. Agency for Healthcare Research and Quality, Rockville, MD, 2008.
7 NHS Enhanced Recovery Partnership. *Fulfilling the Potential: a Better Journey for Patients and a Better Deal for the NHS.* Avaliable at http://www.nhsiq.nhs.uk/8228.aspx

CHAPTER 44
Excessive Nausea and Vomiting after Surgery

Phil Moore

Birmingham Women's NHS Foundation Trust, Birmingham, UK

Case history 1: Following an uneventful diagnostic laparoscopy, a patient begins to retch and vomit. Despite medication, this continues on the gynecology ward, and the patient has to be admitted overnight.

Case history 2: A 55-year-old woman underwent total abdominal hysterectomy through a midline incision. An epidural catheter had been inserted before surgery, but it became clear in recovery that it was not correctly sited, and PCA morphine was commenced for severe abdominal pain. After a number of bolus doses, the woman complained of severe nausea and started to retch.

Background

Postoperative nausea and vomiting (PONV) is a highly unpleasant experience, and "willingness to pay" research has shown that many patients would prefer to avoid it more than pain. In addition to humanitarian reasons for addressing this problem, PONV can also lead to complications such as aspiration, esophageal tears, electrolyte imbalance (particularly low potassium), wound dehiscence, and unplanned overnight hospital stays, with increased healthcare costs. The risk of PONV is influenced by patient factors, surgical factors, and anesthetic factors (Table 44.1).

Table 44.1 Risk factors for postoperative nausea and vomiting.

Patient factors
Previous PONV or motion sickness
Female gender
Non-smoking status
Young age
High levels of anxiety

Surgical factors
Abdominal surgery
Gynecologic surgery
Inner ear surgery
Prolonged surgery
Some antibiotics used for surgical prophylaxis, e.g., penicillins and cephalosporins

Anesthetic factors
Opioid drug use
Inhalational anesthesia
Nitrous oxide use
Neostigmine use
Dehydration

There is overlap of some of these risk factors (e.g., all gynecologic surgery is in women, and many abdominal surgeries require opioids), and cohort studies suggest that a simple score taking into account the four most important items has a good predictive ability. The four items are female gender, a history of motion sickness or PONV, non-smoking status, and the use of perioperative opioids; in patients with zero, one, two, three or four of these factors, PONV rates are 10, 21, 39, 61, and 79%, respectively.

Anatomy and physiology of the vomiting reflex

The vomiting reflex originates in two discrete areas of the brain: the "vomiting center" in the medulla and the higher cortical centers (Figure 44.1). The vomiting center in the medulla is affected by anesthetic agents, opioids and surgery, while the higher cortical centers are affected by sensory input (e.g., smell and sight) and memory, fear, and anticipation. There are also peripheral pathways, with mechanoreceptors in the distal stomach and proximal duodenum, and chemoreceptors in the small bowel.

Management

Assess and treat causes of PONV

The first step in the management is to consider the various causes of PONV and manage these. The key causes to consider are severe pain, opioid use, inadequate hydration, sepsis, and mechanical causes (gastric distension, ileus, constipation, and bowel obstruction). Pain should be treated with adequate analgesia, and opioids do not need to be avoided purely out of concern for PONV. However, opioid dose may need adjusting, and non-opioid analgesics may be preferable. Inadequate hydration and electrolyte imbalances should be corrected. It is important to consider sepsis, particularly urinary tract infection, and investigate and treat in a timely fashion. If a mechanical cause is suspected, appropriate investigations and management will need to be put in place, for example nasogastric suction to decompress gastric stasis.

Use antiemetic drugs

Most antiemetic drugs work by antagonizing the receptors of one of the neurotransmitters involved in the vomiting reflex pathways (Figure 44.1), although steroids work by a more

Gynecologic and Obstetric Surgery: Challenges and Management Options, First Edition. Edited by Arri Coomarasamy, Mahmood I. Shafi, G. Willy Davila and Kiong K. Chan.
© 2016 John Wiley & Sons, Ltd. Published 2016 by John Wiley & Sons, Ltd.

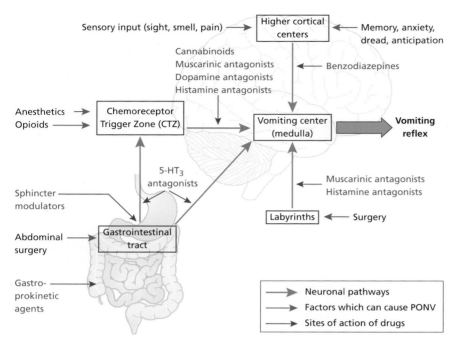

Figure 44.1 Anatomy and physiology of the vomiting reflex.

generalized mechanism. In addition to their primary mode of action, some drugs have additional beneficial effects, for example metoclopramide increases gastric emptying, and cyclizine has an anticholinergic effect. Established PONV is treated with rescue medication of a drug group which has not already been used for prophylaxis. Members of the various drug groups in common clinical use are given in Table 44.2. If one rescue agent is ineffective, further agents should be given until all the groups of drugs have been given in an adequate dose to block all the receptors in the vomiting pathway. However, cyclizine and metoclopramide should not be combined as there is an increased risk of extrapyramidal side effects. Extrapyramidal side effects such as oculogyric crisis and acute dystonia can occur especially in young and very old patients, and can be treated with procyclidine 5–10 mg by slow intravenous injection, with usually rapid response.

Table 44.2 Antiemetic drugs.

Drug type	Examples
5-HT$_3$ (serotonin) antagonists	Ondansetron 4–8 mg i.m./slow i.v. 8-hourly Granisetron 1 mg i.v.
Histamine antagonists	Cyclizine 50 mg i.m. or slow i.v. 8-hourly
Dopamine antagonists	Prochlorperazine 12.5 mg i.m., maximum 25 mg in 24 hours Droperidol 0.625–1.25 mg i.v.
Muscarinic antagonists	Glycopyrrolate 0.2–0.6 mg i.v. Atropine 0.5–1 mg i.v.
Gastroprokinetic agents	Metoclopramide 10 mg i.v./i.m./orally three times daily
Steroids	Dexamethasone 4–8 mg orally/slow i.v. 8-hourly

Prevention

There are a number of interventions other than antiemetic drugs which can be implemented for all patients to minimize the risk of PONV.

- Minimizing anxiety with good preoperative preparation and counseling, with anxiolytic benzodiazepine premedication for the most anxious patients.
- Minimizing the length of starvation and maintaining good hydration by allowing water until 2 hours before surgery. Hydration should be maintained intraoperatively with intravenous fluids.
- Avoiding inhalational general anesthesia by using a local or regional technique, or total intravenous anesthesia (TIVA).
- Avoiding the use of drugs which may increase PONV, including nitrous oxide, neostigmine and certain antibiotics, such as erythromycin, which is particularly emetogenic.
- Minimizing the administration of opioid analgesics by using paracetamol, NSAIDs, and local anesthetic techniques.
- Counseling patients to mobilize slowly on the first occasion after surgery, and to reintroduce diet gradually after major surgery, with bland food initially.

Patients at high risk of PONV will also benefit from prophylactic antiemetic administration, and drugs from more than one group may be used to gain additional benefit. However, the level of risk at which a cost–benefit analysis of prophylactic drug use ceases to support their use remains unclear; as the major benefit is subjective patient satisfaction, this will inevitably vary according to clinician and healthcare system. Many clinicians consider women undergoing gynecologic surgery as suitable for prophylactic antiemetics, as they are already in the moderate to severe risk group, and this is exacerbated further if they are young non-smokers with a previous history of PONV.

Acupressure or "Sea-Bands" have been shown to be effective for some patients, but it is not clear when they should be applied; it would be wise to be cautious about applying them preoperatively or intraoperatively, as they have to be tight around the wrist to apply an effective degree of pressure, and this may be associated with adverse effects in anesthetized patients. However, they may be safely used once the patient is awake.

KEY POINTS

Challenge: Excessive nausea and vomiting after surgery.

Background
- PONV is associated with:
  - Poor patient satisfaction.
  - Risks of complications, such as aspiration, esophageal tears, electrolyte imbalance (particularly low potassium), wound dehiscence, and unplanned overnight hospital stays.
  - Increased healthcare costs.
- The risk factors for PONV are:
  - Patient: previous PONV, history of motion sickness, female gender, young age, non-smoking status, high level of anxiety, and obesity.
  - Surgical factors: abdominal or gynecologic surgery, prolonged surgery, certain antibiotics.
  - Anesthetic factors: opioid use, inhalational anesthesia, nitrous oxide or neostigmine use, and dehydration.
- Drugs may be used both prophylactically and to treat established PONV.
- Drugs with one of six distinct mechanisms of action may be usefully combined.

Prevention
- Minimize anxiety with good preoperative preparation and counseling, with anxiolytic benzodiazepine premedication for the most anxious patients.
- Minimize the length of starvation and maintain good hydration by allowing water until 2 hours before surgery. Hydration should be maintained intraoperatively with intravenous fluids.
- Avoid inhalational general anesthesia by using a local or regional technique, or TIVA.
- Avoid the use of drugs which may increase PONV, including nitrous oxide, neostigmine, and certain antibiotics.
- Minimize administration of opioid analgesics with use of paracetamol, NSAIDs, and local anesthetic techniques.
- Counsel patients to mobilize slowly on the first occasion after surgery, and to reintroduce diet gradually after major surgery, with bland food initially.
- Give prophylactic antiemetics to patients at high risk of PONV.

Management (of established PONV)
- Assess and treat for causes of PONV. The key causes to consider are severe pain, opioid use, inadequate hydration, sepsis, and mechanical causes (gastric distension, ileus, constipation, and bowel obstruction).
- Optimize pain relief, but minimize opioid use.
- Maintain adequate hydration.
- Use antiemetic drugs, in combination therapy:
  - Give drugs in groups not used prophylactically.
  - 5-hydroxytryptamine antagonist, e.g., ondansetron.
  - Dopamine antagonists, e.g., prochlorperazine.
  - Antihistamines, e.g., cyclizine.
  - Anticholinergics, e.g., glycopyrrolate.
  - Prokinetics, e.g., metoclopramide.
  - Steroids, e.g., dexamethasone.
- Do not combine cyclizine and metoclopramide as there is an increased risk of extrapyramidal side effects.

Further reading

Apfel CC. Postoperative nausea and vomiting. In: MillerRD (ed.) *Miller's Anesthesia*, 7th edn, chapter 86. Churchill Livingstone Elsevier, Philadelphia, 2010.

Apfel CC, Läärä E, Koivuranta M, Greim CA, Roewer N. A simplified risk score for predicting postoperative nausea and vomiting: conclusions from cross-validations between two centers. *Anesthesiology* 1999; 91: 693–700.

Chikwe J, Walther A, Jones P. *Perioperative Medicine*, 2nd edn. Oxford University Press, Oxford, 2009.

CHAPTER 45

Excessive Abdominal Pain after Surgery

Manjeet Shehmar

Birmingham Women's NHS Foundation Trust, Birmingham, UK

Case history: Two days after a laparoscopic ovarian cystectomy, a patient is still experiencing abdominal pain requiring increasing analgesia. Her catheter has been reinserted due to urinary retention and she has not yet opened her bowels.

Background

Patients should recover steadily after surgery, with reducing analgesia requirements and increased activity levels. If they do not, a thorough assessment is required to identify possible complications. Increasing or severe abdominal pain after surgery is a sign of an underlying problem. It should never be assumed to be due to a low pain threshold by the patient.

Management

Assess the patient

Assessment begins with gathering the facts of the surgical procedure(s) from the operative notes and surgeons. The type of surgery and any complications or difficulties such as adhesions, use of diathermy and blood loss should be considered. A full assessment of the patient should include a thorough pain history (Table 45.1), paying attention to associated symptoms such as vomiting, urinary and bowel disturbances, and bleeding. Examination of the observation chart rather than just a single set of observations is necessary to look for patterns and timings of abnormal observations such as swinging pyrexia, signifying a pelvic collection. Examination of the abdomen and pelvis should include listening for bowel signs and examining vaginal loss. A full clinical examination will be required if the patient is unwell and an early warning score should be used for observations, which should include respiratory rate and urine output. General investigations include serum amylase, FBC, CRP, U&E, and specific investigations as dictated by the working and differential diagnoses.

Get the necessary expert help

There should be accessible and agreed pathways for opinions from other surgical specialties such as colorectal surgery and urology to help diagnose, exclude and manage complications of bowel, ureter, bladder, and blood vessels. Early opinion should be sought with teams working together to reduce morbidity and mortality. The specific management will depend on diagnosis and associated complications.

Table 45.1 Pain history using the SOCRATES mnemonic.

Pain question	Example responses
Site	Use anatomic quadrants
Onset	Sudden/gradual Initiating factors
Character	Sharp, throbbing, tearing, pulling, colicky, gripping
Radiation	To other areas such as chest, back, legs
Associated symptoms	Bleeding, urinary or bowel dysfunction, vomiting, vaginal bleeding or discharge
Timing	Onset, constant, intermittent
Exacerbating factors	Exacerbating or relieving factors
Severity	Score using patient's perception

Bowel trauma (see Chapter 37)

Bowel trauma may be associated with symptoms of an acute abdomen such as pain, vomiting, anorexia, and inability to open bowels normally. Clinically, there can be abnormal observations depending on the stage of trauma and secondary complications such as peritonitis and sepsis. There can be abdominal tenderness, distension, guarding, rebound, and reduced or high-pitched bowel sounds.

Diagnosis is usually based on clinical history and examination, but abdominal X-ray may show distended loops of bowel and chest X-ray may show gas below the diaphragm. Multirow detector helical CT (MDCT) has sensitivities up to 95% and specificities up to 84% to detect surgically important bowel trauma [1]. The CT will show free fluid, free air, abnormal bowel enhancement, bowel wall thickening, and mesenteric infiltration.

The mortality of generalized postoperative peritonitis is 22–55% and failure to control peritoneal infection is fatal [2], as is failure to control the septic source. With immediate fecal peritonitis source control, residual peritonitis rates are 41% [2]. A planned early repeat laparotomy is associated with a lower mortality rate versus an emergency laparotomy in response to an acutely sick patient (0% vs. 65%, $P = 0.007$) [2]. Hence, early recognition and a low threshold for planned repeat laparotomy is necessary to minimize mortality; this should be done with surgeons in order to repair any bowel trauma. Preparation for theater will include giving broad-spectrum antibiotics, checking renal and liver function, and FBC.

Gynecologic and Obstetric Surgery: Challenges and Management Options, First Edition. Edited by Arri Coomarasamy, Mahmood I. Shafi, G. Willy Davila and Kiong K. Chan.
© 2016 John Wiley & Sons, Ltd. Published 2016 by John Wiley & Sons, Ltd.

Ileus

An ileus is a secondary event to bowel irritation from handling, trauma, or infection. Presentation is similar to bowel trauma with abdominal pain, distension of the abdomen, vomiting, lack of bowel sounds, and constipation. Once more serious causes are excluded, management is by a nasogastric tube, intravenous rehydration, and attention to electrolyte imbalance to avoid hypokalemia (Chapter 56). An ileus is more likely if the patient has experienced prolonged starvation before or after surgery.

Constipation

The psychologic and physiologic stresses of surgery can cause reduced bowel motility, which can be aggravated by drugs such as opiates. Before a diagnosis of constipation is made, other more serious causes such as bowel trauma should be excluded. Constipation is relieved by increased patient mobility, oral hydration and, if necessary, enemas or laxatives. The pain should be relieved once bowels have opened.

Bladder or ureteric trauma

Bladder trauma can present with a pseudosac (swollen bladder on ultrasound with entrapped gas), hematuria, presence of urine in the abdominal or pelvic cavity, and postoperative anuria. With ureteric trauma, there can be flank pain, an ileus, distended abdomen, and pyrexia if there is concomitant sepsis. Management requires involving urologists as soon as the diagnosis is suspected or made, as prompt diagnosis and treatment is crucial in decreasing morbidity [3]. Postoperative bladder injury is best diagnosed with a retrograde cystogram; CT has lower accuracy for diagnosing bladder injuries [4]. Postoperative ureteric injury can be diagnosed with IVU or CT with intravenous contrast. Management of bladder and ureteric injuries, including those diagnosed postoperatively, is discussed in Chapters 35 and 36, respectively.

Urinary retention

Urinary retention can be a complication of a bladder infection, trauma, or decreased bladder function after surgery. A bladder scan is the correct approach to diagnose retention; catheterization should not be used to diagnose retention. Once trauma has been excluded, treatment is with urinary catheter reinsertion to allow the bladder more time to rest before a further trial without catheter can be conducted.

Urinary tract infection

Urinary tract infections are common after surgery and if not treated promptly can cause pain and complications such as pyelonephritis. There can be urinary symptoms such as dysuria and frequency. Pyelonephritis will have associated symptoms of loin pain, vomiting, and high pyrexia. A urine sample should be dipped for the presence of nitrates and appropriate antibiotics should be prescribed in accordance with local microbiology guidelines. If the urine dipstick is equivocal, a midstream urine sample should be sent for microscopy, culture and sensitivity before antibiotics are commenced. If there are complications of a urinary tract infection, such as pyelonephritis or abscess, then a renal ultrasound scan and advice from urologists and microbiologists should be sought to avoid renal damage and septic shock.

Sepsis (see Chapters 47 and 52)

Generally, sepsis will present with pyrexia, tachypnea, tachycardia and, in severe cases, hypotension and septic shock. All sites of infection should be considered from the wound, pelvis, abdomen, urinary tract, and chest; a targeted history can help to identify the focus of infection. A septic screen will be directed by the presentation but may include a urine sample, vaginal swabs, wound swabs, sputum and stool cultures, and chest X-ray and blood cultures, if there is high-grade pyrexia. Antibiotic treatment will be directed to treat the cause and should be governed by local prescribing policy. If patients do not respond, then there should be close liaison with the microbiologist for further advice.

Pelvic collection

A pelvic collection can be blood or pus from an abscess. Although it is common to have fluid in the pelvis after a hysterectomy [5], it should be considered as a focus of sepsis if there is associated pyrexia. The patient will have swinging pyrexia and localized throbbing pain with an abscess. The site of the collection may be complicated with a resulting ileus or peritonitis. The patient may present with diarrhea due to peritonitis and sepsis. Treatment will include antibiotics as dictated by local policy to cover aerobic and anaerobic organisms, and in some cases drainage may be needed, with ultrasound or CT guidance or via open surgery.

Ischemic trauma

This occurs when organs or vasculature are damaged by thermal spread from diathermy. It classically presents 10 days after surgery, with an acute abdomen, peritonitis, and sepsis, and has a high associated mortality. Treatment will be repeat laparotomy to excise the ischemic organ and re-establish blood supply to viable tissue. Broad-spectrum antibiotics will be needed due to the risk of sepsis from ischemic tissues. Preparation for theater will include a septic screen, renal and liver function tests, and clotting studies to ensure that there has not been multiorgan failure and disseminated intravascular coagulopathy. Because of the high risk of mortality, a critical care bed is often needed.

Hemorrhage

As hemorrhage can cause pelvic irritation and peritonitis, it can present with an acute abdomen. There will be associated symptoms of blood loss such as a tachypnea, tachycardia, hypotension, reduced urine output, pallor, and reduced capillary refill. There may or may not be revealed bleeding, and an abdominal scan for free fluid could be useful in the diagnosis. Management of hemorrhagic shock is addressed in Chapters 40 and 52.

Surgically unrelated causes

All other causes of abdominal pain can happen at the time of surgery and these should not be forgotten. Examples include appendicitis, cholestasis or cholecystitis, diverticulitis, gastritis, renal calculi, and pancreatitis. A good surgical history and targeted investigations can help to diagnose or rule out these causes.

Prevention

Adequate pain relief in the postoperative period is a priority, as poor pain relief is associated with various complications such as nausea and vomiting, ileus, chest infection, and DVT. Prevention is always better than management of pain. Pain should be treated promptly, and pain relief should not be withheld while investigating for a diagnosis.

If the patient cannot take oral analgesics, intramuscular or intravascular pain relief needs to be given. If a drug fails to be effective, an alternative drug from a higher rung of the WHO analgesic ladder should be used (Table 45.2). If the pain is severe, it is reasonable to omit rungs 1 and 2, and go straight to rung 3. However, for all patients with severe or worsening pain, an aggressive search for the cause of the pain is important to ensure a serious complication is not missed.

Table 45.2 WHO analgesic ladder.

Rung 3	Strong opioid: morphine, diamorphine, fentanyl
Rung 2	Weak opioid: codeine, dihydrocodeine, tramadol
Rung 1	Non-opioid: paracetamol, NSAID (e.g., diclofenac)

KEY POINTS

Challenge: Severe abdominal pain after surgery.

Background
- Patients should get progressively better after surgery, not worse. If there is severe or worsening pain after surgery, find and manage the cause.

Management
- Assess the patient:
  - Thorough review of operative notes and observation charts.
  - Obtain a complete pain history: onset, character, severity, timing, radiation, associated symptoms, and exacerbating factors.
  - Systematic examination, including abdomen and pelvis.
- Initial general investigations: U&E, FBC, CRP, amylase, urine dipstick and culture.
- Consider differential diagnosis:
  - Bowel: injury, ileus, constipation.
  - Urinary: bladder or ureteric injury, urinary retention, urinary tract infection.
  - Sepsis and abscess.
  - Ischemic trauma.
  - Hemorrhage.

- Unrelated causes, e.g., appendicitis, cholestasis or cholecystitis, diverticulitis, gastritis, renal calculi, and pancreatitis.
- Specific targeted investigations, e.g., abdominal X-ray, ultrasound, CT, IVU, CT with intravenous contrast, blood cultures.
- Involve appropriate specialists in managing any serious complications, e.g., a bowel surgeon for bowel injury, or a urologist for ureteric injury.

Prevention
- Adequate pain relief is essential as poor pain relief is associated with complications such as nausea and vomiting, ileus, chest infection, and DVT.
- Pain should be treated promptly, and pain relief should not be withheld while investigating for a diagnosis.
- If the patient cannot take oral analgesics, intramuscular or intravascular pain relief needs to be given.
- If a drug fails to be effective, an alternative drug from a higher rung of the WHO analgesic ladder should be used:
  - Rung 1: non-opioid (e.g., paracetamol and diclofenac).
  - Rung 2: weak opioid (e.g., codeine, dihydrocodeine, tramadol).
  - Rung 3: strong opioid (e.g., morphine, diamorphine, fentanyl).

References

1 Atri M, Hanson JM, Grinblat L, Brofman N, Chughtai T, Tomlinson G. Surgically important bowel and/or mesenteric injury in blunt trauma: accuracy of multidetector CT for evaluation. *Radiology* 2008; 249:524–533.

2 Mulier S, Penninckx F, Verwaest C *et al.* Factors affecting mortality in generalized postoperative peritonitis: multivariate analysis in 96 patients. *World J Surg* 2003; 27:379–384.

3 Gomez RG, Ceballos L, Coburn M *et al.* Consensus statement on bladder injuries. *BJU Int* 2004; 94:27–32.

4 Hsieh CH, Chen RJ, Fang JF *et al.* Diagnosis and management of bladder injury by trauma surgeons. *Am J Surg* 2002; 184:143–147.

5 Hasson J, Maslovich S, Har-Toov J, Lessing JB, Grisaru D. Post-hysterectomy pelvic fluid collection: is it associated with febrile morbidity? *BJOG* 2007;114: 1566–1568.

CHAPTER 46

Bowel Damage: Postoperative Presentation

Ketan Gajjar and Mahmood I. Shafi

Addenbrooke's Hospital, Cambridge University Hospitals NHS Foundation Trust, Cambridge, UK

Case history 1: A 66-year-old woman with ovarian cancer underwent a laparotomy for interval debulking surgery. The postoperative recovery was slow and complicated with paralytic ileus. On the third postoperative day, the patient develops increasing abdominal pain with distension and has persistent temperature with tachycardia.

Case history 2: A 69-year-old woman with endometrial cancer underwent a laparoscopic-assisted vaginal hysterectomy with bilateral salpingo-oophorectomy. She contacts the gynecology ward on the third postoperative day complaining of nausea, vomiting, and increasing abdominal pain.

Background

Laparoscopic and open abdominal surgery for gynecologic conditions, especially malignancy, carries a risk of bowel injury. Other predisposing factors are increasing age, obesity, previous abdominal and pelvic surgery, adhesions, radiation therapy, pelvic inflammatory disease, and endometriosis [1]. Although the most favorable time to diagnose bowel damage is within the intraoperative period, a smaller proportion may go unrecognized at the time of primary surgery and manifest during the postoperative period. Patients with unrecognized bowel damage develop signs and symptoms in the postoperative period, causing significant diagnostic dilemma, major morbidity and, on occasion, mortality. Bowel surgery may also be a part of gynecologic oncology procedures and early recognition of a failed repair or an anastomotic leak is vital to patient outcome. Mortality is most often the result of overwhelming and prolonged sepsis, leading to multiorgan failure, bleeding diathesis, and adult respiratory distress syndrome.

Most of the unrecognized bowel injuries with delayed presentation are due to thermal damage, while most mechanical damage is recognized at the time of injury. The risk of bowel injury at laparoscopy is small when compared with abdominal surgery; however, at laparoscopy, bowel damage is more likely to remain unrecognized leading to significant morbidity (Chapter 75).

Mode of colonic injury

The left colon and rectum are at risk of injury when dissecting in the pelvis, while the transverse colon may be damaged during omentectomy. Damage to the rectum can occur during radical hysterectomy where the rectum tends to be attached higher on the vagina than one expects, and during dissection of fixed pelvic masses. Intraoperative damage may be difficult to detect, so a high degree of suspicion should be entertained in such circumstances.

Mode of small bowel injury

The small intestine is susceptible to injury particularly when entering the peritoneal cavity or during adhesiolysis. Ischemic injury that interrupts the blood supply to small bowel may not manifest for a few days and is a real challenge for timely diagnosis. Damage to the blood supply of a segment of bowel may result in necrosis and perforation of a segment in the postoperative period.

Presentation

Patients with unrecognized bowel injury tend to present with ileus, gastrointestinal fistula, abscess, or peritonitis. The principal derangements arising from untreated bowel damage are related to infection, fluid and electrolyte imbalance, and their subsequent sequelae. Spiking temperatures, signs of peritonitis, absolute constipation, or diarrhea are some of the common features of anastomotic bowel leak.

During the early postoperative period, patients should experience a steady daily improvement with return to normal activity. Understanding the normal course of postoperative recovery helps to identify any deviation from normal without delay. Patients with bowel damage would experience persistent and worsening pain often associated with nausea, vomiting, or both. However, symptoms could be non-specific and pain could be masked due to use of epidural or opiate pain relief. Patients may complain of chills, weakness, or simply not feeling normal (Table 46.1). Their breathing may be labored. Patients with laparoscopic bowel injuries often have atypical symptoms and are less likely to experience nausea, vomiting, paralytic ileus, and severe pain. This may be because laparoscopy elicits less inflammatory and immune response compared with laparotomy.

To prevent delay in diagnosis, a high index of suspicion is required when the patient does not show steady postoperative improvement. Clear guidance for nursing staff involved in patient monitoring and regular medical review are vital for timely detection of postoperative complication. The Modified Early Warning Score (MEWS) [2] is now commonly used for routine assessment of unwell patients to

Gynecologic and Obstetric Surgery: Challenges and Management Options, First Edition. Edited by Arri Coomarasamy, Mahmood I. Shafi, G. Willy Davila and Kiong K. Chan.
© 2016 John Wiley & Sons, Ltd. Published 2016 by John Wiley & Sons, Ltd.

Table 46.1 Symptoms and signs of bowel damage.

Symptoms
No symptoms or vague abdominal symptoms
Bloating
Persistent nausea and vomiting
Fever, chills
Difficulty in breathing
Weakness
Increasing abdominal pain after initial improvement

Signs
Direct or rebound tenderness
Persistent abdominal distension
Diminished or absent bowel sounds
Elevated temperature
Pallor, hypotension, diminished consciousness
Oliguria, hypotension
Raised MEWS

quickly determine the degree of illness. The observations recorded include heart rate, respiratory rate, systolic blood pressure, level of consciousness, oxygen saturation, and temperature [2]. The vital signs may show a normal, low-grade or subnormal temperature and persistent tachycardia. Respiratory rate of more than 20 breaths per minute could be the first sign, and it suggests diaphragmatic irritation or a reactionary pleural effusion due to intestinal leakage. As the abdominal sepsis progresses further, high-grade temperature or hypothermia and hypotension develop. As renal function deteriorates, urine output decreases. Drainage of fecal material or succus entericus (intestinal fluid) from peritoneal drain makes the diagnosis fairly straightforward. Blood tests may show low, normal or high white cell count, elevated liver profile, and elevated creatinine levels.

Examination may reveal a distended abdomen with direct or rebound tenderness; however, it may be difficult to elicit rebound tenderness, particularly in obese patients. Normal bowel function will have usually returned by the third postoperative day. Physiologic studies have shown return of function and motility of the small bowel in 6–12 hours, of the stomach in 12–24 hours, and of the colon in 48–72 hours. In patients with bowel injury, bowel sounds can be diminished or absent.

Role of imaging
Abdominopelvic CT with contrast (intravenous with or without oral contrast) is the imaging modality of choice in the evaluation of bowel continuity, fistula, and abscess. It may demonstrate loculated fluid collections with air–fluid levels and extravasation of oral contrast material from the area of bowel leak. However, a negative CT (no extraluminal leakage of contrast) could be falsely reassuring and does not exclude all types of bowel damage. If a collection is shown to indicate a localized leak, CT- or ultrasound-guided drainage may be indicated. However, major leakage has a significant mortality (10–15%) and so prompt return to the operating room is indicated. Whenever a small bowel or proximal large bowel problem is suspected, it is important to exclude distal obstruction by a Gastrografin enema [3].

Gastrointestinal fistulae after gynecologic surgery are rare. They occur 10–14 days postoperatively, and may be heralded by spiking temperatures with no clear focus, no response to antibiotics, and a tender but otherwise normal-appearing abdominal wound. When a fistula is present, its site can be determined by either a fistulogram or a CT scan with oral contrast if a small bowel lesion is suspected, or a Gastrografin enema if a large bowel lesion is suspected.

Management (see Chapter 37)

Radiologic or clinical evidence of a bowel perforation and intra-abdominal leak should prompt immediate action. Patients with sepsis should be managed according to the resuscitation care bundle, as recommended in the Surviving Sepsis Campaign (Box 46.1). Immediate re-exploration and segmental resection of the affected bowel are necessary. Gross contamination and peritonitis are high risk factors for anastomotic breakdown in the setting of unrecognized bowel injury and therefore repair of any bowel damage should be accompanied by proximal diversion.

> **BOX 46.1 MANAGING SEPSIS (THE "SEPSIS SIX")**
>
> Give high-flow oxygen
> Take blood cultures
> Give intravenous antibiotics
> Start intravenous fluid resuscitation
> Check hemoglobin and lactate levels
> Measure accurate hourly urine output

Resolution of the case

Both cases were diagnosed to have unrecognized bowel damage. The initial resuscitation of patients included insertion of nasogastric tube, evaluation for parenteral nutrition, broad-spectrum antibiotics, correction of fluid and electrolyte balance, and intravenous hydration. In Case history 1, the inflammatory markers (white cell count and CRP) showed an upward trend. A CT scan with contrast was suggestive of a leak from sigmoid colon. Review of the operative notes highlighted difficult surgery with ovarian mass densely adherent to sigmoid colon and rectum. After initial resuscitation, the patient underwent a laparotomy with resection of sigmoid colon with an end colostomy.

In Case history 2, the patient was asked to attend the hospital immediately. Examination found distended abdomen and rebound tenderness with reduced bowel sounds. Vital signs showed raised temperature and tachycardia. Operative notes suggested the presence of bowel and omental adhesions. Abdominal X-ray showed persistent gas under the diaphragm, and CT revealed a collection in the subphrenic space. Because of a high index of suspicion of bowel injury, a laparotomy was carried out after initial resuscitation. At laparotomy, there was considerable contamination of the peritoneal cavity with leak from a small bowel injury. Patient required resection of unhealthy bowel with an ileostomy.

Postoperative care
Optimal postoperative management requires coordination of appropriate care providers, especially out of routine hours. Multidisciplinary care in HDU in liaison with anesthetists is required to reduce the postoperative morbidity and mortality. If a prolonged postoperative recovery is anticipated (>5 days), then nutritional support should be considered.

Prevention

With increasing utilization of complex laparoscopic surgery, it is likely that some patients will present with signs and symptoms after being discharged early from hospital. Therefore, patient education about normal recovery and deviation from normal is of great value in preventing delays in seeking advice from healthcare practitioners.

KEY POINTS

Challenge: Postoperative presentation of bowel damage.

Background
- Bowel injury is a risk of nearly all abdominal surgeries, including those for gynecologic cancers.
- Patients with unrecognized bowel damage tend to have high mortality rates compared with the group of patients with recognized intraoperative injuries.
- A high level of suspicion is required to detect bowel damage as early as possible. The diagnosis is often delayed because postoperative pain, analgesia, and antibiotics complicate assessment.

Management
- The signs and symptoms of bowel damage can be subtle and overlap with more benign processes, such as postoperative ileus.

- A range of symptoms is possible, including fever, abdominal pain, abdominal distension, delayed return of bowel function, peritonitis, and fistula formation. The most common indicators of bowel damage are persistent unexplained pyrexia, tachycardia, or ileus.
- Abdominal and pelvic CT with contrast is the test of choice in the evaluation of bowel damage and has good accuracy. However, a negative CT (no extraluminal leakage of contrast) could be falsely reassuring and does not exclude all types of bowel damage.
- Unrecognized bowel injuries should always be suspected in patients who develop signs of sepsis postoperatively.
- See Chapters 37 and 75 for operative management of bowel injury.

Prevention
- Familiarity with normal postoperative physiology and understanding the pitfalls of interpreting investigations facilitate management.

References

1 Stany M, Farley J, Complications of gynecologic surgery. *Surg Clin North Am* 2008; 88:343–359.
2 National Institute for Health and Care Excellence. *Acutely ill patients in hospital. Recognition of and response to acute illness in adults in hospital.* NICE Clinical Guideline 50, July 2007. Available at https://www.nice.org.uk/guidance/cg50/
3 Zissin R, Osadchy A, Gayer G. Abdominal CT findings in small bowel perforation. *Br J Radiolol* 2009; 82(974):162–171.

CHAPTER 47

Wound Infection

Pallavi Latthe and James Gray
Birmingham Women's NHS Foundation Trust, Birmingham, UK

Case history: An obese woman who had emergency cesarean section develops seropurulent discharge at the surgical site on the fourth postoperative day.

Background

It is estimated that 3–15% of cesarean sections and 3–8% of abdominal hysterectomies are complicated by an abdominal wound infection [1]. Surgical site infection (SSI) is a healthcare-associated infection (HCAI) in which a wound infection occurs after an invasive (surgical) procedure. SSI is possible with any transabdominal procedure, but especially with those that are contaminated. SSIs can have a significant effect on quality of life for the patient, as well as having medical and economic implications. They account for approximately 14% of all HCAIs, and are estimated to double the length of postoperative stay in hospital, thereby significantly increasing the cost of care [2]. The annual cost to European healthcare systems of SSIs is estimated to be €1.5–19 billion [3].

Risk factors for wound infection
Risk factors can be categorized into patient, wound, and operative factors. General patient factors include advanced age, obesity (BMI >30 kg/m²), malnutrition, endocrine and metabolic disorders (e.g., diabetes), smoking, hypoxia, anemia, malignant disease, and immunosuppression. Wound factors include non-viable tissue in wound, foreign bodies, tissue ischemia, and hematoma formation. Operative factors include poor surgical technique, long operation time (>2 hours), intraoperative contamination, prolonged hospital stay, and hypothermia.

Classification of wound infections
An SSI may range from a self-limiting wound discharge within 7–10 days of an operation to a life-threatening postoperative complication. Most SSIs are caused by contamination of an incision with microorganisms from the patient's own body during surgery [4]. Infection caused by microorganisms from an outside source following surgery is less common. There are three different levels of SSI [2]:
1 superficial incisional infection, involving only the skin or subcutaneous tissue of the incision;

2 deep incisional infection, involving the fascial or muscle layers;
3 intra-abdominal infection, involving intra-abdominal tissues, peritoneum, subphrenic or subdiaphragmatic space.

Wound infections may be early or late in onset. Early-onset infections are characterized by pyrexia and cellulitis that develops within the first 48 hours. These infections are usually caused by a single highly virulent bacterial species such as group A streptococci or sometimes *Clostridium perfringens*. Wound breakdown and dehiscence can occur if treatment is not initiated rapidly. Late-onset infections are associated with persistent (often low-grade) pyrexia together with local wound symptoms and signs, including pain, tenderness, redness, warmth and discharge, which may be purulent. These infections generally present between 4 and 7 days postoperatively, but can occur later. Causative organisms are *Staphylococcus aureus* in 25% of cases and vaginal or gastrointestinal bacteria (often polymicrobial) in 75% of cases.

Management

The management will need to take into account the patient's condition and comorbidities, the extent of the infection, whether the infection is superficial, deep or intra-abdominal, and whether there is an associated abscess.

Inspect
Thorough general examination and wound inspection should be done to assess the depth of wound infection and rule out dehiscence.

Investigate
Investigations depend on the clinical presentation. Mild infections presenting in primary care may be treated empirically without any investigations. For more serious infections a wound swab should be collected for microscopy, culture, and sensitivity. FBC and measurement of CRP may be useful if it is uncertain whether the wound is infected. Where there is uncertainty about the site of infection, urine and vaginal cultures may be useful. Blood cultures are indicated for patients with fever over 38°C [5].

Gynecologic and Obstetric Surgery: Challenges and Management Options, First Edition. Edited by Arri Coomarasamy, Mahmood I. Shafi, G. Willy Davila and Kiong K. Chan.
© 2016 John Wiley & Sons, Ltd. Published 2016 by John Wiley & Sons, Ltd.

Treat abscess

First-line therapy for an abscess is to open the wound to allow drainage and healing by secondary intention. Intra-abdominal abscesses will generally require ultrasound-guided transvaginal drainage (as opposed to just aspiration), or drainage and lavage of the abdomen and pelvis via laparoscopy or laparotomy.

Administer antibiotics

Antibiotics are indicated where there is evidence of cellulitis, lymphangitis, bacteremia, or sepsis. Several factors influence the choice of antibiotics and the route of their administration, including the timing and clinical presentation of the infection, and the likelihood that a patient may have an infection with antibiotic-resistant bacteria (e.g., MRSA).

Management of early-onset infections

Infections that occur in the first 48 hours are usually caused by group A streptococci or anaerobes such as *C. perfringens*. They require prompt and aggressive management with broad-spectrum intravenous antibiotics (ensuring good cover against streptococci and anaerobes) and early surgical review with early excision of necrotic tissue if required. Combined amoxicillin and clavulanic acid (co-amoxiclav) is a suitable agent that carries a lower risk of *C. difficile* infection than the traditional alternative regimen of a cephalosporin such as cefuroxime plus metronidazole. For patients who are severely systemically unwell, piperacillin and tazobactam may be preferred to co-amoxiclav to provide cover against *Pseudomonas aeruginosa*. If the patient is considered to be at risk of infection with a multiresistant Gram-negative bacterium such as an extended spectrum β-lactamase (ESBL)-producing member of the Enterobacteriaceae (coliforms), use a carbapenem (meropenem or imipenem with cilastatin) instead of co-amoxiclav or piperacillin and tazobactam. For patients who have developed septic shock, consider adding a single dose of intravenous gentamicin 6–7 mg/kg body weight; this will provide cover for 24 hours, after which the need for further doses of gentamicin can be reviewed in the light of culture results and the patient's clinical condition. For patients with cellulitis, consider adding clindamycin. For patients at risk of MRSA infection, add a glycopeptide such as vancomycin.

Management of late-onset infections

The majority of late-onset infections can be managed on an outpatient basis with oral antibiotics. As *S. aureus* is the commonest single cause of infection, flucloxacillin may suffice. If broader-spectrum therapy is required, oral co-amoxiclav is appropriate.

Patients with late-onset infections requiring hospital admission for intravenous antibiotics should be treated with broad-spectrum antibiotics as for early-onset infections. More commonly, these patients will have earlier microbiology results to refer to, which can help in the targeting of appropriate therapy.

Review of antibiotic therapy

In all cases, antibiotic therapy should be reviewed after 48 hours or sooner. A patient who is improving should be assessed in the light of any microbiology results to determine whether she might be a candidate for (i) switch to narrower-spectrum agents (reduces the risk of antibiotic resistance, and *C. difficile* infection) and (ii) switch to oral therapy wherever feasible (reduces length of hospitalization).

Failure to respond to antibiotic therapy after 48 hours may be because the patient is infected with an antibiotic-resistant organism, or because the patient has a focus of infection such as an abscess that has not been drained; here the pattern of fever is classically intermittent. The patient should be carefully re-examined, and the results of microbiology cultures reviewed. A scan should be ordered to search for a collection. Where an abscess is found, antibiotic therapy alone is rarely sufficient, but antibiotic therapy should be commenced to stabilize the patient prior to surgical or radiologic drainage.

Common antibiotic regimens used in obstetrics and gynecology are given in Table 47.1.

Table 47.1 A brief guide to antibiotic prescribing in obstetrics and gynecology.

Indication	Intravenous therapy		Oral therapy	
	First choice	Alternatives	First choice	Alternatives
Abdominal wound infection	Co-amoxiclav (expressed as amoxicillin) 1 g t.d.s.	Clarithromycin 500 mg b.d.	Flucloxacillin 500 mg q.d.s.	Erythromycin 500 mg q.d.s.
Perineal wound infection	Co-amoxiclav (expressed as amoxicillin) 1 g t.d.s.	Ciprofloxacin 200 mg b.d. + metronidazole* 500 mg t.d.s.	Co-amoxiclav 250–500 mg (expressed as amoxicillin) t.d.s.	Ciprofloxacin 500 mg b.d. + metronidazole 400 mg b.d.
Cellulitis	Co-amoxiclav or piperacillin/tazobactam or meropenem + gentamicin ± clindamycin (contact a microbiologist for advice in all cases)		Flucloxacillin 500 mg q.d.s.	Erythromycin 500 mg q.d.s.
Postoperative pelvic infection	Co-amoxiclav (expressed as amoxicillin) 1 g t.d.s.	Ciprofloxacin 200 mg b.d. + metronidazole* 500 mg .t.d.s	Co-amoxiclav 250–500 mg (expressed as amoxicillin) t.d.s.	Ciprofloxacin 500 mg b.d. + metronidazole 400 mg b.d.
Prevention of cesarean section surgical site infections	Cefuroxime 750 mg as a single dose 30 min before skin incision	Co-amoxiclav (expressed as amoxicillin) 1 g as a single dose after clamping the cord *or* clarithromycin 500 mg 30 min before skin incision	Not applicable	
Prevention of gynecologic surgical site infections	Co-amoxiclav (expressed as amoxicillin) 1 g as a single dose 30 min before skin incision	Cefuroxime 750 mg + metronidazole 500 mg as single doses 30 min before skin incision. Metronidazole can also be 1 g p.r. 2 hours before surgery	Not applicable	

* Antibiotic regimens used for prophylaxis and treatment may have to be modified for patients with antibiotic-resistant bacteria, such as MRSA and ESBL-producing Enterobacteriaceae (see text).

Wound care

Use an appropriate interactive dressing to manage surgical wounds that are healing by secondary intention; do not use Eusol and gauze, moist cotton gauze, or mercuric antiseptic solutions for debridement or to manage surgical wounds that are healing by secondary intention. Refer to a tissue viability nurse (or another healthcare professional with tissue viability expertise) for advice on appropriate dressings for the management of surgical wounds that are healing by secondary intention.

Although there is no direct evidence to support the provision of specialist wound care services for managing complex surgical wounds, a structured approach to care (including preoperative assessments to identify individuals with potential wound healing problems) is required in order to improve overall management of surgical wounds.

The use of secondary closure of disrupted wounds is 80–100% effective and reduces healing time. Negative pressure wound therapy (NPWT) is a therapeutic technique that uses a vacuum dressing to promote healing in acute or chronic wounds (Figures 47.1 and 47.2). The therapy involves the controlled application of subatmospheric pressure to the local wound environment, using a sealed wound dressing connected to a vacuum pump. Generally, NPWT can be considered in a chronic wound if the wound size decreases by less than 30% after 4 weeks following debridement or if excessive exudate cannot be managed effectively with daily dressing changes. The use

of this system is contraindicated over necrotic, cancerous, and friable tissues. There is evidence, though of poor quality, to suggest that healing of other wounds might also be accelerated with NPWT [6].

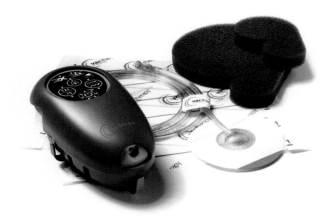

Figure 47.1 Vacuum-assisted closure (V.A.C. Via™) negative pressure wound therapy system. Used with permission, courtesy of KCI. http://www.kci1.com/cs/Satellite?c=KCI_Product_C&childpagename=KCI1%2FKCILayout&cid=1229636483749&p=1229538260417&packedargs=locale%3Den_US&pagename=KCI1Wrapper.

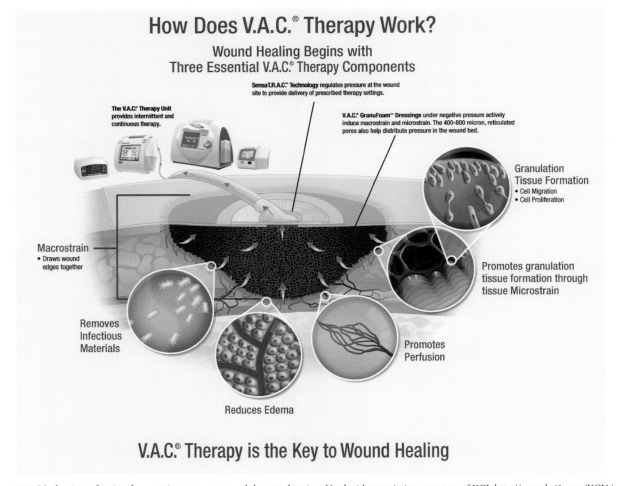

Figure 47.2 Mechanism of action for negative vacuum wound therapy dressing. Used with permission, courtesy of KCI. http://www.kci1.com/KCI1/vactherapysystemfactsheet

Prevention

Various preoperative, intraoperative and postoperative measures have been shown to reduce the risk of SSI. Careful hand-washing techniques preoperatively and when seeing patients postoperatively are associated with a reduction in hospital-associated healthcare infections. Postoperative hospitalization should be limited as far as possible.

Even though preoperative showers reduce the skin's microbial colony counts, they have not definitively been shown to reduce SSI rates [7]. Hair removal should be avoided unless there is abundance of hair at the operation site. Shaving immediately before the operation compared to shaving within 24 hours preoperatively was associated with decreased SSI rates. Thus patients should be discouraged from shaving themselves at home before admission for elective surgery. If hair has to be removed, use electric clippers (rather than razors) with a single-use head on the day of surgery.

It is not advisable to use nasal decontamination with topical antimicrobial agents aimed at eliminating *S. aureus* or use mechanical bowel preparation to reduce the risk of SSI. Give patients specific theater wear that is appropriate for the procedure and clinical setting, and that provides easy access to the operative site and areas for placing devices, such as intravenous cannulae. All staff should wear appropriate theater wear in all areas where operations are undertaken. Staff wearing non-sterile theater wear should keep their movements in and out of the operating area to a minimum. The operating team should remove hand jewellery, artificial nails, and nail polish before operations.

Prophylactic antibiotics

Perioperative single-dose antibiotic prophylaxis, ideally 30 min prior to incision, is now a well-established practice to reduce the risk of wound infections.

All women undergoing elective or emergency cesarean section should receive antibiotic prophylaxis. The choice of prophylactic antibiotic for cesarean section is usually cefuroxime. Note that co-amoxiclav is not recommended before the umbilical cord is clamped. If the patient has a penicillin allergy, clindamycin or erythromycin can be used. The timing of prophylactic antibiotics for cesarean section should be 15–60 min prior to skin incision [8]. In patients with morbid obesity (BMI >35 kg/m^2) undergoing cesarean section, doubling the antibiotic dose should be considered.

Preoperative MRSA screening is mandatory in some countries, including the UK. MRSA screen-positive patients can be decolonized before surgery and/or have intraoperative antibiotic prophylaxis tailored to cover MRSA. Vancomycin should be given in addition to the usual prophylaxis if the patient is known to be colonized with MRSA.

Surgical technique

Meticulous surgical techniques are mandatory to reduce the risk of deep and superficial wound infections. Adequate hemostasis should be achieved and pedicles should be kept short [7]. Closure of the subcutaneous fat may reduce wound complications [9]. Routine prophylactic use of subcutaneous drainage does not prevent significant wound complications after cesarean delivery [10].

The operating team should wear sterile gowns in the operating theater during the operation. Consider wearing two pairs of sterile gloves when there is a high risk of glove perforation and the consequences of contamination may be serious. Do not use wound irrigation or intracavity lavage to reduce the risk of SSI. Do not use intraoperative skin re-disinfection or topical cefotaxime in abdominal surgery to reduce the risk of SSI. Cover surgical incisions with an appropriate interactive dressing at the end of the operation.

KEY POINTS

Challenge: Postoperative wound infection.

Background
- Approximately 1 in 10 cesarean sections and abdominal hysterectomies are complicated by an abdominal wound infection.
- In many SSIs, the responsible pathogens originate from the patient's endogenous flora. The most commonly isolated organisms are *Staphylococcus aureus*, coagulase-negative staphylococci, *Enterococcus* species, and *Escherichia coli*.

Risk factors
- Patient factors: advanced age, obesity (BMI >30 kg/m^2), malnutrition, endocrine and metabolic disorders (e.g., diabetes), smoking, hypoxia, anemia, malignant disease, and immunosuppression.
- Wound factors: non-viable tissue in wound, foreign bodies, tissue ischemia, and hematoma formation.
- Operative factors: poor surgical technique, long operation time (>2 hours), intraoperative contamination, prolonged hospital stay, and hypothermia.

SSI classification
- Superficial incisional infection: involving only the skin or subcutaneous tissue of the incision.
- Deep incisional infection: involving the fascial or muscle layers.
- Intra-abdominal infection: involving intra-abdominal tissues, peritoneum, subphrenic or subdiaphragmatic space.

Management
- Consider patient's condition and comorbidities, the extent of the infection, and whether there is an associated abscess.

Inspect
- To assess the depth of infection and rule out dehiscence.

Investigate
- Wound swab.
- Blood count and CRP if presence of infection is uncertain.
- Urine and vaginal cultures if location of infection is uncertain.
- Blood cultures if temperature >38°C; ultrasound or CT if abscess is suspected.

Treat abscess
- Superficial abscesses: open the wound to allow drainage.
- Intra-abdominal abscesses: decide between ultrasound-guided transvaginal drainage (as opposed to just aspiration), and drainage and lavage of the abdomen and pelvis via laparoscopy or laparotomy.

Administer antibiotics
- Consult local guidelines and microbiologist.
- Consider broad-spectrum antibiotics such as co-amoxiclav as first-line treatment.
- For patients who are severely unwell, consider piperacillin and tazobactam.
- If the patient is considered to be at risk of infection with a multiresistant Gram-negative bacterium, use a carbapenem (meropenem or imipenem with cilastatin) instead of co-amoxiclav or piperacillin and tazobactam.
- For patients who have developed septic shock, consider adding a single dose of intravenous gentamicin 6–7 mg/kg; this will provide cover for 24 hours, after which the need for further doses of gentamicin can be reviewed in the light of culture results and the patient's clinical condition.
- For patients with cellulitis, consider adding clindamycin.
- For patients at risk of MRSA infection, add a glycopeptide such as vancomycin.

Review progress
- Review patient and wound daily. Review response to antibiotic regimen within 48 hours of starting antibiotics. If patient is better, consider narrow-spectrum antibiotics and oral therapy. If patient is not better or worse, review antibiotic sensitivities and investigate for abscesses.
- Seek expert help in wound management from a tissue viability nurse.

Prevention
- Do not remove hair routinely. If hair has to be removed, use electric clippers (rather than razors) with a single-use head on the day of surgery.
- Give single dose of antibiotic prophylaxis intravenously on starting anesthesia.
- Preoperative MRSA screening is mandatory in some countries, including the UK. MRSA screen-positive patients can be decolonized before surgery and/or have intraoperative antibiotic prophylaxis tailored to cover MRSA.
- Prepare the skin at the surgical site immediately before incision using an antiseptic (aqueous or alcohol-based) preparation: povidone iodine or chlorhexidine are most suitable. Do not wipe off the prep, but allow it to dry naturally before making the skin incision.
- During the operation, pay attention to ensure adequate perfusion, oxygenation, and temperature of the patient.
- Maintain sterility and hemostasis through good operative techniques.
- Cover surgical incisions with an appropriate interactive dressing at the end of the operation.

References

1 Sweet RL, Gibbs RS. Infections of abdominal wounds, episiotomies and perineal laceration. In: *Infectious Diseases of the Female Genital Tract*, 5th edn, pp. 350–358. Lippincott Williams & Wilkins, Philadelphia, 2009.
2 Public Health England. *Protocol for the surveillance of surgical site infection.* Available at http://webarchive.nationalarchives.gov.uk/20140714084352/http://www.hpa.org.uk/webc/HPAwebFile/HPAweb_C/1194947388966
3 Leaper DJ, van Goor H, Reilly J *et al.* Surgical site infection: a European perspective of incidence and economic burden. *Int Wound J* 2004; 1:247–273.
4 Cliby WA. Abdominal incision wound breakdown. *Clin Obstet Gynecol* 2002; 45:507–517.
5 Hager WD, Larsen JW. Postoperative infections: prevention and management. In: Rock JA, JonesHW (eds) *Te Linde's Operative Gynecology*, 10th edn, pp. 190–202. Lippincott Williams & Wilkins, Philadelphia, 2008.
6 Xie X, McGregor M, Dendukuri N. The clinical effectiveness of negative pressure wound therapy: a systematic review. *J Wound Care* 2010; 19: 490–495.
7 Mangram AJ, Horan TC, Pearson ML, Silver LC, Jarvis WR. Guideline for prevention of surgical site infection, 1999. Centers for Disease Control and Prevention (CDC) Hospital Infection Control Practices Advisory Committee. *Am J Infect Control* 1999; 27:97–132.
8 van Schalkwyk J, Van Eyk N. Antibiotic prophylaxis in obstetric procedures. *J Obstet Gynaecol Can* 2010; 32:878–892.
9 Anderson ER, Gates S. Techniques and materials for closure of the abdominal wall in caesarean section. *Cochrane Database Syst Rev* 2004;(4):CD004663.
10 Hellums EK, Lin MG, Ramsey PS. Prophylactic subcutaneous drainage for prevention of wound complications after cesarean delivery: a metaanalysis. *Am J Obstet Gynecol* 2007; 197:229–235.

CHAPTER 48
Wound Dehiscence

T. Justin Clark

Birmingham Women's NHS Foundation Trust, Birmingham, UK

Case history 1: A cesarean section wound has partially separated on removal of the continuous subcuticular polypropylene suture. The operation was performed as an emergency 7 days earlier. The patient is slim, fit and well, no hematoma is visible, and the wound appears clean.

Case history 2: An obese 52-year-old woman presents with a foul-smelling, discharging, midline laparotomy wound 10 days following a total abdominal hysterectomy that was complicated by a pelvic hematoma. On inspecting the wound, viable bowel is visible. The patient has no medical problems but is a heavy smoker.

Background

Wound dehiscence is the separating or "bursting" open of a wound along the surgical suture line. The separation of the wound edges may be partial or complete. Abdominal wound dehiscence is estimated to complicate around 1.2% of laparotomies, although the incidence varies between 0.2 and 6.0% according to population and surgical factors [1]. Wound dehiscence is usually superficial but deeper fascial dehiscence may occur with resulting evisceration, where internal organs, namely bowel, protrude slightly or actually spill outside of the open surgical incision. Evisceration is more serious, being associated with prolonged hospitalization, need for reoperations, and increased mortality.

Wound dehiscence usually presents between days 7 and 14 following surgery, usually at the time of staple or suture removal. Although the complication can present without warning, dehiscence is most often preceded by a discharging wound [1]. The complication results from poor wound healing.

Risk factors for wound dehiscence
The following are risk factors for dehiscence.
1 Preoperative patient variables: age over 45 years, smoking, obesity, pulmonary disease, renal disease, liver disease (ascites, jaundice), anemia, and malnutrition.
2 Perioperative surgical variables: emergency operation, midline incision, prolonged surgery over 2.5 hours, and method of wound closure.
3 Postoperative variables: raised intra-abdominal pressure (including postoperative coughing), wound infection, trauma to the wound, and radiation.

Surprisingly, a recent study that developed and validated a prognostic risk model for wound dehiscence did not find hypertension, uremia, corticosteroid use, diabetes mellitus, previous laparotomy, malignancy, sepsis, and postoperative vomiting to be independent risk factors, in contrast to other studies [2].

What has remained consistent across studies is the pre-eminent importance of wound infection. Infection causes a prolonged inflammatory phase and negatively affects deposition of collagen and fibroblast activity.

Management

Care of superficial dehiscence
Case history 1 describes a superficial partial wound separation triggered by suture removal, at a time when wound integrity would have reasonably been anticipated. Faced with this situation, the wound should be carefully inspected and gently probed with a sterile cotton-tipped applicator to exclude a deeper fascial defect that might require surgical intervention. A wound swab should be taken and sent for microbiologic examination, given that infection commonly precipitates wound dehiscence. In the absence of a subcuticular collection, non-viable tissue, or other evidence of infection (e.g., cellulitis, induration, heat, and discharge), the skin edges can be reapproximated to continue wound healing by primary intention. In this case, adhesive strips (Steri-strips™) may suffice; however, with more complete separation in larger women, resuturing under either local or general anesthesia may be preferable. The wound should be reviewed after 7 days.

If infection is suspected, the wound should be cleaned and either packed with gauze or covered with a sterile occlusive dressing, and broad-spectrum antibiotics commenced. Healing can progress by secondary intention, or delayed resuturing can be considered.

Management of full-thickness wound dehiscence
Case history 2 is a more serious complication necessitating urgent intervention because visibly exposed, eviscerated organs can lead to sepsis from bacterial contamination. This woman has risk factors for wound complications, namely age over 45 years, obesity, smoking, hematoma (and probable resulting anemia), and a midline laparotomy. Such a presentation can be very alarming to patients; a calm

Gynecologic and Obstetric Surgery: Challenges and Management Options, First Edition. Edited by Arri Coomarasamy, Mahmood I. Shafi, G. Willy Davila and Kiong K. Chan.
© 2016 John Wiley & Sons, Ltd. Published 2016 by John Wiley & Sons, Ltd.

and reassuring approach is important. No attempt should be made to replace the bowel, but instead it should be covered with a gauze pack soaked with sterile saline and secured over the open wound with a self-adhesive dressing in order to minimize risks of dehydration and bacterial contamination. Flexing the patient's knees can help to reduce wound tension. The patient's clinical condition should be stabilized, including the use of intravenous fluids, blood transfusion if anemic, and a nasogastric tube if significant ileus and vomiting are present. Preparations should be made for a formal examination under general anesthesia to explore the wound. Preoperative broad-spectrum antibiotics should be started and continued postoperatively. These may need to be changed once microbiologic culture and sensitivity results from wound swabs are available. The viability of surrounding tissues should be assessed and the presence of necrotizing fasciitis excluded (Chapter 50). Non-viable tissue should be removed. The involvement of a general and plastic surgeon is advisable where extensive debridement is anticipated.

The options for wound closure are either immediate resuturing or sterile wound packing allowing the wound to heal by secondary intention. Resuturing may be partial (some layers closed) or full (all abdominal wall layers closed). If resuturing is undertaken, mass closure using a heavy, loop PDS suture is advisable. In addition to reapproximating the skin edges, deep retention sutures should be considered, especially in an obese patient, to reinforce the wound closure by minimizing tension on the skin edges. One option is to use nylon "through-and-through" sutures (Figure 48.1); each suture is placed about 2 cm apart, and at least 2 cm from the skin edges. Particular care should be taken to avoid catching the bowel in the suture, and the sutures should be left in place for 3 weeks.

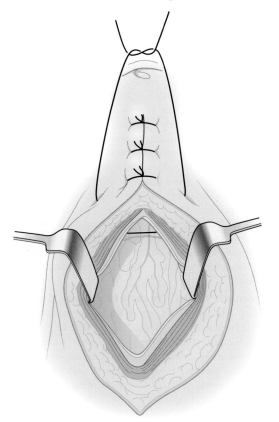

Figure 48.1 "Through-and-through" nylon sutures to manage complete dehiscence.

Superficial wound drains should be considered. In Case history 2, there are clear signs of infection and the tissue perfusion and tensile strength are likely to be compromised in an obese anemic smoker. Thus, the surgeon should consider debriding, cleaning and packing the wound with sterile antiseptic gauze packs, and reassessing after 24–48 hours of antibiotics with a view to surgical closure. Delayed primary closure in this way provides an opportunity for debridement of necrotic tissue, control of local infection, and resolution of bowel edema. On occasions, such as in the presence of extensive necrotizing fasciitis, it may not be technically feasible or safe to close the wound surgically.

Negative pressure wound therapy

For large partial or complete defects of the anterior abdominal wall, healing can be expedited by the use of negative pressure wound therapy (NPWT; see Figures 47.1 and 47.2), which involves the controlled application of subatmospheric pressure to the local wound environment using a sealed wound dressing connected to a vacuum pump [3]. The separated wound tissue is mechanically drawn together, inducing healing by gradually decreasing the wound defect, encouraging granulation tissue formation, increasing local blood perfusion, reducing bacterial colonization, and removing interstitial fluid.

Postoperative care

On discharge the patient needs to be informed about the rationale of the proposed wound management and be made aware that complete healing will take many weeks. Regular domiciliary visits by a nurse qualified in wound care will be necessary, and frequent dressing changes may be necessary, particularly if there is continuous or excessive wound drainage. Regular review by the clinical team in hospital will also be necessary to ensure gradual wound healing is occurring, and to exclude long-term complications such as enterocutaneous fistulae and incisional hernia.

Prevention

Although surgical technique, especially regarding the choice of suture material, and perioperative care have improved, the incidence of abdominal wound dehiscence does not appear to have substantially decreased. This may simply reflect better data capture, but may also be attributable to a higher prevalence of risk factors within patient populations undergoing surgery.

Preoperative work-up should identify women at increased risk of wound dehiscence by identifying known risk factors; use of formally developed predictive models should be considered. Future research on interventions aimed at optimizing wound healing and reinforcing wounds, for example with the use of NPWT devices or placement of biologic meshes, may benefit high-risk women. For now, interventions must include optimizing the preoperative clinical health of high-risk women. Such interventions include correcting anemia, smoking cessation, improving chronic medical conditions, enhancing nutritional state, and weight loss programs.

Minimally invasive surgical approaches should be adopted where possible, even if this necessitates referral to specialist centers. If laparotomy is undertaken, broad-spectrum antibiotics should be used to reduce the likelihood of wound contamination; transverse incisions are preferable to midline approaches and mass closure is preferable to layered closure [4]. Wound dehiscence does not appear to be affected by separate closure of the peritoneum, whether interrupted or continuous suturing is adopted, nor by the type of suture material (absorbable vs. non-absorbable) [5]. However, slowly absorbing monofilament sutures such as polydioxanone (PDS) may be the preferred method for fascial closure in women with risk factors for wound dehiscence because in addition to prolonged suture retention, PDS is associated with less wound pain and sinus formation compared with non-absorbable materials such as nylon (Ethilon) and polypropylene (Prolene) [5]. There is no compelling evidence supporting the routine use of fat stitches.

Removal of sutures before day 4 of a transverse incision after cesarean section may increase the risk of wound separation [6].

Postoperatively, interventions to minimize the risk of developing pneumonia and wound infection are key considerations and these include regular postoperative review, physiotherapy, early mobilization, and recourse to antibiotics when infection is suspected. On discharge, women should be advised to avoid placing undue stress on the incision, to avoid constipation, and to avoid heavy lifting. Patients should also be instructed to brace (i.e., apply gentle counter-pressure to the wound) when coughing, laughing, vomiting or sneezing.

KEY POINTS

Challenge: Wound dehiscence.

Background
- Wound dehiscence is the separating or "bursting" open of a wound along the surgical suture line, and complicates around 1% of laparotomies.
- Wound evisceration can lead to sepsis from bacterial contamination and is a surgical emergency.
- Wound infection is the most important risk factor for wound dehiscence. Other risk factors are:
  - Patient factors: age >45 years, smoking, obesity, pulmonary disease, renal disease, liver disease (ascites, jaundice), anemia, and malnutrition.
  - Perioperative surgical factors: emergency operation, midline incision, prolonged surgery >2.5 hours, and method of wound closure.
  - Postoperative factors: raised intra-abdominal pressure (including postoperative coughing), wound infection, trauma to the wound, and radiation.

Management
- Superficial wound dehiscence can often be managed without recourse to further surgery in an operating room:
  - Explore the wound gently.
  - Swab the wound for aerobic and anaerobic bacteria.
  - Clean the wound.
  - Reapproximate the skin edges. This can sometimes be done with adhesive strips (Steri-strips).
  - Antibiotics should generally be given to treat and/or prevent infection.

- Where infection is present, the wound should be cleaned and packed and allowed to heal over several weeks by secondary intention. Antibiotics should be administered according to wound culture results, and regular wound review and dressing changes are needed.
- In the presence of more extensive wound infection, subcutaneous collections, an unstable patient, or wound evisceration, an urgent formal examination under anesthesia is indicated and the viability of underlying tissues should be assessed, and cleaning and debridement undertaken as necessary.
- Primary wound closure in these circumstances should employ slowly absorbable, heavy monofilament sutures such as loop PDS, and deep tension sutures to reduce the tension on the skin edges should be considered. An alternative approach is the use of nylon "through-and-through" sutures.
- Wound closure may be enhanced by the use of NPWT.
- Consider superficial wound drains.
- Arrange appropriate postoperative care, including the involvement of a nurse qualified in wound care.

Prevention
- Preoperative work-up should identify women at increased risk of wound dehiscence by identifying known risk factors; interventions to correct or minimize the impact of these variables should be instigated.
- Minimally invasive surgical approaches should be adopted where possible.
- Pneumonia and wound infection should be prevented where possible and treated promptly should these conditions develop.

References

1 Carlson MA. Acute wound failure. *Surg Clin North Am* 1997; **77**:607–636.
2 van Ramshorst GH, Nieuwenhuizen J, Hop WC *et al.* Abdominal wound dehiscence in adults: development and validation of a risk model. *World J Surg* 2010; 34: 20–27.
3 Heller L, Levin SL, Butler CE. Management of abdominal wound dehiscence using vacuum assisted closure in patients with compromised healing. *Am J Surg* 2006; 191:165–172.
4 Weiland DE, Bay RC, Del Sordi S. Choosing the best abdominal closure by meta-analysis. *Am J Surg* 1998; 176: 666–670.
5 van't Riet M, Steyerberg EW, Nellensteyn J, Bonjer HJ, Jeekel J. Meta-analysis of techniques for closure of midline abdominal incisions. *Br J Surg* 2002; 89:1350–1356.
6 Mackeen AD, Berghella V, Larsen ML. Techniques and materials for skin closure in caesarean section. *Cochrane Database Syst Rev* 2012;(9):CD003577.

CHAPTER 49

Late Wound Failure: Incisional Hernia

Saloney Nazeer

Geneva Foundation for Medical Education and Research, World Health Organization Collaborating Center in Education and Research in Human Reproduction, Geneva, Switzerland

Case history 1: One year after a cesarean section, a woman presented with severe lower abdominal pain. Diagnostic laparoscopy showed a hernia defect at the Pfannenstiel incision between the rectus abdominis muscle and anterior rectus sheath. Surgical repair was performed with no postoperative complications.

Case history 2: A 55-year-old woman presented with abdominal distension and pain accompanied by nausea and vomiting 6 months after undergoing laparoscopic bilateral salpingo-oophorectomy. Examination, CT scan, and laparoscopy confirmed a small bowel herniation through the umbilical trocar site. The fascial defect was reapproximated to create a tension-free closure. The postoperative recovery was uncomplicated.

Background

The incidence of incisional hernias is reported to be 2–19% for various abdominal incisions. Transverse, oblique, and paramedian incisions cause significantly less incisional hernias when compared with midline incisions, with a reported occurrence of 1% for transverse incisions (Case history 1) as compared with 14% for the midline incisions [1]. The reasons for high incisional hernia rate after midline laparotomy include the contraction of abdominal wall muscles retracting wound edges laterally, the avascular nature of the midline incision, and perpendicular cutting of most of the fibers of the linea alba.

Incisional hernias are a rare complication of laparoscopic surgery, with a reported incidence of less than 1%. Most complications arise in trocar sites that are larger than 10 mm. The reported incidence of trocar-site hernia in diagnostic laparoscopic procedures is approximately 0.2% [2]. These hernias largely occur at the umbilical port site (Case history 2). The risk factors for postoperative hernia are large trocar size, leaving the fascial defect open, and stretching of the port site. Large surveys reporting trocar-site hernias for port sizes less than 8 mm and published case reports describing 5-mm port-site hernias have led some to recommend routine fascial closure when there has been extensive operative manipulation [2].

Management

Incisional hernia repair is associated with significant risk of morbidity and mortality, with reported mortality of elective hernia repair of up to 5.3% [3].

To repair or not to repair

Whether surgical repair is the best option for each patient with incisional hernia remains an open question because of the paucity of clinical research to elucidate their natural course and the incidence of complications of untreated incisional hernias [3].

The main indication for incisional hernia repair is symptoms such as discomfort, pain, and cosmetic complaints. Other indications include the complications associated with untreated incisional hernia, namely visceral incarceration or strangulation, dystrophic skin ulcer at the hernial site, or rupture of hernial sac and impairment of respiratory function. However, the true incidence of these complications has not been documented.

In view of the postoperative risks (infection, adhesions, recurrence, and death), it is generally recommended that monitoring instead of surgical repair be considered for most patients with asymptomatic incisional hernia. In patients unfit for surgery or the elderly, incisional hernias may be treated conservatively using supports such as trusses or belts [4].

Surgical technique

Two surgical approaches are used to treat incisional hernias: conventional open repair or laparoscopic incisional herniorrhaphy. No single technique is the best solution and the choice is indicated by the location and type of defect and the skill of the surgeon. As a rule, large incisional hernias (≥10 cm) are best repaired by the open technique, as are cases with visceral incarceration or strangulation [4]. Extremely obese patients may also require an open procedure because deeper layers of fatty tissue will have to be removed from the abdominal wall. Another advantage of the open technique is the treatment of loss of domain with component separation and restoration of abdominal wall anatomy and function, hence reducing the risk of abdominal compartment syndrome.

Gynecologic and Obstetric Surgery: Challenges and Management Options, First Edition. Edited by Arri Coomarasamy, Mahmood I. Shafi, G. Willy Davila and Kiong K. Chan.
© 2016 John Wiley & Sons, Ltd. Published 2016 by John Wiley & Sons, Ltd.

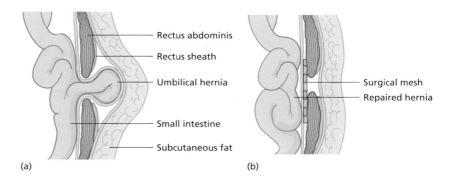

Figure 49.1 Sublay (retromuscular) repair of incisional hernia.

(a)   (b)

For the open procedure the traditional suture repair carries a two to three times greater risk of recurrence than the mesh repair (43% vs. 24%, respectively), and therefore it is not recommended except in the event of infected mesh removal or gross contamination [4]. The mesh can be placed using three techniques: onlay (prefascial), sublay (retro-muscular, i.e., Case history 1, Figure 49.1), or inlay (intraperitoneal). The onlay and sublay are the recommended techniques because of lower morbidity and recurrence rates (4.9% and 3.4%, respectively). A Cochrane review concluded that there was insufficient evidence to show advantage of a particular open technique [5].

The inlay technique, also used with laparoscopic repair, has the disadvantages of inability to restore anatomy and physiology of the abdominal wall, and exposure of viscera to the mesh requiring use of an expensive mesh with inner non-adhesive coating.

The laparoscopic repair approach requires placement of three or more ports inserted away from the hernia site. An intraperitoneal mesh is usually secured by sutures to the abdominal wall (Case history 2). The advantages of the laparoscopic approach include less postoperative complications and reduced hospital stay. The recurrence rate is reported to be 3–15% depending on the experience of the operator [4].

Choice of mesh

At present, the data comparing the clinical advantages of lightweight mesh with standard-weight mesh are limited. Similarly, limited experience exists to define the indications for biologic meshes as opposed to use of surgical steel or polypropylene mesh. To prevent risk of recurrence at the edges of the mesh, the mesh must overlap the hernial defect by several centimeters. Based on estimated mesh shrinkage from animal studies, it is recommended that a 3–5 cm overlap for open repair with complete fascial closure, and a 3-cm overlap for laparoscopic repair, is sufficient [4].

Prevention

The risk factors for the development of incisional hernia include obesity, diabetes, postoperative wound infection, dehiscence, emergency surgery, smoking, and malnutrition.

Prophylactic care to avoid risk of late wound failure [6]

Preoperative measures
- Lose weight; maintain suitable weight for age and height.
- Strengthen abdominal muscles through regular moderate exercise.

- Reduce abdominal pressure by avoiding constipation.
- Learn to lift heavy objects in a safe, low-strain way.
- Control diabetes and poor metabolism.
- Healthy, natural, balanced diet of whole foods, high in essential nutrients.
- Cessation of smoking before and after surgery.
- It is advisable for patients to shower either the day before or on the day of surgery. The skin at the surgical site should be prepared immediately before incision using an aqueous or alcohol-based antiseptic preparation (povidone-iodine or chlorhexidine). At the end of operation, the surgical incision should be covered with an appropriate interactive dressing.

Intraoperative measures

Appropriate selection of operative technique and incision
A significant reduction in incisional hernia can be achieved by using unilateral transverse incisions for small unilateral surgeries and selecting lateral paramedian incisions for most major elective surgeries [1]. The midline incision should be reserved for emergency or exploratory surgery, as it is quicker and allows broader access.

Suture material and suture technique
The choice of suture material for abdominal closure remains controversial. Evidence from randomized clinical trials and meta-analysis shows that continuous running non-absorbable or slowly absorbable suture is the method of choice for abdominal wall closure [7]. A large clinical trial showed that despite the incidence of wound infection being less in the group sutured with Vicryl Plus (braided suture material with antibacterial activity), there was no difference in the incidence of incisional hernia as compared with the group sutured with PDSII (polydioxanone) (15.2% vs. 14.0%, respectively). In the multivariate analysis of this study population, only BMI (>30 kg/m^2) showed a significant influence on the development of incisional hernia [8].

Closure of fascial layers
Based on emerging clinical evidence, routine closure of fascia is now recommended for laparoscopic ports greater than 10 mm and for 5-mm ports with extensive operative manipulation [2].

Postoperative measures
- It is important that surgeons continue to audit incisional hernia rates following different abdominal closure techniques.
- It is recommended that laparoscopy be considered when there is persistent, severe, or atypical pain following an abdominal surgery.

KEY POINTS

Challenge: Minimizing risk of late wound failure and incisional hernia.

Background

- Incisional hernia can occur in 2–19% of abdominal surgeries.
- The risk factors for the development of incisional hernia include obesity, diabetes, emergency surgery, postoperative wound dehiscence, smoking, and postoperative wound infection.
- Laparoscopic and transverse incisions have significantly lower incidence of incisional hernia than midline incisions (>1%, 1%, and 14%, respectively).

Prevention (of complications)

- Lose weight; maintain suitable weight for height and age.
- Strengthen abdominal muscles through regular moderate exercise.
- Reduce abdominal pressure by avoiding constipation.
- Control diabetes and poor metabolism.
- Skin and wound care preoperatively and postoperatively to prevent infection.
- Appropriate choice of incision and suturing technique.

Management (of incisional hernia)

- A careful decision on whether to repair needs to be made; asymptomatic incisional hernias may not need to be repaired.
- Some patients, particularly the elderly or those unfit for surgery, may benefit from conservative managements such as trusses or belts.
- Two surgical approaches are used to treat incisional hernias: laparoscopic incisional herniorrhaphy or conventional open repair.
- Open procedures are recommended for incisional hernias of 10 cm or more and in cases with intestinal incarceration or strangulation.
- Extremely obese patients may also require an open procedure because deeper layers of fatty tissue will have to be removed from the abdominal wall.
- The most effective surgical repair with lower recurrence rate is by using mesh to create little or no tension. The mesh can be placed using one of three techniques:
  - Onlay (prefascial).
  - Sublay (retromuscular).
  - Inlay (intraperitoneal).
- To prevent risk of recurrence at the edges of the mesh, the mesh must overlap the hernial defect by several centimeters (3–5 cm overlap for open repair, and 3-cm overlap for laparoscopic repair).

References

1 Burger JWA, Riet MV, Jeekel J. Abdominal incisions: techniques and postoperative complications. *Scand J Surg* 2002; 91:315–321.

2 Huang M, Musa M, Castillo C, Holcomb K. Postoperative bowel herniation in a 5-mm nonbladed trocar site. *JSLS* 2010; 14:289–291.

3 Nieuwenhuizen J, Halm JA, Jeekel J, Lange JF. Natural course of incisional hernia and indications for repair. *Scand J Surg* 2007; 96:293–296.

4 Kingsworth A, Banerjea A, Bhargava A. Incisional hernia repair: laparoscopic or open surgery? *Ann R Coll Surg Engl* 2009; 91:631–636.

5 den Hartog D, Dur AHM, Tuinebreijer WE, Kreis RW. Open surgical procedures for incisional hernias. *Cochrane Database Syst Rev* 2008;(3):CD006438.

6 Kingsnorth A. The management of incisional hernia. *Ann R Coll Surg Engl* 2006; 88:252–260.

7 Harlaar JJ, Deerenberg EB, van Ramshorst GH *et al*. A multicenter randomized controlled trial evaluating the effect of small stitches on the incidence of incisional hernia in midline incisions. *BMC Surgery* 2011; 11: 20.

8 Justinger C, Slotta JE, Schilling MK. Incisional hernia after abdominal closure with slowly absorbable versus fast absorbable, antibacterial-coated sutures. *Surgery* 2012; 151:398–403.

CHAPTER 50
Necrotizing Fasciitis

Tariq Ahmad

Addenbrooke's Hospital, Cambridge University Hospitals NHS Foundation Trust, Cambridge, UK

Case history: A 49-year-old diabetic patient who underwent abdominal hysterectomy two days previously becomes acutely unwell with intolerable pain in her abdomen, particularly around the incision site. On clinical examination erythema and edema of the abdominal wall are noted, as well as livid discoloration of the suture line and blistering of the skin adjacent to the wound. The erythema spreads within the hour beyond the extent of the initial assessment. The patient quickly deteriorates, becoming hemodynamically unstable with rising temperature and showing signs of fulminant sepsis.

Background

This is a classic description of a case of necrotizing fasciitis, a bacterial infection of the soft tissues that might be difficult to diagnose in its early stage. It is characterized by rapid progression to local tissue necrosis and severe systemic toxicity, often leading to multiorgan failure and death.

Necrotizing fasciitis may be related to surgery or interventional procedures, and the risk is increased in immunocompromised patients (e.g., HIV infection, diabetes, steroid use, alcohol dependency, chronic illness, and malnutrition). Fortunately, necrotizing fasciitis is uncommon, but the mortality rate is high at approximately 20–40%. Immediate surgical debridement remains one of the key factors for improved survival.

Management

Diagnosis

The diagnosis is foremost clinical, and is guided by the quick progression of the disease. The local signs may present as rapidly spreading erythema and edema with epidermolysis and blistering (Figure 50.1). Cyanosis or bronze discoloration of the skin especially near the injury site can be seen, and the subcutaneous tissue may feel indurated or wooden on palpation. Furthermore, crepitus may be present due to gas formation in the fascial plane. The most important symptom is pain, out of proportion to the physical findings or what would commonly be expected as postoperative pain. Pain will usually occur before malaise commences. Anesthesia of the affected area, due to ischemia of the cutaneous nerves, may be a late sign.

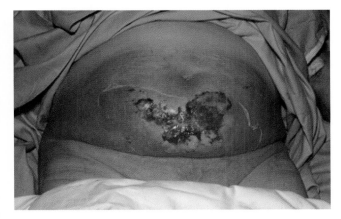

Figure 50.1 Extensive erythema and sloughing skin from necrotizing fasciitis. From Busby & Broome, 2006 [1] with permission from Wiley.

Systemically the patient may show signs of sepsis, shock, and acute renal failure. Scoring systems for laboratory tests (e.g., Laboratory Risk Indicator for Necrotizing Fasciitis or LRINEC), are available but should only be used to support the clinical diagnosis [2].

Mark the extent of the erythema in the initial assessment to monitor progression. Early reassessment of the patient is imperative. Medical photography will be a useful adjunct to the essential detailed description of the findings in the clinical notes.

In cases of suspected necrotizing fasciitis, urgent referral to the plastic surgery department is recommended. Plastic surgeons are familiar with the treatment of necrotizing fasciitis and, if uncertainty remains, might initiate or recommend a diagnostic incision [3]. This diagnostic procedure involves an approximately 2-cm incision down to deep fascia in the affected area, performed with an aseptic technique under local anesthesia. In necrotizing fasciitis, an absence of bleeding in subcutaneous tissue may be seen as a result of thrombosis of the subcutaneous vessels and, occasionally, there is a dishwater-colored fluid discharge. Digital examination will often show that subcutaneous tissues can be easily lifted off the fascia by a simple sweep of the finger.

The diagnostic incision will also allow deep tissue to be obtained; these should be sent for microbiology testing including immediate Gram stain and culture, as well as histology. It is advisable to contact the duty microbiologist in advance in order to provide information

Gynecologic and Obstetric Surgery: Challenges and Management Options, First Edition. Edited by Arri Coomarasamy, Mahmood I. Shafi, G. Willy Davila and Kiong K. Chan.
© 2016 John Wiley & Sons, Ltd. Published 2016 by John Wiley & Sons, Ltd.

about the suspected diagnosis, to facilitate workflow, and to allow discussion of initial empiric antibiotic therapy. Tissue samples of the fascia are to be preferred over skin samples as the latter might be cross-contaminated. Microbiology results may show anaerobic or aerobic bacteria or, commonly, a polymicrobial infection (4).

Ultrasound-guided aspiration and Gram staining can also be undertaken but a diagnostic incision is simple and can often provide an immediate and obvious clinical diagnosis.

Imaging has been described as a diagnostic tool in necrotizing fasciitis and might be used in the reasonably stable patient, though surgery should never be delayed for further diagnostic tests if necrotizing fasciitis is suspected. Currently CT and MRI are the imaging tools of choice to assess the constitution of the fascia and subcutaneous tissues, but even plain X-ray might establish whether gas is present in the deeper tissues.

Clinical management

The key to controlling disease progression in necrotizing fasciitis is early aggressive debridement, supported by appropriate resuscitation and antibiotic therapy. The complexity of the disease will require a multidisciplinary approach that involves the anesthetists, ITU team, microbiologists and, if available, plastic surgeons.

The care of the critically ill patient should follow normal assessment and resuscitation guidelines with respect to fluid management and cardiovascular support. Reassess the patient at short intervals and closely monitor hemodynamic variables. Initiate all routine investigations for the acutely unwell and septic patient including blood gases and cultures.

Early involvement of intensivists and anesthetists to optimize the patient's outcome is recommended as the patient will need to be managed in the ITU. Empiric antibiotic therapy with broad-spectrum antibiotics (e.g., clindamycin) should be commenced under the guidance of the microbiologist, taking into account renal and liver function if the patient is showing signs of organ failure; however, note that antibiotic treatment *alone* will not be successful in treating necrotizing fasciitis.

Contact needs to made with the local or regional plastic surgery unit; however, if no plastic surgery services are available in the hospital, transfer of the patient will most likely be too time-consuming and emergency debridement should not be delayed to allow a transfer. Anticipate that the infection may have spread beyond anatomic boundaries into other areas. Should there be any suspicion preoperatively, liaise with colleagues from other surgical specialties to be available to support the debridement.

Surgical management

The patient should be taken to the operating room as a true life-threatening emergency. Position and drape the patient so that access is allowed well beyond the obvious superficial extent of the necrosis as the disease will most likely have progressed further in the deeper fascial layers. Make your incisions straight onto fascia and peripherally into healthy tissue. If you are uncertain about the viability of the tissue, extend your incision. It might be advisable to carry out a sharp debridement with a blade rather than diathermy to allow assessment: if the skin edges show healthy capillary bleeding, this is a sign that the vasculitis and thrombosis of the subcutaneous vessels have not progressed this far.

Necrotic subcutaneous fat will be seen to have lost its healthy yellow color and consistency. Areas of fascial necrosis will show a yellow-greenish discoloration and your finger will pass with little

resistance, dividing the subcutaneous tissue from the fascia. The extent of the fascial necrosis may extend far beyond the superficial demarcation. Remove any tissue that can be easily lifted off the fascia with gentle pressure [4].

Myonecrosis of the underlying muscle is often only present at a later stage of the disease process or associated with compartment syndrome, but if it has occurred then dead muscle should be removed. The muscle will have lost its pink shine and will not show signs of arterial bleeding but, equally importantly, it will cease to contract on stimulation. Pinching with forceps should evoke a twitching of the muscle fibers, but remember to check with the anesthetist that the patient is not relaxed.

Excision of the affected tissue in necrotizing fasciitis will necessitate structures to be sacrificed that the surgeon would normally strive to preserve (i.e., subcutaneous nerves and vessels), but only a radical debridement will stop the progression of the disease and save the patient's life. Leave nothing behind that shows signs of necrosis (Figure 50.2) [5].

Tissue samples of the deeper necrosis, preferentially the fascia, should be sent for microbiology and histopathology.

Once all necrotic tissue has been excised, the wound cavity should be thoroughly irrigated. We recommend a combination of antiseptic irrigation (e.g., H_2O_2 or Betadine solution) and a wash with several liters of warm saline solution. The final inspection of

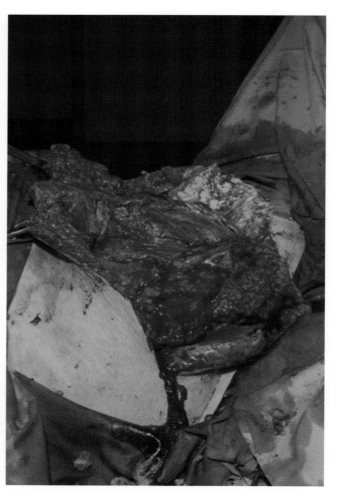

Figure 50.2 Extensive debridement of anterior abdominal wall. From Busby & Broome, 2006 [1] with permission from Wiley.

the wound should include steps to achieve meticulous hemostasis, as clotting may be deranged or the blood pressure may be lower than usual because of the systemic effects of the disease.

The final step is to pack the wounds (e.g., with Betadine- or saline-soaked gauze), but do not attempt to close the defect. Necrotizing fasciitis commonly requires more than one debridement and the patient should be taken back to theater after a maximum of 24–48 hours or sooner if she is clinically unstable or shows failure to improve. It may be necessary to repeat surgical debridement until the

progress of tissue necrosis ceases or signs of healthy healing tissues appear. At a later stage, if the wounds are clean but secondary direct closure is not possible, a negative pressure dressing (VAC dressing) might prove useful (see Figures 47.1 and 47.2); liaise with the local or regional plastic surgery unit to arrange for transfer once the patient is stabilized, and for advice with respect to further management or ancillary therapies (e.g., hyperbaric oxygen).

Intraoperative photo documentation will be a useful adjunct to facilitate the referral and for the patient's clinical notes.

KEY POINTS

Challenge: Necrotizing fasciitis.

Background
- Necrotizing fasciitis is a life-threatening soft tissue infection that requires immediate treatment as only a prompt radical debridement will increase the likelihood of survival.
- It is characterized by rapid progression to local tissue necrosis and severe systemic toxicity, often leading to multiorgan failure and death.
- Risk of this condition is increased in immunocompromised patients (e.g., HIV infection, diabetes, steroid use, alcohol dependency, chronic illness, and malnutrition).

Management
- Diagnosis:
  - Maintain a high index of suspicion. Necrotizing fasciitis is a clinical diagnosis, so thorough assessment and early reassessment are required.
  - A bedside 2-cm incision down to deep fascia (under local anesthesia) can be made to aid diagnosis.
  - No diagnostic tests (or transfer) should delay the surgical intervention if necrotizing fasciitis is suspected.
- Multidisciplinary approach: aggressive emergency resuscitation and antibiotic therapy. Seek early support from anesthetists, ITU, microbiology, and plastic surgery.
- Radical debridement: be "bold, bloody and resolute." Leave no necrotic tissue behind.
- Myonecrosis may necessitate excision of muscle.
- Once all necrotic tissues have been excised, thoroughly irrigate the wound cavity with a combination of antiseptic irrigation (e.g., H_2O_2 or Betadine solution) and several liters of warm saline solution.
- Pack the wounds (e.g., with Betadine- or saline-soaked gauze), but do not attempt to close the defect. Necrotizing fasciitis commonly requires more than one debridement.
- Involve plastic surgeons in ongoing care.

References

1 Busby G, Broome J. Case report: Necrotising fasciitis following unrecognised bladder injury during transobturator sling procedure. *BJOG* 2006; 114:111–112.
2 Swain RA, Hatcher JC, Azadian BS, Soni N, De Souza B. A five-year review of necrotising fasciitis in a tertiary referral unit. *Ann R Coll Surg Engl* 2013; 95:57–60.
3 Andreasen TJ, Green SD, Childers BJ. Massive infectious soft-tissue injury: diagnosis and management of necrotizing fasciitis and purpura fulminans. *Plast Recons Surg* 2001; 107:1023–1035.
4 Edlich RF, Cross CL, Dahlstrom JJ, Long WB III. Modern concepts of the diagnosis and treatment of necrotizing fasciitis. *J Emerg Med* 2010; 39:261–265.
5 Burge TS, Watson JD. Necrotising fasciitis. *BMJ* 1994; 308:1453–1454.

CHAPTER 51
Management of Surgical Drains

Ahmed M. El-Sharkawy and Sherif Awad

School of Clinical Sciences, University of Nottingham, Nottingham, UK

Case history: *At the end of an abdominal myomectomy, the gynecologist was confident about hemostasis, but decided to leave a Robinson drain in the pelvis "as a precaution." By 24 hours after the operation, there was 30 mL of blood in the drain; the nursing staff request the gynecologist when it would be appropriate to remove the drain.*

Background

Using surgical drains dates back to the Hippocratic era when, controversially, empyema and ascites were drained. In today's evidence-based practice, their use remains contentious, mainly consequent on a paucity of controlled trials. Most abdominal surgeons feel that there are certain indications for using drains; however, these should be balanced against potential morbidity from drains. This chapter considers the indications and morbidities of drains, the different types of drains in use, and an algorithm for their daily management.

Indications and morbidities associated with surgical drains

Indications for using drains include:
- draining existing/potential collections (e.g., blood, bile, pus, or reactive inflammatory fluid);
- facilitating irrigation of cavities;
- permitting contrast studies (e.g., tubograms);
- minimizing dead space in a wound cavity (thereby avoiding seroma formation);
- encouraging wound healing through use of vacuum-assisted drains or devices which promote tissue apposition and encourage wound healing.

Although some surgeons consider a drain to be useful when there is oozing from peritoneal surfaces, a drain is not a replacement for achieving adequate hemostasis.

A definite indication for a pelvic drain is after surgery for tubo-ovarian abscess or infection. Where there is evidence of clotting defect, it is advisable to leave a pelvic drain, as it will help with diagnosis of any new pelvic bleeding and reduce the risk of formation of pelvic hematoma and subsequent abscess.

The evidence supporting "prophylactic" use of drains remains controversial, and several studies did not demonstrate drains to be associated with reduced formation of intra-abdominal fluid collections.

Furthermore, use of drains was associated with higher rates of postoperative surgical site infection, skin irritation or discomfort, and longer duration of hospital stay [1,2]. Some studies have even demonstrated prophylactic abdominal drainage to be an independent risk factor for postoperative morbidity [2,3,4]. Finally, Enhanced Recovery After Surgery (ERAS) guidelines currently discourage the routine use of drains as this may hinder patient recovery [5,6]. Other problems associated with use of drains include increased inflammatory fluid formation, migration and tissue irritation (a factor which may aid anastomotic dehiscence and formation of enterocutaneous fistulae), and visceral herniation through the drain tract [7].

Types of surgical drains

Types and classification of drains in common use are shown in Figure 51.1 and Table 51.1. Open drains channel fluid into a wound bag or dressing and are used when output is expected to be low. Fluid flow in these passive drains is encouraged by gravity and the differential pressure gradient between body cavity and the exterior. However, their use is not favored as they may cause skin irritation and unpleasant odor if discharge is offensive. Closed drains channel fluid into a wound bag or container, have a reduced risk of ascending infection, and are easier to manage. Active drains utilize a suction device to create a negative pressure which draws fluid out of the cavity. Sump drains allow active drainage and consist of a double lumen, comprising a small inner and a larger outer lumen. The outer lumen allows air into the cavity, helping displace the fluid out through the inner lumen. Most drains are composed of inert Silastic material that minimizes tissue reaction, enabling rapid closure of the drain tract on removal of the drain. Conversely, red rubber or latex drains induce an intense tissue reaction which forms a tract; the latter is of use in certain clinical situations to form a controlled fistula.

Table 51.1 Types and classification of abdominal drains in common use.

	Active	Passive
Open	—	Penrose drain Corrugated drain Yeates drain
Closed	Redivac® drain Jackson–Pratt drain Sump drain	Silastic tube drains (e.g., Robinson drain) Latex tube drain

Gynecologic and Obstetric Surgery: Challenges and Management Options, First Edition. Edited by Arri Coomarasamy, Mahmood I. Shafi, G. Willy Davila and Kiong K. Chan.
© 2016 John Wiley & Sons, Ltd. Published 2016 by John Wiley & Sons, Ltd.

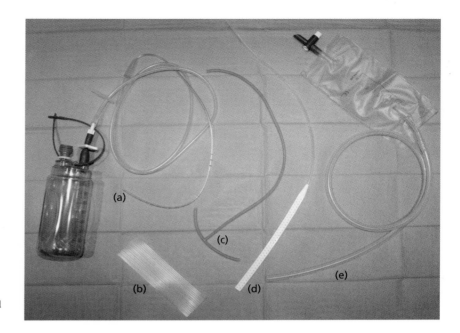

Figure 51.1 Types of abdominal surgical drains in common use: (a) Redivac® drain system; (b) corrugated drain; (c) latex T-tube drain; (d) Jackson–Pratt drain; (e) Robinson drain connected to drain bag.

Management

Review of surgical drains should be performed on (at least) a daily basis to reduce the risks of patient discomfort and morbidity and facilitate timely removal. The useful mnemonic "DRAINS" defines the daily drain checks which should be performed.

- **D**etermine 24-hour volume and type of fluid drained.
- **R**eplace drain fluid losses (if excessive) as part of the patient's fluid balance schedule.
- **A**nchor the drain to the skin if it is loose or displaced.
- **I**mage the drain (e.g., tubogram) if there is a suspicion it is blocked, kinked or dislodged.
- **N**eed to remove the drain when drainage is minimal (<50 mL in 24 hours), the patient is clinically stable, and the indication for drain insertion is no longer present.
- **S**ite of drain and drain itself should be inspected to ensure that all components of the drain have been removed, as retained foreign bodies could lead to infections, sinus formation, and potential litigation.

Drains placed during elective surgery are generally removed within 24–48 hours of the procedure, particularly when output is less than 50 mL in 24 hours. When removing an active drain, the vacuum should be released and output monitored for up to 24 hours prior to removal. Latex drains placed to encourage the formation of a tract are left in place for up to 6 weeks. Adequate understanding of the drain fixation mechanism is essential to ensure safe, pain-free removal and the original operation notes should be reviewed prior to removing drains. While external fixating ligatures to the skin are merely cut to release the drain, other drains (especially percutaneously placed drains) may have internal anchor mechanisms such as inflated balloons or coiled tips, which need to be released to ensure safe removal of all parts of the drain.

Resolution of the case

As the drainage is less than 50 mL in 24 hours, as long as the patient's clinical condition is good, it may be reasonable to remove the drain. However, it is correct to check with the surgeon before removal of a drain.

KEY POINTS

Challenge: Management of surgical drains.

Background
- Indications for surgical drains include:
  - Draining existing/potential collections (e.g., blood, bile, pus, or reactive inflammatory fluid).
  - Facilitating irrigation of cavities.
  - Minimizing dead space in a wound cavity (thereby avoiding seroma formation).
  - Encouraging wound healing through use of vacuum-assisted drains or devices which promote tissue apposition and encourage wound healing.
- A drain may be useful where there is oozing from peritoneal surface, but the priority is to achieve adequate hemostasis.
- Patients who have had surgery for tubo-ovarian abscess or infection should have a pelvic drain.
- It is advisable to leave a pelvic drain in patients with clotting abnormalities.

- The evidence for use of "prophylactic" drainage is unclear.
- Risks of drains include surgical site infection, skin irritation, longer hospital stay, damage to surrounding tissues, and visceral herniation through drain tract.
- Drains can be open or closed, and active or passive:
  - Open and passive: Penrose, corrugated, or Yeates drain.
  - Closed and active: Redivac, Jackson–Pratt or sump drain.
  - Closed and passive: Robinson drain.

Management
- Review drain daily, noting total and preceding 24-hour loss.
- Inspect drain site daily to ensuring the drain is not loose and there is no evidence of infection.
- Remove drain when drainage is minimal (<50 mL in 24 hours) and patient stable; but check with operating notes for drain removal instruction, or consult with the surgeon before removal.
- Remove drains by gentle traction; if there are internal anchoring mechanisms (e.g., balloon or coiled tip), ensure these are released before drain removal.

References

1 Petrowsky H, Demartines N, Rousson V, Clavien PA. Evidence-based value of prophylactic drainage in gastrointestinal surgery: a systematic review and meta-analyses. *Ann Surg* 2004; 240: 1074–1084.

2 Urbach DR, Kennedy ED, Cohen MM. Colon and rectal anastomoses do not require routine drainage: a systematic review and meta-analysis. *Ann Surg* 1999; 229: 174–180.

3 Liu CL, Fan ST, Lo CM *et al.* Abdominal drainage after hepatic resection is contraindicated in patients with chronic liver diseases. *Ann Surg* 2004; 239: 194–201.

4 Jesus EC, Karliczek A, Matos D, Castro AA, Atallah AN. Prophylactic anastomotic drainage for colorectal surgery. *Cochrane Database Syst Rev* 2004;(4):CD002100.

5 Sjetne IS, Krogstad U, Odegard S, Engh ME. Improving quality by introducing enhanced recovery after surgery in a gynaecological department: consequences for ward nursing practice. *Qual Saf Health Care* 2009; 18: 236–240.

6 Lassen K, Soop M, Nygren J *et al.* Consensus review of optimal perioperative care in colorectal surgery: Enhanced Recovery After Surgery (ERAS) Group recommendations. *Arch Surg* 2009; 144: 961–969.

7 Gates S, Anderson ER. Wound drainage for caesarean section. *Cochrane Database Syst Rev* 2005;(1):CD004549.

CHAPTER 52
Shocked Patient

Manjeet Shehmar

Birmingham Women's NHS Foundation Trust, Birmingham, UK

Case history: A woman who had a termination of pregnancy at 6 weeks of gestation 2 days previously collapsed on the ward. She reported vaginal bleeding and abdominal pain before the event.

Background

Shock occurs when the circulatory system fails to meet the metabolic demands of the tissues. It can range from being transient and self-limiting to severe insult resulting in permanent tissue damage. Early recognition and correction are important in minimizing morbidity and mortality. Causes of shock include (Figure 52.1):

- hypovolemic shock from hemorrhage, dehydration, or anaphylaxis;
- vasovagal shock;
- septic shock from endotoxic vasodilation due to Gram-negative infections;
- anaphylactic shock from medications, blood, nuts, or latex;
- cardiogenic shock when more than 50% of the left ventricle is damaged by infarction;
- neurogenic shock from traumatic or pharmacologic blockade of the sympathetic nervous system.

Diagnosis

Stages of shock and the associated physiologic responses are shown in Figure 52.2. General signs of shock include tachycardia, hypotension, decreased urine output, and confusion. However, these may not always be present. Sometimes only weakness and confusion may be present. A tachycardia is usually present but in those who are very fit, on beta-blockade, or in some people with shock due to intra-abdominal bleeding, there may be a normal heart rate or bradycardia. In pregnant women, there is circulatory compensation and hypotension is a late sign of shock, whereas a tachypnea is a relatively early and often missed indicator.

Each type of shock will also have its own specific presentations, such as arrhythmias or an increased jugular venous pressure in cardiogenic shock, and pyrexia in septic shock. The severity and progress of shock and treatment can be measured clinically by monitoring the cardiac output, respiratory rate, and oxygen saturation using a MEWS (Modified Early Warning Score) chart, urine output, central venous pressure, and arterial blood gas analysis.

If shock is not corrected it becomes progressive, causing electrolyte leakage, capillary membrane leakage, and inflammatory response with release of histamine and increased blood osmolality. End organs such as bowel become hypoxic leading to endotoxic shock. The next stage is refractory shock when vital organs fail and shock can no longer be reversed, leading to brain damage and death.

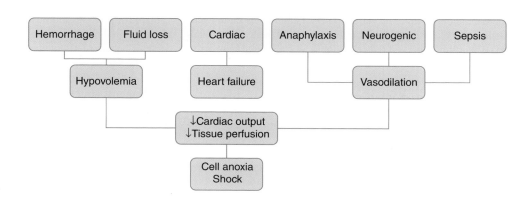

Figure 52.1 Pathogenesis of shock.

Gynecologic and Obstetric Surgery: Challenges and Management Options, First Edition. Edited by Arri Coomarasamy, Mahmood I. Shafi, G. Willy Davila and Kiong K. Chan.
© 2016 John Wiley & Sons, Ltd. Published 2016 by John Wiley & Sons, Ltd.

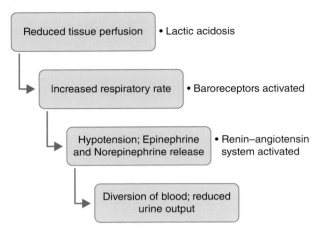

Figure 52.2 Stages of shock.

Management

Management is to search systematically to find the cause of shock and treat it. Initial treatment is resuscitation using the ABCDE (Airway, Breathing, Circulation, Disability, and Exposure/Examination) approach.

Assess airway, breathing, and circulation

The first step is to call out to the patient to assess consciousness, followed by an immediate assessment of airway, breathing, and circulation. If the airway is open and the patient is breathing, oxygen (15 L/min) should be given via a facemask with reservoir bag. If the airway is obstructed, an anesthetist or an arrest team should be immediately summoned. If there is no breathing or pulse, an arrest team should be immediately summoned and resuscitation commenced.

Administer fluids and/or blood

Aggressive fluid resuscitation is needed in most types of shock. There is no evidence on the best type of intravenous fluid [1] and thus crystalloids are usually recommended due to low cost [2]. A typical initial treatment is the intravenous infusion of 500 mL of a crystalloid over 5 min; the maximum crystalloid bolus should generally not exceed 1 L. If initial intravenous fluid resuscitation fails to correct shock, packed red cells should be considered in order to maintain the hemoglobin above 10 g/dL [1].

Consider using a vasopressor

Vasopressors may be considered if hypotension is not improved with fluids alone. There is no evidence for the superiority of any specific vasopressor agent [3], and there is no evidence that vasopressors improve hypovolemic shock from hemorrhage [4], but they may be of use in neurogenic shock. The use of sodium bicarbonate is controversial and is usually only considered if pH is below 7.0.

Treat the cause of shock

Hemorrhage

The classification and management of hemorrhagic patients is summarized in Table 52.1. The source of bleeding (e.g., uterus as in the case history, a bleeding vessel after an operation, or a ruptured

Table 52.1 Classification and management of hemorrhagic patients.

Class	Blood loss	Response	Treatment required
I	<15% (0.75 L)	Mild tachycardia, normal BP	Minimal; supportive
II	15–30% (0.75–1.5 L)	Tachycardia, mild hypotension	Intravenous fluids
III	30–40% (1.5–2 L)	Severe tachycardia, hypotension and confusion	Packed RBCs and fluid
IV	>40% (>2 L)	Critical hypotension and tachycardia	Aggressive interventions

ectopic pregnancy) should be identified and surgically managed as appropriate, after initial resuscitation (Chapter 40).

Septic shock

As well as resuscitative measures, the focus of infection needs to be identified and treated using antimicrobials, with draining or removal of tissue such as products of conception or foreign bodies such as IUCDs. Early introduction of intravenous antibiotics (e.g., co-amoxiclav, or cefuroxime with metronidazole) is associated with reduced mortality [5]. Blood cultures should be taken before administering antibiotics; urine, sputum, stool, wound and vaginal swabs can be taken if clinically indicated.

Anaphylaxis [6,7]

Immediate action is necessary to avert death or serious morbidity that can occur from anaphylactic bronchospasm, laryngeal edema and hypoxia, massive vasodilation, and hypotension. Immediate help should be sought from an anesthetist or an arrest team. The first step is to sit the patient up and give high-flow oxygen immediately at the highest concentration possible using a mask with an oxygen reservoir. Commence the resuscitation of the patient, and without delay the following three drugs should then be administered.

1 Epinephrine (adrenaline): administer 0.5 mL of 1 in 1000 epinephrine (0.5 mg) i.m. into the anterolateral aspect of the middle third of the thigh. Repeat epinephrine at 5-min intervals if there is no improvement in the patient's condition.

2 Antihistamines: administer chlorphenamine 10 mg i.m. or slow i.v., and flush the intravenous line with 5–10 mL of normal saline.

3 Corticosteroids: administer hydrocortisone 200 mg i.m. or slow i.v. injection.

Rapid intravenous administration of 500–1000 mL of crystalloid is often required. If the patient is wheezy, bronchodilator therapy with 5 mg of nebulized salbutamol will be necessary. As an alternative, 1 mg of nebulized epinephrine can be used for bronchodilatation.

Cardiogenic shock

This could be from various causes including arrhythmias, pulmonary embolism, myocardial infarction, fluid overload and heart failure, and tension pneumothorax. Clinical history may include chest pain, dyspnea, and palpitations. Depending on the probable diagnosis, immediate help from an anesthetist, cardiologist, general physician, or the arrest team should be sought. Immediate management includes high-flow oxygen, morphine 2.5 mg i.v. (as an anxiolytic, analgesic, vasodilator, and antiarrhythmic), 12-lead ECG, bloods (troponin, FBC, U&E, clotting, and G&S), arterial blood gases, and chest X-ray. Central venous and peripheral arterial monitoring are often needed. Initial treatment of pulmonary embolism will include LMWH; initial treatment of myocardial infection will include GTN 0.1 mg and oral aspirin

300 mg; and initial treatment of fluid overload will require furosemide 40 mg i.v.

Neurogenic shock

This can typically occur when pregnancy tissues are expelled through the cervix during a miscarriage, or when cervix is dilated with surgical dilators or instruments. The management entails removal of the pregnancy tissues or surgical instruments from the cervical os. This usually treats the underlying problem; however, if neurogenic shock persists, the following steps may be necessary.

- Lay the patient supine with head down, and administer intravenous fluids.
- Perform carotid massage to improve bradycardia.
- If no improvement, call the cardiac resuscitation team.
- If bradycardia persists, administer atropine 0.5 mg i.v. to a maximum dose of 0.03–0.04 mg/kg (3 mg, total cumulative adult dose); depending on the severity of the condition, an atropine dosing interval of 3–5 min can be used [3].

Resolution of the case

Immediate management involves resuscitation using the ABCDE approach and calling the cardiac arrest team. Facial oxygen and intravenous crystalloid fluids should be initiated via two large-bore cannulae. Venous blood should be sent for FBC, U&E, G&S with a view to cross-matching, as guided by degree of hypovolemic hemorrhagic shock.

The cause of shock should be established by a history, review of previous notes and investigations results, and clinical examination. Possible differential diagnoses are:

- neurogenic shock from retained tissue in the cervical os;
- hypovolemic shock from hemorrhage;
- septic shock from infected pregnancy tissues or foreign body;
- anaphylaxis if medication has been administered.

Further management of this patient will depend on the diagnosis and patient's clinical condition.

KEY POINTS

Challenge: Management of a shocked patient.

Background
- Shock can range from transient and self-limiting to severe resulting in permanent tissue damage or death.
- Early recognition and treatment is associated with better outcomes.
- Causes include:
  - Hemorrhage.
  - Fluid loss.
  - Cardiac.
  - Neurogenic (e.g., vasovagal).
  - Anaphylaxis.
  - Sepsis.
- Diagnosis: general signs of shock are tachycardia, hypotension, decreased urine output, and confusion.

Management
- Call for help, including specialist help (e.g., anesthetist and hematologist).
- Assess and manage airway, breathing and circulation:
  - If airway is open, give oxygen (15 L/min) via a facemask with reservoir bag.
  - If airway is obstructed, crash call an anesthetist or an arrest team.
  - If there is no breathing or pulse, crash call an arrest team, and commence resuscitation.
- Administer fluids and blood:
  - Typical initial treatment is intravenous infusion of 500 mL of a crystalloid over 5 min.
  - Give blood with the aim of raising hemoglobin above 10 g/dL.
- Correct clotting defects (Chapter 40).
- Consider vasopressor treatment if hypotension does not improve with fluid or blood administration.
- Treat cause of shock:
  - Hemorrhage: resuscitate the patient, and identify and manage the source of bleeding.
  - Septic shock: take blood cultures, and administer intravenous broad-spectrum antibiotics. Take other infection swabs as clinically indicated. Identify infective focus and manage surgically if necessary.
  - Anaphylaxis: give high-flow oxygen; give 0.5 mL of 1 in 1000 epinephrine (0.5 mg) i.m.; give chlorphenamine 10 mg i.m. or slow i.v.; give hydrocortisone 200 mg i.m. or slow i.v. injection.
  - Cardiogenic shock: manage with high-flow oxygen, morphine 2.5 mg i.v. (as an anxiolytic, analgesic, vasodilator, and antiarrhythmic), 12-lead ECG, bloods (troponin, FBC, U&E, clotting, and G&S), arterial blood gases, and chest X-ray. Involve a cardiologist.
  - Neurogenic shock (e.g., vasovagal attack): resuscitate; perform carotid massage; if bradycardia persists, administer atropine 0.5 mg i.v. Involve anesthetist or cardiologist.

References

1 Tintinalli JE. *Tintinalli's Emergency Medicine: A Comprehensive Study Guide*, 7th edn, pp. 165–172. McGraw-Hill, New York, 2010.

2 Perel P, Roberts I. Colloids versus crystalloids for fluid resuscitation in critically ill patients. *Cochrane Database Syst Rev* 2007;(4):CD000567.

3 Havel C, Arrich J, Losert H, Gamper G, Müllner M, Herkner H. Vasopressors for hypotensive shock. *Cochrane Database Syst Rev* 2011;(5):CD003709.

4 Diez C, Varon AJ. Airway management and initial resuscitation of the trauma patient. *Curr Opin Crit Care* 2009;**15**:542–547.

5 Gaieski DF, Mikkelsen ME, Band RA *et al*. Impact of time to antibiotics on survival in patients with severe sepsis or septic shock in whom early goal-directed therapy was initiated in the emergency department. *Crit Care Med* 2010;**38**:1045–1053.

6 Royal College of Physicians. Emergency treatment of anaphylaxis in adults. Available at http://www.rcplondon.ac.uk/sites/default/files/emergency-treatment-anaphylaxis-concise-guideline_0.pdf (accessed August 2013).

7 Resuscitation Council (UK). Emergency treatment of anaphylactic reactions: Guidelines for healthcare providers. Available at https://www.resus.org.uk/anaphylaxis/emergency-treatment-of-anaphylactic-reactions/

CHAPTER 53

Breathless Patient: Postoperative Pulmonary Complications

Heinke Kunst

Queen Mary University of London, London, UK

Case history: A 35-year-old woman with a known history of asthma presents with acute dyspnea and a productive cough after emergency laparotomy for an ectopic pregnancy. The patient is a non-smoker. Chest examination shows mild wheeze, reduced breath sounds, and increased vocal resonance on the left side. Chest radiograph shows a complete collapse of the left lung.

Background

Compared with upper abdominal surgery, pelvic surgery is less likely to cause postoperative pulmonary complications; however, patients with underlying respiratory disease and the elderly are at risk of conditions such as hospital-acquired pneumonia and pulmonary embolism, as well as exacerbation of underlying chronic lung disease [1]. Postoperative pulmonary complications are associated with increased length of hospital stay, morbidity and mortality; therefore, it is important to assess patients promptly if there are signs of respiratory compromise after surgery [2].

During abdominal surgery many patients develop lung atelectasis, a reversible collapse of alveoli in dependent lung areas, believed to result from surfactant inhibition and lung compression [3]. Atelectasis leads to reduction in functional residual capacity (FRC) and a restrictive lung function pattern, and there is a risk of patients developing respiratory dysfunction. Postoperatively, patients may be less able to cough due to pain, impairing mucociliary clearance; this could be made worse by sedation with analgesic medication and delayed mobilization after surgery, increasing the risk of atelectasis and lung collapse. Patients, particularly the elderly and those with underlying lung disease, are at risk of pneumonia if atelectasis and lung collapse do not resolve within the postoperative period [4]. A history of preoperative symptoms of a lower respiratory tract infection may help to distinguish a community-acquired from hospital-acquired pneumonia.

If a patient presents with acute dyspnea immediately post extubation and there is evidence of an acute lung collapse, especially of the left lung, misplacement of the endotracheal tube into the right main bronchus should be considered. Intense physiotherapy is needed, and sometimes a bronchoscopy will help to remove excessive secretions which will lead to reinflation of the affected lung.

Patients with underlying obstructive airway disease such as asthma and chronic obstructive pulmonary disease (COPD) may develop bronchospasm postoperatively and may present with acute dyspnea and wheeze. Furthermore, even patients without confirmed airway disease, especially smokers, may develop acute bronchospasm in the postoperative period especially if mucociliary clearance is impaired. Incidence of pneumothorax is rare after pelvic surgery [5], but should be excluded if there are signs of respiratory compromise.

Respiratory depression leading to hypoxia and hypercapnia in the postoperative period may occur due to oversedation, especially in obese patients or those with underlying pulmonary disease such as obstructive sleep apnea. Patients may present with acute dyspnea and confusion and may exhibit a flapping tremor suggesting acute hypercapnia.

Pelvic surgery is associated with an increased incidence of thromboembolic events; patients who present with acute dyspnea and pleuritic chest pain should be investigated for pulmonary embolism.

The pattern of onset of dyspnea is very useful in considering the etiology [6].

- Sudden onset: consider pulmonary embolism, pneumothorax, cardiac causes, aspiration, and anaphylaxis [6].
- Onset over a few hours: consider atelectasis, bleeding, asthma, pulmonary edema, and ARDS [6].
- Onset over a few days: consider pneumonia, anemia, pleural effusion, and slowly developing pulmonary edema [6].
- Onset over a few weeks: consider slowly developing anemia [6].

Management

Investigations

An acutely breathless postoperative patient needs to be investigated with ECG, chest radiography, and blood tests including FBC, U&E, and CRP. Arterial blood gases are useful to establish whether the patient is in respiratory failure and to detect hypoxia, hypercapnia, and acidosis (Table 53.1). Chest radiography may show evidence of atelectasis, pneumonia, lung collapse, pneumothorax or signs of a pleural effusion. Patients with no history of underlying lung disease who present with acute dyspnea and wheeze should have spirometry to exclude an underlying airway

Gynecologic and Obstetric Surgery: Challenges and Management Options, First Edition. Edited by Arri Coomarasamy, Mahmood I. Shafi, G. Willy Davila and Kiong K. Chan.
© 2016 John Wiley & Sons, Ltd. Published 2016 by John Wiley & Sons, Ltd.

Table 53.1 Arterial blood gas interpretation.

	Normal range	Abnormalities
pH	7.35–7.45	Low pH with high $PaCO_2$ = respiratory acidosis (respiratory distress)
		High pH with low $PaCO_2$ = respiratory alkalosis (hyperventilation)
		Low pH and low HCO_3^- (negative base excess) = metabolic acidosis (e.g., shock with increased lactate, diabetic ketoacidosis, renal failure)
		High pH and high HCO_3^- (base excess) = metabolic alkalosis (vomiting: loss of acid from gut)
PaO_2	11–13 kPa (83–98 mmHg)	<11 kPa = hypoxemia
		<8 kPa = respiratory failure
$PaCO_2$	4.8–6.0 kPa (36–45 mmHg)	>6.5 kPa = hypercapnia
		<3.5 kPa = hypocapnia
HCO_3^-	22–29 mmol/L	See above
Base excess	−2 to +2	See above

disease such as asthma or COPD. A pneumothorax should be excluded, especially in patients with underlying lung disease who present with acute dyspnea and unilateral chest pain. In the acutely breathless patient who complains of chest pain and has a normal chest radiograph, a diagnosis of pulmonary embolism needs to be excluded by CT pulmonary angiogram, which will show evidence of filling defects in the pulmonary arteries. An ECG will confirm right heart strain and a serum troponin may be raised. D-dimers will not be helpful since they will be invariably elevated in the postoperative period.

Management of pulmonary complications

Patients with acute dyspnea and evidence of atelectasis, lung collapse or consolidation postoperatively should have physiotherapy. Depending on signs and symptoms suggestive of a lower respiratory tract infection, such as fever and rigors, patients should be given broad-spectrum antibiotics to treat a hospital-acquired pneumonia unless symptoms precede surgery, in which case management should include treatment for a community-acquired pneumonia.

Patients with evidence of acute bronchospasm who present with dyspnea and wheeze should be given salbutamol nebulizers and may need a course of steroids. If there is evidence of a lower respiratory tract infection, antibiotics should be added.

Patients with a suspected or confirmed diagnosis of pulmonary embolism are anticoagulated with intravenous heparin if there is a risk of pelvic hemorrhage. If risk of bleeding is low, high-dose low-molecular-weight heparin should be administered. Warfarin should be commenced once diagnosis is confirmed and if there is no significant risk of bleeding. Obese patients and those with underlying obstructive sleep apnea may develop hyercapnic respiratory failure postoperatively and non-invasive ventilation may be needed; in severe respiratory failure invasive ventilation may be required [7].

Various postoperative pulmonary complications and the management principles for them are summarized in Table 53.2.

Resolution of the case

The patient in the case history was intubated with an endotracheal tube which was misplaced into the right main bronchus. Endotracheal intubation led to a mild exacerbation of her asthma. Intensive physiotherapy and bronchodilators resulted in resolution of the left lung collapse within 48 hours.

Table 53.2 Postoperative pulmonary complications and management.

	History	Signs	Investigations	Management
Atelectasis	Dyspnea	Reduced breath sounds, decreased vocal resonance	Chest X-ray: atelectasis ABG	Physiotherapy Deep breathing exercises Consider CPAP
Pneumonia	Fever, productive cough, dyspnea	Unilateral crackles, bronchial breathing, increased vocal resonance	Chest X-ray: consolidation ABG Sputum for microscopy and culture Blood tests: raised neutrophil count and CRP	Antibiotics Physiotherapy
Lobar collapse	Dyspnea	Reduced breath sounds; reduced or increased vocal resonance	Chest X-ray: lobar collapse	Physiotherapy/bronchoscopy
Pulmonary embolism	Acute dyspnea and pleuritic chest pain; hemoptysis	Normal examination	CT pulmonary angiogram: filling defects ECG: right heart strain ABG	Low-molecular-weight heparin Warfarin
Acute bronchospasm	Dyspnea, wheeze	Wheeze or rhonchi	Chest X-ray: hyperinflated lungs Spirometry: obstructive defect ABG	Salbutamol nebulizer Consider steroids
Pulmonary edema	Dyspnea, wheeze and orthopnea	Pink frothy sputum; bilateral crackles; wheeze	Chest X-ray ABG	Fluid restriction Furosemide 20–40 mg i.v.
Hypercapnic respiratory failure	Dyspnea, confusion	Obesity; obstructive sleep apnea; flapping tremor	Chest X-ray ABG	Non-invasive or invasive ventilation
Pleural effusion	Dyspnea	Reduced breath sounds and decreased vocal resonance	Chest X-ray: unilateral or bilateral effusions	Pleural aspirate May need chest drain
Pneumothorax	Acute dyspnea and unilateral chest pain	Absent breath sounds; hyperresonant percussion	Chest X-ray	Pleural aspirate Chest drain

KEY POINTS

Challenge: Assessment of the acutely breathless patient.

Background
- Atelectasis occurs commonly in the postoperative period, especially after laparotomy.
- Decreased cough due to postoperative pain impairs mucociliary clearance, increasing risk of pulmonary complications.
- The pattern of onset of dyspnea is very useful in considering the etiology:
  - Sudden onset: consider pulmonary embolism, pneumothorax, cardiac causes, aspiration, and anaphylaxis.
  - Onset over a few hours: consider atelectasis, bleeding, asthma, pulmonary edema, and ARDS.
  - Onset over a few days: consider pneumonia, anemia, pleural effusion, and slowly developing pulmonary edema.
  - Onset over a few weeks: consider slowly developing anemia.

Management
Investigations
- Arrange chest radiography, ECG, and blood tests including FBC, U&E, and CRP.

- Arrange arterial blood gases to detect hypoxia, hypercapnia, and acidosis.
- In patients with no history of underlying lung disease who present with acute dyspnea and wheeze, arrange spirometry to exclude an underlying airway disease such as asthma or COPD.
- If patient has chest pain in addition to dyspnea, arrange CT pulmonary angiogram to exclude PE; consider cardiac causes.

Treatment
- Arrange physiotherapy if there is evidence of atelectasis, lobar collapse, or pneumonia.
- Give broad-spectrum antibiotics if there is evidence of a chest infection.
- Give bronchodilators (e.g., nebulized salbutamol) if there is evidence of bronchospasm.
- Treat pulmonary edema with fluid restriction and furosemide 20–40 mg i.v.
- Treat PE with low-molecular-weight heparin.
- Arrange chest drain for pneumothorax.
- Consider non-invasive or invasive ventilation for patients with obstructive sleep apnea.

References

1 Joris J, Kaba A, Lamy M. Postoperative spirometry after laparoscopy for lower abdominal or upper abdominal surgical procedures. *Br J Anaesth* 1997;**79**:422–426.

2 Lawrence VA, Cornell JE, Smetana GW. Strategies to reduce postoperative pulmonary complications after noncardiothoracic surgery: systematic review for the American College of Physicians. *Ann Intern Med* 2006;**144**:596–608.

3 Lindberg P, Gunnarsson L, Tokics L *et al.* Atelectasis and lung function in the postoperative period. *Acta Anaesthesiol Scand* 1992;**36**:546–553.

4 Manku K, Bacchetti P, Leung JM. Prognostic significance of postoperative in-hospital complications in elderly patients. I. Long-term survival. *Anesth Analg* 2003;**96**:583–589.

5 Solomon ER, Muffly TM, Barber MD. Common postoperative pulmonary complications after hysterectomy for benign indications. *Am J Obstet Gynecol* 2013;**208**:54e1–5.

6 Chikwe J, Walther A, Jones P. *Respiratory.* In: *Perioperative Medicine: Managing Surgical Patients with Medical Problems*, 2nd edn, pp. 171–210. Oxford University Press, Oxford, 2009.

7 Pompei L, Della RG. The postoperative airway: unique challenges? *Curr Opin Crit Care* 2013;**19**:359–363.

CHAPTER 54
Confused Postoperative Patient

Idnan Yunas
University Medical Practice Edgbaston, Birmingham, UK

Case history: A 45-year-old woman was noted to be "not her usual self" by her family a day after her hysterectomy. The family described her as having short periods of agitation followed by periods of apathy with intervening periods of normality.

Background

Delirium is characterized by disturbances in awareness, thought, and perception. Subtypes include hypoactive (apathy), hyperactive (agitation), and a mixed subtype which displays features of both. The symptoms often fluctuate [1,2].

Delirium complicates up to 20% of all hospital admissions. In the elderly, it is the most frequent complication of hospitalization, and is associated with high levels of morbidity and mortality [3,4]. Although less common in younger patients, it is more likely to point toward severe illness.

Delirium can begin hours after surgery and remain for several days. The peak onset is within the first 72 hours. In some cases the onset may be more insidious. If there are several risk factors present, only a small precipitant is required to result in delirium. The risk factors include [2,3,5–8]:

- age more than 65 years;
- significant comorbidity;
- type of operation (delirium more likely with emergency operations and more extensive surgery);
- drug dependence and abuse;
- poor mobility;
- social isolation;
- preoperative cognitive problems (e.g., dementia, depression);
- sensory deficits (e.g., visual, hearing).

The differential diagnosis for the causes of delirium can be vast [5,6,8].

- Infective: wound infection, sepsis, urinary tract infection, pneumonia, encephalitis, meningitis.
- Vascular: bleeding, deep vein thrombosis, pulmonary embolus, cerebrovascular accident, myocardial infarction.
- Metabolic: hypoxia, anemia, hypoglycemia/hyperglycemia, electrolyte disturbance, hepatic/renal impairment, alcohol intoxication/withdrawal, thiamine/B_{12} deficiency, substance misuse.
- Medication: opioids, benzodiazepines, anticonvulsants, anticholinergics, steroids.

- Pain.
- Trauma: falls, head injury.
- Others: urinary retention, constipation, hyperthermia/hypothermia, idiopathic, brain tumors, dementia.

Management

Assessment
The diagnosis of delirium is clinical. The main diagnostic features are included in the DSM-IV and ICD-10 classifications [9,10].

1 Disturbance of consciousness.
2 Change in cognition.
3 Onset of hours to days and tendency to fluctuate.
4 Behavior may be overactive or underactive with sleep often disturbed and loss of circadian rhythm.
5 Thinking is often slow and confused, but the content may be complex.

Assessment must involve a full history including a collateral history to determine the patient's premorbid mental state and functional ability. A thorough physical examination of all major systems should be performed, including a neurologic examination to look for any focal signs. If the patient is not too unwell, assessment of cognitive function must also be undertaken using available tools such as the Confusion Assessment Method [2] or Mini Mental State Examination (MMSE). This must be reassessed regularly because of the fluctuating nature of delirium. Observations such as heart rate, respiratory rate, temperature, blood pressure, pulse oximetry and BM should be recorded regularly. In all cases airway, breathing, and circulation must be assessed and maintained.

Investigations include ABG, FBC, U&E, LFT, TFT, Ca^{2+}, blood glucose, and MSU. Other investigations such as blood cultures, head CT, chest radiograph, lumbar puncture, and echocardiogram may be necessary depending on clinical suspicion.

If an underlying cause is identified, it should be treated promptly. Generally, non-pharmacologic therapy is the mainstay of delirium treatment, although there may be a role for medication [2]. Although confusion may sometimes be attributable to anesthesia, if the patient was lucid after waking up from anesthesia and then becomes confused, anesthesia can no longer be considered the cause.

Gynecologic and Obstetric Surgery: Challenges and Management Options, First Edition. Edited by Arri Coomarasamy, Mahmood I. Shafi, G. Willy Davila and Kiong K. Chan.
© 2016 John Wiley & Sons, Ltd. Published 2016 by John Wiley & Sons, Ltd.

Conservative management

This involves supporting patients to orientate and "normalize" themselves as much as possible [1–3].

- Maintain normal routine and orientation: give patients information about the time, day, date, and where they are. Provide them with familiar day-to-day objects such as a clock, television, spectacles, hearing aids, and mobility aids if they have any.
- Allow contact with familiar people such as family members, friends, carers, and known medical staff.
- Provide a relaxed environment with appropriate levels of noise, lighting, space, and temperature. Single occupancy rooms are preferred to minimize distress to the patient and others.
- Ensure basic needs are met: toileting, nutrition, hydration, and sleep hygiene with awareness of the day–night cycle.
- Effective, caring, and empathetic communication should be employed.

Medical management

Medications may be the underlying cause of the delirium so they should be used with caution as a treatment. Furthermore, side effects of medications may exacerbate delirium.

Pain is often a contributory factor so effective analgesia is important [2]. Antipsychotics such as haloperidol (0.5–1.5 mg up to a total of 10 mg in 24 hours, given orally, i.m. or i.v.) may be useful in

a minority of patients who display agitation or aggression [2]. They are particularly useful because of their fast onset of action if needed urgently. In cases of delirium due to alcohol withdrawal, a course of benzodiazepines as a reducing-dose regimen may be required [5]. If opioid overdose is suspected to be the cause, discontinue opioids and give intravenous naloxone in 0.4-mg increments up to 1 mg total.

Follow-up

Patients and family members will need ongoing support after discharge as the symptoms of delirium may persist after the underlying cause has been corrected.

Prevention

Identifying patients at risk of developing delirium is crucial. A multidisciplinary approach with prompt assessment of risk factors on admission is recommended [2]. Those at high risk should be provided with an appropriate inpatient environment with regular observation and assessment. Training and education of all hospital staff should focus on the prevention and management of delirium. The management of delirium should be seen as a continuation of preventive measures.

KEY POINTS

Challenge: Confusion in the postoperative patient.

Background
- Postoperative delirium is very common especially in the elderly.
- It is a major cause of inpatient morbidity and mortality.
- Risk factors include age over 65 years, comorbidity, social isolation, and premorbid cognitive problems.
- Causes of delirium include infective, vascular, metabolic, pain, trauma, medications, and others.

Prevention
- At-risk patients should be identified on admission and provided with an appropriate environment with regular assessment.
- Training and education of all hospital staff in recognizing delirium is important.
- The prevention and management of delirium involves a multidisciplinary team approach.

Management
Assessment
- All patients should have airway, breathing, and circulation assessed and stabilized.

- Assessment includes full history, clinical examination, close monitoring of cognitive function, and relevant investigations.
- Clinical examination should include a neurologic examination to look for focal signs; pupils should be examined.
- Investigations should include ABG, FBC, U&E, LFT, TFT, Ca²⁺, blood glucose, MSU, and if appropriate, other investigations such as blood cultures, head CT, abdominopelvic ultrasound, and chest X-ray.

Treatment
- Underlying organic causes should be corrected promptly.
- Conservative management focuses on providing patients with a familiar and supportive environment involving the multidisciplinary team.
- If patient is very agitated or aggressive, consider treatment with haloperidol 0.5–1.5 mg up to a total of 10 mg in 24 hours, given orally, i.m. or i.v.
- In cases of delirium due to alcohol withdrawal, consider a course of benzodiazepines as a reducing-dose regimen.
- If opioid overdose is suspected to be the cause, discontinue opioids and give intravenous naloxone in 0.4-mg increments up to 1 mg total.
- For management of medical complications, involve appropriate specialists.

References

1 Gleason O. Delirium. *Am Fam Physician* 2003;**67**:1027–1034.
2 National Institute for Health and Care Excellence. *Delirium: diagnosis, prevention and management*. NICE Clinical Guideline No. 103, July 2010. Available at https://www.nice.org.uk/guidance/cg103
3 Meagher D. Delirium: optimising management. *BMJ* 2001;**322**:144–149.
4 Young J, Inouye S. Delirium in older people. *BMJ* 2007;**334**:842–846.
5 Burns A, Gallagley A, Byrne J. Delirium. *J Neurol Neurosurg Psychiatry* 2004;**75**:362–367.
6 Dasgupta M, Dumbrell A. Preoperative risk assessment for delirium after noncardiac surgery: a systematic review. *J Am Geriatr Soc* 2006;**54**:1578–1589.
7 Ansaloni L, Catena F, Chattat R *et al*. Risk factors and incidence of postoperative delirium in elderly patients after elective and emergency surgery. *Br J Surg* 2010;**97**:273–280.
8 Bryson G, Wyand A. Evidence-based clinical update: general anesthesia and the risk of delirium and postoperative cognitive dysfunction. *Can J Anaesth* 2006;**53**:669–677.
9 American Psychiatric Association. Delirium. In: *Diagnostic and Statistical Manual of Mental Disorders: DSM-IV*. American Psychiatric Association, Washington, DC, 2000.
10 World Health Organization. Delirium. In: *The ICD-10 Classification of Mental and Behavioural Disorders*. WHO, Geneva, 1992.

CHAPTER 55
Patient with Poor Urine Output

Amelia Davison[1] and Jackie A. Ross[2]
[1] Homerton University Hospital, London, UK
[2] King's College Hospital, London, UK

Case history 1: A 29-year-old healthy woman, who is now 8 hours following an abdominal myomectomy, has poor urine output. On clinical assessment, she has an abdominal drain with 500 mL of blood and a catheter containing 200 mL of concentrated blood-stained urine. She has a pulse rate of 100 bpm and a blood pressure of 105/68 mmHg. On examination her abdomen is tense and distended.

Case history 2: A 70-year-old woman with COPD and mild congestive cardiac failure is now 8 hours following a retropubic tape procedure. She has passed only small volumes of urine since returning from theater. On clinical assessment, she does not have a catheter in situ; all her observations are stable and she is eating and drinking normally. On examination her abdomen is distended.

Case history 3: A 35-year-old woman had an uneventful laparoscopic salpingo-oophorectomy; however, 9 hours following the surgery, she has not passed urine. On examination, she is well and observations are stable. An in-and-out catheter drains 100 mL of clear urine. However, 12 hours later she has still not passed urine. Her temperature is now 38°C. A urine dipstick is nitrite positive and antibiotics are commenced. A repeat in-and-out catheter drains 350 mL of clear urine. Fluid balance is now 4 L in and 450 mL out, so a positive balance of 3550 mL. She is catheterized; 3 hours later (i.e., 24 hours postoperatively) she has right flank pain. Her temperature is now 38.7°C. On examination she is tachycardic and hypotensive. The catheter has drained 60 mL of clear urine and she remains in positive fluid balance.

Background

Normal urine output is estimated at 1 mL/kg per hour, or approximately 70 mL/hour. Oliguria may be defined as urine output that is inadequate to maintain physiologic homeostasis. In practice this equates to a urine output of less than 0.5 mL/kg per hour for at least two consecutive hours or a daily urine output of less than 400 mL (about 15 mL/hour) [1]. Medical review should be sought when patients have gradually reducing hourly urine output, particularly when it becomes less than 30 mL/hour.

Oliguria is not a clinical diagnosis but a sign that indicates an underlying disorder. Management of oliguria must not only be aimed at restoring urine output but also at identifying and treating the underlying disorder. Whatever the underlying cause, if left untreated, oliguria may lead to acute renal failure and its sequelae,

including hyperkalemia, acidosis, and fluid overload. Oliguria of more than 12 hours and oliguria of three or more episodes are associated with an increased mortality rate. Urine output is a sensitive and early marker for acute kidney injury (AKI) and is associated with adverse outcomes in ITU patients [2]. When reviewing the urine output, it is important to consider it in the context of overall fluid balance, taking into account other losses. In postoperative patients, the clinician needs to consider the effects of wound sites, surgical drains, nasogastric tubes, vomiting, diarrhea, sepsis, or an ileus.

Postoperative patients can have complex reasons for low urine output. These, in combination with any pre-existing renal problems, can make it difficult to establish the correct cause of poor urine output. However, making the correct diagnosis is important for a full and quick recovery.

Poor urine output can be broadly classified into three main categories (Box 55.1).

1 Prerenal: poor perfusion of the kidneys due to heart failure or low circulating blood volume.
2 Renal: due to primary or secondary renal failure.
3 Postrenal: due to structural damage, obstruction, or poor function of the ureters, bladder or urethra.

Differentiating between the causes is important for the correct management and recovery of these patients.

Prevention

Optimizing overall health prior to elective surgery, especially in older patients, reduces overall morbidity and mortality related to anesthesia and surgery. Adequate preoperative hydration, such as placing patients on an enhanced recovery pathway [3] whereby they can have clear fluids up to 2 hours before surgery, reduces the risk of dehydration and improves postoperative recovery.

The role of prophylactic ureteric stenting prior to complex pelvic surgery is controversial in reducing the risk of injury [4]. Experts recommend a low threshold for performing cystoscopy if bladder injury is suspected [5].

Postoperative patients should have a fluid input/output chart and this should include all losses including vomiting and drainage. It is essential to calculate total input and output to establish a positive or negative fluid balance and correct as necessary.

Gynecologic and Obstetric Surgery: Challenges and Management Options, First Edition. Edited by Arri Coomarasamy, Mahmood I. Shafi, G. Willy Davila and Kiong K. Chan.
© 2016 John Wiley & Sons, Ltd. Published 2016 by John Wiley & Sons, Ltd.

BOX 55.1 CAUSES OF POSTOPERATIVE OLIGURIA

Prerenal causes

Hypovolemia (most common cause)
- Dehydration, typically because of inadequate perioperative fluid management.
- Fluid depletion, for example caused by vomiting, losses from nasogastric tube, diarrhea, high-output stoma, diuretic therapy, heat, fever, burns
- Sepsis (usually after the second day)
- Hemorrhage from the operative site

Acute heart failure
- Cardiac event including myocardial infarction and arrhythmia (especially atrial fibrillation)
- Iatrogenic fluid overload

Renal hypoperfusion
- Drugs interfering with mechanisms that maintain renal perfusion (NSAIDs, ACE inhibitors, angiotensin II receptor antagonists, cyclooxygenase 2 inhibitors)
- Hepatorenal syndrome

Edema states
- Acute heart failure (see also above)
- Nephrotic syndrome
- Decompensated liver disease

Renal causes

Intrinsic renal disease
- Prolonged period of hypovolemia
- Nephrotoxic drugs (e.g., gentamicin)
- Acute exacerbation of pre-existing renal disease

Postrenal causes

Urinary tract outflow obstruction
- Ureteric or bladder injury
- Obstructed catheter

Source: Behjati & Dvorkin, 2008 [1] with permission from the *British Medical Journal.*

Ensuring the patient voids adequately within 4–8 hours of the removal of a catheter or postoperatively will prevent distension injury.

Management

Review the clinical history

Clinical history and assessment play an important role in differentiating between low urine production and postrenal causes. Establishing a prompt and correct diagnosis limits further complications and aids recovery.

The history should be reviewed, paying particular attention to the type of surgery, any difficulties encountered, and the estimated blood loss. Occasionally, the presentation of oliguria can be delayed and can occur with arduous laparoscopic surgery causing visceral injury [6]. A history of any coexisting medical problems should be obtained. This should include establishing any pre-existing renal or cardiovascular disease.

Preoperative blood results are important as they may show preoperative anemia or abnormal renal or liver function. Albumin is particularly important in patients with malignancy or ovarian hyperstimulation syndrome because a low serum albumin increases third space losses and the risk of peripheral and pulmonary edema; in such patients, fluid resuscitation may not result in improvement in the urine output.

Recent clinical observations should be noted, paying particular attention to any trends. Patients who have regional blocks may have blood pressure values that are misleadingly low. Early warning scores are often useful since they allow careful monitoring of patients' basic observations and prompt nursing staff to seek appropriate and timely medical reviews.

Assessment

Armed with a good knowledge of history and perioperative findings, examining the patient can become more directed (indeed the clinician may have already reached a working diagnosis).
- First appearances count! Does the patient look well or unwell?
- Is the patient in pain? Does he or she look shocked? Feel the peripheries and take the pulse.
- Examine the abdomen for evidence of bleeding, peritonism, abdominal distension, or a palpable bladder.
- Listen to the chest and examine the legs for signs of pulmonary or peripheral edema; this is especially important in patients with low albumin or with a history of cardiac failure and a positive fluid balance. Arrange chest X-ray if indicated.
- Inspect the color of the urine in the catheter, if the patient has one. Is it concentrated, dilute, blood-stained or empty?
- If the catheter is empty or heavily blood-stained, it is worthwhile flushing or changing the catheter because it may be wrongly sited or blocked.
- Finally perform a urine dipstick test. Infection and inflammation can result in poor voiding and are not uncommon following use of a catheter.
- If the patient does not have a laparotomy scar, a bladder scan is useful to check on bladder urine volume.
- Renal function tests for serum urea, creatinine and electrolytes, and hemoglobin levels, may be useful.
- Review operative notes to check whether any technical difficulty was encountered (this might raise the suspicion of bladder or ureteric injury).

Resolution of the cases

Case history 1

The patient appears to be bleeding intra-abdominally and the kidneys are thus not producing urine due to hypovolemia. Blood-stained urine is uncommon after a myomectomy, so consider DIC or over-anticoagulation as possible contributory factors.

Resuscitation is key to preventing further clinical deterioration in the case of hypovolemia. Intravenous access should be obtained and bloods sent for FBC, clotting, U&E, LFT, and G&S. If hemorrhage is suspected, at least 4 units of blood should be cross-matched. The patient should be catheterized and fluid balance should be recorded hourly using a urometer.

Assessment should be made to exclude intra-abdominal hemorrhage, which may necessitate prompt return to theater for hemostasis.

Bladder and ureteric injury should be considered among the differential diagnoses; it may be necessary to arrange investigations such as CT urogram. If ureteric injury causes hydronephrosis, referral to a urologist should be promptly made to consider percutaneous nephrostomy and antegrade stenting prior to planning definitive reconstructive surgery [7].

Case history 2

This patient demonstrates poor urine outflow. She is likely to have a palpable bladder and be in general discomfort but with no evidence of peritonism. Prescribing additional fluids in this case may result in fluid overload, potential cardiac failure, and bladder distension injury.

Once a voiding difficulty has been diagnosed, an in-and-out catheter or indwelling Foley catheter should be inserted. The residual volume should be measured and recorded. If there is less than 500 mL urine in the bladder, the patient should have a strict fluid balance assessment; if she is still unable to pass urine in 4 hours or the residual volume is greater than 150 mL, then an indwelling catheter should be sited. Patients requiring catheterization should be referred to the urogynecology team for further management. Following catheterization for urine retention, a trial without catheter (TWOC) can take place, usually 12–24 hours later. If this fails and residual volumes remain high, the patient can be sent home for 3–7 days with an indwelling catheter, followed by return for TWOC. If this fails and the patient is willing, she is taught clean intermittent self-catheterization (CISC). In older women or those who cannot learn CISC and have long-term voiding difficulties, insertion of a suprapubic catheter can be considered.

Case history 3

In this patient, sepsis due to bowel perforation was suspected and a laparotomy was performed, which demonstrated a large bladder perforation. The patient suffered overwhelming sepsis as a consequence of retroperitoneal urine leakage from a bladder perforation sustained at the time of her laparoscopy. She recovered but required debridement and skin grafting from her upper thigh.

KEY POINTS

Challenge: Postoperative poor urine output.

Background
- Normal urine output is estimated at 1 mL/kg per hour.
- Medical review is required if urine output is consistently less than 30 mL/hour.
- It is important to consider overall fluid balance, including losses related to surgery (e.g., hemorrhage, bladder or ureteric injury, sepsis, drains, and fistulae).
- Differentiation between low urine output and poor voiding is key to successful management and recovery.

Prevention
- Optimize overall health prior to elective surgery, especially in older patients.
- Provide adequate hydration preoperatively, intraoperatively, and postoperatively.
- The role of prophylactic ureteric stenting prior to complex pelvic surgery is controversial in reducing the risk of injury.
- Experts recommend a low threshold for performing cystoscopy if bladder injury is suspected.
- The patient should void adequately within 4–8 hours of the removal of a catheter or postoperatively.

Assessment
Low urine production
- Unwell: pale, dehydrated.
- Signs suggestive of bleeding: external or internal.
- Abnormal clinical observations (e.g., tachycardia and hypotension).
- History of renal impairment or comorbidities.

Poor outflow
- Small frequent volumes of urine.
- Sensation of incomplete voiding.
- Abdominal or pelvic pain.
- Stable observations and renal function.
- Palpable bladder.

Management
- Review clinical history, symptoms, records, observations, and fluid chart.
- Examine for palpable bladder and hemoperitoneum.
- Perform: urine dipstick, serum U&E, creatinine, hemoglobin, albumin; if injury suspected, then also cystoscopy, CT urogram, ultrasound with or without tapping the abdominal fluid for biochemistry to rule out extravasation of urine.

Low urine production
- Provide fluid resuscitation.
- Consider sepsis, dehydration, hemoperitoneum, and return to theater.
- Consider bladder/ureteric injury and investigations such as abdominal ultrasound, intravenous pyelogram, CT urogram, and cystoscopy.

Outflow problems
- Measure residual volume with a bladder scan or in-and-out catheter:
  - If over 500 mL, catheterize with indwelling Foley catheter.
  - If under 500 mL, empty the bladder with a simple in-and-out catheter. After 4 hours, if the patient is still unable to pass urine or residual volume more than 150 mL, insert an indwelling catheter or teach CISC.
- Maintain strict fluid balance.
- Refer the patient to a urogynecology team.
- If hydronephrosis and ureteric injury are suspected, refer the patient to urology and interventional radiology for antegrade stenting and percutaneous nephrostomy.

References

1 Behjati S, Dvorkin LS. Managing postoperative oliguria. *Student BMJ* 2008;1:28–29.
2 Macedo E1, Malhotra R, Bouchard J, Wynn SK, Mehta RL.Oliguria is an early predictor of higher mortality in critically ill patients. *Kidney Int* 2011;80:760–767.
3 Kalogera E, Bakkum-Gamez JN, Jankowski CJ *et al.* Enhanced recovery in gynecologic surgery. *Obstet Gynecol* 2013;122:319–328.
4 da Silva G, Boutros M, Wexner SD. Role of prophylactic ureteric stents in colorectal surgery. *Asian J Endosc Surg* 2012;5:105–110.
5 Dwyer PL. Urinary tract injury: medical negligence or unavoidable complication? *Int Urogynecol J* 2010;21:903–910.
6 Lad M, Duncan S, Patten DK.Occult bladder injury after laparoscopic appendicectomy. *BMJ Case Rep* 2013, doi:10.1136/bcr-2013-200430.
7 Hausegger KA, Portugaller HR. Percutaneous nephrostomy and antegrade ureteral stenting: technique, indications, complications. *Eur Radiol* 2006;16:2016–2030.

CHAPTER 56
Electrolyte Imbalance

Manjeet Shehmar[1] and Arri Coomarasamy[2]

[1] Birmingham Women's NHS Foundation Trust, Birmingham, UK
[2] College of Medical and Dental Sciences, University of Birmingham, Birmingham, UK

Case history: A 48-year-old woman had a hysterectomy for severe endometriosis. Adhesions between large bowel and the pouch of Douglas were divided, but there was no evidence of bowel trauma. However, the patient vomited for 24 hours, with a distended abdomen and reduced bowel sounds. The surgical team reviewed her and a diagnosis of ileus was made; the patient had intravenous fluid hydration and a nasogastric tube. She was hydrated with 0.9% saline with 20 mmol potassium over 8 hours; urea and electrolytes were checked, and her potassium was found to be 2.7 mmol/L.

Background

The British Consensus Guideline on Intravenous Fluid Therapy for Adult Surgical Patients (GIFTASUP) recommends that adult patients should receive 50–100 mmol of sodium and 40–80 mmol of potassium in 1.5–2 L of water by the oral, enteral, or parenteral routes (or in a combination) in order to meet adult daily maintenance requirements [1]. Furthermore, additional amounts should be given to correct deficit or continuing losses. Careful monitoring using clinical examination, fluid balance charts, and regular weighing is recommended. Renal function is monitored using urea and electrolyte blood tests. Urea is produced by the liver as a waste product of amino acid metabolism. Normal urea levels are 2.5–6.7 mmol/L and are raised in dehydration. Creatinine is a waste product of muscle breakdown and can be raised in renal disease or renal obstruction. A normal creatinine level in a non-pregnant adult is 60–100 µmol/L. Normal values and functions of common electrolytes are given in Table 56.1 [2].

Management

Potassium

It is important to maintain normal levels of potassium for neuromuscular function. Potassium imbalance is the most common clinical metabolic abnormality seen and, if severe, both hyperkalemia and hypokalemia can be fatal.

Table 56.1 Normal values and functions of common electrolytes.

Electrolyte (normal levels)	Function	Homeostasis
Potassium (3.5–5.0 mmol/L)	Neuromuscular function	ICF/ECF levels maintained by Na⁺/K⁺ pump. Intake via diet; excretion via kidneys, gastrointestinal tract and sweating
Sodium (135–145 mmol/L)	Controls water distribution and ECF volume	ICF/ECF levels maintained by Na⁺/K⁺ pump. Intake via diet; excretion via kidneys, gastrointestinal tract and sweating
Calcium (2.23–2.57 mmol/L)	Major role in transmission of nerve impulses. Regulates muscle contraction and relaxation	Parathyroid hormone promotes transfer of calcium from bones to plasma and augments intestinal absorption of calcium. Calcitonin inhibits bone resorption (reducing serum levels)
Magnesium (0.65–1.1 mmol/L)	Enzymatic reactions particularly those involving ATP. Neuronal control, neuromuscular transmission, and cardiovascular tone	Intake via diet and excretion via kidneys
Phosphorus (0.81–1.45 mmol/L)	Source of high-energy bonds of ATP. Muscle function, RBCs and nervous system	Intake via diet and excretion via kidneys

Source: Felstead, 2007 [2] with permission from Wiley.

Gynecologic and Obstetric Surgery: Challenges and Management Options, First Edition. Edited by Arri Coomarasamy, Mahmood I. Shafi, G. Willy Davila and Kiong K. Chan.
© 2016 John Wiley & Sons, Ltd. Published 2016 by John Wiley & Sons, Ltd.

The effects of hyperkalemia include ECG changes (severity depends on level of hyperkalemia), peaking of T waves, flattening of P wave, prolonged PR interval, widening of QRS complex and, in severe hyperkalemia, sine wave and cardiac arrest.

The effects of hypokalemia include weakness, leg cramps, paralytic ileus, respiratory difficulties, ECG changes (U waves, T-wave flattening, ST segment changes, and cardiac arrhythmias especially in patients who are ischemic, on digoxin, or in heart failure) and, in patients with severe hypokalemia, rhabdomyolysis and ascending paralysis.

Hyperkalemia

Hyperkalemia is defined as a serum potassium concentration (serum K+) greater than 5.0 mmol/L. High serum potassium levels can be a spurious result due to collection, storage or laboratory errors that cause potassium to leak from cells, or can be the result of blood collection from an intravenous infusion arm. A repeat sample should be checked to confirm the result. True hyperkalemia has many causes, including excessive potassium intake (e.g., in intravenous fluids), renal impairment, tissue necrosis or lysis, insulin deficiency, metabolic acidosis, and pharmacologic agents [3]. The cause should be identified and treated, but hyperkalemia is a medical emergency when levels are above 6.5 mmol/L or if there are ECG changes. In this circumstance, prompt management should be initiated with continuous ECG, intravenous calcium gluconate (10 mL of calcium gluconate 10% over 1–2 min), intravenous insulin with glucose (15 units of insulin in 50 mL 50% glucose), and nebulized salbutamol if required [4]. Calcium gluconate can be repeated every 5 min for up to four doses if ECG abnormalities persist [4]. Furosemide should be given in addition, with consideration for calcium resonium and dialysis [3]. Immediate advice should be sought from the on-call medical team and joint care should be provided. Consideration should be given to where the patient is best managed; because of the need for continuous cardiac monitoring, a medical ward, high-dependency or critical care unit may be better suited than a gynecologic ward. Patients with moderate hyperkalemia (6.0–6.5 mmol/L) should be admitted for supervised lowering of serum potassium.

Hypokalemia

Potassium is lost during prolonged periods of vomiting and diarrhea, and in these situations potassium needs to be replaced according to the patient's U&E levels. A lowering of 1 mmol/L of K+ (e.g., from 4 mmol/L to 3 mmol/L) is associated with a deficit of 200–400 mmol of K+ [4]. Hypokalemia should be corrected using oral or intravenous potassium in fluids. If there are no clinical manifestations, oral therapy is generally the first-line treatment (e.g., Sando-K 12 mmol tablets, two to three tablets, taken 8–12 hourly for 48 hours); K+ should be checked every day. The patient should be encouraged to eat food rich in K+ (e.g., bananas, dried apricot, spinach, and raisins).

If the patient has severe hypokalemia or is unable to tolerate oral medications, intravenous K+ is needed [5]. Great care must be taken when giving intravenous potassium because of the risk of fatal hyperkalemia. It is recommended to use pre-packed KCl, rather than adding KCl by hand. If KCl needs to be added by hand, it is recommended to cross-check the dose with another doctor *and* a nurse. It is advisable to use KCl that is not concentrated more

than 40 mmol/L, and use it no faster than 40 mmol in 6 hours [4]. An exception to this advice needs to be made in a patient at risk of fluid overload; in such patients, concentrated KCl (10–20 mmol in 100 mL of normal saline) can be given slowly via a central line [4]. A daily maintenance dose of potassium is 60 mmol, but if a patient is hypokalemic more potassium may be required to reach normal levels.

Infusion with 0.9% sodium chloride is recommended rather than 5% glucose [5]. Cardiac ECG changes and magnesium should be monitored, and the renal team should be contacted if there is renal impairment. Serum K+ levels should be monitored after every 40 mmol of potassium supplemented and the cardiac resuscitation team should be called if there are unstable arrhythmias.

The causes of hypokalemia are shown in Table 56.2. Management involves addressing the causes, in addition to KCl replacement.

Table 56.2 Causes of hypokalemia.

Drugs: diuretics (thiazides, loop diuretics), laxatives, glucocorticoids, fludrocortisone, penicillins, amphotericin, aminoglycosides, insulin/glucose therapy, salbutamol and other beta-agonists, theophylline

Gastrointestinal losses: diarrhea, vomiting, ileostomy, intestinal fistula

Renal: renal disease with primary hyper-reninism, dialysis

Endocrine disorders: hyperaldosteronism (Conn's syndrome), Cushing's syndrome, adrenal hyperplasia

Trancellular shifts: promoted by alkalemia, insulin, β-adrenergic stimulation, and xanthines such as caffeine [6]

Metabolic: metabolic alkalosis

Magnesium depletion

Decreased intake: unlikely cause [7]

Other electrolyte imbalances

Other key electrolyte imbalances, with their respective causes, clinical features, and principles of management, are provided in Table 56.3 [4].

Resolution of the case

This patient has hypokalemia, increased gastrointestinal losses through vomiting, an ileus leading to dehydration and hypokalemia, and the risk of possible bowel trauma with high-risk surgery. Causes of hypokalemia should be alleviated by effective antiemetics and resolution of the ileus. The hypokalemia should be treated with intravenous supplementation in her fluids. As she is already hypokalemic, she will need additional potassium to her daily maintenance dose, with 40 mmol potassium in 0.9% saline to a maximum dose of 20 mmol/hour. As she has moderate hypokalemia, it would be acceptable for the fluids to run over 6 hours as long as she is not dehydrated and has good urine output and normal renal function. She will need monitoring, with hourly observations of urine output, a fluid balance chart, and her U&E will need to be checked after each 40 mmol potassium supplementation in order to direct further treatment. One would expect improvement in U&E and urine output, reduced vomiting, and reduced abdominal distension with this regimen; if she does not improve, a full clinical review should be undertaken to rule out bowel trauma.

Table 56.3 Management of key electrolyte imbalances.

Electrolyte imbalance	Causes	Clinical features	Management principles
Hypernatremia	Dehydration (e.g., vomiting or diarrhea) Uncontrolled diabetes mellitus Excessive infusion of normal saline	Extreme thirst Confusion Seizures Coma Subarachnoid hemorrhage	Replace the estimated body water deficit; give water 20–50 mL/hour orally or via NGT or as intravenous 5% dextrose, in addition to the standard fluid replacement If hypernatremia is chronic, ensure slow correction. Check urine output hourly, and U&E every 4–6 hours
Hyponatremia	Dehydration (e.g., vomiting or diarrhea) Long-term diuretic therapy Excessive infusion of 5% dextrose Distension media overload (Chapter 63)	Headaches Confusion Seizures Coma Cerebral edema Rate of change of Na^+ more important than actual level; acute drop in Na^+ more likely to cause fatal cerebral edema	*Volume-overloaded patient* Give normal saline, with repeated doses of furosemide 20–40 mg i.v. *Volume-depleted patient* Give normal saline If hyponatremia is acute onset and severe, or if patient has neurologic symptoms, ensure rapid correction; otherwise correct slowly. Check urine output hourly, and U&E every 4–6 hours *Chronic hyponatremia* Exclude SIADH
Hypercalcemia	Primary hyperparathyroidism Bony metastasis Myeloma Excessive vitamin D intake	Abdominal pain Nausea and vomiting Constipation Tiredness Renal stones In severe cases (>3 mmol/L), arrhythmias and coma, often associated with dehydration	Defer elective surgery if Ca^{2+} >3 mmol/L For emergency surgery, seek medical advice on management; treatment is with intravenous hydration and pamidronate; in life-threatening cases, calcitonin treatment should be considered
Hypocalcemia	Hyperventilation Hypoparathyroidism Overhydration Pancreatitis	Tetany Seizures Bronchospasm Perioral paresthesia	If Ca^{2+} >2 mmol/L, give oral calcium supplements If Ca^{2+} <2 mmol/L, seek medical advice; treatment is with calcium gluconate infusion, and possibly calcitriol. Correct any hypomagnesemia
Hypomagnesemia	Reduced food intake Vomiting and diarrhea Can be associated with hypocalcemia and hypokalemia	Tetany Seizures Psychosis Ventricular arrhythmias	Always check magnesium in patients with hypocalcemia or hypokalemia Replace with oral magnesium salts; in symptomatic patients, give magnesium infusion (4 mL of 50% magnesium solution over 15 min)

KEY POINTS

Challenge: Management of perioperative electrolyte imbalance.

Background
- Severe electrolyte imbalance can be life-threatening.
- Adult patients should receive 50–100 mmol of sodium and 40–80 mmol of potassium in 1.5–2 L of water by the oral, enteral, or parenteral routes (or in a combination) to meet daily maintenance requirements.

Normal ranges
- Urea: 2.5–6.7 mmol/L.
- Creatinine: 60–100 μmol/L.
- Potassium: 3.5–5.0 mmol/L.
- Sodium: 135–145 mmol/L.
- Calcium: 2.23–2.57 mmol/L.
- Magnesium: 0.65–1.1 mmol/L.
- Phosphorus: 0.81–1.45 mmol/L.

Management
Hyperkalemia
- Causes: spurious result from blood collection from infusion arm; excessive K^+ infusion, renal disease, tissue necrosis, insulin deficiency, drugs, and metabolic acidosis.
- Clinical features: ECG changes and cardiac arrest.
- Management of severe hyperkalemia (K^+ >6.5 mmol/L or if there are ECG changes):
  - Continuous ECG.
  - Give intravenous calcium gluconate (10 mL of calcium gluconate 10% over 1–2 min); repeat every 5 min for up to four doses if ECG abnormalities persist.
  - Give intravenous insulin with glucose (15 units of insulin in 50 mL 50% glucose).
  - Give nebulized salbutamol (5 mg).
  - Give furosemide, and consider calcium resonium and dialysis.

Hypokalemia
- Causes: drugs (e.g., diuretics, insulin), diarrhea and vomiting, renal disease, and endocrine disease (e.g., Conn's syndrome and Cushing's syndrome).
- Clinical features: weakness, cramps, paralytic ileus, respiratory difficulties, ECG changes.
- Management:
  - If there are no clinical manifestations, oral therapy is first line (e.g., Sando-K 12 mmol tablets, two to three tablets, taken 8–12 hourly for 48 hours); encourage to eat food rich in K^+ (e.g., bananas, dried apricot, spinach, and raisins).
  - If the patient has severe hypokalemia or is unable to tolerate oral medications, intravenous K^+ is needed.
  - Great care must be taken when giving intravenous potassium because of the risk of fatal hyperkalemia.
  - It is advisable to use KCl that is not concentrated more than 40 mmol/L, and use it no faster than 40 mmol in 6 hours. An exception is in a patient at risk of fluid overload; in such patients, concentrated KCl (10–20 mmol in 100 mL of normal saline) can be given slowly via a central line.
  - Infusion with 0.9% sodium chloride is recommended rather than 5% glucose.
  - Check ECG and magnesium levels.

Hypernatremia
- Causes: vomiting, diarrhea, uncontrolled diabetes mellitus, and excessive infusion of normal saline.
- Clinical features: extreme thirst, confusion, seizures, coma, and subarachnoid hemorrhage.
- Management:
  - Replace the estimated body water deficit; give water 20–50 mL/hour orally or via NGT or as intravenous 5% dextrose, in addition to the standard fluid replacement.
  - If hypernatremia is chronic, ensure slow correction. Check urine output hourly, and U&E every 4–6 hours.

Hyponatremia
- Causes: vomiting, diarrhea, long-term diuretic therapy, excessive infusion of 5% dextrose, and distension media overload.
- Clinical features: headaches, confusion, seizures, coma, and cerebral edema.
- Management:
  - Volume-overloaded patient: give normal saline, with repeated doses of furosemide 20–40 mg i.v.
- Volume-depleted patient: give normal saline.
- If hyponatremia is acute onset and severe or patient has neurologic symptoms, ensure rapid correction; otherwise correct slowly. Check urine output hourly, and U&E every 4–6 hours.
- Chronic hyponatremia: exclude SIADH.

References

1 Powell-Tuck J, Gosling P, Lobo DN *et al. British Consensus Guidelines on Intravenous Fluid Therapy for Adult Surgical Patients*. British Association for Parenteral and Enteral Nutrition (BAPEN). Available at http://www.bapen.org.uk/pdfs/bapen_pubs/giftasup.pdf

2 Felstead I. Upper gastrointestinal surgery. In: McArthur-RouseFJ, ProsserS (eds) *Assessing and Managing the Acutely Ill Adult Surgical Patient*, pp. 125–144. Blackwell Publishing Ltd, Oxford, 2007.

3 Nyirenda MJ, Tang JI, Padfield PL, Seckl JR. Hyperkalaemia. *BMJ* 2009;**339**:b4114.

4 Chikwe J, Walther A, Jones P. Renal and urological. In: *Perioperative Medicine: Managing Surgical Patients with Medical Problems*, 2nd edn. Oxford University Press, Oxford, 2009.

5 Palmer BF, Duboise TD Jr. Disorders of potassium metabolism. In: SchrierRW (ed.) *Renal and Electrolyte Disorders*, 7th edn, chapter 5. Lippincott Williams & Wilkins, Philadelphia, 2010.

6 Tannen RL, Hallows KR. Hypo–hyperkalaemia. In: DavisonAM, CameronSJ, GrünfeldJ.-P. *et al.* (eds) *Oxford Textbook of Clinical Nephrology*, 3rd edn, Vol. **1**, pp. 241–267. Oxford University Press, Oxford, 2005.

7 Unwin RJ, Luft FC, Shirley DG. Pathophysiology and management of hypokalemia: a clinical perspective. *Nat Rev Nephrol* 2011;**7**:75–84.

CHAPTER 57
Swollen Leg

Edwin Stephen[1], Indrani Sen[2], and Tim Lees[1]
[1]Freeman Hospital, Newcastle upon Tyne Hospitals NHS Foundation Trust, Newcastle upon Tyne, UK
[2]Christian Medical College, Vellore, Tamil Nadu, India

Case history 1: A 48-year-old female presents with painful right leg swelling 3 days after a pelvic tumor operation. Diagnosis: DVT.

Case history 2: A 52-year-old female treated with pelvic radiation 12 years ago presents with painful left leg swelling, inability to move the foot, and limb paresthesia for 2 hours. She does not have fever or any other systemic illness. She is tachycardic and her pedal pulses are not palpable. Diagnosis: DVT with venous gangrene.

Case history 3: A 48-year-old obese woman underwent laparotomy and tumor debulking surgery. Intraoperative hemostasis was difficult and required extensive packing of the pelvis. Postoperatively, she complains of a painful, swollen, cold right leg. Diagnosis: acute limb ischemia, arterial injury.

Case history 4: A 25-year-old female presents with aching pain, dilated veins, and swelling of both legs following her second pregnancy. She has been using compression stockings which have not provided symptomatic relief. Diagnosis: varicose veins.

Case history 5: A 68-year-old female presents with thickening of the skin around her ankles and swelling (pitting edema) of the leg and foot. Her pedal pulses cannot be felt but she does not complain of pain on walking. She was treated with pelvic radiotherapy in the past. Diagnosis: lymphedema.

Background

Leg swelling is a common clinical problem. Symptomatic treatment is sufficient in the majority of patients but the underlying etiology should be determined; the main concern is a deep vein thrombosis (DVT).

Diagnosis and treatment of refractory swelling can be difficult because of its multifactorial nature and the absence of evidence-based clinical guidelines. Venous disease is very common in females and varicose veins are a common complication of pregnancy [1]. Clinically, there is a broad spectrum of presentation from acute (DVT, including phlegmasia) to chronic conditions (varicose veins, lymphedema). These can often coexist with arterial disease, and awareness of this enables early identification of a threatened limb to avoid amputation [2]. This chapter focuses on areas where early

recognition and treatment are paramount in ensuring good patient outcome.

Causes of leg swelling can be categorized by whether the onset is acute or chronic, and whether one or both legs are affected (Table 57.1).

Table 57.1 Causes of leg swelling.

	Acute	Chronic
Unilateral	DVT	Post-phlebitic limb
	Cellulitis/fasciitis	Chronic venous insufficiency
	Trauma/fracture	Varicose veins
	Ruptured Baker's cyst	Lymphedema
	Muscle tears	Drug induced
	Compartment syndrome	
Bilateral	DVT	Systemic medical disease
	Pre-eclampsia	(liver, heart, renal, thyroid, malnutrition, vasculitis)
		Pregnancy
		Neoplasm, radiation, trauma, infection
		Chronic venous insufficiency
		Lymphedema

Management

Assessment

Patients who present with sudden-onset unilateral painful leg swelling should have investigations for DVT (Case histories 1–3). Venous gangrene (phlegmasia alba/cerulea dolens, Case history 3) presents with paresthesia and paresis; loss of arterial pulses is a sign that the thrombosis is extensive and limb threatening [2]. Other differentials are listed in Table 57.1, and most of these can be arrived at after a complete history and clinical examination (sensory, motor, and pulse examinations are essential). Investigations directed to supplement the clinical diagnosis include FBC, U&E, LFT, TFT, blood sugar, urinalysis, D-dimer, venous duplex, ECG, echocardiogram, chest X-ray, and abdominopelvic imaging.

If a DVT is suspected, an emergency venous ultrasound scan should be performed [3]. If clinical suspicion is high and the initial scan is negative, it should be repeated in 72 hours, or alternative imaging (MR or CT venography) should be considered [3].

Gynecologic and Obstetric Surgery: Challenges and Management Options, First Edition. Edited by Arri Coomarasamy, Mahmood I. Shafi, G. Willy Davila and Kiong K. Chan.
© 2016 John Wiley & Sons, Ltd. Published 2016 by John Wiley & Sons, Ltd.

Management of deep vein thrombosis

If a DVT is confirmed, therapeutic anticoagulation is started after checking the baseline coagulation profile [3]. Low-molecular-weight heparin (LMWH) or unfractionated heparin should be initiated along with oral anticoagulation as per institutional protocol. Duration of anticoagulation is determined by the etiology; unprovoked or ilio-femoral DVT typically requires 6 months of oral anticoagulation with a target INR of 2–3 [3]. Compression garments, early mobilization, and counseling about secondary prevention should be started in parallel. Management of DVT in pregnancy requires an individual management plan for pregnancy, labor, and the postnatal period [4]. Thrombolysis, IVC filter placement, open venous thrombectomy, suction thrombectomy, and venoplasty or stenting are other treatment options [3].

Management of acute arterial insufficiency

Pain, pallor, paresis, paresthesia, and pulselessness are signs of acute arterial insufficiency. The clinical diagnosis in Case history 3 is acute limb ischemia; this necessitates an emergency referral to vascular surgeons. Imaging with CT or MR angiogram may be required, with emergency revascularization [2].

Compartment syndrome can develop after trauma or ischemia. It is characterized by intense pain, worse on flexion of the extremities, woody hard swelling, and paresthesia. Compartment pressures can be measured using a transducer, and fasciotomies can be performed if the pressures are elevated.

Management of varicose veins

Varicose veins can cause leg swelling, pain, bleeding, skin changes, or ulceration (Case history 4). A venous duplex determines which veins are involved. Management is guided by symptoms and duplex results. Compression garments help in relieving symptoms to a certain extent but endovenous ablation (laser or radiofrequency ablation, or foam sclerotherapy) or open operation are often required for a definitive cure.

Management of lymphedema

Swelling involving the dorsum of the foot usually points to lymphedema; skin thickening corroborates this as the primary diagnosis [5]. Assessment of the arterial system with ankle–brachial pressure index (ABPI) is necessary where pulses are not palpable (Case history 5). Pain in these patients points to superinfection; recurrent infections (clinical or subclinical) cause fibrosis, worsening the vicious circle of edema and dermal thickening [6].

Abdominal and pelvic imaging may be necessary to assess the stage or recurrence of pelvic disease. Isotope lymphoscintigraphy can help to confirm the diagnosis. Complex decongestive therapy (exercises, massage, stockings) offers a degree of relief, especially in patients where fibrosis is not advanced [7]. Skin care is of utmost importance. Management of other comorbidities like diabetes needs to be strict as small infections can progress rapidly in these patients.

Prevention of venous thromboembolism

Hospital-associated VTE leads to about 40,000 deaths in England per year, and an estimated 25,000 of these may be preventable through proper risk management and care [8]. All inpatients are potentially at risk of VTE. Assessment should include individual patient risk factors, bleeding risks, contraindications, and procedural risk factors in order to determine the most appropriate thromboprophylaxis plan [9,10].

KEY POINTS

Challenge: Swollen leg.

Background
- Leg swelling is a common clinical problem.
- The main concern is DVT.
- Causes of leg swelling can be categorized by whether the onset is acute or chronic, and whether one or both legs are affected:
  - Acute onset/unilateral: DVT, cellulitis, fasciitis, trauma, ruptured Baker's cyst, muscle tears, compartment syndrome.
  - Acute onset/bilateral: DVT, pre-eclampsia.
  - Chronic onset/unilateral: varicose veins, lymphedema, chronic venous insufficiency, post-phlebitic limb, drug induced.
  - Chronic onset/bilateral: pregnancy, neoplasm, radiation, trauma, infection, chronic venous insufficiency, lymphedema.

Management
- Obtain history: nature of onset, progression, pain, dyspnea, previous DVT.
- Examine the patient: abdominal examination; leg examination, including sensory, motor and pulse examination.
- Investigate: the key investigation is leg Doppler ultrasound; if inconclusive (and a DVT is strongly suspected), arrange MR or CT venography. Other investigations may include FBC, U&E, LFT, TFT, blood sugar, urinalysis, D-dimer, ECG, echocardiogram, chest X-ray, and abdominopelvic imaging.
- Management of DVT:
  - Start LMWH or unfractionated heparin, along with oral anticoagulation.
  - For unprovoked or ilio-femoral DVT, aim for treatment for 6 months with an INR target of 2–3.
  - Arrange compression stockings; encourage early mobilization.
  - Other options: thrombolysis, IVC filter placement, open venous thrombectomy, suction thrombectomy, and venoplasty or stenting.
- Management of acute arterial insufficiency (limb ischemia, compartment syndrome):
  - Symptoms: pain, pallor, paresis, paresthesia, and pulselessness.
  - Arrange CT or MR angiogram.
  - Refer to vascular surgeons.
- Management of varicose veins: compression garments; endovenous ablation (laser or radiofrequency ablation, or foam sclerotherapy) or open operation.
- Management of lymphedema:
  - Isotope lymphoscintigraphy can help to confirm the diagnosis.
  - Complex decongestive therapy (exercises, massage, stockings) offers a degree of relief.
  - Skin care is of utmost importance.
  - Management of other comorbidities like diabetes needs to be strict.

Prevention
- All inpatients are at risk of VTE; assess risk and provide prophylaxis according to local protocols.
- Encourage early hydration and mobilization of the patient after surgery.
- All new leg swellings should be taken seriously, and investigated and managed promptly.

References

1 Boivin P, Cornu-Thenard A, Charpak Y. Pregnancy-induced changes in lower extremity superficial veins: an ultrasound scan study. *J Vasc Surg* 2000; **32**: 570–574.

2 Norgren L, Hiatt WR, Dormandy JA *et al*. Inter-Society Consensus for the Management of Peripheral Arterial Disease (TASC II). *Eur J Vasc Endovasc Surg* 2007;**33**(Suppl 1):S1–S75.

3 National Institute for Health and Care Excellence. *Venous thromboembolic diseases: the management of venous thromboembolic diseases and the role of thrombophilia testing*. NICE Clinical Guideline No. 144, June 2012. Available at https://www.nice.org.uk/guidance/cg144/

4 Royal College of Obstetricians and Gynaecologists. Treatment of venous thrombosis in pregnancy and after birth. Available at http://www.rcog.org.uk/womens-health/clinical-guidance/venous-thrombosis-pregnancy-and-after-birth

5 Stemmer R. Ein klinisches Zeichen zur Früh- und Differentialdiagnose des Lymphödems. *Vasa* 1976; **5**: 261–262.

6 Mayrovitz HN. The standard of care for lymphedema: current concepts and physiological considerations. *Lymphat Res Biol* 2009;7:101–108.

7 Kim S-J, Park Y-D. Effects of complex decongestive physiotherapy on the oedema and the quality of life of lower unilateral lymphoedema following treatment for gynecological cancer. *Eur J Cancer Care (Engl)* 2008; **17**: 463–468.

8 House of Commons Health Select Committee. The prevention of VTE in hospitalised patients. February 2005. Available at http://www.publications.parliament.uk/pa/cm200405/cmselect/cmhealth/99/99.pdf

9 National Institute for Health and Care Excellence. *Venous thromboembolism in adults admitted to hospital: reducing the risk*. NICE Clinical Guideline No. 92, January 2010. Available at http://guidance.nice.org.uk/CG92

10 National Institute for Health and Care Excellence. Venous thromboembolism overview. NICE Pathways. Available at http://pathways.nice.org.uk/pathways/venous-thromboembolism

CHAPTER 58
Cardiorespiratory Arrest

Jennie Kerr
University Hospitals Birmingham NHS Foundation Trust, Birmingham, UK

Case history: A pregnant woman at 32 weeks of gestation is found on the floor of the bathroom on the antenatal ward. She is unresponsive, is making no respiratory effort, and has no pulse.

Background

Cardiorespiratory arrest is identified by no respiratory effort, or agonal gasping breathing, and no pulse or signs of life. Confirmation of cardiac arrest is made by placing your cheek next to the patient's mouth to listen and feel for breath, and looking for chest movement, while simultaneously feeling for a carotid pulse. If there is no respiratory effort (or only agonal gasps) and no pulse, then cardiac arrest is confirmed; cardiopulmonary resuscitation must commence immediately and the cardiac arrest team should be called. The shorter the interval between collapse and commencing chest compressions, the better the chances of survival for both mother and baby [1].

Prevention

The incidence of maternal collapse is estimated at 0.14–6 per 1000 births [2], and so cardiac arrest is rare. Intervening and treating the patient in response to early signs of demise may prevent deterioration to the point of arrest. An early warning score (EWS) can help to identify deteriorating patients and trigger medical attention.

Management of cardiac arrest

The cardiac arrest team should be called, including an obstetrician and a neonatologist. Management of the patient in cardiac arrest follows the Advanced Life Support (ALS) algorithm (Figure 58.1). The algorithm requires determination of whether the rhythm is shockable or not.
- Shockable: pulseless ventricular tachycardia (VT) or ventricular fibrillation (VF).
- Non-shockable: pulseless electrical activity (PEA) or asystole.
Good-quality basic life support (chest compressions and ventilation) should continue throughout the arrest.

Chest compressions and ventilation
Chest compressions [3] should be:
1 performed with two interlocking hands over the center of the chest, allowing the chest to fully recoil after each compression;
2 at a rate of 100–120 per minute;
3 at a depth of one-third of the chest;
4 at a ratio of 30 compressions to 2 ventilations until the airway is secured, when they should be continuous;
5 minimally interrupted for rhythm checking and delivering shocks ("hands on charging" is now recommended);
6 rotated around members of the team every 2 min to prevent fatigue.

Pregnant patient
Three additional issues are important in a pregnant patient.
1 *Tilt.* It is important to use a left lateral tilt of 15° or manual displacement of the uterus in a woman who is more than 20 weeks of gestation to relieve aortocaval compression. This can considerably increase cardiac output [1,2]. A wedge is no longer recommended as the quality of compressions is compromised.
2 *Early intubation.* Often, a laryngeal mask airway (LMA) is used in aiding ventilation in the arrested patient. Intubation with an endotracheal tube by an anesthetist is recommended in pregnant patients as there is more risk of aspiration of gastric contents due to decreased gastric motility and reduced lower esophageal sphincter tone. Intubating a pregnant patient can be more difficult because of airway edema and increased breast tissue.
3 *Positioning of defibrillation pads.* The pads may be positioned in anterior and posterior positions on the left side of the chest as it may be difficult to position the apical pad in a left-tilted position [3].

The Confidential Enquiry into Maternal and Child Health (CEMACH) 2003–2005 Report identified that poor resuscitation skills contributed to substandard care [2,4]. There are many life support courses available (e.g., ALS, ALSO) to increase skills in managing the arrested patient, but good team working, leadership, high-quality CPR, and reversal of the underlying causes are key to success.

Gynecologic and Obstetric Surgery: Challenges and Management Options, First Edition. Edited by Arri Coomarasamy, Mahmood I. Shafi, G. Willy Davila and Kiong K. Chan.
© 2016 John Wiley & Sons, Ltd. Published 2016 by John Wiley & Sons, Ltd.

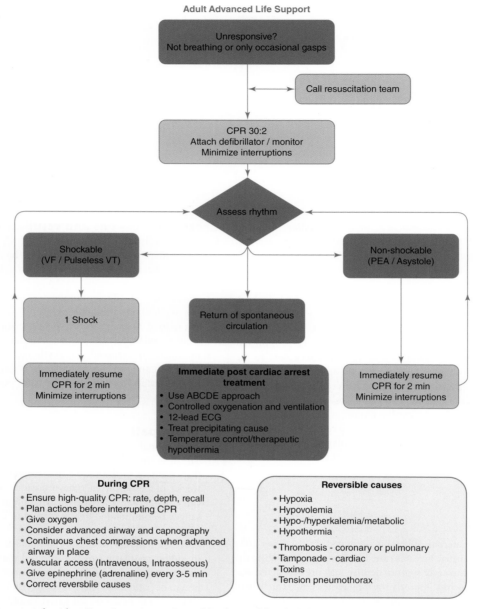

Adult Advanced Life Support

Unresponsive?
Not breathing or only occasional gasps

Call resuscitation team

CPR 30:2
Attach defibrillator / monitor
Minimize interruptions

Assess rhythm

Shockable
(VF / Pulseless VT)

Non-shockable
(PEA / Asystole)

1 Shock

Return of spontaneous
circulation

Immediately resume
CPR for 2 min
Minimize interruptions

**Immediate post cardiac arrest
treatment**
• Use ABCDE approach
• Controlled oxygenation and ventilation
• 12-lead ECG
• Treat precipitating cause
• Temperature control/therapeutic
  hypothermia

Immediately resume
CPR for 2 min
Minimize interruptions

During CPR
• Ensure high-quality CPR: rate, depth, recall
• Plan actions before interrupting CPR
• Give oxygen
• Consider advanced airway and capnography
• Continuous chest compressions when advanced
  airway in place
• Vascular access (Intravenous, Intraosseous)
• Give epinephrine (adrenaline) every 3-5 min
• Correct reversbile causes

Reversible causes
• Hypoxia
• Hypovolemia
• Hypo-/hyperkalemia/metabolic
• Hypothermia

• Thrombosis - coronary or pulmonary
• Tamponade - cardiac
• Toxins
• Tension pneumothorax

Figure 58.1 Adult cardiac arrest algorithm. From Resuscitation Council (UK), 2011 [3] with the kind permission of the Resuscitation Council (UK).

Causes and management

The reversible causes of cardiac arrest are denoted by the four "H"s and four "T"s (Table 58.1) [3]. In the pregnant patient, causes may be pregnancy-related or a result of conditions unrelated to pregnancy. In pregnancy, the most likely causes of cardiac arrest are cardiac disease, hypovolemia due to sepsis, hemorrhage, or thromboembolism [4]. Other pregnancy-related causes include amniotic fluid embolism, drug overdose, anaphylaxis, intracerebral hemorrhage, and eclampsia [2].

Perimortem cesarean section

CPR is less effective in the pregnant patient as the gravid uterus compresses the inferior vena cava and restricts venous return to the heart, and because chest compressions are more difficult to perform in a tilted position [5]. Pregnant patients are more at risk of hypoxic brain injury than non-pregnant patients because of a higher oxygen

consumption and lower oxygen store. Delivering the fetus reduces oxygen consumption and improves venous return, thereby improving cardiac output by up to 80% [1].

A perimortem cesarean section should be performed in women at more than 20 weeks of gestation. The purpose of this is to improve maternal survival. Perimortem cesarean section should start at 4 min into the arrest, so that delivery has been achieved by 5 min [1–3,5,6].

Perimortem cesarean section should occur at the scene of the resuscitation, and equipment (at least a scalpel and two cord clamps) should be immediately available on the cardiac arrest trolley. A classical incision is used as it provides quicker access to the uterus [1] but a transverse incision may be used if the operator is more familiar with this technique [2]. CPR should continue throughout delivery. The baby should be handed to the neonatal team. The outcome for the fetus is improved by prompt commencement of CPR, and by a shorter time between arrest and delivery [1,6].

Table 58.1 Causes of cardiac arrest (4 "H"s and 4 "T"s).

Reversible cause	Pregnancy-related causes	Specific management
Hypovolemia (Chapter 52)	Hemorrhage (Chapter 40)	Blood and blood products; stop bleeding
	Sepsis (Chapter 47)	Broad-spectrum antibiotics; fluids
	High or total spinal	Vasopressors; allow block to recede
Hypoxia (Chapters 3, 8 and 53)	Airway obstruction	Airway maneuvers; intubation
	Failed intubation	LMA; cricothyroid puncture
	Cardiac disease	
	Pulmonary edema	Furosemide; ventilation
Hypokalemia/Hyperkalemia, other electrolyte disturbances (Chapter 56)		Correction of electrolyte abnormality
Hypothermia		Internal and external warming
Thromboembolism (Chapters 15 and 57)	Pulmonary embolus	Thrombolysis and prolonged CPR
	Amniotic fluid embolus	
	Myocardial infarction	Thrombolysis, PCI
Toxicity	Drug overdose	Calcium to treat magnesium toxicity
	Local anesthetic toxicity	Intralipid (protocol available at www.lipidrescue.org)
Tension pneumothorax (Chapter 53)		Needle decompression and chest drain
Tamponade		Pericardiocentesis

Laparoscopic patient

Bradycardias may occur in laparoscopic surgery due to the insufflating gas compressing the inferior vena cava, thereby reducing venous return. Releasing the insufflating gas usually restores venous return and thereby improves heart rate. Atropine or glycopyrrolate may be given by the anesthetist to increase heart rate. If not managed quickly, the bradycardia may slow to asystole.

Post-arrest issues

If a return of spontaneous circulation is achieved, preparations need to be made for the ongoing care of the patient, usually in a critical care setting. It is important to debrief the team, and obtain support. Managing a cardiac arrest, particularly in a pregnant patient, is stressful. The patient and her family will also need a debrief, and may require ongoing support. Documentation is important; assigning a scribe during the arrest will aid accurate documentation of events later.

KEY POINTS

Challenge: Cardiorespiratory arrest.

Background
- Cardiorespiratory arrest in pregnant women is rare.
- Common reasons for cardiac arrest in the pregnant woman include cardiac disease, hemorrhage, sepsis, and thromboembolism. Less common reasons include amniotic fluid embolism, drug overdose, anaphylaxis, intracerebral hemorrhage, and eclampsia.
- Raised intra-abdominal pressure due to insufflation of gas into the abdomen in laparoscopic surgery may cause bradycardia and asystole.

Prevention
- Early recognition of the deteriorating patient with an EWS may prevent deterioration to the point of cardiac arrest.

Management
- The management of all cardiac arrests follows the ALS algorithm. Cardiac arrest team should be called, and cardiopulmonary resuscitation must commence immediately.

- The algorithm requires determination of whether the rhythm is:
  - Shockable: pulseless VT or VF.
  - Non-shockable: PEA or asystole.
- Chest compression and ventilation: chest compression should be at a rate of 100–120 per minute, and at a ratio of 30 compressions to 2 ventilations until the airway is secured, when chest compression should be continuous.
- Pregnant patient:
  - Needs a left tilt or manual displacement of the uterus.
  - Needs early intubation with an endotracheal tube.
  - May need defibrillation pads placed in the left anterior and posterior positions.
  - Should have a perimortem cesarean section started by 4 min into the arrest to improve chances of maternal survival (if the gestation is greater than 20 weeks).
- It is important to consider the reversible causes of cardiac arrest (4 "H"s and 4 "T"s) and treat suspected causes while continuing good-quality chest compressions with minimal interruptions.

References

1 Whitten M, Irvine LM. Postmortem and perimortem caesarean section: what are the indications. *J R Soc Med* 2000; 93:6–9.
2 Johnston TA, Grady K. *Maternal Collapse in Pregnancy and the Puerperium.* RCOG Green-top Guideline No. 56. Royal College of Obstetricians and Gynaecologists, London, 2011. Available at https://www.rcog.org.uk/globalassets/documents/guidelines/gtg_56.pdf (accessed December 2013).
3 Resuscitation Council (UK). *Advanced Life Support,* 6th edn. Resuscitation Council (UK), London, 2011.
4 Cantwell R (ed.) *Saving Mothers Lives:Reviewing Maternal Deaths to Make Motherhood Safer, 2006–2008.* The Eighth Report of the Confidential Enquiries into Maternal Deaths in the United Kingdom (CEMACE). *BJOG* 2011; 118(Suppl 1):1–203.
5 Lipman SS, Daniels KI, Carvalho B *et al.* Deficiencies in provision of cardiopulmonary resuscitation during simulated obstetric crises. *Am J Obstet Gynecol* 2010; 203: 179e1–5.
6 Katz VL, Dotters DJ, Droegemueller W. Perimortem cesarean delivery. *Obstet Gynecol* 1986; 68: 571–576.

PART II

Operations and Challenges

Section 4
General and Minimal Access Gynecology
Editors: T. Justin Clark, Kiong K. Chan, and Arri Coomarasamy

CHAPTER 59

Difficulty in Dilating the Cervix: Cervical Stenosis and Cervical Closure

Arri Coomarasamy

College of Medical and Dental Sciences, University of Birmingham, Birmingham, UK

Case history 1: At the beginning of a diagnostic hysteroscopy, the surgeon is unable to find the cervical canal. The woman has a history of cervical loop excision.

Case history 2: In preparation for a fibroid resection, the surgeon attempts to dilate the cervical canal to 10 mm, but is unable to advance beyond a size 7 Hegar dilator.

Case history 3: An IVF practitioner is unable to perform an embryo transfer as the embryo transfer catheter will not go through the cervical canal.

Background

Cervical dilatation to 10 mm and occasionally even up to 12 mm may be necessary for operative procedures such as surgical management of miscarriage, termination of pregnancy, and resection of submucous fibroids or the endometrium. The surgical instruments need to move freely in and out of the uterus; a tight or stenosed cervix will hinder the operation, and may increase the risk of complications.

Risk factors for cervical stenosis include nulliparity; menopause; prior cervical surgery, particularly loop or cone excision; previous uterine surgery, such as ablation and cesarean section; lower uterine or cervical fibroids; and GnRH treatment.

Cervical stenosis may preclude access to the uterine cavity so that the desired operation cannot be performed. Dilatation of the cervix risks traumatizing the genital tract; cervical laceration, "false passage" creation, and uterine perforation can arise leading to substantial bleeding and damage to adjacent structures (Chapter 60).

Management

Cervical stenosis

If cervical stenosis is identified, a number of management steps can be taken. These include the application of counter-traction by placing a tenaculum forceps on the ectocervix, probing of the cervical canal with a small dilator (preferably under abdominal ultrasound guidance), use of a flexible or rigid mini-hysteroscope to trace the cervical canal under direct vision, and intraoperative installation of intracervical vasopressin. In the presence of ongoing difficulty, an alternative approach for accessing the uterine cavity may need to be considered and the strength of the indication for the procedure reviewed. Rather than persevering, the procedure may need to be rescheduled after cervical preparation using mechanical or chemical agents (e.g., laminaria tents, prostaglandins, and local estrogen).

Cervical counter-traction

Application of a tenaculum on the anterior lip of the cervix can help to apply gentle traction to straighten the cervico-uterine canal and reduce resistance to the insertion of a dilator or mini-hysteroscope. If the patient is awake, she should be warned in advance about a sharp sensation that often results from application of a tenaculum; very slow application of the tenaculum can minimize the discomfort.

Cervical dilatation

Semi-flexible and graduated "os-finding" probes or graduated rigid cervical dilators can be used to dilate the cervix. However, there is a substantial risk of creation of a false passage or perforation, and therefore the procedure should be carried out under abdominal ultrasound guidance. A good "acoustic window" can be created for the abdominal ultrasound by filling the bladder with 200 mL of sterile water or saline. Fine dilators, including lacrimal duct dilators, can be useful for probing a severely stenosed cervix; however, false passages and perforations are more likely with fine dilators, and a slightly larger dilator can sometimes be easier to pass through the cervical canal because it will ride over the small cul-de-sacs in the endocervical canal [1].

Entry with a mini-hysteroscope

Use of a 0° "end-on" flexible or rigid mini-hysteroscope can allow the operator to trace the cervical canal safely and assess any acute contortions in the canal. Diagnostic single-flow mini-hysteroscopy systems are available, typically incorporating a 1.9-mm telescope and with a total outer diameter of around 3 mm. The 0° distal lens allows easier navigation of the cervical canal because the direction of view, with the cervical canal centrally visualized, equates to the

Gynecologic and Obstetric Surgery: Challenges and Management Options, First Edition. Edited by Arri Coomarasamy, Mahmood I. Shafi, G. Willy Davila and Kiong K. Chan.
© 2016 John Wiley & Sons, Ltd. Published 2016 by John Wiley & Sons, Ltd.

line of hysteroscopic advancement. It is important to avoid trauma and bleeding from the endocervical canal as this will impair the views and predispose to false passages and perforations. Slow advancement of the hysteroscope will allow the distension media to open up the canal, thus reducing resistance to the instrument and likelihood of cervical canal injury. As the hysteroscope is advanced, it is important to take note of any turns and twists in the canal, because this knowledge will be informative if blind dilatation is subsequently needed.

Intracervical vasopressin

A randomized trial found that intracervical injection of 20 mL of dilute vasopressin solution (0.05 units/mL) can reduce the force needed to dilate the cervix [2]. In this study, dilute vasopressin was injected at the 4 and 8 o'clock positions into the stroma of the cervix just under the mucosal surface. This approach can be useful when there is limited cervical dilatation.

Use of alternative instruments

Despite various remedial measures, it may not be possible to dilate beyond a certain diameter in some women. In such situations, modifying the approach to use smaller instruments or an altogether different approach may be necessary. For example, for resection, smaller 7-mm resectoscopes are available. For small submucous fibroids, ablation using bipolar electrodes placed down smaller-diameter continuous-flow operating systems (typically <6 mm) can be an alternative to resection. If the purpose of the procedure is to obtain an endometrial sample, then ultrasound-guided transvaginal endometrial aspiration is an alternative option [3].

Cervical closure

If an external os is not identifiable, this could be because there are flimsy adhesions over it or the cervical canal has closed, often following cervical surgery. However, if the woman has a history of menstrual bleeds, then this implies that she has an open cervical canal; examining her during menstruation may help identify the os and the cervical canal.

Gentle probing with a dilator, os finder or hysteroscope (with saline flow turned on) may remove the flimsy adhesions identifying the external cervical os and canal. An abdominal ultrasound can be useful in helping to find the cervical tract and to minimize the risk of creating a false passage. If these approaches are unsuccessful, the likelihood is that the woman has a closed cervical canal. Often a cervical "dimple" is visible and this can be useful to help guide hysteroscopic scissors or bipolar electrodes, which can be used to cut into the ectocervix revealing the cervical canal. Alternative approaches to facilitate access to the endocervical canal can include excision of part of the cervix with diathermy knives [4], loops, or lasers [5]. These procedures should be performed by an experienced surgeon who should take special care not to damage bladder, bowel, or blood vessels. A transabdominal ultrasound will help to minimize complications.

Hemorrhage from cervical trauma

Following cervical dilatation, cervical tears can occur causing brisk persistent bleeding which can usually be managed with tamponade, using swabs or atraumatic tissue forceps. If bleeding continues despite these measures, then placement of one or two cervical sutures will usually resolve the problem. Massive hemorrhage is rare but can result from a ruptured branch of the cervical or uterine arteries. It may be possible to suture if the bleeding vessel(s) can be seen directly or after splitting the cervix to identify the bleeding vessel(s) [1]. If the bleeding vessel(s) cannot be identified, the uterine artery on the side of the injury can be exposed, as in a vaginal hysterectomy, and sutured [1].

A bleeding cervical or uterine artery branch can also cause a hematoma that can extend into the broad ligament. This will necessitate a laparotomy and possibly a hysterectomy.

Resolution of the cases

Case history 1

A thorough pelvic examination to evaluate the size and the position of the cervix and the uterus is needed. Gentle probing with a small dilator, os finder, or mini-hysteroscope (with saline flow turned on) can remove flimsy adhesions and identify the external cervical os. A concomitant pelvic ultrasound scan can provide information on the site and axis of the cervical tract to facilitate these measures. Where the external cervical os is obliterated, cutting into the cervix under direct hysteroscopic vision should be undertaken. Deeper cervical excision to identify the cervical canal should rarely, if ever, be required and only by appropriately experienced practitioners after other options described in this chapter have been exhausted.

Case history 2

Intracervical injection of dilute vasopressin may aid further dilatation. Graded dilators that increase by 0.5-mm increments (e.g., 7.5, 8, 8.5 mm, and so on) rather than 1-mm increments may facilitate dilatation. If dilatation is not possible, then there are two options: (i) use an alternative method to complete the operation (e.g., smaller resectoscopes or use of bipolar electrodes), or (ii) abandon the procedure and rebook the case after cervical preparation with prostaglandins such as misoprostol, or laminaria tents.

Case history 3

The IVF practitioner can use a firmer catheter or a rigid "stylet" to access the uterine cavity under ultrasound guidance. If cervical access is impossible, ultrasound-guided transmyometrial transfer (TMET) is an option.

Prevention

Although it is not possible to identify all patients who may have cervical stenosis, a proportion of patients can be identified from a careful history; if risk factors for cervical stenosis are present, then a number of preoperative measures can be taken to improve outcomes.

Be prepared

Liaise with the operating room staff, and ensure the following are available on the day of operating: mini-hysteroscope (3 mm), ideally with 0° distal end; ultrasound machine with abdominal probe; small dilators, including lacrimal duct dilators; semi-flexible os finders; and small-diameter instruments, such as a 7-mm resectoscope or a 5-mm continuous-flow hysteroscope down which 5 Fr scissors or bipolar electrodes can be used.

Cervical preparation

There is some evidence that misoprostol can soften the cervix and aid cervical dilatation. A typical regimen is 400 μg of oral or vaginal misoprostol 12–24 hours before the procedure [6]. A single 2–4 mm diameter laminaria japonica inserted into the cervical canal on the day before surgery can also be effective in softening and dilating the cervix. In postmenopausal women, application of vaginal estrogen for a month before the procedure may allow easier dilatation by reversing atrophic changes within the lower genital tract.

KEY POINTS

Challenge: Difficulty in dilating the cervix (cervical stenosis and cervical closure).

Background
- Risk factors for cervical stenosis include: history of cervical surgery, particularly loop or cone excision; nulliparity; menopause; previous uterine surgery, such as ablation and cesarean section; and lower uterine or cervical fibroids.
- The risks from cervical stenosis include: inability to perform the desired operation; creation of false passages in the cervix or uterus; cervical laceration with serious risk of cervical or uterine artery bleeding; and uterine perforation.

Prevention
- Identify patients at risk.
- Prepare the cervix with:
  - Local estrogen for a month in postmenopausal women.
  - Misoprostol 400 μg orally or vaginally 12–24 hours before the procedure.
  - Laminaria tent insertion a day before the procedure.

Management
- Use ultrasound guidance to reduce intraoperative complications.
- Enter with a flexible or rigid mini-hysteroscope (3 mm) with a 0° distal lens. Advance slowly, let the distension medium open the cervical canal, and take note of all turns and twists in the canal to aid later dilatation.
- Dilate gently with semi-flexible or rigid probes or dilators. Fine dilators such as lacrimal duct dilators can be useful, but the risk of a false passage or perforation is high with fine dilators.
- Inject 20 mL of dilute vasopressin solution (0.05 units/mL) at 4 and 8 o'clock positions into the stroma of the cervix just under the mucosal surface.
- Use alternative smaller-diameter instruments if possible (e.g., 7-mm resectoscope).

Cervical closure: blind-ending cervical canal
- Examine the patient during menstruation to identify the os and cervical canal.
- Use an os finder probe, small dilator, or mini-hysteroscope to remove flimsy adhesions which may be covering the os.
- A fibrous and densely closed cervix may require cervical excision with diathermy or laser to reveal the endocervical canal.

Massive hemorrhage from cervical or uterine trauma
- Ruptured branches of cervical or uterine artery can cause massive hemorrhage and broad ligament hematoma.
- Suture bleeding artery if it is visible; if it is not visible, the cervix may need to be split to demonstrate the bleeding artery.
- Uterine artery on the side of injury may be isolated and sutured as in a vaginal hysterectomy.
- Broad ligament hematoma will usually necessitate a laparotomy.

References

1 Monaghan JM, Lopes T, Naik R. Operations on the cervix. In: *Bonney's Gynaecological Surgery*, 10th edn, pp. 27–46. Blackwell Science Ltd, Oxford, 2004.

2 Phillips DR, Nathanson HG, Milim SJ, Haselkorn JS. The effect of dilute vasopressin solution on the force needed for cervical dilatation: a randomized controlled trial. *Obstet Gynecol* 1997;89:507–511.

3 Hammoud AO, Deppe G, Elkhechen SS, Johnson S. Ultrasonography-guided transvaginal endometrial biopsy: a useful technique in patients with cervical stenosis. *Obstet Gynecol* 2006;107:518–520.

4 Shankar A, Kassab A, Fox R. Knife entry into the uterine cavity: overcoming severe cervical stenosis at hysteroscopy. *J Obstet Gynaecol* 2007;27:868–869.

5 Luesley DM, Williams DR, Gee H, Chan KK, Jordan JA. Management of postconization cervical stenosis by laser vaporization. *Obstet Gynecol* 1986;67:126–128.

6 Thomas JA, Leyland N, Durand N, Windrim RC. The use of oral misoprostol as a cervical ripening agent in operative hysteroscopy: a double-blind, placebo-controlled trial. *Am J Obstet Gynecol* 2002;186:876–879.Section 4

CHAPTER 60
Uterine Perforation

Arri Coomarasamy

College of Medical and Dental Sciences, University of Birmingham, Birmingham, UK

Case history 1: A postmenopausal woman having a D&C is suspected to have sustained a uterine perforation after the insertion of a size 5 Hegar dilator.

Case history 2: During surgical termination of a pregnancy of 8 weeks, the operator grasped what he thought was pregnancy tissue, twisted and pulled. The removed tissue had the appearance of omentum.

Case history 3: Following a suspected lateral wall uterine perforation at the level of the internal os, the gynecologist noted torrential vaginal hemorrhage.

Background

The risk of uterine perforation varies by the type of surgery: in postpartum surgery, the incidence is estimated to be as high as 5%; in hysteroscopic surgery, 1.6%; in surgical termination of pregnancy, 0.5%; and in postmenopausal investigation, 0.2–2.0% [1].

A key risk factor for uterine perforation is difficult cervical dilation because of cervical stenosis or acute degrees of uterine anteversion or retroversion. The uterus is more prone to being perforated in the presence of congenital uterine abnormalities, adhesions (e.g., Asherman's syndrome), and fibroids. Uterine trauma is also more likely in postpartum or postmenopausal women.

Risks of perforation

Most perforations are small and are not associated with uterine hemorrhage or damage of adjacent organs. Lateral wall perforations in the cervix or lower uterus are often serious as they can cause hemorrhage from the uterine vessels and broad ligament hematomas. Anterior wall perforations can cause injury to the bladder. Use of thermal, grasping or suction devices can cause injury to bowel, bladder, ureter, or major blood vessels. Uterine rupture in a future pregnancy is possible and some authors have suggested a low threshold for cesarean sections in women with a past history of uterine perforations [1].

Uterine perforation can result in rapid accumulation of large volumes of distension media in the abdomen (Chapter 63). The use of a transcervical catheter, inserted into the abdomen through the uterine perforation, to aspirate the fluid under ultrasound guidance has been described [2].

Management

The first step in management is to recognize that a uterine perforation has occurred. A sudden loss of resistance from the instrument, a loss of uterine distension, or the appearance of peritoneal cavity contents on hysteroscopy can indicate a perforation. The location of the intrauterine instrument at the time of perforation should be noted, and the procedure should be halted. If continuous video recording is the usual practice, then this can be viewed in slow motion to help identify exactly when the perforation took place, and whether any thermal or avulsion instruments were used after the perforation occurred [2].

Immediate management will depend on the complications arising from the uterine trauma, namely the degree of hemorrhage and the likelihood of injury to adjacent pelvic organs. An appreciation of the instruments used (e.g., blunt dilators vs. avulsion forceps), the type of procedure being carried out (e.g., diagnostic hysteroscopy vs. diathermy resection), and the location of the injury (fundal/anterior/posterior vs. cervical/lateral) will inform clinical decision-making.

Perforation with non-thermal and non-grasping instruments

Perforation with blunt instruments such as a Hegar dilator, a closed forceps (that has not yet been used for any grasping), a hysteroscope, a non-activated resectoscope, or a non-activated suction device will not generally cause any serious harm, and expectant management can be appropriate. There is usually no need for surgical closure of the perforation. Antibiotics, observation for 2–4 hours, and if necessary, admission for 24 hours may be all that is required, as long there is no evidence of hemorrhage. If the perforation involves the lateral uterine walls, then the risk of severe intra-abdominal hemorrhage needs to be considered.

If bowel adhesions to the uterus are suspected or known to be present, it is possible for the perforating instrument to have damaged the bowel that is directly over the uterine perforation site; in this situation, a laparoscopy to assess for potential bowel injury is necessary.

Gynecologic and Obstetric Surgery: Challenges and Management Options, First Edition. Edited by Arri Coomarasamy, Mahmood I. Shafi, G. Willy Davila and Kiong K. Chan.
© 2016 John Wiley & Sons, Ltd. Published 2016 by John Wiley & Sons, Ltd.

Perforation with thermal, avulsion, or suction instruments

The risk of hemorrhage and adjacent organ injury are significant, and thus an examination of the abdomen with laparoscopy or laparotomy is required. A full assessment of the bowel, bladder, broad ligaments, and ureters is required, and if necessary assistance from general surgeons or urologists should be sought. The uterine perforation and any organ damage can be repaired by laparoscopy or laparotomy. Antibiotics and admission will be necessary. Bowel injury may be difficult to identify intraoperatively and postoperatively, and may only manifest 1 or 2 weeks later. Patients should therefore be warned of danger symptoms (vomiting, abdominal pain, bloating, changed bowel habits, and fever) and instructed to contact emergency services without delay.

Lateral wall cervical or lower uterine perforations

Such perforations can result in uterine artery injury and broad ligament hematoma. The patient's condition should be evaluated and she should be resuscitated with fluids and blood as appropriate. A laparotomy is needed if the patient is unstable or if the adnexal mass from broad ligament hematoma continues to extend (on ultrasound scan), and a hysterectomy may be necessary to avert catastrophic outcomes.

Completion of the original procedure

When perforation occurs it will be difficult to achieve proper uterine distension, and thus non-urgent original procedures (e.g., D&C or IUCD insertion) should be abandoned. The patient can be reviewed later and plans can be made for alternative non-surgical options or rescheduling of surgery after at least 6 weeks to allow time for tissue healing. Occasionally it may be possible to complete the operation with direct laparoscopic guidance, after repair of the uterine perforation.

Resolution of the cases

Case history 1

Abandon the procedure, and administer broad-spectrum intravenous antibiotics. Observe the patient for 2–4 hours; if the patient is well, she can be discharged, with clear instructions on what symptoms should trigger her to seek medical review. The D&C can be rescheduled 6–8 weeks later and the use of cervical preparation with a course of local estrogen considered. A hysteroscopy should

be carried out prior to blind uterine instrumentation; where this is not possible or feasible, the D&C should be performed under direct ultrasound guidance.

Case history 2

Abandon the procedure, and administer broad-spectrum intravenous antibiotics. The removed tissue can be sent for urgent histopathologic examination. Perform laparoscopy or laparotomy to repair the uterine perforation and any bowel damage. Complete the termination of pregnancy with laparoscopic or laparotomic visualization of the uterus.

Case history 3

The likely diagnosis is injury of the uterine artery, and broad ligament hematoma is likely. A laparotomy is needed, and a hysterectomy may be necessary.

Prevention

Careful risk assessment and pelvic examination (for uterine size and position) will help to minimize the risk of perforation. Avoidance of forceful cervical dilatation is key to preventing a perforation. Consideration should be given to the use of tapered (Hawkins–Amber) dilators. Cervical preparation with prostaglandins or laminaria can help with cervical dilatation where difficulties are anticipated (Chapter 59).

Difficult cervical dilatation and endometrial or fibroid resection are best carried out under ultrasound guidance. Some use laparoscopic guidance in an effort to avoid an injury during resection, but laparoscopy merely confirms an injury after it has occurred; ultrasound, on the other hand, can give contemporaneous information about uterine wall thickness as the resection progresses [2]. Transabdominal scanning requires an acoustic window and this can be achieved by filling the bladder with sterile saline [2].

Complex cases, for example a second-trimester surgical termination, should be performed by a senior surgeon. Non-surgical alternatives, for example medical management of terminations at advanced gestations, could avoid many complications. Ultrasound-guided approaches are particularly suited to surgical management of miscarriages and terminations.

It is important to activate a diathermy or suction instrument as it is withdrawn down from the fundus to minimize the risk of perforation and injury to adjacent organs.

KEY POINTS

Challenge: Uterine perforation.

Background
- The risk of uterine perforation varies by the type of surgery.

Risk factors
- Cervical stenosis or difficult cervical dilation.
- Termination of pregnancy in advanced gestations.
- Acutely anteverted or retroverted uterus.
- Postmenopausal uterus.
- Postpartum uterus.
- Congenital or acquired uterine abnormalities.
- Scarred uterus (Asherman's syndrome or previous cesarean section).
- Fibroid uterus.
- Poor visualization during hysteroscopy.

Risks of uterine perforation
- Most perforations are minor, and do not result in hemorrhage or organ damage.
- Lateral wall perforations in the cervix or lower uterus can cause hemorrhage from the uterine vessel and broad ligament hematomas.
- Anterior wall perforations can cause injury to the bladder.
- Use of thermal, grasping or suction devices can cause injury to bowel, bladder, ureter, and major blood vessels.
- Uterine rupture in a future pregnancy is possible.

Prevention
- Risk assessment and pelvic examination for uterine size and position.
- Avoidance of forceful cervical dilatation.
- Cervical preparation with prostaglandins or laminaria when difficulties are anticipated.

- Ultrasound guidance for cervical dilation, surgical management of termination or miscarriage, and endometrial or fibroid resection.
- Consider alternatives to surgery (e.g., medical management for terminations at advanced gestations).

Management
- Consider the likelihood and location of injury and any associated organ damage.

Perforation with non-thermal and non-grasping instruments
- Abandon the procedure.
- Give intravenous broad-spectrum antibiotics.
- Observe for a minimum of 2–4 hours; admit overnight if ongoing pain or systemically unwell.

Perforation with thermal, avulsion or suction instruments
- Abandon the procedure and give antibiotics.
- Laparoscopy or laparotomy to assess for injury to the bowel, bladder, broad ligaments, and ureters.
- Instruct the patient to look out for symptoms and signs of bowel injury for at least 2 weeks after the procedure, and to seek immediate medical review if symptoms develop.

Lateral wall cervical or lower uterine perforations
- If hemodynamically unstable, resuscitate the patient.
- Laparoscopy or laparotomy (if torrential hemorrhage) is needed; a hysterectomy may be required.

References

1 Shakir F, Diab Y. The perforated uterus. *Obstetrician & Gynaecologist* 2013;15: 256–261.

2 Wortman M. Complications of hysteroscopic surgery. In: IsaacsonK (ed.) *Complications of Gynecologic Endoscopic Surgery*, pp. 185–200. Saunders Elsevier, Philadelphia, 2006.

CHAPTER 61

Surgical Uterine Evacuation: Excessive Bleeding

Rajesh Varma

Guy's and St Thomas' Hospitals NHS Foundation Trust, London, UK

Case history: *A 25-year-old woman presents with a malodorous vaginal discharge for 3 days. She is apyrexial. A pelvic ultrasound identifies a miscarriage consistent with a pregnancy of 10 weeks of gestation. She is scheduled for surgical evacuation of retained products of conception (ERPC) on the same day. At operation, excessive uterine bleeding is noted following withdrawal of the plastic suction catheter at the end of the procedure.*

Background

Surgical evacuation of the uterus is a commonly performed gynecologic procedure. ERPC is indicated in the treatment of miscarriage, termination of pregnancy, and secondary postpartum hemorrhage. Although non-surgical treatments such as misoprostol regimens exist, surgical ERPC is particularly indicated in those women experiencing excessive bleeding, hemodynamic instability, evidence of infected retained tissue, and suspected gestational trophoblastic disease.

In the vast majority of cases, ERPC is performed as a day-case procedure under general anesthesia without complication. However, in a minority (<1%) of ERPC procedures, excessive genital tract bleeding (i.e., >500 mL) may occur during or immediately following uterine evacuation. The timing of onset of the excessive bleeding in relation to the ERPC procedure may help indicate the likely cause.

Management

General measures

It is important to provide circulatory support through intravenous fluid replacement and, if necessary, blood transfusion. Other essential steps include alerting the anesthetist of the situation, requesting an urgent cross-match of 2–4 units of blood, and inserting a urinary catheter. An experienced senior gynecologist ought to be involved at an early stage.

Diagnose and treat cause

Excessive genital tract bleeding occurring soon after insertion of suction catheter or early in suction evacuation procedure

This may indicate uterine perforation as the causative mechanism. Importantly, the degree of circulatory shock may exceed the degree of revealed genital tract bleeding because uterine perforation may result in concealed intra-abdominal bleeding. Clinical features indicative of uterine perforation include fat or bowel tissue identified in suction catheter specimens and uterine instruments (e.g., suction catheter, polyp forceps) extending beyond the expected border of the uterus. If perforation is suspected, urgent laparoscopy is needed to confirm or refute the diagnosis and appropriate surgical treatment instituted (Chapter 60). Further management depends on whether the uterine evacuation is complete or incomplete. If incomplete, uterine suction catheter evacuation should only be completed under laparoscopic guidance. Thereafter, the uterine perforation may be surgically sealed with laparoscopic or laparotomic suturing or application of a surgical hemostat.

Excessive genital tract bleeding occurring on completion of ERPC immediately after withdrawal of plastic suction catheter

This may indicate persisting uterine products of conception, or uterine atony, or a combination of both. It is difficult to clinically distinguish the two processes reliably, so a combination of the following interventions is advised.

1 Careful exploration of the uterine cavity using "blunt" polyp forceps or sponge holders. A useful tip is to introduce the closed polyp forceps until the uterine fundus is reached and thereafter undertake instrument "sweeps," opening and closing the instrument in a direction toward the cervix from this maximum uterine depth. A sponge holder is more suitable for exploring uterine cavities exceeding 12 weeks of gestation in size.

2 Undertake ultrasound-guided polyp forceps or suction catheter retrieval of retained products of conception. Ultrasound can reliably localize retained placental product tissue, enabling polyp forceps or suction catheters to be safely "steered" into the target uterine location under continuous ultrasound guidance. Ultrasound is unable to reliably diagnose uterine perforation.

3 Mechanical uterine compression and uterotonic drugs. Assuming the uterine cavity is checked to be empty (preferably confirmed by transabdominal ultrasound), and uterine perforation is considered unlikely, then uterine massage and mechanical bimanual uterine compression should achieve rapid cessation of uterine bleeding. Intravenous oxytocin (initial dose 10 IU, repeat bolus 10 IU permitted) and ergometrine (0.5 mg) may be administered to induce and sustain uterine contraction.

Gynecologic and Obstetric Surgery: Challenges and Management Options, First Edition. Edited by Arri Coomarasamy, Mahmood I. Shafi, G. Willy Davila and Kiong K. Chan.
© 2016 John Wiley & Sons, Ltd. Published 2016 by John Wiley & Sons, Ltd.

Excessive genital tract bleeding occurring on removal of cervical vulsellum instruments at completion of operation but not noted following completion of suction catheter uterine evacuation

This suggests a bleeding cervical laceration as the cause, which is readily identifiable on speculum clinical examination. The vulsellum instrument, used to stabilize and grasp the cervix during ERPC, is usually responsible. Treatment options include mechanical application of sponge holders for 2–3 min at the cervical laceration, or suturing the laceration using an absorbable suture (e.g., Vicryl).

Excessive genital tract bleeding not responding to above measures

Assuming uterine perforation is unlikely, and the uterine cavity is empty (checked by polyp instrument examination or ultrasound), then intrauterine balloon tamponade may be appropriate. For a uterus exceeding 10 weeks of gestation in size, 100 mL of warmed saline instilled into the intrauterine balloon is sufficient to generate adequate uterine tamponade to arrest bleeding caused by uterine atony or an inflamed/traumatized endometrial surface. However, excessive saline instillation of the balloon may predispose to uterine perforation or complicate an existing perforation. A useful tip is to instill saline into the balloon up to the point where the syringe plunger tends to recoil when depressed and released.

Should all these measures fail, then a laparotomy is required and consideration may be given to either uterine compression using a brace suture or hysterectomy. An alternative option is to undertake a diagnostic laparoscopy in order to exclude uterine perforation, and thereafter conduct emergency uterine artery embolization.

Prevention

Although a rare event, excessive genital tract bleeding at ERPC is difficult to prevent. The following may be useful to consider.

1 Any alternative to ERPC: conservative treatment and medical management (e.g., mifepristone and misoprostol regimens) are acceptable treatment choices in the medical management of miscarriage and termination of pregnancy.

2 Awareness of at-risk women: the following groups of women are at heightened risk of bleeding at ERPC: size of uterus exceeding 13 weeks of gestation, molar pregnancies, uterine sepsis, repeat ERPC procedures, postpartum ERPC procedures, uterine fibroids, obesity, acutely anteverted or retroverted uterus, and women with previous uterine or cervical surgery (e.g., cesarean section, myomectomy, or cervical excision/ablation for CIN). Women with morbidly adherent placental tissue or uterine arteriovenous malformations are rarely encountered; however, such women may experience significant hemorrhage at ERPC.

3 Preoperative preparation of the cervix: use of preoperative intravaginal prostaglandin will increase the ease of performing gradated cervical dilatation and thereby decrease the risk of creating false cervical/uterine passage and uterine perforation.

4 Routinely performing all ERPC procedures under simultaneous ultrasound guidance: although there are resource implications, there is an argument that this approach maximizes patient safety by reducing the risk of uterine perforation and persisting retained products of conception following ERPC.

5 Routine use of intravenous uterotonics (oxytocin with or without low-dose ergometrine) administered immediately after insertion of the plastic suction catheter. There are limited observational data to suggest that earlier administration of uterotonics reduces the risk of uterine atony complicating the ERPC.

6 Routinely group and save all women undergoing ERPC, prior to the scheduled procedure, to enable rapid cross-match of blood should excessive bleeding occur.

KEY POINTS

Challenge: ERPC and excessive uterine bleeding.

Background
- Uncommon event: less than 1% risk of excessive uterine bleeding (>500 mL) at ERPC.
- Timing of onset of the excessive bleeding may help to indicate the likely cause.

Prevention
- Consider whether surgical ERPC is indicated or whether alternative conservative or medical treatments are more appropriate.
- Maintain awareness of at-risk groups: uterus >13 weeks of gestation in size, postpartum, uterine sepsis, repeat ERPC.
- Undertake preoperative cervical preparation with intravaginal prostaglandins.
- Perform ERPC procedures under simultaneous transabdominal ultrasound guidance.
- Administer intravenous oxytocin (with or without low-dose ergometrine) just after insertion of the uterine suction catheter at the start of the surgical ERPC.

Management
General measures
- Intravenous fluid resuscitation.
- Order blood cross-match.
- Involve a senior gynecologist.

Diagnose and treat cause(s)
- Recognize uterine perforation: if suspected undertake a laparoscopy to diagnose and dictate further management.
- If uterine evacuation remains incomplete, then completion of the procedure should be undertaken under laparoscopic or ultrasonographic guidance (assuming perforation has been excluded).
- Uterine atony: uterine massage, bimanual compression, and uterotonic drugs.
- Cervical laceration: tamponade or surgically repair the laceration.

Intractable uterine bleeding not responding to above measures
- Consider intrauterine balloon tamponade (assuming uterine perforation is excluded), laparotomy and a uterine compression brace suture, hysterectomy or uterine artery embolization.

Further reading

Haddad L, Delli-Bovi L. Uterine artery embolization to treat hemorrhage following second-trimester abortion by dilatation and surgical evacuation. *Contraception* 2009;79:452–455.

Madden T, Burke AE. Successful management of second-trimester postabortion hemorrhage with an intrauterine tamponade balloon. *Obstet Gynecol* 2009;113:501–503.

Royal College of Obstetricians and Gynaecologists. *The Management of Early Pregnancy Loss*. RCOG Green-top Guideline No. 25. Royal College of Obstetricians and Gynaecologists, London, 2006. Available at https://www.rcog.org.uk/en/guidelines-research-services/guidelines/gtg25/

Steinauer JE, Diedrich JT, Wilson MW, Darney PD, Vargas JE, Drey EA. Uterine artery embolization in postabortion hemorrhage. *Obstet Gynecol* 2008;111:881–889.

CHAPTER 62

Surgical Uterine Evacuation in a Woman with Multiple Fibroids

Rajesh Varma

Guy's and St Thomas' Hospitals NHS Foundation Trust, London, UK

Case history: A woman presents with a miscarriage at 12 weeks of gestation. She is known to have a large posterior uterine wall fibroid. She opts for medical management (vaginal misoprostol), but this is unsuccessful. A decision for surgical evacuation of uterus is made. Examination under general anesthesia shows a stenosed "dimple" cervix displaced anteriorly and inaccessible to vulsellum grasping forceps. On bimanual examination the uterus is estimated to be 18–20 weeks of gestation in size.

Background

Around 25–40% of women of reproductive age have uterine fibroids. In the vast majority, the uterine fibroids are not excessive in size (individually not more than 3 cm) and do not significantly distort the cervix or uterine cavity. However, the location of fibroids may significantly impact on fertility and pregnancy outcome.

Fibroids that are submucosal (intracavity) or intramural (particularly those that compress or deviate the uterine cavity) in location are associated with increased risks of infertility, miscarriage, and preterm delivery. Fibroids located near the cervix may compromise visualization of the cervix and obstruct access to the endocervical canal, making surgical ERPC technically difficult. Furthermore, enlargement and distortion of the uterine cavity by fibroids can restrict access to retained products of conception by conventional suction catheters and mechanical instruments. Fortunately, these cases are rare, complicating less than 2% of planned surgical ERPC procedures, and available techniques are capable of overcoming such challenges.

Management

The effectiveness of interventions is limited if mechanical obstruction is identified at the commencement of the ERPC procedure; hence emphasis ought to be placed on preventive strategies (see Prevention further on). The following steps are likely to facilitate a successful ERPC procedure when fibroid obstruction is identified or suspected.

Conduct the surgical ERPC under continuous ultrasound surveillance

The use of transabdominal and transvaginal pelvic ultrasound can precisely locate fibroids, align the endocervical canal with the uterine cavity, and identify pregnancy tissue prior to introducing surgical instruments. Ultrasound can be used to help achieve safe insertion of the suction catheter into the uterine cavity and reach the target pregnancy tissue; thereafter, the suction evacuation may be conducted under continuous transabdominal ultrasound surveillance. Post ERPC, a check transvaginal ultrasound may be performed to confirm the absence of residual pregnancy tissue.

Maximize surgical access and identify the cervix

In cases where the cervix is not visualized by speculum examination because of fibroid displacement or stenosis, bimanual examination may reveal where the cervix is likely to reside. In addition, an assistant using lateral vaginal wall retractors may aid exposure of the cervix. A technique of intermittently grasping and retracting tissue adjacent to the displaced cervix and then "walking" the instrument closer to the cervix using an additional grasper will often achieve identification of the external cervical os.

Employ strategies to overcome cervical obstruction

Once cervical stenosis is diagnosed, a decision needs to be made as to whether the ERPC procedure should be abandoned or alternative surgical techniques used. The risk of false passage creation and uterine perforation are markedly increased with cervical stenosis, particularly when pre-procedure cervical preparation with intravaginal prostaglandin has not been undertaken. Graded, fine-bore, rigid cervical dilators can incrementally traverse most cases of cervical stenosis, especially if the inserted dilator ends are lubricated with sterile gel. An alternative strategy is to insert a narrow-bore, 2–3 mm, single-channel diagnostic hysteroscope with continuous saline irrigation to identify the endocervical canal under direct vision. Occasionally, where there is complete occlusion of the stenosed ectocervix, mechanical or electrosurgical incisions can be made (usually over an identifiable "dimple" delineating the opening to the endocervical canal) to allow hysteroscopic access.

Consider use of flexible uterine catheter insertion under concurrent ultrasound guidance

Commonly used rigid plastic catheters may not be able to negotiate distorted non-linear cervical canals and uterine cavities, and persistent attempts may result in uterine perforation, even when

Gynecologic and Obstetric Surgery: Challenges and Management Options, First Edition. Edited by Arri Coomarasamy, Mahmood I. Shafi, G. Willy Davila and Kiong K. Chan.
© 2016 John Wiley & Sons, Ltd. Published 2016 by John Wiley & Sons, Ltd.

concurrent ultrasound guidance is being used. Narrow-diameter flexible plastic catheters inserted into the uterine cavity under concurrent ultrasound guidance may be able to overcome issues related to distorted and longer-length uterine cavities to reach the target pregnancy tissue. Alternative "improvised" strategies include the use of narrow-bore nasogastric tubes for increased length, or endotracheal tubes for increased rigidity and maneuverability compared with flexible cannulae; or utilizing a narrow-bore curved rigid dilator or intubation bougie first and then inserting a flexible suction catheter over this "guidewire," analogous to the Seldinger technique for vascular access.

Contemplate hysterotomy or hysterectomy

These procedures are considered "last resort" measures and should only be embarked upon if alternative medical and conventional surgical therapies have been exhausted and the woman has provided informed consent. Although there is a degree of surgical morbidity associated with hysterotomy, it is better to undertake this as a planned procedure rather than as an emergency.

Prevention

Pelvic examination prior to ERPC

It is likely that the fibroids will be diagnosed by ultrasound prior to surgical evacuation of the uterus. However, it is not always possible to predict whether fibroids will obstruct the surgical ERPC until the procedure has commenced with the woman under general anesthesia. If the ultrasound shows a cervical fibroid, distorted or poorly visualized uterine cavity, or eccentrically positioned pregnancy tissue in a larger-sized uterus, then clinical pelvic examination is recommended to determine the likelihood of an obstructed surgical uterine evacuation. Women may then be appropriately counseled as to their treatment choices and alternatives to surgical uterine evacuation.

Medical management

Medical management for miscarriage or pregnancy termination is an established and highly effective method of uterine evacuation.

Protocols incorporating oral mifepristone 200 mg followed 48 hours later by vaginal misoprostol 600–800 μg are recommended by RCOG induced abortion guidelines (November 2011) and NICE miscarriage guidelines (December 2012). Women with large-sized uteri or multiple fibroids that complicate access to the cervix, uterine cavity, or gestational sac are better suited to medical rather than surgical uterine evacuation in the first instance. Even a failed attempt at medical ERPC may have a beneficial effect, because it is likely to induce a degree of cervical softening and uterine canal bleeding that will facilitate safer suction catheter insertion under ultrasonographic guidance. Medical uterine evacuation regimens may also be considered as safer alternatives for women with fibroids requiring postpartum ERPC procedures, repeat ERPC procedures or septic miscarriages, because surgery in such cases carries increased surgical morbidity and risk.

Pre-procedure cervical softening

There is robust evidence to support the use of pre-procedure cervical softening agents to increase the ease of surgical cervical dilatation and uterine catheter insertion, to reduce the risk of failed surgical ERPC and persisting products of conception, and to potentially reduce the risk of uterine perforation. A protocol comprising 400–800 μg intravaginal misoprostol inserted around 3 hours prior to the surgical ERPC is capable of achieving adequate cervical softening, even in cases of cervical stenosis. Synthetic cervical osmotic dilators (e.g., laminaria) have also been demonstrated to be effective cervical softening agents, although they generally require a longer time (6–12 hours) to achieve their peak effect.

Arrange for availability of portable ultrasound and flexible suction catheters for time of planned ERPC

It is prudent to organize the availability of necessary fine-bore cervical dilators, flexible suction catheters, and portable ultrasound for the time of planned ERPC, if it is considered likely that the procedure would be complicated by fibroid obstruction, uterine cavity distortion, or substantial enlargement of the uterine cavity.

KEY POINTS

Challenge: ERPC in a woman with multiple fibroids.

Background
- Women with multiple fibroids are at increased risk of infertility, miscarriage, and preterm delivery.
- Surgical ERPC in such women may be complicated because of fibroids distorting or obstructing the cervix and uterine cavity and the target pregnancy tissue being inaccessible to conventionally used suction catheters because of increased uterine length and uterine cavity distortion.

Management
- Use transabdominal or transvaginal ultrasound to localize fibroids, uterine cavity, and pregnancy tissue; undertake surgical evacuation under continuous ultrasound guidance.
- Employ surgical techniques to identify a deviated cervix and overcome cervical stenosis. Contemplate the use of graded, fine-bore, rigid cervical dilators and/or miniature diagnostic hysteroscopes.

- Consider using a flexible suction catheter (or "improvised" long flexible catheter system, e.g., narrow-bore nasogastric or endotracheal tubes) and evacuate the uterus under continuous ultrasound guidance.
- If medical and conventional surgical strategies for uterine evacuation are unsuccessful, consider hysterotomy (or hysterectomy) but these procedures should be considered a "last resort" and it is important to obtain informed consent in those women where such action is deemed a possibility.

Prevention
- Identify fibroid obstruction prior to ERPC by employing pelvic ultrasound and clinical pelvic examination as part of routine diagnostic work-up.
- In the case of fibroid obstruction or uterine enlargement with multiple fibroids, consider:
  - Planned medical management.
  - Pre-procedure cervical softening (e.g., vaginal misoprostol).
  - Portable ultrasound and flexible suction catheters during surgical ERPC.

Further reading

Borgatta L, Sayegh R, Betstadt SJ, Stubblefield PG. Cervical obstruction complicating second-trimester abortion: treatment with misoprostol. *Obstet Gynecol* 2009;113:548–550.

Dalton VK, Lebovic DI. Use of a flexible cannula to bypass an obstructing fibroid during a first-trimester surgical abortion. *J Reprod Med* 2003;48:551–552.

Meirik O, My Huong NT, Piaggio G, Bergel E, von Hertzen H. Complications of first-trimester abortion by vacuum aspiration after cervical preparation with and without misoprostol: a multicentre randomised trial. *Lancet* 2012;379:1817–1824.

National Institute for Health and Care Excellence. *Ectopic pregnancy and miscarriage: diagnosis and initial management in early pregnancy of ectopic pregnancy and miscarriage.* NICE Clinical Guideline No. 154, December 2012. Available at https://www.nice.org.uk/guidance/cg154

Royal College of Obstetricians and Gynaecologists. *The Care of Women Requesting Induced Abortion.* RCOG Evidence-based Clinical Guideline No. 7. RCOG Press, London, 2011. Available at https://www.rcog.org.uk/en/guidelines-research-services/guidelines/the-care-of-women-requesting-induced-abortion/

CHAPTER 63
Use of Excessive Distension Media at Hysteroscopy

Arri Coomarasamy

College of Medical and Dental Sciences, University of Birmingham, Birmingham, UK

Case history 1: At the end of a hysteroscopic resection of a submucous fibroid with a saline distension medium, a total deficit of 1.2 L is noted. Postoperative serum sodium is 132 mmol/L and the patient is noted to be well.

Case history 2: At the end of a hysteroscopic resection of a submucous fibroid with a glycine distension medium, a total deficit of 1.8 L is noted. Postoperative serum sodium is 119 mmol/L and the patient is noted to be disoriented.

Background

Excessive absorption of distension media is documented to occur in approximately 0.5% of women undergoing operative hysteroscopy, and in as many as 5% of those having a hysteroscopic myomectomy [1].

Hysteroscopic distension media can contain electrolytes (e.g., normal saline or lactated Ringer's solution) or be electrolyte-free (e.g., glycine, sorbitol, or mannitol). Electrolyte-containing solutions cannot be used with monopolar diathermy as the electricity will be dispersed, resulting in an ineffective electrode. For monopolar diathermy, electrolyte-free solutions are needed as they are non-conductive. Bipolar diathermy can be carried out with electrolyte-free or electrolyte-containing media.

Normal serum osmolality is 290 mOsmol/L. In comparison, the osmolality of glycine 1.5% is 200 mOsmol/L, sorbitol 3% or mannitol 0.5% is 178 mOsmol/L, and mannitol 5% is 280 mOsmol/L [2]. Massive intravasation is more likely with hypotonic solutions such as glycine and sorbitol. Isotonic solutions such as mannitol 5%, normal saline, and lactated Ringer's solution do not create powerful osmotic gradients across the cell membrane, and thus intravasation complications are less likely. However, fluid overload and complications can occur with any distension medium. Vigilance to allow early recognition of overload and prompt management is necessary to avoid serious complications.

Complications of excessive distension media

The primary risk with an electrolyte-containing solution such as saline is fluid overload. Electrolyte-free solutions such as glycine have a particular association with the serious complication of dilutional

hyponatremia, in addition to fluid overload. Dilutional hyponatremia may lead to critical complications, such as intravascular hemolysis, hepatorenal failure, respiratory arrest, cardiac arrest, cerebral edema, coma, and death. A serum sodium concentration of 135–142 mmol/L is normal; a concentration of 130–135 mmol/L indicates mild hyponatremia, 120–130 mmol/L moderate hyponatremia, and less than 120 mmol/L severe hyponatremia, a critical situation associated with encephalopathy and cardiovascular complications. A concentration below 115 mmol/L is associated with brainstem herniation, seizures, coma, respiratory arrest, and mortality rates of up to 85% [3]. As an approximate rule, for every liter of hypotonic fluid that is absorbed, the serum sodium concentration drops by 10 mmol/L [4].

Glycine is an amino acid that metabolizes into ammonia; thus excessive glycine can lead to hyperammonemia and encephalopathic complications, in addition to the other complications already described. Hyperammonemia symptoms include nausea, vomiting, altered mental status, muscle aches, and decreased visual acuity [5]. Ammonia toxicity should be considered in patients with severe neurologic symptoms that are not explained by the degree of hyponatremia [5].

Management

Once the maximum permitted distension medium deficit level is achieved (see Prevention further on), an operative hysteroscopic procedure should be stopped. If an excessive deficit has occurred, a full assessment of the patient's condition is required, including urgent serum urea and electrolytes, with particular attention paid to the sodium level.

The immediate treatment for water intoxication and dilutional hyponatremia is to remove the excess water with diuretics and correct the hyponatremia with intravenous hypertonic saline solution. Rapid diuresis is usually achieved with intravenous furosemide 10 mg; a total dose of 20 mg of furosemide is usually sufficient, unless the patient has renal insufficiency. With moderate to severe hyponatremia, hypertonic sodium chloride (514 mmol/L) can be used to increase the sodium concentration by 1–2 mmol/L per hour, to a maximum of 6–12 mmol/L in the first 24 hours [6]. Both the degree and the speed with which hyponatremia should be corrected is debated, but expectant management is certainly not an option [5].

Gynecologic and Obstetric Surgery: Challenges and Management Options, First Edition. Edited by Arri Coomarasamy, Mahmood I. Shafi, G. Willy Davila and Kiong K. Chan.
© 2016 John Wiley & Sons, Ltd. Published 2016 by John Wiley & Sons, Ltd.

Electrolyte levels should be checked at least every 4 hours during sodium replacement and special attention should be given to avoid overcorrection [6]. The aim is to reach an endpoint of slight hyponatremia because overcorrection is associated with permanent brain injury [6].

l-Arginine may be given to aid the metabolism of ammonia in patients with ammonia toxicity [5]. Mannitol 10–20% should be considered as an osmotic diuretic. It may be effective at reducing cerebral edema.

Resolution of the cases

Case history 1
If the postoperative sodium concentration is above 130 mmol/L (mild hyponatremia) and the patient is well, no treatment is generally required.

Case history 2
This patient requires intensive management, with the involvement of an intensivist. She will need intravenous furosemide 10–20 mg to induce diuresis, and gradual correction of her severe hyponatremia with hypertonic saline solution. The glycine deficit is higher than permitted safe levels; thus a critical incident form, root cause analysis, and review of policies and procedures are warranted.

Prevention

A multidisciplinary guideline on fluid management, agreed by anesthetists, gynecologists, and nursing staff, is essential. The anesthetist should limit preoperative and intraoperative hydration in patients having procedures that require use of extensive distension media.

Isotonic electrolyte-containing solutions (e.g., saline) are safer than hypotonic electrolyte-free solutions such as glycine. Therefore use of bipolar diathermy, which allows use of isotonic electrolyte-containing solutions, should be standard practice. If monopolar diathermy is necessary, consider using 5% mannitol rather than 1.5% glycine. However, regardless of the choice of distension medium, a high level of vigilance and adherence to guidelines are necessary.

Fluid can intravasate directly into blood vessels during endometrial or fibroid resection, and the intravasation is likely to be greater when intrauterine fluid pressures are high. The use of automated pumps can maintain preset intrauterine pressures; in the absence of such technology, avoidance of excessive inflow pressures from distension media delivery systems, or intentional over-dilatation of the cervix, can help to reduce intrauterine fluid pressures.

Timely recognition of excessive fluid absorption is fundamental to the avoidance of complications. This requires accurate measurement of fluid input and output. An automated fluid management system that tracks fluid balance in real time is the ideal standard. If this is not available, a designated member of the operating room should be assigned the task of monitoring fluid input and output, and informing the surgeon and the anesthetist every 5 min [6]. It is important to minimize unaccounted-for fluid losses (on the floor and drapes) because such losses falsely elevate the total fluid deficit, resulting in unnecessarily premature termination of the operation. As general guidance, for non-isotonic distension media such as glycine, the total intravasation should be no more than 1 L, and for isotonic normal saline, less than 2 L. There should be a strict policy of terminating the operation once the preset threshold for intravasation is achieved. Another useful threshold to consider is the cessation of operation within 1 hour of starting.

KEY POINTS

Challenge: Use of excessive distension media at hysteroscopy.

Background
- Excessive fluid absorption complicates 0.5% of operative hysteroscopies, but can be as high as 5% in hysteroscopic resection of fibroids.
- Hysteroscopic distension media can be:
  - Electrolyte-containing (e.g., normal saline or lactated Ringer's solution).
  - Electrolyte-free (e.g., glycine, sorbitol, or mannitol).
- The key risk with electrolyte-containing solutions is fluid overload.
- Electrolyte-free solutions (e.g., glycine) can cause serious hyponatremia and hypervolemia resulting in critical complications such as intravascular hemolysis, hepatorenal failure, respiratory arrest, cardiac arrest, cerebral edema, coma, and death.
- A serum sodium concentration of less than 120 mmol/L is classified as severe hyponatremia, and is associated with serious complications.

Prevention
- A clear guideline on fluid management for operative hysteroscopy is essential.
- The anesthetist should limit preoperative and intraoperative hydration in anticipation of fluid absorption from the distension media.
- Isotonic electrolyte-containing solutions are safer than hypotonic electrolyte-free solutions.
- The use of automated pumps to maintain a set intrauterine pressure, or if unavailable the avoidance of high inflow pressures and intentional slight

over-dilatation of the cervix creating a natural outflow, may help to avoid excessive intrauterine fluid pressures that aggravate intravasation of fluids.
- Timely information on fluid input and output is necessary. An automated fluid tracking system is ideal. If this is not available, a designated person should be assigned the task of fluid monitoring.
- The maximum permissible deficit should be defined before the procedure and should be strictly adhered to:
  - For glycine, the maximum fluid absorption should not be more than 1 L.
  - For saline, the maximum fluid absorption should not be more than 2 L.

Management
- Assess the patient's condition and request urgent serum urea and electrolytes (with particular attention to the sodium level, which will dictate management).
- Remove excess water with a diuretic; intravenous furosemide 10–20 mg is the usual drug of choice.
- If the sodium concentration is above 130 mmol/L and the patient is well, conservative management is appropriate.
- If the sodium concentration is below 130 mmol/L, and particularly less than 120 mmol/L, involve an intensivist to develop a plan of management which will include the infusion of hypertonic saline. The correction of hyponatremia needs to be gradual to avoid overcorrection.
- l-Arginine may be useful to treat ammonia toxicity from excessive glycine absorption.
- Mannitol 10–20% may be useful as an osmotic diuretic to reduce cerebral edema.

References

1 Propst AM, Liberman RF, Harlow BL, Ginsburg ES. Complications of hystero-scopic surgery: predicting patients at risk. *Obstet Gynecol* 2000;96:517–520.

2 Indman PD, Brooks PG, Cooper JM, Loffer FD, Valle RF, Vancaillie TG. Compli-cations of fluid overload from resectoscopic surgery. *J Am Assoc Gynecol Laparosc* 1998;5:63–67.

3 Morrison DM. Management of hysteroscopic surgery complications. *AORN J* 1999;69:194–197, 199–209; quiz 210, 213–215, 221.

4 Isaacson KB. Complications of hysteroscopy. *Obstet Gynecol Clin North Am* 1999;26:39–51.

5 Swedarsky LM, Isaacson K. Complications related to hysteroscopic distension media. In: IsaacsonK (ed.) *Complications of Gynecologic Endoscopic Surgery*, pp. 201–207. Saunders Elsevier, Philadelphia, 2006.

6 Wortman M. Complications of hysteroscopic surgery. In: IsaacsonK (ed.) *Compli-cations of Gynecologic Endoscopic Surgery*, pp. 185–200. Saunders Elsevier, Phila-delphia, 2006.

CHAPTER 64

Hysteroscopy: Endometrial Resection and Ablation in the Abnormal Uterine Cavity

Alessandro Conforti and Adam Magos

The Royal Free Hospital, London, UK

Case history: *A 49-year-old woman, having had two spontaneous vaginal deliveries, presents with painless heavy menstrual bleeding which had not been controlled by medical treatment. She wishes to preserve her uterus despite having no desire for future pregnancy and a desire for amenorrhea. She has no identifiable risk factors for endometrial cancer. Clinically, the uterus is enlarged to an 8–10 week gestational size and pelvic ultrasound shows several small uterine fibroids. At hysteroscopy, the uterine cavity is found to be enlarged and distorted with a 3-cm type II submucous fibroid on the posterior wall. Endometrial histology is normal.*

Background

The resectoscope was originally introduced into gynecologic practice by Robert Neuwirth in 1978 for the excision of submucous fibroids. Subsequently, in the 1980s, another American, Alan DeCherney, used the resectoscope loop to burn (ablate) the endometrium in women with intractable heavy menstrual bleeding (HMB) who were too ill for hysterectomy. Thus was born the first technique for endometrial ablation under direct vision, all previous attempts being blind methods (e.g., the use of intrauterine steam). The concept of hysteroscopic endometrial ablation quickly spread to Europe and the indications were extended to include otherwise healthy women with HMB who either failed with medical treatment or did not want hysterectomy.

The initial technique involved ablating the endometrium with the cutting loop. In the mid-1980s the cutting loop started to be the method of choice for excising the endometrium, a procedure commonly referred to as transcervical resection of the endometrium or TCRE, Hamou in France being one of its pioneers. The single-flow resectoscope combined with high-viscosity uterine distension media (e.g., Hyskon) as used by Neuwirth and DeCherney was also changed in favor of a continuous-flow instrument and the use of low-viscosity distension media (e.g., 1.5% glycine solution) due to the influence of another Frenchman, Hallez. In 1989, Vancaillie suggested ablating the endometrium using a rollerball electrode rather than the resectoscope loop and this technique became commonly known as rollerball ablation. Historically, both techniques are considered the first-generation endometrial ablation techniques, and are the gold standard by which the newer second-generation techniques are judged.

The popularity of these techniques quickly spread worldwide as they offered women a safe, day-case surgical procedure with rapid recovery as opposed to major surgery in the form of hysterectomy. Unfortunately, this also meant that gynecologists not familiar with hysteroscopy or hysteroscopic surgery started to carry out endometrial resections and ablations after minimal training. It quickly became apparent that the technique, while safe and highly effective in skilled hands, was also associated with potentially serious morbidity from uterine perforation, fluid overload, and hemorrhage. These safety and technical considerations were the impetus for the more recent development of safer, less skill-dependent ablation techniques that are now referred to as second-generation ablation procedures.

However, while second-generation techniques confer some advantages, the resectoscope is still the best instrument for excising submucous fibroids, a common finding in women with HMB. Many second-generation ablative techniques cannot be used effectively unless the uterine cavity is of a relatively normal size and shape. In contrast, TCRE can be used in enlarged and abnormally shaped uterine cavities, namely in the presence of submucous fibroids, adhesions or congenital (unicornuate, bicornuate, or subseptate) uterine anomalies. In addition, TCRE provides all the endometrium for histologic evaluation.

Management

Choice of surgical technique

In the case history, a traditional first-generation technique is optimal because (i) the uterine cavity is enlarged and distorted, and (ii) there was a significant submucous fibroid which was suitable for resection. This patient therefore fulfills National Institute for Care and Health Excellence (NICE) criteria for endometrial ablation in terms of an appropriate uterus size (<10 weeks) and absence of an intracavitary lesion more than 3 cm in diameter [1]. Her age over 45 years also places her in a good prognostic group in terms of HMB treatment outcomes [2]. An alternative approach is to perform the hysteroscopic myomectomy in isolation, without continuing with ablating the endometrium, as this has been shown to be an effective treatment in women with fibroid-related HMB. However, this patient preferred to have a chance of amenorrhea, which is more likely with a concomitant endometrial ablation.

Endometrial preparation

Preparation of the endometrium using GnRH agonists or the selective progestogen receptor modulator ulipristal acetate for up to 3 months before the procedure can aid surgery. Pretreatment

Gynecologic and Obstetric Surgery: Challenges and Management Options, First Edition. Edited by Arri Coomarasamy, Mahmood I. Shafi, G. Willy Davila and Kiong K. Chan.
© 2016 John Wiley & Sons, Ltd. Published 2016 by John Wiley & Sons, Ltd.

in this way improves the operating conditions for the surgeon by reducing fibroid volume, thinning the endometrium, and reducing endometrial debris which can otherwise compromise the operative view. Furthermore, there is some evidence that a superior short-term postoperative outcome in terms of amenorrhea may result following pretreatment [3]. The procedure should be planned for the immediate post-menstrual phase in those cases where pretreatment is not practical or desired.

Treatment setting

The procedure has been well described in journals and textbooks. Although hysteroscopic resection can be done under local anesthesia, most patients opt for a general anesthetic and this is especially preferable when the operating time is expected to be longer than average because of the need to carry out a myomectomy as well as an endometrial ablation. If women opt to be awake, a combination of intracervical, paracervical, and intrauterine anesthesia using dilute lidocaine with 1 in 200,000 epinephrine (adrenaline) is highly effective when combined with conscious sedation [4].

Technique

The patient is placed in the lithotomy position with the buttocks over the edge of the operating table, thighs at 45°, with slight head-down tilt to encourage bowel to fall away from the uterine fundus, and therefore avoid danger should the procedure be complicated by uterine perforation. After cleaning with a sterile medium, a fluid-collection drape should be placed under the pelvis to facilitate the measurement of fluid balance. Most gynecologists prefer to use a 26 Fr gauge (8.7 mm) resectoscope as it allows faster surgery, but smaller ones are available; historically, the first resectoscope manufactured specifically for gynecologists was 21 Fr gauge (Hallez resectoscope).

The monopolar resectoscope has been all but superseded by bipolar instruments, which allow the use of more physiologic electrolyte-containing uterine distention solutions rather than the slightly hypotonic non-ionic irrigants necessary with the older monopolar technology, which risk hyponatremia and other adverse metabolic changes. However, fluid overload remains a potential problem and means that careful monitoring of fluid balance is still required during surgery. It is for this reason that the intrauterine pressure should be adequate but not excessive, which in practical terms means an intrauterine operating pressure of 100–150 mmHg.

After the cervix has been dilated, the resectoscope is inserted and the surgery can begin. A systematic approach is recommended; many surgeons choose to treat the fundus first, either with a rollerball or, if the endometrium is unduly thickened, by resecting it with a slightly forward angled loop. Particular care has to be taken at the cornu where the myometrial thickness can be only a few millimeters. Grade 0 and I fibroids are easier to resect as the majority of the fibroid is visible within the uterine cavity. One approach is to resect the fibroid using the technique of "cold-knife dissection," which dissects and delivers the intramural portion of the fibroid into the uterine cavity without electrosurgery, thereby reducing the risk of perforation or inadvertent thermal injury.

Once the fibroid has been completely excised, the rest of the uterine cavity can then be systematically resected from the fundus to the internal cervical os, undercutting the endometrium by 2–3 mm to ensure complete endometrial excision as far as possible. If the resected tissue begins to obscure the view, which it may well

do when a fibroid has also been resected, a sponge holder can be used to remove the tissue chips before continuing the ablation. When ablation or resection of the uterine cavity is complete, many surgeons choose to resect the upper half of the endocervical canal in order to minimize the risk of continued menstruation in those women who desire amenorrhea. In women with a cesarean section scar, resection or ablation of the lower anterior uterine wall is best avoided for fear of perforation or bladder injury.

Fastidious attention to fluid balance is of prime importance during hysteroscopic surgery (Chapter 63); fluid inflow and outflow should be monitored continuously during the surgery. Even now, 30 years on from the inception of the technique, the medical literature still reports morbidity and mortality from fluid overload. The operating surgeon should be kept regularly informed about fluid balance, and warned when fluid deficit (absorption) reaches 1 L. Fluid deficits beyond 1–1.5 L necessitate cessation of the surgery when non-osmotic distension media are used. Fluid deficits up to 2 L may be acceptable in healthy women undergoing bipolar procedures where physiologic saline media are employed. Once substantial fluid overload is recognized, careful observation is mandated, serum electrolytes checked, and urine output monitored. Intravenous diuretics and supportive measures, including high-dependency care, may become necessary especially in the presence of severe hyponatremia and hemodynamic compromise (Chapter 63).

KEY POINTS

Challenge: Hysteroscopic endometrial resection and ablation of the abnormal cavity.

Background
- Hysteroscopic techniques for endometrium ablation were introduced more than 30 years ago and are still used in the conservative management of HMB.
- In experienced hands, hysteroscopic resection and/or ablation are suitable techniques whatever the shape and conformation of the uterine cavity, and give results comparable to second-generation techniques.
- Endometrial resection/ablation can be combined with hysteroscopic myomectomy in patients with submucous fibroids.

Management
- Preoperative thinning of endometrium improves the hysteroscopic view and may result in a better surgical outcome.
- With few exceptions, the loop or ball electrode should only be activated as it is being moved away from the uterine fundus toward the cervix.
- It is essential that fluid balance is carefully monitored during surgery to avoid fluid overload even if a bipolar resectoscope is used.
- The versatility and diagnostic capability of the resectoscope makes it a valuable tool in the management of women with HMB.

References

1 National Institute for Care and Health Excellence. *Heavy menstrual bleeding.* NICE Clinical Guideline No. 44, January 2007. Available at http://www.nice.org.uk/guidance/cg44
2 Sharp HT. Endometrial ablation: postoperative complications. *Am J Obstet Gynecol* 2012;207:242–247.
3 Sowter MC, Lethaby A, Singla AA. Pre-operative endometrial thinning agents before endometrial destruction for heavy menstrual bleeding. *Cochrane Database Syst Rev* 2002;(3):CD001124.
4 Magos AL, Baumann R, Lockwood GM, Turnbull AC. Experience with the first 250 endometrial resections for menorrhagia. *Lancet* 1991;337:1074–1078.

CHAPTER 65
Laparoscopy in a Pediatric Patient

Suketu Mansuria[1], Cara R. King[1], and Arri Coomarasamy[2]
[1] University of Pittsburgh Medical Center, Pittsburgh, Pennsylvania, USA
[2] College of Medical and Dental Sciences, University of Birmingham, Birmingham, UK

Case history 1: *A neonate is found to have a complex adnexal mass; following appropriate investigations, a multidisciplinary team recommends laparoscopic removal of the mass.*

Case history 2: *An 11-year-old girl with an 8-cm simple cyst has symptoms consistent with ovarian torsion. Laparoscopic treatment is recommended.*

Background

A child may need laparoscopic surgery for ovarian masses, appendectomy, cholecystectomy, splenectomy, abdominal exploration in trauma, and operations for uterovaginal abnormalities. Laparoscopy may be indicated in a neonate for ovarian and other pelvic or abdominal masses.

Neonatal and pediatric surgery should ideally be centralized, and be carried out by an experienced team, to ensure best outcomes are obtained and risks are minimized [1].

Pediatric surgery is considered a newcomer within the field of laparoscopy. It was not until the production of high-quality miniaturized instruments that surgeons began to look for applications of laparoscopy in the pediatric population. Few procedures were performed laparoscopically in this age group before 1970, primarily because the smaller scopes being used resulted in unacceptable visualization. With the advent of fiber-optic light sources and advanced camera systems, excellent optical performance could now be provided by smaller laparoscopes, overcoming the obstacles to use in a pediatric population.

Management

Diagnostic work-up has to be complete, and the need for surgery should be established by a multidisciplinary team that may include a pediatrician, pediatric surgeon, gynecologist, anesthetist, and nurses.

Consenting

The team caring for children should have specific expertise in looking after children, specifically in communication, consenting, and child protection issues. A girl under 16 years of age cannot legally consent, and therefore her parent or guardian will need to provide consent; however, the girl should be fully involved in the decision-making about her care. If there is a need for vaginal examination or instrumentation during the operation, this should be discussed preoperatively with the girl and the parent.

Instruments

Veress needle should be avoided (due to short distance from abdominal wall to major vessels) and an open technique (e.g., Hasson) should be used to gain access into the abdomen. Radially expanding trocars may be useful in neonates and small children to minimize the risk of CO_2 leakage from around the port site and slippage of trocar from the abdominal wall [2]. For neonatal and infant surgery, special 3–5 mm trocars and 2.7–4.5 mm instruments are available (Figure 65.1). Not only is trocar diameter important, but the length should also be taken into consideration. Trocars that are too long can inhibit free range of motion inside the abdomen in smaller patients. On the other hand, shorter trocars may not be able to traverse the entire length of the subcutaneous tissue.

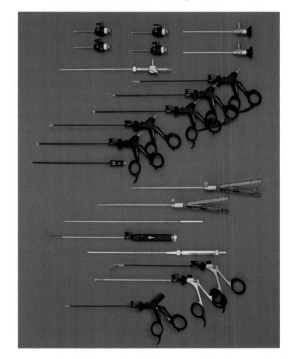

Figure 65.1 Pediatric laparoscopic instruments (© Karl Storz – Endoskope, Germany).

Gynecologic and Obstetric Surgery: Challenges and Management Options, First Edition. Edited by Arri Coomarasamy, Mahmood I. Shafi, G. Willy Davila and Kiong K. Chan.
© 2016 John Wiley & Sons, Ltd. Published 2016 by John Wiley & Sons, Ltd.

For older children, adult laparoscopic instruments may be appropriate [3]. Harmonic scalpel may be safer to use, and could shorten operative time [2].

Patient positioning

Whenever possible, positioning in Allen stirrups allows unencumbered access to the vagina during the procedure (Figure 65.2). Care must be taken to ensure proper leg placement within the stirrups to avoid peripheral neuropathies secondary to nerve compression. In patients with intact hymens, preparing the vagina can be accomplished with minimal trauma to the hymen through the use of a large 60-mL syringe. This avoids the use of sponges, which can cause trauma to the hymen during insertion and can also cause abrasions to the delicate vaginal mucosa during scrubbing.

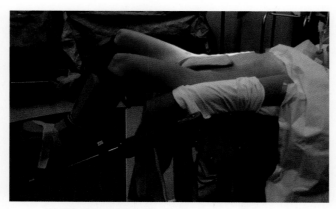

Figure 65.2 Proper patient positioning with legs secured in Allen stirrups and arms tucked at the side.

An additional key step in the preoperative set-up is bilateral tucking of the patient's arms by her side during the procedure. Given the smaller stature of patients in this population, the shorter distance between the arms and pelvis limits the surgeon's maneuverability. By tucking the patient's arms, the surgeon is able to more ergonomically position himself or herself above the level of the shoulder. Securing arms in this way is also a safety precaution, as inadvertent leaning on an outstretched arm can have dire consequences. When tucking the arms, the surgeon should protect the fingers so that they are not injured during articulation of the foot of the bed or the stirrups. Also, the arms should be placed at the patient's side in their anatomic position to further reduce the risk of a median nerve injury (Figure 65.2).

Risks of laparoscopy and management

In addition to the general risks of anesthesia and laparoscopy, there are several specific risks that need to be considered with neonates and children [3,4].

Ventilation and perfusion abnormalities

Infants rely on diaphragmatic excursion for effective ventilation. High insufflation pressures will increase intra-abdominal and intrathoracic pressures and compromise diaphragmatic movement, causing ventilation and perfusion abnormalities. An insufflation

pressure of 8 mmHg with a gas flow rate of 0.5 L/min is recommended for neonates or infants [3]. For small children, an insufflation pressure of 12–15 mmHg may be appropriate. Older children can be managed by similar insufflation protocols to those of adults.

Patients with pulmonary or cardiac compromise may not tolerate the increased intra-abdominal pressure of insufflation or the Trendelenburg position; in such patients, mini-laparotomy should be considered.

Hypercapnia and metabolic acidosis

CO_2 insufflation can give rise to these complications quickly in a neonate or child; end-tidal CO_2 and oxygen saturations should therefore be closely monitored, and minute ventilation maintained to keep end-tidal CO_2 between 30 and 45 mmHg.

Dehydration and hypothermia

Neonates and infants are at particular risk of these complications. Appropriate preoperative and intraoperative hydration is necessary, and the use of humidified gas (at 37°C) is recommended to reduce the risk of hypothermia. In a neonate, continuous rectal monitoring of temperature is advisable [2]. Newer insufflators (e.g., Stryker, Kalamazoo, Michigan) are equipped with the ability to insufflate with warmed air to reduce fogging during the case and prevent hypothermia in the patient.

High risk of injury from Veress needle and trocar

The short distance between the abdominal wall and the major vessels puts children at risk of catastrophic vessel injury. The risk of such injury should be minimized with the use of open (Hasson) entry technique; the use of Veress needle is best avoided in children. Umbilical vessels may still be patent in neonates; these will need to be identified and ligated before abdominal entry and this can be achieved through a small umbilical incision. An obvious difference between adults and children is the smaller surface area in which to enter the abdomen and the smaller working space within the abdominal, pelvic, and retroperitoneal spaces. The decreased cross-sectional area in turn decreases the distance between the inferior epigastric vessels, which should be noted prior to placing accessory ports. Identification of the inferior epigastric vessels is often quite easily accomplished in pediatric patients as the lack of extraperitoneal fat makes transperitoneal visualization quite clear. If there is difficulty in identifying these vessels, the medial umbilical ligaments (also known as the obliterated umbilical arteries) can be used as landmarks. The inferior epigastric vessels are invariably located just lateral to these ligaments. Also, the rectus muscles can be used as a guide for lower trocar placement. The inferior epigastric vessels run along the lateral edge of the rectus muscles, and as long as trocars are inserted lateral to the muscle, injury to these vessels is rare. Given the elastic nature of young patients' tissue, placing accessory ports can be quite difficult due to tenting of the abdominal wall. This can be ameliorated by (i) transiently increasing the insufflation pressure to provide increased counter-traction by the abdominal wall, or (ii) providing counter-traction against the abdominal wall with another laparoscopic instrument. The tip of the trocar should remain in view at all times during insertion.

The abdominal viscera are closer to the anterior abdominal wall in children, and the liver often extends below the ribcage. It is advisable to deflate the stomach with a nasogastric tube as this maneuver assists in expanding the intra-abdominal workspace and protects the stomach.

Bladder injury
Neonates and infants have a substantial part of the bladder in the abdomen. Emptying the bladder before trocar insertion is therefore essential to avoid bladder injury. Care needs to be exercised in the use of suprapubic ports.

Port-site herniation
There is a high likelihood of herniation due to weak fascia and muscles in children. The fascia of all ports 5 mm and larger should be closed in pediatric patients because of the high risk of omental herniation.

Femoral nerve injury
Hyperflexion of the hips can result in this complication (Chapter 181); if access to vagina is needed, then an appropriately sized stirrups with good padding is necessary to avoid injury. For most pediatric patients, access to vagina is not needed, and thus the patient can be placed in the supine position (after catheterization).

Resolution of the cases

Case history 1
An experienced anesthetic and surgical team will need to carry out the procedure with all the necessary precautions outlined above.

Case history 2
A careful assessment for risk of malignancy should be made, including necessary imaging and tumor markers (AFP, HCG and LDH, as germ cell tumors are a possibility). Every effort should be made to preserve the ovary, and therefore laparoscopic detorsion should be the aim.

Prevention

Prevention of complications requires careful preoperative assessment, multidisciplinary decision-making, and diligent adherence to the specific requirements for pediatric laparoscopic surgery as outlined. It is important to consider what support services are needed and involve them early. The multidisciplinary team should audit its results to ensure excellent outcomes are the norm, and that there is continuous learning and improvement.

KEY POINTS

Challenge: A neonate or child requiring laparoscopic surgery.

Background
- Laparoscopic approach can be a reasonable alternative to laparotomy for many neonatal and pediatric operations.
- Pediatric surgery should ideally be centralized.

Management
- Age-appropriate communication with child and parent or guardian, and obtain consent from parent or guardian for children under 16 years.
- If intraoperative vaginal examination or instrumentation is required, obtain prior consent from the child and parent or guardian.
- Entry: use open (Hasson) technique. Avoid Veress needle entry.
- Use low insufflation pressures to minimize ventilation and perfusion abnormalities:
  - Neonates or infants: 8 mmHg.
  - Small children: 12–15 mmHg.
  - Older children: generally the same insufflation protocols as adults.

- Radially expanding trocars minimize CO_2 leakage from port site and are less likely to slip from the abdominal wall of a neonate or infant, and are thus recommended.
- For neonatal and infant surgery, special 3–5 mm trocars and 2.7–4.5 mm instruments can be used.
- Monitor end-tidal CO_2 and oxygen saturation to assess for hypercarbia and acidosis.
- Maintain good hydration.
- Use humidified gas (at 37°C) to avoid hypothermia; monitor continuous rectal temperature in neonates.
- As fascia and muscles are weak in a child, close all ports 5 mm or larger in size.

Prevention
- Prevention of complications requires careful preoperative assessment, multidisciplinary decision-making, and diligent adherence to the specific requirements for pediatric laparoscopic surgery.

References

1 Royal College of Surgeons of England. *Surgery for Children: Delivering a First Class Service.* RCS, London, 2007. Available at https://www.rcseng.ac.uk/publications/docs/CSF.html
2 Fujimoto T, Segawa O, Lane GJ, Esaki S, Miyano T. Laparoscopic surgery in newborn infants. *Surg Endosc* 1999;13:773–777.
3 Templeman C, Paige Hertweck S. Pediatric laparoscopy. In: Pasic RP, Levine RL (eds) *A Practical Manual of Laparoscopy and Minimally Invasive Gynecology*, 2nd edn, pp. 339–346. CRC Press, Boca Raton, FL, 2007.
4 Michala L, Creighton SM, Cutner A. Minimal access surgery in paediatric and adolescent gynaecology. In: Cutner A, Vyas S (eds) *Laparoscopic Surgery for Benign Gynaecology*. RCOG Press, London, 2011.

CHAPTER 66

Safe Laparoscopic Entry in a Thin Patient

Janesh Gupta and Justin Chu

Birmingham Women's NHS Foundation Trust, Birmingham, UK

Case history: *A 33-year-old with a BMI of 18 is admitted for a diagnostic laparoscopy. She has previously undergone a cesarean section.*

Background

Safe laparoscopic entry is pivotal for completing a laparoscopic procedure. If this first hurdle is not accomplished safely, the intended operation may need to be abandoned because of an unintended complication which is associated with morbidity and sometimes mortality. Although complications associated with laparoscopic surgery are rare, a significant proportion of these occur at the time of laparoscopic entry. Pooled risks of vascular and bowel injury at the time of laparoscopic entry are estimated to be 0.2 per 1000 and 0.4 per 1000 procedures, respectively. These complications are compounded if such injuries are not detected at the time of original surgery, particularly in the case of bowel injury.

There are several methods of laparoscopic entry.

1 Closed entry, which involves creation of a pneumoperitoneum at the umbilicus (or at Palmer's point);
2 Open (Hasson) entry, which is associated with a lower risk of vascular injury but does not reduce risk of bowel injury;
3 Other techniques, used less frequently and with limited supporting evidence, such as direct entry, optical access trocars, and radially expanding trocars.

According to current evidence, based mainly on observational studies, no one laparoscopic entry method has demonstrated clear superiority over another. This has led to wide variations among clinicians on the entry methods used.

Women who are extremely thin, obese (Chapter 67), or known to have abdominal adhesions (Chapters 7 and 27) are at increased risk for laparoscopic entry-related injury at the umbilical entry point. In the thin patient, visceral injury complications are more common because of the short distance between the anterior abdominal wall and the organs below.

Management

Safe transumbilical laparoscopic entry

Evidence shows that there are specific steps that can be used to reduce the risks of intra-abdominal injury at the time of laparoscopy [1,2]. A survey of clinical practice in the UK in 2002 showed wide variation in the methods actually practiced [3]. The widespread variation in practice was confirmed in subsequent publications [4,5], one of which also detailed the 10 steps required for safe laparoscopic entry [5], with further endorsement from RCOG guidelines [6].

The main steps for safe entry include the following.
- The use of deep vertical umbilical incision starting at the umbilical pit.
- Stabilization or elevation of the umbilicus so that the Veress needle can be inserted at right angles to the skin. It should be pushed vertically inward, the point of entry being deep in the umbilicus, until it has just penetrated the fascia and peritoneum. The "give" of the tissues should be sensed and the insertion should be stopped as soon as the cavity is entered. This is often detected by hearing and sensing a double "click" sound.
- Correct placement of the Veress needle in the peritoneal cavity should be checked by either the Palmer's test or by observing a low gas flow pressure (<8 mmHg).
- Movement of the Veress needle after insertion should be minimized to prevent a needlepoint injury becoming a large complex tear.
- The initial abdominal insufflation pressure should be set at 25 mmHg to create an increased splinting tympanic effect on the abdominal wall, maximizing the largest safe distance between the abdominal wall and underlying bowel, without compromising respiratory function or venous return. This pressure should then be reduced to a working pressure of 12–15 mmHg *after* all the trocars have been inserted.
- The primary umbilical trocar should be inserted in a vertical *controlled* manner using a two-handed screwing technique through the thinnest part of the abdominal wall in the pit of the umbilicus. Insertion should be stopped immediately the trocar is through the abdominal wall skin and fascia and just inside the abdominal cavity.
- Once the laparoscope has been introduced down the primary trocar, it should be rotated through 360° to check visually for adherent and potentially damaged bowel and for evidence of hemorrhage.
- Secondary trocars should be inserted in a controlled manner using a two-handed screwing technique with an intra-abdominal pressure of 25 mmHg and under direct vision.

Special considerations in a thin patient

The prime concern in patients with a BMI of 18 or less is that the distance between the anterior abdominal wall and the abdominal organs (in particular the great vessels) is shorter than a patient with

Gynecologic and Obstetric Surgery: Challenges and Management Options, First Edition. Edited by Arri Coomarasamy, Mahmood I. Shafi, G. Willy Davila and Kiong K. Chan.
© 2016 John Wiley & Sons, Ltd. Published 2016 by John Wiley & Sons, Ltd.

a normal BMI or one who is obese. Special considerations need to be taken in order to further reduce the risks of laparoscopic entry.

Patient positioning for transumbilical insufflation

All patients should have Veress needle entry in the flat supine position; this is particularly important in thin patients. Great care should be taken to ensure that there is no rotation or Trendelenburg positioning of the patient on the operating table, as such positions can lead to alignment of the abdominal aorta or inferior vena cava with the axis of insertion of the Veress needle (Figure 66.1). Rotation of the hips and spine can bring the iliac vessels into the path of the needle [7].

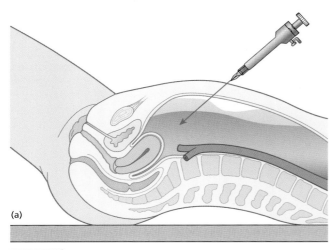

(a)

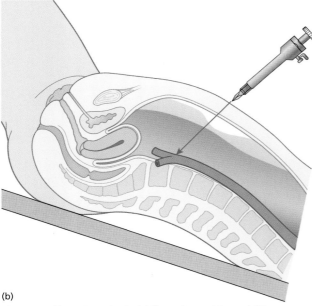

(b)

Figure 66.1 Trocar insertion in (a) flat supine position and (b) Trendelenburg position.

Angle of needle insertion for transumbilical insufflation

In very thin patients, the bifurcation of the abdominal aorta may be directly below the umbilicus. Therefore care should be exercised when considering the angle at which the Veress needle is inserted. The needle should be inserted firstly in a vertical axis, but when the

fascia has been breached any further advance of the needle should be toward the sacral promontory at a 45° angle [8] (see Chapter 76, Figure 76.2).

Palmer's point entry

Patients with very low BMI should be considered for insertion of the insufflation needle at an alternative site from the umbilicus. Again, this is to reduce the risk of injury to the great vessels. Entry in the left upper quadrant through Palmer's point is the usual alternative to an intraumbilical entry.

Palmer's point entry is gained by making an incision in the mid-clavicular line just below the costal margin on the left side. The Veress needle can then be inserted in a vertical direction; three clicks should be felt as the needle pierces the anterior abdominal wall. It is important to ask the anesthetist to drain all gastric contents with a nasogastric tube before Palmer's point entry.

Open (Hasson) entry

As the main concern in thin patients is that of vascular injury, direct visualization may aid the insertion of the primary trocar [9]. This technique requires a 2-cm skin incision to the umbilical skin. Dissection of the abdominal wall is performed with Kelly clamps and small retractors. When the abdominal fascia is reached, it is dissected and two sutures are placed on either side. The peritoneum is then incised and the peritoneal cavity entered with a blunt open laparoscopy trocar. The sutures from the fascia are tied to the trocar to prevent gas leak. The peritoneal cavity can then be insufflated directly through the trocar.

Resolution of the case

This patient has a BMI of 18 and therefore has an increased risk of intra-abdominal injury, in particular to the great vessels. This patient has also had previous open surgery, further increasing the risk of complications due to the presence of intra-abdominal adhesions and leading to inadvertent bowel injury. The surgeon should ensure that she is lying in a flat supine position. If intraumbilical closed laparoscopic entry is to be attempted, then the insufflation needle should first be inserted in a vertical axis with change in vector toward the sacral promontory once the abdominal fascia has been pierced. Alternatively, non-umbilical entry sites or open entry technique can be considered.

KEY POINTS

Challenge: Safe laparoscopic entry.

Background
- Vascular and bowel injury at the time of laparoscopic entry occur mainly at the time of laparoscopic abdominal wall entry.
- Women who are extremely thin, obese, or known to have abdominal adhesions are at increased risk for laparoscopic entry-related injury at the umbilical entry point.

Management
Ten steps for safe laparoscopic entry
1. Suitability criteria: consider risk factors (e.g., low or high BMI).
2. Safety criteria: flat, empty bladder, abdominal palpation, equipment check.
3. Incision: 10 mm vertical intraumbilical.

4. Insertion of Veress needle: 90° to skin, insert 2 cm through mid-umbilical point.
5. No movement: avoid unnecessary movement of Veress needle.
6. Safety check for Veress: intra-abdominal pressure (IAP) <8 mmHg.
7. Safety check for IAP: insufflate to 25 mmHg.
8. Insertion of primary trocar: two-handed controlled screw.
9. Injury check: 360° check.
10. Insertion of secondary trocars: direct vision, two-handed, 90° to skin.

The thin patient

- Vascular injury to the great vessels is the prime concern in women with a BMI of 18 or less. In these women special considerations include the following.
- The patient should be placed in a flat supine position with no Trendelenburg tilt or rotation.
- Angle of Veress needle insertion: initial vertical entry, but when fascia is breached further advance at 45° toward the sacral promontory.
- Alternative insufflation sites should be considered (e.g., Palmer's point).
- Open laparoscopic entry should be considered to allow direct visualization of trocar insertion.

References

1 Garry R. Towards evidence-based laparoscopic entry techniques: clinical problems and dilemmas. *Gynaecol Endosc* 1999;8:315–326.

2 A consensus document concerning laparoscopic entry techniques: Middlesborough, March 19–20, 1999. *Gynaecol Endosc* 1999;8:403–406.

3 Lalchandani S, Phillips K. Laparoscopic entry technique: a survey of practices of consultant gynaecologists. *Gynecol Surg* 2005;2:245–249.

4 Ahmad G, Duffy JMN, Watson AJS. Laparoscopic entry techniques and complications. *Int J Gynecol Obstet* 2007;99:52–55.

5 Varma R, Gupta JK. Laparoscopic entry techniques: clinical guideline, national survey and medicolegal ramifications. *Surg Endosc* 2008;22:2686–2697.

6 Royal College of Obstetricians and Gynaecologists. *Preventing Entry-related Gynaecological Laparoscopic Injuries.* RCOG Green-top Guideline No. 49. RCOG, *London, 2008. Available at* https://www.rcog.org.uk/en/guidelines-research-services/guidelines/gtg49/

7 Isaacson K. *Complications of Gynecologic Endoscopic Surgery.* Saunders Elsevier, Philadelphia, 2006.

8 Ahmad G, O'Flynn H, Duffy JM, Phillips K, Watson A. Laparoscopic entry techniques. *Cochrane Database Syst Rev* 2012;(2):CD006583.

9 Vilos GA, Ternamian A, Dempster J, Laberge PY. Laparoscopic entry: a review of techniques, technologies, and complications. *J Obstet Gynaecol Can* 2007;29:433–465.

CHAPTER 67
Laparoscopy: Unable to Gain Entry

Mohamed Mehasseb
Glasgow Royal Infirmary, Glasgow, Scotland, UK

Case history 1: A 28-year-old woman with suspected endometriosis and subfertility is undergoing a diagnostic laparoscopy. She has a high BMI (38). The surgeon uses a Veress needle to induce the pneumoperitoneum. The pressures during insufflation were high, but the abdomen was distending. On attempt to insert the umbilical port, the operator realizes that the insufflation was extraperitoneal. Three attempts fail to penetrate the peritoneal cavity.

Case history 2: A 40-year-old woman presents as an emergency with a clinical picture supported by imaging of torsion of a 12-cm left ovarian cyst. She has a past surgical history of a midline laparotomy because of intra-abdominal trauma following a previous road traffic accident. The gynecologist proceeds with a laparoscopy using the open Hasson technique. However, she cannot access the peritoneal cavity in view of extensive bowel and omental adhesions at the site of the umbilical port.

Background

There is wide variation in the techniques used by laparoscopic surgeons to gain primary entry into the peritoneal cavity. Gynecologists have tended to favor the transumbilical Veress needle (closed) entry technique, whereby the abdominal cavity is insufflated with carbon dioxide gas prior to introduction of the primary trocar and cannula. In contrast, general surgeons have preferred the open (Hasson) approach. This method uses a small periumbilical incision to enter the peritoneal cavity under direct vision. Direct trocar insertion is an acceptable alternative method; in experienced hands, it is the most rapid method of entry and can be safely used if the cases are carefully selected, but the technique is not widely used within gynecologic practice [1].

Management

Failed entry into the peritoneal cavity can arise because of improper placement of Veress needle or extraperitoneal insufflation of CO_2, resulting in inability to gain surgical access through the anterior abdominal wall. Where entry using a standard closed technique has failed, the options available to the surgeon are (i) conversion to an open or direct entry technique, (ii) use of alternative entry point (e.g., Palmer's point), (iii) conversion to laparotomy, or (iv) abandonment of the procedure.

The morbidly obese woman

In a morbidly obese woman, proper placement of the Veress needle and pneumoperitoneum may be difficult to achieve. If the needle "tunnels" the subcutaneous fat below the umbilicus, the surgeon may induce extraperitoneal insufflation. In obese patients, a 90° angulation of the needle relative to the peritoneal cavity (i.e., perpendicular to the umbilicus) is necessary to avoid "tunneling" (see Chapter 76, Figure 76.2). It is important to make the vertical incision in the pit at the base of the umbilicus. In this area where the skin, deep fascia and parietal peritoneum of the anterior abdominal wall meet, there is little opportunity for the parietal peritoneum to tent away from the Veress needle tip.

The open (Hasson) technique (which can prove technically difficult) or needle insertion at Palmer's point (3 cm below the left costal margin in the mid-clavicular line) is recommended for the primary entry in women with morbid obesity [2].

If these techniques fail, insufflation through the cul-de-sac of Douglas (Figure 67.1) or transfundal insufflation (Figure 67.2) are options. These techniques avoid the excess adipose tissue found

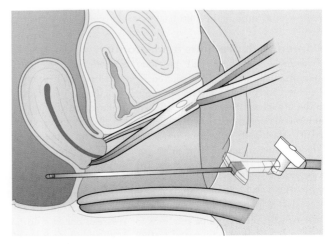

Figure 67.1 Insufflation through the cul-de-sac of Douglas.

Gynecologic and Obstetric Surgery: Challenges and Management Options, First Edition. Edited by Arri Coomarasamy, Mahmood I. Shafi, G. Willy Davila and Kiong K. Chan.
© 2016 John Wiley & Sons, Ltd. Published 2016 by John Wiley & Sons, Ltd.

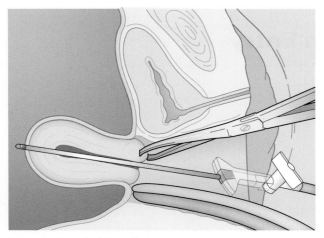

Figure 67.2 Transfundal insufflation.

at the anterior abdominal wall in obese patients and can lead to successful insufflations. However, they are rarely used in practice due to the risk of inadvertent bowel injury, especially in patients with rectovaginal endometriosis or those with previous pelvic surgeries [3]. If these techniques are to be used, then the surgeon must be certain that the pouch of Douglas and the uterine fundus are free of any adhesions or masses.

Insufflation through the cul-de-sac of Douglas is achieved by placing the patient in Trendelenburg position and grasping the posterior lip of the cervix and applying anterior traction (Figure 67.1). A long insufflation needle is then inserted through the posterior fornix of the vagina.

As a last resort, transfundal insufflations can be attempted (Figure 67.2). The uterus must be normal in structure with no fibroids so that the uterine cavity is not distorted. A long insufflation needle is inserted with the cervix held in axial traction. The needle pierces through the fundus of the uterus with a click or pop felt in the needle; ultrasound guidance can also be used to trace the path of the needle through the uterus.

Women with previous laparotomy (Chapter 27)
In women who have had previous laparotomies, the intra-abdominal anatomy may be altered by adhesions. Attachment of the bowel and omentum to the abdominal wall usually occurs distal to the umbilicus. However, in patients who have had complicated abdominal operations, the bowel may be attached under, very close to, or occasionally above the umbilicus. In general, women with prior midline incisions have more adhesions compared to those with prior low transverse incisions. The number of prior incisions does not have a bearing on the incidence of adhesions. Women with prior gynecologic pelvic procedures have more adhesions compared with those who have undergone a cesarean section. Patients with prior midline incisions for cesarean delivery do not have more adhesions compared to those with the more common low transverse access [4]. Extensive adhesions are frequently encountered in women with a history of generalized peritonitis, bowel resection after intestinal obstruction, oncologic procedure with omentectomy, and previous irradiation or intraperitoneal chemotherapy [2]. Open laparoscopic entry or Palmer's point entry

are preferred in women with a history of previous surgery and in women where intra-abdominal adhesions are anticipated.

Palmer's point is situated 3 cm below the left costal margin in the mid-clavicular line. A small incision is made and a sharp Veress needle inserted vertically. After the pneumoperitoneum is established, a 2–5 mm endoscope is used to inspect the undersurface of the umbilical region. If this is free of adhesions, the trocar and cannulae can be inserted under direct laparoscopic vision. If there are many adhesions present, it is possible to dissect these free via secondary ports [2].

Multiple alternative entry device systems are available commercially. Some radially expanding devices include visual access systems (optical trocars) that accommodate a 0° laparoscope and allow real-time visualization of the abdominal wall layers being penetrated [2].

Prevention

Multiple safety tests have been described to help confirm the correct placement of the Veress needle prior to CO_2 insufflation. However, no one test has been shown to be clearly superior [5].

Aspiration test
This is the most widely used safety test. It is performed with the aid of an empty syringe or a syringe that contains physiologic saline. This test consists of three steps.
1 Aspiration: the syringe should not retrieve air, fluid, blood, or bowel contents, thus ascertaining the absence of vascular, urinary, or intestinal perforation.
2 Injection: 20 mL of air or fluid is injected and no resistance should be encountered.
3 Re-aspiration: it should not be possible to re-aspirate the injected air or liquid into the syringe, confirming the proper placement of the needle and the dispersion of air or saline intraperitoneally. If the needle is placed within adhesions or the preperitoneal space, the air or fluid will be recovered by aspiration.

Hanging drop test
A few drops of physiologic saline are poured over the needle hub after insertion. The abdominal wall should be slightly lifted, establishing negative pressure within the abdomen. If the tip of the Veress needle is properly placed, the saline should be drained inside the peritoneal cavity.

Gas insufflation test
The confirmation of low intraperitoneal pressure is generally considered the most reliable method to confirm Veress needle placement. The intraperitoneal pressure should be no greater than 8 mmHg. If higher pressures are encountered, this may indicate that the needle tip is lodged in the omentum; gentle elevating and shaking of the lower abdominal wall may dislodge the needle. If neither of these techniques relieves the increased recorded pressure, the Veress needle is removed and reinserted. Whenever the Veress needle is withdrawn because of high recorded pressures, the surgeon should check its patency as tissue can become lodged in the tip of the needle during passage through the different layers of the abdomen.

Resolution of the cases

Case history 1

In this case of failed entry in an obese patient, the surgeon should either attempt entry using open technique (although this may be technically challenging due to the extraperitoneal gas and increased adiposity) or insufflate through Palmer's point entry.

Case history 2

In this patient with subumbilical adhesions, Palmer's point entry should be used. The anesthetist should be notified so that he or she can evacuate the stomach with a nasogastric tube before insertion of the insufflation needle. The subumbilical adhesions can then be assessed and divided to allow insertion of an umbilical 10-mm port.

KEY POINTS

Challenge: Failure to enter and insufflate the peritoneal cavity during laparoscopic surgery.

Background
- There is wide variation in the techniques used by laparoscopic surgeons to gain primary entry in the peritoneal cavity (transumbilical Veress needle entry technique, the open approach, and direct trocar insertion).
- The literature has no consistent definition for failed entry.

Management
Options following failed entry with needle insufflation
- Conversion to an open or direct entry technique.
- Use of an alternative entry point (e.g., Palmer's point).
- Conversion to laparotomy.
- Abandonment of the procedure.

Morbidly obese women
- Proper placement of the Veress needle may be difficult.
- Use of the open (Hasson) technique (although this may prove difficult) or needle insertion at Palmer's point may be necessary.

- In selected women, Veress needle entry through the posterior cul-de-sac of Douglas or the uterus may be possible.

Women who have had previous laparotomies
- Intra-abdominal anatomy may be altered by adhesions.
- Open laparoscopic entry or Palmer's point entry is preferred.

Prevention
- Entry complications may be minimized by:
  - Use of alternative entry sites (Palmer's point).
  - Use of alternative entry devices or open entry technique.
  - Use of safety tests to confirm the correct placement of the Veress needle prior to insufflation (e.g., aspiration test, hanging drop test, gas pressure test).
- The surgeon should be cognizant of the fact that the likelihood of complications increases with increasing number of attempts with Veress needle. If Veress needle insertion is unsuccessful, the surgeon should consider requesting help from a senior colleague, consider an alternative site entry, revert to an open technique, perform a laparotomy, or abandon the procedure altogether.

References

1 Vilos GA, Ternamian A, Dempster J, Laberge PY. Laparoscopic entry: a review of techniques, technologies, and complications. *J Obstet Gynaecol Can* 2007;29:433–465.
2 Ahmad G, O'Flynn H, Duffy JM, Phillips K, Watson A. Laparoscopic entry techniques. *Cochrane Database Syst Rev* 2012;(2):CD006583.
3 Rosen DM, Lam AM, Chapman M, Carlton M, Cario GM. Methods of creating pneumoperitoneum: a review of techniques and complications. *Obstet Gynecol Surv* 1998;53:167–174.
4 Vilos GA. The ABCs of a safer laparoscopic entry. *J Minim Invasive Gynecol* 2006;13:249–251.
5 Teoh B, Sen R, Abbott J. An evaluation of four tests used to ascertain Veres needle placement at closed laparoscopy. *J Minim Invasive Gynecol* 2005;12:153–158.

CHAPTER 68
Surgical Emphysema

Arri Coomarasamy

College of Medical and Dental Sciences, University of Birmingham, Birmingham, UK

Case history 1: Midway through a laparoscopic hysterectomy, the surgeon notices vulval and lower abdominal subcutaneous emphysema.

Case history 2: Midway through a laparoscopic hysterectomy, the anesthetist notices neck and facial swelling consistent with subcutaneous emphysema. End-tidal CO_2 steadily rose from 30 mmHg after intubation to 60 mmHg despite an increase in minute ventilation.

Background

Subcutaneous surgical emphysema occurs in 0.3–3% of laparoscopic operations [1]. Risk factors for surgical emphysema include advanced age, the use of multiple ports, high-pressure pneumoperitoneum, prolonged surgery, and extraperitoneal laparoscopic procedures [2,3]. Surgical emphysema has been categorized into three groups [4].

1 Mild: emphysema at the trocar insertion sites or in the groin.
2 Marked: emphysema extending to the abdomen and thighs.
3 Massive: emphysema extending to the chest, neck, and face.

Complications of surgical emphysema

Mild or marked surgical emphysema normally subsides without any complications. However, massive surgical emphysema can result in potential complications such as severe acidosis, hypercarbia, upper airway obstruction, pneumomediastinum, pneumopericardium, pneumothorax, and gas embolism (Chapter 69). Neck swelling and paratracheal emphysema can result in upper airway obstruction. Acidosis from hypoventilation and excessive CO_2 can result in arrhythmias, increased intracranial pressure, and depressed central nervous system [5]. Pneumomediastinum, characterized by impaired cardiovascular and pulmonary functions, can be life-threatening.

Management

Diagnostic features

High end-tidal CO_2 is an early sign. If this is noted, then the patient should be examined, including palpation of the anterior chest and neck for crepitus. Tachycardia, loss of cardiac dullness, decreased

heart sounds, and crunching sounds over the precordium (a friction rub called Hamman's sign) can be signs of pneumomediastinum. X-ray and CT are useful for ascertaining the extent of surgical emphysema, particularly if mediastinal involvement or pneumothorax is suspected.

Treatment

Close communication between the surgeon and the anesthetist is essential. Initial measures should include reduction of the CO_2 insufflation pressures and enlargement of the laparoscopic port-site skin incisions to allow CO_2 to escape. Anesthetic measures include an increase in minute ventilation and several manual breaths to help with alveolar recruitment. If no improvement in $PaCO_2$ and acidosis occurs, then termination of the operation or conversion to laparotomy must be considered.

If there is any evidence of pharyngeal compression and airway compromise, or if significant neck swelling is present, then it will be necessary to keep the patient sedated and intubated until the neck swelling and compression settle and hypercarbia is corrected. When the patient's condition improves, the endotracheal tube cuff can be deflated (cuff leak test) to assess if there is a leak around the endotracheal tube [4]; if there is, then significant pharyngeal compression is unlikely, and it may be safe to extubate the patient. When extubating the patient, it is necessary to ensure that there is someone with the skills and materials for establishing a surgical airway should this become necessary.

In the rare event of critical cardiorespiratory compromise, mediastinotomy may be necessary to relieve tension pneumomediastinum [6]. Infraclavicular "blowholes" (bilateral skin incisions under the clavicles) to allow the trapped air to escape have also been described [7].

Resolution of the cases

Case history 1

The surgical and anesthetic team should now be vigilant for the extension of the surgical emphysema and the development of serious mediastinal or airway complications; end-tidal CO_2 monitoring and frequent examination of the chest and neck by the anesthetist are indicated. The insufflation pressure should be dropped to 10–12 mmHg. The laparoscopic surgery may be continued and

Gynecologic and Obstetric Surgery: Challenges and Management Options, First Edition. Edited by Arri Coomarasamy, Mahmood I. Shafi, G. Willy Davila and Kiong K. Chan.

completed as long as the surgical emphysema is not compromising the patient's condition. The operative time should be minimized and the most experienced surgeon should complete the operation.

Case history 2

The laparoscopic approach should be abandoned if the patient's condition does not improve rapidly. The operation can be completed via a laparotomy. Investigations including a chest X-ray and arterial blood gases are needed to understand the extent of the complication. Postoperatively, the patient should be kept intubated and mechanically ventilated until the $PaCO_2$ returns to normal and the surgical emphysema resolves, which may take several hours. If airway compromise is suspected, ventilation will need to be continued for longer. After extubation, admission to ITU will be necessary for close surveillance and management of any complications.

Prevention

Vigilance, prompt diagnosis, and management are of prime importance to avoid complications. The risk of interstitial insufflation can be minimized by careful placement of the Veress needle and trocar at exactly the base of the umbilicus where all layers of the anterior abdominal wall fuse. Further measures to avoid inadvertent introduction of CO_2 into preperitoneal subcutaneous tissues include keeping the pneumoperitoneal pressure below 12 mmHg after initial entry, minimizing the number of ancillary ports, and shortening the operative time (which may require the presence of experienced surgeons for complex cases and the availability of sufficient numbers of operative assistants and appropriate equipment). End-tidal CO_2 should be carefully monitored by the anesthetist.

KEY POINTS

Challenge: Surgical emphysema during laparoscopy.

Background
- Incidence: 0.3–3% of laparoscopic procedures.
- Risk factors: advanced age, multiple ports, high insufflation pressures, prolonged surgery, and extraperitoneal procedures.
- Grades:
  - Mild: emphysema around trocar site or groin.
  - Marked: emphysema around abdomen and thighs.
  - Massive: emphysema extending to chest, neck and face.
- Complications: mild or marked emphysema does not normally result in complications. Massive emphysema can result in severe acidosis, hypercarbia, upper airway obstruction, pneumomediastinum, pneumopericardium, pneumothorax, and gas embolism.

Prevention
- Prompt diagnosis and management of massive emphysema is key to avoiding complications.
- Aim to avoid inadvertent introduction of CO_2 into preperitoneal subcutaneous tissues. Enter exactly at the base of umbilicus where all layers of the abdomen fuse.

- Keep the pneumoperitoneum pressure below 12 mmHg (after initially higher 25 mmHg pressure for trocar entry).
- Minimize the number of ports and operative time.

Management
Diagnosis
- Palpate for chest and neck crepitus.
- Monitor end-tidal CO_2 and vital signs.
- Chest X-ray.
- Consider CT to assess for mediastinal emphysema.

Treatment
- Enlarge the laparoscopic port-site skin incision to allow CO_2 to escape.
- Reduce insufflation pressures.
- Increase minute ventilation.
- If emphysema extends to the upper body, consider termination of the operation or conversion to laparotomy.
- Pharyngeal compression and airway compromise is very rare, but if this happens keep the patient sedated and ventilated until swelling settles and hypercarbia is corrected.
- If critical cardiorespiratory compromise from mediastinal emphysema ensues, then mediastinotomy may be necessary to relieve tension pneumomediastinum; consider infraclavicular "blowholes" to allow the trapped air to escape.

References

1 Gutt CN, Oniu T, Mehrabi A *et al.* Circulatory and respiratory complications of carbon dioxide insufflation. *Dig Surg* 2004;21:95–105.

2 Singh K, Singhal A, Saggar VR, Sharma B, Sarangi R. Subcutaneous carbon dioxide emphysema following endoscopic extraperitoneal hernia repair: possible mechanisms. *J Laparoendosc Adv Surg Tech A* 2004;14:317–320.

3 Murdock CM, Wolff AJ, Van Geem T. Risk factors for hypercarbia, subcutaneous emphysema, pneumothorax, and pneumomediastinum during laparoscopy. *Obstet Gynecol* 2000;95:704–709.

4 Worrell JB, Cleary DT. Massive subcutaneous emphysema and hypercarbia: complications of carbon dioxide absorption during extraperitoneal and intraperitoneal laparoscopic surgery. Case studies. *AANA J* 2002;70:456–461.

5 Lindsey S. Subcutaneous carbon dioxide emphysema following laparoscopic salpingo-oophorectomy: a case report. *AANA J* 2008;76:282–285.

6 Kandiah S, Iswariah H, Elgey S. Postpartum pneumomediastinum and subcutaneous emphysema: two case reports. *Case Rep Obstet Gynecol* 2013; Article ID 735154.

7 Herlan DB, Landreneau RJ, Ferson PF. Massive spontaneous subcutaneous emphysema. Acute management with infraclavicular "blow holes". *Chest* 1992;102:503–505.

CHAPTER 69

Venous Air Embolism

Anneke Chu[1] and Jennie Kerr[2]

[1] City Hospital, Sandwell and West Birmingham Hospitals NHS Trust, Birmingham, UK

[2] University Hospitals Birmingham NHS Foundation Trust, Birmingham, UK

Case history 1: A 52-year-old female is undergoing a laparoscopic hysterectomy. Midway through the procedure there is a sudden drop in the end-tidal CO_2 trace; the patient is hypotensive and tachycardic. The anesthetist suspects she may have a venous air embolism.

Case history 2: A 30-year-old female is undergoing an elective cesarean section under spinal anesthesia for a breech presentation. She starts to complain of severe chest pain and shortness of breath. She is hypotensive despite frequent phenylephrine boluses and the ECG shows ischemic changes.

Background

Venous air embolism (VAE) is the introduction of air bubbles into the venous circulation [1]. Arterial air embolism (AAE) and paradoxical air embolism (PAE), where an embolus from the venous circulation crosses to the arterial blood system, can also occur but are not discussed in this chapter. VAE is a potential risk when the venous pressure is lower than atmospheric pressure, such as when an open vein is raised above the level of the heart [1]. Air is the commonest gas entrained; however, embolism from carbon dioxide and nitrous oxide can also occur [2]. Carbon dioxide used for laparoscopic abdominal insufflation is more soluble than other gases, and thus any carbon dioxide gas embolism will dissolve over time [3].

There are various risk factors associated with VAE. They can be classified as patient-related, anesthesia-related, and surgery-related (Table 69.1). Obstetric and gynecologic procedures associated with VAE include cesarean section (incidence as high as 40–50%, especially if the uterus is exteriorized [4]), termination of pregnancy, removal of the placenta, laparoscopic procedures that involve creating a pneumoperitoneum [2], and use of the Trendelenburg position [4].

Pathophysiology

Morbidity and mortality are dependent on the volume of air entrained and the rate of accumulation [1]. Intravascular gas may travel from its site of entry to the right atrium and subsequently to the right ventricle, where it can produce an "airlock" obstructing outflow to the pulmonary circulation and increasing pulmonary vascular resistance [3]. Cardiovascular instability and ultimately cardiac arrest can rapidly ensue. This presentation is more common following introduction of a large bolus of air (approximately 5 mL/

Table 69.1 Risk factors associated with venous air embolism.

Patient
Patent foramen ovale (found in 27% of the adult population)[a] [2]

Anesthesia
Spontaneous ventilation
Hypovolemia
Pressurized infusions
Insertion or removal of CVP lines
Epidural anesthesia when using the loss of resistance to air technique during insertion
Nitrous oxide use
Venous injection of air

Surgery
Obstetric and gynecologic surgery
  Cesarean section
  Termination of pregnancy
  Removal of placenta
  Laparoscopy
  Trendelenburg positioning
Neurosurgery
Orthopedic surgery
Head and neck surgery

[a] Associated with an increased risk of paradoxical air embolism (PAE).

kg) into the venous circulation [2,5]. If sufficient pressure builds up in the right ventricle, the air trapped in the right ventricle can be pushed through the pulmonary circulation and into the left atrium, producing a paradoxical air embolism [2].

More gradual air entrainment leads to microemboli, which not only obstruct flow but also stimulate neutrophils, fibrin, red blood cells, fat globules, and platelets to bind to the air bubbles [2]. These physical and chemical responses can lead to increased basement membrane permeability and subsequently pulmonary edema [2,6]. A systemic inflammatory response syndrome (SIRS) may also develop [7].

Moderate gas entrainment can lead to significant right ventricular outflow obstruction with subsequent reduction in cardiac output, resulting in hypotension and myocardial and cerebral ischemia [5].

Diagnosis

Clinical signs and symptoms vary and presentations can range from subclinical suspicion to acute life-threatening events. Presentation is reported to occur with as little as 0.5 mL/kg per min of intravascular gas [3]. Volumes between 100 and 300 mL can be fatal [2,5].

Gynecologic and Obstetric Surgery: Challenges and Management Options, First Edition. Edited by Arri Coomarasamy, Mahmood I. Shafi, G. Willy Davila and Kiong K. Chan.
© 2016 John Wiley & Sons, Ltd. Published 2016 by John Wiley & Sons, Ltd.

Although the signs and symptoms of VAE are non-specific, they are generally features of cardiovascular, respiratory, and neurologic dysfunction. The awake patient may complain of severe chest pain, breathing difficulties, light-headedness, and a sense of impending doom [2,5]. In the anesthetized patient VAE may present with a tachyarrhythmia or evidence of myocardial ischemia on ECG, a reduction in end-tidal CO_2, tachypnea, and progressive hypoxia. The first presentation may also be a cardiac arrest. Having a high index of suspicion is important.

The classical "millwheel" murmur heard on precordial auscultation is insensitive and is often a late sign. It is indicative of a massive VAE with imminent cardiovascular collapse [3,8].

Transesophageal echocardiography (TEE) is the most sensitive monitoring device and may detect as little as 0.02 mL/kg of air, and bubbles as small as 5 μm in diameter [8]. Furthermore, TEE allows localization of the air to a specific chamber and also enables assessment of cardiac function [5], but it is a relatively invasive intervention and requires expertise to insert and interpret [8]. Transthoracic echocardiography (TTE) is less sensitive than TEE but may be more readily available and easier to use and interpret [8].

Prevention

A thorough preoperative assessment is vital in identifying at-risk patients. (Table 69.1). Patients should be well hydrated prior to surgery and intravenous fluids prescribed where necessary. The use of nitrous oxide in anesthesia should be avoided (nitrous oxide can dramatically increase the size of an air embolus as it is 35 times more soluble than nitrogen [5]). Additional monitoring, such as an arterial line, CVP line and TEE/TTE, should be considered in high-risk patients. Where possible the level of the operative site in relation to the heart should be lowered and the time the venous circulation is open to the atmosphere minimized.

Management

VAE is a surgical emergency, which should be declared to the team. The immediate management should follow a structured ABCDE approach. Senior surgical and anesthetic assistance should be sought without delay. Specific management is targeted at preventing further gas entrainment, limiting the spread of central progression, and minimizing the systemic cardiovascular effect [3,5].

It is important to ensure that 100% oxygen is administered and the use of any nitrous oxide is discontinued. A definitive airway (endotracheal tube) will be required if not already *in situ*. In laparoscopic procedures, the pneumoperitoneum should be immediately decompressed. The surgical site should be flooded with sterile saline or covered with saline-soaked drapes. Any visible open vessels should be compressed or ligated. If possible, the surgical site should be depressed below the level of the heart. Alternatively, placing the patient in the left lateral position with a slight head-down tilt may trap the embolism in the right atrium [8]. The operation should be terminated as soon as it is safe to do so.

Increasing venous pressure aims to prevent embolus progression to the heart. This can be achieved by rapid intravenous infusion (warmed if possible), creating moderate continuous positive airway pressure (CPAP) or positive end-expiratory pressure (PEEP), and by performing a Valsalva maneuver.

In severe cases cardiovascular instability will require management with inotropes and vasopressors. Presentation with pulseless electrical activity (PEA) or pulseless ventricular tachycardia or fibrillation should be treated following standard Resuscitation Council (UK) ALS algorithms, remembering to exclude other causes of cardiac arrest (4 "H"s/4 "T"s; see Chapter 58).

If a CVP line is *in situ*, then an attempt to aspirate the line may be made. If there is no CVP line *in situ*, preparation can be made to site one but this should not delay any ongoing resuscitation [8].

Once the patient is stabilized, arrangements should be made for ITU transfer for ongoing supportive treatment.

Following any VAE, the incident should be fully documented in the patient's notes, a critical incident report form completed, and the occurrence of the event communicated to the patient at a suitable time.

Resolution of the cases

Case history 1

A structured ABCDE approach should be followed, including the administration of 100% oxygen and discontinuation of any nitrous oxide. Rapid intravenous fluid boluses should be administered in an attempt to increase venous pressure. The surgeon should decompress the pneumoperitoneum and flood the pelvis with sterile saline. The Trendelenburg position should be reversed and the patient placed in a partial left lateral decubitus position (Durant maneuver [5]). The surgery should be concluded as quickly and safely as possible and ITU transfer arranged for ongoing supportive treatment.

Case history 2

A structured ABCDE approach should be followed. As this patient is awake it may be reasonable to convert to general anesthesia in order to facilitate delivery of the baby and adequately resuscitate the patient.

KEY POINTS

Challenge: Venous air embolism.

Background
- VAE is the introduction of air bubbles into the venous circulation.
- Risk factors are patient-related, anesthetic-related, and surgery-related.
- Obstetric and gynecologic factors associated with VAE include cesarean section, termination of pregnancy, removal of the placenta, laparoscopic surgery, and use of the Trendelenburg position.
- Morbidity and mortality are dependent on the volume of air entrained and the rate of accumulation.
- A large embolus can produce an "airlock" in the right ventricle resulting in rapid cardiovascular instability and/or cardiac arrest.
- Gradual gas entrainment can lead to microemboli, which can cause increased basement membrane permeability and subsequent pulmonary edema and/or SIRS.

Diagnosis
- Symptoms and signs are non-specific, ranging from subclinical to fatal, and are those of cardiovascular, respiratory, and neurologic dysfunction.
- The classical "millwheel" murmur is a late and insensitive sign.
- TEE is the most sensitive diagnostic tool; however, it is invasive and requires expertise in insertion and interpretation. TTE could be considered.

Prevention
- Identify at-risk patients and consider additional monitoring in high-risk groups (arterial line, CVP line, and TEE or TTE).
- Ensure the patient is adequately hydrated prior to surgery.

- Where possible keep the surgical site below the level of the heart and minimize the time the circulation is open to the atmosphere.

Management

- VAE is a surgical emergency.
- A structured ABCDE approach should be adopted.
- Specific management is targeted at preventing further gas entrainment, preventing central progression, and minimizing cardiovascular effects.
- In a laparoscopic case:
  - Decompress pneumoperitoneum immediately.
  - Reverse Trendelenburg position immediately (i.e., flatten the table).
  - Flood surgical site with sterile saline.
  - Ligate or compress any open vessels.
  - If possible, place the patient in left lateral position.
  - Terminate the operation as soon as it is safe to do so.
- Once the patient is stable arrange transfer to ITU.
- Fully document the event in the patient's notes, complete a critical incident report form, and when possible communicate the event to the patient.

References

1 Yentis SM, Hirsch NP, Smith GB. *Anaesthesia and Intensive Care A–Z: An Encyclopaedia of Principles and Practice*, 4th edn. Churchill Livingstone, London, 2009.

2 Webber S, Andrzejowski J, Francis G. Gas embolism in anaesthesia. *Br J Anaesth CEPD Rev* 2002;2:53–57.

3 Allman KG, Wilson IH. *Oxford Handbook of Anaesthesia*, 3rd edn. Oxford University Press, New York, 2011.

4 Handler JS, Bromage PR. Venous air embolism during cesarean delivery. *Reg Anesth* 1990;15:170–173.

5 Mirski A, Lele AV, Fitzsimmons L, Toung TJ. Diagnosis and treatment of vascular air embolism. *Anesthesiology* 2007;106:164–177.

6 Chandler WF, Dimcheff DG, Taren JA. Acute pulmonary edema following venous air embolism during a neurosurgical procedure. Case report. *J Neurosurg* 1974;40:400–404.

7 Kapoor T, Gutierrez G. Air embolism as a cause of the systemic inflammatory response syndrome. A case report. *Crit Care* 2003;7:R98–R100.

8 Spoors C, Kiff K. *Training in Anaesthesia: The Essential Curriculum*. Oxford University Press, New York, 2010.

CHAPTER 70

Laparoscopy: Problems with Monopolar Diathermy

Thomas G. Lang[1] and Resad Pasic[2]
[1] Bethesda Memorial Hospital, Boynton Beach, Florida, USA
[2] University of Louisville, Louisville, Kentucky, USA

Case history: During a diagnostic laparoscopy for chronic pelvic pain, a patient was found to have many adhesions on the left adnexa and descending colon. She underwent extensive lysis of the adhesions and enterolysis with monopolar scissors. On postoperative day 5 she called her physician's office with complaints of increasing nausea with occasional vomiting. She also noticed that her abdomen has been getting increasingly tender. In the office, her physical examination demonstrated rebound tenderness and she was admitted to the hospital. Her CT scan showed a possible perforation of the bowel, and she underwent a laparoscopy which revealed an area of bowel with obvious thermal injury and perforation. She underwent a bowel resection with colostomy. She improved clinically and was discharged home 5 days later.

Background

Electrosurgical equipment can cause thermal injury for a number of reasons. A good understanding of the basic principles of electrosurgery can drastically reduce this risk. Unfortunately, many surgeons do not have a good understanding of the electrosurgery instruments they use, and therefore increase their potential for thermal injury.

Basics of energy

Instead of electrosurgery, the term "electrocautery" is often used in the operating room, but the use is incorrect. Electrocautery involves the use of a direct current to heat up a metal conductor with a high impedance to flow so that the metal becomes hot. Electrosurgery involves manipulating electrons through living tissue by using an alternating current with enough current density to create heat within a cell to destroy the tissue [1].

To understand the basics of energy, Ohm's law needs to be understood. Ohm's law states that $V = IR$, where V represents voltage, or the force required to push the electrons; I represents current, or the quantitative measurement of this electron flow; and R represents resistance, or the opposition to this flow by the medium. The standard unit of current is amperes (A), or coulombs per second, while the standard unit of resistance is ohms (Ω).

The formula $W = IV$ represents power, or the rate of work being done, measured in watts. This corresponds to the specific power setting that is entered into the electrosurgical generator. This formula can be expressed alternatively using Ohm's law:

$$W = I^2 \times R \text{ or}$$
$$W = V^2 IR$$

It can now be understood why when the electrosurgical generator is set at a specific and constant power (W), applied to tissue with high impedance (R), such as fat or carbonized tissue, that the voltage will increase. This increase in voltage allows an increase in thermal spread and possible adjacent tissue injury.

The electrosurgical generator supplies power. Why then would a patient not experience an electric shock? A typical electrical outlet current oscillates at 50–60 Hz (depending on where in the world you live) which causes depolarization of the neuromuscular junction and can lead to tetanic contractions. This is overcome by electrosurgical generators using a frequency that is greater than 100,000 Hz, more specifically 300–600 kHz. At these frequencies the energy is dissipated, converted into heat by tissue impedance and does not cause tetanic contractions [2]. The circuit involved in monopolar electrosurgery is shown in Figure 70.1.

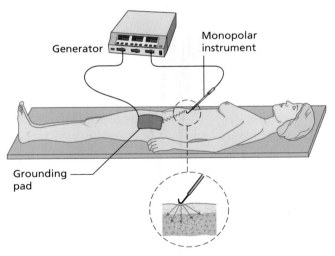

Figure 70.1 Monopolar circuit: the electrosurgical generator, the active electrode, the patient's tissue, the return electrode (grounding pad), and back to the ground in the generator.

Gynecologic and Obstetric Surgery: Challenges and Management Options, First Edition. Edited by Arri Coomarasamy, Mahmood I. Shafi, G. Willy Davila and Kiong K. Chan.
© 2016 John Wiley & Sons, Ltd. Published 2016 by John Wiley & Sons, Ltd.

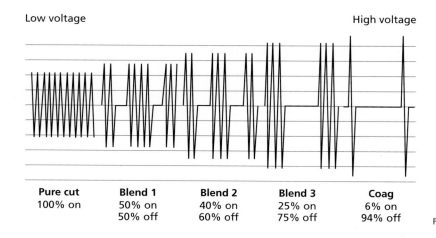

Low voltage   High voltage

Pure cut	Blend 1	Blend 2	Blend 3	Coag
100% on	50% on	40% on	25% on	6% on
	50% off	60% off	75% off	94% off

Figure 70.2 Electrosurgery waveforms.

The original generators relied on grounding from a wall outlet (ground-referenced generators), which had the potential to allow the energy to follow alternative pathways (as it follows the path of least resistance). These could cause burns, and most of the burns were at the site of the return electrode if part of the electrode was peeled off or was not in full contact with the patient. Modern generators use an isolated ground circuitry system. In this type of system, current in the transformers as well as the return current is insulated from the frame of the generator. Unlike ground-referenced systems, these systems will not work if there is a break in the circuit. Another safety feature built into the grounding pads is having two pads that are side by side and which have built-in monitors that can measure contact stability and power density. If there is poor pad-to-skin contact, the generator will not work [1].

Several variables can be altered to achieve different tissue effects when using monopolar electrosurgery, such as changing the waveform, the size or shape of the electrode (power density), and the speed at which the instrument is moved.

- *Waveform.* The power generator has settings for Coag, Cut, and Blend (Figure 70.2). The waveform of the Coag setting is not continuous and is only on 6% of the time; however, it is set to a higher voltage/amplitude. The Cut waveform in comparison is continuous, and because of this the voltage is lower to achieve the same wattage. The Blend waveform is also non-continuous but is on for a longer duration depending on the setting. Blend 1, 2, and 3 are on for 50%, 40%, and 25% of the time, respectively (Figure 70.2). The longer the current is on, the lower the voltage to achieve the same wattage. It is advisable to use the lowest power setting possible to achieve the desired tissue endpoint [2].
- *Surface area.* The tissue effects of coagulation and cutting can be achieved simply by changing the power density or size of the electrode (surface area) used. If the surgeon uses a smaller surface area, cutting will occur; if a larger surface area is used, coagulation occurs.

Prevention

Preoperative measures
The most common complication from monopolar electrosurgery is burns from improper placement of grounding pads. As discussed, split "smart" pads will not allow the generator to work if a proper

ground is not made. Burns in other sites can occur where cardiac monitor leads and body jewellery are located; jewellery should be removed if possible or taped down so that the surface area increases, minimizing any current density. If jewellery is located in a direct line from the surgical field to the grounding electrode and it cannot be removed, the grounding pad should be placed in a different position [2].

If a patient has an implanted electronic device, such as a pacemaker, cochlear implants, or an infusion pump, it is safer to avoid monopolar diathermy and use bipolar diathermy instead (Chapter 71). If monopolar diathermy needs to be used, the return electrode should be placed as far from the implanted device and as close to the surgical site as possible. If the implantable device is an implantable cardioverter defibrillator (ICD), the device should be deactivated beforehand so as to prevent a possible discharge to the patient [3].

Intraoperative measures
Inadvertent thermal injuries from monopolar electrosurgical instruments during laparoscopy are caused by direct coupling, inadvertent tissue contact, insulation failure, or capacitive coupling (Figure 70.3) [4].

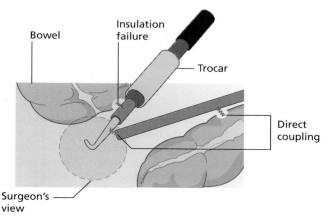

Figure 70.3 Inadvertent thermal injury from monopolar electrosurgical instruments.

Insulation failure

Insulation failure presents a danger in electrosurgery because of the introduction of an alternative current pathway. Smaller breaks are more dangerous than larger breaks because the power density is higher. Insulation failure injuries can be reduced by thorough inspection of the instruments, by limiting high-voltage waveforms, and by decreasing unnecessary removal and entry of the instrument through the trocar.

Direct coupling

When one instrument is active it is important that the surgeon remains vigilant to the location of all instruments and that the appropriate field of view is maintained. When the electrode is activated and a metal accessory instrument is near or touching it, the accessory instrument will become energized as well. This presents a danger because thermal injury can occur to the viscera if the power density is high enough. This type of injury can often go unrecognized because the contact point is often out of the field of view of the surgeon when the injury occurs (Figure 70.3). As with any other thermal injury, the signs of the injury may not be apparent at the time of injury and may present several days following surgery. Injury can occur not only with direct contact to the tissue but also secondary to electrical sparks or arcing.

Capacitive coupling

Capacitive coupling is a known electrical phenomenon where electricity can be capacitated in a secondary conductor when two conductors are separated by an insulator and the primary conductor is charged. This phenomenon occurs in laparoscopic surgery when the electrode in a monopolar device is surrounded by an insulator and introduced through the metal sheath. No insulator is able to completely shield the flow of electrons from the electrode to the surrounding sheath. If the sheath is composed of metal, it may then store energy as a capacitor, and this energy will always be discharged to the abdominal wall. If there is a plastic collar shielding the abdominal wall and isolating the metal sheath, there is a higher capacitive effect, which increases potential for a higher power density since the capacitated electricity is stored in the metal cannula. The possible tissue injury occurs when the cannula touches the bowel. A possible second scenario would be if electrosurgical scissors were introduced through the channel of the operative scope and the scope introduced through a plastic cannula. The risk of tissue injury from capacitive coupling can be minimized by avoiding open circuit activation and by using the lowest power setting necessary to achieve the desired tissue effect [2].

Resolution of the case

The exact mechanism of the thermal injury to the bowel is unclear because the trauma was not recognized during surgery. Any of the mechanisms described in this chapter could be implicated, although in this instance a direct surgical injury is possible given the complexity of the surgery, which involved division of bowel adhesions. The subsequent need for a colostomy highlights the substantial morbidity associated with electrosurgical injuries and emphasizes the need for surgeons to appreciate the scientific and surgical principles underpinning safe practice during laparoscopic surgery.

KEY POINTS

Challenge: Problems of monopolar diathermy during laparoscopy.

Background
- Electrosurgery involves manipulating electrons through living tissue by using an alternating current with enough current density to create heat within a cell to destroy the tissue.
- Several variables can be altered to achieve different tissue effects when using monopolar electrosurgery, such as changing the waveform, the size/shape of the electrode (power density), and the speed with which an instrument is moved.
- The most common inadvertent thermal injuries caused by a monopolar surgical instruments during laparoscopic surgery arise because of:
  - Inadvertent tissue contact.
  - Insulation failure.
  - Direct coupling.
  - Capacitive coupling.

Prevention
- The most common complication from monopolar electrosurgery is return electrode and alternate site burns from improper placement of grounding pads; good pad-to-skin contact should be maintained.
- A modern electrosurgical generator incorporating an isolated ground circuitry system should be used; such a system will not work if there is a break in the circuit.
- Split grounding pads (two pads side by side) should be used because they have built-in monitors that can measure contact stability and power density and will not work if there is poor pad-to-skin contact.
- Insulation failure injuries can be reduced by:
  - Thorough inspection of the instruments.
  - Limiting high-voltage waveforms.
  - Decreasing unnecessary removal and entry of the instrument through the trocar.
- It is advisable to use the lowest power setting possible to achieve the desired tissue endpoint.
- Burns can occur where cardiac monitor leads and body jewellery are located; jewellery should be removed if possible or taped down. If jewellery is located in a direct line from the surgical field to the grounding electrode and it cannot be removed, the grounding pad should be placed in a different position.
- In a patient with an implanted electronic device, such as a pacemaker, cochlear implants, or an infusion pump:
  - Avoid monopolar diathermy and use bipolar diathermy instead (Chapter 71).
  - If monopolar diathermy needs to be used, place the return electrode as far from the implanted device and as close to the surgical site as possible.
  - If the implantable device is an ICD, deactivate the device before surgery (Chapter 5).

References

1 Rock JA, Jones HW (eds) *Te Linde's Operative Gynecology*, 10th edn. Lippincott Williams & Wilkins, Philedelphia, 2008.

2 Brill AI. *Electrosurgery: Principles and Practice.* APGO Educational Series on Women's Health Issues. Association of Professors of Gynecology and Obstetrics, Crofton, MD, 2011.

3 Fickling J, Loeffler CR. Electrosurgery safety update: pacemakers and implantable cardiac defibrillators. *ValleyLab* 2002;7(3).

4 Shirk GJ, Johns A, Redwine DB. Complications of laparoscopic surgery: how to avoid them and how to repair them. *J Minim Invasive Gynecol* 2006;13:352–359.

CHAPTER 71

Laparoscopy: Problems with Bipolar Diathermy

Thomas G. Lang[1] and Resad Pasic[2]
[1] Bethesda Memorial Hospital, Boynton Beach, Florida, USA
[2] University of Louisville, Louisville, Kentucky, USA

Case history: *A woman underwent an uneventful total laparoscopic hysterectomy, and the colpotomy was closed with a series of figure-of-eight sutures. On final inspection it was noted that the right uterine pedicle was oozing. The pedicle was grasped with a bipolar electrosurgical device in an attempt to stop the bleeding. It was noted that the pedicle was still bleeding and a larger grasp of the pedicle was taken and desiccated. Hemostasis was achieved. On postoperative day 6, the patient re-presented complaining of severe back pain on the right. On examination she was found to have tenderness over the right costovertebral angle (loin) and was admitted for further work-up. Her serum creatinine was mildly elevated and a CT scan demonstrated partial obstruction of the right ureter. At surgical repair a thermal injury to the ureter on the right was confirmed.*

Background

Bipolar electrosurgery differs from monopolar electrosurgery in that the only part of the patient's body that is part of the circuit is the tissue between the instrument's graspers. Bipolar instruments are designed to have two opposing electrodes that can grasp the desired tissue that needs to be coagulated. These instruments work by receiving energy from a generator (the same generator used for monopolar devices). This energy is conducted down the two-poled electrode ("bipolar") instrument; the current first passes to one of these electrodes, then passes through the interposing grasped tissue to return to the generator via the opposing electrode (Figure 71.1). Bipolar electrosurgery therefore does not require a large dispersive return electrode to be attached to the patient as in monopolar electrosurgery, and consequently decreases the possibility of cross-interference with implanted electrical devices such as cardiac pacemakers [1]. Because of this bidirectional circuit in the instrument itself, the risks of direct coupling and capacitive coupling are not present in bipolar electrosurgery [2]. Power requirements are also much less than those of monopolar electrosurgery because the distance between the active electrodes is much smaller and therefore the low-voltage "cut" waveform is the default output current. However, this does limit its uses to desiccation and coagulation of tissue [3]. In contrast to monopolar electrodes, the bipolar instrument can readily conduct electricity in saline solution, an advantage used in modern hysteroscopic surgery [3].

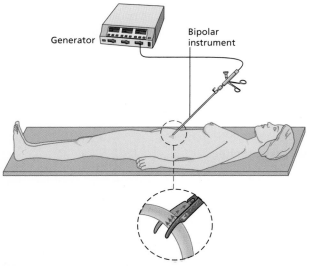

Figure 71.1 A bipolar electrical circuit.

Prevention

Application of bipolar energy

There are several advantages of bipolar electrosurgery. It is a good method for sealing and occluding blood vessels, and because of the limited area of interaction with the tissue and decreased voltage requirements, thermal spread is decreased. Smoke production is also considerably less than that found in monopolar electrosurgery [4]. That said, thermal spread can still occur beyond the electrode paddles. This happens because water is heated during tissue desiccation and percolates into the surrounding tissue. If the energy is continued past the desired endpoint, a secondary thermal bloom may occur that can send steam to the surrounding tissues. Another issue with "overcooking" the tissue is that it can form a carbonized layer and cause the instrument to become stuck to the tissue. A common mistake is that the surgeon uses force to pull the instrument off the tissue, and this often pulls the carbon layer off, causing bleeding to resume. The way to avoid this complication is to prevent carbonization in the first place, by stopping the current when tissue whitens and water vapor is no longer seen [4]. If carbonization does occur, the activated instrument can be

Gynecologic and Obstetric Surgery: Challenges and Management Options, First Edition. Edited by Arri Coomarasamy, Mahmood I. Shafi, G. Willy Davila and Kiong K. Chan.
© 2016 John Wiley & Sons, Ltd. Published 2016 by John Wiley & Sons, Ltd.

removed from the tissue with the current still applied, which allows the generated steam bubbles to aid in dislodging the instrument without tearing the carbonized layer from the desiccated tissue. An ammeter is incorporated into some generator devices to aid in determining the optimal tissue sealing endpoint; however, such generators have been shown to promote over-desiccation. Reliance on the visual cues to judge when tissues are adequately sealed remains the best approach [5].

It must be remembered that when the bipolar device is manipulated in the surgical field after being activated it can still retain a substantial amount of heat. This heat may cause damage to surrounding tissues such as bowel, bladder, and ureter, and may go unrecognized if it occurs out of the surgeon's field of view.

Advanced bipolar instruments

Traditional bipolar devices rely solely on the surgeon's discretion regarding power and "burn time." Newer "smart" bipolar devices have decreased lateral thermal spread and provide a consistently reliable form of hemostasis [3], including the ability to seal vessels up to 7 mm in diameter. However, they do not use traditional generator units and require power from proprietary units. These devices have been referred to as "smart" because they integrate impedance (resistance) feedback technology that can deliver either pulsed or continuous electrical output with constant voltage by only moderating the output current [4]. These devices can therefore create the desired endpoint with considerably less energy delivery.

The Plasmakinetics® Cutting Forceps (Gyrus ACMI, a division of Olympus Corporation) constantly receives resistance information from the tissue, and delivers pulsed energy using traditional tissue grasping. This is a common energy device used in robotics. Another device from Olympus called Thunderbeat® integrates advanced bipolar technology and ultrasonic energy to form a device that can provide controlled rapid dissections and reliably seal vessels. It also has the added feature of using the advanced bipolar mode alone for hemostasis without cutting if so desired.

The Ligasure® Vessel Sealing Device differs from traditional bipolar technology; not only does it utilize impedance feedback and low constant voltage, but it differs in instrument design as it has a jaw that is shaped similarly to Heaney forceps. This allows the development of large amounts of coaptive pressure to the tissue. The mixture of impedance feedback and high mechanical pressure makes this device a good vessel sealer [4]. A version of the Ligasure® device is also equipped with a monopolar tip to aid in dissection and formation of a colpotomy during a total laparoscopic hysterectomy.

Management

While there have been many devices created to decrease unwanted tissue endpoints, the surgeon must have a good understanding of how the instruments work and how to troubleshoot the instruments given instrument error. The area undergoing treatment should be adequately visualized to precisely apply bipolar energy and the surgeon should appreciate the margins of thermal spread, even with advanced "smart" bipolar technologies.

In the case history, the ureter was thermally damaged during retreatment of the bleeding right uterine vascular pedicle. The ureter is in close proximity to the uterine artery, especially when the uterine vessels retract within the pelvic sidewall. If the ureter cannot be visualized at an adequate distance away from the bleeding vessel, then retroperitoneal dissection into the broad ligament is necessary to identify the ureter so that it can be displaced away from the bleeding uterine vessels (Chapter 36). Only then should the bleeding tissues be grasped and bipolar electrical energy applied to achieve hemostasis.

KEY POINTS

Challenge: Problems with bipolar diathermy during laparoscopy.

Background
- Bipolar electrosurgery differs from monopolar electrosurgery in that the only part of the patient's body that is part of the circuit is the tissue grasped within the forceps of the instrument.
- Because of this bidirectional circuit in the instrument itself, the risks of direct coupling and capacitive coupling are not present in bipolar electrosurgery.
- The bipolar instrument can readily conduct electricity in saline or non-electrolyte solutions.

Prevention
- Use bipolar energy. Compared with monopolar energy, bipolar diathermy is a better method for sealing and occluding blood vessels, and because of the limited area of interaction with the tissue and decreased voltage requirements, thermal spread is decreased.
- Do not overtreat the tissues. If the energy is continued past the desired endpoint, a secondary thermal bloom may occur that can send steam to the surrounding tissues, risking thermal injury. "Overcooking" the tissue can also form a carbonized layer and cause the instrument to become stuck to the tissue.
- Maintain visualization and appreciate thermal spread margins. When the bipolar device is manipulated in the surgical field after being activated it can still retain a substantial amount of heat. This heat may cause damage to surrounding tissues such as bowel, bladder, and ureter, and may go unrecognized if it occurs out of the surgeon's field of view.

Management
- Familiarity with bipolar instrumentation. There are a number of instruments available that each have their own subtleties. The surgeon must have a good understanding of how the instruments work and how to troubleshoot the instruments given instrument error.
- Good surgical technique is of paramount importance. Understanding the anatomy of the female pelvis and being proficient in tissue dissection to precisely identify and isolate bleeding vessels is crucial in avoiding inadvertent thermal injury to closely approximated vital pelvic structures such as the ureter.

References

1 Harrell AG. Energy sources in laparoscopy. *Semin Laparosc Surg* 2004;11:201–209.
2 Odell RC. Pearls, pitfalls and advancement in the delivery of electrosurgical energy during laparoscopy. *Probl Gen Surg* 2002;19:5–17.
3 Brill AI. Bipolar electrosurgery: convention and innovation. *Clin Obstet Gynecol* 2008;51:153–158.
4 Brill AI. *Electrosurgery: Principles and Practice*. APGO Educational Series on Women's Health Issues. Association of Professors of Gynecology and Obstetrics, Crofton, MD, 2011.
5 Phipps JH. Thermometry studies with bipolar diathermy during hysterectomy. *Gynaecol Laparosc* 1994;3:5–7.

CHAPTER 72
Laparoscopy: Bladder Injury

Peter L. Rosenblatt
Mount Auburn Hospital, Cambridge, Massachusetts, USA

Case history: A woman with heavy menstrual bleeding and a fibroid uterus elected to have a total laparoscopic hysterectomy. She has a history of three cesarean deliveries, and the bladder was found to be densely adherent to the lower uterine segment. The surgeon found mobilization of the bladder difficult and was concerned about making an inadvertent cystotomy.

Background

Estimates of bladder injury during gynecologic laparoscopic surgery range between 0.2 and 8.3% [1,2]. Compared with open hysterectomy, laparoscopic hysterectomy has a higher incidence of cystotomy, with some studies reporting a greater than twofold higher risk of urinary tract injury [3,4]. This rate is dependent on many factors, including complexity of the laparoscopic procedure, patient pathology, and whether cystoscopy is performed.

Although bladder injuries are more likely to be identified intraoperatively than ureteral injuries, the true rate of bladder injuries is unknown due to the difficulty in identifying these injuries during the perioperative period. Lack of intraoperative diagnosis can lead to significant morbidity, including the need for additional procedures, loss of renal function, and even fistula formation [1,5].

Iatrogenic bladder injuries most often occur during laparoscopic-assisted vaginal hysterectomy (LAVH) compared with other gynecologic laparoscopic procedures [6]. This is thought to be secondary to electrosurgical dissection and most commonly occurs at the bladder dome [2]. Patients with a history of previous cesarean delivery are at higher risk of cystotomy during an LAVH [7]. Trocar injury is another cause of bladder damage during laparoscopy. The injury can occur with either primary trocar placement (usually when the surgeon fails to empty the bladder before placing the trocar) or secondary suprapubic trocar placement. Thermal injuries can also affect the bladder with procedures such as endometriosis surgery in the anterior cul-de-sac [6]. Foreign bodies such as tacks, staples, or permanent sutures introduced during laparoscopy can also cause bladder damage.

Prevention

Prevention can be at three levels: primary prevention is aimed at avoiding the injury; secondary prevention is intraoperative recognition and repair; tertiary prevention is postoperative diagnosis and treatment of urinary tract injury, and therefore the least desirable form of prevention of long-term sequelae [8]. Although bladder injury can occur with any laparoscopic procedure, there are risk factors that increase the likelihood of these complications and these should be identified before the procedure to allow for primary and secondary prevention.

Primary prevention

Operative set-up is important in primary prevention. Patients should be positioned in dorsal lithotomy to allow access to the urinary tract for possible cystoscopy or vaginal manipulation. Bladder injury during laparoscopy is most likely to occur when the bladder is not being properly drained; urinary bladder volumes as small as 100 mL can increase the risk of bladder injury during laparoscopy. Bladder catheterization should be performed prior to beginning any laparoscopic procedure and strong consideration should be given to the use of an indwelling catheter. Another advantage of placing an indwelling catheter is the ability to retrofill the bladder if it becomes difficult to delineate its margins during surgery. This technique can be used during procedures that require the bladder to be mobilized off the lower uterine segment, as with hysterectomy, or off the vaginal cuff, as with laparoscopic sacrocolpopexy. Adding a dye such as indigo carmine to the fluid back-filled into the bladder can also assist in preventing or detecting bladder injury as the dye can usually be seen under the bladder if the dissection plane is too close to the mucosa.

Visualization is paramount during surgical dissection and factors such as bleeding and adhesions can obscure or distort normal anatomic landmarks. Meticulous attention to hemostasis is essential to permit proper visualization throughout laparoscopic surgery. When lysing adhesions between the bladder and other structures such as the anterior abdominal wall, a sharp dissection technique should be used to avoid tearing of the bladder with excessive tension. Hydrodissection is another common technique used to prevent bladder injuries if the surgeon needs to excise

Gynecologic and Obstetric Surgery: Challenges and Management Options, First Edition. Edited by Arri Coomarasamy, Mahmood I. Shafi, G. Willy Davila and Kiong K. Chan.
© 2016 John Wiley & Sons, Ltd. Published 2016 by John Wiley & Sons, Ltd.

or coagulate endometriosis overlying the bladder. A small cut is made in the peritoneum and an irrigating instrument is placed through the incision. This will separate the peritoneum from the underlying structure, allowing for safer removal of endometriosis lesions.

Secondary prevention (see Chapter 35)

Intraoperative recognition of bladder injuries reduces morbidity associated with complications such as urine ascites, bladder stone formation, recurrent urinary tract infection, voiding dysfunction, or even fistula formation. Easily recognized intraoperative signs that should lead the surgeon to suspect bladder injury include urine leakage from the cystotomy or cannula site or the presence of air in the Foley bag. Hematuria is certainly a sign that should prompt intraoperative investigation to rule out urinary tract injury.

A bladder perforation injury can be confirmed during laparoscopy by instilling indigo carmine-stained solution or sterile milk in a retrograde manner through the catheter and observing spillage through the cystotomy. This also allows precise localization of the injured area. Inability to distend the bladder with 200–300 mL is another sign of bladder perforation. With a larger cystotomy, the bladder mucosa, Foley balloon, or trigone may be directly visualized with the laparoscope. If injury is suspected near the trigone, alternative techniques can be used to better visualize the injured area laparoscopically. Wohlrab *et al.* [9] describe creating an intentional cystotomy at the bladder dome, then placing a pursestring suture around the intentional cystotomy and tightening it around the laparoscope to allow further distension and better visualization of the injured area. This also allows the surgeon to place a suprapubic catheter if desired. Bladder injury near the trigone may require ureteral stenting in order to avoid kinking or obstructing the ureter(s) during the repair. Cystoscopy can also be performed to check for the presence of bladder injuries.

Tertiary prevention

Unfortunately, the majority of bladder injuries are not diagnosed intraoperatively [1]. Delayed bladder injuries should be considered when patients complain of malaise, lethargy, nausea, vomiting, or abdominal pain. Oliguria or anuria may also be reported by the patient. On examination, the patient's abdomen may be distended from urinary ascites or a urinoma, in which urine collects retroperitoneally after procedures such as a Burch or paravaginal repair. Laboratory results often will be notable for elevated serum renal function tests. A trial of conservative therapy with continuous bladder drainage should be attempted to allow spontaneous closure of the bladder defect prior to surgical intervention. These patients should also be monitored closely for infection or ileus [9].

Vesicovaginal fistulae generally develop during the first few weeks after surgery but can occur in the immediate postoperative period. Fistulae should be suspected in any postoperative patient with a new complaint of urinary leakage or constant vaginal discharge. There are several ways to diagnose this complication, including cystoscopy, intravenous pyelogram, or a tampon test. The tampon test consists of placing a tampon in the vagina and back-filling the bladder with indigo carmine-stained saline through a Foley catheter. The patient walks for at least 10 min and the tampon is then removed and examined; if blue fluid is located on the proximal end of the tampon, this confirms a vesicovaginal fistula.

Management (see Chapter 35)

Management of a bladder injury depends on the type of injury (thermal or perforation), size, location, and timing of diagnosis. Cystotomies up to 10 mm in size, often resulting from needles and laparoscopic trocars, have been successfully treated with bladder drainage for 7–14 days postoperatively [10]. To confirm bladder integrity after continuous drainage, a retrograde cystogram can be performed prior to catheter removal. Alternatively, a preformed suture loop (e.g., Endoloop®) can be used laparoscopically for injuries less than 5 mm in size. The tissue is elevated with a laparoscopic grasper and the suture loop is placed around the defect in the bladder. Bladder integrity is tested with retrograde filling through an indwelling catheter [11]. A catheter should remain for 7–10 days after the repair and can be followed by retrograde cystogram to confirm healing.

Transperitoneal cystotomies greater than 10 mm should always be treated by primary surgical repair. This repair can be open or laparoscopic depending on the surgeon's preference. Numerous case reports and series have demonstrated the effectiveness of laparoscopic repairs [12,13]. In addition, laparoscopic repair has the benefit of a shorter recovery period, improved cosmesis, and often better visualization. As with secondary prevention, the first step in the repair of a bladder injury is to determine the location of the injury, particularly in relation to the trigone and ureteral openings. The surgeon should also remove any necrotic tissue, adhesions, or endometriosis before repairing the defect.

Either polyglactin (Vicryl) or polydioxanone (PDS) sutures can be used in an interrupted or continuous full-thickness manner to repair the bladder injury. Previous teaching recommended closing the bladder wall in two layers, mucosa and muscularis [12]. More recently, a one-layer mass closure with incorporation of mucosa, muscularis, and serosa has been reported with success [13,14,15].

In order to facilitate laparoscopic suturing, devices such as Lapra-Ty® can be used if the surgeon has difficulty with laparoscopic knot tying. Orvieto *et al.* [16] used porcine models to demonstrate the safety of the Lapra-Ty in cystotomy repair. They found fibrous capsules surrounding the Lapra-Ty at 8 weeks postoperatively and no incidences of migration or erosion into the bladder. The literature regarding the use of V-Loc barbed suture (Covidien, Mansfield, MA) and Quill self-retaining suture (Angiotech Pharmaceuticals, Vancouver, BC, Canada) in cystotomy repair is sparse, and therefore the use of these materials is not yet recommended.

Cystoscopy should be performed at the completion of the repair to confirm ureteral integrity and watertight closure. Again, the bladder should be drained for 7–14 days after repair, and this may be followed by a retrograde cystogram to confirm healing. A non-watertight closure and inadequate postoperative drainage are additional risk factors for fistula formation [9]. If there is leakage on cystogram, the bladder should be allowed an additional week of continuous drainage.

KEY POINTS

Challenge: Bladder injury during laparoscopy (see also Chapter 35).

Background
- Estimates of bladder injury during gynecologic laparoscopic surgery range between 0.2 and 8.3%.
- Iatrogenic bladder injuries most often occur during laparoscopic-assisted vaginal hysterectomy.

Prevention
- Arrange appropriate preoperative planning including adequate patient history and necessary imaging studies.
- Position the patient in dorsal lithotomy and have an indwelling catheter during surgery.
- Pay meticulous attention to hemostasis to allow adequate visualization.
- Have a low threshold for cystoscopy.

Management
- Identify the location of the bladder injury and its relation to the trigone and ureters.
- Cystotomies up to 10 mm in size can be treated with 7–14 days of continuous bladder drainage.
- Cystotomies greater than 10 mm can be repaired with a one-layer mass closure with absorbable suture, or with a two-layer closure.
- Repairs should be watertight.
- Prior to removal of Foley catheter, retrograde cystogram should be obtained to confirm healing.

References

1 Gilmour DT, Das S, Flowerdew G. Rates of urinary tract injury from gynecologic surgery and the role of intraoperative cystoscopy. *Obstet Gynecol* 2006;107:1366–1372.

2 Ostrzenski A, Ostrzenska KM. Bladder injury during laparoscopic surgery. *Obstet Gynecol Surv* 1998;53:175–180.

3 Hulka JF, Levy BS, Parker WH *et al.* Laparoscopic-assisted vaginal hysterectomy: American Association of Gynecologic Laparoscopist's 1995 membership survey. *J Am Assoc Gynecol Laparosc* 1997;4:2–6.

4 Johnson N, Barlow D, Lethaby A, Tavender E, Curr L, Garry R. Methods of hysterectomy: systematic review and meta-analysis of randomized controlleld trials. *BMJ* 2005;330:1478.

5 Gilmour DT, Baskett TF. Disability and litigation from urinary tract injuries at benign gynecologic surgery in Canada. *Obstet Gynecol* 2005;105:109–114.

6 Shirk GJ, Johns A, Redwine DB. Complications of laparoscopic surgery: how to avoid them and how to repair them. *J Minim Invasive Gynecol* 2006;13:352–359.

7 Rooney CM, Cawford AT, Vassallo BJ, Kleeman SD, Karram MM. Is previous cesarean section a risk for incidental cystotomy at time of hysterectomy? A case-controlled study. *Am J Obstet Gynecol* 2005;193:2041–2044.

8 Thompson JD. Operative injuries to the ureter: prevention, recognition, and management. In: RockJA, ThompsonJD (eds) *Te Linde's Operative Gynecology*, 8th edn, pp. 1135–1174. Lippincott-Raven, Philadelphia, 1997.

9 Wohlrab KJ, Sung VW, Rardin CR. Management of laparoscopic bladder injuries. *J Minim Invasive Gynecol* 2011;18:4–8.

10 Angle HS, Young SB. Conservative management of incidental cystotomy at laparoscopy: a report of two cases. *J Reprod Med* 1995;40:809–812.

11 Azziz R, Murphy AA. *Practical Manual of Operative Laparoscopy and Hysteroscopy*, 2nd edn. Springer-Verlag, New York, 1997.

12 Taskin O, Wheeler JM. Laparoscopic repair of bladder injury and laceration. *J Am Assoc Gynecol Laparosc* 1995;2:227–229.

13 Nezhat CH, Seidman DS, Nezhat F, Rottenberg H, Nezhat C. Laparoscopic management of intentional and unintention cystotomy. *J Urol* 1996;156:1400–1402.

14 Amuzu BJ. Single-layer closure of a bladder laceration during laparoscopy. A case report. *J Reprod Med* 1998;43:593–594.

15 Kim FJ, Chammas MF Jr, Geweher EV, Campagna A, Moore EE. Laparoscopic management of intraperitoneal bladder rupture secondary to blunt abdominal trauma using intracorporeal single layer suturing technique. *J Trauma Injury Infect Crit Care* 2008;65:234–236.

16 Orvieto MA, Lotan T, Lyon MB *et al.* Assessment of the LapraTy clip for facilitating reconstructive laparoscopic surgery in a porcine model. *Urology* 2007;69:582–585.

CHAPTER 73

Laparoscopy: Ureteric Injury

Peter L. Rosenblatt

Mount Auburn Hospital, Cambridge, Massachusetts, USA

Case history: During a total laparoscopic hysterectomy, the patient is found to have significant endometriosis and adhesions in the pelvis. The surgeon is unable to identify the ureter on the left side during the dissection and is concerned about a possible ureteric injury.

Background

The incidence of ureteric injury during laparoscopic gynecologic surgery is estimated to be less than 1%, although some studies report rates up to 2% [1,2,3]. Published data have shown a higher risk of ureteric injury with laparoscopic hysterectomies compared with open or vaginal approaches [4,5], although this apparently increased risk is not universally accepted. For example, a prospective analysis conducted in 2005 demonstrated that the incidence of ureteric injury is similar whether laparoscopic, open, or vaginal hysterectomy is performed [6]. In a membership survey of the American Association of Gynecologic Laparoscopists (AAGL) in 1995, ureteric injury was found to occur at a rate of 3 per 1000 laparoscopic-assisted hysterectomies [7].

Anatomy of the ureters

Anatomic consideration is essential not only for the performance of advanced laparoscopic procedures, but also to reduce the likelihood of intraoperative complications. Each ureter measures 25–30 cm in length. The ureters are divided into abdominal and pelvic components, which are approximately equal in length. The abdominal ureters course along the anterior surface of the psoas muscles retroperitoneally and enter the pelvis by crossing over the bifurcation of the common iliac vessels at the pelvic brim. Each ureter courses superficially along the medial leaf of the broad ligament. The ureters then pass under the uterine artery in a connective tissue tunnel within the cardinal ligament, about 1.5 cm lateral to the cervix, and finally enter the bladder at the trigone.

The blood supply to the ureter is variable and can include branches directly from the aorta in addition to renal, ovarian, and internal iliac arteries. Histologically, the ureter has an inner transitional epithelial layer, a middle muscle layer, and an outer layer of adventitial tissue, which contains the arterial blood supply, nerve supply, and lymphatics.

Prevention

Identification of the ureters

The first step to prevent ureteric injury during laparoscopy is identification of the course of the ureter. This should be done at the start of the procedure because later on the peritoneum becomes more opaque, making structures difficult to identify. The ureter is found along the pelvic sidewall, anterior to the uterosacral ligaments, and posterior to the adnexa. If the ureter cannot be identified on the pelvic sidewall, it is often helpful to examine the pelvic brim, where the ureter crosses over the bifurcation of the common iliac artery, and trace its path more distally. The left ureter is often more difficult to identify than the right because of congenital adhesions of the descending colon to the pelvic sidewall. Visualization of peristalsis can help confirm identification of the ureter.

The ureter can also be identified in the retroperitoneal space if transperitoneal detection is difficult. This space can be entered by making an incision in the peritoneum, lateral and parallel to the infundibulopelvic ligament and bluntly dissecting the retroperitoneal connective tissue until the ureter is visualized. This identification will help prevent ureteric damage during infundibulopelvic ligament ligation. During a hysterectomy, adequate skeletonization of the uterine vessel at the level of the cardinal ligaments and cranial deviation of the uterus will help lateralize the ureters from the area of coagulation and transection.

Risk reduction

Multiple risk factors can increase the chance of a ureteric injury, and these should be identified prior to, and during, the procedure. As in open surgery, bleeding can obscure anatomic landmarks, and in an effort to achieve hemostasis, inadvertent clamping or suture ligation may fully or partially obstruct the ureter. For this reason, meticulous attention to hemostasis is essential for proper visualization.

Pelvic infections, endometriosis, or tumors can also distort anatomy and may involve important structures such as the ureters. These pathologies can also lead to scarring of tissue, making dissection and visualization difficult. Other risk factors include congenital genitourinary tract abnormalities such as duplicated collecting systems and ectopic ureters. Among high-risk patients, preoperative

Gynecologic and Obstetric Surgery: Challenges and Management Options, First Edition. Edited by Arri Coomarasamy, Mahmood I. Shafi, G. Willy Davila and Kiong K. Chan.
© 2016 John Wiley & Sons, Ltd. Published 2016 by John Wiley & Sons, Ltd.

imaging of the genitourinary tract may be helpful (Chapter 36). However, it is important to recognize that most cases of ureteral injury have no identifiable predisposing risk factors [8].

Ureteral stenting

When there is concern about identifying the ureter, particularly in cases where normal anatomy has been distorted, ureteric stents can be considered [9]. Although they carry minimal morbidity and take on average less than 10 min to insert, their usefulness is questionable [10]. Routine use of stents is not recommended as complications such as infection and damage to the ureters from the stents themselves can occur [11]. A randomized controlled trial of nearly 3000 major gynecologic operations found no significant difference in the incidence of ureteric injury between patients who underwent prophylactic ureteral catheterization and those who did not [12]. Lighted stents (see Chapter 32, Figure 32.1) are helpful in visualizing the ureter as it courses along the pelvic sidewall; however, the light is usually not visible as the ureter enters the cardinal ligament.

Surgical techniques

Often the surgeon needs to treat a lesion of endometriosis or malignancy in proximity to the course of the ureter. In such cases, the surgeon can make a peritoneal relaxing incision between the lesion and the ureter, with or without hydrodissection, to provide more distance between the lesion and the ureter. This allows separation between the lesion and the ureter. This technique can also be used for uterosacral ligament suspension for prolapse if the ureter lies close to the ligament.

Management (see Chapter 36)

Detection

Injury to the ureter most often occurs at one of three locations in open or laparoscopic surgery: (i) near the infundibulopelvic ligament, (ii) within the cardinal ligament at the level of the uterine artery, and (iii) at the anterolateral fornix of the vagina [13]. Early recognition of ureteric injury significantly reduces morbidity associated with this complication. Unfortunately, only approximately one-third of the injuries are recognized intraoperatively [14].

Cystoscopy is an important tool for the surgeon to identify possible ureteric compromise intraoperatively. In a prospective study of 471 hysterectomies undertaken for benign disease in 2004, visual inspection only identified one out of the eight ureteric injuries that were recognized on cystoscopy [6]. Intravenous indigo carmine can be administered by the anesthetist during surgery, which facilitates identification of ureteric function during cystoscopy. In most cases, a 30° or 70° cystoscope is necessary to visualize the ureteric orifices. Visualization of brisk blue jets of urine from each orifice confirms ureteric patency, but does not rule out delayed injury from thermal damage. If ureteric jets are not visualized bilaterally, the surgeon should suspect obstruction and take the necessary steps to relieve the obstruction. In cases such as uterosacral ligament suspension, removal of suspected sutures can be undertaken and repeat cystoscopy should confirm ureteric

patency. If ureteric function is still not visualized after removal of sutures, a retrograde pyelogram or placement of ureteric stents can be performed with the involvement of a urologist. Early recognition of injury often allows for more conservative treatment when compared with delayed diagnosis [15].

When ureteric injury is not diagnosed intraoperatively, patients may re-present with symptoms of flank pain, fevers, chills, or signs of peritonitis within several days after surgery. Urinalysis may reveal hematuria and/or leukocytosis. Patients should be imaged with either intravenous urography (IVU) or CT to determine whether a partial or complete obstruction is present, and to identify its location. There have also been reports of ureterovaginal fistulae complicating laparoscopic hysterectomy [16]. Immediate treatment following diagnosis may not be possible, and the patient will often undergo retrograde ureteric catheter placement if possible and/or nephrostomy drainage prior to later repair [13].

Treatment (see Chapter 36)

In most cases, a urologist should be consulted when a ureteric injury is suspected. Injuries identified intraoperatively can usually be treated immediately. Minor injuries such as partial ligation and some crush injuries of the ureter can often be treated with temporary ureteric stent placement followed by an IVU at 6 weeks with stent removal if IVU is normal [13]. When repairing a ureteric injury, care should be taken to avoid compromising the ureteric blood supply during dissection. Some authors have described using an omental flap over the injured site to help promote healing and vascularity [17]. All repairs should be made tension-free to ensure proper healing [18].

Complete ligation, crush injuries, or thermal injuries are most often repaired with resection followed by immediate or delayed re-anastomosis. The re-anastomosis location depends on the level of injury. Distal injuries in the pelvic ureter can be repaired with ureteroneocystostomy (Chapter 36). Sometimes a psoas hitch, in which the bladder is sewn to the psoas tendon, may be needed to add length and ensure a tension-free repair (see Figure 36.3). A ureteroureterostomy is often appropriate for injuries in the middle third of the ureter, with care taken to ensure a tension-free repair and use of a Boari flap if needed. A Boari flap consists of tubularizing a full-thickness flap of the bladder wall to bridge the gap from the injured ureter (see Figure 36.4). The ureteral ends that are eventually reapproximated should be spatulated at a 45° angle to help with approximation and decrease the risk of stenosis [17]. Similarly, injuries to the upper third of the ureter are also repaired via ureteroureterostomy.

Trans-ureteroureterostomy (see Figure 36.5) should be avoided if possible given concern for damage to both ureters. Typically, repairs are done over double-J catheters to aid suturing. These stents generally remain in place for 4–6 weeks. Following the closure, a drain is placed near the anastomotic site and is removed when the output is low (<50 mL over 24 hours) or when the creatinine level in the drain is equal to serum creatinine [18]. Ureteric repairs can often be safely accomplished laparoscopically [18]. When a repair is not possible, a last resort treatment is a nephrectomy. Delayed recognition injuries generally require 6 weeks of tissue healing with percutaneous nephrostomy tubes until repair is attempted [9].

KEY POINTS

Challenge: Ureteric injury during laparoscopy.

Background

- Ureteric injuries are estimated to occur in less than 1 to 2% of all laparoscopic gynecologic procedures.
- Knowledge of the anatomic course of the ureter is helpful for avoiding injury.

Prevention

- The ureter should be identified as early as possible during laparoscopic surgery.
- When the ureter cannot be identified transperitoneally, the retroperitoneal space should be opened to find it.

- Risk factors for injury include bleeding, endometriosis or other factors that obscure normal anatomy, and anatomic genitourinary anomalies. However, the majority of injuries occur in patients without any identifiable risk factors.
- Ureteric stents should not be used routinely but can be considered in cases where the ureter is difficult to identify.

Management

- When possible, intraoperative identification of the injury is preferred, and cystoscopy is a useful (though not foolproof) test for injury identification.
- Delayed injuries typically present 7–10 days following surgery with flank pain, fevers, hematuria, and leukocytosis.
- Repair of ureteric injuries usually requires urologic consultation and may be done using minimally invasive surgical techniques.
- See Chapter 36 for surgical approaches to repair of ureteric injury.

References

1 Tamussino KF, Lang PF, Brein E. Ureteral complications with operative gynecologic laparoscopy. *Am J Obstet Gynecol* 1998;178:967–970.

2 Oztrzenski A, Radolinski B, Ostrzenska KM. A review of laparoscopic ureteral injury in pelvic surgery. *Obstet Gynecol Surv* 2003;58:794–799.

3 Saidi MH, Sadler RK, Vancaillie TG, Akright BD, Farhart SA, White AJ. Diagnosis and management of serious urinary complications after major operative laparoscopy. *Obstet Gynecol* 1996;87:272–276.

4 Härrki-Sirén P, Sjöberg J, Tiitinen A. Urinary tract injuries after hysterectomy. *Obstet Gynecol* 1998;92:113–118.

5 Garry R, Fountain J, Mason S et al. The eVALuate study: two parallel randomised trials, one comparing laparoscopic with abdominal hysterectomy, the other comparing laparoscopic with vaginal hysterectomy. *BMJ* 2004;328:129.

6 Vakili B Chesson RR, Kyle BL et al. The incidence of urinary tract injury during hysterectomy: a prospective analysis based on universal cystoscopy. *Am J Obstet Gynecol* 2005;192:1599–1604.

7 Hulk JF, Levy BS, Parker WH et al. Laparoscopoic-assisted vaginal hysterectomy: American Association of Gynecologic Laparoscopist's 1995 membership survey. *J Am Assoc Gynecol Laparosc* 1997;4:2–6.

8 Liapis A, Bakas P, Giannopoulos V, Creatsas G. Ureteral injury in gynecologic surgery. *Int Urogynecol J* 2001;12:391–394.

9 Manoucheri E, Cohen SL, Sandberg EM, Kibel AS, Einarsson J. Ureteral injury in laparoscopic gynecologic surgery. *Rev Obstet Gynecol* 2012;5:106–111.

10 Tanaka Y, Asada H, Kuji N, Yoshimura Y. Ureteral catheter placement for prevention of ureteral injury during laparoscopic hysterectomy. *J Obstet Gynaecol Res* 2008;34:67–72.

11 Wood ED, Maher P, Pelosi MA. Routine use of ureteric catheters at laparoscopic hysterectomy may cause unnecessary complications. *J Minim Invasive Gynecol* 1995;3:393–397.

12 Chou MT, Want CJ, Lien RC. Prophylactic ureteral catheterization in a gynecologic surgery: a 12-year randomized trial in a community hospital. *Int Urogynecol J* 2009;20:689–693.

13 Chan JK, Marrow J, Manetta A. Prevention of ureteral injuries in gynecologic surgery. *Am J Obstet Gynecol* 2003;188:1273–1277.

14 Drake MJ, Noble JG. Ureteric trauma in gynecologic surgery. *Int Urogynecol J* 1998;9:108–117.

15 Wu HH, Yang PY, Yeh GP, Chou PH, Hsu JC, Lin KC. The detection of ureteral injuries after hysterectomy. *J Minim Invasive Gynecol* 20016;13:403–408.

16 Nouira Y, Oueslati H, Reziga H, Horchani A. Ureterovaginal fistulas complicating laparoscopic hysterectomy: a report of two cases. *Eur J Obstet Gynecol Reprod Biol* 2001;96:132–134.

17 Tulikangas PK, Goldberg JM, Gill IS. Laparoscopic repair of ureteral transection. *J Am Assoc Gynecol Laparosc* 2000;7:415–416.

18 Cholkeri-Singh A, Narepalem N, Miller CE. Laparoscopic ureteral injury and repair: case reviews and clinical update. *J Minim Invasive Gynecol* 2007;14:356–361.

CHAPTER 74

Bowel Injury During Laparoscopy: Intraoperative Presentation

Alan Lam

Center for Advanced Reproductive Endosurgery, University of Sydney, St Leonards, Australia

Case history: A woman underwent laparoscopy for assessment of chronic pelvic pain. She had previously undergone two laparoscopies for treatment of endometriosis, and a vertical midline laparotomy for myomectomy. The surgeon chose to perform a visual entry at the left upper quadrant using an optical trocar. Although seemingly certain of the abdominal wall layers under direct vision, the surgeon recognized the view of the bowel lumen (Figure 74.1).

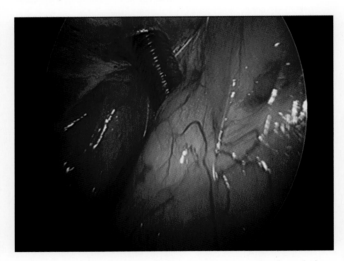

Figure 74.1 Laparoscopic view of a 5-mm trocar penetrating through the wall of large bowel which is adherent to the anterior abdominal wall.

Background

Bowel injury is an uncommon but serious risk of laparoscopic surgery, with a reported incidence varying from 0.1% in diagnostic to 0.5% in operative laparoscopy. As less than half of the injuries are recognized during surgery, the intrinsic fear is that a delay in diagnosis can result in the consequent risks of peritonitis, septicemia, multiorgan failure, and death.

It is estimated that up to half of traumatic bowel injuries occur during the insertion of Veress needle, trocar, or a secondary port. Patients with a history of laparotomies, intra-abdominal or pelvic adhesions, inflammatory bowel conditions, severe endometriosis, and extremes of BMI are particularly at risk. The remainder may

be due to bowel trauma during surgery, adhesiolysis, excision of endometriosis, removal of entrapped ovaries, or from delayed thermal injuries from energy sources, herniation though port sites or leakage after bowel resection.

Large bowel injury is generally associated with greater morbidity than small bowel injury due to the higher bacterial density from the colon. A high index of clinical awareness along with prompt recognition and appropriate management are key factors in the prevention and avoidance of serious complications and death from bowel injuries (Chapter 37).

Management (see Chapter 37)

Recognition of bowel injury

The case history illustrates that it remains possible to injure the loops of bowel adherent to the anterior abdominal wall despite taking precautions; in this case, selection of the left upper quadrant as an alternative site to the umbilicus for insertion of the primary port, and the use of an optical trocar for entry under direct vision, did not prevent an injury. Hence, in every diagnostic or operative laparoscopy, the surgeon should routinely inspect the bowels and this should be carried out not only during first entry, but also during exchange of instrumentation, during adhesiolysis, and at the completion of the laparoscopic procedure. The surgeon should also be aware that bowel injury may occur outside the field of surgery, from bowel retraction or stray electrical current. The surgeon should therefore be vigilant for the possibility of bowel injury at all times during laparoscopy, no matter whether entering the abdomen using a closed or open entry technique.

Steps after recognizing the bowel injury

Once a bowel injury is recognized, there are several decisions that the surgeon needs to make: (i) whether to repair the injury or to call for assistance from a colorectal surgeon; (ii) whether to undertake the repair laparoscopically or via a laparotomy; and (iii) whether to proceed with the originally planned surgery, to postpone it, or to re-evaluate the ongoing indication for the procedure in light of the enhanced risks. Outside of these surgical considerations, intravenous antibiotics should be administered promptly to minimize infective sequelae.

Gynecologic and Obstetric Surgery: Challenges and Management Options, First Edition. Edited by Arri Coomarasamy, Mahmood I. Shafi, G. Willy Davila and Kiong K. Chan.
© 2016 John Wiley & Sons, Ltd. Published 2016 by John Wiley & Sons, Ltd.

Repairing through a laparotomy

In order to facilitate easy identification of the injured bowel, many surgeons would recommend approaching the injured loop of bowel through a laparotomy, with the trocar left *in situ*. Once inside the abdominal cavity, the injured loop of bowel should be carefully dissected and mobilized using fine, sharp dissecting scissors such as Metzenbaum scissors. Care should be taken to exclude a "through-and-through" bowel injury and to avoid causing further injury to other adherent loops of bowels.

If the injury involves the serosal layer only, this may not need to be repaired. Where the injury extends to muscularis layer, the seromuscular layer can be repaired with a continuous or interrupted 4-0 silk or PDS suture on a small tapered needle in one layer. For full-thickness bowel perforation, the repair should be completed in two layers using similar suture materials. It is important to ensure that the suture line is perpendicular to the bowel length, to avoid narrowing the bowel lumen.

In general, where colorectal surgical expertise is available, the gynecologic surgeon should have a low threshold to call for help. A full-thickness bowel injury will usually necessitate input from a color-ectal surgeon. It is advisable to get help from an experienced colorectal surgeon where the injury is large and involves (i) unprepared large bowel, (ii) multiple loops of bowels, or (iii) mesenteric blood vessels, raising the concern of potential devascularization. In these circumstances the nature of the most appropriate repair will need to be decided; this may involve a formal bowel resection with primary or delayed closure after defunctioning the bowel and formation of a stoma.

Repairing by laparoscopic surgery

It is possible to repair the injured bowel laparoscopically where there is adequate surgical dissection and suturing skill. Before this can be done, the surgeon must safely place additional 5-mm ports into the peritoneal cavity away from possible adhesions elsewhere. The injured loop of bowel and surrounding adhesions should be mobilized by sharp scissor dissection. Under magnification, the injured loop of bowel can be repaired by laparoscopic suturing with 4-0 silk or PDS suture, using intracorporeal knot tying, in the same manner as through laparotomy.

Mini-laparotomy

Where the surgeon is sufficiently confident to conduct bowel adhesiolysis but not intracorporeal suturing and knot tying, the injured bowel can be exteriorized through a 3-cm incision over the site of the injury and repaired externally. In order to reduce the risk of bowel content spillage inside the abdomen, an Endoloop® may be used to ligate around the perforation and the cut long suture used to facilitate delivery of the bowel loop through the mini-laparotomy incision. This injury can then be repaired in a similar fashion as at laparotomy using a 4-0 PDS suture on a small tapered needle.

Postoperative care

The patient should be clearly informed of the nature of the complication and asked to report any symptoms. Investigations including observation of vital signs, blood tests, and radiologic imaging should be arranged appropriately to monitor recovery and detect early signs of clinical deterioration. Antibiotics will need to be continued in liaison with a microbiologist.

Prevention

In high-risk patients such as this woman, all measures should be taken to not only minimize the chances of encountering bowel injury but also to allow immediate recognition of the injury. While there is no evidence to show that open entry is any safer than closed entry techniques from a bowel injury point of view, it is generally accepted that bowel injury may be more readily recognized with methods of entry under visual control such as open entry or the use of optical trocar as illustrated in this case.

Choosing alternative primary port placement sites away from the umbilicus, such as the left upper quadrant, may reduce the chance of encountering bowel injury from midline adhesions in high-risk cases. Before placement of a port in the left upper quadrant, however, it is important to ensure that the spleen is not palpable and that the stomach is empty. If in doubt, a nasogastric tube should be inserted to ensure the stomach is empty before commencing the port insertion in the left upper quadrant.

Ultimately, it is important to be vigilant for the possibility of inadvertent bowel injury during laparoscopic entry and surgery because the most serious morbidity and mortality from bowel injuries arise not from the initial insult but rather from delayed recognition and inappropriate initial management.

KEY POINTS

Challenge: Entry-related bowel injury during laparoscopy (see Chapter 37).

Background
- Up to half of traumatic bowel injuries occur during insertion of Veress needle, trocar, or secondary port. The remainder may occur during surgery or outside the operative field.
- As less than half of bowel injuries are recognized during surgery, this can result in delayed presentations and serious or even fatal complications.
- A high index of clinical awareness, prompt recognition, and appropriate response are key factors in the prevention and avoidance of serious complications and death from bowel injuries.

Prevention
- Appreciate which patients are at a higher risk of bowel injury during a laparoscopic procedure; risks include past laparotomies, known adhesions, inflammatory bowel conditions, severe endometriosis, and extremes of BMI.

- Consider using open techniques, optical trocars, and alternative sites to the umbilicus to increase the chances of safe laparoscopic entry in women at high risk of bowel adhesions.
- Routinely assess the bowels at entry, during, and on completion of laparoscopy.
- A high index of clinical awareness, prompt recognition, and instigation of appropriate management are key factors in preventing and avoiding serious complications from bowel injuries.

Management
- Immediate recognition of an entry-related bowel injury allows the surgeon time to consider the best way to manage the injury.
- An early bowel injury may be repaired via laparoscopic surgery, the use of mini-laparotomy to exteriorize the bowel, or traditional open surgery.
- A colorectal surgeon should be consulted when bowel injury is discovered or suspected.

Further reading

Lam A, Kaufman Y, Khong SY, Liew A, Ford S, Condous G. Dealing with complications in laparoscopy. *Best Pract Res Clin Obstet Gyanecol* 2009; 23:631–646.

Chapron C, Pierre F, Harchaoui Y *et al.* Gastrointestinal injuries during gynaecological laparoscopy. *Hum Reprod* 1999;14:333–337.

Perkins JD, Dent LL. Avoiding and repairing bowel injury in gynaecologic surgery. *OBG Management* 2004;16(8):15–28.

Brosens I, Gordon A, Campo R, Gordts S. Bowel injury in gynecologic laparoscopy. *J Am Assoc Gynecol Laparosc* 2003;10: 9–13.

Li TC, Saravelos H, Richmond M, Cooke ID. Complications of laparoscopic pelvic surgery: recognition, management and prevention. *Hum Reprod Update* 1997;3:505–515.

CHAPTER 75
Bowel Injury After Laparoscopy: Late Presentation

Alan Lam
Center for Advanced Reproductive Endosurgery, University of Sydney, St Leonards, Australia

Case history: A woman underwent laparoscopic excision of endometriosis involving the pouch of Douglas (Figure 75.1). She was well when discharged from hospital the following morning. Four days later, while at home, she experienced sudden onset of severe abdominal pain following a bowel movement. On admission to the emergency department, she looked unwell and was tachycardic, with a low-grade temperature of 37.5°C. She had a mildly distended abdomen with minimal guarding and audible bowel sounds.

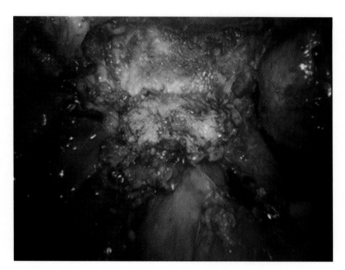

Figure 75.1   Deep nodular endometriosis in the pouch of Douglas infiltrated onto rectal wall.

Background

Bowel injury, while rare, is one of the most feared complications following laparoscopy. The majority of bowel injuries are not readily recognizable during surgery, and may manifest at any time from 1 to 30 days after surgery, with a median delay of 4–5 days. Unless promptly recognized and appropriately managed, the clinical situation may progress quickly from local to generalized peritonitis with septicemia and eventually multiorgan failure. The reported mortality rate from fecal peritonitis is estimated to be between 2 and 20%.

Factors which may account for delayed diagnosis of bowel perforation include unrecognized intraoperative bowel trauma, injury outside of the operative field, thermal injury with delayed tissue necrosis, and pericolic abscess formation with subsequent perforation. Atypical clinical presentations and the use of postoperative narcotic medications masking pain may also hinder prompt diagnosis.

While the diagnosis is not difficult in patients presenting with classical symptoms of sudden onset of acute abdominal pain, fever, tachycardia, and abdominal rigidity, more often than not the clinical picture may be unclear due to variable, atypical or subtle symptoms such as low-grade fever, mild abdominal distension, few peritoneal signs, or mild ileus. At times, respiratory distress, mild hypoxia, and chest consolidation may falsely lead to a diagnosis of pulmonary embolism or pneumonia. At times, the delay may be due to the surgeon's unwillingness to consider the diagnosis of bowel injury, fuelled by fear or ego, or reluctance to ask for a second opinion.

In general, the longer the delay from the time of injury to diagnosis, the greater the morbidity and mortality associated with bowel complications.

Management (see Chapter 37)

The woman presented in the case history should be admitted for further clinical assessment and management with a provisional diagnosis of bowel injury until proven otherwise. She should be kept nil by mouth, commenced on intravenous fluids and broad-spectrum antibiotics, and undergo urgent investigations and colorectal surgical assessment without delay. While her condition appears stable on admission and indeed may improve with these initial conservative management interventions, the nature of bowel injury is such that the clinical picture can change abruptly with rapid clinical deterioration.

Investigations

Hematologic, microbiologic, and radiologic investigations will help the overall clinical assessment. A full blood count may be normal or show mild leukocytosis in early sepsis, while leukopenia and neutropenia may reflect more severe sepsis. Despite their limitations, CRP and procalcitonin have been found to be useful as sensitive early diagnostic biomarkers for sepsis. Liver function test may

Gynecologic and Obstetric Surgery: Challenges and Management Options, First Edition. Edited by Arri Coomarasamy, Mahmood I. Shafi, G. Willy Davila and Kiong K. Chan.
© 2016 John Wiley & Sons, Ltd. Published 2016 by John Wiley & Sons, Ltd.

show hypoalbuminemia, which is caused by increased capillary permeability. Blood cultures should be performed but bacteremia may be found in less than half of patients with sepsis, depending on previous antibiotic treatment.

An abdominopelvic CT scan is the test of choice over other alternative imaging techniques such as abdominal X-ray, ultrasound, and MRI. The decision to add oral, rectal, or intravenous contrast media prior to the CT scan should be made in consultation with a colorectal surgeon and a radiologist. The CT findings may find extraluminal contrast material consistent with a bowel "leak." A large amount of free intraperitoneal air or fluid indicates a high probability for the presence of a bowel perforation, whereas a small amount of air, air and fluid collections, or soft-tissue thickening in the presacral space suggests a lower probability for a bowel perforation.

Ultimately, the diagnosis is made on clinical grounds; the results of all investigations should be interpreted in association with clinical symptoms and signs as there may be considerable overlap between patients with and without a clinically significant bowel injury.

Conservative management

Conservative management with judicious use of analgesia, careful observations, and regular clinical reviews may be adopted initially, provided the woman's clinical condition remains stable, while awaiting investigation results and surgical opinions.

Role of laparoscopy

A diagnostic laparoscopy may be an appropriate course of action if the clinical picture remains unresolved following investigations and surgical consultations. If there is high clinical suspicion of a bowel injury, it may be wiser to err on the side of carrying out an exploratory laparoscopy rather than risk an unnecessary or late laparotomy. If laparoscopy is pursued, an open entry is the preferred entry method into the abdominal cavity because there may be distended loops of bowel adherent to the anterior abdominal wall. The surgeon should pay particular attention to any foul, feculent odor on entry. Once inside, a thorough and systematic inspection of the entire abdomen and pelvis should be carried out with the use of soft bowel grasping forceps to look for signs of fecal contamination or abscess formation. Peritoneal fluid may be collected for microscopy and culture.

In the absence of a bowel perforation, the abdominal and pelvic cavity should be washed out with warm saline, and an active (e.g., Jackson–Pratt) or passive (e.g., Robinson) drain placed through the laparoscopic port sites. In the presence of a bowel injury, the approach to management of the injury depends on the extent, site, likely cause of the injury, the viability of the bowels involved, and the experience of the surgeon.

Laparotomy

An exploratory laparotomy should be promptly carried out by an experienced colorectal surgeon if there is a high index of suspicion of a bowel injury based on clinical and radiologic grounds. Prior to surgery, the patient may require a central line for resuscitation, fluid replacement and antibiotics, a nasogastric tube to deflate the stomach, and an indwelling catheter to monitor urine output. Upon entry, an assessment may immediately reveal the presence of enteric or fecal content in the peritoneal cavity and the site of perforation. However, at times, checking and finding a tiny bowel perforation can be a most challenging and frustrating task that may involve meticulous and delicate removal of fibrinous material covering the surface areas of the bowels adherent to the anterior abdominal wall or the pelvis.

Small bowel injury

In the case of a small bowel perforation, careful inspection of the wound edges, and debridement of devitalized tissue, followed by primary closure of the defect in two layers with 4-0 silk or PDS sutures on a tapered needle, may be considered if the freshened edges of the perforation readily bleed, thus signifying viability. However, if the bowel perforation is edematous, if multiple perforations are found, if more than 50% of the circumference of the bowel wall is involved, or if there is concern with segmental vascularity, primary closure should be avoided and resection with hand-sewn or stapled anastomosis should be considered.

Large bowel injury

Delayed presentation and diagnosis in colonic injuries have a far worse prognosis than small bowel injuries because of higher bacterial exposure from fecal contamination. The decision of how best to manage the bowel injury should be made by the colorectal surgical team. The options include primary closure or resection of affected bowel with either re-anastomosis or fecal diversion via a stoma. Thorough peritoneal lavage and placement of large-bore drains are of utmost importance to reduce the risk of intra-abdominal and pelvic abscess postoperatively.

Prevention

Thorough observation and assessment of the bowels should be done routinely on entry, during instrument exchange, during adhesiolysis, or during excision of pathology close to or from the bowel wall. Potential rectal injury should be checked with a rectal insufflation test, although this test is not foolproof for tiny leaks or delayed bowel injury. The patient should be warned of possible delayed presentation of a bowel injury due to the uncertain nature of tissue healing following surgery; she should be told to report any abnormal symptoms such as increasing abdominal pain, fever, vomiting and respiratory distress while still an inpatient or after hospital discharge. During the early postoperative period, any unexpected excessive pain that requires opiates warrants further investigations and delay in hospital discharge.

Clinical assessment should include observation of the temperature chart, pulse rate, blood pressure, and specifically oxygen saturation. While not commonly recognized, a drop in oxygen saturation is one of the earliest signs of bowel injury, as contamination and infection decreases oxygenation at the alveolar–capillary membrane caused by inflammatory mediators.

Blood tests for CRP and procalcitonin in conjunction with imaging with an abdominopelvic CT scan can assist the early detection of bowel injury.

KEY POINTS

Challenge: Management of late bowel injury after laparoscopy (see Chapter 37).

Background
- Delayed diagnosis of bowel perforation results in greater risks of morbidity and mortality.
- The classical clinical presentation of fecal peritonitis is with sudden onset of acute abdominal pain associated with fever, tachycardia, and abdominal rigidity. Respiratory distress, mild hypoxia, and chest consolidation can also occur.

Management
- Hematologic, microbiologic, and radiologic investigations will help the overall clinical assessment.
- Blood tests should include FBC, U&E, liver function tests, and blood cultures. CRP and procalcitonin have been found to be useful as sensitive early diagnostic biomarkers for sepsis.
- An abdominopelvic CT scan is the test of choice to detect evidence of a bowel perforation; extraluminal contrast material, and free intraperitoneal air or fluid can indicate bowel injury.

- Urgent assessment and assistance from the colorectal surgical team should be sought.
- A diagnostic laparoscopy may be useful where the patient's clinical status is stable but the clinical picture remains unresolved after hematologic and imaging investigations.
- A laparotomy should be performed promptly if the clinical suspicion of bowel injury is high, to locate and repair the bowel injuries.

Prevention
- Thorough observation and assessment of the bowels should be done routinely upon entry, during instrument exchange, during adhesiolysis, or during excision of pathology close to or from the bowel wall.
- Check for potential rectal injury with rectal insufflation test.
- Ask the patient to report any abnormal symptoms such as increasing abdominal pain, fever, or respiratory distress while still an inpatient or after hospital discharge.
- During the early postoperative period, any unexpected excessive pain that requires opiates warrants further investigations and delay in hospital discharge.
- Clinical assessment should include temperature chart, pulse rate, blood pressure, and specifically oxygen saturation.

Further reading

Wacker C, Prkno A, Brunkhorst F, Schlattmann. Procalcitonin as a diagnostic marker for sepsis: a systematic review and meta-analysis. *Lancet Infect Dis* 2013;13:426–435.

Power N, Atri M, Ryan S, Haddad R, Smith A. CT assessment of anastomotic bowel leak. *Clin Radiol* 2007;62:37–42.

Khoury W, Ben-Yahuda A, Ben-Haim M, Klausner JM, Szold O. Abdominal computed tomography for diagnosing postoperative lower gastrointestinal tract leaks. *J Gastrointestinal Surg* 2009;13:1454–1458.

Agresta F, Ciardo LF, Mazzarolo G et al. Peritonitis: laparoscopic approach. *World J Emerg Surg* 2006;1:9.

Kirshtein B, Roy-Sharpira A, Lantsberg L, Mandel S, Avinoach E, Mirzah S. The use of laparoscopy in abdominal emergencies. *Surg Endosc* 2003;17:1118–1124.

Nelson R, Singer M. Primary repair for penetrating colon injuries. *Cochrane Database Syst Rev* 2003;(3):CD002247.

Lam A, Kaufman Y, Khong SY, Liew A, Ford S, Condous G. Dealing with complications in laparoscopy. *Best Pract Res Clin Obstet Gynecol* 2009;23:631–646.

CHAPTER 76
Blood Vessel Injury at Laparoscopy

Elizabeth Ball
Queen Mary University of London, London, UK

Case history: *A patient is placed in Trendelenburg position for a diagnostic laparoscopy but her sacrum overlaps the lower edge of the operating table, encouraging lumbar lordosis. After Veress needle insertion frank blood is withdrawn. In view of stable vital signs, the pelvis is inspected laparoscopically through Palmer's point, and 1.5 L of blood is evacuated from the pelvis; the large vessels are thoroughly inspected and intact. Following this, the retroperitoneal space and mesentery are systematically examined. Obvious bruising is identified over the mesenteric vein but bleeding has already ceased. Hemostasis is maintained even with low insufflation pressures.*

Background

Injury of the inferior epigastric vessels in the abdominal wall is the most common laparoscopic vascular injury and accounts for 2% of all laparoscopic complications. If undetected, it can cause considerable blood loss into the soft tissues, but it can usually be repaired without conversion to laparotomy.

In contrast, injury of the large intra-abdominal vessels is a rare laparoscopic complication, with an estimated incidence of 0.1 per 1000 cases [1], but it carries a high mortality of around 15% [2]. Large vessel injury may occur during laparoscopic entry or, more commonly, during operative manipulation, especially with sharp instruments, electrosurgery, or lasers. Because of the limited visual field in laparoscopy, up to 30% of vascular injuries are missed intraoperatively [2], especially when bleeding occurs retroperitoneally. Delays in diagnosis and instituting effective treatments cost lives [3].

Prevention

Anatomic considerations at entry
Good anatomic knowledge is a prerequisite to safe and proficient surgery. The surgeon should be mindful of the course of the right common iliac artery (Figure 76.1) and the distal aorta beneath the umbilicus. With increasing BMI, the umbilicus lies more caudally to the aortic bifurcation [4]. Special care needs to be taken in slim patients, where the aorta bifurcates almost at the same level as the umbilicus (Chapter 66). The surgeon should adjust the angle of insertion of the Veress needle at the umbilicus from the usual 90° to 45° toward the pelvis in very slim patients (Figure 76.2).

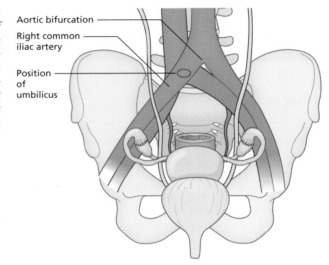

Figure 76.1 Aortic bifurcation and right common iliac artery. Adapted from Krishnakumar & Tambe, 2009 [5], Figures 1 and 3, with permission from Medknow Publications and Media PVT, Ltd.

Anatomic considerations at secondary port placement
Two veins ("tram tracks") flank the inferior epigastric arteries, which should be positively identified running from the inguinal ring toward the anterior abdominal wall. Transillumination will usually only show superficial rather than deep epigastric vessels.

General preoperative considerations
A laparoscopic surgeon should perform a mental "dry run" before the operation and plan a rough "route map" of the procedure. This includes ensuring familiarity with the laparoscopic equipment including energy modalities to be used and an appreciation of what actions to take if complications should arise. Surgeons need to be aware of their patients' individual risk factors, such as anatomic distortion from endometriosis or previous surgery. Surgery should be undertaken or supervised by a suitably experienced, competent laparoscopic surgeon.

Gynecologic and Obstetric Surgery: Challenges and Management Options, First Edition. Edited by Arri Coomarasamy, Mahmood I. Shafi, G. Willy Davila and Kiong K. Chan.
© 2016 John Wiley & Sons, Ltd. Published 2016 by John Wiley & Sons, Ltd.

Non-obese

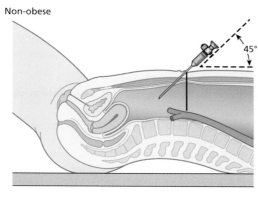

Overweight

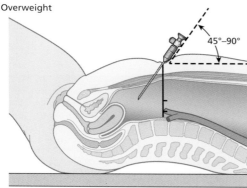

Obese

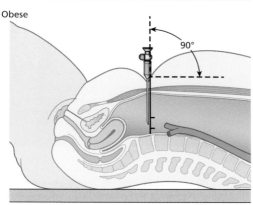

Figure 76.2 Variation of angle of Veress needle for different body weights.

Positioning of the patient
The patient's sacrum should not be hanging over the end of the table; this causes exaggerated lumbar lordosis, which pushes the retroperitoneal spaces closer to the abdominal wall. The same error occurs if the Trendelenburg position is erroneously assumed before trocar entry.

Choice of mode of access
There is no difference in the rate of vascular complications when comparing various entry techniques, including Veress needle insufflation before trocar entry, open (Hasson) entry, or optical trocar entry [6]. The most common gynecologic approach in the UK is Veress needle insufflation, followed by blind trocar insertion. I prefer an optical trocar for the primary port, but this is only useful if the camera head is properly oriented during trocar insertion and the trocar movement is controlled. Patients with a reduced BMI may

benefit from a Palmer's point entry, which is 3 cm below the subcostal border in the mid-clavicular line. The Palmer's point port can usually be used as an operating port in the course of the operation.

Veress needle and trocar insertion
There remains some uncertainty about the relative risks of large vessel injury from lifting or not lifting the peritoneum during Veress needle insertion [6]. I always lift the abdominal wall because it measurably increases the distance from the retroperitoneum [7]. With an umbilical entry, the Veress needle should not be advanced further after two "clicks" have been felt, indicating entry into the abdominal cavity through the rectus fascia and peritoneum. Any side-to-side movement must be avoided because it would further enlarge any vascular or bowel puncture.

In order to avoid an uncontrolled thrust of the trocar toward the retroperitoneum, the surgeon needs to ensure that reusable trocars are sharp, the skin incision is adequate, insufflation pressures are 20–25 mmHg in order to splint the abdominal wall [8], the trocar angle is appropriate for the patient's BMI, and advancement of the trocar is carefully controlled.

Intraoperative anatomic and spatial awareness
Good camera driving can help to overcome the limited laparoscopic field; this includes a change between magnified close-up and panoramic views and keeping the active instruments centered to avoid blind manipulation, especially when activating energy sources. Holding the camera head upright at all times aids anatomic and spatial orientation.

Insertion of the secondary ports
The secondary port should be inserted lateral to the deep epigastric vessels, and tunneling medially through the anterior abdominal wall during entry toward them must be avoided; this is best achieved by advancing the trocar perpendicularly through an adequate skin incision until the peritoneum is tenting. Only then should the trocar be angled into the pelvis. Secondary ports must always be removed under vision to detect potential bleeding. Bruising at the port site on transillumination can help to identify suspected trauma.

Operating near large vessels
Lymphadenectomy, presacral neurectomy, and surgery for deep endometriosis all carry a high risk of trauma to large vessels, especially in the presence of anatomical distortion. In adnexal surgery the surgeon must be aware of the course of the internal iliac vessel along the pelvic sidewall and resist the temptation to rest adnexal tissue on this area during dissection; instead, adnexal tissues should be lifted away from the sidewall.

Management (see Chapters 38, 40 and 121)

What should be done when large vessel injury occurs?
It is important not to panic, but to communicate well and act swiftly and systematically in order to save the patient's life. If a laparoscope is in place, efforts should be made to maintain visualization by placing the distal lens outside the angle of the spurting blood vessel. If the trauma has occurred during Veress needle placement (as indicated by the aspiration of blood in the case history), the needle should be left in place so that the puncture can be identified easily at further exploratory surgery.

The anesthetist needs to be informed to anticipate the need for cardiovascular stabilization, to appreciate the increased risk of CO_2 embolism (Chapter 69), and to allow immediate ordering of necessary blood products. Immediate involvement of a vascular surgeon should be sought. The operative team needs to prepare for a midline laparotomy, which will be necessary in almost all cases. Until the vascular surgeon arrives, direct pressure ought to be applied to the traumatized vessel.

In some situations, as judged by the vascular surgeon, large veins may be ligated, but large arteries always require repair. Repair can be undertaken with clips, fine sutures such as 5-0 Prolene, re-anastomosis, or by using grafts. The patient must be closely monitored for postoperative thromboembolic events.

Only very accomplished laparoscopic surgeons should attempt laparoscopic vessel repair. The bowel and ureter need to be isolated first. If bipolar electrodesiccation is used to occlude a large blood vessel, the vessel should be encircled with the forceps, compressed,

and fused at the lowest degree of heating (20–25 W), in order to fuse the elastic fibers and collagen within the wall of the vessel [3]. Other techniques include the laparoscopic application of clips or oversuturing while the leak is compressed with a non-traumatic grasper.

What should be done when an abdominal wall injury occurs?

If there is bleeding at trocar removal, bipolar electrosurgery should be attempted. Failing this, a suture can be placed across the lesion and tied extracorporeally below the skin surface within the incision. This is best achieved under laparoscopic vision with an Endoclose system or a J-needle. Alternatively, a catheter balloon can be inflated and compressed against the internal abdominal wall with an artery forceps for several hours to tamponade the puncture (see Chapter 38, Figure 38.2). In all cases hemostasis has to be confirmed at low insufflation pressures.

KEY POINTS

Challenge: Laparoscopy and blood vessel injury.

Background
- Large vessel trauma is a rare but potentially catastrophic laparoscopic complication that can occur with all techniques of laparoscopic access or during the operative laparoscopic procedure.
- Delay in detection and in instituting effective treatment to rectify the situation, usually through undertaking a midline laparotomy, greatly increases mortality.

Prevention
- Avoid lordosis and Trendelenburg position during umbilical Veress needle and primary trocar placement.
- Very slim women are at higher risk of vascular injury; the operating surgeon should insert the Veress needle at a 45° angle toward the pelvis, or alternatively use Palmer's point entry.
- Good knowledge of anatomy and energy sources is a prerequisite for operative procedures. Adnexal structures should always be pulled away from the sidewall vessels for dissection.

- Care should be taken to identify the inferior epigastric vessels when inserting secondary trocars; they should be placed laterally, and tunneling in a medial direction should be avoided.

Management
- Good communication and swift action help save patients' lives.
- The anesthetist and operative team should be informed immediately of the suspected complication. The patient is at acute risk of exsanguination and CO_2 embolism.
- A vascular surgeon should be summoned. While waiting for the vascular surgeon, the vascular puncture should be compressed.
- If Veress needle caused the injury, it should be left in place, where possible. Apart from selected cases, midline laparotomy is usually necessary.
- First the injured vessel is isolated. The lesion is then repaired by occlusion (ligation or bipolar desiccation) for some veins, or repair (clips, fine sutures) for veins and all arteries.
- The patient requires close monitoring for thromboembolic events.
- Inferior epigastric vascular injury can usually be repaired without converting to laparotomy; techniques include extracorporeal suturing using a J-needle, Endoclose suturing, or catheter balloon tamponade.

References

1 Jansen FW, Kapiteyn K, Trimbos-Kemper T, Hermans J, Trimbos JB. Complications of laparoscopy: a prospective multicentre observational study. *Br J Obstet Gynaecol* 1997;104:595–600.
2 Chandler JG, Corson SL, Way LW. Three spectra of laparoscopic entry access injuries. *J Am Coll Surg* 2001;192:478–490; discussion 490–491.
3 Nezhat C, Childers J, Nezhat F, Nezhat CH, Seidman DS. Major retroperitoneal vascular injury during laparoscopic surgery. *Hum Reprod* 1997;12:480–483.
4 Hurd WW, Bude RO, DeLancey JO, Pearl ML. The relationship of the umbilicus to the aortic bifurcation: implications for laparoscopic technique. *Obstet Gynecol* 1992;80:48–51.
5 Krishnakumar S, Tambe P. Entry complications in laparoscopic surgery. *J Gynecol Endosc Surg* 2009;1:4–11.
6 Ahmad G, O'Flynn H, Duffy JM, Phillips K, Watson A. Laparoscopic entry techniques. *Cochrane Database Syst Rev* 2012;(2):CD006583.
7 Roy GM, Bazzurini L, Solima E, Luciano AA. Safe technique for laparoscopic entry into the abdominal cavity. *J Am Assoc Gynecol Laparosc* 2001;8:519–528.
8 Phillips G, Garry R, Kumar C, Reich H. How much gas is required for initial insufflation at laparoscopy? *Gynaecol Endosc* 1999;8:369–374.

CHAPTER 77

Laparoscopy for Large Ovarian Cyst

T. Justin Clark

Birmingham Women's NHS Foundation Trust, Birmingham, UK

Case history 1: A slim 19-year-old woman presents with a history of abdominal distension. A urinary pregnancy test is negative. An ultrasound scan shows a 20-cm anechoic adnexal cyst thought to be of ovarian origin. The cyst is felt to be mobile on clinical examination and a CA125 level is 10 units/mL.

Case history 2: A 25-year-old woman is referred with a 2-year history of intermittent pelvic pain. A transvaginal ultrasound scan shows a 12-cm left ovarian mass consistent with a benign dermoid cyst. Serum levels of CA125 antigen, α-fetoprotein (AFP), and human chorionic gonadotropin (HCG) are within normal limits.

Background

In premenopausal women almost all ovarian masses and cysts are benign [1]. Differentiation between the benign and the malignant ovarian mass in premenopausal women relies on assessment by transvaginal ultrasound and CA125 antigen levels. If a germ cell tumor is suspected, other serum markers such as AFP and HCG need to be checked. While many ovarian masses in premenopausal women can be managed conservatively given their generally benign nature and the high likelihood of spontaneous resolution, surgical intervention is indicated in both case histories presented. This is because spontaneous resolution is unlikely in cysts over 10 cm in size and both women are symptomatic [2].

Management

In Case history 1, the presence of the large mass is causing the abdominal distension and while the origin of the cyst is uncertain, it is likely to be ovarian or tubal. The ultrasound appearances are suggestive of a benign lesion and this view is supported by a low CA125 level. In Case history 2, while the intermittent pain may be arising from the presence of the mass (e.g., episodic torsion), it may simply be an incidental finding. However, in light of its size and complex ultrasonic appearance, albeit in keeping with a commonly encountered benign teratoma (and reassuringly normal serum tumor markers), surgical removal is necessary to obtain histology, treat symptoms, and prevent ovarian cystic accidents.

At any point where borderline or frank malignancy is suspected, the involvement of a gynecologic oncologist should be sought and laparoscopic management may be contraindicated, although interestingly there are no differences in rates of intraoperative cyst rupture between laparotomy and laparoscopy [1].

The large, benign, ovarian mass presents surgical challenges for the laparoscopic surgeon. Once the decision for laparoscopy has been made, it is important to warn the patient that a laparotomy may become necessary if laparoscopic approach is technically unfeasible or complications arise at laparoscopy. Patients should also be aware that oophorectomy is a possibility if no normal ovarian tissue is identified, to stem bleeding, or where malignancy is suspected. Prior to surgery, the approach to laparoscopic entry needs to be planned. A decision should be made on whether removal of the intact cyst is desired, and the method of cyst extraction from the peritoneal cavity should be devised.

Management of a simple cyst

In Case history 1, the appearances are in keeping with a benign, mobile, simple cyst and the patient is slim so laparoscopic surgery should be feasible. The mass should be easily palpable and laparoscopic entry performed a few centimeters above the limits of the lesion centrally (which in the described case is likely to be above the umbilicus) or using Palmer's point in the left subcostal region. The choice of open or closed entry should be according to the individual surgeon's discretion. The mass should be inspected carefully to determine its origin, mobility, and nature. The contralateral ovary should be identified and inspected to confirm normality should oophorectomy rather than cystectomy become necessary. The rest of the abdominal cavity including the liver, omentum and peritoneum will need inspection and any free fluid should be aspirated and sent for cytologic evaluation. The cyst should be incised to allow decompression, with all fluid contents removed via suction and sent for cytology. Ovarian cystectomy should then be undertaken using standard laparoscopic techniques. Despite the simple nature of the collapsed cyst, its sheer size is likely to make extraction of the material from the abdomen difficult. Options include the use of a standard retrieval bag though an enlarged port site with or without further decompression or debulking, a mini-laparotomy,

Gynecologic and Obstetric Surgery: Challenges and Management Options, First Edition. Edited by Arri Coomarasamy, Mahmood I. Shafi, G. Willy Davila and Kiong K. Chan.

or a posterior culdotomy through which large traumatic grasping forceps or retrieval bags are passed under direct laparoscopic visualization and the cyst removed through the more distensible vaginal mucosa.

Management of a dermoid cyst

The surgical approach for Case history 2 is more challenging because intraperitoneal spillage of the dermoid cyst contents can potentially result in chemical peritonitis. Indeed, in one published series of 600 dermoid cystectomies, spillage occurred in 65% of cases although chronic granulomatous peritonitis developed in only one patient [4]. Three different surgical approaches for cystectomy or oophorectomy are justifiable: (i) laparotomy, (ii) laparoscopy with mini-laparotomy for exteriorization of the ovary, or (iii) laparoscopy alone. In light of the potential sequelae of rupturing a dermoid cyst, a laparotomy may not be unreasonable. However, a careful laparoscopic approach to mobilize, dissect and enucleate the cyst, the use of additional ports as required, and the judicious use of an endoscopic bag during surgery can avoid or reduce any leakage of cyst material into the peritoneal cavity [3,4]. In contrast to many "functional" ovarian cysts, the cyst wall of a benign teratoma is fairly robust and the avoidance of cyst rupture during enucleation is feasible in most cases. The intact cyst can then be removed from the abdominal cavity by puncturing and evacuating the cyst within a retrieval bag. However, laparoscopic pelvic access is restricted with larger cysts and the bag apertures often of insufficient dimension to accommodate such a cyst. Placement of an open retrieval bag under the dermoid cyst during dissection, with the aim of minimizing the risk of abdominal spillage of intracystic material, has been advocated along with preliminary cystic puncture prior to intraperitoneal cystectomy or oophorectomy depending on the size of the cyst and the preference of the surgeon [4]. At the end of the procedure, in addition to the usual checks for adequate hemostasis, a thorough washout of the abdominal cavity is indicated, especially where intraperitoneal spillage of cystic contents has occurred. All specimens should be sent for histologic assessment and most patients can be discharged within 24 hours of surgery.

KEY POINTS

Challenge: Laparoscopy for large ovarian cyst.

Background
- In premenopausal women almost all ovarian masses and cysts are benign.
- Large cysts are less likely to spontaneously resolve and ovarian cyst accidents can impact adversely on future fertility.
- Laparotomy can be avoided for most large ovarian cysts in premenopausal women.

Management
- Meticulous preoperative planning of the surgical approach is necessary, including site and mode of laparoscopic access and method of specimen retrieval.
- Advanced laparoscopic surgical skills are needed to manage large ovarian masses, especially with dermoid cysts, endometriomas, and abdominopelvic adhesions.
- The use of lesion debulking, endoscopic retrieval bags, additional port sites, and posterior culdotomy along with appropriate energy modalities, such as advanced bipolar technologies and ultrasonic technologies, can aid successful laparoscopic surgery for large ovarian cysts.

References

1 Royal College of Obstetricians and Gynaecologists. *Management of Suspected Ovarian Masses in Premenopausal Women*. RCOG Green-top Guideline No. 62, November 2011. Available at http://www.rcog.org.uk/womens-health/clinical-guidance/ovarian-masses-premenopausal-women-management-suspected-green-top-62
2 American College of Obstetricians and Gynecologists (ACOG). *Management of Adnexal Masses*. ACOG Practice Bulletin No. 83. ACOG, Washington, DC, 2007.
3 Shawki O, Ramadan A, Askalany A, Bahnassi A. Laparoscopic management of ovarian dermoid cysts: potential fear of dermoid spill, myths and facts. *Gynecol Surg* 2007;4:255–260.
4 Kondo W, Bourdel N, Cotte B *et al*. Does prevention of intraperitoneal spillage when removing a dermoid cyst prevent granulomatous peritonitis? *BJOG* 2010; 117:1027–1030.

CHAPTER 78

Laparoscopy for an Ovarian Cyst in Pregnancy

T. Justin Clark

Birmingham Women's NHS Foundation Trust, Birmingham, UK

Case history 1: A slim 35-year-old woman attends antenatal clinic at 10 weeks of gestation. Her dating scan confirms her gestation and detects a 12-cm anechoic simple-looking left-sided ovarian cyst. The woman is asymptomatic and complains of no problems so far in her pregnancy. On abdominal palpation a smooth pelvic mass is palpable up to the umbilicus.

Case history 2: A 28-year-old parous woman who is 15 weeks pregnant presents with central and right-sided pelvic pain which is colicky in nature. She has been an inpatient for 2 days but her pain has persisted and she has required regular morphine for analgesia. Her observations including urinalysis are normal and she has a soft non-distended abdomen with mild tenderness in the right iliac fossa. An abdominal ultrasound demonstrates an 8-cm adnexal hyperechoic adnexal mass with little intraovarian venous flow seen on Doppler and free fluid within the pelvis. At booking 4 weeks previously, she was noted to have a 5-cm right-sided adnexal mass with features suggestive of a dermoid cyst.

Background

Ovarian cysts are detected by ultrasound in approximately 1% of pregnancies in the first trimester [1]. The cysts are usually benign: dermoids (7–37%), cystadenomas (5–28%), endometriomas (1–27%), or functional cysts (13–20%) [2,3]. The majority of cysts resolve, but it is estimated that up to 25% of cysts persist [4] and this is more likely with larger and more complex cysts [5]. Malignant ovarian cysts, including borderline cysts, are less common [2]. Most ovarian cysts are found incidentally on ultrasound during early pregnancy, but some women will present with acute or chronic pain and discomfort. As with adnexal cysts outside of pregnancy, pelvic ultrasound is useful to delineate morphology and describe cyst characteristics. The utility of the epithelial cell tumor marker CA125 is limited because reference ranges to define normality do not apply [6].

Outside of pregnancy, in women of reproductive age, most guidelines recommend surgical removal of ovarian cysts that are symptomatic, large (usually above 5–10 cm in diameter), enlarging on serial scanning, or appearing complex sonographically, especially if CA125 levels are raised or other risk factors for ovarian malignancy are present [7,8]. However, in the pregnant woman, the threshold

at which surgical removal is indicated may be different. Pregnancy increases the general risks associated with anesthesia and surgery (e.g., venous thromboembolism). Laparoscopic entry and surgical access to the adnexae may be compromised as the gravid uterus enlarges and becomes an abdominal organ, and there is a risk of inducing fetal loss. These additional considerations need to be weighed against the usual risks of adopting an expectant approach to management, namely failing to detect a malignant cyst or the occurrence of a cyst accident (i.e., hemorrhage or torsion).

Management (see Chapter 25)

Management decisions

In all cases where ovarian cysts are encountered in pregnancy, a decision needs to be made as to the appropriateness of adopting an expectant approach with clinical observations and serial ultrasound scanning versus surgical or radiologic intervention. If intervention is chosen, then the most appropriate techniques need to be considered. In the case of radiologic intervention, should ultrasound-guided aspiration be performed via a transvaginal or transabdominal approach? For surgical intervention, should access to the pelvis be acquired via laparoscopy (umbilical – open or blind – vs. subcostal Palmer's point) or laparotomy (midline or transverse) and once the ovarian cyst is identified, should it be treated via aspiration, cystectomy, or oophorectomy?

Conservative management

In general, a conservative approach to managing ovarian cysts in pregnancy is preferable, supported by evidence from the literature that malignancy is uncommon and serious sequelae to mother or baby are rare [2,8,9]. Moreover, early pregnancy may be compromised if the cyst arises from the corpus luteum, which has a pivotal role in maintaining pregnancy in the first trimester before the placenta has developed sufficiently to supersede it. In Case history 1, the woman is asymptomatic and has a simple, albeit relatively large, ovarian cyst. The likelihood of malignancy is thus minimal and so the danger of non-intervention seems restricted to enlargement, hemorrhage, or torsion. If the cyst continues to enlarge, then this would be detected on serial ultrasound with or without pain symptoms. The risk of hemorrhage or rupture is

Gynecologic and Obstetric Surgery: Challenges and Management Options, First Edition. Edited by Arri Coomarasamy, Mahmood I. Shafi, G. Willy Davila and Kiong K. Chan.
© 2016 John Wiley & Sons, Ltd. Published 2016 by John Wiley & Sons, Ltd.

small but torsion is more common, with an estimated incidence of 8–15% [8,10,11]. Risk factors for torsion include a persistent corpus luteal cyst or dermoid cyst, size above 6 cm, and gestation between 10 and 17 weeks [11]. The woman should be told to re-present if she develops pain or bleeding.

Surgical management

Ovarian surgery is predominantly undertaken laparoscopically in light of the reduced morbidity and enhanced recovery associated with this approach. This also holds true within pregnancy, but it is generally considered safest to conduct laparoscopic pelvic surgery in the first and second trimesters before the gravid uterus becomes too large, restricting surgical access and thereby necessitating laparotomy. There is no evidence of harm to human fetuses from carbon dioxide pneumoperitoneum. The advantages of laparoscopic surgery in pregnancy include reduced narcotic requirements, in turn minimizing fetal respiratory suppression, as well as minimized risk of wound complications and VTE. The traditional notion that the risk of miscarriage is reduced if surgery is delayed to the second trimester is not supported by recent evidence [8]. However, non-emergency cases should probably be scheduled at 16–20 weeks to allow time for spontaneous resolution of the cystic mass (especially functional corpus luteal cysts) while still allowing access to the pelvis beyond the gravid uterus [2]. It has been suggested that diminished uterine manipulation with laparoscopy as compared with laparotomy may decrease uterine irritability and risk of miscarriage or preterm labor [8].

Resolution of the cases

Case history 1

It would seem sensible to repeat the ultrasound within 4–6 weeks as long as the patient remains asymptomatic. If the balance tips toward intervention because of pain or significant enlargement of the adnexal mass, then laparoscopic surgery can be undertaken at an optimal time within the second trimester. If this becomes necessary, a cystectomy would be the procedure of choice because the cyst is likely to be benign and, given its size, recurrence would be a substantial possibility with simple aspiration (use of which should be restricted to radiologically guided approaches). If the cyst remains static, then monitoring with serial scans throughout the remainder of the pregnancy and at 6 weeks postnatally would be prudent. The further the pregnancy progresses, the lower the risk of torsion [11]. The risk of obstructed labor is negligible and if a cesarean section is undertaken, then the cyst could be removed at that point.

Case history 2

Laparoscopic surgical intervention is indicated in light of the woman's persistent symptoms, reliance on narcotic analgesia, and the change in the size and morphology of the previously identified dermoid cyst. While her observations and clinical examination findings do not suggest an acute surgical abdomen, the working diagnosis has to be one of ovarian torsion. This contention is supported by the colicky, episodic, and persistent nature of her pain. Torsion in pregnancy is commonly associated with dermoid cysts [11]. A laparoscopic approach to surgery is indicated at this gestation. On confirmation of the diagnosis, the viability of the tube and ovary should be evaluated. If the adnexa is clearly non-viable and gangrenous, then a salpingo-oophorectomy should be undertaken.

Otherwise, the ovarian ligament and tube should be untwisted and the viability of the adnexa re-evaluated. A cystectomy should be performed to prevent recurrence. Oophoropexy is not indicated without a recurrent history of ovarian torsion. It is especially important with a dermoid cyst to try to avoid inadvertent spillage of cyst contents, in order to minimize the risk of chemical peritonitis. This is best done by adopting a careful surgical approach and using a specimen retrieval bag. Indeed, some authors recommend placement of an opened surgical retrieval bag via a fourth port underneath the ovary during dissection of the cyst to avoid spillage into the abdominal cavity [12]. If cyst contents are spilt, then a meticulous saline washout is indicated. Presence of the fetal heart should be confirmed before discharge.

KEY POINTS

Challenge: Laparoscopy for ovarian cyst in pregnancy.

Background
- Ovarian cysts are common in pregnancy, being found in 1% of booking scans; the majority of women are asymptomatic. The risk of malignancy is low.
- Most ovarian cysts will resolve during the pregnancy, and even those that persist rarely cause problems. However, complications including hemorrhage, rupture, and torsion can occur, and as well as causing maternal morbidity, ovarian cyst accidents may increase the likelihood of pregnancy loss.
- The risk of torsion is estimated to be approximately 8–15%, and is most commonly found in association with dermoid cysts.

Management
- An expectant approach to the management of ovarian cysts in pregnancy is recommended for most women in the absence of pain.
- Serial ultrasound is useful to monitor cysts, but CA125 is not helpful in pregnancy since it can be elevated due to pregnancy itself.
- Surgical intervention should be considered for symptomatic women and those with complex and/or enlarging ovarian cysts. MRI is useful where there is doubt regarding the nature of an ovarian cyst in pregnancy.
- Where ovarian torsion is suspected, urgent surgery is indicated to minimize the risk of ischemia.
- Laparoscopy is preferable to laparotomy in the first and second trimesters of pregnancy for the treatment of benign adnexal pathology. The mode and site of laparoscopic entry should be adjusted according to the size of the gravid uterus (at least 6 cm above the uterine fundus or in the left upper quadrant) (Chapter 25).
- Whatever management approach is adopted, the plan should be discussed with the woman so she understands the relevant risks and benefits to both her and her baby.

References

1 Nelson MJ, Cavalieri R, Graham D, Sanders RC. Cysts in pregnancy discovered by sonography. *J Clin Ultrasound* 1986;14:509–512.
2 Hoover K, Jenkins TR. Evaluation and management of adnexal mass in pregnancy. *Am J Obstet Gynecol* 2011;205:97–102.
3 Koo YJ, Lee JE, Lim KT, Shim JU, Mok JE, Kim TJ. A 10-year experience of laparoscopic surgery for adnexal masses during pregnancy. *Int J Gynaecol Obstet* 2011;113:36–39.
4 Condous G, Khalid A, Okaro E, Bourne T. Should we be examining the ovaries in pregnancy? Prevalence and natural history of adnexal pathology detected at first-trimester sonography. *Ultrasound Obstet Gynecol* 2004;24:62–66.
5 Bernhard LM, Klebba PK, Gray DL, Mutch DG. Predictors of persistence of adnexal masses in pregnancy. *Obstet Gynecol* 1999;93:585–589.

6 Aslam N, Ong C, Woelfer B, Nicolaides K, Jurkovic D. Serum CA125 at 11–14 weeks of gestation in women with morphologically normal ovaries. *BJOG* 2000;107:689–690.

7 Marret H, L'homme C, Lecuru F *et al.* Guidelines for the management of ovarian cancer during pregnancy. *Eur J Obstet Gynecol Reprod Biol* 2010;149:18–21.

8 Society of American Gastrointestinal and Endoscopic Surgeons. *Guidelines for diagnosis, treatment, and use of laparoscopy for surgical problems during pregnancy.* SAGES, Los Angeles, CA. Available at http://www.sages.org/publications/guidelines/guidelines-for-diagnosis-treatment-and-use-of-laparoscopy-for-surgical-problems-during-pregnancy/

9 Zanetta G, Mariani E, Lissoni A *et al.* A prospective study of the role of ultrasound in the management of adnexal masses in pregnancy. *BJOG* 2003;110:578–583.

10 Aggarwal P, Kehoe S. Ovarian tumours in pregnancy: a literature review. *Eur J Obstet Gynecol Reprod Biol* 2011;155:119–124.

11 Yen CF, Lin SL, Murk W *et al.* Risk analysis of torsion and malignancy for adnexal masses during pregnancy. *Fertil Steril* 2009;91:1895–1902.

12 Kondo W, Bourdel N, Cotte B *et al.* Does prevention of intraperitoneal spillage when removing a dermoid cyst prevent granulomatous peritonitis? *BJOG* 2010;117:1027–1030.

Laparoscopic Removal of Rectovaginal Endometriosis

Alan Lam
Center for Advanced Reproductive Endosurgery, University of Sydney, St Leonards, Australia

Case history: A 27-year-old woman with debilitating dysmenorrhea, dyspareunia, and deep rectal pain is found to have a firm nodule in the posterior fornix on vaginal examination. At subsequent laparoscopy, the pouch of Douglas appeared obliterated with the rectosigmoid firmly adherent to the left pelvic sidewall and the posterior uterine surface. A diagnosis of severe endometriosis was made, and the patient wished for fertility-preserving surgery.

Background

Rectovaginal endometriosis (RVE) should be suspected in women presenting with a combination of dysmenorrhea, dyspareunia, deep rectal pain, and dyschezia. The finding of tender scar tissues or nodularity in the pouch of Douglas and rectovaginal septum on pelvic examination should raise the clinical suspicion of this condition. The prevalence of RVE is higher than generally appreciated, with reported rates estimated to be between 5 and 30% [1].

Management

Diagnosis

Several imaging tests are available with varying sensitivity and specificity to aid the diagnosis of RVE. Transvaginal ultrasound has been shown to be a highly sensitive and specific investigation that can estimate the extent of muscularis infiltration, but it does require specialized training and bowel preparations. Alternative imaging modalities such as rectal endoanal ultrasound, MRI, and multislice CT enteroclysis have also been shown to be useful in assessing the depth of endometriosis infiltration. In contrast, bowel endometriosis is rarely seen on colonoscopy, as the lesions typically infiltrate from the serosal to the submucosal layer and infrequently through the bowel mucosa. The choice of imaging test would depend on availability, expertise, costs, and individual preference.

Expectant management

Expectant management with periodic surveillance is a reasonable treatment option for asymptomatic women with RVE, or for women with minimal pelvic pain or bowel symptoms.

Medical treatment

In symptomatic women (as in the case presented), medical treatment to suppress menstruation should be considered. Available hormonal treatments include continuous combined contraceptive pills, systemic or local progestogens, and GnRH agonists. However, pain symptoms may persist, side effects or contraindications may preclude such treatments and, even if effective, symptoms are likely to recur when treatment is discontinued and menstruation returns.

Surgical management

Surgery for removal of rectovaginal and bowel endometriosis has been shown to be feasible, safe, and effective through either open or laparoscopic surgery. However, thorough preoperative counseling is required prior to undertaking surgery so that the patient can weigh the potential clinical outcomes against the serious potential complications that may arise from this technically challenging surgery. Surgical removal of rectovaginal and bowel endometriosis should be undertaken by experienced surgeons in well-equipped operating theaters after proper planning and with multidisciplinary support, preferably within dedicated endometriosis centers.

There are several options open to the gynecologists who treat women with RVE. These include (i) see and discuss, (ii) see and refer, (iii) see and treat at the same time, or (iv) see, discuss and treat at a later time. Ideally, all these potential options should have been discussed with the patient presented in the case history in advance of the laparoscopy in view of the clinically detected endometriotic nodule in the vagina.

See and discuss

As the actual nature and extent of the pathology will not be apparent until the time of surgery, the surgeon will only be able to confirm the diagnosis, determine the extent of the disease, and assess the potential risks of surgery at the time of laparoscopy. In the presence of extensive RVE, the surgeon may decide not to proceed with surgery but instead document the operative findings clearly and arrange an outpatient follow-up visit. At this appointment the operative findings can be explained in more detail and the treatment options discussed and further written information provided to help the patient decide her preferred choice of management.

Gynecologic and Obstetric Surgery: Challenges and Management Options, First Edition. Edited by Arri Coomarasamy, Mahmood I. Shafi, G. Willy Davila and Kiong K. Chan.
© 2016 John Wiley & Sons, Ltd. Published 2016 by John Wiley & Sons, Ltd.

See and refer

After taking the opportunity for discussion of the laparoscopic findings and management options, the surgeon may make a judicious clinical decision to refer the patient to a more experienced surgical colleague or a center where there is appropriate expertise to care for her condition.

See and treat

Faced with significant RVE, surgeons should not proceed with removing the disease unless (i) they have the necessary skills and experience; (ii) the patient has been made fully aware of the potential benefits and risks of extensive RVE surgery; (iii) there is adequate theater time available; (iv) optimal theater equipment is present; and (v) colorectal surgical expertise is available. The chances of completing the surgery safely will be maximized if these prerequisites are satisfied.

Surgical treatment

A clear strategy is required to remove RVE. The essential steps include the following.

Appropriate port placement

In addition to the two lateral 5-mm ports, the surgeon should consider where to place the third operative port so as to make it easy to dissect the rectosigmoid adhesions, the ureters if required, and approach the pouch of Douglas in order to the dissect out the rectovaginal disease.

Mobilization of rectosigmoid adhesions

This is an essential step to allow visualization of the left ureter, access to the left adnexa, excision of endometriosis from the left broad ligament if present, and dissection of the pararectal spaces if required.

Identification of the ureters

Mobilization of the left ureter is required to remove an endometrioma or excise endometriotic implants from the broad and uterosacral ligaments. This step is essential to reduce the risk of ureteric injury (Figure 79.1).

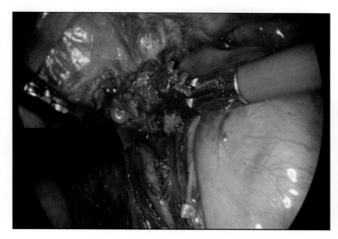

Figure 79.1 Left ureter being dissected away from the endometriosis infiltrating into the left uterosacral ligament.

Dissection of the rectovaginal endometriosis

With the ureters identified, dissection to identify the pararectal spaces medial to the ureters and uterosacral ligaments allows the lateral border of the rectum to be delineated. From here, the rectovaginal nodule can be dissected off the posterior uterine surface, the uterosacral junction, and posterior fornix.

From the pararectal spaces, and with the aid of rectal and vaginal probes as reference points, the lesion can be dissected and reflected onto the anterior rectal wall. If the lesion penetrates the posterior vaginal fornix, the dissection will result in a colpotomy (Figure 79.2). By placing a surgical glove or gauze pack inside the vagina, the pneumoperitoneum can be maintained to allow the rectovaginal lesion to be dissected from the posterior vaginal wall. The colpotomy can be closed with continuous 0-Vicryl suture.

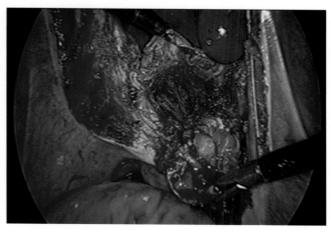

Figure 79.2 The rectovaginal nodule is being reflected onto the anterior rectal wall. The lesion penetrates through the posterior vaginal fornix. The green glove inside the vagina maintains the pneumoperitoneum.

Evaluation of the extent of bowel involvement

Once the rectovaginal lesion is completely dissected free from the vagina and reflected onto the anterior rectum, its volume, extent of infiltration, and the degree of circumferential spread can then be assessed to determine the extent of bowel surgery.

Removal of rectal disease

- Superficial rectal lesions involving the serosal layer can be excised with sharp scissors without electrodiathermy so as to avoid delayed thermal damage. Any potential weakness of the bowel wall is carefully buttressed with interrupted 2-0 or 3-0 absorbable sutures (Figure 79.3).

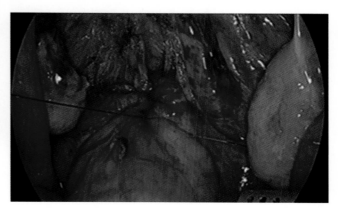

Figure 79.3 After removal of rectal endometriosis, the rectal wall is buttressed with 3-0 absorbable sutures.

- For deep lesions infiltrating into the muscularis and submucosal layer of the rectum, a full-thickness disk resection can be achieved by one of the following methods. The first method involves placing two stay sutures on either side of the rectal nodule, followed by sharp scissor excision without electrodiathermy, and two-layer continuous suture closure of the bowel wall defect with 2-0 or 3-0 Vicryl. The second method involves removing the lesion transanally by invaginating the anterior rectal wall nodule into a fully opened circular stapler, thus negating the need for intracorporeal suturing (Figure 79.4).

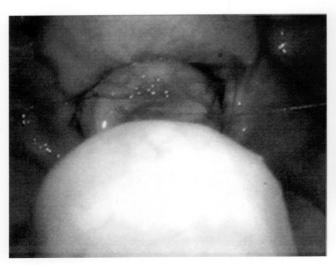

Figure 79.4 The rectal nodule is being invaginated into the hollow of the endoscopic circular stapler using the stay sutures placed on either side of the lesion.

- While opinions may differ as to when segmental bowel resection should be performed, it is generally indicated in symptomatic women with a large single nodule or multifocal disease with deep infiltration into the muscularis layer of the bowel, or involving more than half of the bowel wall circumference, with surrounding severe fibrosis. This procedure involves full mobilization of the rectum below the rectal nodule (Figure 79.5).

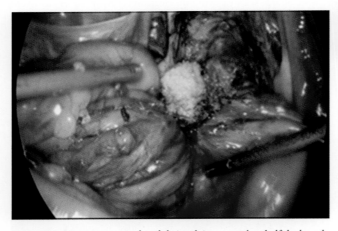

Figure 79.5 Large rectovaginal nodule involving more than half the bowel circumference.

- The rectum is then resected distal to the lesion using an Endo GIA stapler. The proximal diseased segment, exteriorized through a suprapubic mini-laparotomy incision, is then resected (Figure 79.6). After ensuring adequate blood supply, the proximal bowel stump with the anchored anvil is re-anastomosed with the distal rectal stump using the transanal endoscopic circular stapler (Figure 79.7).

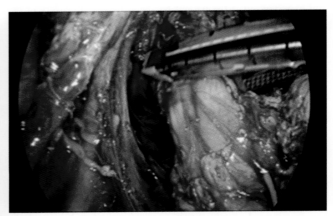

Figure 79.6 Resection of the rectum distal to the rectal nodule using an Endo GIA stapler.

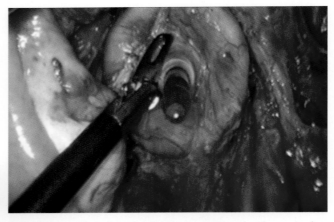

Figure 79.7 Distal rectal stump is being re-anastomosed to the proximal segment using endoscopic circular stapler.

Assessment of rectal integrity

A leak test, while not infallible, should be carried out after any surgery for the removal of RVE to check for air leak. This involves insufflating the rectum with air using a bulb syringe while occluding the rectum, immersed under water, proximal to the site of bowel resection. Any potential leakage should be sutured tightly with 3-0 Vicryl and the test repeated until the surgeon is completely satisfied.

KEY POINTS

Challenge: Laparoscopic removal of rectovaginal endometriosis.

Background

- RVE should be suspected in women presenting with a combination of dysmenorrhea, dyspareunia, deep rectal pain, and dyschezia.
- Surgery for the removal of rectovaginal and bowel endometriosis has been shown to be feasible, safe and effective through either open or laparoscopic surgery.
- As surgery is often technically challenging and carries potential for significant morbidities, surgical removal of rectovaginal and bowel endometriosis should be considered in symptomatic women after thorough preoperative counseling, by experienced surgeons, in well-equipped operating theaters, with proper planning and multidisciplinary support.

Management

- There are several options open to gynecologists who see women with RVE. These include (i) see and discuss, (ii) see and refer, (iii) see and treat at the same time, or (iv) see, discuss and treat at a later time.

- The decision about whether to see and treat at the time of the initial laparoscopic surgery or to treat at a later time depends on the extent of preoperative counseling, the surgeon's experience, the adequacy of theater time, the availability of instrumentation and equipment, and the level of colorectal support and assistance.
- Surgery for excision of RVE should be performed when optimal conditions exist so as to maximize the chance of completing the surgery required, and to minimize the risks associated with surgery. The essential steps for laparoscopic removal of RVE include:
  - Appropriate port placement.
  - Mobilization of rectosigmoid adhesions.
  - Identification of the ureters.
  - Dissection of the rectovaginal endometriosis.
  - Evaluation and removal of rectal disease based on the size, depth, location, and number of bowel lesions.
  - Bowel integrity check following removal of endometriosis using the rectal leak test.

Reference

1 Remorgida V, Ferrero S, Fulcehri E, Ragni N, Martin DC. Bowel endometriosis: presentation, diagnosis, and treatment. *Obstet Gynecol Surv* 2007;62:461–470.

Further reading

Abrao MS, Gonçalves MO, Dias JA Jr, Podgaec S, Chamie LP, Blasbalg R. Comparison between clinical examination, transvaginal sonography and magnetic resonance imaging for the diagnosis of deep endometriosis. *Hum Reprod* 2007;22:3092–3097.

Johnson N, Hummelshoij L. Consensus on current management of endometriosis. *Hum Reprod* 2013;28:1552–1568.

Kwok A, Lam A, Ford R. Deeply infiltrating endometrosis: implications, diagnosis and management. *Obstet Gynecol Surv* 2001;56:168–177.

Minelli L, Fanfani F, Fagotti A *et al.* Laparoscopic colorectal resection for bowel endometriosis: feasibility, complications and clinical outcome. *Arch Surg* 2009;144:234–239.

CHAPTER 80
Laparoscopic Myomectomy

Ertan Saridogan

University College London Hospitals NHS Foundation Trust, London, UK

Case history: A 29-year-old nulliparous woman presented with heavy menstrual bleeding and anemia, and was diagnosed with a 12-cm intramural fibroid distorting the uterine cavity. On examination, the uterus was palpable just below the umbilicus. She elected to have her fibroid removed and requested to have a laparoscopic myomectomy.

Background

Myomectomy is still the most preferred treatment for symptomatic fibroids in women who wish to retain their fertility. Since its first description in 1977, laparoscopic myomectomy (LM) has gained considerable popularity and is now performed by a large number of clinicians worldwide. However, it remains a challenging procedure and requires advanced laparoscopic skills.

There are now a significant number of publications, including randomized controlled trials comparing LM with open myomectomy, which demonstrate the feasibility and safety of LM [1,2]. These studies suggest that LM is associated with reduced blood loss, lower hemoglobin drop, less postoperative pain, shorter hospital stay and recovery period, and lower risk of complications [1]. Although the likelihood of missing small fibroids may be higher because of the lack of tactile sensation during laparoscopy, this does not seem to be of any clinical consequence. Thus, it can be concluded that the laparoscopic approach is a better choice than the open approach in appropriately selected patients.

Management

A 12-cm intramural fibroid may be difficult to remove laparoscopically because of its bulk and lack of space to work comfortably with the laparoscopic instruments in the lower abdominal cavity. In addition, bleeding from a large and deep incision to enucleate the fibroid may be somewhat challenging. The strategies to overcome these restrictions include appropriate patient selection, preoperative medical treatment to reduce the size of the fibroid, intraoperative optimization of port placement, use of vasoconstrictive agents, and good surgical technique to enucleate the fibroid and repair the myometrial defect.

Preoperative patient selection

The number and size of fibroids that can be removed laparoscopically depend on the surgeon's experience and expertise. The number, size, and location of fibroids must be carefully mapped preoperatively. This is an essential requirement, as there is no possibility of palpating the uterus intraoperatively. Mapping not only helps determine the feasibility of LM versus an open approach, but also guides in planning the uterine incision(s) and reduces the risk of residual fibroids. In experienced hands, transvaginal ultrasound examination using high-quality machines is usually adequate for evaluating fibroids preoperatively. When ultrasound findings are equivocal, MRI may help to confirm the diagnosis and to differentiate fibroids from adenomyosis. This is an important distinction to be made because adenomyosis presents an added challenge during laparoscopy owing to the lack of a clearly defined dissection plane.

Saline infusion sonohysterography and hysteroscopy may also assist in identifying submucosal fibroids and may be particularly useful when there is significant uterine distortion from several other fibroids. The final decision as to whether LM is feasible may only be possible at the time of surgery. It is therefore imperative that the woman is warned of the possibility of an open approach and that this is reflected in the preoperative consultation and consent.

Preoperative medical treatment to reduce the size of fibroids

The preoperative use of GnRH analogs is known to reduce the size of fibroids and uterus [3]. This may be beneficial by creating more space to work around the uterus with the relatively small laparoscopic instruments. A smaller fibroid may be easier to handle laparoscopically and would later take less time to morcellate. GnRH analogs also reduce the blood loss at operation. However, they may obscure the plane between the fibroid and myometrium and this may make fibroid enucleation more difficult. In addition, smaller fibroids may be easier to miss during the operation, increasing the risk of fibroid recurrence postoperatively. Ulipristal acetate can also be used to shrink fibroids preoperatively, without the menopausal side effects [4]. Its impact on the tissue planes is not known. Both GnRH analogs and ulipristal acetate are helpful in correcting anemia before surgery.

Gynecologic and Obstetric Surgery: Challenges and Management Options, First Edition. Edited by Arri Coomarasamy, Mahmood I. Shafi, G. Willy Davila and Kiong K. Chan.
© 2016 John Wiley & Sons, Ltd. Published 2016 by John Wiley & Sons, Ltd.

Port placement

At surgery, port placement should be planned to create enough space between the laparoscope and the uterus. Using an epigastric port for the telescope would help with this purpose; the other ports should be positioned according to the location of fibroid(s), type of incision(s), and the suturing technique of the surgeon.

Intraoperative vasoconstrictive agents

Prior to incising the serosa, a dilute solution of synthetic vasopressin is injected into the myometrium, and possibly into the broad ligaments. Vasopressin causes vasoconstriction and reduces blood loss significantly [2]. It may cause untoward cardiovascular complications, making it important to forewarn the anesthetist prior to its instillation. The use of a synthetic vasopressin for myomectomies is not permitted in some countries. Possible alternatives are vaginal misoprostol and epinephrine.

Surgical technique

The location and direction of uterine incision(s) will depend on the location of fibroid(s) and the surgeon's preference; those who use ipsilateral suturing may prefer transverse incisions whereas those who use contralateral suturing would find longitudinal or oblique incisions easier to suture. The location of the fallopian tubes and ovarian ligaments in relation to the fibroids should also be taken into account before making the incision [5].

Ultrasonic scalpels, monopolar diathermy attached to a hook or scissors, and laser may all be used to incise the overlying serosa and myometrium. It is helpful to cut deep into the fibroid so that the actual plane between the fibroid and the myometrium is easier to identify (Figures 80.1 and 80.2). Once the plane is determined, the incision is then enlarged to the required size and a combination of instruments such as myomectomy screws, claw forceps, and tooth graspers is used to enucleate the fibroids. Traction and counter-traction using these instruments, as well as the counter-traction applied by a second assistant via a vulsellum on the cervix, together with division of the myometrial and fibrous bands utilizing the energy source used for the initial incision would eventually result in removal of the fibroid. Care should be taken to avoid pushing laparoscopic instruments into the uterine cavity if possible; similarly, the second assistant should refrain from using excessive force on the uterine manipulator as that can cause uterine perforation (Figure 80.3).

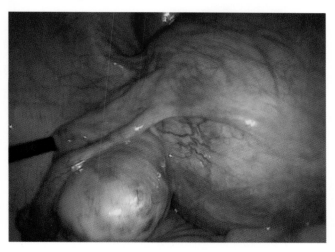

Figure 80.1 An enlarged uterus due to a large deep intramural/submucosal fibroid in the left posterolateral wall.

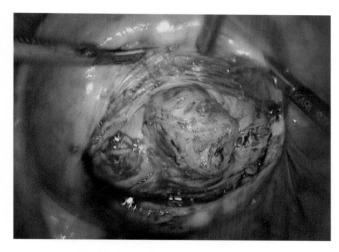

Figure 80.2 A posterior wall transverse incision is made over the fibroid to expose the fibroid and the plane between the fibroid and myometrium.

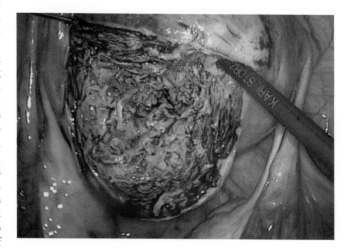

Figure 80.3 The myometrial defect after enucleation of the fibroid. The endometrium is reached but not breached.

Once removed, the smaller fibroids should be placed in the pouch of Douglas (POD) to avoid difficulty in locating them later. Larger fibroids may be placed in the upper abdomen as they will be difficult to fit into the POD and easier to locate.

Hemostasis is usually achieved by targeted electrocoagulation and suturing. Indiscriminate and excessive diathermy should be avoided as this is probably one of the main factors contributing to uterine rupture in future pregnancies, along with inadequate suturing.

The repair of the myometrial defect should be similar to the repair at open myomectomy. If the uterine cavity is breached, separate repair of the endometrium may be beneficial in preventing the rare future cases of myometrial pregnancy. The myometrium should be repaired using large curved needles to avoid leaving significant "dead-spaces" within the defect (Figure 80.4). The suture material could be either delayed absorbable conventional products or so-called "barbed sutures" that reduce the operating time as they do not require knot-tying. The serosa could also be closed with similar sutures; however, if barbed sutures are used it is probably useful to cover the incision with an anti-adhesion agent to reduce risk of bowel adherence, which may result in postoperative mechanical ileus (Figure 80.5).

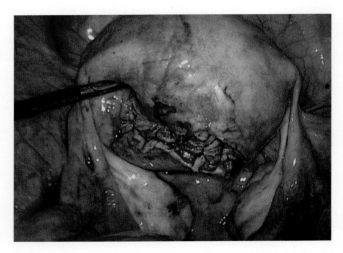

Figure 80.4 Myometrial defect repaired using barbed suture in two layers.

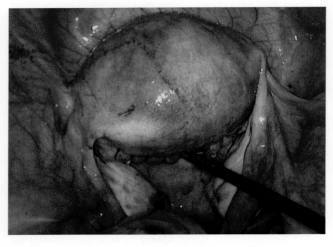

Figure 80.5 Serosal incision closed using barbed suture. The incision is later covered with a barrier anti-adhesion agent.

The fibroid is usually removed using a single-use or reusable electromechanical morcellator. It is important to have a complete view of the morcellator when it is activated, taking extreme care that its tip is free of the abdominal wall, bowel, and any other adjacent structures. After removing the fibroid, complete inspection of the abdominopelvic cavity is necessary to remove any fibroid fragments, as morcellated fragments of fibroid can cause disseminated peritoneal leiomyomatosis.

After thorough irrigation and confirmation of hemostasis, an anti-adhesion agent may be applied to the incision(s). At the end of the procedure it is important to repair the rectus sheath defects of larger ports, particularly the one used for the morcellator, to avoid later herniation (Chapter 90).

Prevention of complications

Appropriate patient selection and detailed preoperative mapping of fibroids are important for reducing the likelihood of surgeons embarking on operations that may be too challenging for their level of experience. Consideration should be given to the preoperative use of GnRH analogs or ulipristal acetate to reduce the size of larger fibroids and correct anemia. The benefits should be weighed against the cost, side effects, possibilities of difficult fibroid enucleation, and increased risk of recurrence in the presence of multiple small fibroids.

The use of intraoperative vasoconstrictive agents reduces excessive blood loss. Hemostasis should be targeted, and excessive or indiscriminate use of diathermy should be avoided. A good repair technique that resembles the reconstitution of myometrium at open surgery will also help with hemostasis and reduce the possibility of uterine rupture in future pregnancies.

Surgeons should follow the principles of appropriate training before attempting the procedure and receive mentoring during the initial stages of their learning curve.

KEY POINTS

Challenge: Laparoscopic removal of a very large symptomatic intramural fibroid.

Background
- Laparoscopic myomectomy is associated with reduced blood loss, lower hemoglobin drop, less postoperative pain, shorter hospital stay and recovery period, and lower risk of complications in comparison with open myomectomy.
- However, it remains a challenging procedure and requires advanced laparoscopic skills.

Prevention
- Comprehensive preoperative assessment for feasibility and planning, including ultrasound, MRI, and hysteroscopy to help appropriate patient selection.
- Preoperative shrinkage of very large fibroids, with either GnRH analogs or ulipristal acetate treatment, is likely to be beneficial.

Management
- The following approaches are likely to improve the success of operation and reduce risk of complications:
  - Appropriate port placement to leave a good distance between the laparoscope and uterus.
  - Intraoperative use of vasoconstrictive agents.
  - Use of large curved needles to repair the myometrial defect, in multiple layers if necessary.
  - Use of electromechanical morcellators.
- Avoiding use of excessive diathermy and a good repair of the myometrial defect should reduce future risk of uterine rupture.

References

1 Jin C, Hu Y, Chen XC *et al.* Laparoscopic versus open myomectomy: a meta-analysis of randomized controlled trials. *Eur J Obstet Gynecol Reprod Biol* 2009;145:14–21.
2 Sizzi O, Rossetti A, Malzoni M *et al.* Italian multicenter study on complications of laparoscopic myomectomy. *J Minim Invasive Gynecol* 2007;14:453–462.
3 Lethaby A, Vollenhoven B, Sowter M. Pre-operative GnRH analogue therapy before hysterectomy or myomectomy for uterine fibroids. *Cochrane Database Syst Rev* 2001;(2):CD000547.
4 Donnez J, Tomaszewski J, Vázquez F *et al.* Ulipristal acetate versus leuprolide acetate for uterine fibroids. *N Engl J Med* 2012;366:421–432.
5 Homer H, Saridogan E. Laparoscopic myomectomy. In: CutnerA, VyasS (eds) *Laparoscopic Surgery for Benign Gynaecology.* RCOG Press, London, 2012.

CHAPTER 81
Total Laparoscopic Hysterectomy

Alan Farthing
Imperial College Healthcare NHS Trust, London, UK

Case history: A 48-year-old nulliparous woman with chronic pelvic pain is listed for a total laparoscopic hysterectomy. The uterus is estimated to be 12-week size with reduced mobility. She had a ruptured appendix as a child removed through an incision in the right iliac fossa.

Background

Total laparoscopic hysterectomy (TLH), as the name suggests, requires all the surgery to be done laparoscopically; currently this technique is gaining prominence at the expense of laparoscopic-assisted vaginal hysterectomy (LAVH) and abdominal hysterectomy. This change is at least partly because of advances in instrumentation along with surgical skills and experience.

Systematic review data from available trials comparing routes of hysterectomy for benign disease support the first-line use of vaginal hysterectomy where possible over laparoscopic hysterectomy, which in turn is preferred over abdominal hysterectomy [1]. It is likely that this hierarchy will be challenged with increasing proficiency and experience of surgeons in advanced laparoscopic procedures. Laparoscopy also facilitates salpingectomy at the time of hysterectomy, which is likely to become more routinely performed in light of recent evidence that the fallopian tube may be the origin of many high-grade serous ovarian cancers.

Where adhesions are anticipated, a laparoscopic hysterectomy is a good option, as it provides good visualization to facilitate adhesiolysis and restoration of normal pelvic anatomy. Although an enlarged uterus can be removed vaginally by surgeons skilled in this technique (Chapter 110), the laparoscopic approach will often simplify the removal of the bulky uterus for many surgeons (Chapter 82); as a general principle, if the surgery is easier for the surgeon, it is safer for the patient. TLH for the treatment of patients with endometrial cancer is now becoming the gold standard. In endometrial cancer, it is important to obtain a good view of the peritoneal cavity, peritoneal washings should be taken, and occasionally a lymphadenectomy needs to be performed; all of these are possible with TLH.

Management

Different surgeons will find different ways of performing the same operation. A variety of instruments can be used but I use an ultrasonic scalpel to divide most tissues, with bipolar diathermy

used for ensuring hemostasis when transecting larger blood vessels. Alternatively, advanced bipolar technologies with integrated cutting systems (Chapter 71) can also be used. A method for performing a TLH based on the approach of a pioneer laparoscopic surgeon, Professor Tony McCartney, is summarized here.

- An umbilical port is inserted for the camera and subsequently, under direct vision, two 5-mm ports are inserted as the operating ports. It is my preference to stand on the left side of the patient and insert the first port lateral to the left inferior epigastric vessels with the second 5-mm port inserted medial to the inferior epigastric blood vessels on the right. Although this gives an asymmetric series of scars, it allows for a more comfortable stance for the surgeon.
- The round ligament is then divided and the broad ligament is opened. Hemostasis of the ovarian artery and veins is secured if an oophorectomy is to be performed; the vessels medial to the ovary within the ovarian ligament are secured if the ovaries are to be preserved. Recent evidence suggests that the fallopian tube may be responsible for many high-grade serous "ovarian cancers" so it is rational to remove the tubes whether the ovaries are being preserved or not.
- After taking the upper pedicles, the peritoneum in the uterovesical fold is incised and the bladder reflected caudally from the cervix. The posterior broad ligament peritoneum is then divided, skeletonizing the uterine vessels. These are secured and divided before the McCartney tube (or similar device) is inserted into the vagina to outline the cervico-vaginal junction (Figure 81.1). This is then divided around its full circumference and the cervix placed in the tube and delivered vaginally.

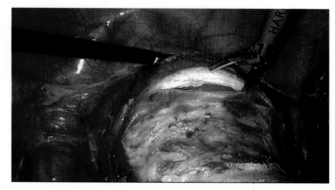

Figure 81.1 A colpotomy being performed around the edge of a McCartney tube.

Gynecologic and Obstetric Surgery: Challenges and Management Options, First Edition. Edited by Arri Coomarasamy, Mahmood I. Shafi, G. Willy Davila and Kiong K. Chan.
© 2016 John Wiley & Sons, Ltd. Published 2016 by John Wiley & Sons, Ltd.

245

• A large uterus can be morcellated if the pathology is benign, although most uteri of 12-week size or less can be easily passed through the vagina intact. The vault of the vagina is repaired laparoscopically (Figure 81.2), using a standard suture or barbed self-locking suture.

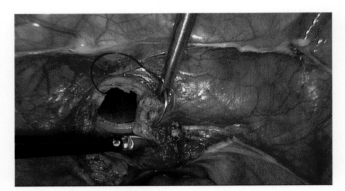

Figure 81.2 Suturing of the vaginal vault.

On occasions, and especially when teaching a trainee, an additional right lateral 5-mm port may be necessary. This can also be helpful if there are adhesions or if the woman is obese. This port can be useful for retracting the bowel out of the pelvis. Steep Trendelenburg tilt will be required to allow pelvic access despite the difficulty with ventilation and build-up of carbon dioxide in the patient's bloodstream; close collaboration of an experienced anesthetist is important.

Evidence

With the development of laparoscopic hysterectomy, several randomized controlled trials were undertaken to evaluate the evidence for benefit or otherwise of these new techniques. However, the main confounder in surgical trials is generally the surgeon, and a disadvantage of many of these early trials was that many of the surgeons lacked experience in advanced laparoscopic techniques. Thus, these trials may have been biased toward the conventional alternative techniques, explaining the findings that laparoscopic hysterectomy, while associated with faster recovery, did so at the expense of longer operating times and a higher number of complications.

A Cochrane review of 4495 benign hysterectomies [1] showed that when laparoscopic hysterectomy was compared with abdominal hysterectomy, the recovery was on average 13.6 days faster, with 2 days less spent in hospital. However, the laparoscopic operation took on average 20 min longer and the relative risk of bladder or urinary tract injury was 2.4 times higher. In the last few years, some of the more experienced surgeons have published up-to-date records of their morbidity; in one series of 1577 total laparoscopic hysterectomies [2], the minor complication rate was 1.14% and major complication rate 0.51%. A recent meta-analysis of patients treated by TLH for endometrial cancer showed a decreased risk of complications in comparison with abdominal hysterectomy, with a relative risk (RR) of 0.53 for major complications and an RR of 0.59 for all complications [3]. In my series of 200 patients with endometrial cancer, over 25% had a BMI over 40, but the

overall complication and conversion rate was low at 1% and similar between those women with extreme obesity and the rest of the cohort [4].

KEY POINTS

Challenge: Total laparoscopic hysterectomy.

Background
• Total laparoscopic hysterectomy, as the name suggests, requires all the surgery to be done laparoscopically.
• TLH is the operation of choice for endometrial cancer and one of the better options for patients with benign disease.
• The technique is gaining increasing prominence at the expense of LAVH and abdominal hysterectomy.
• This observed change in surgical trends is probably because of advances in instrumentation along with surgical skills and experience.

Prevention
• Complication rates are very low in centers where large numbers of these operations are being performed.
• Surgeons conducting TLH should equip themselves with the required skills and maintain their experience.

Management
• TLH may be preferable to vaginal hysterectomy when:
  • Vaginal access is restricted (e.g., nulliparous women).
  • Adhesions are anticipated.
  • The uterus is enlarged.
  • The fallopian tubes and/or ovaries are to be removed.
• In addition to an experienced surgeon and anesthetist, TLH requires good endoscopic equipment including imaging systems, access to good-quality energy modalities (e.g., bipolar diathermy, advanced bipolar electrosurgical systems, or ultrasonic scalpel), vaginal tubes to assist with colpotomy, laparoscopic needle holders and sutures according to the surgeon's preference.
• A typical TLH has the following steps:
  • Insertion of a 10-mm umbilical port, and two or three operating ports (5 mm).
  • Division of round ligament and opening of broad ligament.
  • Identification of the ureters.
  • Electrocoagulation and transection of the infundibulopelvic ligament (if ovaries are being removed) or the ovarian ligament (if ovaries are being preserved).
  • Incision of the peritoneum of the uterovesical fold, and reflection of the bladder caudally away from the cervix.
  • Skeletonization of the uterine vessels, followed by electrocoagulation and division of the vessels.
  • Following outlining of the cervico-vaginal junction with a McCartney tube (or similar device), circumferential incision of the vagina.
  • Removal of the specimen vaginally, or with the aid of a morcellator.
  • Closure of the vaginal vault using a standard suture or barbed self-locking suture.

References

1 Nieboer TE, Johnson N, Lethaby A et al. Surgical approach to hysterectomy for benign gynaecological disease. *Cochrane Database Syst Rev* 2009;(3):CD003677.
2 Donnez O, Jadoul P, Squifflet J, Donnez J. A series of 3190 laparoscopic hysterectomies for benign disease from 1990 to 2006: evaluation of complications compared with vaginal and abdominal procedures. *BJOG* 2009;116:492–500.
3 Hui-Ling Wang, Yan-Fang Ren, Jun Yang, Rui-Ying Qin, Kai-Hua Zhai. Total laparoscopic hysterectomy versus total abdominal hysterectomy for endometrial cancer: a meta-analysis. *Asian Pac J Cancer Prev* 2013;14:2515–2519.
4 Farthing A, Chatterjee J, Joglekar-Pai P, Dorney E, Ghaem-Maghami S. Total laparoscopic hysterectomy for early stage endometrial cancer in obese and morbidly obese women. *J Obstet Gynaecol* 2012;32:580–584.

CHAPTER 82

Laparoscopic Hysterectomy for a Large Fibroid Uterus

Alan Lam

Center for Advanced Reproductive Endosurgery, University of Sydney, St Leonards, Australia

Case history: A woman with an 18-week size multiple fibroid uterus requested a laparoscopic hysterectomy. After insertion of the Veress needle and trocar at the umbilicus, and placement of the operative ports in the left and right iliac fossa and suprapubic region, the surgeon noticed bleeding from the fundus of the uterus.

Background

Removal of a large, multiple fibroid uterus that fills the pelvic cavity and extends to the pelvic sidewalls is a challenging operation whether performed as an open or laparoscopic operation. There is often great difficulty seeing and accessing the ovaries, bladder, ureters, and uterine vessels.

While the benefits of laparoscopic hysterectomy are well recognized, the surgeon needs to fully discuss and inform the woman of potentially higher risks of (i) intraoperative blood loss, (ii) bowel, bladder, and ureteric complications, (iii) conversion to laparotomy, (iv) extra time required for specimen removal, and (v) longer operative time. Ultimately, the surgeon needs to keep in mind that the woman's safety is the foremost consideration in deciding if it is feasible to undertake a laparoscopic hysterectomy [1].

The experienced laparoscopic surgeon will recognize that the potential challenges arising from the restricted surgical access and manipulation that may be experienced at open surgery are likely to be magnified during laparoscopic surgery; the operative field and the range of laparoscopic movements are limited, increasing the likelihood of inadvertent damage to the ovaries, uterine arteries, bladder, ureters, and bowels.

Management

With judicious planning, laparoscopic hysterectomy can be performed safely and efficiently [2,3] with the following special considerations in mind.

Entering the abdomen without causing trauma to the uterus

Because of the proximity of a large uterus to the umbilicus, a routine entry using a Veress needle and trocar at the umbilicus is likely to cause trauma to the uterus with consequent bleeding. An open entry followed by direct insertion of a blunt 10-mm port into the abdominal cavity allows the surgeon to evaluate the pathology being treated with a clear, bloodless operative field. This would allow the surgeon time to decide whether and how to proceed with intended laparoscopic surgery.

Maximizing view of the operative field and range of instrumentation

To improve view of the operative field, the surgeon should consider positioning the primary port halfway between the umbilicus and the xiphisternum rather than at the umbilicus. In addition, by using a 30° telescope instead of the 0° telescope, the surgeon will have a better view above and around the protruding fibroids, to recognize the bladder anteriorly, the ureters on the pelvic sidewalls, and the pouch of Douglas (Figure 82.1).

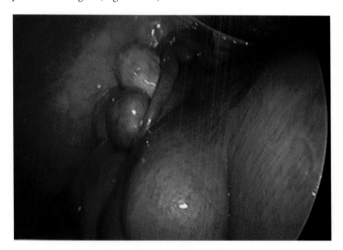

Figure 82.1 The left tube and ovary are displaced into the left paracolic gutter. Note that visualization of the uterovesical peritoneum, pelvic sidewall, and pouch of Douglas is enhanced with the use of a 30° laparoscope.

The operative ports should also be positioned above the level of the umbilicus and toward the flank of the abdomen rather than in the lower abdomen to allow an optimal range of instrument movement above the fundus and around the body of the enlarged uterus. This will facilitate access to the ovaries, the bladder, and the pelvic sidewalls.

Gynecologic and Obstetric Surgery: Challenges and Management Options, First Edition. Edited by Arri Coomarasamy, Mahmood I. Shafi, G. Willy Davila and Kiong K. Chan.
© 2016 John Wiley & Sons, Ltd. Published 2016 by John Wiley & Sons, Ltd.

Ensuring adequate uterine maneuverability

To ensure adequate vision and access to the ovaries, uterine vessels, bladder and ureters, the surgeon should use a robust uterine manipulator to maneuver the heavy uterus from side to side and from front to back. Without adequate uterine maneuverability, the surgeon may not be able to safely dissect and protect the ureters, bladder, and rectum.

Avoiding back-bleeding from the uterus

Care and patience is required to secure the round ligaments, the ovarian ligaments (where ovaries are preserved), or the infundibulopelvic ligaments (where ovaries are to be removed). This can be achieved with bipolar diathermy (Chapter 71) and/or suture ligation before transection. When the uterus is heavy, it is important to avoid excessive traction on the divided pedicles due to the risk of troublesome back-bleeding from the engorged uterus during the procedure.

Ensure adequate bladder dissection off the cervix

Use of the 30° telescope helps to obtain visibility over and around the protruding anterior fibroids so that the uterovesical peritoneum can be sharply dissected with either a pair of laparoscopic scissors with monopolar diathermy or laparoscopic ultrasonic curved shears. The latter is an excellent tool allowing tactile, precise, and hemostatic dissection of tissues in this situation.

Ensuring adequate ureteric dissection before coagulation of the uterine arteries

With fibroids extending out to the pelvic sidewall, the ureters may no longer follow their normal course. Therefore, the surgeon should not assume that "hugging" the body of the uterus will avoid risk of ureteric injury in this situation. Rather, the uterine arteries should be identified by retroperitoneal dissection either anteriorly by following the obliterated umbilical artery or posteriorly from the pelvic brim by following the ureter (Figure 82.2).

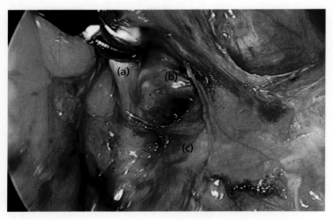

Figure 82.2 Retroperitoneal dissection following the left obliterated umbilical artery (a) to identify the left uterine artery (b) and the ureter (c).

Once the ureters are clearly identified, the uterine vessels may be secured lateral or medial to the ureters depending on individual circumstances with bipolar diathermy, vascular clips, or sutures

before transection. Once the ovarian and uterine vessels are safely secured, the prospect of successfully completing the operation laparoscopically is greatly enhanced. On the other hand, failure to access or identify the ureters and the uterine vessels clearly should make the surgeon consider conversion to laparotomy.

Colpotomy under laparoscopic visualization

Once the uterus is devascularized, it is advantageous to perform colpotomy under laparoscopic visualization so as to avoid a separate vaginal set-up. This can be done by using laparoscopic scissors with monopolar diathermy or preferably by using laparoscopic ultrasonic curved shears because this latter energy modality avoids excessive smoke plume. Using a colpotomy tube, the anterior vaginal fornix may be entered in the midline followed by circumferential incision until the entire cervix is dissected.

Removal of the specimen

Depending on the individual surgeon's preferences, the uterus may be removed vaginally or abdominally by morcellation. However, if there is any suspicion of sarcomatous change within a fibroid, especially in women of postmenopausal age, then morcellation should be avoided because of concerns over potential dissemination of disease [4,5].

As the woman in the case presented is nulliparous, access through the vagina may be limited and it may be easier and quicker to remove the huge fibroid uterus abdominally through a 3–4 cm incision either suprapubically or at the umbilicus through an Alexis retractor. It is advisable to re-insufflate the abdomen to check for hemostasis and complete removal of all specimens. A cystoscopy may also be performed to ensure bladder and ureteric integrity.

Prevention

Careful preoperative evaluation is required to determine the method of hysterectomy and the route of specimen removal if laparoscopic hysterectomy is considered [2]. Compared with physical, ultrasound, or CT examination, MRI is particularly useful and more reliable in assessing the number, location, and size of the fibroids where the uterine mass rises into the abdomen.

The use of GnRH analogs or ulipristal acetate for 3 months should be considered if the surgeon feels uncomfortable taking on such a large uterus. This therapy may not only improve the woman's preoperative hemoglobin if she is anemic, but also may help shrink the fibroids, thereby reducing the risks of intraoperative bleeding, specimen retrieval and operating times, making laparoscopic hysterectomy a more feasible option [3].

Because of the size of the uterus, the surgeon needs to give special consideration to higher port positioning and the use of a laparoscope with an offset distal lens to help overcome problems presented by the restricted operative field and limited maneuverability of ancillary instruments.

At all stages, the woman's safety is the foremost factor in determining whether the surgeon should proceed with the planned laparoscopic hysterectomy or convert to open surgery.

KEY POINTS

Challenge: Problems in laparoscopic removal of a huge fibroid uterus.

Background
- Removal of a large fibroid uterus is a challenge whether performed as open or laparoscopic surgery.
- Restricted operative fields, limited instrumentation, difficult access, and proximity to vital structures increase the operative time, risk of bleeding, and surgical morbidities associated with laparoscopic hysterectomy.
- Laparoscopic hysterectomy in this setting is for the experienced surgeon, after adequate preoperative counseling of the patient.

Prevention
- Thorough preoperative evaluation, counseling and self-examination of the surgeon's own skills are important in determining whether laparoscopic hysterectomy should be offered.
- GnRH analogs or ulipristal acetate for 3 months may improve feasibility and safety of laparoscopic hysterectomy for large fibroid uteri.

- Decision about the mode of specimen retrieval should be made prior to surgery. If there is any suspicion of sarcomatous change within a fibroid, especially in women of postmenopausal age, then morcellation should be avoided because of concerns over potential dissemination of disease.

Management
- Enter the abdomen without causing trauma to the uterus: consider open entry; consider positioning the primary port halfway between the umbilicus and the xiphisternum rather than at the umbilicus.
- Maximize the view around corners: consider using a 30° telescope instead of the 0° telescope.
- Ensure adequate uterine maneuverability: use a robust uterine manipulator.
- Ensure adequate bladder dissection off the cervix.
- Ensure adequate ureteric dissection before coagulation of the uterine arteries.
- Perform a colpotomy under laparoscopic visualization.
- Remove the specimen vaginally, or abdominally by morcellation.
- Do not hesitate to convert to an open procedure if patient safety dictates this.

References

1 Chang WC, Huang SC, Sheu BC et al. Successful laparoscopically assisted vaginal hysterectomies for large uteri of various sizes. *Acta Obstet Gynecol Scand* 2008;87:558–563.

2 Ferrari MM, Berlanda N, Mezzopane R, Ragusa G, Cavallo M, Pardi G. Identifying the indications for laparoscopically assisted vaginal hysterectomy: a prospective, randomised comparison with abdominal hysterectomy in patients with symptomatic uterine fibroids. *BJOG* 2000;107:620–625.

3 Wu KY, Lertvikool S, Huang KG, Su H, Yen CF, Lee CL. Laparoscopic hysterectomies for large uteri. *Taiwan J Obstet Gynecol* 2011;50:411–414.

4 American College of Obstetricians and Gynecologists. Power morcellation and occult malignancy in gynecologic surgery. A special report. ACOG, May 2014. Available at http://www.acog.org/Resources-And-Publications/Task-Force-and-Work-Group-Reports/Power-Morcellation-and-Occult-Malignancy-in-Gynecologic-Surgery

5 American Association of Gynecologic Laparoscopists. Morcellation during uterine tissue extraction. Available at http://www.aagl.org/wp-content/uploads/2014/05/Tissue_Extraction_TFR.pdf

CHAPTER 83

Laparoscopy: Difficulty in Tissue Retrieval

Su-Yen Khong[1] and Alan Lam[2]

[1] University of Malaya Medical Center, Kuala Lumpur, Malaysia
[2] Center for Advanced Reproductive Endosurgery, University of Sydney, St Leonards, Australia

Case history: A woman undergoes a laparoscopic ovarian cystectomy for a 12-cm dermoid cyst with calcification suggestive of teeth or bony formation. The specimen is shelled out intact from the ovary. The surgeon now faces the challenge of removing the large dermoid cyst containing solid components.

Background

The use of laparoscopic surgery has become accepted as the "standard" approach for removal of benign pathology such as ovarian cysts or fibroids. This is because minimal access surgery, compared with open surgery, is associated with smaller skin incisions, better cosmetic results, less postoperative pain, shorter hospital stay, faster recovery, and earlier return to normal activities [1,2].

Retrieval of tissue specimens by laparoscopic surgery is intrinsically more difficult compared with open surgery, presenting a number of challenges. Firstly, when the surgical specimen cannot be removed via a 5- or 10-mm port, it must be reduced in size either within the abdomen, or placed inside a tissue retrieval bag to be removed in a piecemeal fashion or by morcellation through an extended port-site incision. These steps prolong the operative and anesthetic time. Secondly, there is a higher risk of specimen rupture or spillage during laparoscopic dissection and specimen removal. Thirdly, the use of endoscopic retrieval bags can minimize the risk of spillage but will add to the procedural costs because of the requirement for these consumables. Fourthly, extension of the incision site may aid retrieval of large specimens but this can increase the risks of port herniation (Chapter 90), hematoma formation, and postoperative pain [3].

The suitability for laparoscopic specimen retrieval is dependent on various factors.

- *Size of the specimen.* The size of the specimen will likely influence the size of the retrieval bag and the degree of difficulty in manipulating the cyst into the bag. Once inside the retrieval bag, the larger specimen is also likely to require aspiration to reduce cyst volume before it can be debulked or morcellated for removal from the peritoneal cavity. In the case of large uterine fibroids or uteri after subtotal hysterectomy, the surgeon needs to select a 15-mm morcellator or remove the specimen via a mini-laparotomy incision.

- *Consistency of the specimen.* Cystic specimens which can be decompressed by aspiration either intra-abdominally or within the retrieval bag are easier to remove than cysts which contain thick or solid contents such as sebum, hair, or calcified materials (Figure 83.1). On the other hand, soft friable tissues such as degenerative fibroids may be impossible to grasp, while heavily calcified fibroids may be impossible to morcellate and may require a mini-laparotomy to extract from the peritoneal cavity.

- *Tissue pathology.* Benign specimens can be removed piecemeal but the surgeon should be aware of special circumstances where specimen retrieval may lead to complications if the cyst ruptures or if the tissue comes into contact with the port-site skin incisions during the process of removal from the peritoneal cavity. Examples include the risks associated with tissue spillage and dissemination of malignancy (ovarian carcinoma, uterine leiomyosarcoma), pseudomyxoma peritonei (mucinous cystadenoma), chemical peritonitis (ruptured dermoid cyst), and tissue seedling (endometriosis and fibroids implanting onto distant sites within the peritoneal cavity or port sites).

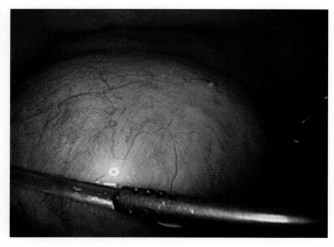

Figure 83.1 A huge dermoid cyst containing solid components can present challenges when trying to remove the specimen from the peritoneal cavity.

Gynecologic and Obstetric Surgery: Challenges and Management Options, First Edition. Edited by Arri Coomarasamy, Mahmood I. Shafi, G. Willy Davila and Kiong K. Chan.
© 2016 John Wiley & Sons, Ltd. Published 2016 by John Wiley & Sons, Ltd.

Management

In order to optimize the chances of specimen retrieval during laparoscopic surgery while ensuring that this process is carried out safely and efficiently, it is important that the surgeon is aware of the different methods and routes available. The following options should be considered.

1 Direct retrieval of excised specimen through the 5- or 10-mm laparoscopic port(s) by cutting the tissue into long strips. This method is suitable for simple large ovarian cysts, endometriomas, and small dermoid cysts with no solid components. The disadvantages with this method include tissue spillage and seedling.

2 Large benign ovarian cysts can be decompressed intraoperatively under direct vision before cystectomy. Decompression can be achieved under direct vision by inserting a 5- or 10-mm trocar directly into the cyst (Figure 83.2). To minimize spillage of the cyst contents, an Endoloop® can be used to tie around the punctured cyst opening while grasping the perforation edges with forceps, after initial aspiration. Alternatively, large unruptured cysts, once dissected free, can be placed inside a retrieval bag and decompressed by exteriorizing the bag through the port site. Preoperative decompression of cysts under imaging guidance (e.g., ultrasound or CT) has been described. However, the disadvantages include another intervention with associated resource use and inflated costs as well as the lack of direct final inspection and assessment of the pathology before surgical intervention.

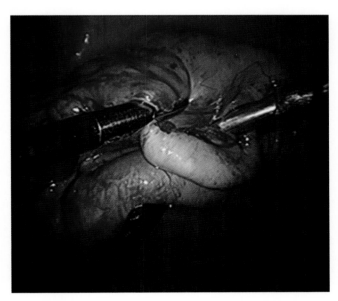

Figure 83.2 Direct decompression of the cystic area of a large dermoid cyst through a 5-mm trocar.

3 Through a 2–3 cm mini-laparotomy incision, a large benign ovarian cyst can be decompressed in a similar fashion to the intra-abdominal decompression method described by first placing a pursestring suture and then inserting a sharp trocar into the cyst wall. This maneuver will minimize spillage of the fluid content during suction drainage. Once decompressed, the cyst may be exteriorized (Figure 83.3) through the abdominal wall for removal by cystectomy or oophorectomy.

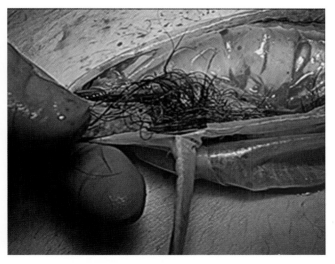

Figure 83.3 A dermoid cyst placed inside a specimen retrieval bag is exteriorized via an umbilical incision.

4 Tissue morcellation can be performed manually or with an electrical morcellator. The advantages include performing the procedure under direct vision while utilizing the same port incision, albeit larger. This method of tissue retrieval is suitable for firm masses such as uterine fibroids but inappropriate for cystic masses such as ovarian dermoid cysts, degenerative fibroids, and potentially premalignant or malignant cysts. Risks include internal organ injury from uncontrolled or inappropriate use of the morcellator and from repeated introduction and removal of sharp laparoscopic graspers. Port-site herniation and hematoma can occur with the larger incisions (10–15 mm) required for the morcellator (Chapter 90).

5 Colpotomy with laparoscopic guided removal of specimen with or without a specimen retrieval bag is an option [4]. Risks include vaginal hematoma, vaginal scarring potentially resulting in dyspareunia, pelvic infection, and rectal injury. This method is contraindicated in cases where the pouch of Douglas is obliterated or vaginal access is very limited.

6 Specimen retrieval bags can be used to avoid spillage and wound contamination. Introduction of these bags into the peritoneal cavity requires at least a 10-mm port. A popular method is to introduce the retrieval bag via the 10-mm umbilical port [5] with the guidance of a 5-mm laparoscope inserted via a lateral port. This allows clear visualization of the pelvis and enables the excised tissues to be fed directly into the bag. Exteriorization of the retrieval bag via the 10-mm port allows cyst contents to be decompressed by aspiration with a large-bore needle, or incision into the cyst wall and aspiration using laparoscopic suction. However, transvaginal specimen retrieval using tissue retrieval bags is associated with less pain than removal through a more conventional umbilical port [6]. Solid tissues, such as fibroids, can be manually morcellated and bony calcification within dermoid cysts broken up with a bone crusher within a retrieval bag. However, specimen retrieval bags can be expensive and those made with less durable material may tear during surgical manipulation.

Prevention

Even though the laparoscopic route is widely used for the surgical management of gynecologic conditions, there are certain factors which make this route inappropriate. A surgeon has to consider certain prerequisites before determining the route of surgery. These can be categorized into patient, surgeon, and equipment-related factors.

Preoperative assessment of the patient is essential. History, clinical examination, and investigations such as ultrasonography and tumor markers will allow the surgeon to formulate a likely diagnosis. The suitability of laparoscopic surgery will depend on the size, consistency and pathology of the pelvic mass. In addition, any existing patient comorbidities have to be identified preoperatively. Those with cardiorespiratory compromise may not be able to tolerate a steep Trendelenburg tilt or a CO_2 pneumoperitoneum.

The surgeon should have undergone specialized training and possess good technical skills and knowledge. Careful patient selection and understanding the limitations of laparoscopic surgery, such as the difficulties which can be encountered in specimen retrieval, are important.

Appropriate equipment and an experienced theater team are essential for surgery to be performed in a safe and efficient manner. Without the correct facilities and trained personnel for laparoscopic surgery, it would be more appropriate to proceed with the traditional open surgery.

KEY POINTS

Challenge: Difficult tissue retrieval during laparoscopy.

Background
- Laparoscopic retrieval of tissue specimens can be challenging via small operative ports, resulting in longer operative and anesthetic time.
- Concerns exist regarding specimen rupture or spillage during laparoscopic dissection and specimen removal.
- The suitability for laparoscopic specimen retrieval should depend on the size and consistency of the tissue specimen as well as its pathology.

Management
- Methods to aid laparoscopic specimen retrieval include:
- Direct retrieval of excised specimens through the 5- or 10-mm laparoscopic port(s) by cutting the tissue into long strips.
- Mini-laparotomy.
- Decompression of cysts performed intraoperatively, or preoperatively under imaging.
- Tissue morcellation performed manually or with an electrical morcellator.
- Colpotomy with laparoscopic-guided removal of specimens.
- Use of specimen retrieval bags inserted via a transabdominal or transvaginal route.

Prevention
- The suitability of laparoscopic surgery will depend on the nature, size, and consistency of the pelvic mass. Preoperative assessment of the patient including history, clinical examination, and investigations such as ultrasonography and serum tumor markers will help formulate a likely diagnosis.
- The surgeon performing laparoscopic surgery should have specialized training and experience not just in the technical aspects of the procedure but also in appreciating appropriate patient selection and recognizing the limitations of laparoscopic surgery.
- The availability of appropriate equipment and an experienced theater team are essential for surgery to be performed in a safe and effective manner.

References

1 Garry R. Laparoscopic surgery. *Best Pract Res Clin Obstet Gynaecol* 2006;20:89–104.

2 Sciarra JJ. Endoscopy in gynecology: past, present and future. *J Minim Invasive Gynecol* 2006;13:367–369.

3 Stavroulis A, Memtsa M, Yoong W. Methods for specimen removal from the peritoneal cavity after laparoscopic excision. *Obstetrician & Gynaecologist* 2013;15:26–30.

4 Pillai R, Yoong W. Posterior colpotomy revisited: a forgotten route for retrieving larger benign ovarian lesions following laparoscopic excision. *Arch Gynecol Obstet* 2010;281:609–611.

5 Ghezzi F, Cromi A, Uccella S, Siesto G, Bergamini V, Bolis P. Transumbilical surgical specimen retrieval: a viable refinement of laparoscopic surgery for pelvic masses. *BJOG* 2008;115:1316–1320.

6 Ghezzi F, Cromi A, Uccella S, Bogani G, Serati M, Bolis P. Transumbilical versus transvaginal retrieval of surgical specimens at laparoscopy: a randomized trial. *Am J Obstet Gynecol* 2012;207:112e1–6.

CHAPTER 84

Surgery for Cornual or Interstitial Pregnancy

Ayesha Mahmud and Yousri Afifi
Birmingham Women's NHS Foundation Trust, Birmingham, UK

Case history: A woman diagnosed with a tubal pregnancy on ultrasound scan undergoes laparoscopy. She had previously been managed with methotrexate therapy, but had failed to respond. The surgeon finds an intact left-sided cornual ectopic pregnancy.

Background

Cornual or interstitial pregnancies account for up to 2–4% of all ectopic pregnancies [1]. The various factors predisposing to development of a cornual pregnancy are pelvic inflammatory disease (PID), tubal surgery, smoking, increasing maternal age, previous ectopic pregnancy, uterine anomalies, and *in vitro* fertilization [2,3]. The associated maternal mortality rate is estimated to be as high as 2.5%. This is seven times greater than the mortality rate for ectopic pregnancies in general [2,4]. According to the Confidential Enquiry into Maternal and Child Heath Report (2000–2002), a total of 11 maternal deaths were reported secondary to ruptured ectopic pregnancies; four of these were cornual ectopic pregnancies [5]. A more recent Confidential Enquiry into Maternal Deaths has shown that while the incidence of ectopic pregnancy remained static in the triennium 2006–2008, the case mortality rate was reduced and there were no deaths from ectopic pregnancies sited in the uterine cornu [6]. This is a welcome observation because it may imply better diagnosis and treatment. However, cornual pregnancy remains a life-threatening condition which can be more complex to manage than the more common tubal ectopic pregnancy.

Prevention

Barrier contraception helps to prevent PID. Early diagnosis and treatment of PID and smoking cessation also lower the risk of ectopic pregnancy. Investigations such as high-resolution transvaginal ultrasonography (TVS) and sensitive β-human chorionic gonadotropin (bHCG) assays have made early detection of cornual ectopic pregnancies possible. Detection is possible as early as 6–8 weeks, but requires a very high index of clinical suspicion. Prompt diagnosis allows the use of conservative medical or endoscopic surgical techniques to achieve satisfactory outcomes, avoiding the morbidity associated with laparotomy. However,

despite these advances, cornual pregnancies remain a diagnostic challenge and are often missed. In a series by Soriano *et al.* [3], preoperative diagnosis was made in only 56% of the reported cases.

Management

Cornual ectopic pregnancies can be treated medically using methotrexate. Although relatively non-invasive, medical management is not without side effects, and can put the patient at risk of requiring secondary surgical treatment. Surgical treatment is also not without consequences. The traditional approach has been surgical management with exploratory laparotomy, ending in either cornual resection or hysterectomy. This can be complicated by catastrophic hemorrhage resulting in significant patient morbidity and mortality. However, in recent years, minimally invasive laparoscopic and hysteroscopic techniques have been used with favorable outcomes (Table 84.1). Ultimately, the patient's wishes and compliance with follow-up are key factors in the management of such cases.

Table 84.1 Surgical approaches to cornual ectopic pregnancy [7].

Laparotomy
Hysterectomy
Cornual resection

Laparoscopic approach
Cornual wedge resection
Cornual resection or excision
Cornuostomy or salpingotomy
Microcornual excision

Hysteroscopic approach
Endometrial resection with laparoscopy
Cornual evacuation with laparoscopy or ultrasound

Laparoscopic approach

Laparoscopy offers several advantages over laparotomy, such as significantly reduced blood loss, reduced hospital stay, and quick recovery, but requires clinical expertise and good laparoscopic techniques. In hemodynamically unstable patients this approach may not be suitable. Nonetheless, laparoscopic approach is safe and effective if adequate technical skills are available.

Gynecologic and Obstetric Surgery: Challenges and Management Options, First Edition. Edited by Arri Coomarasamy, Mahmood I. Shafi, G. Willy Davila and Kiong K. Chan.
© 2016 John Wiley & Sons, Ltd. Published 2016 by John Wiley & Sons, Ltd.

One of the key technical skills required for surgical management of a cornual ectopic pregnancy relates to achieving a bloodless field with minimal tissue trauma. Various techniques have been described over the years to achieve a bloodless field. This aids excision, preserves fertility, and helps prevent excessive blood loss (Table 84.2).

Table 84.2 Hemostatic techniques for cornual ectopic pregnancy [7].

Technique	Mechanism
Vasopressin injection	10 units diluted in 50–100 mL of 0.9% saline solution provides vasoconstriction
Pursestring suture	Placed around the base of the cornual ectopic. Requires laparoscopic suturing. Reduces blood loss but may occlude tube
Square suture	Suture carried through the posterior and anterior cornual walls, and then carried back through the anterior and then the posterior wall at a point 2 cm lateral to the initial knot. The knot is tied intracorporeally, achieving hemostasis by compression effect
Encircling suture	Placed around the base of the cornual ectopic. Requires laparoscopic suturing. Acts like a tourniquet
Endoloop®	Similar mechanism as above. No need for laparoscopic suturing
Electrocoagulation	Achieves hemostasis by coagulation, with devices such as bipolar diathermy and harmonic instruments. These can cause thermal damage to the myometrium
Occlusion of ascending branch of uterine artery	Occlusion by electrocoagulation or suture ligation. May not achieve complete hemostasis
Fibrin glue	Used to seal myometrium and achieve hemostasis
Automatic stapler	Endo GIA stapler simultaneously excises and stitches the uterine cornua
Double impact devascularization technique (Figure 84.1)	A stitch with two bites, one at the fundus (medial margin of the cornual mass) and the second in the mesosalpinx (below the cornual mass). This compresses the ascending uterine artery and reduces collateral blood supply by compression effect

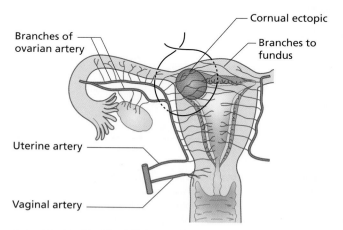

Figure 84.1 Double impact devascularization. Adapted from Mahmud A, *et al*, 2015 [7].

In the clinical scenario, the surgeon could employ any of the above-mentioned hemostatic techniques. It is also reasonable to use vasopressin alongside other techniques for better results. This would then be followed by a linear cornuotomy to aid evacuation of the cornual mass. Afterwards, the myometrial defect should be closed [8]. We recommend two-layer closure, with serosal edge inversion to reduce the risk of adhesions and allow myometrial strengthening.

Hysteroscopic approach

This approach can be undertaken using either a hysteroscope under ultrasound guidance or concomitant laparoscopy. The main principle behind this approach is to identify and evacuate the contents of the cornual ectopic. However, complete evacuation is often avoided to reduce the risk of uterine perforation. Therefore, subsequent follow up with bHCG is necessary to ascertain complete resolution. This approach may be suitable in cases where patients wish to avoid extensive surgery or in cases where methotrexate treatment has failed. It also offers a quicker recovery, with a shorter hospital stay and subsequent normal delivery with no expectation of an increased risk in uterine rupture.

Postoperative management

All patients should be followed up in an outpatient setting for serial bHCG levels to confirm complete resolution of the pregnancy. In some cases persistent trophoblastic tissue may require further treatment. Appropriate debriefing of surgical events with advice on future pregnancies should be provided. In cases managed laparoscopically, although subsequent term deliveries have been reported, it is necessary to highlight the importance of consultant-led antenatal care alongside the possibility of a planned cesarean section at term to avoid the risk of uterine rupture. The risk of subsequent ectopic pregnancy is estimated at 10% and an early antenatal booking scan should be advised.

KEY POINTS

Challenge: Surgery for cornual or interstitial pregnancy.

Background
- Cornual pregnancy can present as a diagnostic and therapeutic challenge with considerable risk of hemorrhage-related patient morbidity and mortality.
- Surgical management options are dependent on operator skills, experience, and patient wishes.

Prevention
- High clinical index of suspicion with comprehensive clinical assessment, using transvaginal ultrasound and serial bHCG can aid early diagnosis.
- Early diagnosis allows use of less invasive management options.
- Risk reduction can be encouraged by early treatment of pelvic infections, smoking cessation, and use of barrier contraception.

Management
- Use an appropriate surgical method depending on expertise of the operator.
- Use a combination of hemostatic techniques. Options include vasopressin injection, pursestring suture, square suture, encircling suture, occlusion of ascending branch of uterine artery, and double impact devascularization technique.
- Once hemostatic measures have been taken, a linear cornuotomy can be performed to evacuate the cornual mass.
- Close the myometrial defect in two layers.
- Arrange follow-up serial bHCG after discharge. The patient may require additional treatment with methotrexate.
- Discuss the impact of surgery on future pregnancy, the risk of subsequent ectopic pregnancy, uterine rupture, and possibility of planned cesarean section.
- Advise booking under consultant-led care for future antenatal care.

References

1 Tulandi T, Al-Jaroudi D. Interstitial pregnancy: results generated from the Society of Reproductive Surgeons Registry. *Obstet Gynecol* 2004;103:47–50.

2 Lau S, Tulandi T. Conservative medical and surgical management of interstitial ectopic pregnancy. *Fertil Steril* 1999;72:207–215.

3 Soriano D, Vicus D, Mashiach R, Schiff E, Seidman D, Goldenberg M. Laparoscopic treatment of cornual pregnancy: a series of 20 consecutive cases. *Fertil Steril* 2008;90:839–843.

4 Walker J. Ectopic pregnancy. *Clin Obstet Gynecol* 2007;50:89–99.

5 Lewis G (ed.) *Why Mothers Die 2000–2002. The Sixth Report of the Confidential Enquiries into Maternal Death in the United Kingdom.* RCOG Press, London, 2004.

6 Cantwell R (ed.) *Saving Mothers Lives: Reviewing Maternal Deaths to Make Motherhood Safer, 2006–2008.* The Eighth Report of the Confidential Enquiries into Maternal Deaths in the United Kingdom (CEMACH). *BJOG* 2011;118(Suppl 1).

7 Mahmud A, Fatma A, Afifi Y. Haemostatic techniques for laparoscopic management of cornual pregnancy. *J Minim Invasive Gynecol* 2015: doi: 10.1016/j.jmig.2015.09.002. [Epub ahead of print]

8 Moawad N, Mahajan S, Moniz M, Taylor S, Hurd W. Current diagnosis and treatment of interstitial pregnancy. *Am J Obstet Gynecol* 2010;202:15–29.

CHAPTER 85

Surgery for Cervical Ectopic Pregnancy

Bassel H. Al Wattar[1] and Yousri Afifi[2]
[1] Blizard Institute, Queen Mary University of London, London, UK
[2] Birmingham Women's NHS Foundation Trust, Birmingham, UK

Case history: A woman who was 8 weeks pregnant attended an emergency room with intermittent, painless, and light vaginal bleeding. Speculum examination showed an enlarged and globular cervix with active bleeding through the os. Her β-human chorionic gonadotropin (bHCG) on admission was 25,000 mIU/mL. An urgent transvaginal ultrasound scan confirmed a live cervical ectopic pregnancy with a characteristic "hourglass"-shaped uterus. She opted for medical treatment with methotrexate. Her serum bHCG levels 1 week later showed a 30% reduction, but the follow-up scan showed a persistent mass in the cervix although there was now no identifiable fetal heart activity. In view of the scan findings, she opted to undergo hysteroscopic resection of the cervical pregnancy sac. The procedure was successful and she had an uneventful recovery.

Background

Epidemiology

Cervical ectopic pregnancy is rare, with estimates ranging between 1 in 95,000 and 1 in 1000 pregnancies [1,2,3,4]. The etiology of the condition is not completely understood. Predisposing factors include an IUCD, Asherman's syndrome, previous uterine surgery such as endometrial curettage and cesarean section, *in vitro* fertilization, pelvic inflammatory disease, and endometriosis [5–9].

Diagnosis

Cervical ectopic pregnancy classically manifests with painless vaginal bleeding. Advances in ultrasonography, color Doppler, and rapid bHCG testing have had a substantial impact on the speed and accuracy of diagnosis, facilitating treatment at early gestations [10–14].

The following ultrasound criteria have been suggested for standardizing the diagnosis of cervical ectopic pregnancy [15].
1 Gestational sac in the endocervix.
2 Presence of an intact portion of the cervical canal between the sac and the endometrium.
3 Local invasion of endocervical tissue by the trophoblast.
4 Visualization of embryonic or fetal structures in the ectopic gestational sac, in particular cardiac activity.
5 Empty uterine cavity.

6 Endometrial decidualization.
7 "Hourglass" uterus.

Two additional criteria for diagnosing cervical ectopic pregnancy on ultrasound [16] have been proposed.
1 The "negative sliding organ sign": the products of conception of a miscarriage will slide against the endocervical canal when the sonographer applies gentle pressure on the cervix with the transvaginal probe.
2 Peritrophoblastic blood flow in the cervical canal: color Doppler can be used to identify this vascular flow, which can help differentiate between cervical ectopic implantation and products of conception passing through the cervical canal during early miscarriage.

In addition to pelvic ultrasound, MRI is increasingly being employed to aid the diagnosis of cervical ectopic pregnancy. The technology is considered particularly useful in identifying the position of the gestational sac and any involvement of neighboring organs, which can help in planning surgical interventions [17].

Management

The traditional management of this condition was urgent laparotomy and frequently hysterectomy to manage severe vaginal hemorrhage. However, the ability to detect the condition earlier through improvements in diagnostic imaging has enabled the safe and effective use of more conservative fertility-sparing approaches [18].

Medical management

Methotrexate is now considered the first line of management for cervical ectopic pregnancy in early gestation with no fetal heart activity. Success rates are reported to be between 81 and 96% [14,16,19], although in about one-fifth of cases additional procedures are necessary to resolve the pregnancy [14]. The dose of methotrexate is 1–1.5 mg/kg and women should be counseled regarding the possible risk of systemic adverse effects, such as thrombocytopenia, leukopenia, elevated serum liver enzymes, fever, and gastrointestinal symptoms [20].

A higher failure rate is expected with medical management when one of the following features is present: serum bHCG concentrations

Gynecologic and Obstetric Surgery: Challenges and Management Options, First Edition. Edited by Arri Coomarasamy, Mahmood I. Shafi, G. Willy Davila and Kiong K. Chan.
© 2016 John Wiley & Sons, Ltd. Published 2016 by John Wiley & Sons, Ltd.

of more than 10,000 IU/L; gestational age over 9 weeks; positive fetal heart activity; or crown–rump length greater than 10 mm.

For cervical pregnancies with fetal heart activity, local injection of chemotherapeutic agents into the gestation sac under ultrasound guidance is considered to be a more effective treatment with fewer side effects [12–14,21,22]. Methotrexate is the agent most commonly used for local injection, with a reported success rate of almost 90% [18]. However, a number of other agents (e.g., etoposide, actinomycin D and KCl) can also be used [15]. Mechanical disruption of the pregnancy by aspirating the sac products is possible before injecting methotrexate; the dose suggested by many authors is 50 mg [13].

Surgical management

Laparotomy

Surgical interventions are reserved as a second line of management in cases of failure of medical management, or where diagnosis is late with an impending risk of rupture and torrential hemorrhage. Laparotomy and hysterectomy, or interventional radiology, should be considered for a patient at risk of torrential hemorrhage. In a clinically stable patient, fertility-sparing surgical procedures or arterial embolization are now feasible alternatives to hysterectomy when medical management fails or is inappropriate.

Dilatation and curettage

Dilatation and curettage (D&C) is the simplest form of surgical treatment, but when practiced alone can precipitate excessive bleeding [16]. Thus, D&C has been combined with other interventions designed to reduce the blood supply to the cervical pregnancy; these include chemotherapy; local injection of vasoconstrictive agents such as vasopressin [23,24]; cervical cerclage with Mersilene tape; Foley catheter tamponade; vaginal ligation of the cervical arteries; uterine artery or internal iliac artery ligation; and angiographic embolization of the cervical, uterine or internal iliac arteries [20].

Hysteroscopy

The use of operative hysteroscopy to resect the gestation sac under direct vision has been described. Modern bipolar resectoscopes can be used with normal saline medium, reducing the risk of electrolyte imbalance from fluid overload (Chapter 63). Hemostasis is achieved by cauterizing the surrounding vasculature [25]. As with D&C, hysteroscopic surgery can be combined with hemostatic interventions such as ligation of the cervical branch of the uterine artery [26] and laparoscopic uterine artery ligation [27].

The following criteria have been suggested for determining when to consider the use of hysteroscopic resection after a failed medical treatment [12].

1 There is a satisfactory decline in the serum bHCG level.
2 There is no fetal heart activity.
3 There is decreased peritrophoblastic flow.
4 There is no active massive hemorrhage.

Interventional radiology

Interventional radiology should be considered in both the stable and unstable patient. Embolization of the major pelvic arteries has been successfully used in conjunction with medical or surgical treatments. The radiologic procedure can also be used to control acute hemorrhage in association with a laparotomy.

KEY POINTS

Challenge: Surgery for cervical ectopic pregnancy.

Background
- Cervical ectopic pregnancy is rare.
- Predisposing factors may include:
  - IUCD.
  - Asherman's syndrome.
  - Previous uterine surgery.
  - *In vitro* fertilization.
  - Pelvic inflammatory disease.
  - Endometriosis

Management
- Early diagnosis is the key for successful and safe management.
- Transvaginal ultrasound and color Doppler have a key role in diagnosis and in formulating a management plan.
- Medical management should be considered as first-line treatment in stable patients.
- Surgical management is reserved for unstable patients, late diagnosis, and where initial medical management has failed.
- Surgical options include:
  - Laparotomy and hysterectomy (reserved for patients with torrential hemorrhage).
  - D&C (can be associated with excessive bleeding, and therefore needs to be combined with other approaches).
  - Bipolar hysteroscopic resection of ectopic tissues: surgical method of choice.
- Adjuvant pharmacologic, radiologic, and surgical methods for reducing intraoperative bleeding should be considered:
  - Chemotherapy.
  - Local injection of vasoconstrictive agents (e.g., vasopressin).
  - Cervical cerclage (e.g., with Mersilene tape).
  - Foley catheter tamponade.
  - Vaginal ligation of the cervical arteries.
  - Uterine artery or internal iliac artery ligation.
- Consider interventional radiology (e.g., embolization of the cervical, uterine or internal iliac arteries) by itself or together with medical or surgical treatment.

References

1 Cerveira I, Costa C, Santos F, Santos L, Cabral F. Cervical ectopic pregnancy successfully treated with local methotrexate injection. *Fertil Steril* 2008;90:2005e7–10.
2 Shinagawa S, Nagayama M. Cervical pregnancy as a possible sequel of induced abortion. *Am J Obstet Gynecol* 1969;105:282–284.
3 Parente JT, Ou CS, Levy J, Legatt E. Cervical pregnancy analysis: a review and report of five cases. *Obstet Gynecol* 1983;62:79–82.
4 Frates MC, Benson CB, Doubilet PM *et al.* Cervical ectopic pregnancy: results of conservative treatment. *Radiology* 1994;191:773–775.
5 Kraemer B, Abele H, Hahn M, Wallwiener D, Rajab TK, Hornung R. Cervical ectopic pregnancy on the portio: conservative case management and clinical review. *Fertil Steril* 2008;90:2011e1–4.
6 Spitzer D, Steiner H, Graf A, Zajc M, Staudach A. Conservative treatment of cervical pregnancy by curettage and local prostaglandin injection. *Hum Reprod* 1997;12:860–866.
7 Fylstra DL, Coffey MD. Treatment of cervical pregnancy with cerclage, curettage and balloon tamponade. *J Reprod Med* 2001;46:71–74.
8 Dicker D, Feldberg D, Samuel N, Goldman JA. Etiology of cervical pregnancy. *J Reprod Med* 1985;30:25–27.
9 Ginsburg ES, Frates MC, Rein MS, Fox JH, Hornstein MD, Friedman AJ. Early diagnosis and treatment of cervical pregnancy in an in vitro fertilization program. *Fertil Steril* 1994;61:966–969.
10 Weyerman PC, Verhoeven AT, Alberda AT. Cervical pregnancy after in vitro fertilization and embryo transfer. *Obstet Gynecol* 1989;161:1145–1146.
11 Verma U, Goharkhay N. Conservative management of cervical ectopic pregnancy. *Fertil Steril* 2009;91:671–674.
12 Hirakawa M, Tajima T, Yoshimitsu K *et al.* Uterine artery embolization along with the administration of methotrexate for cervical ectopic pregnancy: technical and clinical outcomes. *Am J Roentgenol* 2009;192:1601–1607.

13 Lin CY, Chang CY, Chang HM, Tsai EM. Cervical pregnancy treated with systemic methotrexate administration and resectoscopy. *Taiwanese J Obstet Gynecol* 2008;47:443–447.

14 Jeng CJ, Ko ML, Shen J. Transvaginal ultrasound-guided treatment of cervical pregnancy. *Obstet Gynecol* 2007;109:1076–1082.

15 Kirk E, Condous G, Haider Z, Syed A, Ojha K, Bourne T. The conservative management of cervical ectopic pregnancies. *Ultrasound Obstet Gynecol* 2006;27:430–437.

16 Ushakov FB, Elchalal U, Aceman PJ, Schenker JG. Cervical pregnancy: past and future. *Obstet Gynecol Surv* 1996;52:45–59.

17 Jurkovic D, Hacket E, Campbell S. Diagnosis and treatment of early cervical pregnancy. *Ultrasound Obstet Gynecol* 1996;8:373–380.

18 Jung SE, Byun JY, Lee JM, Choi BG, Hahn ST. Characteristic MR findings of cervical pregnancy. *J Magn Reson Imaging* 2001;13:918–922.

19 Sijanovic S, Vidosavljevic D, Sijanovic I. Methotrexate in local treatment of cervical heterotopic pregnancy with successful perinatal outcome: case report. *J Obstet Gynaecol Res* 2011;37:1241–1245.

20 Hung TH, Shau WY, Hsieh TT, Hsu JJ, Soong YK, Jeng CJ. Prognostic factors for an unsatisfactory primary methotrexate treatment of cervical pregnancy: a quantitative review. *Hum Reprod* 1998;13:2636–2642.

21 Leeman LM, Wendland CL. Cervical ectopic pregnancy: diagnosis with endovaginal ultrasound examination and successful treatment with methotrexate. *Arch Fam Med* 2009;9:72–77.

22 Marcovici I, Rosenzweig BA, Brill AI, Khan M, Scommegna A. Cervical pregnancy: case reports and a current literature review. *Obstet Gynecol Surv* 1994;49:49–55.

23 Hwang JL, Hsieh BC, Huang LW, Seow KM, Pan HS, Chen HJ. Successful treatment of a cervical pregnancy by intracervical vasopressin. *BJOG* 2004;111:387–388.

24 Hsieh BC, Lin YH, Huang LW et al. Cervical pregnancy after in vitro fertilization and embryo transfer successfully treated with methotrexate and intracervical injection of vasopressin. *Acta Obstet Gynecol Scand* 2004;83:112–114.

25 Di Spiezio Sardo A, Alviggi C, Zizolfi B et al. Cervico-isthmic pregnancy successfully treated with bipolar resection following methotrexate administration: case report and literature review. *Reprod Biomed Online* 2013;26:99–103.

26 Ash S, Farrell SA. Hysteroscopic resection of a cervical ectopic pregnancy. *Fertil Steril* 1996;66:842–844.

27 Kung FT, Lin H, Hsu TY et al. Differential diagnosis of suspected cervical pregnancy and conservative treatment with the combination of laparoscopy-assisted uterine artery ligation and hysteroscopic endocervical resection. *Fertil Steril* 2004;81:1642–1649.

CHAPTER 86
Surgery for Cesarean Scar Pregnancy

T. Justin Clark

Birmingham Women's NHS Foundation Trust, Birmingham, UK

Case history: A woman presents to an early pregnancy unit complaining of light, painless vaginal bleeding. Clinical observations are normal and examination reveals no abdominal masses or tenderness. A transvaginal ultrasound scan detects the presence of a gestation sac containing a fetal pole with cardiac activity consistent with a 7-week pregnancy in the anterior part of the uterine isthmus. The uterine cavity and cervical canal are noted to be empty and without any apparent contact with the gestation sac. No adnexal mass or free fluid in the pouch of Douglas is seen. A cesarean scar pregnancy is diagnosed. The serum β-human chorionic gonadotropin (bHCG) is 19,755 mIU/mL.

Background

Implantation of the embryo within a previous cesarean scar can result in a cesarean scar pregnancy (CSP) and this phenomenon is becoming an increasingly recognized type of ectopic pregnancy. The increased reporting of CSP reflects better diagnosis as a result of heightened awareness and the more extensive use of high-resolution transvaginal ultrasound imaging. The apparent increased incidence also mirrors the inexorable rise in cesarean delivery. Estimates of the incidence of CSP are imprecise but it is thought to complicate around 1 in 2000 pregnancies, with a rate of 0.15% in women with a previous cesarean section (CS). The gestational age at diagnosis appears to range from 5+0 to 12+4 weeks with a mean of 7.5 weeks. CSP has been reported in both spontaneous and assisted conceptions [1]. The time interval between previous CS and a CSP has been observed to vary between 6 months and 12 years, and it is uncertain whether the risk of CSP is related to the number of previous cesarean sections [2].

In CSP, the gestation sac is completely surrounded by myometrium and the fibrous tissue of the scar, quite separate from the endometrial cavity [3]. Diagnosis is made by transvaginal ultrasound although detection by MRI, hysteroscopy, and histologic diagnosis has been reported [4]. Diagnosis of a CSP by ultrasound is relatively easy in early pregnancy, but as the pregnancy advances the distinction between CSP, cervical pregnancy, and low implantation of an intrauterine pregnancy becomes more difficult [5]. How best to manage CSP is unclear, with most of the published literature confined to case reports and small case series. There is a consensus, however, that termination of the ectopic pregnancy in the first trimester is indicated because there is a high risk of subsequent uterine rupture, massive bleeding, and life-threatening complications.

Management

Treatment objectives should be to remove the gestation sac and its contents while retaining the woman's future fertility. In the case history there are no symptoms or signs to indicate impending or actual CSP rupture: no severe pain, no profuse bleeding, a non-tender uterus, and hemodynamic stability. Thus, in such circumstances, as for other types of ectopic pregnancy, surgical management is an option alongside or in conjunction with expectant and medical approaches. Systemic use of methotrexate and/or local injection of embryocides including methotrexate, potassium chloride, hyperosmolar glucose, and crystalline trichosanthin have been described [4] usually under transvaginal imaging, although hysteroscopy has also been employed. While medical approaches are less invasive compared with surgery, they may simply interrupt the pregnancy, such that trophoblast remains and symptoms continue with heavy bleeding. Furthermore, it can be difficult to exclude scar dehiscence developing during the process of treatment.

Early medical or surgical intervention is indicated to prevent the consequences of CSP rupture. Moreover, early intervention is associated with less morbidity given that the embryo is more fragile and, importantly, the vascularity of the placental bed, the depth of placental implantation, and the risk of bladder invasion are all considerably reduced compared with a CSP at a later gestation.

Surgically, the uterine isthmus is accessible via vaginal, uterine, hysteroscopic, laparoscopic, and laparotomic routes. In addition, surgical disruption or removal of a CSP can be performed in conjunction with the aforementioned medical approaches.

Medical treatment combined with surgical sac aspiration

Here the contents of the gestation sac are disrupted and aspirated usually under ultrasound guidance after prior medical treatment. The minimal invasiveness of this enhanced "medical" technique needs to be weighed against the probability of incomplete treatment and ongoing symptoms.

Gynecologic and Obstetric Surgery: Challenges and Management Options, First Edition. Edited by Arri Coomarasamy, Mahmood I. Shafi, G. Willy Davila and Kiong K. Chan.
© 2016 John Wiley & Sons, Ltd. Published 2016 by John Wiley & Sons, Ltd.

Uterine curettage

Blind mechanical curettage or suction aspiration is not recommended because the approach lacks a clear rationale as the gestation sac of a CSP is not actually within the uterine cavity. Moreover, this approach can cause severe bleeding. Various adjuvant hemostatic measures have been described to prevent or control hemorrhage and these include local injection of vasopressin, intrauterine balloon tamponade, placement of a Shirodkar suture, selective bilateral uterine artery embolization, and even bilateral uterine artery ligation [4]. The procedure has been advocated by some if the gestation is less than 7 weeks and myometrium is seen to overlie the CSP. However, rupture of the uterine scar where the chorionic villi of the ectopic pregnancy have implanted remains a major risk that would necessitate immediate laparoscopy or laparotomy to rectify.

Hysteroscopic evacuation

This approach has been rarely reported [4]. Advanced hysteroscopic skills are required to visualize and coagulate the blood vessels at the implantation site to prevent severe intraoperative hemorrhage. Adequate distension and visualization of the surgical field at the level of the uterine isthmus may be problematic and uterine rupture, although unreported with this technique, remains a possibility. A CSP that grows inwards into the uterine cavity is most suitable for a hysteroscopic approach.

Vaginal removal

The anterior vaginal mucosa is incised, the bladder reflected, and the anterior vesical pouch entered to reveal the CSP mass which is then excised, and the defect repaired with sutures. This technique is suitable for those with appropriate vaginal surgical skills.

Laparoscopic removal

The CSP mass is easily identifiable at laparoscopy as a bulging vascular lesion arising from the anterior isthmic part of the uterus at the previous cesarean scar. The area is incised, dissected and removed. Bleeding can be minimized by local injection of vasopressin and meticulous hemostasis using bipolar diathermy. The uterine defect is then closed with laparoscopic sutures. This technique is safe and associated with minimal blood loss in trained hands. Postoperative recovery is rapid. With wider acquisition of advanced laparoscopic skills, this technique may become the one of choice, especially for CSPs which are deeply implanted and protruding into the abdominal cavity and toward the bladder.

Open surgical removal

The surgical method is as described using a laparoscopic approach. The open approach is more invasive with prolonged hospital stay compared with vaginal and laparoscopic techniques, but is within the skill set of most practicing gynecologists. A laparotomy may allow a more extensive "wedge" resection of the lesion and complete excision of the old cesarean scar. Thus with this technique the risk of persistent trophoblastic tissue is minimized and some have argued the more invasive approach may minimize the risk of recurrent CSP.

Hysterectomy

All women must be aware of the small risk of hysterectomy should other treatment options fail and the pregnancy advances or, more commonly, where bleeding becomes profuse and uncontrollable. In the latter circumstance, fertility-sparing hemostatic interventions such as bilateral uterine artery ligation or embolization should be considered prior to removing the uterus. Hysterectomy has been performed as a primary procedure, but if CSP is diagnosed early this intervention should be avoidable.

Prevention

It is unlikely that rates of CS will fall in contemporary obstetric practice and so the small risk of subsequent CSP will remain. Until the etiology and pathophysiology of CSP is better understood, effective preventive strategies will not be possible. It has been suggested that scar implantation arises as a result of myometrial invasion through a micro-tubular tract between the CS scar and the endometrial canal. The importance of the technique, number and spacing interval between CS, the impact of trauma arising from other intervening uterine procedures, and the recurrence risk of CSP is at present unknown. Similarly, the significance of the relatively common finding of a cervical "niche" (a filling defect arising from deficient myometrium in the vicinity of the uterine isthmus) in the non-pregnant state at outpatient hysteroscopy or saline infusion sonography in women with a previous CS is unclear. Thus, early detection and therapeutic intervention in the first trimester is of prime importance to minimize subsequent morbidity. This requires heightened vigilance in all women presenting in early pregnancy with a previous delivery by CS. Timely, skilled and standardized transvaginal ultrasound with close inspection of the CS scar should be undertaken, and management decisions overseen by senior team members following diagnosis.

KEY POINTS

Challenge: Surgery for cesarean scar pregnancy.

Background
- In CSP, the gestation sac is completely surrounded by myometrium and the fibrous tissue of the scar, quite separate from the endometrial cavity.
- Women with CSP may be asymptomatic or present in the first trimester with bleeding or pain, and with or without local scar tenderness.
- Diagnosis is usually made by transvaginal ultrasound scan.

Management
- Treatment objectives should be to remove the gestation sac and its contents while retaining the woman's future fertility.
- Medical, surgical, or combined treatment approaches are available and should be undertaken without undue delay to minimize morbidity.

- Surgical removal of a CSP can be effected via intrauterine, vaginal, laparoscopic, or open routes.
- Medical (methotrexate) treatment with surgical aspiration of the gestation sac is a reasonable first option in women with CSP of early gestation.
- In later gestations, laparoscopic removal of CSP is generally the treatment of choice, but can be combined with medical treatment to improve safety and effectiveness.
- Blind D&C should be avoided.

Prevention
- Awareness of the small possibility of CSP is important in all women presenting in early pregnancy with a previous CS delivery.
- Timely, skilled, and standardized transvaginal ultrasound with close inspection of the CS scar should be undertaken and management decisions overseen by a multidisciplinary team.

References

1 Seow K-M, Huang L-W, Lin YH, Yan-Sheng Lin M, Tsai Y-L, Hwang J-L. Caesarean scar pregnancy: issues in management. *Ultrasound Obstet Gynecol* 2004;23:247–253.

2 Rotas MA, Haberman S, Levgur M. Cesarean scar ectopic pregnancies: etiology, diagnosis and management. *Obstet Gynecol* 2006;107:1373–1377.

3 Coniglio C, Dickinson JE. Pregnancy following prior Caesarean scar pregnancy rupture: lessons for modern obstetric practice. *Aust NZ J Obstet Gynaecol* 2004;44:162–166.

4 Ash A, Smith A, Maxwell D. Caesarean scar pregnancy. *BJOG* 2007;114:253–263.

5 Jurkovic D, Hillaby K, Woelfer B, Lawrence A, Salim R, Elson CJ. First trimester diagnosis and management of pregnancies implanted into the lower uterine Caesarean section scar. *Ultrasound Obstet Gynecol* 2003;21:220–227.

CHAPTER 87

Surgery for Adnexal Torsion

Mohamed Otify and Jackie A. Ross

King's College Hospital, London, UK

Case history: A 27-year-old woman presented to the emergency department 48 hours after sudden onset of lower abdominal pain, mainly on the right side and radiating to her thigh. She described the pain as severe with acute exacerbations coming in waves and associated with nausea and vomiting. An ultrasound scan performed 3 months previously for intermittent abdominal pains had shown an enlarged right ovary (7 cm) containing three dermoid cysts, with no visible left ovary. She had a past gynecologic history of a laparoscopic left ovarian cystectomy for a dermoid cyst.

On examination, the abdomen was soft, with tenderness and guarding in the right lower quadrant. She had neither costovertebral angle tenderness nor hepatosplenomegaly. Rovsing's, psoas, and obturator signs were negative and bowel sounds were audible. Bimanual pelvic examination revealed cervical motion tenderness and a suspected mass in the right adnexa with tenderness on that side. The patient's β-human chorionic gonadotropin (bHCG) was negative. She was admitted to the gynecology ward with a suspected ovarian torsion. A transvaginal ultrasound was performed the following day that showed a 9-cm right adnexal mass containing echogenic material consistent with dermoid cysts.

The patient was taken to theater for a laparoscopic detorsion of her right ovary. By the time this was done she had been in pain for over 72 hours and the ovary was congested and appeared friable and necrotic. Only a streak of ovarian tissue was visible on the left side due to her previous ovarian cystectomy. The right ovary was detorsed and the decision made that, on balance, it was worth attempting to preserve the right ovary rather than risk an iatrogenic menopause and infertility. However, at clinical review 12 days later the patient complained of feeling feverish and on scan the ovary appeared non-viable, with no detectable perfusion on Doppler examination. A second procedure was performed that necessitated a laparotomy and oophorectomy. Postoperatively, she did not resume taking her combined contraceptive pill and her periods resumed a couple of months later. A small left ovary was seen on follow-up scan, and the patient conceived naturally after a year.

Background

Adnexal torsion is an uncommon but significant cause of acute lower abdominal pain in women. Any cause of ovarian enlargement predisposes to torsion, though occasionally a normal ovary may torse. Torsion causes reduced venous return from the ovary and, as a result, is associated with stromal edema and congestive hemorrhage into any underlying ovarian lesion. The ovary and fallopian tube are typically involved. Approximately 60% of cases of torsion occur on the right side [1].

The clinical presentation is often non-specific with few distinctive clinical signs, commonly resulting in delay in diagnosis and surgical management. The clinical history is typically very similar to that of renal colic and the pain is often associated with nausea and vomiting [2]. True ovarian cysts (i.e., neoplastic cysts rather than functional cysts) do not tend to cause acute pelvic pain unless they twist, so the index of clinical suspicion should be high if a patient is already known to have an ovarian cyst, particularly a dermoid cyst as these make the ovary heavier. Torsion may occur at any age, with an underlying ovarian lesion being more common with increasing age [3]. A quick and confident diagnosis is required to save the adnexal structures from infarction and irreversible tissue necrosis, particularly in women who wish to retain their fertility. Ultrasound (and other imaging modalities) have high positive predictive values for torsion, but relatively poor negative predictive values, and are also highly operator dependent. This means that if the ultrasound scan is suggestive of torsion, then it is very likely to be present, but a negative scan does not exclude torsion [4], so a diagnostic laparoscopy may be necessary.

Management

Preoperative preparation

Before embarking on surgery for suspected adnexal torsion, there should be a clear plan.

1 Which grade of surgeon should be performing the procedure? Does he or she have the surgical skills necessary to deal with torsion if it is confirmed?

2 How important is preservation of the affected ovary? There is little to be gained in attempting to preserve the ovary of a woman who is certain that her family is complete or who is over 45 years of age. This will also affect decision-making regarding the urgency and timing of surgery.

3 How likely is it that any underlying ovarian lesion is malignant? This is particularly a consideration in a postmenopausal woman as a staging procedure may be the optimum treatment.

Gynecologic and Obstetric Surgery: Challenges and Management Options, First Edition. Edited by Arri Coomarasamy, Mahmood I. Shafi, G. Willy Davila and Kiong K. Chan.

© 2016 John Wiley & Sons, Ltd. Published 2016 by John Wiley & Sons, Ltd.

Surgical approach

The laparoscopic approach to surgery for adnexal torsion has consistently shown to result in a faster recovery and shorter hospital stay [1,5], and so should be the preferred technique if feasible based on the skill of the surgeon, the patient's comorbidities, and the clinical findings.

Surgical treatment options

Oophorectomy or adnexectomy

This remains the treatment of choice for women with no fertility concerns, a normal underlying ovary or benign-looking cyst, and a normal contralateral ovary. Removing the ovary avoids the risk of recurrent ipsilateral torsion or ovarian necrosis.

Detorsion with or without cystectomy

Several studies have shown that the degree of ovarian necrosis cannot be predicted by the appearance or color of the ovary at the time of surgical diagnosis, and that approximately 90% of cases have evidence of resumption of ovarian function following detorsion [6,7]. Better outcomes have been shown in rats if surgical intervention occurs within 36 hours of ovarian torsion [8]. Additionally, although data are sparse, there is no evidence of an increased risk of thromboembolic events with detorsion. At the time of detorsion, the tissues may be friable, and either hyperemic or ischemic depending on how quickly perfusion is restored to the ovarian tissue, so handling or manipulation may be best kept to a minimum. Functional cysts may resolve spontaneously without further intervention. The decision must be made whether to proceed with a cystectomy at the time of diagnosis or whether to perform an interval procedure, should a cyst persist, a couple of weeks later once the ovarian edema has resolved [9]. Interval surgery, cystectomy, and possible oophoropexy should be performed within 6–8 weeks to minimize the risk of recurrent torsion [10].

Oophoropexy

The need to fix or suspend the ovary after torsion is widely debated in the literature, as there is no guarantee that it will prevent recurrence and there have been reported cases of ovarian failure. There is also a concern that oophoropexy may affect tubal blood supply and adversely affect the anatomic relation of the ovary to the fimbrial end of the tube. However, in cases of recurrent torsion, oophoropexy has been shown to reduce the risk of recurrence. Methods for oophoropexy described in the literature include suturing the ovary to the pelvic sidewall, plication or shortening of the utero-ovarian ligament, and suturing the ovary to the posterior serosal surface of the uterus [11]. A non-absorbable suture should be used.

Staging procedure

This is appropriate when an ovarian malignancy is suspected preoperatively, most commonly in a postmenopausal woman. If surgery can be planned alongside a surgeon with expertise in gynecologic oncology, then it can potentially spare the patient having a second procedure. In the emergency situation it would be reasonable to remove the ovary and perform definitive surgery at a later date.

Follow-up

The risk of recurrent ipsilateral ovarian torsion or asynchronous contralateral ovarian torsion is difficult to quantify with any degree of precision but is thought to be relatively low at around 2–5%.

Follow-up with ultrasound is indicated if the affected ovary has been conserved to check for resolution of edema and assess ovarian viability.

KEY POINTS

Challenge: Surgery for adnexal torsion.

Background
- The prognosis of ovarian torsion is excellent with early diagnosis and appropriate treatment. Delayed diagnosis may result in ovarian infarction and necrosis.
- Ultrasound and Doppler are useful tests; however, scans have high positive predictive values (i.e., if a scan is suggestive of torsion, then it very likely to be present), but relatively poor negative predictive values (i.e., a scan does not exclude torsion).

Prevention of problems
- Have a high index of suspicion in a woman presenting with abdominal pain associated with vomiting and a known ovarian cyst.
- Intervene promptly. Do not delay the decision to go to theater, even if it means operating outside hours.
- Make a plan for the surgery that is most appropriate for the patient given her age, fertility wishes, and any ovarian pathology underlying the torsion. Do this before getting to the operating room.

Management
- Detorsion can be achieved regardless of the color or number of twists of the ovary. Even gangrenous-appearing adnexa may not need to be removed because it is impossible to predict the chances of the ovary reviving after detorsion.
- Concerns over the risk of ovarian vein thrombosis and release of thrombogenic factors into the circulation have no foundation in the literature.
- If fertility is not a concern, and the other ovary is normal, remove the ovary to prevent recurrence or a second procedure.
- Oophoropexy is recommended in cases of repeat torsion.

References

1 Balci O, Icen MS, Mahmoud AS, Capar M, Colakoglu MC. Management and outcomes of adnexal torsion: a 5-year experience. *Arch Gynecol Obstet* 2011;284:643–646.

2 Huchon C, Panel P, Kayem G, Schmitz T, Nguyen T, Fauconnier A. Does this woman have adnexal torsion? *Hum Reprod* 2012;27:2359–2364.

3 Chiou S-Y, Lev-Toaff AS, Masuda E, Feld RI, Bergin D. Adnexal torsion: new clinical and imaging observations by sonography, computed tomography, and magnetic resonance imaging. *J Ultrasound Med* 2007;26:1289–1301.

4 Mashiach R, Melamed N, Gilad N, Ben-Shitrit G, Meizner I. Sonographic diagnosis of ovarian torsion: accuracy and predictive factors. *J Ultrasound Med* 2011;30:1205–1210.

5 Cohen SB, Wattiez A, Seidman DS *et al.* Laparoscopy versus laparotomy for detorsion and sparing of twisted ischemic adnexa. *JSLS* 2003;7:295–299.

6 Oelsner G, Cohen SB, Soriano D, Admon D, Mashiach S, Carp H. Minimal surgery for the twisted ischaemic adnexa can preserve ovarian function. *Hum Reprod* 2003;18:2599–2602.

7 Huchon C, Fauconnier A. Adnexal torsion: a literature review. *Eur J Obstet Gynecol Reprod Biol* 2010;150:8–12.

8 Taskin O, Birincioglu M, Aydin A *et al.* The effects of twisted ischaemic adnexa managed by detorsion on ovarian viability and histology: an ischaemia–reperfusion rodent model. *Hum Reprod* 1998;13:2823–2827.

9 Spinelli C, Buti I, Pucci V *et al.* Adnexal torsion in children and adolescents: new trends to conservative surgical approach. Our experience and review of literature. *Gynecol Endocrinol* 2013;29:54–58.

10 Cass DL. Ovarian torsion. *Semin Pediatr Surg* 2005;14:86–92.

11 Fuchs N, Smorgick N, Tovbin Y *et al.* Oophoropexy to prevent adnexal torsion: how, when, and for whom? *J Minim Invasive Gynecol* 2010;17:205–208.

CHAPTER 88
Laparoscopic Appendectomy

Edward Rawstorne[1], Christopher Smart[2], and Chris Keh[3]
[1] Heart of England NHS Foundation Trust, Birmingham, UK
[2] East Lancashire Hospitals NHS Trust, Blackburn, UK
[3] University Hospitals Birmingham NHS Foundation Trust, Birmingham, UK

Case history: A 25-year-old female is admitted for laparoscopy to investigate chronic right iliac fossa and pelvic pain. At laparoscopy, in the absence of other significant pathology, the gynecologist elects to remove the appendix, which is covered in fibrous adhesions.

Background

Appendicitis has an incidence of 11 per 10,000 in the USA [1]. Laparoscopic appendectomy is now the technique of choice over open surgery for acute appendicitis. Laparoscopic appendectomy is associated with a reduced length of hospital stay, decreased incidence of postoperative wound infection [2], and improved cosmesis in comparison with open appendectomy.

The management of chronic as opposed to acute right iliac fossa pain is complex but studies have shown an improvement in pain scores after elective laparoscopic appendectomy [3]. Patients with chronic right iliac fossa pain do have significant rates of microscopic pathology within the appendix [3,4].

Management

Surgical technique

The patient should be positioned supine and preferably placed directly onto the gel mat of the operating table. The principal surgeon should stand on the patient's left, joined on that side by the assistant. The Hasson or open Scandinavian technique can be used to gain entry to the abdomen. There is no difference in major vascular or visceral injury when compared with the closed Veress needle technique. However, there is a reduced risk of failed entry, extraperitoneal insufflation, and omental injury if an open technique is employed [5]. A pneumoperitoneum at 12–15 mmHg should be established.

A 5-mm laparoscope should be used if available as this allows for it to be placed in any of the three ports. A 30° laparoscope is recommended as it permits views that are not possible with a standard 0° laparoscope.

To achieve triangulation in the right iliac fossa, a 10-mm umbilical port should be established and should be accompanied by a further 5-mm port in the left iliac fossa and a 5-mm suprapubic port in the midline, placed under direct vision (Figure 88.1). Optimal triangulation is achieved by the laparoscope in the left iliac fossa port. If triangulation with a 10-mm laparoscope through the umbilical port is challenging, the left iliac fossa or suprapubic port can be converted to 10 mm.

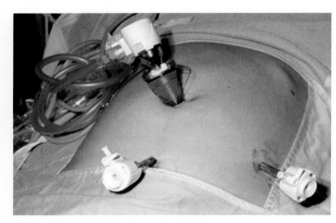

Figure 88.1 Port positions for laparoscopic appendectomy.

The appendix should be identified at the cecal pole. Tilting the table right side up will help to keep the terminal ileum in the left side of the abdomen. It may be necessary to follow the tinea coli in a retrograde direction to find the base of the appendix. The appendix is retrocecal in 65% of cases and gentle medial mobilization of the cecal pole will aid localization. Care should be taken to avoid traction on the appendix while dissecting it to minimize accidental perforation or injury. The bloodless fold of Treves can make identifying the base difficult but traction here should be avoided as it is most often far from bloodless.

Once the appendix with its mesentery is free and the base is visible, it should be held straight with a grasper in the left hand. The appendicular artery runs parallel, but separate, to the appendix from its base to its tip. The appendix itself is supplied by small branches (Figure 88.2).

Gynecologic and Obstetric Surgery: Challenges and Management Options, First Edition. Edited by Arri Coomarasamy, Mahmood I. Shafi, G. Willy Davila and Kiong K. Chan.
© 2016 John Wiley & Sons, Ltd. Published 2016 by John Wiley & Sons, Ltd.

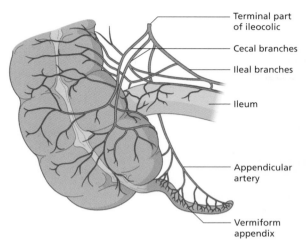

Terminal part
of ileocolic

Cecal branches

Ileal branches

Ileum

Appendicular
artery

Vermiform
appendix

Figure 88.2 Blood supply to the appendix. Adapted from Gray H. Anatomy of the Human Body, published 1918.

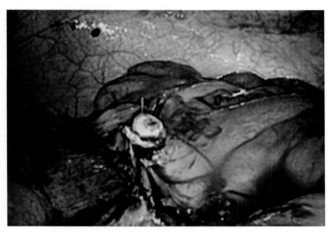

Figure 88.4 Endoloop® placed on the remaining base of the excised appendix.

There are two methods for controlling the appendicular artery.
1 Using the monopolar diathermy hook and starting distally, work parallel to the appendix between the appendicular artery and the appendix itself. Continue toward the level of the base of the appendix. This cauterizes the small branches sequentially. An Endoloop® (Ethicon Endo-Surgery) or extracorporeal (Roeder's) knot can be placed over the mesentery if required.
2 Identify and clear the appendicular artery at the level of the base appendix. Create a window between the artery and the appendix (Figure 88.3) and clip, staple or diathermy the artery at this level.

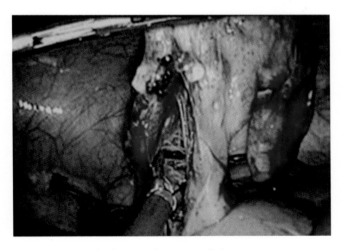

Figure 88.3 Appendicular artery being controlled.

An Endoloop® or ligature with an extracorporeal knot is placed over the appendix and moved down to the base of the appendix. While sufficient tension is applied to ligate the appendix, care must be taken not to "cheesewire" through. A second Endoloop® can be placed distally and the appendix transected between the two sutures (Figure 88.4).

With the 5-mm laparoscope now in the left iliac fossa or suprapubic port, the appendix can be removed via the 10-mm port with or without a specimen bag. If only a 10-mm laparoscope is available the suprapubic port should be converted to a 10-mm port in order to remove the appendix. Suction can be performed and a drain inserted via the suprapubic port if necessary. Studies have shown no reduction in abscess rate or other benefit if irrigation over suction alone is used for perforated appendicitis [6]. We lay the omentum over the appendix stump and deflate the pneumoperitoneum under direct vision. Closure of the port sites can be undertaken in the standard fashion.

Complicated appendicitis or appendicular anatomy
If difficulty in locating the appendix is encountered or appendicitis is expected, early involvement of a general surgeon is mandatory.

Appendicitis with an associated abscess
The abscess can be drained laparoscopically, and a thorough washout is needed. It is advisable to leave a drain in this situation. It is reasonable to convert to an open procedure if there is any doubt that the sepsis has not been adequately drained.

Necrotic and friable appendicitis
It is important that all sections of the appendix are removed if it is in multiple pieces. The base must be identified and closed or oversewn to avoid recurrent sepsis and a fistula. It is advisable to leave a drain. It may be necessary to convert to an open procedure to confidently gain control of the sepsis.

Prevention

Potential iatrogenic injury
Iatrogenic injuries can occur during elective and emergency appendectomy, especially during port entry and with the use of diathermy. The two main sites for thermal injury are the cecum and terminal ileum.

The appendix and its mesentery should be tented up, to allow dissection or diathermy close to the appendix as described. It is essential that the operating surgeon remembers the bulging cecal pole and base behind the mesentery, and does not injure it during this procedure.

The terminal ileum is also at risk as it enters the cecum. If the area is inflamed and the fold of Treves is masking the base of the appendix, careful dissection is required so as not to damage it at this point. Tilting the table can help keep the ileum away but one should remember that the mesentery to the appendix can take a variable course and can lie on the terminal ileum in some cases.

KEY POINTS

Challenge: Laparoscopic appendectomy.

Background
- "A common operation for a common condition": traditionally an appendectomy has been performed through a laparotomy incision but this approach is no longer routine, being superseded by less invasive laparoscopic techniques.

Management
- The important steps in performing laparoscopic appendectomy include:
  - Identification of the base of the appendix.

- Controlling the appendicular artery.
- Securing the appendix stump.

Prevention
- Complications can be minimized by:
  - Converting to a laparotomy if there is inadequate control of bleeding or an inability to adequately demonstrate anatomy.
  - Involving a general surgeon early.
  - Adopting a careful and gentle technique at entry and during surgery to reduce the likelihood of iatrogenic injury.
  - Ensuring vigilance when using diathermy to minimize inadvertent thermal injury to the adjacent cecum or terminal ileum.

References

1 Addiss D, Shaffer, N Fowler B, Tauxe R. The epidemiology of appendicitis and appendectomy in the United States. *Am J Epidemiol* 1990;132:910–925.
2 Sauerland S, Jaschinski T, Neugebauer EAM. Laparoscopic versus open surgery for suspected appendicitis. *Cochrane Database Syst Rev* 2004;(10):CD001546.
3 Roumen R, Groenedijk R, Sloots C, Duthoi K, Scheltinga M, Bruijnickx C. Randomized clinical trial evaluating elective laparoscopic appendicectomy for chronic right lower-quadrant pain. *Br J Surg* 2008;95:169–174.
4 Mussack T, Schmidbauer S, Nerlich A, Schmidt W, Hallfeldt KK. [Chronic appendicitis as an independent clinical entity]. *Chirurg* 2002;73:710–715.
5 Ahmad G, O'Flynn H, Duffy J, Phillips K, Watson A. Laparoscopic entry techniques. *Cochrane Database Syst Rev* 2012;(2):CD006583.
6 St Peter S, Adibe O, Iqbal C *et al.* Irrigation versus suction alone during laparoscopic appendectomy for perforated appendicitis: a prospective randomized trial. *Ann Surg* 2012;256:581–585.

CHAPTER 89

Laparoscopic Surgery: When to Convert to Laparotomy?

Mohamed Mehasseb
Glasgow Royal Infirmary, Glasgow, Scotland, UK

Case history 1: *A woman undergoing a total laparoscopic hysterectomy is found to have marked pelvic endometriosis and adhesions, obscuring the planes of surgery. The surgeon perseveres with the procedure, but ends up with a perforation in the rectosigmoid colon, necessitating a laparotomy to repair.*

Case history 2: *A 65-year-old woman is having a total laparoscopic hysterectomy for early-stage endometrial cancer. The uterus is noted to be bulky during the procedure. The operator decides to go ahead and conclude the hysterectomy laparoscopically. However, he is unable to deliver the uterus through the narrow vaginal vault and has to deliver it through a transverse suprapubic incision.*

Background

Over the last three decades, surgeons and patients have increasingly chosen laparoscopic surgery over abdominal procedures. The scope and complexity of procedures performed have widely expanded well beyond diagnostic purposes. Conversion means changing the surgical approach from an intended laparoscopic to an open procedure because of intraoperative difficulties. The surgeon's experience is an important factor for successful laparoscopy. Many laparoscopy-related complications, as well as conversion rates and morbidity and mortality rates, decrease with increasing experience. However, patient-related difficulties and technical problems can be faced at any level of expertise, and could interfere with completing the procedure laparoscopically [1,2].

Management

Although increased postoperative morbidity and mortality associated with conversions are recognized [3], a conversion should not be considered a defeat, but should rather be seen as choosing the most appropriate way of safely achieving the procedure [4]. It is best considered as an alteration of the operative plan to overcome difficulties and avoid further problems [5,6]. If there is a doubt about safety or effectiveness of the laparoscopic procedure, it should be converted to an open approach, irrespective of possible feelings of failure in decision-making, disappointment, and discouragement on the surgeon's side.

Laparoscopic procedures are converted to laparotomy for three main reasons: (i) complications during the laparoscopy, (ii) technical difficulty, and (iii) change in the planned treatment (e.g., malignancy encountered unexpectedly) [7,8]. Some reported predictors are previous laparotomy, obesity, and coexisting medical conditions (e.g., anticoagulant use) [9].

Adhesions

Unclear anatomy because of adhesions is one of the most frequent causes of conversion [4]. Prior abdominal surgery may result in an inability to obtain adequate exposure for the critical region of interest, and this is a predictor for open conversion and complications [10]. Severe pelvic inflammatory disease and previous abdominal surgeries causing poor visualization with dense adhesions obliterating the cul-de-sac increase the risk of bowel injury during laparoscopy [7], and subsequent conversion for repair.

Very large pelvic mass (see Chapter 82)

A large pelvic mass, for example a fibroid uterus, may fill the entire pelvis and limit vision and access to the ovaries, uterine vessels, bladder, and ureters. If uterine manipulation, from side to side or front to back, is not possible, the surgeon may not be able to safely dissect and protect the ureters, bladder, and rectum; in such a situation conversion to laparotomy is justified.

Obesity

Obesity is one of the main problems leading to conversion. Higher conversion rates (14–36%) have been described in obese women compared with non-obese women (5–6%), depending on the type of, and indication for, surgery [11]. Conversion risks are higher with a BMI greater than 30, and dramatically increase with a BMI greater than 50 [1,3]. Intraoperative complications, including poor exposure and access, are also more frequent in obese patients [8].

Hemorrhage

Excessive intraoperative bleeding has been cited as a reason for conversion and is more likely during technically difficult and lengthy procedures such as laparoscopic myomectomy (conversion rate up to 41%), or in women with deranged coagulation [12,13].

Gynecologic and Obstetric Surgery: Challenges and Management Options, First Edition. Edited by Arri Coomarasamy, Mahmood I. Shafi, G. Willy Davila and Kiong K. Chan.
© 2016 John Wiley & Sons, Ltd. Published 2016 by John Wiley & Sons, Ltd.

Anesthesia

Anesthesia-related conversions to laparotomy are infrequent, although ventilation in Trendelenburg position in women with high BMI can be problematic. Pre-existing chronic obstructive and restrictive lung diseases may have challenges in laparoscopy. Significant hypoxemia, hypercapnia, and respiratory acidosis are the major reported pulmonary complications during laparoscopy [14].

Prolonged intraperitoneal carbon dioxide insufflation and changes in patient positioning might cause hemodynamic, pulmonary, and endocrine problems. Alterations in arterial blood pressure and cardiac output (i.e., hypotension or hypertension), arrhythmias, and cardiac arrest have all been reported [6,15]. Significant decrease in cardiac performance has been shown with peritoneal insufflation during laparoscopic procedures even in young patients [16].

Prevention

Thorough and prudent preoperative assessment and planning should take into consideration the patient's comorbidities and the anticipated intraoperative difficulties, thus avoiding wasteful laparoscopic attempts. Sound knowledge of the factors associated with success or failure of the laparoscopic approach allows the surgeon to weigh these options. Recognized risk factors for conversion of laparoscopic hysterectomy into laparotomy include pelvic adhesions, large uterine size, complications (bladder injury, bowel injury, vascular injury, or ureteral injury), previous cesarean section (two or more), BMI over 30, and history of previous myomectomy. All women undergoing laparoscopy should be counseled that unintended laparotomy is a known risk and has additional morbidity over laparoscopy alone. Less experienced surgeons attempting complicated procedures significantly increase the risk of conversion.

KEY POINTS

Challenge: Changing the surgical approach from an intended laparoscopy to an open procedure because of intraoperative difficulties (conversion).

Background
- The scope and complexity of laparoscopic procedures have widely expanded well beyond diagnostic purposes.
- The surgeon's experience is an important factor for successful laparoscopy.
- Laparoscopic procedures are converted to laparotomy for three main reasons:
  - Complications during laparoscopy.
  - Technical difficulty.
  - Change in the planned treatment.
- Conversions are associated with significantly increased postoperative morbidity and mortality.

Management
- The surgeon should choose the most appropriate way of safely achieving the procedure and alter the operative plan to overcome difficulties.
- Some reported predictors of conversion include unclear anatomy because of adhesions, large pelvic mass, obesity, previous laparotomy, and coexisting medical conditions.
- Problems related to anesthesia and excessive intraoperative bleeding can also be reasons for conversion.

Prevention
- Preoperative planning should take into consideration the patient's comorbidities and anticipated intraoperative difficulties.
- Recognized risk factors for conversion of laparoscopic procedure into laparotomy should be discussed with the woman.
- All women undergoing laparoscopy should be counseled that unintended laparotomy is a known risk and has additional morbidity over laparoscopy alone.

References

1 Tekkis PP, Senagore AJ, Delaney CP. Conversion rates in laparoscopic colorectal surgery: a predictive model with, 1253 patients. *Surg Endosc* 2005;19:47–54.
2 Tekkis PP, Senagore AJ, Delaney CP, Fazio VW. Evaluation of the learning curve in laparoscopic colorectal surgery: comparison of right-sided and left-sided resections. *Ann Surg* 2005;242:83–91.
3 Marusch F, Gastinger I, Schneider C et al. Experience as a factor influencing the indications for laparoscopic colorectal surgery and the results. *Surg Endosc* 2001;15:116–120.
4 Agresta F, De Simone P, Bedin N. The laparoscopic approach in abdominal emergencies: a single-center 10-year experience. *JSLS* 2004;8:25–30.
5 Simopoulos C, Botaitis S, Polychronidis A, Tripsianis G, Karayiannakis AJ. Risk factors for conversion of laparoscopic cholecystectomy to open cholecystectomy. *Surg Endosc* 2005;19:905–909.
6 Reissman P, Spira RM. Laparoscopy for adhesions. *Semin Laparosc Surg* 2003;10:185–190.
7 Chi DS, Abu-Rustum NR, Sonoda Y et al. Ten-year experience with laparoscopy on a gynecologic oncology service: analysis of risk factors for complications and conversion to laparotomy. *Am J Obstet Gynecol* 2004;191:1138–1145.
8 Walker JL, Piedmonte MR, Spirtos NM et al. Laparoscopy compared with laparotomy for comprehensive surgical staging of uterine cancer: Gynecologic Oncology Group Study LAP2. *J Clin Oncol* 2009;27:5331–5336.
9 Jansen S, Jorgensen J, Caplehorn J, Hunt D. Preoperative ultrasound to predict conversion in laparoscopic cholecystectomy. *Surg Laparosc Endosc* 1997;7:121–123.
10 Karayiannakis AJ, Polychronidis A, Perente S, Botaitis S, Simopoulos C. Laparoscopic cholecystectomy in patients with previous upper or lower abdominal surgery. *Surg Endosc* 2004;18:97–101.
11 Lamvu G, Zolnoun D, Boggess J, Steege JF. Obesity: physiologic changes and challenges during laparoscopy. *Am J Obstet Gynecol* 2004;191:669–674.
12 Delis S, Bakoyiannis A, Madariaga J, Bramis J, Tassopoulos N, Dervenis C. Laparoscopic cholecystectomy in cirrhotic patients: the value of MELD score and Child-Pugh classification in predicting outcome. *Surg Endosc* 2010;24:407–412.
13 Dubuisson JB, Fauconnier A, Fourchotte V, Babaki-Fard K, Coste J, Chapron C. Laparoscopic myomectomy: predicting the risk of conversion to an open procedure. *Hum Reprod* 2001;16:1726–1731.
14 Brody FJ, Chekan EG, Pappas TN, Eubanks WS. Conversion factors for laparoscopic splenectomy for immune thrombocytopenic purpura. *Surg Endosc* 1999;13:789–791.
15 Bhayani SB, Pavlovich CP, Strup SE et al. *Laparoscopic radical prostatectomy: a multi-institutional study of conversion to open surgery.* Urology 2004;63:99–102.
16 Harris SN, Ballantyne GH, Luther MA, Perrino AC Jr. Alterations of cardiovascular performance during laparoscopic colectomy: a combined hemodynamic and echocardiographic analysis. *Anesth Analg* 1996;83:482–487.

CHAPTER 90

Laparoscopy: Port-site Herniation

Ayesha Mahmud and Yousri Afifi
Birmingham Women's NHS Foundation Trust, Birmingham, UK

Case history: A woman underwent laparoscopic cervical cerclage at 13 weeks of pregnancy. The laparoscopic procedure required four ports: one 10-mm umbilical port and three 5-mm ancillary ports in the suprapubic region and both iliac fossae. The port-site incisions were closed with interrupted sutures without fascial or peritoneal closure. Eight hours after surgery the patient developed omental herniation through the umbilical port and she was taken back to theater for surgical correction.

Background

Port-site herniation (PSH) is defined as herniation through a fascial defect created by the laparoscopic entry of trocars. It is a recognized complication of laparoscopic surgery, with an estimated incidence of 0.2–3% according to the size of port and associated risk factors [1–5]. The complication can cause considerable morbidity requiring additional surgical intervention. Life-threatening complications of PSH include bowel obstruction, strangulation, and perforation [4–7].

PSH has been classified into three types (Figure 90.1).

1 Early-onset type usually develops within 2 weeks. Features include dehiscence of the fascial plane and the peritoneum, and this most commonly presents with small bowel obstruction.

2 Late-onset type usually presents 3–4 months after the procedure. Features include dehiscence of the fascia with intact peritoneum, constituting a hernia sac.

3 Complex type has features consistent with dehiscence of the abdominal wall along with protrusion of the intestine or the omentum [6].

Risk factors

The following risk factors have been associated with increased risk of herniation [3,6,8,9].

- Use of large-size trocars (≥10 mm).
- Excessive manipulation of the cannula site with long surgery or frequent insertion.
- Excessive traction on the defect during specimen retrieval.
- Pre-existing umbilical defects or hernias.
- General risk factors, including ascites, obesity, poor nutrition, and increased intra-abdominal pressure.

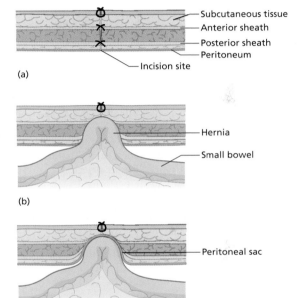

(a)

Subcutaneous tissue
Anterior sheath
Posterior sheath
Peritoneum
Incision site

(b)

Hernia
Small bowel

(c)

Peritoneal sac

Figure 90.1 Classification trocar site hernias: (a) normal trocar-site wound; (b) early-onset hernia; (c) late-onset hernia.

- Medical conditions such as diabetes and connective tissue disorders.
- Postoperative wound and chest infections.

The umbilicus is the most common site for PSH. Most reported PSH outside of the umbilical region occur at sites where larger than 10-mm ports have been used. There are a few case reports of herniation with 5-mm port, and a handful of cases with 3-mm port [10]. The interval between the laparoscopy and diagnosis of PSH ranges from a few days to 3 years [11]. In the majority of cases, PSH is not associated with any bowel obstruction or strangulation. In cases of strangulation, the hernia is typically of a Richter's type, where the omentum rather than the bowel is the herniated tissue.

Gynecologic and Obstetric Surgery: Challenges and Management Options, First Edition. Edited by Arri Coomarasamy, Mahmood I. Shafi, G. Willy Davila and Kiong K. Chan.
© 2016 John Wiley & Sons, Ltd. Published 2016 by John Wiley & Sons, Ltd.

CT is a useful investigation to differentiate port-site hematoma from incarcerated small bowel.

Prevention

Port insertion and closure techniques

For primary port insertion, a higher incidence of PSH has been reported with closed entry techniques compared with open techniques. However, the reported risks were similar when fascial closure was undertaken [12]. Although fascial closure tends to reduce the risk of PSH, it does not eliminate it.

It is recommended that all port sites of 10 mm or more in adults, and 5 mm or more in children (Chapter 65), be closed. It is also recommended to incorporate the peritoneum with fascial closure. At present, there is no strong evidence to support a particular method of fascial closure. However, the inclusion of the peritoneum and fascia in the sutures is considered to be good practice [11].

Port closure techniques can be classified into three groups [13,14].

1 Techniques that use assistance from inside the abdomen (requiring two additional ports). Examples include Maciol needle, Grice needle, catheter or spinal needles, Endoclose device, and Gore-Tex device.
2 Techniques that use extracorporeal assistance (requiring one additional port). Examples include Carter–Thomason device, Endo-Judge device, and Tahoe Ligature device.
3 Closure techniques that can be performed with or without visualization (i.e., without additional ports). Examples include suture carrier, dual-hemostat technique, Lowsley retractor with hand closure, and standard technique of hand-sutured closure.

Any of these techniques can be used when undertaking port-site closure. However, the choice of approach should be influenced by the clinical expertise of the operator, the availability of suitable instruments, and appropriate assistance.

Van Sickle *et al.* [15] reported an animal model investigation of tensile strength and breaking strength of the fascia, based on closure type. They found that both are significantly better with sutures placed using the figure-of-eight technique as opposed to simple interrupted sutures.

Operative factors

There is evidence to suggest that use of trocars of 10-mm diameter or more increases the risk of PSH. Other factors such as extension of port sites, excessive manipulation or traction at port sites, and repeated reinsertions of ports have been implicated in increasing the risk of PSH. Therefore, caution should be taken during surgery to reduce the risk of PSH [9,11]. Careful choice of port-site location and incision in relation to the intended surgical procedure can reduce the need for excessive manipulation or traction, thus lowering the incidence of PSH. It is also good practice to keep the endoscope inside the port cannula while removing the primary port, to prevent inadvertent entrapment of omentum or bowel.

Wound infection

Wound infection has also been implicated in the pathogenesis of umbilical hernia. Local antibiotics have been suggested to reduce such risk but the evidence is sparse [6,9,11].

Detection of undetected hernia

Identification of any previously undetected hernia by digital examination of the fascia at the time of surgery is an important preventive measure. If any defect is identified, proper repair should be undertaken. It is important to document fascial defects and inform the patient after surgery.

Management

In the case history, in order to avoid bowel damage, a Palmer's point laparoscopic entry can be performed. This will allow replacement of the omentum herniating through the umbilicus, with the aid of blunt laparoscopic forceps, and subsequent port closure using an Endoclose device (Figure 90.2). The closure should be performed using the figure-of-eight technique with 0 PDS or similar suture, incorporating the fascia and peritoneum.

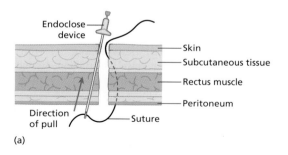
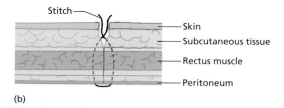

Figure 90.2 Endoclose suture device: (a) insertion; (b) end result.

KEY POINTS

Challenge: Port-site herniation.

Background
- PSH is a recognized complication of laparoscopic surgery, with an estimated incidence of 0.2–3%.
- PSH can lead to considerable morbidity requiring surgical intervention; the life-threatening complications are bowel obstruction, strangulation, and perforation.

- Risk factors for PSH include:
  - Use of large-size trocars (≥10 mm).
  - Excessive manipulation of the cannula site with long surgery or frequent insertion.
  - Excessive traction on the defect during specimen retrieval.
  - Pre-existing umbilical defects or hernias.
  - General risk factors, including ascites, obesity, poor nutrition, and increased intra-abdominal pressure.
  - Medical conditions such as diabetes and connective tissue disorders.
  - Postoperative wound and chest infections.

Prevention
- Assess and reduce preoperative risks.
- Reduce intraoperative risks through use of careful port-site insertion, avoidance of excessive port-site manipulation, and suitable port-site closure.
- Close all port sites of 10 mm or more in adults, and 5 mm or more in children (Chapter 65).
- Include the peritoneum and fascia in port-site closures.
- Identify and repair any previously undetected hernia by digital examination of the fascia at the time of surgery.

Management
- Identify the type of herniation: early, late, or complex herniation.
- Enter abdomen via a virgin area (e.g., Palmer's point).
- Replace any herniating omentum or bowel with the aid of a blunt laparoscopic forceps; examine bowel for any injury.
- Close the port site with figure-of-eight sutures, using 0 PDS or similar suture material, ensuring both the fascia and peritoneum are incorporated into the sutures; an Endoclose device is helpful to achieve good closure.
- For late or complex type hernias, involve general surgeons.

References

1 Kadar N, Reich H, Liu CY, Manko GF, Gimpelson R. Incisional hernias after major laparoscopic gynecologic procedures. *Am J Obstet Gynecol* 1993;168:1493–1495.

2 Nezhat C, Nezhat F, Seidman DS, Nezhat C. Incisional hernias after operative laparoscopy. *J Laparoendosc Adv Surg Tech A* 1997;7:111–115.

3 Azurin DJ, Go LS, Arroyo LR, Kirkland ML. Trocar site herniation following laparoscopic cholecystectomy and the significance of an incidental preexisting umbilical hernia. *Am Surg* 1995;61:718–720.

4 Montz FJ, Holschneider CH, Munro MG. Incisional hernia following laparoscopy: a survey of the American Association of Gynecologic Laparoscopists. *Obstet Gynecol* 1994;84:881–884.

5 Lajer H, Widecrantz S, Heisterberg L. Hernias in trocar ports following abdominal laparoscopy, a review. *Acta Obstet Gynecol Scand* 1997;76:389–393.

6 Tonouchi H, Ohmori Y, Kobayashi M, Kusunoki M. Trocar site hernia. *Arch Surg* 2004;139:1248–1256.

7 Maio A, Ruchman R. CT diagnosis of post laparoscopic hernia. *J Comput Assist Tomogr* 1991;15:1054–1055.

8 Hussain A, Mahmood H, Singhal T, Balakrishnan S, Nicholls J, El-Hasani S. Long-term study of port-site incisional hernia after laparoscopic procedures. *JSLS* 2009;13:346–349.

9 Nassar AH, Ashkar KA, Rashed AA, Abdulmoneum MG. Laparoscopic cholecystectomy and the umbilicus. *Br J Surg* 1997;84:630–633.

10 Plaus WJ. Laparoscopic trocar site hernias. *J Laparoendosc Surg* 1993;3:567–570.

11 Coda A, Bossotti M, Ferri F *et al*. Incisional hernia and fascial defect following laparoscopic surgery. *Surg Laparosc Endosc Percutan Tech* 2000;10:34–38.

12 Mayol J, Garcia-Aguilar J, Ortiz-Oshiro E, De-Diego Carmona JA, Fernandez-Represa JA. Risks of the minimal access approach for laparoscopic surgery: multivariate analysis of morbidity related to umbilical trocar insertion. *World J Surg* 1997;21:529 –533.

13 Shaher Z. Port closure techniques. *Surg Endosc* 2007;21:1264–1274.

14 Ng WT. A full review of port-closure techniques. *Surg Endosc* 2007;21:1895–1897.

15 Van Sickle KR, Nanda Kumar HR, Parikh A, Ayon AA, Cohn SM. Development of an animal model to investigate optimal laparoscopic trocar site fascial closure. *J Surg Res* 2013;184:126–131.

CHAPTER 91
Uterine Septum

Basim Abu-Rafea[1] and Khaldoun Sharif[2]
[1] Dalhousie University, Halifax, Nova Scotia, Canada
[2] Istishari Fertility Center, Amman, Jordan

Case history: A 30-year-old woman with a history of four consecutive first-trimester losses was diagnosed as having a complete uterine septum on saline infusion sonography (Figure 91.1).

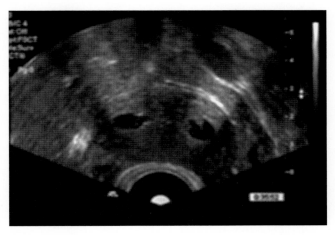

Figure 91.1 Saline infusion sonography demonstrating a uterine septum.

Background

Septate uterus, resulting from failure of apoptotic resorption of the medial segment of the Mullerian ducts, is the most common congenital uterine anomaly, accounting for approximately 35% of all uterine anomalies [1]. Septate uterus affects reproductive health by impairing fertility, and increasing miscarriages and adverse pregnancy outcomes [2,3].

The mechanism by which a uterine septum causes these adverse effects remains speculative. Hypotheses include excessive amount of fibroelastic tissue and decreased blood supply to the septum which may adversely affect placentation, but these ideas remain controversial.

Management

Diagnosis

The diagnosis of septate uterus is made by a variety of imaging techniques or by direct endoscopic visualization. Hysterosalpingography or two-dimensional ultrasound may be used as initial screening tools, but contrast infusion sonography and three-dimensional ultrasound are more accurate for a definitive diagnosis. MRI is also highly accurate in detecting septate uteri, but because it is time-consuming and expensive, its routine use in clinical practice remains controversial. Combined laparoscopic and hysteroscopic examination is considered the gold standard for assessing congenital uterine anomalies, establishing a correct diagnosis, and possibly applying the principle of "see and treat."

When to treat?

The main indications for treating a septate uterus are unexplained infertility and recurrent pregnancy loss in the presence of a uterine septum. Hysteroscopic metroplasty (septal incision) is presently considered the standard of care. This minimally invasive approach offers many advantages, including outpatient surgery with or without anesthesia, reduced risk of intraoperative and postoperative morbidity, and no risk of postoperative pelvic adhesions, when compared with laparotomic transfundal correction.

Preoperative preparation

Preoperative thinning of the endometrial lining is not necessary prior to hysteroscopic septal incision. However, it may be advantageous in the presence of a wide septum or a complete septum as it helps in improving visibility and reducing bleeding [4]. Endometrial preparation can be achieved by either booking the procedure in the early proliferative phase of the menstrual cycle or administration of GnRH agonist or progestins [5].

Concomitant laparoscopy

Laparoscopy is recommended to complete the evaluation of patients with infertility, including assessment and possible concomitant treatment of tubal disease and other conditions including endometriosis. Laparoscopy also differentiates between a septate and a bicornuate uterus and it may be of value in aspirating excessive intra-abdominal irrigant fluid and provide safety during hysteroscopic metroplasty. The only situation in which it may be unnecessary is when the patient has undergone previous laparoscopic evaluation documenting the normal shape of the fundus of the uterus and the surgery is monitored by ultrasound.

Gynecologic and Obstetric Surgery: Challenges and Management Options, First Edition. Edited by Arri Coomarasamy, Mahmood I. Shafi, G. Willy Davila and Kiong K. Chan.
© 2016 John Wiley & Sons, Ltd. Published 2016 by John Wiley & Sons, Ltd.

Choice of instrument

Incision of the uterine septum is best achieved hysteroscopically [3] using a 0° or 12° scope. Hysteroscopic septal incision can be done using scissors, electrosurgery (radiofrequency energy) or fiber-optic laser (neodymium/YAG). The scissors are generally preferred in the case of a thin septum. However, a resectoscope with a knife electrode is preferred in the case of a wide septum as bleeding may be anticipated. It is important to note that the theoretical risk of thermal damage to the endometrium using electrocautery or laser has never been proven to be a real risk.

Operative technique

Two techniques have been described in the literature for hysteroscopic septal incision. The first is referred to as the shortening technique, mainly used in long septa. In this technique, the septum is incised initially at its apex and then shortened in a cephalad direction (Figure 91.2). The second technique is usually best utilized for wide septa. Here the septum is incised along its side in a longitudinal manner starting at the cornual end moving caudally. The incisions are made on each side of the septum alternately. However, in a wide and long septum, a combination of both techniques is usually required to achieve the desired result.

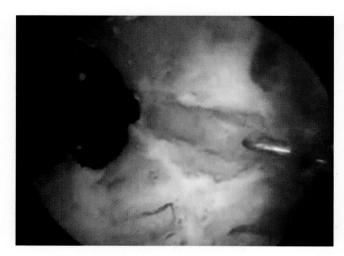

Figure 91.2 Septal division.

Completion of the procedure: when to stop?

The objective of metroplasty is to obtain normality of the uterine cavity. If a residual septum remains, it should be no more than 1 cm in length in order to obtain optimal clinical outcomes [6]. Normality of the uterine cavity is usually achieved when the hysteroscope can be moved freely from one cornual recess to the other without obstruction, or when both tubal ostia can be viewed simultaneously. In cases where ultrasound guidance is used during septal incision, fundal thickness should be no less than 10 mm at completion [7].

Postoperative care

Many surgeons advocate routine use of antibiotic prophylaxis after hysteroscopic metroplasty. However, a beneficial role of routine antibiotic therapy during hysteroscopy has not been firmly established. In a study of 2116 hysteroscopic surgical procedures over a 10-year period, there were no infections in the 90 women who had septum division [8].

Attempts to epithelialize the denuded septal surface have been made with the use of exogenous estrogen. However, the efficacy of postoperative hormone therapy using estrogen and terminal progesterone has not been demonstrated [9,10]. A prospective randomized trial that evaluated the use of estrogen alone versus no estrogen concluded that estrogen has no apparent role after hysteroscopic incision of the septum [11].

Splinting the uterine cavity with Foley catheter or IUD following hysteroscopic septum incision has no effect on septum reformation, clinical pregnancy rate, and pregnancy outcomes [12,13,14].

Routine second-look hysteroscopy and breakdown of adhesions has been advocated by some investigators [3]. However, this practice remains controversial [10].

KEY POINTS

Challenge: Uterine septum.

Background
- Uterine septum is associated with infertility, recurrent miscarriages, and adverse pregnancy outcomes.
- The mechanisms of its effects remain speculative, but could be related to excessive amount of fibroelastic tissue and decreased blood supply to the septum, which in turn may affect placentation.

Management
- Diagnosis:
  - Ultrasound and hysterosalpingography are useful screening tests.
  - Three-dimensional ultrasound, infusion sonography, and MRI have high accuracy to diagnose septum.
  - Combined laparoscopic and hysteroscopic examination is considered the gold standard for diagnosing uterine anomalies, and can be combined with a "see and treat" approach.
- Preoperative thinning of the endometrial lining is not generally necessary. However, in the presence of a wide or long septum, endometrial thinning with GnRH agonist or progestins can reduce bleeding and improve visibility. Another approach is to perform the procedure in early proliferative phase when the endometrium is thin.
- Instruments:
  - Use 0° or 12° hysteroscope.
  - Use scissors for a thin septum.
  - Use a knife electrode or laser for a thick septum.
- Technique:
  - Use "shortening technique" for a long septum (starting at the apex and advancing in the cephalad direction).
  - For a wide septum, consider incising along its side in a longitudinal manner starting at the cornual end and moving caudally. The incisions are made on each side of the septum alternately.
  - For a long and thick septum, a combination of both approaches may be necessary.
- Following hysteroscopic metroplasty, a residual septum should be no more than 1 cm in length.
- In cases where ultrasound guidance is used, fundal thickness should be no less than 10 mm at completion.
- There appears to be no role for postoperative antibiotics, estrogen and/or uterine stenting by IUD or Foley catheter.

References

1 Chan YY, Jayaprakasan K, Zamora J, Thornton JG, Raine-Fenning N, Coomarasamy A. The prevalence of congenital uterine anomalies in unselected and high-risk populations: a systematic review. *Hum Reprod Update* 2011;17: 761–771.

2 Raga F, Bauset C, Remohi J, Bonilla-Musoles F, Simón C, Pellicer A. Reproductive impact of congenital Müllerian anomalies. *Hum Reprod* 1997;12:2277–2281.

3 Homer H, Li T, Cooke I. The septate uterus: a review of management and reproductive outcome. *Fertil Steril* 2000;73:1–14.

4 Mencaglia L, Tantini C. Hysteroscopic treatment of septate and arcuate uterus. *Gynaecol Endosc* 1996;5:151–154.

5 Tantini C, Tiso E, Napolitano A, Mencaglia L. GnRH analogues for preparation for hysteroscopic metroplasty. *Gynaecol Endosc* 1996;5:161–163.

6 Fedele L, Bianchi S, Marchini M, Mezzopane R, Di Nola G, Tozzi L. Residual uterine septum of less than 1 cm after hysteroscopic metroplasty does not impair reproductive outcome. *Human Reprod* 1996;11:727–729.

7 Querleu D, Brasme TL, Parmentier D. Ultrasound-guided transcervical metroplasty. *Fertil Steril* 1990;54:995–998.

8 Agostini A, Cravello L, Shojai R, Ronda I, Roger V, Blanc B. Postoperative infection and surgical hysteroscopy. *Fertil Steril* 2002;77:766–768.

9 Vercellini P, Fedele L, Arcaini L, Rognoni MT, Candiani GB. Value of intrauterine device insertion and estrogen administration after hysteroscopic metroplasty. *J Reprod Med* 1989;34:447–450.

10 Assaf A, Serour G, Elkady A, El Agizy H. Endoscopic management of the intrauterine septum. *Int J Gynaecol Obstet* 1990;32:43–51.

11 Dabirashrafi H, Mohammad K, Moghadami-Tabrizi N, Zandinejad K, Moghadami-Tabrizi M. Is estrogen necessary after hysteroscopic incision of the uterine septum? *J Am Assoc Gynecol Laparosc* 1996;3:623–625.

12 Tonguc EA, Var T, Yilmaz N, Batioglu S. Intrauterine device or estrogen treatment after hysteroscopic uterine septum resection. *Int J Gynaecol Obstet* 2010;109: 226–229.

13 Fedele L, Bianchi S, Frontino G. Septums and synechiae: approaches to surgical correction. *Clin Obstet Gynecol* 2006;49:767–788.

14 Abu Rafea BF, Vilos GA, Oraif AM, Power SG, Cains JH, Vilos AG. Fertility and pregnancy outcomes following resectoscopic septum division with and without intrauterine balloon stenting: a randomized pilot study. *Ann Saudi Med* 2013;33:34–39.

CHAPTER 92

Surgery for Intrauterine Adhesions

Mohan Kumar

Good Hope Hospital, Heart of England NHS Foundation Trust, Sutton Coldfield, West Midlands, UK

Case history: A woman with secondary subfertility has a history of a miscarriage requiring surgical evacuation of the uterus twice. Since the miscarriage operation, she reported her menstrual bleeds were light, and an ultrasound showed an endometrial pattern suggestive of intrauterine adhesions.

Background

Intrauterine adhesions commonly develop as a result of trauma to the uterine cavity. Most of the cases of severe intrauterine adhesions occur due to curettage for pregnancy conditions such as termination, miscarriage, or postpartum hemorrhage for retained placental tissues [1]. The basalis layer of the endometrium is susceptible to damage in the first four postpartum or post-abortion weeks [2]. Adhesions can also develop in the non-gravid uterus as a result of endometrial injury from procedures such as myomectomy or non-puerperal curettage [2]. In the developing world, genital tuberculosis is a cause of intrauterine adhesions that are often severe with complete obliteration of the uterine cavity [3].

Adhesions can arise from the endometrium, myometrium, or connective tissue. They vary in size and thickness, from thin and fragile to thick and dense. They may occur at the margins of the endometrial cavity or diffusely; in severe cases they can completely obliterate the cavity. Intrauterine adhesions can be asymptomatic with no clinical significance or may present with several clinical features including menstrual irregularities (hypomenorrhea, amenorrhea), cyclical pelvic pain, infertility, or recurrent pregnancy loss.

Transvaginal ultrasound, hysterosalpingography (HSG), or contrast sonography can be useful for screening for this condition. However, hysteroscopy is the gold standard for diagnosing this condition as it can detect even the smallest adhesions, and can also allow a "see and treat" approach.

Management

The main aim of the management of intrauterine adhesions is the removal of adhesions within the uterine cavity, followed by the prevention of re-formation of adhesions. Removal of intrauterine adhesions is expected to restore the uterine cavity shape and promote regeneration of destroyed endometrium, thereby aiding the restoration of endometrial function and fertility.

The standard treatment is lysis under direct visualization by hysteroscopy. Care must be taken while dilating the cervix because it is easy to create false passages and perforate the uterus. In patients with severe and dense adhesions it is recommended to perform lysis under ultrasound or laparoscopic guidance to prevent perforation of the uterus.

Adhesiolysis technique

Each surgical case for this procedure may be unique and this requires a careful understanding of uterine anatomy as well as skilled dissection. Sometimes more than one operation is required to eliminate the adhesions completely if the adhesions are very thick and occupying the entire cavity. Aggressive dissection that might enter the myometrium should be avoided.

The procedure should begin by advancing the hysteroscope to the internal cervical os, and lysing the adhesions by sharp dissection using rigid hysteroscopic scissors. Careful dissection should be continued until the entire cavity is clear of adhesions and a normal cavity shape is achieved. This procedure can also be performed using bipolar electrocautery [4], while the marginal adhesions are best dealt with using a resectoscope with a pointed knife. When using electrocautery, low energy should be used to minimize further damage to the endometrium. Fluoroscopy can also be used in severe cases to guide direction in the uterine cavity [5].

Adhesion prevention after adhesiolysis

Once all the adhesions are completely released, management should be focused on preventing the re-formation of adhesions. One approach is to introduce a non-hormonal intrauterine device (IUD) or intrauterine balloon into the uterus. If an IUD is inserted, it should be left *in situ* for 3 months. The intrauterine balloon approach involves either a pediatric Foley catheter inflated with 5 mL of fluid or a triangular-shaped intrauterine balloon (developed by Cook Medical) that maintains the normal configuration of the uterine cavity (Figure 92.1). The balloon should be left *in situ* for 5 to 10 days [6]. Antibiotics should be given to reduce the risk of infection while the balloon remains *in situ*. In a non-randomized comparative study comparing IUD with Foley catheter, Foley balloon catheter was associated with a greater proportion of women achieving normal menses (81% vs. 63%), higher conception rates (34% vs. 23%), and a reduced need for repeat procedure [6]. Another approach is to introduce an

Gynecologic and Obstetric Surgery: Challenges and Management Options, First Edition. Edited by Arri Coomarasamy, Mahmood I. Shafi, G. Willy Davila and Kiong K. Chan.
© 2016 John Wiley & Sons, Ltd. Published 2016 by John Wiley & Sons, Ltd.

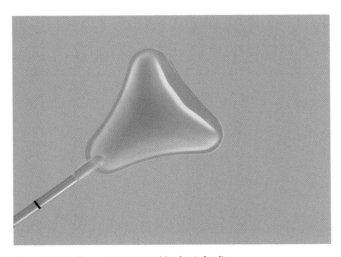

Figure 92.1 Balloon uterine stent (Cook Medical).

anti-adhesion barrier (e.g., Hyalobarrier®) into the uterine cavity after division of adhesions.

Regenerating endometrium

It is good practice to use high-dose estrogen postoperatively to help regeneration of the endometrium over the denuded areas created by the adhesions. One possible regimen is estradiol valerate 6 mg/day for a total of 6 weeks, with the concurrent use of progestogen in the form of medroxyprogesterone acetate 10 mg three times daily during the fifth and sixth weeks to complete the process of shedding of endometrium. Following this treatment serial ultrasonography at different stages of the cycle may be used to assess endometrial development [7].

Test of treatment

It is recommended to assess the uterine cavity postoperatively for recurrence of adhesions [8]. This can be done by HSG, hystero-contrast sonography, or hysteroscopy. Second-look hysteroscopy provides an opportunity to treat any residual adhesions.

Prevention

Many miscarriages can be managed either expectantly or medically, rather than resorting to surgery. There is an argument that surgical evacuation of the uterus should be reserved only for selected cases, or for failed expectant or medical management. Where evacuation of the uterus is carried out, suction evacuation should be performed rather than metal curettage; if metal curettage is required, it must be performed gently without undue trauma to the uterine cavity. Resection of a submucous fibroid can also lead to intrauterine adhesion formation. Therefore while resecting a submucous fibroid, low electrical energy must be used or mechanical devices like morcellators can be used to prevent damage to the endometrium. There are at least two different types of morcellators available, one designed by Smith & Nephew (Truclear®) and the other designed by Hologic (MyoSure®). The role of intrauterine balloon or anti-adhesion gel in preventing primary adhesions is uncertain.

KEY POINTS

Challenge: Surgery for intrauterine adhesions.

Background
- Most cases of intrauterine adhesions are due to curettage for pregnancy complications such as miscarriage or postpartum hemorrhage. Other causes include endometrial injury from myomectomy and genital tuberculosis.
- Clinical presentations include secondary amenorrhea, cyclical pelvic pain, infertility, and recurrent pregnancy losses.
- Ultrasound, hystero-contrast sonography, and HSG are useful tests, but hysteroscopy is the gold standard test for diagnosing intrauterine adhesions.

Management
- The standard treatment is lysis under direct visualization using hysteroscopy.
- Care must be taken when dilating the cervix as it is easy to make false passages and perforations; ultrasound or laparoscopic or fluoroscopic guidance may be necessary with difficult cases.
- Mechanical devices like hysteroscopic scissors should be used to release adhesions. If bipolar electrocautery is used, a low-energy setting is preferable.
- For prevention of adhesions after adhesiolysis, the options are:
  - Non-hormonal IUD: can be left *in situ* for 3 months.
  - Pediatric Foley catheter inflated with 5 mL of fluid: leave *in situ* for 5–10 days.
  - Triangular balloon (Cook Medical): leave *in situ* for 5–10 days.
  - Consider intrauterine instillation of anti-adhesion barrier (e.g., Hyalobarrier).
- To aid regeneration of endometrium, give estrogen (estradiol valerate 6 mg daily) for 6 weeks, and concurrently use progestogen (medroxyprogesterone acetate 10 mg three times daily during fifth and sixth weeks) to induce withdrawal bleed.
- Test effectiveness of treatment with second-look hysteroscopy; this also allows treatment of any adhesions.

Prevention
- Surgical evacuation of the uterus for management of miscarriage should generally be performed when either expectant or medical management is unsuitable or has failed.
- Vigorous uterine curettage should be avoided.

References

1 Schenker JG. Etiology of and therapeutic approach to synechia uteri. *Eur J Obstet Gynecol Reprod Biol* 1996;65:109–113.

2 Al-Inany H. Intrauterine adhesions. An update. *Acta Obstet Gynecol Scand* 2001;80:986–993.

3 Netter A, Musset R, Lambert A, Salomon Y, Montbazet G. [Tuberculous endo-uterine symphysis: an anatomo-clinical and radiologically characteristic syndrome]. *Gynecol Obstet (Paris)* 1955;54:19–36.

4 Fernandez H, Gervaise A, de Tayrac R. Operative hysteroscopy for infertility using normal saline solution and a coaxial bipolar electrode: a pilot study. *Hum Reprod* 2000;15:1773–1775.

5 Thomson AJ, Abbott JA, Kingston A, Lenart M, Vancaillie TG. Fluoroscopically guided synechiolysis for patients with Asherman's syndrome: menstrual and fertility outcomes. *Fertil Steril* 2007;87:405–410.

6 Orhue AA, Aziken ME, Igbefoh JO. A comparison of two adjunctive treatments for intrauterine adhesions following lysis. *Int J Gynaecol Obstet* 2003;82:49–56.

7 Bromer JG, Aldad TS, Talor HS. Defining the proliferative phase endometrial defect. *Fertil Steril* 2009;91:698–704.

8 AAGL Advancing Minimally Invasive Gynecology Worldwide. AAGL practice report: practice guidelines for management of intrauterine synechiae. *J Minim Invasive Gynecol* 2010;17:1–7.

CHAPTER 93
Myomectomy: Breach of the Endometrial Cavity

Masoud Afnan[1] and Arri Coomarasamy[2]
[1] Beijing United Family Hospital, Beijing, China
[2] College of Medical and Dental Sciences, University of Birmingham, Birmingham, UK

Case history: A woman with an ultrasound-diagnosed single anterior wall fibroid measuring 5 cm in diameter and indenting the uterine cavity underwent abdominal myomectomy. During the "shelling out" process of the "fibroid," no cleavage plane was noted. It was quickly appreciated that this was an adenomyoma, and not a fibroid. In view of the focal nature of the lesion, it was decided to continue with the removal of the adenomyoma. Unfortunately, as often happens in cases of adenomyoma in which there is no clear capsule cleavage plane, the endometrial cavity was breached. This was identified and the endometrium was repaired with fine non-absorbable sutures.

Background

Controversy remains as to how best to treat women who are infertile (a common condition) and who have fibroids (also a common condition). A systematic review [1] concluded that generally the studies were few and of poor methodologic quality. Acknowledging this rider, the studies suggested that myomectomy in patients with submucosal fibroids could improve clinical pregnancy rates, that there is no clear evidence as to how best manage infertile patients with intramural fibroids, and that myomectomy for subserosal fibroids is not indicated. A subsequent systematic review concluded that intramural fibroids reduced the chance of a live birth following IVF (RR 0.79, CI 0.70–0.88) [2]. A more recent Cochrane review [3] examined only randomized controlled trials and found no benefit in favor of myomectomy, though with few studies and wide confidence intervals. There were no RCTs of hysteroscopic myomectomy.

Breaching the uterine cavity is always a risk when performing a myomectomy. There is little written on the risk of adhesions following a breach of the uterine cavity; however, following hysteroscopic resection of intracavity fibroids, this risk has been reported to be as high as 30% for a single fibroid [4].

Management

Transvaginal ultrasound is the mainstay of diagnosis of fibroids, even though it has the lowest sensitivity and specificity, because the alternatives are more invasive and expensive [5]. Other techniques, such as MRI, hysterosonography, or hysteroscopy, are indicated when more precise mapping of the fibroids is required, such as prior to fibroid embolization. MRI is better able to differentiate between fibroids and adenomyoma. Usually, adenomyosis is not treated surgically, although if there is a discrete adenomyoma it is a reasonable option in view of the limited treatment options available.

Repair of endometrial cavity

In order to minimize the risk of adhesions, it is important to recognize the opened cavity and to repair the endometrium, approximating the edges without tension to facilitate the healing process. Identification is not always easy, especially if there is much bleeding. Methylene blue can be injected transcervically to stain the endometrium, making identification easier.

The appropriate choice of suture for the endometrium is not known. Non-absorbable sutures theoretically decrease the risk of adhesions in the uterine cavity, but with the risk of leaving a "foreign body" in the uterine cavity.

Testing the uterine cavity

In view of the significant risk of adhesions, it is prudent to check the uterine cavity after the procedure if fertility is a desired outcome. Ideally this should be done after one complete menstrual cycle in order to allow complete regeneration of the endometrium, but without waiting too long for adhesions to become fibrotic. This will allow any adhesions to be divided easily, or for any visible sutures to be cut and removed.

Prevention

Constant awareness of the possible location of the endometrial cavity and meticulous approach to dissection are important in minimizing the risk of uterine cavity breach. Preoperative MRI mapping of fibroids can aid with the awareness of fibroid and cavity location.

Some surgeons routinely place a Foley catheter in the uterine cavity before myomectomy [6]. This can confer four advantages.
1 Palpation of the Foley catheter balloon through the myometrium can provide the surgeon with information about the location of the cavity.
2 The Foley catheter can be used to inject methylene blue into the uterine cavity, aiding diagnosis of cavity breach.
3 Repair of the endometrium is facilitated by the presence of the Foley balloon [6].

Gynecologic and Obstetric Surgery: Challenges and Management Options, First Edition. Edited by Arri Coomarasamy, Mahmood I. Shafi, G. Willy Davila and Kiong K. Chan.
© 2016 John Wiley & Sons, Ltd. Published 2016 by John Wiley & Sons, Ltd.

4 If a cavity breach occurs following repair of the defect, the Foley balloon can be left in the uterine cavity for 10 days to minimize the risk of intrauterine adhesion formation [6].

If a myomectomy involved large or multiple incisions on the myometrial wall, an elective cesarean section should be considered in a future pregnancy, regardless of whether the endometrial cavity itself was breached or not.

KEY POINTS

Challenge: Endometrial cavity breach during a myomectomy.

Background
- Endometrial cavity breach is a risk of myomectomy, with a significant risk of subsequent intrauterine adhesions.

Prevention
- Preoperative MRI mapping to understand the location of fibroids and their relationship to the uterine cavity.
- Constant awareness of the location of endometrial cavity during the operation.
- Meticulous dissection, especially when there is no clear capsule plane.
- Insertion of Foley catheter in the uterine cavity before myomectomy has at least four benefits:
  - Palpation of the Foley balloon through the myometrium helps to identify the endometrial cavity.
  - Foley catheter allows the injection of methylene blue, which can be useful for identifying the endometrial edges.
  - Repair of the endometrial defect is facilitated by the presence of the Foley catheter.

- The Foley balloon can be left in the uterine cavity for 10 days to minimize the risk of intrauterine adhesions.

Management
- Inject methylene blue to identify the presence of endometrial defect and endometrial edges.
- Appropriate sutures for repair are not known; many prefer non-absorbable fine sutures as they are associated with a decreased risk of adhesion formation; however, they can act as "foreign bodies" and cause problems of their own.
- Repair should be performed with approximation of endometrial edges, but without tension. Repair over an intrauterine Foley balloon can be helpful.
- Given the risk of intrauterine adhesions following repair of a breached endometrial cavity, a hysteroscopy after one complete menstrual cycle is recommended. This allows any visible sutures to be cut and removed, and for any intrauterine adhesions to be divided before they become fibrotic.
- If a myomectomy involved extensive incisions (in terms of length or number) on the myometrial wall, an elective cesarean section should be considered in a future pregnancy, regardless of whether the endometrial cavity was breached or not at the time of myomectomy.

References

1 Pritts EA, Parker WH, Olive DL. Fibroids and infertility: an updated systematic review of the evidence. *Fertil Steril* 2009;91:1215–1223.
2 Sunkara SK, Khairy M, El-Toukhy T, Khalaf Y, Coomarasamy A. The effect of intramural fibroids without uterine cavity involvement on the outcome of IVF treatment: a systematic review and meta-analysis. *Hum Reprod* 2010;25:418–429.
3 Metwally M, Cheong YC, Horne AW. Surgical treatment of fibroids for subfertility. *Cochrane Database Syst Rev* 2012;(11):CD003857.
4 Taskin O, Sadik S, Onoglu A, et al. Role of endometrial suppression on the frequency of intrauterine adhesions after resectoscopic surgery. *J Am Assoc Gynecol Laparosc* 2000;7:351–354.
5 Griffin KW, Ellis MR, Wilder L, DeArmond L. Clinical inquiries. What is the appropriate diagnostic evaluation of fibroids? *J Fam Pract* 2005;54:458, 460, 462.
6 Hatasaka HH. Acquired uterine factors and infertility. In: CarrellDT, PetersonCM (eds) *Reproductive Endocrinology and Infertility*, pp. 235–263. Springer, New York, 2010.

CHAPTER 94

Myomectomy: Multiple Large Fibroids

Justin Chu[1] and Arri Coomarasamy[2]
[1] Birmingham Women's NHS Foundation Trust, Birmingham, UK
[2] College of Medical and Dental Sciences, University of Birmingham, Birmingham, UK

Case history: A patient with a uterus enlarged with multiple fibroids is scheduled to have myomectomy. The fundus is noted to be 6 cm above the umbilicus.

Background

Fibroids are very common, affecting approximately 50% of women of reproductive age [1,2]. Half of these women will have symptoms from their fibroids [3], including abnormal uterine bleeding leading to anemia, pressure on surrounding structures (bowel, bladder and ureters), and infertility [4]. Fibroids can also increase the risk of miscarriage. The removal of fibroids can lead to better reproductive outcomes in selected patients [5,6,7].

Myomectomy can be performed hysteroscopically, laparoscopically (Chapter 80), vaginally (Chapter 96), or abdominally depending on the size and location of the fibroids. Type 0 fibroids are pedunculated myomas within the uterine cavity; type 1 fibroids are those which extend less than 50% into the myometrium; and type 2 fibroids are those with greater than 50% extension into the myometrium [8]. Type 0 and 1 fibroids can be removed hysteroscopically. Type 2 fibroids are generally best removed abdominally via laparoscopy or laparotomy.

In the case of multiple large fibroids, the standard approach is an abdominal myomectomy. In this chapter, we address the preoperative, intraoperative, and postoperative considerations required to perform an abdominal myomectomy in a patient with multiple fibroids.

Management

Preoperative considerations
Imaging
MRI is useful for evaluating the number, size, and location of the fibroids. Ultrasound can also be used to map the fibroids, but is of limited value when multiple fibroids are present; in such patients, ultrasound gives poor views of the endometrium and deeper fibroids.

Counseling
It is necessary to provide appropriate counseling about the benefits and risks of surgery. Immediate risks include bleeding, blood transfusion, injury to other abdominal organs, infection, and venous thromboembolism. Late complications include adhesions and recurrence of fibroids, which is common when multiple fibroids are removed [9]. Adhesions can compromise fertility and be associated with chronic pelvic pain. Counseling should include the small risk (approximately 1%) of conversion of myomectomy to hysterectomy should there be uncontrollable hemorrhage during surgery.

Correction of anemia
Many patients with multiple large fibroids also suffer with menorrhagia and are therefore more likely to have iron-deficiency anemia. The hemoglobin level should therefore be checked and iron treatment initiated. Adequate time should be given for iron therapy to elevate the hemoglobin level. On the day of surgery the surgeon should ensure that there are blood products available.

Reducing the size of fibroids
Three months of GnRH agonist therapy should be considered in order to reduce the size and vascularity of fibroids before open myomectomy [10]. The selective progesterone receptor modulator ulipristal acetate 5 mg orally once daily for 3 months has also been found to reduce the size of fibroids before surgical intervention [11].

Intraoperative considerations
Adequate access
The key step to surgical success is to achieve adequate exposure. For a large multiple fibroid uterus, it may be necessary to perform a midline laparotomy. Some gynecologic surgeons insist that any myomectomy can be performed through a lower transverse incision. The approach they propose is to remove the lower uterine fibroids first, and bring the upper uterus into view. However, such an approach can still be associated with poor views and access, and compromise the safety of the operation; if a vertical midline incision is required, a gynecologist should not hesitate to perform this (Chapter 26). The incision may end at the umbilicus or may need to be extended above the level of the umbilicus depending on the size of the uterus. After adequate access is achieved the uterus is usually exteriorized so that access to the whole uterus can be gained and a thorough visual examination and palpation of all the tumors can be performed. The use of a myoma screw can be helpful for exteriorizing the uterus [12]. The bowel should be kept away from the operating site with warm moist large swabs.

Gynecologic and Obstetric Surgery: Challenges and Management Options, First Edition. Edited by Arri Coomarasamy, Mahmood I. Shafi, G. Willy Davila and Kiong K. Chan.
© 2016 John Wiley & Sons, Ltd. Published 2016 by John Wiley & Sons, Ltd.

option (Chapter 162); if hemorrhage persists, hysterectomy is the last life-saving resort. Occasionally uterine artery embolization can be performed to reduce intraoperative bleeding; however, this requires interventional radiology to be set up in the operating room.

Laparoscopic myomectomy

Excessive intraoperative hemorrhage can be dealt with by local injection of vasopressin as described, or by laparoscopic uterine vessel occlusion. The use of V-loc sutures during laparoscopic myomectomy is likely to reduce blood loss. Occasionally one may need to convert a laparoscopic procedure to an open procedure if the above measures fail.

Hysteroscopic myomectomy

For excessive intraoperative bleeding, local vasopressin can be injected at the base of the myoma. A preventive approach is the injection of diluted vasopressin (4 units pitressin in 80 mL of normal saline) into the stroma of the cervix (10 mL each into 4 and 8 o'clock positions), before starting the resection of fibroid [12]. Intrauterine balloon tamponade for 24 hours can help to stop the bleeding from hysteroscopic resection of fibroids.

Prevention

Intraoperative bleeding and associated morbidity can be minimized by the preventive measures taken prior to and during surgery (Table 95.1). Ongoing communication between the gynecologist and the anesthetist is important to ensure accurate assessment of blood loss, and appropriate and timely implementation of management steps.

Table 95.1 Measures to prevent massive intraoperative bleeding and morbidity associated with myomectomy.

	Hemodynamic stability	Reduction of fibroid volume	Reduction of bleeding
Preoperative	Optimize preoperative hemoglobin Check sickle cell status if Afro-Caribbean	GnRHa or SPRM for 3 months before surgery	Pharmacologic agents to reduce heavy menstrual bleeding: progesterone, GnRHa, SPRM
Perioperative	Cross-match blood Arrange blood products Organize cell salvage		Vaginal prostaglandin E₂, e.g., misoprostol 400 µg rectally 30–60 min before the operation [13,14]
Intraoperative	Ongoing communication with the anesthetist Blood and blood product transfusion		Maintain MAP at around 60 mmHg Use tourniquet Use vasopressin Close an incision before making a new incision Rapid and adequate suturing Consider intravenous tranexamic acid and gelatin-thrombin matrix sealant

GnRHa, gonadotropin releasing hormone agonist; SPRM, selective progesterone receptor modulator.

Preoperative MRI mapping of uterine fibroids may allow a degree of planning in terms of uterine incisions, although key decisions about the number and length of incisions can only be made intraoperatively, after careful palpation of the fibroids. Around the fundal area, transverse incisions are better than vertical incisions, as

the arcuate vessels in the fundus run transversely, and these are less likely to be damaged with a transverse incision.

Some gynecologists shell out all fibroids before commencing the process of closure of the myometrial dead spaces; however, this can result in substantial blood loss. It is therefore generally advisable to close an incision before making a new incision, or at least close all incisions in an area (e.g., anterior wall) before making incisions in another area (e.g., posterior wall).

During myomectomy, maintaining mean arterial pressure (MAP) at approximately 60 mmHg can minimize blood loss. However, the MAP should be raised at the end of the operation and the incision sites carefully observed for bleeding before closing the abdomen [12].

KEY POINTS

Challenge: Myomectomy: massive intraoperative hemorrhage.

Background
- Intraoperative hemorrhage of over 1000 mL occurs in one in five patients undergoing myomectomy.
- Massive hemorrhage can occur from slow but constant ooze from vessel plexuses around fibroids, or less commonly from an injury to a key vessel.

Prevention
- Optimize preoperative hemoglobin.
- Reduce fibroid volume by using a GnRH agonist or selective progesterone receptor modulator for 3 months before the operation.
- Cross-match blood and arrange blood products.
- Organize cell salvage.
- Administer vaginal prostaglandin E₂, e.g., misoprostol 400 µg rectally 30–60 min before the operation.
- Maintain MAP at around 60 mmHg.
- Use vasopressin injections into the myometrium before uterine incisions are made. Diluted vasopressin can be administered into cervical stroma before hysteroscopic resection of fibroids.
- Close one uterine incision before making a new one.

Management
- Alert anesthetist and operating room staff.
- Use tourniquet around uterine arteries if not already in place.
- Consider using tourniquet around the ovarian vessels if not already in place.
- Rapid and adequate suturing of the myometrial wall.
- Consider gelatin-thrombin matrix administration to uterine incisions.
- Consult with hematologist: consider intravenous tranexamic acid, and recombinant factor VIIa infusion.
- For intractable hemorrhage:
  - Consider uterine artery or internal iliac artery ligation.
  - Consider embolization.
  - Consider hysterectomy as the last life-saving option.

References

1 Berkeley AS, DeCherney AH, Polan ML. Abdominal myomectomy and subsequent fertility. *Surg Gynecol Obstet* 1983;156:319–322.

2 Fletcher H, Frederick J, Hardie M, Simeon D. A randomized comparison of vasopressin and tourniquet as hemostatic agents during myomectomy. *Obstet Gynecol* 1996;87:1014–1018.

3 Kongnyuy EJ, Wiysonge CS. Interventions to reduce haemorrhage during myomectomy for fibroids. *Cochrane Database Syst Rev* 2011;(11):CD005355.

4 Caglar GS, Tasci Y, Kayikcioglu F, Haberal A. Intravenous tranexamic acid use in myomectomy: a prospective randomized double-blind placebo controlled study. *Eur J Obstet Gynaecol Reprod Biol* 2008;137:227–231.

5 Raga F, Sanz-Cortes M, Bonilla F, Casan EM, Bonilla-Musoles F. Reducing blood loss at myomectomy with use of a gelatin-thrombin matrix hemostatic sealant. *Fertil Steril* 2009;92:356–360.

6 Benassi L, Lopopolo G, Pazzoni F *et al.* Chemically assisted dissection of tissues: an interesting support in abdominal myomectomy. *J Am Coll Surg* 2000;191: 65–69.

7 Angioli R, Plotti F, Montera R *et al.* A new type of absorbable barbed suture for use in laparoscopic myomectomy. *Int J Obstet Gynecol* 2012;117:220–223.

8 Taylor A, Sharma M, Tsirkas P, Di Spiezio Sardo A, Setchell M, Magos A. Reducing blood loss at open myomectomy using triple tourniquets: a randomized controlled trial. *Int J Obstet Gynecol* 2005;112:340–345.

9 Ikechebelu JI, Ezeama CO, Obiechina NJ. The use of tourniquet to reduce blood loss at myomectomy. *Nig J Clin Pract* 2010;13:154–158.

10 Monaghan J. Myomectomy and management of fibroids in pregnancy. In: MonaghanJ (ed.) *Bonney's Gynaecological Surgery*, 9th edn, pp. 87–94. Bailliere Tindall, London, 1986.

11 Zullo F, Palomba S, Corea D *et al.* Bupivacaine plus epinephrine for laparoscopic myomectomy: a randomized placebo-controlled trial. *Obstet Gynecol* 2004;104:243–249.

12 Hatasaka HH. Acquired uterine factors and infertility. In: CarrellDT, PetersonCM (eds) *Reproductive Endocrinology and Infertility*, pp. 235–263. Springer, New York, 2010.

13 Frederick S, Frederick J, Fletcher H, Reid M, Hardie M, Gardner W. A trial comparing the use of rectal misoprostol plus perivascular vasopressin with perivascular vasopressin alone to decrease myometrial bleeding at the time of abdominal myomectomy. *Fertil Steril* 2013;100:1044–1049.

14 Shokeir T, Shalaby H, Nabil H, Barakat R. Reducing blood loss at abdominal myomectomy with preoperative use of dinoprostone intravaginal suppository: a randomized placebo-controlled pilot study. *Eur J Obstet Gynaecol Reprod Biol* 2013;166:61–64.

CHAPTER 96
Vaginal Myomectomy

Adam Magos

The Royal Free Hospital, London, UK

Case history: A woman with a history of increasingly heavy periods is found to have a 7-cm anterior transmural fibroid on ultrasound scan. A diagnostic hysteroscopy confirmed a type II submucous fibroid with less than 10% of the fibroid protruding into the uterine cavity. Vaginal access was deemed sufficient for a vaginal myomectomy.

Background

We tend to forget that the first myomectomies ever carried out in the 1840s by pioneers such as Amussat in France and Atlee in the USA were done via the vagina. Standard textbooks of gynecologic surgery a 100 years or so ago included whole chapters on vaginal myomectomy, not only for the prolapsed vaginal fibroid but for myomas sited virtually anywhere in the uterus, be they submucous, intramural, or subserous. Today, all that seems to have survived is the avulsion of a fibroid which has prolapsed through the cervix into the vagina, and some of today's standard textbooks do not mention vaginal myomectomy at all.

This is a pity because removing fibroids via the vagina is an attractive alternative to hysteroscopic, laparoscopic and, in some cases, even open myomectomy [1]. Patient selection is key, and as with any vaginal procedure, adequate vaginal access, good uterine mobility, and reasonable uterine size are essential prerequisites for successful surgery. If these criteria are fulfilled, then fibroids can be removed vaginally using a variety of techniques, a Dührssen's (cervical) incision, hysterotomy or colpotomy being the basic approaches to gain access to fibroids which are situated in the cervix or uterus [2]. The various techniques used for vaginal myomectomy are classified in Table 96.1.

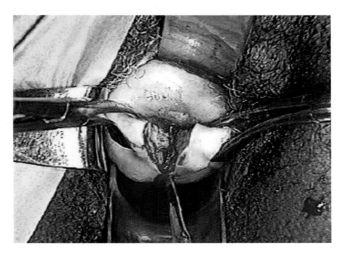

Figure 96.1 Type 3a vaginal myomectomy: a posterior Dührssen's incision being made to gain access to the uterine cavity and a submucous fibroid.

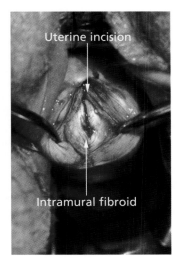

Figure 96.2 Type 4 vaginal myomectomy: the uterus has been pulled through an anterior colpotomy and incised over the fibroid prior to enucleation.

Table 96.1 Classification of vaginal myomectomy.

Type	Technique
1	Avulsion of prolapsed pedunculated submucous fibroid
2	Non-incisional access to intracervical or intracavity fibroid
3a	Incisional access to intracavity fibroid (Dührssen cervical incision) (Figure 96.1)
3b	Incisional access to intracavity/intramural/subserous fibroid (incision continued as hysterotomy)
4	Colpotomy access to intramural/subserous fibroids (Figure 96.2)

Source: Thomas & Magos, 2011 [1] with permission from Elsevier.

Gynecologic and Obstetric Surgery: Challenges and Management Options, First Edition. Edited by Arri Coomarasamy, Mahmood I. Shafi, G. Willy Davila and Kiong K. Chan.
© 2016 John Wiley & Sons, Ltd. Published 2016 by John Wiley & Sons, Ltd.

Management

In the case history, although there is only a single fibroid, it is not suitable for hysteroscopic resection because of its size and site. It could be removed laparoscopically (or of course by laparotomy), but vaginal myomectomy is another option. Removing the fibroid vaginally would have the advantages of avoiding any abdominal incisions and being able to use conventional instruments to repair the uterus just as at laparotomy with, logically, a reduced risk of uterine rupture in any future pregnancy compared with laparoscopic myomectomy [3].

Vaginal myomectomy procedure

The first step is to perform an EUA to evaluate the pelvis, in particular vaginal access, and uterine size and mobility. The bladder is then emptied, and 20 mL of 1% lidocaine with 1 in 200,000 epinephrine is injected into the periphery of the cervix. For the woman in the case history, an approach to the fibroid via an anterior colpotomy (type 4 vaginal myomectomy) is appropriate, and so an anterior semicircular incision can be made at the cervico-vaginal junction and the vagina then reflected cephalad. The lower margin of the bladder is dissected away from the cervix and uterus, and the uterovesical peritoneum is opened. A vaginal retractor is inserted into the peritoneal cavity and the uterus pulled into the incision by a combination of backward pressure on the cervix using a tenaculum and forward pressure on the anterior uterine wall using No. 1 Prolene sutures. Once the anterior uterine wall overlying the fibroid is in view through the colpotomy, a vertical midline incision can be made and the fibroid shelled out using a combination of sharp and digital dissection and morcellation. Once the fibroid has been removed, the uterus is pulled through the colpotomy incision to facilitate its repair in layers before being replaced into the peritoneal cavity. Finally, the vagina is closed and the bladder emptied to confirm its integrity.

The alternative approach to removing the fibroid in this case would have been to make a Dührssen's incision into the cervix, and extend it into a hysterotomy until the fibroid is reached; the fibroid can then be removed by dissection and morcellation (type 3a vaginal myomectomy). The bladder would have to be dissected away from the cervix and uterus just as with the colpotomy technique. Unlike when a colpotomy is used, however, hysterotomy invariably involves opening the uterine cavity with future implications on pregnancy, so may not be the preferred technique in this case. On completion of the myomectomy, the uterine and cervical incisions are closed, followed by repair of the vaginal incision.

Drains are not used routinely with either technique, but if there is concern about postoperative oozing such as following multiple myomectomies or if the fibroid is particularly large, a Foley catheter can be left in the pouch of Douglas overnight. It is our standard practice to give all our patients intraoperative and postoperative prophylactic antibiotics for 5 days and low-molecular-weight heparin after surgery until they are fully mobile.

Conclusion

Most of today's gynecologists have probably not only never seen or done a vaginal myomectomy, but probably not even heard of these operations which were so familiar to our forefathers. And yet, if we are able to remove a whole uterus via the vagina when doing a

hysterectomy, why should we not remove fibroids vaginally as well? A review of the medical literature shows that there is increasing interest in these operations worldwide, particularly in removing fibroids via an anterior or posterior colpotomy, and comparative trials with laparoscopic myomectomy have favored the vaginal operation in terms of quicker operating time, less blood loss, and shorter hospitalization [4,5]. As concluded by Faivre *et al.* [6] in their review published in 2010, "A vaginal approach may be considered an alternative to laparotomy or laparoscopy in surgery to treat accessible myomas, and seems to be the simplest method." We would extend this sentiment to hysteroscopic myomectomy as well for the larger submucous fibroid where accidental uterine perforation and fluid overload are avoided when operating vaginally.

KEY POINTS

Challenge: Removing fibroids via the vagina.

Background
- The first myomectomies were performed via the vagina, and not done by laparotomy.
- Vaginal myomectomy can be accomplished using a variety of techniques which were popular in the late 1800s and early 1900s as evidenced by standard textbooks of the time.
- Patient selection is important and criteria for the procedure should include adequate vaginal access, normal uterine mobility, and no more than moderate uterine enlargement.

Management
- Techniques for removing the fibroid via the vagina range from avulsion of prolapsed fibroids in the vagina or endocervical canal to colpotomy access to intramural or subserosal fibroids.

Vaginal myomectomy technique
- Perform an EUA to assess vaginal access, and uterine size and mobility.
- Empty the bladder.
- Infiltrate the periphery of the cervix with 20 mL of 1% lidocaine with 1 in 200,000 epinephrine.
- For an anterior wall fibroid, perform an anterior colpotomy: make an anterior semicircular incision at the cervico-vaginal junction; reflect the vagina cephalad; dissect the lower margin of the bladder away from the cervix; and finally open the uterovesical peritoneum.
- Insert a vaginal retractor into the peritoneal cavity, and pull the uterus into the incision using No. 1 Prolene sutures.
- Once the anterior uterine wall is in view through the colpotomy, make a vertical midline incision on the uterus, and shell out the fibroid with sharp and digital dissection.
- Once the fibroid has been removed, pull the uterus through the colpotomy, and repair the myometrium in layers.
- Replace uterus into the peritoneal cavity and close the vagina.
- An alternative technique is an approach through a Dührssen's incision into the cervix and extension into a hysterotomy until the fibroid is reached.

References

1 Thomas B, Magos A. Subtotal hysterectomy and myomectomy: vaginally. *Best Pract Res Clin Obstet Gynaecol* 2011;25:133–152.

2 Crossen HS. Vaginal myomectomy. In: *Operative Gynaecology*, pp. 277–283. C.V. Mosby Company, St Louis, 1907.

3 Rovia PH, Heinonen PK. Pregnancy outcomes after transvaginal myomectomy by colpotomy. *Eur J Obstet Gynaecol Reprod Biol* 2012;161:130–133.

4 Yu X, Zhu L, Li L, Shi HH, Lang JH. Evaluating the feasibility and safety of vaginal myomectomy in China. *Chin Med J (Engl)* 2011;124:3481–3484.

5 Yi YX, Zhang W, Guo WR, Zhou Q, Su Y. Meta-analysis: the comparison of clinical results between vaginal and laparoscopic myomectomy. *Arch Gynecol Obstet* 2011;283:1275–1289.

6 Faivre E, Surroca MM, Deffieux X, Pages F, Gervaise A, Fernandez H. Vaginal myomectomy: literature review. *J Minim Invasive Gynecol* 2010;17:154–160.

CHAPTER 97
Surgery for Proximal Tubal Blockage

Spyros Papaioannou
Heart of England NHS Foundation Trust, Birmingham, UK

Case history: *Infertility investigations for a couple found all tests to be normal, except for HSG that reported "Normal uterine cavity. No fill or spill of dye was seen from either fallopian tube."*

Background

The proximal third of the fallopian tube, which includes the intramural tubal segment, should be seen as a structure which has important differences to the rest of the fallopian tube. Sulak *et al.* [1] found the presence of amorphous material forming a cast in the tubal lumen of women who underwent segmental tubal resection as a treatment for proximal tubal blockage. Histologically, the tubal wall itself could be entirely normal. This finding suggested that tubal segmental resection in such cases, common practice for decades, not only represented overtreatment but also converted a "normal" oviduct into a scarred one. The logical next step was to try to treat proximal tubal blockage by applying pressure directly to the tubal ostia in an attempt to flush the obstructing material or break the minor tubal synechiae, in a process described as selective salpingography. If that fails to clear the tube, then a guidewire can be forwarded into the tube through the selective salpingography cannula, using basic principles of interventional radiology. This is called tubal catheterization. The whole process can be completed as an outpatient procedure under fluoroscopic control (Figure 97.1). Alternatively, tubal catheterization can also be performed through an operative hysteroscope, with or without concurrent laparoscopy.

Management

Preoperative management
Women are asked to call the X-ray department on the first day of a menstrual period. Appointments are booked within the following 14 days. They are advised to take paracetamol or ibuprofen approximately 2 hours before the procedure. Informed consent is obtained prior to all examinations.

Equipment
All examinations are carried out in a radiologic examination room. A digital fluoroscopic unit with a C-arm and a large view image intensifier is used. Radiographic parameters (roentgenogram tube voltage and current) are controlled automatically. The fluoroscope is operated by a foot switch, which provides the operator with the flexibility to obtain images whenever and for as long as it is judged to be necessary. The radiation dose to the patient is measured as a dose–area product (DAP) with a fitted calibrated meter. The DAP is a measure of the total energy imparted to the patient for the complete examination.

Ideally, the set-up should provide equipment for the assessment of tubal perfusion pressure (TPP). Before commencing the procedure the distal end of the selective salpingography catheter is connected, by polyethylene tubing, to a syringe pump and by means of a three-way stopcock to a pressure-sensitive transducer, which conveys information to a computer. The pump is then activated to flush the catheter with contrast agent so that the encountered resistance is displayed, as a pressure curve, on the computer screen. In this way, the background system pressure is recorded and air is expelled from the system. Water-soluble contrast medium at a constant flow rate of 10 mL/min is used.

The Cook selective salpingography system, shown in Figure 97.2, is a standard kit for selective salpingography and tubal catheterization.

Patient preparation
The patient is placed on the radiology examination table in the lithotomy position. A sterile drape is placed underneath the buttocks. The cervix is visualized using a Cusco's speculum and is thoroughly cleaned with 0.05% chlorhexidine gluconate aqueous sterile solution. Local anesthesia and lubrication are provided by instillation of 2% lidocaine gel into the cervical canal. After waiting for about 3 min, a single-toothed tenaculum is applied at the 12 o'clock position of the cervix.

Technique
The inner cannula is inserted into the selective salpingography catheter so that a suitable distal catheter angle is formed. Using a gentle rotational motion, the catheter is then forwarded through the cervical canal. Its passage is facilitated by simultaneous gentle traction on the tenaculum, which helps to straighten the uterocervical junction. Once inside the uterine cavity, contrast medium can be injected so that the uterine cavity can be assessed first. The selective salpingography catheter is then gently rotated so that its tip is pointing to one of the uterine cornua and is advanced,

Gynecologic and Obstetric Surgery: Challenges and Management Options, First Edition. Edited by Arri Coomarasamy, Mahmood I. Shafi, G. Willy Davila and Kiong K. Chan.
© 2016 John Wiley & Sons, Ltd. Published 2016 by John Wiley & Sons, Ltd.

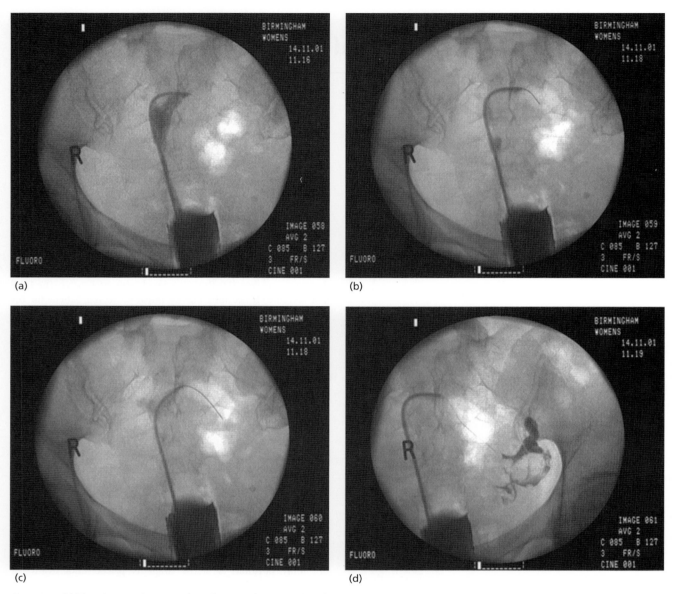

Figure 97.1 (a) The selective salpingography catheter can be seen at the left tubal orifice. Contrast medium back-flows into the uterus as the tube shows minimal fill and high resistance. (b) The guidewire has been passed successfully into the left fallopian tube. (c) The fallopian tube fills with contrast medium. (d) Fill and spill can now be observed.

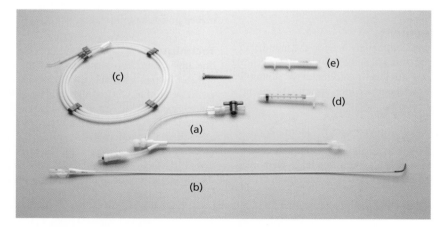

Figure 97.2 The Cook selective salpingography system: (a) uterine introducer; (b) selective salpingography catheter, which is forwarded toward the fallopian tube uterine opening through the uterine introducer; (c) roadrunner guidewire, which is threaded through the selective salpingography catheter into the fallopian tube; (d) syringe to inflate the balloon of the uterine introducer; (e) guidewire handler (attached to the guidewire to assist with manipulation).

by tactile sensation, toward the tubal ostium. Its position is checked fluoroscopically and, if satisfactory, dye is injected. If the obstruction is overcome the tubal contour is outlined. The isthmus, ampulla, and infundibulum are studied and the pattern of peritoneal spill of dye is observed. The TPP is recorded.

If the obstruction persists or the TPP is raised (>350 mmHg), the roadrunner guidewire is threaded through the inner cannula and is advanced toward the blockage. When the blockage is reached, gentle push is applied to overcome it. If recanalization is achieved, this becomes radiologically visible, since the guidewire follows the expected contour of the tube. The guidewire is then withdrawn and contrast is injected through the selective salpingography catheter to confirm patency and measure the TPP. In case of perforation of the fallopian tube, the patient may report a sharp pain, while a collection of contrast, in the form of a pseudo-diverticulum (perforations are submucosal most of the time), would be evident.

Postoperative care

After the procedure, antibiotics are prescribed only for patients who were diagnosed with distal tubal disease. A combination of co-amoxiclav (amoxicillin 250 mg and clavulanic acid 125 mg) 8-hourly and doxycycline 100 mg 12-hourly, both for 7 days, is used. Penicillin-sensitive patients can receive erythromycin 250 mg three times daily for 7 days, instead of co-amoxiclav. Pain relief is prescribed as required.

Tubal spasm

Proximal tubal blockage has been observed to be, in many cases, intermittent; one tubal patency test might demonstrate it, while the next will not. The concept of tubal spasm, defined as normal variation of the function of the uterotubal junction or a physiologic response to uterine distension created during diagnostic procedures, was suggested as the possible explanation. However, there is evidence that proximal tubal blockage is a sign of tubal dysfunction. The multicenter transcervical balloon tuboplasty study [2] demonstrated that pregnancy rate in a group of women diagnosed with tubal spasm was disappointing. Furthermore, TPPs measured during selective salpingography in patients diagnosed with tubal spasm were found, with few exceptions, to be elevated. Intermittent tubal blockage cannot therefore be considered a normal physiologic variation [3].

Pregnancy results

Survival analysis of spontaneous conceptions following selective salpingography has shown a cumulative pregnancy rate of 40% at 3 years follow-up for women less than 35 years of age, with the decline in the possibility of a pregnancy during the study period being minimal [4]. The safety of the procedure in terms of ovarian radiation exposure has been studied, with reassuring results [5]. Perforation of the tube can occur in up to 4% of cases; however, a perforation does not require any treatment, although further treatment in that tube is best avoided.

KEY POINTS

Challenge: Management of proximal tubal blockage.

Background
- There are substantial differences between the proximal and distal fallopian tubes, and their pathologies. Distal tubes are often blocked by an infective cause, while proximal tubes can be blocked by amorphous casts.
- Once proximal tubal blockage is relieved, the fallopian tube often returns to normal.
- Selective salpingography and tubal catheterization is an outpatient procedure designed to treat proximal tubal blockage.
- Up to 40% cumulative natural pregnancy rate over 3 years has been reported with selective salpingography and tubal catheterization treatment for women aged 35 years or less.

Treatment
This is best performed in a radiology room under fluoroscopy control; however, it can be done hysteroscopically with laparoscopy at the same time to confirm that recanalization of the tube has been achieved.

Equipment
- Use standard selective salpingography kits such as the one manufactured by Cook Medical.
- Use a digital fluoroscopic unit with a C-arm and a large view image intensifier.
- Equipment to measure TPP will add value to the diagnostic information.

Procedure
- Conduct the procedure in the follicular phase of the menstrual cycle.
- Place patient in lithotomy position, and clean the cervix.
- Instill 2% lidocaine gel into the cervical canal, and apply a single-toothed tenaculum to the cervix.
- Insert the selective salpingography catheter through the cervix into the uterus, and inject contrast to view the uterine cavity contour.
- Then rotate the selective salpingography catheter to face a cornua and advance the tip of the catheter to sit at the tubal ostium.
- Inject contrast to assess the fallopian tube, to unblock it, and record TPP.
- If the tube is unblocked or has high TPP (>350 mmHg), proceed with tubal catheterization with the roadrunner guidewire.

Postoperative care
- Prescribe broad-spectrum antibiotics and pain relief.

References

1 Sulak PJ, Letterie GS, Coddington CC, Hayslip CC, Woodward JE, Klein TA. Histology of proximal tubal occlusion. *Fertil Steril* 1987;48:437–440.

2 Gleicher N, Confino E, Corfman R *et al* The multicenter transcervical balloon tubaplasty study: conclusions and comparison to alternative technologies. *Hum Reprod* 1993;8:1264–1271.

3 Papaioannou S. The pathophysiology and natural history of proximal tubal blockage. Opinion paper. *Hum Reprod* 2004;19:481–485.

4 Papaioannou S, Afnan M, Girling AJ *et al*. Long-term fertility prognosis following selective salpingography and tubal catheterization in women with proximal tubal blockage. *Hum Reprod* 2002;17:2325–2330.

5 Papaioannou S, Afnan M, Coomarasamy A *et al*. Long term safety of fluoroscopically guided selective salpingography and tubal catheterisation. *Hum Reprod* 2002;17:370–372.

CHAPTER 98
Surgery for Distal Tubal Disease

Lynne Robinson, Hemant N. Vakharia, and Yousri Afifi
Birmingham Women's NHS Foundation Trust, Birmingham, UK

Case history: A woman with a history of pelvic inflammatory disease and infertility is found to have a terminal hydrosalpinx. She wishes tubal surgery in preference to assisted conception treatment.

Background

Tubal disease is prevalent in 25% of subfertile couples [1]. The common causes of distal tubal disease are infection, in particular chlamydia, endometriosis, and adhesions due to previous surgery. Distal tubal surgery was the mainstay of treatment for tubal infertility until the advent of *in vitro* fertilization (IVF) in the 1970s. Since then, tubal surgery has been superseded by assisted reproductive technology (ART) treatment; as a result, there is currently limited expertise in tubal surgery.

Patients with hydrosalpinges are commonly recommended to have a salpingectomy or tubal occlusion prior to ART because of the deleterious effect of the fluid in the fallopian tube on the developing embryo caused by several possible mechanisms: mechanical effects, embryotoxicity and gametotoxicity, alterations in endometrial receptivity resulting in poor implantation, and a possible direct effect on the endometrium [2]. However, salpingectomy precludes future tubal surgery, which a couple may come to regret if ART treatment were unsuccessful.

Tubal surgery has seen a resurgence in popularity in recent years, and this may be partly related to the cost of ART treatment. In the absence of other causes of subfertility, tubal surgery allows repeated attempts at natural conception, in contrast to the restriction of a limited number of ART attempts. Success rates of tubal surgery vary widely but a large series [3] found a 53% intrauterine pregnancy rate after tubal surgery for hydrosalpinges. A Cochrane review [4] identified no randomized trials comparing different tubal surgery techniques.

Classification of tubal disease

The type and extent of tubal disease is important in advising patients on the best treatment option. Several studies have shown that the best prognostic factor for successful tubal surgery is the degree of tubal damage [5,6,7,8,9]. The severity of tubal disease can be assessed and classified (Table 98.1).

Management

A proposed management algorithm is shown in Figure 98.1. However, treatment for a specific couple should be individualized based on anticipated outcome (Table 98.1), other fertility problems (e.g., low sperm count), and the couple's preferences. Women with mild to moderate tubal disease could consider tubal surgery in the first instance. Women with severe tubal disease may have a better chance of pregnancy with ART. However, many women with hydrosalpinges will require surgery before ART treatment to occlude or remove their tube. Undergoing surgery to open the fallopian tube(s) can treat their hydrosalpinx while also giving them a chance of natural conception if ART is not successful. At present, occlusion or removal of the tube is the gold standard treatment before ART. More evidence is needed to explore the effectiveness of salpingostomy before ART, instead of salpingectomy or tubal occlusion.

Types of tubal surgery

There are several techniques available for distal tubal surgery, and the choice of a specific technique will depend on the tubal pathology and patient characteristics.

Adhesiolysis

Distal tubal obstruction can be caused by peritubal adhesions. These can be released using monopolar and bipolar diathermy

Table 98.1 Classification of tubal disease.

Poor outcome (<10% CPR)	Acceptable outcome (10–30% CPR)	Favorable outcome (30–60% CPR)	Excellent outcome (>60% CPR)
Dense adhesions	Lack of poor outcome features	Lack of poor outcome features	Lack of all other features
Thick walls and tubal diameter	Full diameter of tube >3 cm	Full diameter of tube 1.5–3 cm	Full diameter of tube <1.5 cm
Atrophy of mucosa	Fimbrial damage	Partial fimbrial damage	
Intra-ampullary adhesions		Filmy adhesions	

CPR, clinical pregnancy rate.

Gynecologic and Obstetric Surgery: Challenges and Management Options, First Edition. Edited by Arri Coomarasamy, Mahmood I. Shafi, G. Willy Davila and Kiong K. Chan.
© 2016 John Wiley & Sons, Ltd. Published 2016 by John Wiley & Sons, Ltd.

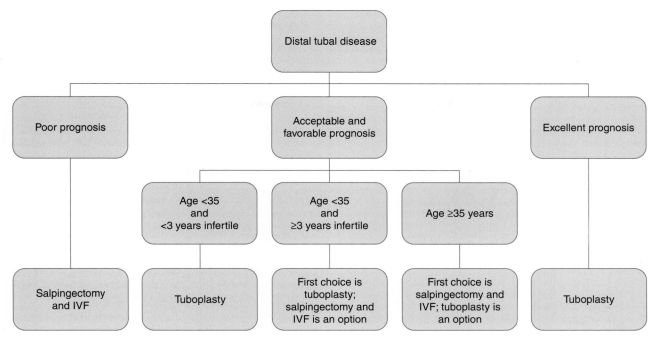

Figure 98.1 A proposed management algorithm for tubal disease.

(Figure 98.2). Adhesiolysis can be performed alone or in conjunction with salpingostomy to achieve tubal patency.

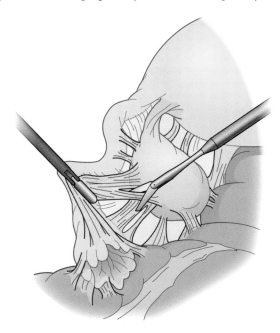

Figure 98.2 Division of peritubal adhesions with laparoscopic scissors. Adapted from Gomel & Brill, 2010 [12] with permission from Informa Healthcare.

Salpingostomy

There are various methods for salpingostomy, but the commonest one involves making incisions over the distal end of the tube with laparoscopic scissors or monopolar needle diathermy, and then making a cuff (Figure 98.3). A typical method involves making a Y- or X-shaped incision at the thinnest and ideally avascular portion of the clubbed distal end of the tube (Figure 98.3a), after injecting dye via the cervix to achieve tubal distension. If any bleeding occurs, the precise location of the point(s) of bleeding should be identified with the help of an irrigation jet, and the bleeding point(s) should be controlled with needlepoint diathermy or microbipolar forceps. The mucosa is then everted (Figure 98.3b), and the cuff is secured with three or four fine (7-0 or 8-0) monofilament sutures (Figure 98.3c). A dye test is then performed to ensure patency.

Some surgeons use methods such as Bruhat's technique. Bruhat's technique involves "flowering" of the distal end of the fallopian tube to evert it. In the 1980s and 1990s, prostheses were often used at salpingostomy although there is no evidence to support this approach [10]. A Cochrane review found no evidence of benefit or harm in using microsurgery over standard techniques, laparoscopic approach over laparotomy, and the use of CO_2 laser or other salpingostomy techniques [2,9,10,11]. However, trials using currently available advanced laparoscopic techniques are absent.

Prevention

Chlamydia is the most common sexually transmitted disease in Western society; however, because it can be asymptomatic, it can lead to undiagnosed extensive tubal disease. The use of barrier contraception can prevent the transmission of the disease and good sex education can help to increase awareness. Approximately one-fifth of women with symptomatic *Chlamydia* infection suffer from infertility. Other causes of PID, such as gonorrhea and syphilis, are on the increase. In all these cases, referral to a genitourinary clinic will provide the best treatment and help limit any tubal damage.

Avoidance of open surgery can help decrease the risk of adhesions causing tubal disease. Laparoscopic surgery causes significantly less adhesion formation and therefore is the preferred approach whenever possible, to decrease the risk of tubal damage.

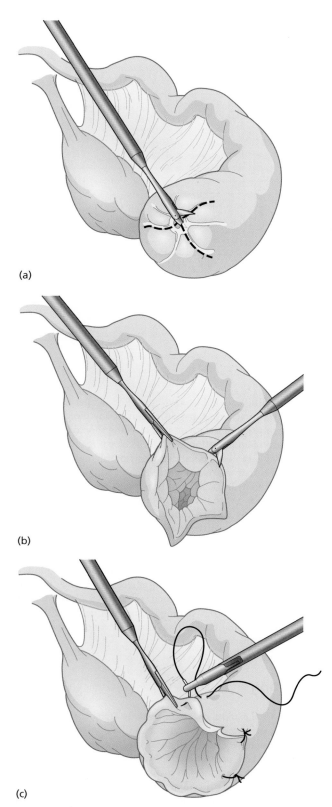

(a)

(b)

(c)

Figure 98.3 Salpingostomy: (a) a Y-shaped incision is made at the fimbrial end of the clubbed fallopian tube; (b) a cuff is created at the fimbrial end using graspers; (c) the cuff is secured with monofilament stitches. Adapted from Gomel & Brill, 2010 [12] with permission from Informa Healthcare.

KEY POINTS

Challenge: Surgery for distal tubal disease.

Background
- Tubal disease is prevalent in 25% of subfertile couples.
- The common causes for distal tubal disease are infection, endometriosis, and previous surgery.
- Tubal surgery has variable success rates depending mainly on the severity of tubal damage. Hydrosalpinges are known to decrease the success of ART and therefore require removal or disconnection before IVF treatment.

Prevention
- Barrier contraception to reduce risk of *Chlamydia* and other PID pathogens.
- Prompt treatment of pelvic infection.
- A preference for laparoscopic surgery whenever possible to reduce the risk of pelvic adhesions and tubal disease.

Management
- Women with mild to moderate tubal disease could consider tubal surgery in the first instance, if there are no other fertility factors.
- Women with severe tubal disease may have a better chance of pregnancy with ART.
- It may be possible to treat hydrosalpinges by salpingostomy before ART, but the effectiveness of this approach needs to be confirmed in a clinical trial. For hydrosalpinges before IVF treatment, the gold standard treatment currently is the occlusion or removal of the fallopian tube.
- Tubal surgery can be in the form of adhesiolysis, fimbrioplasty, and salpingostomy.
- Tubal adhesiolysis: peritubal adhesions can be released with monopolar and bipolar diathermy.
- Salpingostomy:
  - Perform adhesiolysis around the tube if necessary.
  - Inject dye via the cervix to achieve tubal distension for ostia site selection.
  - Make a Y- or X-shaped incision on an avascular area at the thinnest portion of the clubbed distal portion of the tube, using laparoscopic scissors or monopolar energy.
  - Evert the edges of the mucosa using interrupted monofilament sutures.
  - Perform a dye test to ensure patency.

References

1   Posaci C, Camus M, Osmanagaoglu K, Devroey P. Tubal surgery in the era of assisted reproductive technology: clinical options. *Hum Reprod* 1999;14(Suppl 1):120–136.

2   Johnson N, van Voorst S, Sowter MC, Strandell A, Mol BW. Surgical treatment for tubal disease in women due to undergo in vitro fertilisation. *Cochrane Database Syst Rev* 2010;(1):CD002125.

3   Dubuisson JB. [Are there still indications for tubal surgery in infertility?] *Presse Med* 1998;27:1793–1794.

4   Pandian Z, Akande VA, Harrild K, Bhattacharya S. Surgery for tubal infertility. *Cochrane Database Syst Rev* 2008;(3):CD006415.

5   Kitchin JD III, Nunley WC Jr, Bateman BG. Surgical management of distal tubal occlusion. *Am J Obstet Gynecol* 1986;155:524–531.

6   Dubuisson JB, Bouquet de Joliniere J, Aubriot FX, Darai E, Foulot H, Mandelbrot L. Terminal tuboplasties by laparoscopy: 65 consecutive cases. *Fertil Steril* 1990;54:401–403.

7   Winston RM, Margara RA. Microsurgical salpingostomy is not an obsolete procedure. *Br J Obstet Gynaecol* 1991;98:637–642.

8   Sasse VV, Karageorgieva E, Keckstein J. Laparoscopic treatment of distal tubal occlusion-reocclusion and pregnancy rate. *J Am Assoc Gynecol Laparosc* 1994;1(4 Part 2):S32.

9   Oh ST. Tubal patency and conception rates with three methods of laparoscopic terminal neosalpingostomy. *J Am Assoc Gynecol Laparosc* 1996;3:519–523.

10   Ahmad G, Watson A, Vandekerckhove P, Lilford R. Techniques for pelvic surgery in subfertility. *Cochrane Database Syst Rev* 2006;(2):CD000221.

11   Chong AP. Pregnancy outcome in neosalpingostomy by the cuff vs Bruhat technique using the carbon dioxide laser. *J Gynecol Surg* 1991;7:207–210.

12   Gomel V, Brill A. *Reconstructive and Reproductive Surgery in Gynecology: Principles and Practice.* Informa Healthcare, London, 2010.

CHAPTER 99
Reversal of Sterilization

Hemant N. Vakharia, Lynne Robinson, and Yousri Afifi
Birmingham Women's NHS Foundation Trust, Birmingham, UK

Case history: A woman who is in a new relationship is requesting reversal of sterilization. She previously had sterilization with Filshie clips.

Background

Tubal ligation is a safe and effective method of contraception. Although rates of female sterilization have declined, there were still 14,900 sterilization procedures (by any method) recorded during the 2012/2013 fiscal year in the UK [1].

Sterilization is intended to be a permanent procedure. However, regret and requests for reversal of sterilization are common [2,3]. Data suggest that between 2 and 30% of patients regret the decision [4], with age less than 30 years and change in relationship being identified as common reasons [2,3]. UK data from the 2012/2013 fiscal year show that 17% of sterilizations were performed in those aged 20–29 years [1]. Currently, reversal of sterilization is not funded on the National Health Service and this should be made very clear when counseling patients requesting sterilization.

Female sterilization can be performed via a number of methods, with laparoscopic application of Filshie clips and tubal ligation at the time of cesarean section being the most common methods. Hysteroscopic sterilization techniques are increasingly being used, and are regarded as irreversible.

Management

Reversal of sterilization has been approached via open (laparotomy), laparoscopic, and robotic methods [5,6,7,8]. Irrespective of mode of entry, microsurgical principles have to be followed strictly; these include magnification, point hemostasis, gentle tissue handling, irrigation, fine suturing, and use of anti-adhesion therapy.

Historically, reversal was achieved with laparotomy, with microsurgical techniques to perform the anastomosis [5]. The introduction of laparoscopic technology with benefits such as detailed magnification of tissues, reduction in adhesions, and quick recovery times led to clinicians adopting laparoscopic reversal. However, advanced laparoscopic skill is required for sterilization reversal, and therefore it should only be attempted by those appropriately trained [6].

Reversal technique

Regardless of the approach, the first step is to identify the sterilization site, mobilize it, excise the blocked segment, and prepare the proximal and distal stumps for anastomosis (Figure 99.1). Following the stump preparation, mesosalpingeal approximation is performed with interrupted stitches, bringing the tubal ends into close proximity (Figure 99.2). Dye is passed via the cervix prior to anastomosis. Tubal anastomosis can now be performed with a fine suture (6-0) in one or two layers, using four stitches as shown in Figure 99.3. We would endorse the one-layer technique using four stitches (Figure 99.4), although some authors have described a two-layer techniques. The stitch can either be full thickness or submucosal to spare the mucosa. In addition, the use of clips, glue, and tubal splints has also been described [9,10,11,12]. When tubal splints are employed we recommend tubal catheterization hysteroscopically as this is less traumatic to the proximal stump. Following anastomosis, dye is passed again to ensure the tube is patent.

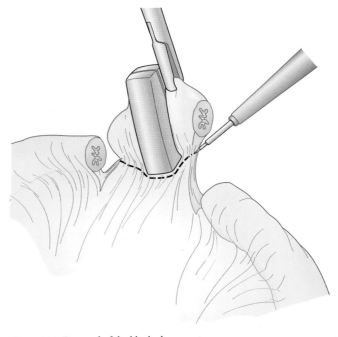

Figure 99.1 Removal of the blocked segment.

Gynecologic and Obstetric Surgery: Challenges and Management Options, First Edition. Edited by Arri Coomarasamy, Mahmood I. Shafi, G. Willy Davila and Kiong K. Chan.
© 2016 John Wiley & Sons, Ltd. Published 2016 by John Wiley & Sons, Ltd.

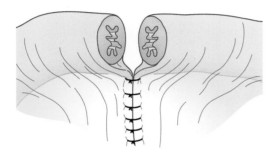

Figure 99.2 Mesosalpingeal approximation with interrupted stitches.

Outcomes

Rates of intrauterine pregnancy following reversal of sterilization have been reported to be between 57 and 84%, with data suggesting similar rates can be achieved both laparoscopically and via the traditional open approach [6,9,10,13]. The rate of ectopic pregnancy has been found to be 2–10% [6,11,13].

Prognostic factors

Age

Age is a key prognostic factor in tubal anastomosis [14]. A retrospective study evaluating patients who underwent reversal of sterilization in one hospital in Belgium found a cumulative intrauterine pregnancy rate of 81% for women aged under 36 years, compared with 67% for those aged 36–39 years, 50% for those aged 40–43 years, and 12.5% for those aged over 43 years [13]. While this comes as no surprise given that female fecundity declines with age, it is important to note this when counseling patients considering reversal.

Type of sterilization

The type of sterilization the patient has undergone appears to have an effect on pregnancy rates, with one study finding that reversal resulted in live births in 41% of women with a previous tubal electrocautery, in 50% of those who had a Pomeroy technique, in 75% of those in whom rings were used, and in 84% of those who had a clip-based sterilization [6]. Another retrospective study showed similar findings, with pregnancy rates of 78%, 72%, 68%, and 67% with reversal after clip, ring, electrocautery, and Pomeroy, respectively [13]. The data from these studies failed to reach statistical significance, possibly due to their small sample size, but they do suggest that the prognosis is better for women who had sterilization with clips.

Tubal length

Rock *et al.* [15] suggested that a length of 4 cm or less was associated with an inferior pregnancy rate. However, a large study on 1118 cases failed to reproduce this finding [16]. A committee opinion paper prepared by the Practice Committee of the American Society for Reproductive Medicine has recommended that tubal anastomosis should not be performed when the final tubal length is less than 4 cm [17].

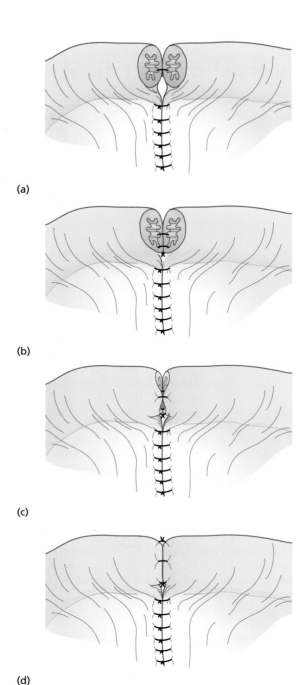

(a)

(b)

(c)

(d)

Figure 99.3 Tubal anastomosis with four stitches: (a) an interrupted suture is applied to the midpoint of the posterior tube; (b) a second suture is placed at the base of the tube; (c) a third suture is placed anteriorly; (d) a final suture is placed at the top.

Assisted conception

When reversal has been unsuccessful, recourse to assisted conception is required. One could argue that with no guarantee of success, the costs associated with reversal of sterilization might make assisted conception a more attractive option, but recent

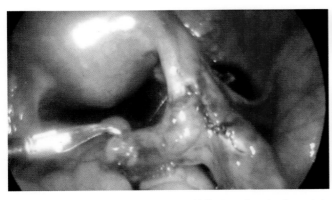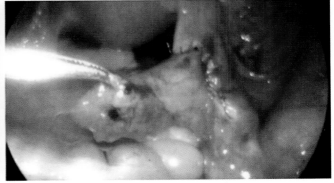

Figure 99.4 Laparoscopic re-anastomosis of fallopian tube using four stitches in one-layer suturing technique.

data have shown that in those who have had previous clip or ring sterilization and are under the age of 40 years, laparoscopic tubal re-anastomosis is a cost-effective option [18]. Reversal of sterilization offers a chance of natural conception(s) over time; patients who have undergone previous sterilization who choose assisted conception will have to self-fund each cycle and be subject to the risk of ovarian hyperstimulation and increased incidence of multiple pregnancies.

Prevention

Given that regret has been identified as the main reason for requesting reversal of sterilization [2,3], appropriate counseling at the time of sterilization is important. Younger patients (under the age of 30 years) are a particularly important cohort in whom clear counseling is essential; a strong preference for long-term reversible contraception (e.g., Mirena IUS or hormonal implant) is justifiable in younger women.

KEY POINTS

Challenge: Reversal of sterilization with the aim of achieving adequate tubal patency with re-anastomosis of the fallopian tube.

Background
- Female sterilization is regarded as a permanent and effective method of contraception, with 14,900 procedures being performed in 2012–2013 [1]. It is most commonly performed laparoscopically with the application of Filshie clips. More recently, hysteroscopic techniques are being used and can be performed on an outpatient basis.
- Requests for reversal of sterilization are common, especially in those who were under the age of 30 at the time of the procedure, with regret being cited as a common reason [2,3].
- Currently in the UK, reversal of sterilization is not available on the National Health Service.

Prevention
- Adequate counseling before sterilization to avoid regret and the need for reversal of the procedure is essential.

- In those under the age of 30, the use of long-acting reversal contraceptives should be given serious consideration.

Management
- Careful preoperative assessment is imperative. Assessment of the patient's age, length of tube, and type of sterilization procedure will mean the patient can be counseled appropriately and given an indication as to the likelihood of success.
- Various surgical techniques have been described with little evidence to favor one technique in particular.
- We favor the laparoscopic one-layer suture technique using up to four interrupted stitches.
- The technique of sterilization reversal involves:
  - Mobilization of sterilization site.
  - Excision of sterilization segment and preparation of stumps.
  - Mesosalpingeal approximation is performed with interrupted stitches.
  - Tubal anastomosis can now be performed with a 6-0 suture in one or two layers, using four stitches.

References

1 Health and Social Care Information Centre. NHS Contraceptive Services: England 2012/13, Community Contraceptive Clinics. Available at http://www.hscic.gov.uk/catalogue/PUB12548

2 Trussell J, Guilbert E, Hedley A. Sterilization failure, sterilization reversal, and pregnancy after sterilization reversal in Quebec. *Obstet Gynecol* 2003;101:677–684.

3 Grubb GS, Peterson HB, Layde PM, Rubin GL. Regret after decision to have a tubal sterilization. *Fertil Steril* 1985;44:248–253.

4 Schmidt JE, Hillis SD, Marchbanks PA, Jeng G, Peterson HB. Requesting information about and obtaining reversal after tubal sterilization: findings from the U.S. collaborative review of sterilization. *Fertil Steril* 2000;74:892–898.

5 Gomel V. Microsurgical reversal of female sterilization: a reappraisal. *Fertil Steril* 1980;33:587–597.

6 Yoon TK, Sung HR, Kang HG, Lee CN, Cha KY. Laparoscopic tubal anastomosis: fertility outcome in 202 cases. *Fertil Steril* 1999;72:1121–1126.

7 Rodgers AK, Goldberg JM, Hammel JP, Falcone T. Tubal anastomosis by robotic compared with outpatient minilaparotomy. *Obstet Gynecol* 2007;109:1375–1380.

8 Dharia Patel S, Steinkampf MP, Whitten SJ, Malizia BA. Robotic tubal anastomosis: surgical technique and cost effectiveness. *Fertil Steril* 2008;90:1175–1179.

9 Goldberg J, Falcone T. Laparoscopic microsurgical tubal anastomosis with and without robotic assistance. *Hum Reprod* 2003;18:145–147.

10 Dubuisson JB, Swolin K. Laparoscopic tubal anastomosis (the one stitch technique): preliminary results. *Hum Reprod* 1995;10:2044–2046.

11 Cha SH, Lee MH, Kim JH, Lee CN, Yoon TK, Cha KY. Fertility outcome after tubal anastomosis by laparoscopy and laparotomy. *J Am Assoc Gynecol Laparosc* 2001;8:348–352.

12 Wiegerinck MA, Roukema M, van Kessel PH, Mol BW. Sutureless re-anastomosis by laparoscopy versus microsurgical re-anastomosis by laparotomy for sterilization reversal: a matched cohort study. *Hum Reprod* 2005;20:2355–2358.

13 Gordts S, Campo R, Puttemans P, Gordts S. Clinical factors determining pregnancy outcome after microsurgical tubal reanastomosis. *Fertil Steril* 2009;92:1198–1202.

14 Boeckxstaens A, Devroey P, Collins J, Tournaye H. Getting pregnant after tubal sterilization: surgical reversal or IVF? *Hum Reprod* 2007;22:2660–2664.

15 Rock JA, Guzick DS, Katz E, Zacur HA, King TM. Tubal anastomosis: pregnancy success following reversal of Falope ring or monopolar cautery sterilization. *Fertil Steril* 1987;48:13–17.

16 Kim SH, Shin CJ, Kim JG, Moon SY, Lee JY, Chang YS. Microsurgical reversal of tubal sterilization: a report on 1,118 cases. *Fertil Steril* 1997;68:865–870.

17 The Practice Committee of the American Society for Reproductive Medicine. Committee opinion: role of tubal surgery in the era of assisted reproductive technology. *Fertil Steril* 2012;97:539–545.

18 Hirshfeld-Cytron J, Winter J. Laparoscopic tubal reanastomosis versus in vitro fertilization: cost-based decision analysis. *Am J Obstet Gynecol* 2013;209:56e1–6.

CHAPTER 100
Surgery for Congenital Abnormalities of the Genital Tract

Naomi S. Crouch

St Michael's Hospital, Bristol, UK

Case history 1: *A 13-year-old girl presents with worsening dysmenorrhea. Her periods have always been painful since her menarche aged 12, but have become increasingly intolerable requiring days off school each month. On examination a pelvic mass is identified.*

Case history 2: *A 16-year-old girl presents with primary amenorrhea. She has normal secondary sexual characteristics and is otherwise well. Ultrasound shows normal ovaries but no uterus or cervix. Her chromosomal pattern is 46XX. On perineal inspection you notice the vagina is short and blind-ending.*

Background

Congenital abnormalities of the genital tract, often known as Müllerian anomalies, are considered to be any anomaly that may occur in the Müllerian duct. Incidence is hard to ascertain, as many anomalies may be asymptomatic, but may range from 0.1 to 10% of all women. The American Society for Reproductive Medicine classification of Müllerian anomalies is the most widely used for uterine anomalies (Figure 100.1) [1]. It allows comparison of

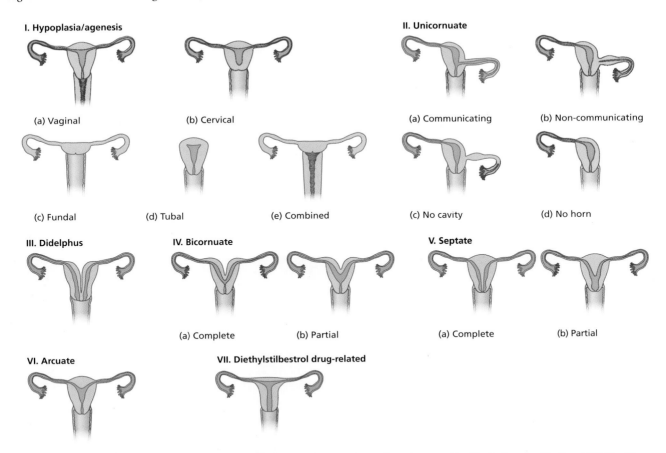

I. Hypoplasia/agenesis

(a) Vaginal (b) Cervical

(c) Fundal (d) Tubal (e) Combined

II. Unicornuate

(a) Communicating (b) Non-communicating

(c) No cavity (d) No horn

III. Didelphus

IV. Bicornuate

(a) Complete (b) Partial

V. Septate

(a) Complete (b) Partial

VI. Arcuate

VII. Diethylstilbestrol drug-related

Figure 100.1 American Fertility Society classification of Müllerian anomalies. Redrawn from American Fertility Society classification, 1988 [1] with permission from Elsevier.

Gynecologic and Obstetric Surgery: Challenges and Management Options, First Edition. Edited by Arri Coomarasamy, Mahmood I. Shafi, G. Willy Davila and Kiong K. Chan.
© 2016 John Wiley & Sons, Ltd. Published 2016 by John Wiley & Sons, Ltd.

anomalies for research purposes. However, it is not exhaustive and does not include vaginal anomalies. There is a clear need for a similar system for vaginal anomalies to aid understanding of these rare conditions [2].

Normal development

In normal fetal development, the two paired Müllerian (paramesonephric) ducts fuse to form the female reproductive tract. The cranial free ends develop into the fallopian tubes, with the remaining tract forming the uterus, cervix, and upper two-thirds of the vagina. The lower third of the vagina is derived from an invagination of the urogenital sinus which meets the Müllerian descending duct. The resulting junction forms the hymen.

Failure of the normal development of the Müllerian ducts may result in a bicornuate uterus, a complete uterus didelphys, or a persisting longitudinal uterine or vaginal septum. A horizontal vaginal septum may result from a lack of descent of the Müllerian ducts, or a failure for a lumen to develop in the hymen.

Obstructive anomalies

Those anomalies which cause an obstruction to menstrual flow are usually associated with worsening dysmenorrhea. Where there is total obstruction, for example with an imperforate hymen, the diagnosis is usually straightforward. However, where the obstruction occurs on one side, with an unobstructed contralateral system, the diagnosis can be harder to reach [3]. The presence of a pelvic mass may be the only clue, representing the obstructed uterus. The girl in Case history 1 has an obstructed uterine horn, with an unobstructed uterus draining into the normal cervix and vagina. Current practice would be for the obstructed horn to be removed laparoscopically, leaving the unaffected contralateral uterus for future fertility. Metroplasty has been advocated in the past, but infection and stenosis may occur and may risk the function of the unaffected side.

Care should be taken in the diagnosis of horizontal vaginal septa, which may range from the simple, such as an obstructed hymen, to the more complex, such as an absent middle third of the vagina. The hymen may also be variously septate or cribriform and be associated with difficulties with tampon use or penetrative intercourse.

Vaginal and uterine agenesis

Case history 2 describes a girl with Müllerian agenesis, and a failure of development of the Müllerian ducts. The chromosomal pattern of 46XX confirms this is a congenital absence of the uterus and upper two-thirds of the vagina, variously known as Mayer–Rokitansky–Kuster–Hauser (MRKH) syndrome or Rokitansky syndrome. A similar absence of the uterus and vagina is seen in girls with disorders of sex development (DSD), such as congenital androgen insensitivity syndrome (CAIS) where the chromosomal pattern would be 46XY.

Management

Diagnosis

As both cases illustrate, an accurate diagnosis is imperative in order to plan management. Care should be given by a multidisciplinary team consisting of a pediatric and adolescent gynecologist, a gynecologist with advanced minimal access skills, and a radiologist with experience in interpreting Müllerian anomalies.

Over the last decade MRI has become the gold standard for imaging Müllerian anomalies [4]. The emergence of three-dimensional ultrasound also provides an alternative option for imaging the uterus, and may be more readily available in an outpatient clinic. However, it has limitations in assessing vaginal anatomy and cannot be performed in younger girls. Diagnostic laparoscopy and hysteroscopy are not indicated, as less information is yielded in comparison with MRI, along with inherent anesthetic and surgical risks.

Renal anomalies occur in up to 30% of those with a Müllerian anomaly [5]. MRI allows the assessment of the number and site of the ureters and kidneys, thereby facilitating the surgical approach.

Management of obstructive anomalies

Once a diagnosis of an obstructive Müllerian anomaly is made, GnRH analogs may be used to downregulate the endometrium while referral to appropriate services and preoperative steps are arranged.

Laparoscopic removal of the obstructed uterus is current standard practice (Figure 100.2), but should be performed by a surgeon with advanced laparoscopic skills. There may be significant

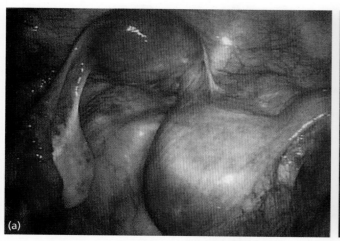
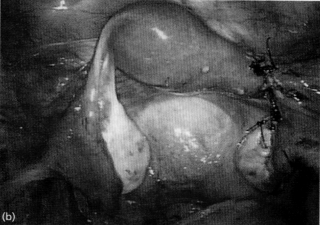

Figure 100.2 Removal of an obstructed uterine horn: (a) an accessory uterine horn on the right; (b) the accessory uterine horn on the right has been removed. Images from Michala *et al.*, 2011 [11] with permission from Cambridge University Press.

endometriosis development from months and years of obstructed menstrual flow. However, ipsilateral renal agenesis is often present, at least avoiding the possibility of ureteric injury on the affected side.

Long-term fertility data are sparse but show an increase in preterm deliveries and breech presentations [6]. Further data on fertility outcomes are needed.

Management of uterine and vaginal septa

Uterine septa are asymptomatic, but are associated with fertility difficulties or recurrent miscarriage. For this reason they are often identified within the context of fertility investigations. Current advice is for the septum to be removed hysteroscopically, and is associated with an improvement in fertility [7].

Vaginal septa are often more apparent clinically, and are usually amenable to a perineal approach at surgery. An imperforate or cribriform hymen may have a simple incision performed with trimming of excess tissue. A vertical vaginal septum may be removed to allow tampon use and comfortable intercourse. The use of vaginal dilators postoperatively may be indicated if the individual is not currently sexually active, in order to prevent adhesion formation. An obstructed hemivagina tends to present with a mass in the vagina. Because of the nature of the tissue, the vagina is able to expand significantly to accommodate menstrual flow. As with a longitudinal vaginal septum, this may be removed vaginally.

Surgery for an absent middle third of the vagina traditionally involved a combined abdominal perineal approach. This surgery is now possible laparoscopically but requires considerable expertise. If the upper vagina does not stretch to meet the perineal portion, a section of bowel may be isolated and used as a cuff of vagina. Again, vaginal dilators should be used postoperatively to reduce the incidence of vaginal stricture formation.

Management of vaginal agenesis

For those with vaginal agenesis, a psychologist forms an essential part of the team, along with a clinical nurse specialist.

Current management involves the use of vaginal dilators. These are a graded series of dilators which are placed against the vaginal dimple for 30 min every day. Evidence shows this is effective in creating a lengthened vagina suitable for penetrative intercourse in up to 85% of women [8]. The average length of time for vaginal development is 3–6 months with daily use. If the individual is not sexually active, once the vagina is developed the dilators should be used twice a week to maintain vaginal length. Vaginal agenesis is understandably a devastating diagnosis for a girl and her family and is associated with a significant reduction in emotional and sexual well-being [9]. Psychological input is essential in the management of understanding the diagnosis and engaging in dilator therapy.

For those where dilator therapy is not successful, the laparoscopic Vecchietti technique offers an alternative (Figure 100.3) [10]. This involves a small threaded acrylic bead or mold being placed in the introitus, and the threads being passed through the top of the vagina into the abdominal cavity, and out onto the abdominal wall. These are attached to a small winching mechanism that rests on the abdomen, and the vagina is lifted up by 1 cm each day. A vagina may be developed over 1 week, after which the threads are cut and the bead removed. Again, if there is coital infrequency, the dilators will need to be used to maintain vaginal length.

Previously, sections of bowel or skin grafts were utilized to create a neovagina. Although there may be rare indications for these techniques, such as in the presence of other complex anomalies or where there is extensive scarring, poor long-term outcomes restrict this approach. Excessive mucus production and contractures are common, with carcinoma formation in the neovagina also reported.

Current fertility options for those with Rokitansky syndrome consist of surrogacy, following an IVF cycle, or adoption. The ovaries develop normally in Rokitansky syndrome and are therefore amenable to egg harvesting. Currently, within UK law the woman is required to adopt the baby formally after delivery.

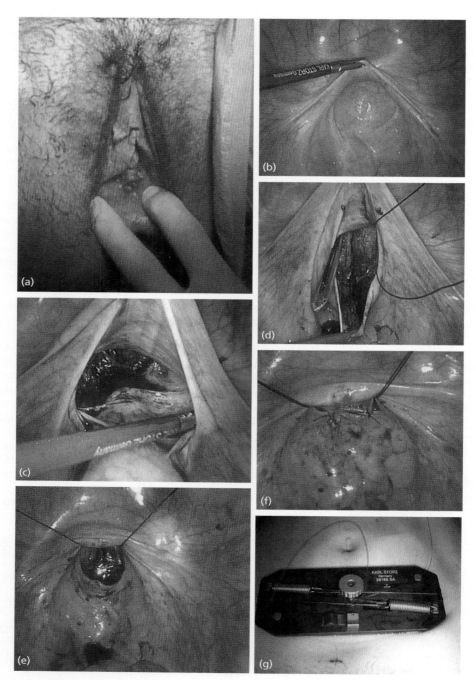

Figure 100.3 Laparoscopic Vecchietti procedure: (a) perineum before surgery; (b) laparoscopic view of pelvis; (c) vesicorectal space opened; (d) first suture passed; (e) both sutures passed; (f) peritoneal defect closed; (g) traction device placed on the abdomen. Images from Michala *et al.*, 2011 [11] with permission from Cambridge University Press.

References

1 The American Fertility Society classifications of adnexal adhesions, distal tubal occlusion, tubal occlusion secondary to tubal ligation, tubal pregnancies, müllerian anomalies and intrauterine adhesions. *Fertil Steril* 1988;49:944–955.

2 Creighton SM, Hall-Craggs MA. Correlation or confusion: the need for accurate terminology when comparing magnetic resonance imaging and clinical assessment of congenital vaginal anomalies. *J Pediatr Urol* 2012;8:177–180.

3 Strawbridge LC, Crouch NS, Cutner AS, Creighton SM. Obstructive mullerian anomalies and modern laparoscopic management. *J Pediatr Adolesc Gynecol* 2007;20:195–200.

4 Santos XM, Krishnamurthy R, Bercaw-Pratt JL, Dietrich JE. The utility of ultrasound and magnetic resonance imaging versus surgery for the characterization of müllerian anomalies in the pediatric and adolescent population. *J Pediatr Adolesc Gynecol* 2012;25:181–184.

5 Hall-Craggs MA, Kirkham A, Creighton SM. Renal and urological abnormalities occurring with Mullerian anomalies. *J Pediatr Urol* 2013;9:27–32.

6 Heinonen PK. Pregnancies in women with uterine malformation, treated obstruction of hemivagina and ipsilateral renal agenesis. *Arch Gynecol Obstet* 2012;287:975–978.

7 Shokeir T, Abdelshaheed M, El-Shafie M, Sherif L, Badawy A. Determinants of fertility and reproductive success after hysteroscopic septoplasty for women with unexplained primary infertility: a prospective analysis of 88 cases. *Eur J Obstet Gynecol Reprod Biol* 2011;155:54–57.

8 Gargollo PC, Cannon GM Jr, Diamond DA, Thomas P, Burke V, Laufer MR. Should progressive perineal dilation be considered first line therapy for vaginal agenesis? *J Urol* 2009;182(4 Suppl):1882–1889.

9 Liao LM, Conway GS, Ismail-Pratt I, Bikoo M, Creighton SM. Emotional and sexual wellness and quality of life in women with Rokitansky syndrome. *Am J Obstet Gynecol* 2011;205:117e1–6.

10 Fedele L, Bianchi S, Frontino G, Fontana E, Restelli E, Bruni V. The laparoscopic Vecchietti's modified technique in Rokitansky syndrome: anatomic, functional, and sexual long-term results. *Am J Obstet Gynecol* 2008;198:377e1–6.

11 Michala L, Creighton SM, Cutner AS. Minimal access surgery in paediatric and adolescent gynaecology. In: CutnerA, VyasS (eds) *Laparoscopic Surgery for Benign Gynaecology*, chapter 14. RCOG Press, London, 2011.

CHAPTER 101

Surgical Sperm Retrieval

David Muthuveloe and Y. Zaki Almallah

University Hospitals Birmingham NHS Foundation Trust, Birmingham, UK

Case history: During fertility investigations, a man is found to have azoospermia on two tests. On examination he is well virilized, with testes smaller than expected in size.

Background

Absence of sperm from the ejaculate (azoospermia) is present in 5% of all couples investigated for infertility [1]. Azoospermia was considered to be untreatable until the advent of surgical sperm retrieval and intracytoplasmic sperm injection (ICSI) treatment. Sperm can be retrieved from many men with azoospermia, either from the epididymis (percutaneous epididymal sperm aspiration, PESA) or from the testicles (testicular sperm aspiration, TESA, or microdissection testicular sperm extraction, micro-TESE). Micro-TESE is now recognized to be an effective treatment for men with azoospermia, with sperm retrieval rates reported at 50–60% [2].

Etiology

The cause of azoospermia can be pre-testicular, testicular, or post-testicular [1]. Pre-testicular causes include all cases of hypogonadotropic hypogonadism (e.g., Kallmann syndrome), and often respond well to hormone therapy. Testicular causes can be congenital (Klinefelter's syndrome or Y-deletion), acquired (chemotherapy, radiotherapy, torsion, or mumps), or developmental (testicular maldescent); surgical sperm retrieval results in sperm in 60% of cases [1]. Post-testicular causes include ductal obstruction (vasectomy, infection or absence of vas) or dysfunction (retrograde ejaculation). Surgical correction of the duct or surgical sperm retrieval will result in sperm in almost all men with ductal obstruction. For retrograde ejaculation, first-line treatment is medical with sympathomimetics to induce antegrade ejaculation, and if that fails, sperm can often be obtained from post-ejaculatory urine [1].

Management

For patients with post-testicular azoospermia secondary to vasal and epididymal obstruction, the best treatment would be microsurgical reconstruction. The success rate of these procedures varies. Microsurgical vasovasostomy has a success rate of 70–99% whereas microsurgical vasoepididymostomy success is reported

as 40–90% [3]. This is the most cost-efficient management and permits natural conception. In addition, if natural conception does not occur, ICSI can still be performed from ejaculated sperm, without the need for surgical sperm retrieval.

If surgical sperm retrieval is required in men with testicular or post-testicular azoospermia, it is usually advanced from the least invasive to the most invasive in a stepwise fashion. The first procedure is usually PESA, which involves attempts at aspiration of sperm from the epididymis with a small-diameter butterfly needle, either under local or general anesthesia. If this procedure is not successful, the next step is often TESA, which involves attempts at aspiration of sperm from the testicle with a large-diameter butterfly needle, often from multiple locations and from both testicles, again under local or general anesthesia. If aspiration does not succeed, then the next step is open biopsy comprising conventional TESE or micro-TESE. Biopsy is often performed under general anesthesia.

Microdissection testicular sperm extraction

If an open testicular biopsy is needed, the surgical retrieval method of choice is micro-TESE. Microsurgical methods are used to recognize tubules with undamaged spermatogenesis (Figure 101.1). Once the sperm are harvested it can be used in conjunction with ICSI to treat male infertility [4].

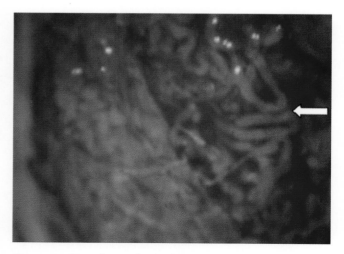

Figure 101.1 Normal seminiferous tubules (white arrow) among damaged and hyalinated tubules

---

Gynecologic and Obstetric Surgery: Challenges and Management Options, First Edition. Edited by Arri Coomarasamy, Mahmood I. Shafi, G. Willy Davila and Kiong K. Chan.

Micro-TESE is advantageous and often superior to other techniques because more areas of the testis can be examined and one can find the areas most likely to contain sperm. Being highly selective, it reduces the need to take testicular biopsies from multiple locations on the testes, so there is less damage to the testicles.

During the management of men with primary testicular failure and azoospermia, it is important to keep in mind the long-term well-being of these men. They have low testosterone production reserve and the surgeon should be very careful when handling testicular tissue by keeping sampling to a minimum to avoid expediting early male menopause. This is a particular advantage of micro-TESE over standard testicular biopsy.

Surgical technique

The procedure is usually performed under general anesthesia but in some centers it is being performed under local anesthesia with sedation [5]. The first step is opening the tunica albuginea. An extended incision is made to reveal the testicular parenchyma. A surgical microscope is used to examine the seminiferous tubules directly *in vivo*. The surgeon can then see which areas have fibrous seminiferous tubules and are expected to be without sperm, and which areas have healthy tubules and are expected to contain sperm (Figure 101.1). Healthy regions are biopsied and examined for sperm by isolating and dissecting the seminiferous tubules using micro-instruments under a high-power surgical microscope. Samples are then transferred to an andrology laboratory in one of the fertility centers for further examination and sperm isolation. The tunica albuginea is repaired with a running Prolene suture. The scrotal skin is closed with interrupted fine dissolvable stitches.

KEY POINTS

Challenge: Surgical sperm retrieval.

Background
- Azoospermia is present in 5% of all couples investigated for infertility.
- Etiology of azoospermia:
  - Pre-testicular: hypogonadotropic hypogonadism (e.g., Kallmann syndrome).
  - Testicular: congenital (Klinefelter's syndrome or Y-deletion); acquired (chemotherapy, radiotherapy, torsion, or mumps); and developmental (testicular maldescent).
  - Post-testicular: ductal obstruction (vasectomy, infection or absence of vas) and ductal dysfunction (retrograde ejaculation).

Management
- If some sperm is isolated from whatever method, treatment can be provided with ICSI.
- Pre-testicular azoospermia: hormone treatment with FSH and HCG (LH equivalent).
- Testicular azoospermia: surgical sperm retrieval; sperm found in approximately 60% of cases.

Post-testicular azoospermia
- Ductal obstruction: vasovasostomy or vasoepididymostomy; if not successful, surgical sperm retrieval.
- Retrograde ejaculation: sympathomimetics, and if that fails, sperm can often be obtained from post-ejaculatory urine.

Surgical sperm retrieval
- PESA: sperm aspiration from the epididymis with a small-diameter butterfly needle.
- TESA: sperm aspiration from the testicles with a large-diameter butterfly needle.
- TESE: conventional open biopsy of the testicles or micro-TESE.

Micro-TESE
- The procedure is usually performed under general anesthesia.
- Open tunica albuginea.
- Extend the incision to reveal testicular parenchyma.
- Use a surgical microscope to recognize and biopsy healthy seminiferous tubules.
- Transfer biopsied samples to an andrology laboratory for examination and storage.
- Close tunica albuginea with a running Prolene suture.
- Close scrotal skin with interrupted dissolvable stitches.

References

1 Sharif K. The azoospermic patient. In: Sharif K, Coomarasamy A (eds) *Assisted Reproduction Techniques: Challenges and Management Options*, pp. 340–343. Wiley-Blackwell, Chichester, 2012.

2 Bryson CF, Ramasamy R, Sheehan M, Palermo GD, Rosenwaks Z, Schlegel PN. Severe testicular atrophy does not affect the success of microdissection testicular sperm extraction. *J Urol* 2014;191:175–178.

3 Goldstein M, Tanrikut C. Microsurgical management of male infertility. *Nat Clin Pract Urol* 2006;3:381–391.

4 Dabaja AA, Schlegel PN. Microdissection testicular sperm extraction: an update. *Asian J Androl* 2013;15:35–39.

5 Shah R. Surgical sperm retrieval: techniques and their indications. *Indian J Urol* 2011;27:102–109.

Section 6
Urogynecologic Surgery
Editors: Pallavi Latthe and G. Willy Davila

CHAPTER 102
Sling Procedures: Bladder Injury

Fidan Israfil-Bayli and Philip Toozs-Hobson
Birmingham Women's NHS Foundation Trust, Birmingham, UK

Case history: During tension-free vaginal tape (TVT) operation for stress urinary incontinence (SUI), after the insertion of trocars, a cystoscopy confirms bladder perforation on both sides.

Background

Bladder perforation (Figure 102.1a) is a common intraoperative complication of retropubic mid-urethral sling placement, occurring in 2.7–10% of cases [1,2]. In some studies, operative perforation rates of up to 24% have been reported [2]. Bladder perforation during retropubic sling placement occurs more commonly in patients with past anti-incontinence procedures, likely due to scarring within the retropubic space [3]. Compared with the retropubic approach, bladder perforations are less common with the transobturator approach, with reported rates of bladder perforation between 0 and 1.5% with this technique [4]. Cadaveric dissections have shown that a correctly placed TVT trocar is just lateral to the bladder and urethra, and an average of 3.2 cm medial to the obturator neurovascular bundle, 3.9 cm medial to the superficial and inferior epigastric vessels, and 4.9 cm medial to the external iliac vessels [5].

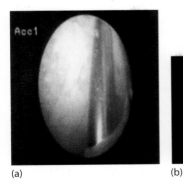
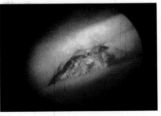

(a) (b)

Figure 102.1 (a) Bladder perforation during TVT procedure and (b) mesh erosion into the bladder several months after TVT procedure.

Bladder injury itself should not be serious if noted and managed during surgery [6]. Unrecognized bladder injury may result in persistent urinary infection postoperatively, *de novo* detrusor overactivity, or formation of bladder calculi.

Mesh extrusion, erosion, or exposure is the appearance of the mesh in a different tissue plane to where it was originally placed. This complication is typically detected in the postoperative period when the sling material is found in the urinary tract (Figure 102.1b) or exposed in the vagina. While extrusions are often considered a postoperative complication, it is important to recognize that many of these are actually the result of undetected perforations that occurred at the time of surgery.

Management

Bladder perforation
Video cystourethroscopy with 70° lens should identify the points at which the needles pass adjacent to the bladder; the needles should be rotated and moved to check, firstly, bladder integrity and, secondly, bladder tethering when the needle is pulled upward.

There are two main techniques for correcting a bladder perforation. The "classic" technique involves removing the trocar on the side of the perforation, emptying the bladder, and reinserting the Foley catheter with the bladder guide. Then after deflecting the bladder and urethra to the same side as the sling placement, the trocar can be repositioned. Finally, the cystoscopy is repeated to confirm that the tape is placed correctly. The "alternative" technique involves removing and repositioning the tape under direct vision using cystoscopy.

With both approaches, it is important to leave an indwelling Foley catheter on free drainage for the subsequent 24–48 hours.

Late sling erosion (see Chapter 107)
The patient may present with urinary urgency and frequency. Initial management will include assessment for urinary tract infections, including details of microbiology. In these circumstances cystourethroscopy is mandatory. If mesh is identified and the patient is symptomatic, the exposed mesh will require excision either via cystotomy or with an operative cystoscope. Suprapubic telescopy with a 5-mm laparoscopic trocar can aid the placement of either a grasping instrument or laparoscopic scissors, with the other needed instrument being placed through a cystoscopic operating channel. The exposed mesh can be excised, with the goal of removing all exposed mesh fibers. This technique obviates the need to perform open suprapubic exploration.

Gynecologic and Obstetric Surgery: Challenges and Management Options, First Edition. Edited by Arri Coomarasamy, Mahmood I. Shafi, G. Willy Davila and Kiong K. Chan.
© 2016 John Wiley & Sons, Ltd. Published 2016 by John Wiley & Sons, Ltd.

Delayed presentation may result in stone formation which requires crushing prior to removal. Urethroscopy is also important for excluding unrecognized urethral injury or later tape extrusion into the urethra.

Prevention

In order to avoid or minimize the risk of bladder injury one should consider the following.

1 Proper preoperative assessment of the patient and identification of risk factors that could potentially complicate the surgery. Examples include previous pelvic surgery, problems with hip joints, and obesity.
2 Proper infiltration of the tissues prior to lateral dissection below the inferior pubic ramus toward endopelvic fascia. Bladder catheterization and use of a guidewire to mobilize the bladder neck and urethra are recommended.

3 Attention should be paid to the hand position on the trocar and appropriate orientation of the trocar. Videocystoscopy is mandatory after passing the needle because it is important to recognize bladder perforation before pulling the needle through the tissues. A 70° lens or flexible scope is recommended. During cystoscopy, it is important to ensure that the needle moves independent of the bladder wall, as intramural placement of the tape can increase the risk of erosion. Additional cystoscopy at the end of the procedure may be helpful for detecting the occult bladder injury which might have happened after the initial cystoscopy.
4 Appropriate training should be provided. The likelihood of bladder perforation decreases with the surgeon's experience. An annual workload of at least 20 cases of each primary procedure for SUI is recommended [7].

All surgeons providing these procedures should maintain ongoing audit data. In the UK, this can be done through use of the British Society of Urogynaecology (BSUG) database (www.bsug.org.uk).

KEY POINTS

Challenge: Bladder injury in sling procedures.

Background
- Sling procedures are usually safe.
- Intraoperative bladder or urethral perforation can happen in 3–24% of cases.
- Bladder injury itself should not be serious if noted and managed during surgery; unrecognized bladder injury may result in persistent urinary infection postoperatively, *de novo* detrusor overactivity, or formation of bladder calculi.

Prevention
- Appropriate patient and sling selection.
- Proper tissue infiltration and dissection.
- Empty the bladder completely. Guidewire should be placed down the Foley catheter to deviate the urethra and bladder neck to ipsilateral side as trocar placement occurs.
- Trocar should be passed close to the posterior surface of the symphysis.
- Cystoscopy (300 mL optimum fill) with 70° lens is mandatory to confirm bladder integrity in retropubic sling surgery; cystoscopy should also ideally be done after transobturator sling placement.

Management
- The "classic" method involves emptying the bladder, repositioning the tape, and repeating cystoscopy to confirm that the tape has been placed correctly.
- The "alternative" technique involves repositioning the tape under direct vision during cystoscopy.
- Free catheter drainage for 24–48 hours postoperatively with or without prophylactic antibiotic cover.

References

1 Kuuva N, Nilsson C. A nationwide analysis of complications associated with the tension-free vaginal tape (TVT) procedure. *Acta Obstet Gynecol Scand* 2002;81:72–77.
2 Andonian S, Chen T, St-Denis B, Corcos J. Randomized clinical trial comparing suprapubic arch sling (SPARC) and tension-free vaginal tape (TVT): one-year results. *Eur Urol* 2005;47:537–541.
3 Tamussino KF, Hanzal E, Kolle D, Ralp G, Riss PA. Tension-free vaginal tape operation: results of the Austrian registry. *Obstet Gynecol* 2001;98:732–736.
4 Latthe PM, Foon R, Toozs-Hobson P. Transobturator and retropubic procedures in stress urinary incontinence: a systematic review and metaanalysis of effectiveness and complications. *BJOG* 2007;114:522–531.
5 Muir TW, Tulikangas PK, Paraiso MF, Walters MD. The relationship of tension-free vaginal tape insertion and the vascular anatomy. *Obstet Gynecol* 2003;101:933–936.
6 Gold RS, Groutz A, Pauzner D, Lessing J, Gordon D. Bladder perforation during tension-free vaginal tape surgery: does it matter? *J Reprod Med* 2007;52:616–618.
7 National Institute for Health and Care Excellence. *Urinary incontinence: the management of urinary incontinence in women*. NICE Clinical Guideline No. 171, September 2013. Available at https://www.nice.org.uk/guidance/cg171

CHAPTER 103
Sling Procedures: Urethral Injury

Gamal M. Ghoniem

Long Beach Memorial Medical Center, Long Beach, California, USA

Case history: A patient with a past history of a hysterectomy (3 years ago), an unsuccessful mini-sling procedure (1.5 years ago), and a retropubic mid-urethral sling (1 year ago) developed left lower abdominal pain, which with time became more centralized to the pelvis. The pain was worse with physical activity, a full bladder, and sexual intercourse, and less on lying down. She also developed recurrent urinary tract infections. On examination there was an area of hard localized tenderness along the mid-urethra.

Background

Urethral mesh erosion is a rare complication that is almost exclusively related to using synthetic mid-urethral slings (Figures 103.1 and 103.2). The rate of reoperation because of urethral erosion has been reported to be 0.08% [1]; however, providing reliable rates for the incidence of urethral injury with various sling procedures is not possible, as valid denominators are rarely available [2].

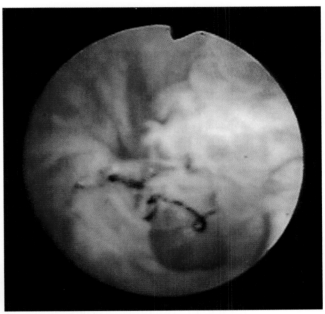

Figure 103.2 Urethroscopy showing the mesh crossing the urethral lumen.

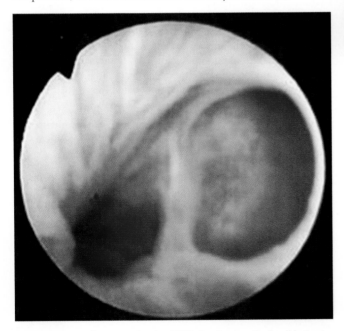

Figure 103.1 Urethroscopy showing TVT sling into urethral wall but not into the lumen, with formation of small diverticulum distal to it.

A standardized terminology and classification was developed by both the International Urogynecology Association (IUGA) and the International Continence Society (ICS) for those complications arising directly from the insertion of synthetic (prostheses) and biological (grafts) materials in female pelvic floor surgery. The category (C), time (T), and site (S) classes and divisions have a sensitivity to encompass all conceivable scenarios for insertion complications and healing abnormalities. The CTS code for each complication, involving mostly three letters and three numerals, is suitable for any surgical audit, particularly one that is procedure-specific [3]. A CTS code calculator is available at www.ics.org/complication.

Presentation

Patients usually present with voiding dysfunction, urinary urgency or incontinence, dysuria, recurrent urinary tract infections, and abdominopelvic pain.

Gynecologic and Obstetric Surgery: Challenges and Management Options, First Edition. Edited by Arri Coomarasamy, Mahmood I. Shafi, G. Willy Davila and Kiong K. Chan.
© 2016 John Wiley & Sons, Ltd. Published 2016 by John Wiley & Sons, Ltd.

Risk factors

Risk factors may include old age, diabetes, smoking, urethral atrophy, history of radiation [2,4], previous sling surgery, and abnormal anatomy (e.g., large cystocele). Poor surgical technique including improper placement, passing the trocars too close to the urethra, excessive sling tension, and deep vaginal dissection can increase the risk of urethral erosion. Traumatic catheterization and urethral dilation are also risk factors.

Management

Intraoperatively diagnosed urethral injury

If urethral injury is noticed at cystourethroscopy after insertion of the trocars, remove the trocar and reinsert in the correct position, preferably away from the site of urethral injury.

If the injury is noticed to be large, then abort the procedure and leave an indwelling catheter for 14 days, after repairing the injury with multilayer closure using 3-0 Vicryl. However, small injuries may heal on their own with urethral rest.

Postoperatively diagnosed urethral injury

Postoperative urethral erosion can be diagnosed by cystourethroscopy. Excision and removal of eroded sling is the key aim of management. Different surgical techniques for achieving this aim have been reported in the literature, including transvaginal, transurethral, and retropubic (laparoscopic or open) approaches.

Transurethral approach

Transurethral resection of the eroded tape can be performed under tactile traction with placement of Halsted clamps on the eroded mesh within the urethra and ultralateral resection with Metzenbaum scissors [5]. However, this resection is done largely blindly and may lead to urethral injury. In order to improve visualization, a nasal speculum has been proven useful to direct grasping and excision of the eroded mesh segment [6]. Alternatively, intra-urethral excision using hysteroscopic scissors can be performed with the use of extraperitoneal laparoscopic ports for lateral retraction of the mesh [7].

Transvaginal approach

Transvaginal urethrotomy results in a urethral defect that requires multilayered closure [8]. It may be necessary to use a Martius graft or fascia lata patch to prevent fistula formation [9].

Laparoscopic approach

Extraperitoneal laparoscopy with intentional cystotomy has been described [10], and can be an option for those surgeons with the necessary skills.

Combined approach

Our technique combines both a visually guided transurethral and an open transvaginal approach. Use of the optical urethrotome allows transection within the view of the operative scope under direct vision and control without excessive manipulation of the urethra (Figure 103.3). The vaginal dissection allows retraction of the mesh away from the urethra without the need for an intentional urethrotomy or urethral repair. If the sling material is embedded in the detrusor or bladder neck muscles, unintentional cystotomy may be unavoidable. Partial excision of the exposed mesh is usually sufficient and complete excision of the mesh is only needed in cases of infection. Our surgical approach adds to the available management strategies for urethral mesh erosion, and benefits include (i) limited urethral manipulation, (ii) incision of the mesh done under direct endoscopic vision and control at all times, (iii) no urethral incision, and (iv) the ability to resect the mesh laterally without the need for an abdominal approach.

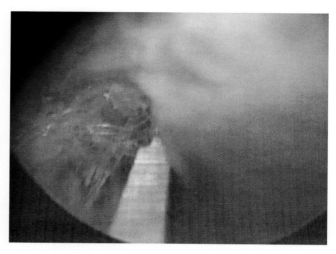

Figure 103.3 Cutting sling close to urethral wall by urethrotome.

Resolution of the case

On examination, the patient had localized tenderness to the urethra. Cystourethroscopy revealed urethral erosion and formation of bladder stone over anterior bladder wall sling erosion (Figure 103.4). We followed a similar technique to that described above, combined with holmium laser lithotripsy and cutting of bladder sling very close to the mucosa. In addition de-epithelialized vaginal wall pedicled flap [8] was used to reinforce the repair by adding robust layer for the repair. Alternatively, a Martius graft could be used [10].

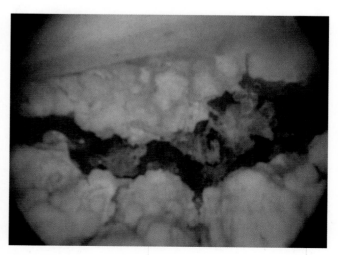

Figure 103.4 Bladder stone over sling erosion anteriorly close to bladder neck (treated with holmium laser lithotripsy and cutting of bladder sling very close to mucosa).

Prevention

It is important to empty the bladder prior to trocar insertion. During sling surgery, a catheter needs to be left in the urethra during passage of trocars to guide them safely away from the urethra. Rotating the urethra away from the passageway is another technique to avoid injury. Careful cystourethroscopy under mild bladder distension is recommended for all mid-urethral tape procedures [2].

Excessive tension is the main force causing bladder outlet obstruction, partial erosion into the urethral wall (Figure 103.1), or complete urethral erosion (Figure 103.2). It is important to leave the sling tension-free.

It is advisable not to use urethral dilatation to manage postoperative urinary retention after mid-urethral slings. Urethral dilatation causes force directed toward the ventral urethra that is compressed by the excessive mesh tension, resulting in erosion. Urethral dilatation has some success for urinary retention after traditional fascial pubovaginal slings, which possess different biological and vesicoelastic properties.

KEY POINTS

Challenge: Urethral injury.

Background
- Urethral erosion is a rare complication but may be encountered given the widespread use of synthetic mid-urethral slings for SUI.
- Where urethral perforation occurs, fistula, diverticulum formation and symptomatic outflow obstruction are serious consequences, and persistent or recurrent SUI is common.
- Symptoms include retention, new-onset urgency or incontinence, recurrent urinary tract infections, dysuria, and pelvic pain.

Prevention
- Insert a catheter during dissection for tactile guidance.
- Empty the bladder before passing trocars/needles.
- Lift the anterior vaginal wall if there is significant prolapse.
- Avoid excessive sling tension.
- Perform cystourethroscopy with 200–300 mL in the bladder as part of any sling procedure.
- If large urethral injury is recognized, abandon the sling insertion, close the defect as appropriate, and leave a urethral catheter *in situ* for 1–2 weeks.
- Do not perform urethral dilatation postoperatively for the management of postoperative retention or voiding difficulty.

Management
- Perform a careful cystoscopy and urethroscopy.
- Perform surgical excision of the exposed urethral mesh using a minimally traumatic procedure, if possible, as described by the various techniques in this chapter. One technique combines both a visually guided transurethral and an open transvaginal approach:
  - Use of the optical urethrotome allows transection within the view of the operative scope under direct vision and control without excessive manipulation of the urethra.
  - Vaginal dissection allows retraction of the mesh away from the urethra without the need for an intentional urethrotomy or urethral repair.

References

1 Nguyen JN, Jakus-Waldman SM, Walter AJ, White T, Menefee SA. Perioperative complications and reoperations after incontinence and prolapse surgeries using prosthetic implants. *Obstet Gynecol* 2012;119:539–546.
2 Morton H, Hilton P. Urethral injury associated with minimally invasive mid-urethral sling procedures for the treatment of stress urinary incontinence: a case series and systematic literature search. *BJOG* 2009;116:1120–1126.
3 Haylen BT, Freeman RM, Swift SE *et al.* An International Urogynecological Association (IUGA)/International Continence Society (ICS) joint terminology and classification of the complications related directly to the insertion of prostheses (meshes, implants, tapes) and grafts in female pelvic floor surgery. *Int Urogynecol J* 2011;22:3–15.
4 Amundsen CL, Flynn BJ, Webster GD. Urethral erosion after synthetic and non-synthetic pubovaginal slings: differences in management and continence outcome. *J Urol* 2003;170:134–137; discussion 137.
5 Quiroz L, Cundiff G. Transurethral resection of tension-free vaginal tape under tactile traction. *Int Urogynecol J* 2009;20:873–875.
6 Plowright L, Davila GW. Endoscopic transurethral resection of urethral mesh erosion with the use of a pediatric nasal speculum. *Obstet Gynecol* 2013;121:440–443.
7 McLennan MT. Transurethral resection of transvaginal tape. *Int Urogynecol J Pelvic Floor Dysfunct* 2004;15:360–362.
8 Koelbl H, Stoerer S, Seliger G, Wolters M. Transurethral penetration of a tension-free vaginal tape. *BJOG* 2001;108:763–765.
9 Al-Wadi K, Al-Badr A. Martius graft for the management of tension-free vaginal tape vaginal erosion. *Obstet Gynecol* 2009;114:489–491.
10 Rehman J, Chugtai B, Sukkarich T, Khan A. Extraperitoneal laparoscopic removal of eroded midurethral sling: a new technique. *J Endourol* 2008;22:365–368.

CHAPTER 104
Sling Procedures: Retropubic Hematoma

Fidan Israfil-Bayli and Philip Toozs-Hobson
Birmingham Women's NHS Foundation Trust, Birmingham, UK

Case history: A woman who had a TVT procedure had some suprapubic discomfort in the immediate postoperative period. Over the following 2 hours her pain increased and developed into severe low abdominal pain. Her blood pressure dropped and she developed tachycardia. Abdominal examination revealed suprapubic tenderness, bruising, and swelling.

Background

Mid-urethral slings are the gold standard treatment of SUI. Insertion of mid-urethral slings may be associated with a small amount of intraoperative bleeding, which usually settles with application of pressure or insertion of a vaginal pack. The incidence of hemorrhagic complications is 2.5–3.5% [1] and a meta-analysis estimated the rate of pelvic hematoma to be 1.7% [2].

Bleeding leading to the formation of a suprapubic hematoma is usually triggered by trocar passage leading to paravesical venous plexus damage [3–5]; other damaged vessels can include the recurrent obturator artery (found in 10% of the population), and the external iliac, inferior epigastric, and femoral vessels [6]. Sometimes hematomas may spread to the paravesico-urethral space between the levator ani and the bladder neck [7]. The evidence generated from a study of cadavers shows that the major vascular structures in the retropubic space and anterior abdominal wall are lateral to the usual placement of the TVT needle [8].

Patients with hematoma present with pain, as in the Case history, or bladder symptoms such as urgency and frequency due to pressure from hematoma. Depending on the extent of blood loss, symptoms may vary. Where the blood loss is large, the woman may have signs of hypovolemic shock including tachycardia and hypotension (Chapter 52).

Management

Diagnostic evaluation

A full blood count and cross-match of blood will need to be arranged. An ultrasound, MRI or CT scan of the pelvis can identify the exact location and extent of the hematoma. Apart from identifying the size of hematoma, ultrasound can also be used for assessing post-void residual urine volume and any obstruction of ureters [7].

Treatment

Hematoma may or may not require surgical intervention depending on the patient's symptoms, the volume of the hematoma, and degree of hemodynamic compromise.

Conservative treatment

Most hematomas are less than 250 mL in volume, and may not require active intervention as they resolve within several months [9]. In these cases, observe the vital signs, provide adequate pain relief, and reassure the patient that the symptoms should gradually subside.

It is important to ensure that the woman is not in urinary retention; if there is evidence of urinary retention, she will need continuous or intermittent bladder drainage. In such cases there is the option of hematoma drainage under ultrasound guidance when the hematoma liquefies.

If the patient is at high risk of infection, a course of oral antibiotics is advisable.

Surgical management

If the hematoma is causing significant hemodynamic changes, as in the Case history, acute surgical intervention is required. The options for managing the hematoma include the following.

- A drain can be inserted into the retropubic space under ultrasound guidance to drain the hematoma.
- If the patient's condition is deteriorating, an immediate exploratory laparotomy with ligation of the bleeding vessel in the retropubic space is recommended. An overt bleeding site may not be identifiable on entering the space of Retzius, despite methodical examination of the trocar passage tracts. Thus, use of coagulation-promoting substances and packing the space of Retzius and vagina should be a consideration.
- Retziusscopy can be used to confirm the presence of the hematoma and arrange its evacuation [10]. The alternative is an extraperitoneal approach via laparoscopy to access the cave of Retzius.
- Embolization of the bleeding vessel by interventional radiology has been reported [11,12], and has become the preferred approach in the USA.

Gynecologic and Obstetric Surgery: Challenges and Management Options, First Edition. Edited by Arri Coomarasamy, Mahmood I. Shafi, G. Willy Davila and Kiong K. Chan.
© 2016 John Wiley & Sons, Ltd. Published 2016 by John Wiley & Sons, Ltd.

Reduction in intraoperative blood loss

After access to the uterus is gained, vasopressin is injected into the myometrium surrounding the fibroids, inducing vasoconstriction and thus reducing blood loss [13]. Care must be exercised to avoid intravascular injection of vasopressin, and adequate warning should be given to the anesthetist prior to injection. Some operators prefer to also use mechanical means to reduce blood flow to the uterus. This can be achieved by using instruments such as Bonney's myomectomy clamp or a rubber catheter to act as a tourniquet around the paracervical region, to reduce bleeding from the uterine arteries [12] (Chapter 95). The use of intraoperative cell salvage should also be considered to reduce the requirements for heterologous blood products [14].

Uterine incision

The site and size of uterine incisions must be carefully considered. The incision should be made to allow for maximum access to as many fibroids as possible for enucleation; however, the incision should also be sited away from the fallopian tubes to reduce the risk of tubal damage. The orientation of uterine incisions can also reduce blood loss; it has been suggested that horizontal incisions lead to reduced blood loss (by avoiding the uterine arcuate vessels) when compared with vertical incisions [15,16]. In reality, the choice of uterine incision will depend on the surgeon's experience, and the size and site of the fibroids. Multiple incisions directly over each fibroid can lead to greater adhesion formation; on the other hand, attempting to reach multiple fibroids through a single uterine incision can cause greater bleeding due to the trauma of digital tunneling through the myometrium. A balance on the number of incisions is therefore necessary.

Dissection of the fibroid

Following uterine serosal incision, the cleavage plane at the fibroid's false capsule must be reached in order to enucleate each fibroid. This level is often deeper than many operators expect and can be found by securing the fibroid with the myoma screw or tenaculum and advancing the incision deeper until the fibroid comes into view. Blunt and sharp dissection are then used to dissect the fibroid from its capsule.

Uterine closure

It is essential that all dead space from each enucleated fibroid is closed to reduce the risk of bleeding and hematoma formation. This often needs to be done in layers from inside out, beginning with the fibroid capsule and then the myometrium, and can be done with figure-of-eight or mattress sutures. Layered myometrial closure may be required in order to achieve obliteration of the dead space. The serosa can then be repaired with either interrupted or continuous sutures. It is advisable to suture each uterine incision after dissection of each fibroid to reduce ongoing blood loss. An alternative is to close the intramyometrial dead space region by region (e.g., closing all anterior incisions before commencing posterior incisions).

Postoperative considerations

Postoperative care should ensure adequate analgesia and hydration. Early mobilization should be the aim, with the removal of urinary catheter once mobility is achieved. Thromboprophylactic measures should be in place during the recovery period. The routine use of antibiotics postoperatively has not been found to be advantageous over the use of single-dose broad-spectrum antibiotics intraoperatively [17].

KEY POINTS

Challenge: Myomectomy in a patient with multiple fibroids.

Background
- Uterine fibroids are common, affecting 50% of women.
- Myomectomy can be performed abdominally, laparoscopically, or hysteroscopically depending on the site and size of the fibroids.
- Patients with multiple large fibroids wishing to conserve fertility will generally require abdominal myomectomy.

Management
Preoperative steps
- Appropriate counseling about alternative treatments, risks of surgery, and consequences of myomectomy.
- Map fibroids by MRI.
- Correct anemia.
- Reduce the size of the fibroids by 3 months of GnRH agonist injections or 3 months of daily oral ulipristal acetate 5 mg.
- Cross-match blood.
- Arrange cell salvage.

Intraoperative considerations
- Adequate access is key; consider midline laparotomy. Perform laparotomy to the umbilicus, and extend above umbilicus if necessary.
- Exteriorize the uterus if possible; the use of a myoma screw can aid the mobilization of the uterus.
- Blood loss during myomectomy should be kept to a minimum by use of vasopressin or mechanical methods (clamp or tourniquet).
- Choose uterine incisions judiciously. Choose incisions that allow access to the maximum number of fibroids, but without undue "tunneling"; use horizontal incisions if possible; avoid incisions near the fallopian tubes.
- Close myometrial dead space layer by layer. Close incisions in one uterine area (e.g., anterior surface of the uterus) before making incisions in another area (e.g., posterior surface of the uterus).

References

1 Ezzati M, Norian J, Segars J. Management of uterine fibroids in the patient pursuing assisted reproductive technologies. *Womens Health (Lond Engl)* 2009;5:413–421.

2 Payson M, Leppert P, Segars J. Epidemiology of myomas. *Obstet Gynecol Clin North Am* 2006;33:1–11.

3 Buttram VC, Reiter RC. Uterine leiomyomata: etiology, symptomatology, and management. *Fertil Steril* 1981;36:433–445.

4 Sarris I, Bewley S, Agnihotri S (eds) *Training in Obstetrics and Gynaecology. The Essential Curriculum.* Oxford University Press, Oxford, 2009.

5 Pritts EA, Parker WH, Olive DL. Fibroids and infertility: an updated systematic review of the evidence. *Fertil Steril* 2009;91:1215–1223.

6 Olive DL, Pritts EA. Fibroids and reproduction. *Semin Reprod Med* 2010;28:218-227.

7 Casini ML, Rossi F, Agostini R, Unfer V. Effects of the position of fibroids on fertility. *Gynecol Endocrinol* 2006;22:106–109.

8 Cohen LS, Valle RF. Role of vaginal sonography and hysterosonography in the endoscopic treatment of uterine myomas. *Fertil Steril* 2000;73:197–204.

9 Malone LJ. Myomectomy: recurrence after removal of solitary and multiple myomas. *Obstet Gynecol* 1969;34:200–203.

10 Lethaby A, Vollenhoven B, Sowter M. Pre-operative GnRH analogue therapy before hysterectomy or myomectomy for uterine fibroids. *Cochrane Database Syst Rev* 2001;(2):CD000547.

11 Donnez J, Tatarchuk TF, Bouchard P *et al.* Ulipristal acetate versus placebo for fibroid treatment before surgery. *N Engl J Med* 2012;366:409–420.

12 Mukhopadhaya N, De Silva C, Manyonda IT. Conventional myomectomy. *Best Pract Res Clin Obstet Gynaecol* 2008;22:677–705.

13 Fletcher H, Fredrick J, Hardie M *et al.* A randomized comparison of vasopressin and tourniquet as hemostatic agents during myomectomy. *Obstet Gynecol* 1996;87:1014–1018.

14 West S, Ruiz R, Parker WH. Abdominal myomectomy in women with very large uterine size. *Fertil Steril* 2006;85:36–39.

15 Guarnaccia MM, Rein MS. Traditional surgical approaches to uterine fibroids: abdominal myomectomy and hysterectomy. *Clin Obstet Gynecol* 2001;44:385–400.

16 Igarashi M. Value of myomectomy in the treatment of infertility. *Fertil Steril* 1993;59:1331–1332.

17 Larsson PG, Carlsson B. Does pre- and post-operative metronidazole treatment lower vaginal cuff infection rate after abdominal hysterectomy among women with bacterial vaginosis? *Infect Dis Obstet Gynecol* 2002;10:133–140.

CHAPTER 95

Myomectomy: Massive Intraoperative Hemorrhage

Neelam Potdar[1] and Arri Coomarasamy[2]

[1] University Hospitals of Leicester NHS Trust, Leicester, UK

[2] College of Medical and Dental Sciences, University of Birmingham, Birmingham, UK

Case history: A woman with multiple uterine fibroids and palpable uterus of 24-week size is undergoing abdominal myomectomy for heavy menstrual bleeding and infertility. Twenty minutes into the procedure, the surgeon observes massive intraoperative bleeding.

Background

Intraoperative bleeding during myomectomy is a major challenge to a gynecologist. Massive bleeding can occur from slow but constant ooze from the vessel plexuses that feed the fibroids, or less commonly from inadvertent injury to a key vessel (e.g., uterine artery) which is more likely when there is extreme distortion of uterine anatomy by fibroids. The extent of the bleeding depends on the size and location of the fibroids and also on the preoperative and perioperative preventive measures. About 20–23% of myomectomy patients experience blood loss of over 1000 mL during the procedure, with high blood transfusion rates [1,2]. Uncontrolled hemorrhage can lead to hysterectomy (~2%) and severe morbidity.

Interventions used to limit intraoperative bleeding include controlling the uterine arteries [3] (pericervical tourniquet, embolization, or temporary clipping of uterine artery); vasopressive drugs (e.g., pitressin); uterotonic drugs (e.g., misoprostol and dinoprostone); and pharmacologic interventions that alter the coagulation cascade (tranexamic acid [4] and gelatin-thrombin sealant [5]). Alteration in myoma dissection techniques, for example use of laser and chemical agents such as sodium 2-mercaptoethane sulfonate (mesna) [6], may also reduce blood loss. For laparoscopic surgery the barbed suture (V-loc, TM 90, Covidien, Mansfield, MA) may help to reduce blood loss significantly [7].

Management

When massive bleeding is encountered, the first action is to alert the anesthetist and operating room staff so that steps to stabilize the patient can be taken, and necessary blood tests and blood products can be arranged (Chapter 40). Consultation with a hematologist will be necessary if clotting defects develop, or advanced treatment such as factor VIIa infusion is being considered. A standard regimen for recombinant factor VIIa is 50–100 µg/kg given intravenously, and

its effect is usually seen within half an hour. A second dose may be administered 2 hours after the first.

Management of intraoperative bleeding during myomectomy is tailored according to the route of the procedure (abdominal, laparoscopic, or hysteroscopic).

Abdominal myomectomy (laparotomy)

If a tourniquet has not been used initially, a Foley or silicon catheter can be used and tied around the pericervical region to stem bleeding from the uterine arteries. This has been shown to be a cheap, safe, and effective method which reduces blood loss during myomectomy [2,8,9]. The tourniquet can be released and retied every 20 min to aid perfusion [10].

The triple tourniquet technique is a more advanced approach but allows occlusion of the uterine arteries and the right and left ovarian vessels, and has been shown to be effective in reducing blood loss without obvious adverse effect on uterine perfusion and ovarian function [8]. The first step with this technique is to open the broad ligament anteriorly and reflect the bladder inferiorly. Next a small opening is made in the avascular area in the posterior leaf of the broad ligament on both sides, above the level of the uterine vessels [8]. A No. 1 polyglactin tie is then threaded through the two openings and tied anteriorly at the level of the internal os. Thin Foley catheter tubing can be used to achieve the two temporary ovarian tourniquets, placed around the infundibulopelvic ligament lateral to the fallopian tube and ovary [8].

Local perivascular injection of vasopressin 20 units (i.e., 1 mL, diluted in 19 mL normal saline) around vessels in the broad ligament or at the base of the largest fibroid helps with vasoconstriction and uterine contraction, thereby reducing bleeding (vasopressin V1a receptors are ubiquitously present in the myometrium). However, one has to be extremely cautious to avoid intravascular injection of vasopressin since this can lead to severe hypotension secondary to coronary artery spasm. Its use is contraindicated in women with cardiac disease. If vasopressin is not available, local injection of bupivacaine with epinephrine into the myometrium can help reduce blood loss by their vasoconstrictive effects [11].

Swiftness in suturing and closure of the myometrial dead space is the key to stopping massive hemorrhage. If these measures do not work, the next step is ligation of the uterine artery (Chapter 162). Care needs to be taken to avoid trauma to the ureters. If this does not control bleeding, internal iliac artery ligation is the penultimate

Gynecologic and Obstetric Surgery: Challenges and Management Options, First Edition. Edited by Arri Coomarasamy, Mahmood I. Shafi, G. Willy Davila and Kiong K. Chan.
© 2016 John Wiley & Sons, Ltd. Published 2016 by John Wiley & Sons, Ltd.

abdominal or pelvic surgery with potential adhesions that may interfere with trocar positioning. Consider transobturator sling if the patient has had multiple laparotomies.
- Some authors consider body habitus an important risk factor in predicting risk of bowel injury. In obese and overweight women, positioning of the trocars may be tricky; on the other hand, petite women may have anatomically narrowed space within the pelvis, which can make bowel perforation more likely [4]. In such cases, it may be more appropriate to consider a transobturator sling.
- Ultrasound scan can be performed on the table to exclude bowel underlying the predicted exit points, as per National Patient Safety Agency (NPSA) guidance on insertion of suprapubic catheters [5].
- Some authors [6] recommend avoidance of regional anesthesia at the time of sling insertion as Valsalva maneuvers at the time

of trocar positioning may lead to bowel loop displacement and subsequent bowel injury.
- Steep Trendelenburg position may help to shift the bowel away from the operative field (out of the pelvis).
- Retropubic infiltration of the space of Retzius, taking care of the hand position on the trocar, and appropriate orientation during insertion of the trocars will ensure that the trocars stay close to the symphysis pubis and exit just above the pubis.

The surgeon's experience is important and appropriate training should be provided. The likelihood of any visceral injury during sling procedures decreases with the surgeon's experience. An annual workload of at least 20 cases of each primary procedure for SUI is recommended by NICE and BSUG [7]. All surgeons providing these procedures should have audit data. In the UK they should be registered and use the BSUG database (www.bsug.org.uk).

KEY POINTS

Challenge: Bowel injury in sling procedures.

Background
- Sling procedures are usually safe.
- Bowel injury is a very rare complication but can be life-threatening.
- Incidence of bowel perforation during mid-urethral sling insertion is 0.03–0.7%.

Prevention
- Preoperative imaging in selected cases (patients with previous abdominal surgery and high likelihood of intra-abdominal adhesions).
- Avoidance of regional anesthesia: to avoid Valsalva effect.
- Proper tissue infiltration and tissue dissection.
- Patient positioning in steep Trendelenburg position.
- Hand position on the trocar, and proper trocar placement close to the posterior surface of the symphysis.

Management
- Be cognizant of risk and suspect if intraoperative or postoperative course is not typical.
- Perform exploratory laparoscopy or laparotomy, as appropriate.
- Consider bowel resection with or without anastomosis depending on site and extent of injury (Chapter 37).
- Prescribe postoperative antibiotics.

References

1 Kobashi KC, Govier FE. Perioperative complications: the first 140 polypropylene pubovaginal slings. *J Urol* 2003;170:1918–1921.
2 Kuuva N, Nilsson CG. Long-term results of the tension-free vaginal tape operation in an unselected group of 129 stress incontinent women. *Acta Obstet Gynecol Scand* 2006;85:482–487.
3 Huffaker RK, Yandell PM, Shull BL. Tension-free vaginal tape bowel perforation. *Int Urogynecol J* 2010;21:251–253.
4 Leboeuf L, Mendez LE, Gousse AE. Small bowel obstruction associated with tension-free vaginal tape. *Urology* 2004;63:1182–1184.
5 National Patient Safety Agency. Minimising risks of suprapubic catheter insertion (adults only). Available at http://www.nrls.npsa.nhs.uk/resources/?EntryId45=61917
6 Gruber DD, Wiersma DS, Dunn JS, Meldrum KA, Krivak TC. Cecal perforation complicating placement of a transvaginal tension-free vaginal tape. *Int Urogynecol J Pelvic Floor Dysfunct* 2007;18:671–673.
7 National Institute for Health and Care Excellence. *Urinary incontinence: the management of urinary incontinence in women.* NICE Clinical Guideline No. 171, September 2013. Available at https://www.nice.org.uk/guidance/cg171

CHAPTER 106

Sling Procedures: Voiding Dysfunction after Stress Urinary Incontinence Surgery

Margarita M. Aponte and Victor W. Nitti
New York University Langone Medical Center, New York, USA

Case history 1: A woman has TVT for stress urinary incontinence; postoperatively, she is unable to void at all.

Case history 2: A woman undergoes transobturator tape for stress predominant mixed urinary incontinence. She presents at 3 months after the operation with urgency, urgency incontinence, and sensation of incomplete emptying. She has had four urinary infections since her operation.

Background

There are a variety of surgical procedures to treat stress urinary incontinence (SUI), but recently the mid-urethral sling (MUS) has become the most popular surgical treatment for the management of SUI. A well-known complication of these procedures is iatrogenic outlet obstruction leading to voiding dysfunction, which can occur even in the hands of the most experienced surgeon. The true incidence of voiding dysfunction following surgery to correct SUI is unknown, and the reported rates vary widely in the literature, from 2.5 to 24% of cases [1]. The wide discrepancy may be explained by various factors, such as underdiagnosis due to incomplete evaluation and follow-up of patients. Even tension-free procedures such as retropubic or transobturator MUS have an estimated voiding dysfunction incidence of up to 3% [2]. Obstruction after anti-incontinence surgery (AIS) may be a result of technical factors, such as improper placement, excessive tensioning, or sling migration. However, patients with preoperative impaired detrusor contractility or patients who habitually void by abdominal straining may have difficulty emptying after sling surgery due to the increase in urethral resistance.

Clinical presentation

Voiding dysfunction is a term used to describe various problems related to the bladder's inability to empty adequately. The evaluation of a patient with voiding dysfunction after incontinence surgery begins with a focused history. Key issues in the history are the patient's preoperative voiding status and the temporal relationship of the lower urinary tract symptoms to the surgery. Patients may present with obstructive symptoms such as straining, slow or interrupted urinary stream, positional voiding, hesitancy or sensation of incomplete emptying, feeling of needing to revoid soon after emptying, and in the most extreme cases urinary retention.

Patients may also complain of *de novo* or worsening storage symptoms like urgency, frequency, nocturia, and urge incontinence.

Management

Evaluation

A physical examination should be performed which may reveal urethral hypersuspension, a palpable band on the anterior vaginal wall across the urethra, vaginal exposure of mesh or significant prolapse, pointing to the cause of obstruction. Urine analysis and culture should be done.

Non-invasive uroflow and post-void residual (PVR) volume determination are good non-invasive methods to screen for disorders of bladder emptying. A PVR should be done routinely in all patients after MUS to assess bladder emptying and rule out incomplete emptying. A single elevated PVR should be confirmed with a repeat measurement on a follow-up visit and should be interpreted within the clinical context.

There is no consensus on urodynamic criteria to diagnose obstruction, and urodynamics may fail to diagnose obstruction after AIS [3]. In patients with voiding symptoms or urinary retention after AIS, urodynamics may not be necessary since findings are not predictive of outcomes after intervention(s) to relieve obstruction. However, in cases of *de novo* or worsened storage symptoms, especially if emptying appears relatively normal, a formal urodynamic evaluation is preferred and may be valuable for patient counseling [4]. Therefore normal urodynamic findings should not be used to exclude patients from surgery, and studies may be performed selectively.

Cystourethroscopy should also be performed when indicated. Findings such as urethral scarring, kinking, or deviation as well as foreign bodies such as retained sutures, mesh, or stones can be the cause of symptoms.

Translabial ultrasound may also be used to determine sling location and may aid in the diagnosis of a malpositioned sling or persistent mesh after sling excision or urethrolysis.

Treatment

A clinical algorithm to guide the management of voiding dysfunction after MUS surgery is proposed in Figure 106.1.

Gynecologic and Obstetric Surgery: Challenges and Management Options, First Edition. Edited by Arri Coomarasamy, Mahmood I. Shafi, G. Willy Davila and Kiong K. Chan.
© 2016 John Wiley & Sons, Ltd. Published 2016 by John Wiley & Sons, Ltd.

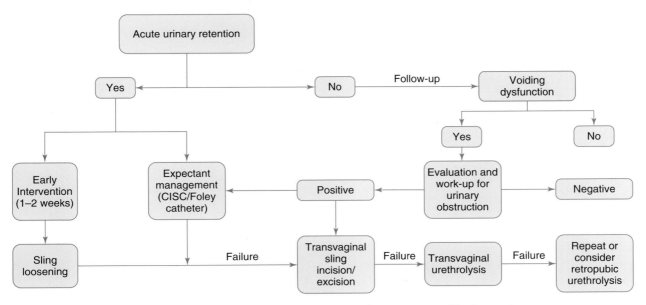

Figure 106.1 Management of voiding dysfunction after mid-urethral slings. CISC, clean intermittent self-catheterization.

Treatment is usually dictated by the degree of postoperative symptoms. Transient voiding dysfunction is frequent after many types of AIS. For patients with predominantly storage or overactive bladder symptoms, with negative urine culture and normal PVR, one can initiate a trial of behavioral therapy and/or medications such as antimuscarinics or β_3-adrenergic agonists.

If a patient has a significantly elevated PVR or urinary retention, she may need to facilitate bladder emptying with clean intermittent self-catheterization (CISC) or an indwelling catheter. Patients can record the amount voided and their PVR by self-catheterization. The process is usually temporary and once residuals are low (e.g., <150 mL), the patient can stop catheterizing. Most women will begin normal emptying within 1 week after MUS surgery, but some may take longer to resume normal voiding if they had a concomitant prolapse repair or have been chronically obstructed. Storage symptoms may take even longer to resolve. For traditional procedures such as Burch colposuspension and pubovaginal slings, normal voiding may be delayed for up to 1–3 months. In the case of MUS, symptoms persisting beyond 6 weeks are unlikely to improve, and require surgical intervention. For patients with complete urinary retention after MUS, 7–10 days is a reasonable time to wait for spontaneous voiding to resume and intervention may be considered if this does not happen. However, the decision to intervene early should be discussed with the patient. Occasionally, a woman with severe preoperative SUI, who is not bothered by catheterization, may prefer CISC to repeat surgery and a risk of recurrent SUI. However, most patients with significant symptoms choose definitive treatment. The type of surgical intervention will depend on several factors, including

patient's presentation, history of a previously failed urethrolysis, and surgeon's preference.

The use of urethral dilation may be detrimental, and is of limited use. If there is complete retention or incomplete emptying requiring CISC, early intervention (within 1–2 weeks) of sling loosening could potentially be performed in the office or in the operating room [5]. In cases of obstructive symptoms with elevated PVR, but not requiring catheterization, we would recommend a longer period of observation. Most commonly, obstructive slings (synthetic or biologic) are treated initially by sling incision with or without removal of the suburethral segment. It is crucial to identify the sling prior to cutting or excising it. In cases of biologic slings (autologous or other), if the sling cannot be identified (usually due to autolysis), one can proceed directly to urethrolysis; however, synthetic slings should always be identified. Success rates following incision or excision of sling vary between 70 and 100% [6,7]. In the case of MUS incision, resumption of normal emptying after incision is closer to 100%.

Urethrolysis involves mobilizing the urethra to varying degrees. The approach can be transvaginal, suprameatal, or retropubic; success rates are variable and, extrapolated from other anti-incontinence procedures, range from 65 to 92% [8,9]. It has been our practice to perform a transvaginal procedure for a sling incision with suburethral slings (Figure 106.2), and transvaginal urethrolysis for sling incisions that have failed. Retropubic urethrolysis is usually reserved for previously failed transvaginal procedures. The risk of recurrent SUI after urethrolysis, sling division or revision has been reported to be up to 19% [6,10,11].

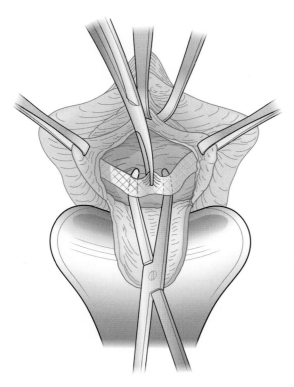

Figure 106.2 Sling incision: after an inverted U-shaped or midline incision is made, the sling is isolated in the midline and incised. A right-angle clamp may be placed between the sling and the periurethral fascia to avoid injury to the urethra. From Goldman, 2011 [12] with permission from Elsevier.

KEY POINTS

Challenge: Voiding dysfunction after stress incontinence surgery.

Background
- The risk of voiding dysfunction varies by the type of surgery. The true incidence of voiding dysfunction following surgery to correct SUI is unknown, but reported rates vary from 2.5 to 24% of cases.
- Up to 3% of cases may need loosening of sling or urethrolysis after sling surgery.
- Risk factors for voiding dysfunction are improper placement, excessive tensioning, sling shrinkage, or sling migration.

Prevention
- Perform appropriate preoperative risk assessment and counseling.
- Use minimally invasive synthetic suburethral slings rather than traditional suburethral slings [13].
- Consider use of the obturator route for MUS in women at high risk of voiding dysfunction, but counsel patients that long-term data are unavailable to support the procedure [13].
- Follow the manufacturer's instructions, and ensure that the sling is mid-urethral rather than proximally placed.

- Keep the sling tension-free with space between the sling and the urethra.
- At the time of a Burch colposuspension, pubovaginal sling or in a patient with voiding dysfunction, a suprapubic catheter can be left *in situ* to manage voiding dysfunction if it happens in the immediate postoperative period.

Management
- Perform a physical examination to feel for the band of the sling and scarring.
- Conduct a urinalysis, and PVR bladder scan.
- Manage postoperative acute retention with indwelling catheter for up to 1 week. CISC is an alternative which carries less risk of UTI.
- Do not perform urethral dilatation.
- If the voiding dysfunction has not resolved within 1–2 weeks, in cases of synthetic slings, it is appropriate to consider office or operating room procedure to loosen the sling under local anesthesia, by opening the same vaginal incision as the one used for the initial operation.
- Obstructive slings (synthetic or biologic) with delayed presentation can be treated initially with suburethral sling incision, with or without removal of the suburethral segment. It is crucial to identify the sling prior to cutting or excising it; a transurethral Hegar dilator can help localize the sling accurately.
- Urethrolysis involves mobilizing the urethra to varying degrees, and can be an option when suburethral sling incision has failed to relieve the voiding dysfunction. The potential risks of urethrolysis are infection, bleeding, injury to urethra, and up to 20% risk of recurrent SUI.

References

1 Dunn JS Jr, Bent AE, Ellerkman RM, Nihira MA, Melick CF. Voiding dysfunction after surgery for stress incontinence: literature review and survey results. *Int Urogynecol J Pelvic Floor Dysfunct* 2004;15:25-31.
2 Albo ME, Litman HJ, Richter HE *et al.* Treatment success of retropubic and transobturator mid urethral slings at 24 months. *J Urol* 2012;188:2281–2287.
3 Nitti VW, Raz S. Obstruction following anti-incontinence procedures: diagnosis and treatment with transvaginal urethrolysis. *J Urol* 1994;152:93–98.
4 Aponte MM, Shah SR, Hickling D, Brucker BM, Rosenblum N, Nitti VW. The utility of urodynamics in clinically suspected obstruction after anti-incontinence surgery in women. *J Urol* 2013;190:598–602.
5 Nguyen JN. Tape mobilization for urinary retention after tension-free vaginal tape procedures. *Urology* 2005;66:523–526.
6 Rardin CR, Rosenblatt PL, Kohli N, Miklos JR, Heit M, Lucente VR. Release of tension-free vaginal tape for the treatment of refractory postoperative voiding dysfunction. *Obstet Gynecol* 2002;100:898–902.
7 Game X, Soulie M, Malavaud B *et al.* [Treatment of bladder outlet obstruction secondary to suburethral tape by section of the tape]. *Prog Urol* 2006;16:67–71.
8 Petrou SP, Brown JA, Blaivas JG. Suprameatal transvaginal urethrolysis. *J Urol* 1999;161:1268–1271.
9 Scarpero HM, Dmochowski RR, Nitti VW. Repeat urethrolysis after failed urethrolysis for iatrogenic obstruction. *J Urol* 2003;169:1013–1016.
10 Goldman HB, Rackley RR, Appell RA. The efficacy of urethrolysis without re-suspension for iatrogenic urethral obstruction. *J Urol* 1999;161:196–198; discussion 198–199.
11 Foster HE, McGuire EJ. Management of urethral obstruction with transvaginal urethrolysis. *J Urol* 1993;150:1448–1451.
12 Goldman H. Urethrolysis. *Urol Clin North Am* 2011;38:31–37.
13 Ogah J, Cody JD, Rogerson L. Minimally invasive synthetic suburethral sling operations for stress urinary incontinence in women. *Cochrane Database Syst Rev* 2009;(4):CD006375.

CHAPTER 107

Sling Procedures: Tape Erosion into Bladder

Samuel J.S. Grimsley[1] and Y. Zaki Almallah[2]
[1] Doncaster and Bassetlaw Hospitals NHS Foundation Trust, Doncaster, UK
[2] University Hospitals Birmingham NHS Foundation Trust, Birmingham, UK

Case history: A 50-year-old female presents with a year's history of recurrent urinary tract infections, storage lower urinary tract symptoms (LUTS), and an episode of visible hematuria. The patient underwent TVT insertion 3 years prior to presentation for stress urinary incontinence (SUI) refractory to conservative management, which significantly improved after surgery. Flexible cystoscopy reveals a portion of the tape eroded into the bladder with an attached calculus.

Background

Since their introduction in the 1990s [1], mid-urethral slings (MUS), both retropubic (TVT) and transobturator (TOT/TVTO), have become the gold standard surgical management for SUI, with long-term success rates of up to 93% over 10 years [2]. Bladder perforation, if intraoperatively recognized, can be managed by re-passage of the trocar and prolonged catheter drainage of the bladder postoperatively (Chapters 35 and 102). In a series of 313 TVT patients, 16 (5.1%) suffered an intraoperative bladder injury; the diagnosis was delayed and erosion encountered in only two of these patients, one at 3 months and the other at 15 months [3].

Erosion is the postoperative appearance of tape material in the bladder or the urethra. Bladder erosion usually represents an undiscovered intraoperative perforation; urethral erosion, on the other hand, is usually due to migration of foreign material, with presentation typically after a long period [4].

Clinical presentation

Symptoms include chronic storage LUTS, recurrent UTI, hematuria, and voiding dysfunction. In one series of 14 patients, presentation was with dysuria, hematuria, urge incontinence, urinary frequency, and pelvic pain [5]. Encrustation and stone formation on exposed tape is common. Pelvic collections and vesicovaginal fistula are also possible.

Prevention

Avoidance of the retropubic space in patients with previous surgery in that area is a sensible precaution. Intraoperative detection of a bladder perforation is the standard method of minimizing the risk of erosion. Routine cystoscopy can identify otherwise undetected bladder perforations in 5% of TVT patients [6]. If corrected intraoperatively, bladder perforation does not impact on TVT outcome.

Management

Diagnosis

Examination with a 70° cystoscope will reveal the site of perforation and erosion; typically, these are at the 2 or 10 o'clock position with retropubic MUS, and at the 4 or 8 o'clock position with TOT. Foreign material extruding into the bladder has also been described following mesh repair of pelvic organ prolapse, and following the use of non-absorbable sutures at colposuspension.

Treatment

Symptomatic exposed intravesical tape is unlikely to resolve without operative treatment. Infections should be treated while the patient is waiting to have surgery. Surgery is best done by a urologist or a urogynecologist with experience in reconstructive surgery.

Transurethral management

Various methods for transurethral removal of eroded vesical tape have been described. The material can be resected using either diathermy or holmium laser [7]. Eroded foreign material can be elevated, with holmium laser resecting the margins close to the bladder mucosa. Endoscopic resection using operative cystoscope and hysteroscopic scissors, laparoscopic endoshears and lighted nasal speculum has also been described [2,8]. Endoscopic techniques are minimally invasive and have low morbidity; however, endoscopic resection is more limited than open techniques in the amount of material accessible for removal, and persistent or recurrent tape exposure is more common.

Techniques to maximize the length of excised tape include traction on the extruding tape utilizing hemostatic clip or other clamps. Suprapubic telescopy using a 5-mm laparoscopic trocar placed into the bladder dome allows for use of laparoscopic scissors or a grasper while the opposite instrument can be placed through the cystoscopic sheath to allow excision of the exposed tape.

Transurethral cystolitholapaxy, or pneumatic or laser lithotripsy can be utilized if significant encrustation or calculus formation has occurred on the exposed tape.

Gynecologic and Obstetric Surgery: Challenges and Management Options, First Edition. Edited by Arri Coomarasamy, Mahmood I. Shafi, G. Willy Davila and Kiong K. Chan.
© 2016 John Wiley & Sons, Ltd. Published 2016 by John Wiley & Sons, Ltd.

Transvaginal management

Transvaginal resection of eroded tape can be performed if the erosion is in the bladder base [9]. With local anesthetic and epinephrine as hemostatic agents, a midline or inverted-U vaginal incision is made suburethrally to the bladder base, exposing the tape to be dissected free. If the erosion is trigonal, temporary ureteric stenting is appropriate. The bladder can be closed in two layers and integrity checked with back-filling.

Laparoscopic management

Laparoscopic transvesical resection of eroded bladder tape has been described by several authors. One technique involves filling the bladder with carbon dioxide and placing three 5-mm ports in the lower abdomen directly into the bladder, excising the tape extruding from the bladder muscle layer completely, and removing it with any adherent calculi [10]. Bladder mucosa is sutured using a continuous 4-0 Vicryl suture. Alternate techniques have used a combination of an operating cystoscope and 5-mm suprapubic ports [11].

Open surgery

Erosions at the bladder dome are more easily exposed via an open approach. A low Pfannenstiel incision allows retropubic extraperitoneal access to enable cystotomy at the dome revealing the exposed mesh [12]. Intravesical mesh should be excised to at least 1 cm beyond the bladder epithelium. Developing the retropubic space aids access in this dissection.

The bladder defect caused by tape excision and the cystotomy will need to be separately sutured with two-layer watertight closures using 3-0 Vicryl. The bladder is kept catheterized and on free drainage for 7–14 days.

KEY POINTS

Challenge: Tape erosion into bladder.

Background
- Tape erosion may be due to a missed intraoperative perforation, or subsequent tape migration through the bladder wall or urethra.
- Presentation could be with storage or irritative LUTS, recurrent UTIs, hematuria, or voiding dysfunction.

Prevention
- Detection of perforation using intraoperative cystoscopy during any type of sling surgery is important to prevent erosion. The bladder should be filled to 200–300 mL to facilitate detection of small perforations.
- If there is no perforation, but tethering of the bladder wall is noted, the tape should be repositioned so that it is away from the mucosa.

Management
- Urine microscopy and culture, free flow rate, and residual volume estimate are the basic tests performed in women presenting with recurrent UTIs.
- Cystourethroscopy is mandatory.

- Conservative management is not appropriate with tape erosion in symptomatic patients.
- The complication is best managed by an experienced urologic surgeon.
- The route of surgery (transurethral, transvaginal, laparoscopic, or open) depends on the location of the erosion within the bladder and the surgeon's expertise:
  - Transurethral resection or ablation of the tape can be performed using diathermy, holmium laser or endoscopic shears, with or without suprapubic teloscopy.
  - If the erosion is in the urethra or near bladder base, transvaginal inverted-U incision can be performed to access the urethra and the bladder base.
  - Laparoscopic transvesical approach can be used, with or without the use of concurrent operative cystoscope.
  - For erosion at dome, open excision via a Pfannenstiel incision and a cystotomy can be a good option.
- Delayed presentation may result in the formation of stones, which require crushing prior to removal.
- After removal of eroded tape, the bladder is sutured in two layers with 3-0 Vicryl and drained continuously for 7–14 days to allow healing of the repaired defect.

References

1 Ulmsten U, Henriksson L, Johnson P, Varhos G. An ambulatory surgical procedure under local anesthesia for treatment of female urinary incontinence. *Int Urogynecol J* 1996;7:81–85.

2 O'Sullivan O, Martyn F, O'Connor R, Jaffery S. Novel endoscopic management of a late complication following TVT insertion for stress urinary incontinence. *Am J Case Rep* 2013;14:459–461.

3 Levin I, Groutz A, Gold R, Pauzner D, Lessing JB, Gordon D. Surgical complications and medium-term outcome results of tension-free vaginal tape: a prospective study of 313 consecutive patients. *Neurourol Urodyn* 2004;23:7–9.

4 Rapoport D, Fenster HN, Wright JR. Reported complications of tension-free vaginal tape procedures: a review. *BC Med J* 2007;49:490–494.

5 Oh T-H, Ryu D-S. Transurethral resection of intravesical mesh after midurethral sling procedures. *J Endourol* 2009;23:1333–1337.

6 Duckett J, Aggarwal I, Basu M, Vella M, Patil A. The value of cystoscopy and bladder biopsy taken at the time of tension-free vaginal tape insertion. *J Obstet Gynaecol* 2007;27:297–299.

7 Doumouchtsis SK, Lee FY, Bramwell D, Fynes MM. Evaluation of holmium laser for managing mesh/ suture complications of continence surgery. *BJU Int* 2011;108:1472–1478.

8 McLennan MT. Transurethral resection of transvaginal tape. *Int Urogynecol J* 2004;15:360–362.

9 Firoozi F, Ingber MS, Goldman HB. Pure transvaginal removal of eroded mesh and retained foreign body in the bladder. *Int Urogynecol J* 2010;21:757–760.

10 Yoshizawa T, Yamaguchi K, Obinata D, Sato K, Mochida J, Takahashi S. Laparoscopic transvesical removal of erosive mesh after transobturator tape procedure. *Int J Urol* 2011;18:861–863.

11 Kim JH, Doo SW, Yang WJ, Song YS. Laparoscopic transvesical excision and reconstruction in the management of mid-urethral tape mesh erosion and stones around the bladder neck: initial experiences. *BJU Int* 2012;110:E1009–1013.

12 Barber MD. Surgical techniques for removing problematic mesh. *Clin Obstet Gynecol* 2013;56:289–302.

CHAPTER 108

Sling Procedures: Sexual Dysfunction

Swati Jha[1] and Ranee Thakar[2]
[1] Sheffield Teaching Hospitals NHS Foundation Trust, Sheffield, UK
[2] Mayday University Hospital, London, UK

Case history: A 42-year-old woman underwent a mid-urethral minimally invasive sling (MUS) for stress urinary incontinence (SUI) 12 months ago. She commenced sexual activity 3 months after the procedure, but reports that she has pain on intercourse. In addition, her partner also complains of discomfort during penetration. Although she does not experience incontinence any longer, she is unhappy.

Background

MUS surgery has revolutionized the management of SUI and has now virtually replaced colposuspension [1]. A systematic review evaluating the impact of MUS continence surgery on sexual function found that the proportion of those with no change in sexual function was 56.7%, whereas an improvement in sexual function was found in 33.9% and a deterioration in sexual function in 9.4% [2]. The chance of improvement was therefore three times as likely as the chance of deterioration. These studies specifically included *de novo* or worsening coital incontinence as a cause of deterioration of sexual function, but did not therefore look solely at painful sex that occurred or worsened after the operation. The review found no difference between retropubic and obturator approaches for surgery. Recent studies have reported varying degrees of sexual impairment after TVT and TOT insertion, ranging from 1.9 to 13.5% at 6 months after surgery [3].

The exact mechanism of dyspareunia or deterioration in sexual function following sling surgery is poorly understood, but there are several hypotheses.

- MUS is inserted approximately in the location of the G-spot on the anterior vaginal wall, which in some women is believed to be responsible for arousal and sensory stimulation.
- Studies have demonstrated that insertion of the MUS, particularly when placed in the retropubic region, interferes with clitoral blood flow [4] which may impact on stimulation and the ability to reach an orgasm.
- It has also been shown that MUS impacts on libido, which may contribute to deteriorating sexual function [5]. This may be due to psychological issues related to surgery.
- Coital incontinence contributes to sexual dysfunction. Although after insertion of MUS coital incontinence significantly improves

in most women, failure of the technique may lead to persistence of coital incontinence and deteriorating sexual function.
- Mesh extrusion, however minimal, may cause significant discomfort to both the patient (dyspareunia) and the partner (hispareunia) during intercourse. The risk of mesh exposure with the MUS is 1–2% [6]. When the mesh is extruded, the patient is usually aware of a gritting feel in the vagina, although this is not always the case; up to 35% of mesh exposures are asymptomatic [7]. Careful examination is required to identify an extrusion.
- Other issues with MUS surgery include narrowing or scarring of the vagina, the tape being inserted too tight, and psychological concerns (e.g., fear that intercourse may damage the surgical result).

Management

It is important to elicit a detailed history of preoperative sexual function, and any postoperative changes. There can be other symptoms such as vaginal discharge or spotting in case of mesh extrusion. A careful examination of the patient in both lithotomy and left lateral position with good exposure and lighting is required. To rule out an extrusion, adequate visualization of the vaginal incision used for sling insertion is necessary. Extrusion may be hidden by folds of the vaginal epithelium and it may be necessary to lift vaginal rugae using a small swab to aid visualization. The examination will also identify if the tape feels superficial, particularly if it is palpable during the digital examination, even in the absence of an extrusion. Scarring and tenderness may be evident during the examination.

Mesh exposure

If there is mesh exposure, the usual principles of treatment of exposed vaginal mesh are followed (Chapter 107). For small exposures, conservative treatment with local estrogens is reasonable in the first instance. If this treatment fails, surgical excision of the mesh may be necessary. When excision is required this is usually limited to the area exposed; postoperatively, the use of estrogen cream promotes healing.

Depending on the presence or absence of mesh extrusion, this complication of TVT would be classified as 2B/T3/S1 or 1B/T3/S1 (Chapter 103) [8].

Gynecologic and Obstetric Surgery: Challenges and Management Options, First Edition. Edited by Arri Coomarasamy, Mahmood I. Shafi, G. Willy Davila and Kiong K. Chan.
© 2016 John Wiley & Sons, Ltd. Published 2016 by John Wiley & Sons, Ltd.

Non-exposed mesh

For dyspareunia associated with non-exposed mesh, treatment is more complicated. Initial treatment is to use topical estrogen to improve vascularization to the area. If this is unsuccessful, topical local anesthetics can be tried. Dryness can be easily dealt with by use of oil-based lubricants.

As the underlying etiology can often be psychological, psychosexual issues may need to be explored and, if identified, appropriate referral should be made to a counsellor. Occasionally certain positions are more uncomfortable than others and changing position during intercourse may help alleviate the symptom. If these approaches fail, medications for vulvodynia (e.g., amitriptyline) may be considered. If all conservative or medical therapies are unsuccessful, the final option is excision of the mesh.

Careful consideration and counseling are needed before proceeding to sling excision, as it does not guarantee a resolution of the symptoms. Patients need to be warned of the risk of recurrence of SUI with tape removal, since up to 20% of women will have recurrence. Sexual function in patients with *de novo* dyspareunia is likely to improve after sling removal. Desire, arousal, lubrication, satisfaction, and pain are significantly improved after removal but orgasm scores can remain low [3].

When the tape is excised, removal of the suburethral portion of the mesh up to the lateral sulci by sharp dissection is performed. Urethral injury is a possibility and this requires considerable caution.

If present, excessive scar tissue should be excised and the vaginal epithelium is closed in one to two layers using Vicryl 2-0 interrupted sutures. Where the excision is close to the urethra, an indwelling catheter should be left *in situ* for 7–10 days to prevent formation of a fistula [3].

Prevention

When performing any procedure that involves the use of mesh, certain basic precautions should be undertaken.

1 In women with vaginal atrophy, topical estrogen should be prescribed for 6 weeks prior to insertion of the tape.
2 Adequate hydrodissection will ensure placement of the tape deep to the vaginal epithelium and fibromuscular fascial layer.
3 Careful attention should be paid to hemostasis to prevent infection and malposition of the tape.
4 The vaginal epithelium should be closed without tension and should not be tethered to the tape prior to closure of the incision.

KEY POINTS

Challenge: Sexual dysfunction following sling surgery.

Background
- Patients need to be warned of a 1 in 10 risk of deterioration of sexual function after MUS surgery.
- Causes of sexual problems may be related to failure of the procedure, alteration of nerve or blood supply, scarring of the vagina, tape erosion, or psychological issues. Sexual dysfunction may also predate the incontinence surgery.

Prevention
- Adequate hydrodissection before tape insertion and placement under vaginal fascia to avoid it being superficial and felt during intercourse.
- Good surgical hemostasis.
- Closure of vaginal epithelium without tension or tethering.

Management
- Identification of any possible causes of sexual dysfunction, related or unrelated to tape placement, is important.
- Early management of mesh extrusion includes topical estrogen, with or without excision of the extruded portion of the mesh and closure of the vagina.
- Patients with *de novo* dyspareunia after MUS may benefit from conservative therapy including topical estrogen, local anesthetics, and lubricants.
- Sling removal may be necessary when other options fail. Patients need to be informed that sexual function is likely to improve but an improvement cannot be guaranteed. They should also be warned of the risk of recurrence of SUI.

References

1 Nilsson CG, Palva K, Aarnio R, Morcos E, Falconer C. Seventeen years' follow-up of the tension-free vaginal tape procedure for female stress urinary incontinence. *Int Urogynecol J* 2013;24:1265–1269.
2 Jha S, Ammenbal M, Metwally M. Impact of incontinence surgery on sexual function: a systematic review and meta-analysis. *J Sex Med* 2012;9:34–43.
3 Kuhn A, Burkhard F, Eggemann C, Mueller MD. Sexual function after suburethral sling removal for dyspareunia. *Surg Endosc* 2009;23:765–768.
4 Caruso S, Rugolo S, Bandiera S, Mirabella D, Cavallaro A, Cianci A. Clitoral blood flow changes after surgery for stress urinary incontinence: pilot study on TVT versus TOT procedures. *Urology* 2007;70:554–557.
5 Maaita M, Bhaumik J, Davies AE. Sexual function after using tension-free vaginal tape for the surgical treatment of genuine stress incontinence. *BJU Int* 2002;90:540–543.
6 Mahon J, Cikalo M, Varley D, Glanville J. *Summaries of the Safety/Adverse Effects of Vaginal Tapes/Slings/Meshes for Stress Urinary Incontinence and Prolapse.* York Health Economics Consortium/University of York. MHRA Final Report, November 2012. Available at http://www.mhra.gov.uk/home/groups/comms-ic/documents/websiteresources/con205383.pdf
7 Hammad FT, Kennedy-Smith A, Robinson RG. Erosions and urinary retention following polypropylene synthetic sling: Australasian survey. *Eur Urol* 2005;47:641–646.
8 Haylen BT, Freeman RM, Swift SE *et al.* An International Urogynecological Association (IUGA)/International Continence Society (ICS) joint terminology and classification of the complications related directly to the insertion of prostheses (meshes, implants, tapes) and grafts in female pelvic floor surgery. *Int Urogynecol J* 2011;22:3–15.

CHAPTER 109

Sling Procedures: Persistent Urine Leakage

Luis Manuel Espaillat-Rijo and G. Willy Davila
Cleveland Clinic Florida, Weston/Fort Lauderdale, Florida, USA

Case history 1: A patient presents with complaints of persistent leakage of urine 6 months after a transobturator tape (TOT) sling operation. Before the sling was placed, she had more than 10 daily incontinent events, more pronounced when she laughed or coughed. She now has only one to two stress incontinent events per week, but is unhappy with the surgical results.

Case history 2: A patient presents with persistent leakage of urine 6 months after a tension free retropubic tape (TVT) sling was placed. She has had significant improvement in the total number of leakage events. However, she now gets a sudden urge to void and barely has enough time to reach the toilet. In addition, when she voids, her stream is slower than what it was before surgery, and she may require three or four attempts to fully empty her bladder.

Background

Mid-urethral slings (MUS) are used in the treatment of stress urinary incontinence (SUI). Their long-term success rates have been reported as high as 90% [1].

The literature on failed slings is difficult to interpret, because the outcome measures used in the different studies are so varied that it makes it difficult to group them for comparison [2]. Proposed definitions of sling failure are described in Box 109.1 [3]. It is important to distinguish persistent leakage against recurrence; any leakage within 12 months after surgery is considered persistence of leakage, whereas onset of leakage after a 12-month period of continence is considered recurrent. In addition, voiding dysfunction, especially *de novo*, whether associated with urgency symptoms or not, may affect a patient's perception of success and satisfaction (Case history 2).

> **BOX 109.1 DEFINITIONS OF SLING FAILURE (NOT MUTUALLY EXCLUSIVE)**
>
> - Failure to cure symptoms of stress incontinence
> - Stress incontinence cured, but *de novo* OAB symptoms with or without voiding symptoms
> - Stress incontinence not cured, and emergence of OAB symptoms with or without voiding symptoms
> - Other new symptoms or complications

Since continence and voiding dysfunction are multifactorial issues, it may be difficult for a patient to define precisely her symptoms and their duration. It is key to define why a patient is dissatisfied with her surgical outcome, and focus on evaluating and addressing such symptoms. Preoperative discussions to develop a realistic expectation of the operation (although not typically carried out) are important for reducing the risk of postoperative patient dissatisfaction.

Potential causes for sling failure

Insufficient tension on the sling

Although many surgeons may think a tight sling is better than a loose sling, this is not the case, especially given the fact that voiding abnormalities can result from even slight over-tightening of a suburethral sling. When faced with a patient with a failed sling, a surgeon should refrain from simply offering to place a "tighter" sling; a complete urogynecologic evaluation will be needed to determine what intervention will have the highest likelihood of improving the patient's symptoms.

Failure of the sling to fix and anchor into tissue

It is unclear exactly how long it takes for the sling arms to fix into the supporting connective tissues. If the arms of the sling do not fixate into the abdominal wall aponeurosis and urogenital diaphragm (retropubic slings) or the obturator membrane (TOT slings), then the sling may indeed be too loose.

Misplacement or migration of the sling (or lack of urethral fixation)

A sling not placed along the mid-urethra is not likely to function effectively. This could represent problems in (i) sling implantation (surgeon factor); (ii) soft-tissue fixation of a properly placed sling; and (iii) sling material not allowing soft-tissue fixation. Only type I large-pore monofilament polypropylene mesh material should be used for synthetic slings. This is in large part to achieve appropriate fixation into soft tissues and reduce the risk of infections. Post-implantation infection can also lead to lack of sling fixation. Thus, technical factors are not simply surgeon-related, although surgeon's experience is certainly important.

Intrinsic sphincteric functional issues

Urethral continence requires appropriate neuromuscular function of the sphincteric mechanism. Urethral closure during stressful

Gynecologic and Obstetric Surgery: Challenges and Management Options, First Edition. Edited by Arri Coomarasamy, Mahmood I. Shafi, G. Willy Davila and Kiong K. Chan.
© 2016 John Wiley & Sons, Ltd. Published 2016 by John Wiley & Sons, Ltd.

activities requires the coordination of multiple interactive factors. Thus, denervation injuries, sphincter muscle trauma, scar tissue from previous surgeries and resultant limitation of physiologic urethral movement (or a combination of the above) can lead to sling failure. TVT slings have a success rate of less than 70% in women with intrinsic urethral sphincter deficiency (ISD) [4]. Women diagnosed with ISD on preoperative urodynamics should be advised that their failure rate from a primary sling (and certainly from a repeat sling) is significantly greater than in women without ISD [5]. This is particularly true if the sling chosen is a TOT sling, where the reduced urethral compression leads to an unacceptably high failure rate and higher rate of repeat sling insertion [6,7].

Presence of complex incontinence

The presence of coexistent detrusor overactivity (DO) or voiding dysfunction jeopardizes the success rate of any sling procedure. Slings in women with mixed incontinence are associated with a 70% success rate for the stress component and approximately 40–60% for the urge component [7]. However, the heterogeneous nature of this patient population makes precise prognostic counseling very difficult. It is our practice to determine which factor is primary in terms of symptomatology (stress > urge, urge > stress) and treat the primary factor first. Thus, if the assessment demonstrates urge over stress, we will treat the urge incontinence with anticholinergics, neuromodulation, or a combination. The presence of dysfunctional voiding (bladder atony, dyssynergic voiding, or another form of outflow obstruction) jeopardizes the result of a sling procedure. This is particularly true with repeat slings, where the previous sling may already be causing at least partial outflow obstruction.

Management

Assessment

Specific assessment is needed to uncover the underlying reason for sling failure. The assessment should include all the following.

History

It is important to establish a detailed description of the patient's symptoms, whether the stress component still exists, or whether it has been modified by the operation. Any new overactive bladder (OAB) symptoms should be elicited. It is important to find out what were her treatment goals prior to her original surgery, and what they are now. Her goals may not be the same as the treating physician's goals.

Examination

The goal of the examination is to look for potential physical causes contributing to sling failure. The vaginal examination should include evaluation of the urethra and the bladder neck for hypermobility and bladder base support (vaginal examination using POP-Q system as well as a Q-tip test). It is important to palpate the sling, assessing for location, mesh erosion, and tenderness. An important assessment is to ask the patient to perform a Valsalva maneuver, after voiding, in the lithotomy position (empty supine stress test). Leakage under these circumstances denotes severity and is a good screening test for ISD.

Three-dimensional ultrasound

This can be used to evaluate for sling to tissue fixation and potential migration, dynamic action with increases in intra-abdominal pressure, and loss of mid-urethral support. In addition, an obstructive sling may be visible as excessive angulation with Valsalva maneuver.

Cystoscopy

Cystoscopy is important to evaluate for tape erosion or other causes of bladder irritation leading to incontinence episodes.

Multichannel urodynamics

This will evaluate almost all components of the urine storage and voiding function. It is important to evaluate bladder compliance, any DO, low maximum urethral closure pressure, Valsalva leak point pressures to identify ISD, and voiding pressures and dynamics to identify any underlying voiding dysfunction.

Treatment

It is important to establish what the patient's expectations are regarding any possible therapy, making sure they are realistic. Once an underlying problem is identified, treatment should be targeted, taking into account the patient's preferences. Treatments such as pelvic floor rehabilitation, drug therapy for DO or OAB, and invasive and non-invasive surgical treatment for SUI can be offered. A proposed algorithm for management of patients with failed sling operation is given in Figure 109.1.

Non-surgical therapy

Depending on patient expectations, conservative options include pelvic floor exercises and physiotherapy, vaginal devices such as pessaries and tampons, and pharmacotherapy with duloxetine or α-agonists such as imipramine. Non-surgical therapy may improve quality of life to an extent that a patient may not request additional surgical therapy.

Placement (or replacement) of a tension-free retropubic sling

TVT, when placed for recurrent SUI, has been shown to be effective [8,9]. Data would suggest that TVT is superior to TOT as repeat surgery, especially in patients who have a diagnosis of ISD or limited hypermobility [4–6]. Only small studies have evaluated the role of retropubic slings for the treatment of SUI with failed slings; Petrou and Frank [10] reported that the efficacy of a repeat sling is 50% by objective measures and 86% by subjective measures in their small series (N = 14).

Bulking agents

Literature is scant regarding the use of bulking agents in patients with a failed sling. However, it is still one of the most rational approaches to persistent SUI. This is especially true in those patients who have a well-supported non-hypermobile urethra with ISD, or in those who decline to undergo another surgical procedure. Bulking agents are typically administered in the office setting under local anesthesia. Extrapolating from a systematic review on Macroplastique® (polydimethylsiloxane injection) bulking agent, long-term cure and improvement rates are 36% and 64%, respectively [11].

Prevention

A proper preoperative assessment of the patient is important to identify risk factors which could potentially complicate the surgery. Examples include previous pelvic surgery, problems with hip joints, obesity, and anticoagulation therapy. Anecdotally, patients with prominent lower abdominal wall vasculature, especially unilateral, may also have prominent retropubic vasculature and require special attention preoperatively and intraoperatively. Transobturator approach may reduce incidence of vascular injury.

Proper infiltration of the tissues (especially the space of Retzius) prior to lateral dissection and insertion of the trocars is important in reducing complications. Trocar placement close to the posterior surface of the symphysis and avoidance of trocar needle deviation laterally are important aspects of good technique. Intraoperative blood loss can be managed by electrocoagulation, manual compression, tamponade by indwelling catheter, and vaginal packing.

Appropriate training and maintenance of competence are key to safety. The likelihood of any complications associated with mid-urethral sling insertions decreases with the surgeon's experience. An annual workload of at least 20 cases of each primary procedure for SUI is recommended [13].

KEY POINTS

Challenge: Retropubic hematoma after sling procedures.

Background
- Retropubic sling procedures are usually safe.
- Retropubic hematoma after sling placement is a rare complication but can be life-threatening.

Prevention
- Proper tissue infiltration and tissue dissection.
- Proper trocar placement close to the posterior surface of the symphysis. Avoid placement close to the urethra (periurethral or perivesical venous plexus damage) or too lateral (external iliac vessel injury).

Management
Conservative management
- Observe vital signs and check FBC.
- Transfuse blood as necessary.
- Provide adequate pain relief.
- Arrange continuous or intermittent bladder drainage in cases of urinary retention.
- Consider antibiotics in patients at higher risk of infection (e.g., diabetic or immunosuppressed patients).

Surgical intervention
- Options include the following.
  - Insertion of drains into retropubic space under ultrasound control to drain the hematoma.
  - Retziusscopy to confirm presence of the hematoma and arrange its evacuation.
  - Immediate exploratory laparotomy with ligation of the bleeding vessel.
  - Use of coagulation-promoting substances and packing of the space of Retzius and vagina.
  - Embolization of the bleeding vessel by interventional radiology.

References

1 Flock F, Reich A, Muche R, Kreienberg R, Reister F. Hemorrhagic complications associated with tension-free vaginal tape procedure. *Obstet Gynecol* 2004;104:989–994.
2 Novara G, Galfano A, Boscolo-Berto R *et al*. Complication rates of tension-free midurethral slings in the treatment of female stress urinary incontinence: a systematic review and meta-analysis of randomized controlled trials comparing tension-free midurethral tapes to other surgical procedures and different devices. *Eur Urol* 2008;53:288–308.
3 Daneshgari F, Kong W, Swartz M. Complications of midurethral slings: important outcomes from future clinical trials. *J Urol* 2008;180:1886–1887.
4 Vierhout ME. Severe hemorrhage complicating tension-free vaginal tape (TVT): a case report. *Int Urogynecol J Pelvic Floor Dysfunct* 2001;12:139–140.
5 Kobashi KC, Govier FE. Perioperative complications: the first 140 polypropylene pubovaginal slings. *J Urol* 2003;170:1918–1921.
6 Center for Devices and Radiological Health. Food and Drug Administration Manufacturer and User Facility Device Experience Database. https://www.accessdata.fda.gov/scripts/cdrh/cfdocs/cfmaude/search.cfm
7 Giri SK, Wallis F, Drumm J, Saunders JA, Flood HD. A magnetic resonance imaging-based study of retropubic haematoma after sling procedures: preliminary findings. *BJU Int* 2005;96:1067–1071.
8 Muir TW, Tulikangas PK, Fidela Paraiso M, Walters MD. The relationship of tension-free vaginal tape insertion and the vascular anatomy. *Obstet Gynecol* 2003;101:933–936.
9 Rajan S, Kohli N. Retropubic hematoma after transobturator sling procedure. *Obstet Gynecol* 2005;106:1199–1202.
10 Flock F, Kohorst F, Kreienberg R, Reich A. Retziusscopy: a minimal invasive technique for the treatment of retropubic hematomas after TVT procedure. *Eur J Obstet Gynecol Reprod Biol* 2011;158:101–103.
11 Vidin E, Jahn C, Saussine C, Jacqmin D. Retroperitoneal haematoma and retropubic suburethral TVT tape. Report of two cases. *Prog Urol* 2004;14:1188–1190.
12 Zorn KC, Daigle S, Belzile F, Tu Mai Le. Embolization of a massive retropubic hemorrhage following a tension-free vaginal tape (TVT) procedure: case report and literature review. *Can J Urol* 2005;12:2560–2563.
13 National Institute for Health and Care Excellence. *Urinary incontinence: the management of urinary incontinence in women*. NICE Clinical Guideline No. 171, September 2013. Available at https://www.nice.org.uk/guidance/cg171

CHAPTER 105
Sling Procedures: Bowel Injury

Fidan Israfil-Bayli and Philip Toozs-Hobson
Birmingham Women's NHS Foundation Trust, Birmingham, UK

Case history 1: A woman was discharged home after insertion of TVT and a cystoscopy to confirm bladder integrity. She was admitted 2 days later feeling unwell, with nausea, vomiting, and abdominal pain. On examination she had extensive abdominal distension and guarding. Some bowel contents were noticed draining through TVT tape exit sites.

Case history 2: A woman came to the emergency department 2 years after a TVT procedure complaining of abdominal pain, distension, nausea, and vomiting. She eventually underwent laparotomy which revealed an adhesive band obstructing part of ileum. Inside the band was a remnant of the TVT sling. The affected part of the bowel was resected, and an anastomosis was performed.

Background

Sling procedures are generally safe but there have been a number of complications identified including death [1]. Complications such as bladder perforations, urethral damage and mesh exposure, vessel injury, nerve damage, and hematoma formation are well reported [2]. Bowel injury is a rare complication; the incidence of bowel perforation during mid-urethral sling insertion is 0.03–0.7% [1,2].

Presentation

The majority of bowel injuries occur in patients with previous abdominal surgery and presence of bowel adhesions in the peritoneal cavity. Usually bowel injuries are due to perforation of the bowel by the trocars, and are diagnosed within hours or days after the sling procedure.

Patients usually present, as in Case history 1, with symptoms of acute abdomen: abdominal pain, nausea and vomiting, sometimes fever and possibly drainage of bowel contents from skin incisions [3]; on occasion, however, tachycardia may be the first sign (Chapter 37).

Patients may rarely present several years after sling procedure, as in Case history 2, which confirms the possibility of asymptomatic bowel perforation and adhesion formation that could be attributed to erosion of the tape through the bowel wall [4]. Sometimes patients may present with symptoms of bowel obstruction without peritonitis.

Bowel perforation should be suspected in any case of unexplained abdominal symptoms after sling procedures, especially where there is an unexplained tachycardia.

Management (see Chapter 37)

Patients presenting with unusually severe postoperative pain should always be investigated as this is not typical and would indicate an untoward event such as urethral, vascular, or visceral injury. Likewise, unexplained abdominal symptoms hours and days after procedure should be managed promptly with a high index of suspicion of bowel injury, which potentially could be life-threatening.

Immediate intraoperative management

If bowel perforation is suspected during insertion of the sling, prompt involvement of a general or bowel surgeon is mandatory. If an abnormally large amount of pressure is required to pass the trocar through the space of Retzius or the abdominal wall fascia, one must suspect possible soft-tissue or visceral damage.

Exploratory laparoscopy or laparotomy should be performed with the trocar in place (for easy identification of the site of injury) and the affected segment of bowel resected with creation of primary anastomosis, as appropriate (Chapter 37). Postoperative intravenous antibiotics should be given for at least 72 hours to prevent or treat associated sepsis.

Management of late bowel perforation

If the tape was adherent to the bowel wall and eventually eroded, as in Case history 2, that part of the mesh needs to be removed. Depending on the extent of bowel damage, resection should be performed with primary anastomosis or stoma formation (Chapter 37).

Prevention

Preoperative risk assessment begins with counseling of the patient before surgery and individualizing the risk for a patient.
• One of the major risk factors for the development of bowel perforation during mid-urethral sling surgery is previous

Gynecologic and Obstetric Surgery: Challenges and Management Options, First Edition. Edited by Arri Coomarasamy, Mahmood I. Shafi, G. Willy Davila and Kiong K. Chan.
© 2016 John Wiley & Sons, Ltd. Published 2016 by John Wiley & Sons, Ltd.

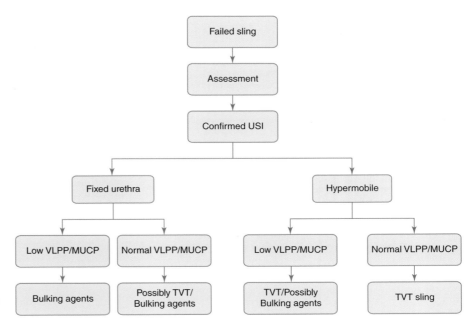

Figure 109.1 An algorithm for management of patients with failed sling operation. MUCP, maximal urethral closure pressure; USI, urodynamic stress incontinence; TVT, tension-free vaginal tape; VLPP, Valsalva leak point pressure.

Management of complex incontinence (mixed incontinence and incontinence due to voiding abnormalities)

If uninhibited detrusor contractions are identified associated with symptomatic urine loss events, then therapy should be directed toward the OAB component, with proven effective therapies such as pharmacotherapy or rehabilitative therapy. If obstructed voiding is identified, medical therapy with alpha blockers or baclofen may be useful but, frequently, relief of outflow obstruction is needed. The most effective means of addressing post-sling outflow obstruction is sling transection (Chapter 103).

Artificial urinary sphincter

Although there are few current data on the use of the artificial sphincter in women, this can be a viable option in the hands of experienced surgeons.

Adjustable slings

Suprapubically adjustable slings allow the tension to be adjusted postoperatively. The currently available sling (Remeex, Neomedic, Spain) has a growing evidence base in primary and recurrent SUI. Improvements in continence can be expected particularly in women with more severe degrees of persistent SUI [12].

Burch colposuspension

An abdominal retropubic approach is not an unreasonable approach to a woman with persistent SUI. The presence of ISD may make it less attractive as success rates are recognized to be lower. Careful dissection into the space of Retzius and a larger abdominal incision will facilitate exposure, given the context of probable scarring along the tape tracts [13].

KEY POINTS

Challenge: Recurrent or persistent stress incontinence after sling surgery.

Background
- Long-term success rate for sling operations for SUI is 90%.
- Patient expectations are key when determining preoperative goals for SUI therapy.
- Potential causes for sling failure include:
  - Failure of the sling to fix and anchor into tissue.
  - Misplacement or migration of the sling (or lack of urethral fixation).
  - Intrinsic sphincter deficiency (ISD).
  - Presence of complex incontinence (coexistent DO or voiding dysfunction).

Prevention
- Primary retropubic monofilament polypropylene slings have the highest success rate, and thus should be performed with the goal of optimizing success.

Management
- Assess the patient:
  - History, including the nature and extent of urinary symptoms, changes since the operation, and any new OAB symptoms.
  - Examination, including evaluation of the urethra and the bladder neck for hypermobility, sling assessment (location, mesh erosion, and tenderness), and the empty supine stress test.
  - Investigations, including three-dimensional ultrasound, cystoscopy, and multichannel urodynamics.
- Identify patient's treatment goals so as to individualize the management to the patient's unique circumstances.
- Medical management can include pelvic floor exercises and physiotherapy, and pharmacotherapy with duloxetine or α-agonists such as imipramine.
- Currently, most commonly available treatment is placement of a retropubic sling (e.g., TVT) or injection of bulking agents.
- Retropubic slings are more effective than transobturator slings for repeat operations.
- If there are concerns with mesh material in the vagina, the alternative of Burch colposuspension or pubovaginal sling can be discussed.
- Referral to a urologist to consider artificial urethral sphincter is an option with failed sling.

References

1 Nilsson CG, Palva K, Rezapour M, Falconer C. Eleven years prospective follow-up of the tension-free vaginal tape procedure for treatment of stress urinary incontinence. *Int Urogynecol J Pelvic Floor Dysfunct* 2008;19:1043–1047.

2 Castillo PA, Espaillat-Rijo LM, Davila GW. Outcome measures and definition of cure in female stress urinary incontinence surgery: a survey of recent publications. *Int Urogynecol J* 2010;21:343–348.

3 Smith A, Artibani W, Drake M. Managing unsatisfactory outcomes after mid-urethral tape insertion. *Neurourol Urodyn* 2011;30:771–774.

4 Rezapour M, Falconer C, Umsten U. Tension-free vaginal tape (TVT) in stress incontinent women with intrinsic sphincteric deficiency (ISD): a long-term follow-up. *Int Urogynecol J Pelvic Floor Dysfunct* 2001;12(Suppl 2):S12–S14.

5 Smith AL, Karp DR, Aguilar VC, Davila GW. Repeat versus primary slings in patients with intrinsic sphincter deficiency. *Int Urogynecol J* 2013;24:963–968.

6 Schierlitz L, Dwyer P, Rosamilla A *et al*. Three year follow-up of tension-free vaginal tape compared with transobturator tape in women with stress urinary incontinence and intrinsic sphincteric deficiency. *Obstet Gynecol* 2012;119:321–327.

7 Guerette NL, Bena JF, Davila GW. Transobdurator slings for stress incontinence: using urodynamic parameters to predict outcomes. *Int Urogynecol J* 2008;19(1):97–102.

8 Pradhan A, Jain P, Latthe PM. Effectiveness of midurethral slings in recurrent stress urinary incontinence: a systematic review and meta-analysis. *Int Urogynecol J* 2012;23:831–41.

9 Rezapour M, Ulmsten U. Tension-free vaginal tape (TVT) in women with recurrent stress urinary incontinence: a long term follow-up. *Int Urogynecol J Pelvic Floor Dysfunct* 2001;12(Suppl 2):S9–S11.

10 Petrou SP, Frank I. Complications and initial continence rates after a repeat pubovaginal sling procedure for recurrent stress urinary incontinence. *J Urol* 2001;165:1979–1981.

11 Ghoneim GM, Miller, CJ. A systematic review and meta-analysis of Macroplastique for treating female stress urinary incontinence. *Int Urogynecol J* 2013;24:27–36.

12 Giberti C, Gallo F, Cortese P, Schenone M. The suburethral adjustable sling (Remeex system) in the treatment of female urinary incontinence due to "true" intrinsic sphincteric deficiency: results after 5 year of mean follow-up. *BJU Int* 2011;108:1140–1144.

13 Maher C, Dwyer P, Carey M, Gilmour C. The Burch colposuspension for recurrent stress urinary incontinence following retropubic continence surgery. *Br J Obstet Gynaecol* 1999;106:719–724.

CHAPTER 110
Difficult Vaginal Hysterectomy

G. Willy Davila
Cleveland Clinic Florida, Weston/Fort Lauderdale, Florida, USA

Case history: An obese 43-year-old woman with two previous cesarean sections is scheduled to undergo a vaginal hysterectomy for abnormal bleeding. Prior to her pregnancies, she had a history of severe endometriosis in the posterior cul de sac and had undergone an abdominal uterine suspension. On examination she has an immobile uterus and a narrow introitus. She is insisting on a vaginal approach. Should you acquiesce to her wishes?

Background

Suspicion that a vaginal hysterectomy may be technically difficult is very important to allow the pelvic surgeon to plan for potential means of optimizing completion of the procedure, to maintain safety, and to obtain appropriate preoperative informed consent. Unfortunately, a surgeon does not often realize the TVH will be difficult until positioning the patient after anesthesia induction, or until the procedure has been started. Experienced surgeons use the preoperative history and pelvic examination to assess for the likelihood of a TVH being technically challenging (or impossible).

Preoperative consent for possible laparoscopic or open approach is important in maintaining realistic expectations from the patient's perspective. In this particular case, alternatives to hysterectomy such as endometrial ablation, progesterone IUD insertion, and systemic hormonal therapy should be seriously considered and attempted before proceeding with TVH.

Preoperative imaging is crucial for identifying and mapping uterine or adnexal masses. Although most can be readily managed vaginally, certain masses can contraindicate a vaginal approach. Certainly, any mass suspicious for cancer should be managed with a staging procedure in mind, typically abdominally.

There are multiple findings on preoperative assessment that can raise the surgeon's index of suspicion that the surgery will be difficult (or even contraindicated) (Box 110.1). On vaginal examination, mucosal scarring along the anterior or posterior fornices strongly suggests the presence of submucosal scarring.

Management

Intraoperative factors which can help facilitate TVH include the presence of knowledgeable and experienced assistants and use of Allen stirrups to provide a safe high lithotomy position. The patient's

> **BOX 110.1 FACTORS SUGGESTIVE OF A DIFFICULT TVH**
>
> - Immobile uterus: lack of descent or fixed in position
> - Markedly retroverted uterus, suggesting obliterated posterior cul de sac
> - Palpable adnexal/uterine mass: imaging recommended for evaluation
> - Hypertrophied and/or very narrow cervix
> - Inability to reach lateral cervico-uterine junction (uterine vessels)
> - Abdominal wall scars: suggestive of pelvic adhesions or possible uterine suspension
> - Reduced patient hip/leg mobility
> - Obese patient with a deep vagina
> - Previous cesarean section(s)
> - Nulliparity
> - Uterine procidentia

buttocks should be at the edge of the table when the foot of the bed is removed. The patient's thighs should be flexed and abducted, and the knees should be flexed with minimal external rotation.

To avoid neuropathy, it is important to consider whether padding the lateral aspect of the lower extremity is needed to avoid compression against the stirrup. Surgical equipment can make the difference between a difficult hysterectomy looking rather routine or adding further challenge. Surgical tools of value include focused surgical field lighting and lighted suction cannulae or speculae, energy sources (cautery, Ligasure™) for maintaining hemostasis and aiding in the ligation of pedicles, Haney-type angled needle drivers, weighted speculae, and Brietsky-Navratil and Deaver retractors. A self-retaining retractor can help with visualization when additional assistance is not available. Two types are available: the Lone Star Retractor System (Cooper-Surgical, Inc., Trumbull, CT) and the Magrina-Bookwalter Vaginal Retractor (Codman, Raynham, MA). Injecting submucosal lidocaine with epinephrine can reduce soft tissue oozing and bleeding. Initiating the TVH with posterior cul de sac entry (main ligaments) facilitates the procedure by transecting the main supportive ligaments and allowing safer entry than the anterior cul de sac approach.

Enlarged uterus

Fibroids per se are not a contraindication to TVH. If large fibroids are present, preoperative hormonal shrinkage with GnRH analogs or ulipristal acetate can be achieved. Lower uterine segment fibroids (especially when located in a lateral position) can impede ligation of the uterine vessels; if hemostasis cannot be achieved by ligation of the uterine vessels, most surgeons would advise against proceeding with the surgery.

Gynecologic and Obstetric Surgery: Challenges and Management Options, First Edition. Edited by Arri Coomarasamy, Mahmood I. Shafi, G. Willy Davila and Kiong K. Chan.
© 2016 John Wiley & Sons, Ltd. Published 2016 by John Wiley & Sons, Ltd.

Midline, fundal and intramural fibroids can usually be managed vaginally with uterine debulking techniques. These should only be performed after hemostasis is confirmed and the anterior and posterior cul de sacs have been entered and retractors placed to protect the bladder and rectum. Debulking techniques include the following.

1. Uterine bivalving, with or without cervical amputation;
2. Subserosal circumscription and intramyometrial coring (Figure 110.1);
3. Bisection of the posterior cervix into the posterior cul de sac.

During debulking, multiple myomectomies can be performed. As the uterine volume is reduced, anatomic asymmetry is also reduced, and the surgeon can follow routine TVH techniques to complete the procedure. A fibroid corkscrew can be useful to put fibroids under traction to aid in removal.

Cervical fibroids may make the procedure extremely difficult due to limited access to the uterine vessels.

Undescended uterus

An undescended uterus in the office may indeed descend remarkably under anesthesia. However, if previous uterine suspension has been performed, or if multiple thick adhesions fixating the uterus are suspected (or known), it is unlikely that there will be increased uterine mobility under anesthesia. Typically, a fixated uterus will promptly recoil back up after being put under traction during a pelvic examination. I prefer to use a long Allis clamp to place traction on the uterus, rather than a single tooth tenaculum.

In order to optimize the odds of completing a TVH of an undescended uterus, intraoperative massage of the uterosacral and cardinal ligaments with the uterus under traction, making sure the bladder is not overly distended, and cutting a generous episiotomy (which reduces vaginal depth) can help reduce the surgery's complexity.

The focus of TVH should be to enter the posterior and anterior cul de sacs as soon as possible, thus allowing ligation of the uterine vessels and sequential bites along the broad and utero-ovarian ligaments in order to complete the procedure.

Previous cesarean section(s)

Previous cesarean section need not be a contraindication to TVH. However, multiple cesarean sections lead to greater degrees of scarring and bladder adherence to the lower uterine segment. Imaging with ultrasound may help in assessing the vesico-uterine reflection, and evaluating the thickness of the bladder wall.

Intraoperatively, care should be taken to identify the correct layer for dissecting the bladder off the lower uterine segment. The subfascial yellow fatty layer is typically readily identifiable with sharp dissection (Figure 110.2). Care should be taken not to initiate the incision above the bladder reflection.

Keeping the bladder somewhat distended during the TVH can help identify the bladder location and clearly identify any cystotomy if it occurs. I personally do not insert a Foley catheter until after I have entered the anterior cul de sac and clamped the uterine vessels bilaterally. The posterior entry approach can also help the surgeon identify the anterior bladder reflection by inserting the index finger into the posterior cul de sac and wrapping it around the uterus onto the anterior uterine surface (Figure 110.3). If a cystotomy occurs, the surgeon can use the clearly visible bladder wall to guide in subsequent dissection, and the defect can be repaired once the anterior cul de sac is entered and/or the TVH is further advanced (or completed).

Obliterated anterior or posterior cul de sac

An obliterated anterior cul de sac, especially if the bladder is adherent to or over the uterine fundus, can make the risk of cystotomy very high. Care should be taken to avoid bluntly dissecting the bladder off the uterine surface, with the use of a gauze sponge. Once the incision is made on the vaginal wall along the anterior bladder reflection, a Deaver retractor is used to retract the bladder anteriorly as the incision is carried onto the level of the pre-peritoneal fatty layer. This layer allows the surgeon to palpate the anterior surface of the uterus and further retract the bladder with the retractor until the peritoneal reflection off the uterus is clearly seen. I leave the bladder full during this process.

Posterior cul de sac obliteration is less common. Options for accessing the posterior cul de sac are reviewed in Chapter 111.

Cervical hypertrophy

The presence of a very narrow, long cervix can trick an inexperienced surgeon into thinking that the procedure will be a very easy "fall out" hysterectomy. The narrower the cervix, the more difficult the TVH may be. Amputation of the cervix during TVH can be a serious complication as the uterus can retract into the pelvic cavity and the tissue layers can become difficult to identify.

This interesting anatomic variation leads to the posterior cul de sac being multiple centimeters above the external cervical os while the bladder reflection can be in very close proximity to the external os. The surgeon must remember that the ureters can be pulled down along the lateral cervix as the uterus prolapses, putting them at risk of ligation, especially in cases of cervical hypertrophy.

It is important to dissect the bladder off the hypertrophied cervix as the TVH is performed. The anterior cul de sac is typically not entered until multiple tissue bites have been taken. The careful surgeon will be stoical in taking small tissue bites in a stepwise fashion, as long as the anterior retractor is holding the bladder out of harm's way, during this type of TVH. If continued difficulty is encountered in identifying the peritoneal reflection, the uterus may be bisected (preferably along its posterior surface) once the surgeon is confident that the uterine arteries have been ligated. This will eventually allow identification of the peritoneal reflection. Amputations of the long cervix may be needed to allow better traction on the uterus. If this maneuver is performed, the surgeon must be certain to maintain traction on the proximal cervical stump in order to not lose anatomic orientation.

Very large bulky cervix

A vault-filling cervix can make any of the initial TVH steps difficult to perform. In order to facilitate this procedure, a LEEP volume reduction procedure can be performed. This can include the distal external os and cervical mass.

Adnexal masses

Large or suspicious ovarian or tubal masses may contraindicate a vaginal approach to TVH. If a mass is found incidentally during TVH, the surgeon must make a decision as to whether the mass would be best removed abdominally. Cystic paratubal cysts are not uncommonly found and can be rather large. If the mass cannot be removed as an intact cyst, the fluid can be aspirated but only if the visual appearance is that of a completely benign cyst.

Fortunately, experienced surgeons can remove most adnexae (when planned) vaginally (see Chapter 112).

After completing the removal of the uterus, I typically grasp the ovary with a Babcock clamp and gently massage its base to help it descend as much as possible. I then pack the bowels with gauze and grasp the tube with smooth pickups. The infundibulopelvic ligament can then be cut and doubly ligated.

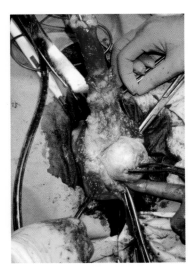

Figure 110.1 Uterine debulking: intramyometrial coring and myomectomy.

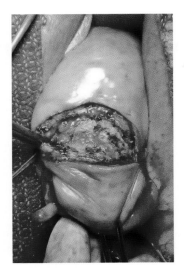

Figure 110.2 Normal planes for anterior reflection of the bladder from the lower uterine segment.

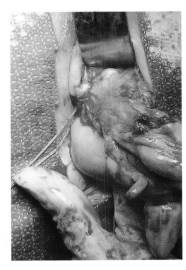

Figure 110.3 Uterine anterior-fundal adhesions lysed with the index finger brought through the posterior colpotomy after the uterus is delivered posteriorly.

Thick pelvic adhesions

Pelvic adhesions involving the pelvic organs are not uncommon. Fortunately, most are thin and can be readily cut or broken down bluntly. Thick omental or bowel adhesions obliterating the posterior cul de sac can be very problematic, and make posterior entry difficult. In such a case, anterior entry should be considered. The surgeon should refrain from cutting through omentum-like fatty tissue as it can be very vascular.

Thick adhesions in the anterior cul de sac are typically the result of cesarean section, as discussed earlier. Thick adhesions to the uterine fundus are less problematic.

Nulliparity

Absence of a preceding vaginal delivery is not in itself a contraindication to TVH. However, the surgeon must be ready to deal with the reduced vaginal caliber and lack of uterine descent. Narrower retractors can facilitate visualization. Performing a large episiotomy can enlarge a restricted introitus, but more importantly shorten the posterior vaginal wall and bring the cervix closer to the introitus. Methodical traction on the uterus, and directed massage of the uterosacral and cardinal ligaments, can further bring the uterus closer to the introitus. Since the uterosacral ligaments will be readily identifiable during cuff closure, the use of energy sources such as Ligasure™ to ligate supportive ligaments has a more important role in this type of TVH.

Anatomic barriers to TVH

A narrow subpubic arch limits uterine descent and may, by itself, pose a significant barrier to TVH. Not much can be done about this.

Reduced patient mobility, especially of the hips or lower spine, can make achieving a satisfactory lithotomy position challenging, and may make TVH impossible. Practice patient positioning in the office can indicate whether intraoperative positioning will be comfortable for the patient. It is key to avoid hip dislocation or vertebral disk trauma during TVH (or in positioning prior to the procedure).

Adjunctive procedures of value

Posterior cul de sac teloscopy, after peritoneal cavity CO_2 insufflation (umbilical, posterior cul de sac or through the uterine fundus), can help visualize the posterior cul de sac, uterine fundus, and other pelvic structures. This simple technique using laparoscopic or hysteroscopic instruments can reassure the surgeon as to intraperitoneal anatomy. In addition, insufflation will distend the peritoneal cavity and facilitate posterior (and even anterior) entry.

Laparoscopy can help evaluate intraperitoneal anatomy when adhesions or other pelvic or adnexal problems are suspected. Laparoscopically assisted TVH with laparoscopic ligation of infundibulopelvic ligaments and broad ligaments can facilitate TVH. The anterior bladder dissection can also be created. Most surgeons leave the lower uterine supports to be ligated vaginally in order to facilitate vault suspension procedures such as McCall culdoplasty.

KEY POINTS

Background
- Despite the best preparation, a vaginal hysterectomy can prove to be technically difficult.

Management
- Preoperative assessment is key to surgical planning for vaginal hysterectomy. The few absolute contraindications to vaginal hysterectomy include severe endometriosis and advanced pelvic malignancy.
- Relative contraindications are multiple cesarean deliveries, suspected abdominal adhesions, pathologic processes of the adnexa, and the necessity to perform bilateral salpingo-oophorectomy. In these cases, laparoscopic assistance might be appropriate.
- Uterine size greater than 14–16 weeks requires the expertise of a vaginal surgeon comfortable with uterine debulking techniques including coring and bivalving.
- Appropriate positioning of the patient, adequate lighting, retraction and patience are essential.

Prevention
- If examination under anesthesia suggests that vaginal hysterectomy is going to be fraught with risks, it will be better to convert the route in the interests of patient safety.

Further reading

ACOG Committee Opinion No. 444. Choosing the route of hysterectomy for benign disease. *Obstet Gynecol* 2009;114:1156–1158.

Kulkarni MM, Rogers RG. Vaginal hysterectomy for benign disease without prolapse. *Clin Obstet Gynecol* 2010;53:5–16.

Lucero M, Shah AD. Vaginal hysterectomy for the prolapsed uterus. *Clin Obstet Gynecol* 2010;53:26–39.

Figueiredo Netto O, Figueiredo O. Difficult vaginal hysterectomy. In: Figueiredo O, Figueiredo Netto O (eds) *Histerectomia Vaginal: Novas Perspectivas*, pp. 133–143. Novo Conceito, Brazil, 2002.

CHAPTER 111

Vaginal Hysterectomy: Difficulty in Entering the Posterior Pouch

Alfredo Jijon and G. Willy Davila

Cleveland Clinic Florida, Weston/Fort Lauderdale, Florida, USA

Case history: A woman with a history of endometriosis and a grade 3 uterine prolapse elects to have a vaginal hysterectomy. The surgeon intends to access the peritoneal cavity through a posterior approach, but intraoperatively he realizes the posterior cul-de-sac is not easily accessible and there are some nodules in the posterior part of the cervix.

Background

There are a variety of commonly used techniques for vaginal hysterectomy. These include initial anterior cul-de-sac (bladder reflection) entry, circumscription of the vaginal mucosa at the cervico-uterine junction and blunt dissection off the uterus prior to anterior or posterior entry, and initial entry into peritoneal cavity via the posterior cul-de-sac (which is usually easier than anterior access) [1]. Surgeons tend to select one approach based on training and personal experience. We prefer to initiate a vaginal hysterectomy via a posterior colpotomy incision as it is associated with less blood loss and risk of trauma to viscera, and facilitates identification of the uterosacral ligaments for subsequent vault suspension prior to cuff closure.

There is a significant difference in surgery progression when there is a difficult approach into the posterior cul-de-sac, compared with the anterior bladder reflection, which does not influence surgery progression as much [2]. It is very unusual to not be able to readily enter the posterior cul-de-sac. However, a surgeon should be familiar with alternatives to simple colpotomy entry, as anatomic or pathologic conditions may necessitate an alternative approach.

Consequences of not readily entering the posterior cul-de-sac include bleeding and inaccurate identification and isolation of uterosacral ligaments, which are needed to provide vaginal support and prevent post-hysterectomy vault prolapse. Among the few accepted relative contraindications to vaginal hysterectomy is the lack of uterine mobility or descent, as in the case with past history of endometriosis, pelvic inflammatory disease, myomectomy, or multiple cesarean sections [3]. Obliteration of the posterior cul-de-sac by adhesions, endometriosis or fat can be found even in the absence of a suggestive history.

When there is a non-mobile uterus, one must suspect that there are adhesions in the area surrounding the uterus, uterine fibroids or some type of adnexal mass that is not allowing the uterus to move freely. When this occurs, the vaginal approach becomes difficult because the peritoneal cavity cannot be easily entered, either anteriorly or posteriorly.

Significant cervical pathology results in multiple anatomic alterations, especially when associated with a large cystocele.

Management

Assessment

The first step in any successful vaginal surgery is the performance of a complete and methodical pelvic examination to carefully assess the anatomic characteristics of the pelvis. Vaginal and rectal examinations are needed, and ultrasound imaging can be considered to help anticipate any adverse situation, such as cervical fibroids or bowel filling the posterior cul-de-sac. These assessments can provide the surgeon with a fairly precise idea of the ability to enter the appropriate operative spaces, such as the posterior cul-de-sac. If difficulties are anticipated, the surgery can be performed by a different approach, or the patient can be referred to a more experienced or specialized surgeon.

Posterior cul-de-sac entry

The first step is identifying the site of peritoneal reflection of the posterior cul-de-sac peritoneum from the cervix, seen as a shift of vaginal mucosa fixed to the cervix and becoming more mobile (Figure 111.1). This area can be readily identified by lifting the vaginal skin using teeth pickups and observing the cul-de-sac edge (Figures 111.2 and 111.3). A full-thickness incision can be made with curved Mayo scissors and the full thickness of peritoneum to vaginal mucosa tagged with a suture (Figures 111.4 and 111.5). Care must be taken to not incise the posterior reflection too distal along the posterior vaginal wall, as vaginal fore-shortening can result. In addition, once a mucosal incision is performed, the surgeon should refrain from pushing the peritoneal reflection off the posterior uterine surface, as that will increase the distance of the peritoneum from the incision.

Gynecologic and Obstetric Surgery: Challenges and Management Options, First Edition. Edited by Arri Coomarasamy, Mahmood I. Shafi, G. Willy Davila and Kiong K. Chan.
© 2016 John Wiley & Sons, Ltd. Published 2016 by John Wiley & Sons, Ltd.

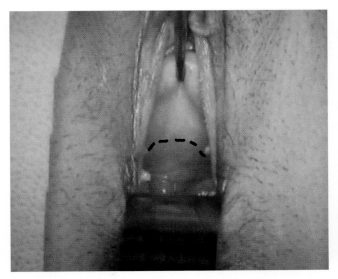

Figure 111.1 Observation of the posterior fornix vaginal mucosa can demonstrate the peritoneal reflection.

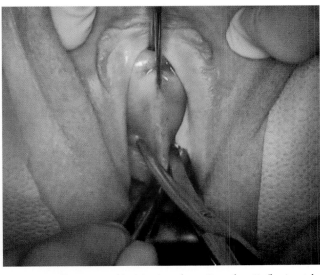

Figure 111.4 Transmucosal incision into the peritoneal cavity (horizontal approach).

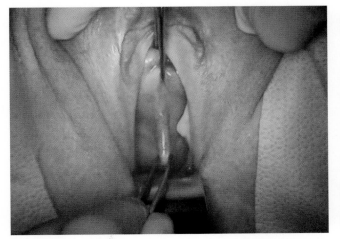

Figure 111.2 Vertical tenting for horizontal approach: tenting the vaginal wall vertically with teeth pickups demonstrates the peritoneal reflection and preferred site for incision.

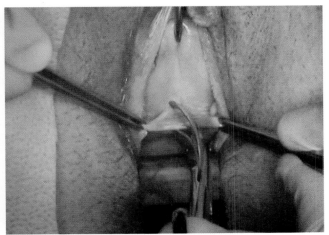

Figure 111.5 Transmucosal incision into the peritoneal cavity (vertical approach).

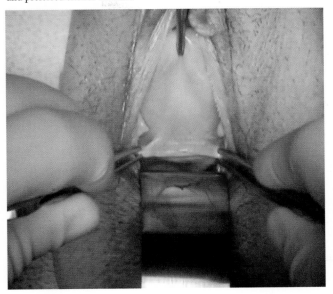

Figure 111.3 Horizontal tenting for vertical approach: tenting the vaginal wall horizontally with teeth pickups demonstrates the peritoneal reflection.

Entry into the posterior cul-de-sac can be challenging if there is an alteration in anatomy, or the space is filled with structures that are not usually found there. Obliteration of the posterior cul-de-sac by adhesions, endometriosis or fat can be found even in the absence of a suggestive history. A surgeon must always be wary of this finding. Lack of prompt entry into the peritoneal cavity should prompt plans for alternative entry techniques (see Alternative options below).

If there is a suspicion that there are alterations in the posterior cul-de-sac anatomy, the vaginal mucosal incision may be made vertically (Figure 111.5) rather than horizontally, from the mid-cervix up to the point where the posterior cul-de-sac becomes more apparent. Care must be taken to not make the incision too far vertically to avoid incising into the rectum. In addition, the surgeon must be careful to not dissect the peritoneal membrane further toward the uterine fundus via digital blunt dissection.

Regardless of the technique used (horizontal or vertical incision), care must be taken to not incise deeply into the uterus. If increased bleeding occurs and no obvious tissue plane is identified, the surgeon should determine if the peritoneal reflection is actually adherent to the vaginal epithelium and efforts should be made to confirm this suspicion by gently pulling soft tissue off the underside of the vaginal wall.

Once in the peritoneal cavity, clamping of the uterosacral and cardinal ligaments is easily performed. Once ligated, these ligaments should be tagged for ready identification and utilization for apical suspension.

The difficult-to-enter posterior cul-de-sac

If entering the posterior cul-de-sac is not possible, extraperitoneal clamping of the uterosacral and cardinal ligaments can be performed with or without a partial colpotomy incision. The cardinal and uterosacral ligaments can be divided first, thus enabling greater mobility of the uterus and easier identification of the posterior peritoneal fold. It must be noted that the safe ligation of the uterine vessels requires the incorporation of the anterior and posterior broad ligament peritoneum, otherwise significant bleeding can result from incomplete tying of the vessels. Even though there are several authors who recommend this maneuver, this can also make the surgery more complex by further altering normal anatomy. This may lead to a higher propensity for bleeding or difficulty performing a uterosacral ligament suspension.

The vaginal hysterectomy can be started by making a circumferential vaginal mucosal incision at the cervico-vaginal junction, and the vaginal mucosa bluntly dissected superiorly until reaching the peritoneal reflection anteriorly and posteriorly. This is intended to facilitate entry into both anterior and posterior cul-de-sacs. The disadvantage of this technique is that if the initial incision is made too deeply, there could be a considerable amount of bleeding. Pre-incision injection of hemostatic agents such as vasopressin or epinephrine may help reduce blood loss. In addition, surgeons tend to fear accidental entry into the bladder and make a shallow incision, leading to further bleeding and surgeon anxiety.

If the posterior cul-de-sac cannot be entered, one option is to enter through the anterior peritoneum (Chapter 110). This may allow the surgeon to digitally palpate up to, and possibly around, the uterine fundus and identify the presence of adhesions or other abnormalities in the posterior cul-de-sac [4].

Alternative options

Suggested means of achieving access to the posterior cul-de-sac when the other approaches have failed include the following.

- Insufflation of the peritoneal cavity, to distend the posterior cul-de-sac. This procedure may allow the surgeon to gain a more precise idea of where the cavity is located, and decrease the risk of perforating other organs. It may be achieved with a Veress needle placed through the abdominal wall, into the posterior cul-de-sac, or through the uterine fundus.
- Rectal examination may offer the surgeon a broader perspective of the situation, inform the decision of how to proceed, and determine whether a perforation has occurred during attempts to dissect the rectovaginal septum.

- If the posterior and anterior approaches fail, a rectal examination may be helpful to mobilize the anterior rectal wall away from the uterus and posterior vaginal wall. With sharp dissection between the anterior rectal wall and the posterior cervix, the peritoneal reflection may be reached and incised. Care must obviously be taken to avoid contamination of the surgical field.
- Laparoscopy: if neither posterior nor anterior peritoneal approach is possible, the likely best option, and what experienced surgeons recommend, may be laparoscopic exploration to identify and resolve the causes of technical challenges such as adhesions, or conversion to laparoscopic or laparoscopic-assisted vaginal hysterectomy, or simply open abdominal hysterectomy.

KEY POINTS

Challenge: Difficulty in entering the posterior pouch during vaginal hysterectomy.

Background
- Initial entry into the peritoneal cavity during a vaginal hysterectomy can be via the anterior or posterior cul-de-sac.
- Vaginal hysterectomy via a posterior colpotomy incision is associated with less blood loss and risk of trauma to viscera, and facilitates identification of the uterosacral ligaments for subsequent vault suspension prior to cuff closure.
- Preoperative case selection is important.
- Risk factors for difficult entry into the peritoneal cavity include endometriosis, PID, myomectomy, multiple cesarean sections, adhesions, or a large cervical fibroid.
- When peritoneal access proves to be challenging, the surgeon's experience becomes a critical prognostic factor.

Management
- If there is a suspicion that there are alterations in the posterior cul-de-sac anatomy, make the vaginal mucosal incision vertically rather than horizontally.
- When the peritoneum cannot be entered posteriorly, try anteriorly.
- If neither posterior nor anterior approach is possible, options are:
  - Extraperitoneal division of cardinal and uterosacral ligaments, to enable greater mobility of the uterus and possibly easier identification of the posterior peritoneal fold.
  - Laparoscopic assessment of the pelvis to guide further management.
  - Conversion to laparoscopic or open hysterectomy.

References

1 Sheth SS. Preoperative assessment. In: Sheth S, Studd J (eds) *Vaginal Hysterectomy*. Isis Medical Media, Oxford, 2002.
2 Hong DG, Seong WJ, Lee YS, Cho YL. Analysis of factor affecting vaginal hysterectomy. *Minim Invasive Ther Allied Technol* 2009;18:317–321.
3 Allahbadia GN, Sheth SS. Access to vesicouterine and rectouterine pouhes. In: Sheth S, Studd J (eds) *Vaginal Hysterectomy*. Isis Medical Media, Oxford, 2002.
3 Stovall TG, Mann WJ. Vaginal hysterectomy. *UpToDate*, April 2012. Available at http://www.uptodate.com/contents/vaginal-hysterectomy

CHAPTER 112

Salpingo-oophorectomy at the Time of Vaginal Hysterectomy

Alfredo Jijon and G. Willy Davila
Cleveland Clinic Florida, Weston/Fort Lauderdale, Florida, USA

Case history: *A vaginal hysterectomy (TVH) with bilateral salpingo-oophorectomy (BSO) is planned for a 64-year-old woman with third-degree uterine prolapse. During the preoperative evaluation, a transvaginal ultrasound revealed a normal-sized uterus and normal right adnexa, but the left ovary contained a single 4-cm simple cyst.*

Background

Vaginal hysterectomy is the recommended surgical approach for benign uterine pathology [1]. For various reasons, the main approach to hysterectomy in the USA is abdominal, with only approximately 20% being performed vaginally [2]. A 2008 ACOG Practice Bulletin stated that when performing a routine hysterectomy in perimenopausal or menopausal women, the vaginal approach should be preferred, and a BSO should be considered after a detailed discussion regarding the risks and benefits of the procedure [3].

The purpose of performing a BSO at the time of TVH, especially in postmenopausal women, is reduction of ovarian cancer risk. In a UK study involving women aged 55–60 years undergoing hysterectomy, BSO was accomplished in 92% of those undergoing total abdominal hysterectomy (TAH) but in only 9.4% of those undergoing TVH [4]. It would seem surgeons are not as comfortable performing BSO vaginally as they are abdominally, even though reported success rates are high and complications low [5–7]. Although a laparoscopic approach can be used along with TVH to assist in removing the ovaries, the vaginal approach takes less time (approximately 15 min) and is more cost-effective [5,8].

One of the most likely causes for the lack of comfort in performing vaginal surgery, including BSO, is lack of training. In an attempt to remedy this situation, a recent study involved purposefully emphasizing the vaginal approach to hysterectomy during residency training. The percentage of TVH increased significantly relative to laparoscopic and abdominal hysterectomies, without an increase in the rate of complications [9].

If BSO cannot be performed at the time of TVH, or is not desired due to factors such as patient's age, bilateral salpingectomy should be strongly considered. Recent evidence has demonstrated that a large proportion of adnexal cancers actually originate from the mucosa of the fallopian tubes, rather than the ovarian surface [10]. Favoring this recommendation is the fact that tubes are typically much easier to remove vaginally than ovaries.

Factors influencing success of BSO at the time of TVH

Various studies have tried to identify predictive factors for the performance of BSO at the time of TVH. Poor prognostic factors for the performance of vaginal BSO include advanced age, high BMI, cervical length greater than 7 cm, lower uterine weight, previous pelvic surgery, uterine prolapse, anterior vaginal prolapse, endometriosis, and the presence of pelvic adhesions [9–11].

Kammerer-Doak *et al.* [12] reported that BSO could not be accomplished in 10% of 490 patients, when the procedure was attempted. Key factors included ovarian position in 76% and pelvic adhesions in 11%. The Baden–Walker scale has been used to describe the degree of ovarian descent once the hysterectomy has been completed (Box 112.1). Although this scale has not been widely used, it is helpful for describing ovarian support anatomy.

> **BOX 112.1 MODIFIED BADEN-WALKER GRADING OF OVARIAN DESCENT AT THE TIME OF HYSTERECTOMY [13]**
>
> 0 No descent defined. IPL little or no stretchability. Ovaries above ischial spine and cannot be brought down with traction.
> 1 IPL stretchability allows ovaries to be brought between ischial spines and mid-vagina
> 2 IPL stretchability allows ovaries to be brought between mid-vagina and hymen
> 3 IPL stretchability allows ovaries to be brought down past hymen

Management

Techniques used for vaginal BSO

Various techniques have been described for performing BSO following a TVH. All techniques require a clear operative field to allow visualization of the pelvic contents and mobilization of the adnexal structures. We describe the techniques used at our institution, with which we have reported high success rates for BSO performance [11].

Gynecologic and Obstetric Surgery: Challenges and Management Options, First Edition. Edited by Arri Coomarasamy, Mahmood I. Shafi, G. Willy Davila and Kiong K. Chan.
© 2016 John Wiley & Sons, Ltd. Published 2016 by John Wiley & Sons, Ltd.

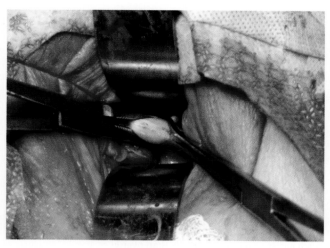

Figure 112.1 Vaginal oophorectomy performed on safe exposure of ovary with a Babcock clamp.

Once the uterus has been removed, and all pedicles are properly secured, a moistened open gauze sponge is inserted into the pelvic cavity to keep the intestines and omentum out of the operative field. The tail of the sponge is left externalized and held in place with the contralateral uterosacral ligament pedicle tag. A curved Deaver-type retractor is placed along the anterior cuff, to hold the bladder out of harm's way. This will also help maintain the ureters along the lateral pelvis. A second Deaver retractor may be needed along the posterior vaginal cuff. A long Babcock clamp is used to grasp both the ovary and oviduct. The distal fimbriated end is gently pulled into the operative field so the entire tube is visualized. A curved Heaney clamp is then placed along the infundibulopelvic ligament (IPL) and mesosalpinx (Figure 112.1). It is critical that the distal edge of the clamp is clearly visualized before clamping it down. The adnexa can then be excised, and the pedicle twice ligated. If the pedicle is too wide for a single bite, multiple bites may be required. The clamps should be kept as close to the base of the ovary as possible, in order to minimize the risk of ureteral damage. The tied suture should not be cut until hemostasis is confirmed, as it can be used to provide gentle traction to the base of the adnexa.

A hydrosalpinx or benign-appearing ovarian cyst can be needle-drained prior to removal in order to reduce bulk. Any suspicious adnexal mass should be removed intact, or consideration given to laparoscopic or open removal.

Various energy sources and instruments are available to facilitate vaginal BSO. The surgeon should be able to handle any residual bleeding if a non-suture-based technique is used. Among the commonly used devices is Ligasure™, which has been shown to reduce surgical time, estimated blood loss, and hospital stay [14]. Laparoscopically, this energy source has been shown to be equivalent to conventional bipolar cautery for BSO [15]. Other reported devices which may assist in vaginal BSO include the Endoloop® suture device to facilitate pedicle ligation. The traditional clamp, cut and suture techniques are quite fast, effective and cheap.

Complications of vaginal BSO

Bleeding from pedicles

Bleeding from a BSO pedicle can occur due to tissue or knot slippage, suture breakage, or soft-tissue tearing. It can usually be addressed vaginally, without the need to resort to an open or laparoscopic approach. The surgeon should be methodical and not simply apply cautery to areas which appear to be bleeding. Gentle tissue handling is key to managing unexpected bleeding. Appropriate use of retractors and gauze packing will help improve visualization. A long tonsil clamp can be placed on the ligated pedicle in order to provide some traction. The surgeon can then "walk up" the pedicle and visualize proximal and distal segments for bleeding sites. Typically, a venous bleeder can be seen along the proximal segment of the pedicle, and can be clamped and separately ligated. In addition, judicious cautery or surgical clips can be used.

Ureteral injury

Ureteral injury is always a concern for the vaginal surgeon. The proximity of the ureter to the ovarian vessels should be kept in mind, especially if anatomy is altered. Although the risk of ureteral injury at the time of TVH is known to be low, few data are available regarding the risk of ureteral injury at the time of vaginal BSO. The anterior cuff/bladder retractor should be held securely in place once the anterior cul-de-sac is entered. This is especially true in patients with exteriorized uterine prolapse, where a large cystocele will lead to the descent of the ureters as well [16]. Some surgeons recommend routine cystoscopy at the time of TVH, as with any advanced prolapse repair, in order to ascertain ureteral function [17]. Certainly, if anatomy was significantly altered, or the surgery did not proceed completely routinely, cystoscopy should be considered at the conclusion of the procedure.

Adnexal malignancy

Occult or overt adnexal malignancy as an incidental surgical finding during TVH should be followed by confirmation and appropriate follow-up. Intraoperative consultation with a gynecologic oncologist, if available, should be considered if a suspicious mass is identified. If the mass is freely mobile and can be removed without tissue spillage, it can be removed and appropriate postoperative evaluation performed. The contralateral ovary should be removed as well. The finding of a simple ovarian cyst is common. Cysts up to 6–7 cm in diameter can usually be removed intact. In order to help pull down an enlarged ovary, a reverse Asepto (or 10 mL) syringe attached to suction can be used to facilitate clamping. Cysts larger than 7 cm usually require aspiration prior to removal.

Transvaginal endoscopy

Inserting an endoscope through the vaginal incision to visualize the upper pelvic contents has been reported to be helpful for vaginal BSO. Insufflation is not needed, but good bowel retraction and Trendelenburg position may be helpful. Cooperation from the anesthesiologist in allowing for abdominal wall relaxation is key to permitting clear visualization with this technique.

KEY POINTS

Challenge: Performance of BSO at time of TVH.

Background
- The performance of BSO should be discussed and encouraged in every postmenopausal woman undergoing TVH.

- Planning to perform a BSO in patients undergoing hysterectomy for benign pathology should not change the approach planned for the procedure.
- Poor prognostic factors for the performance of vaginal BSO include advanced age, high BMI, cervical length over 7 cm, lower uterine weight, previous pelvic surgery, uterine prolapse, anterior vaginal prolapse, endometriosis, and the presence of pelvic adhesions.

- The Baden–Walker scale can be used to describe degree of ovarian descent.

Management
- If adnexal tissue extends below the ischial spines, then vaginal BSO can almost certainly be performed.
- Safe vaginal BSO requires careful tissue handling and a methodical approach.

- The clamps on the IPL should be kept as close to the base of the ovary as possible to minimize risk of ureteral injury.
- A hydrosalpinx or benign-appearing ovarian cyst can be needle-drained prior to removal in order to reduce bulk.
- Any suspicious adnexal mass should be removed intact, or consideration given to laparoscopic or open removal.
- Transvaginal endoscopy to visualize the pelvis may be helpful in selected cases.

References

1 AAGL Advancing Minimally Invasive Gynecology Worldwide. AAGL Position Statement: route of hysterectomy to treat benign uterine disease. *J Minim Invasive Gynecol* 2011;18:1–3.
2 Jacoby VL, Autry A, Jacobson G, Domush R, Nakagawa S, Jacoby A. Nationwide use of laparoscopic hysterectomy compared with abdominal and vaginal approaches. *Obstet Gynecol* 2009;114:1041–1048.
3 American College of Obstetricians and Gynecologists. Elective and risk-reducing salpingo-oopherectomy. ACOG Practice Bulletin No. 89, January 2008. Available in *Obstet Gynecol* 2008;111:231–241.
4 Maresh MJ, Metcalfe MA, McPherson K *et al.* The VALUE national hysterectomy study: description of the patients and their surgery. *BJOG* 2002;109:302–312.
5 Davies A, O'Connor H, Magos AL. A prospective study to evaluate oopherectomy at the time of vaginal hysterectomy. *Br J Obstet Gynaecol* 1996;103:915–920.
6 Shain Y. Vaginal hysterectomy and oopherectomy in women with 12–20 weeks size uterus. *Acta Obstet Gynecol Scand* 2007;186:1359–1369.
7 Magrina J, Cornella L, Lee R. Vaginal salpingo-oopherectomy surgical techniques. *J Pelvic Surg* 1999;5:348–354.
8 Sheth SS, Malpani A. Routine prophylactic oopherectomy at the time of vaginal hysterectomy in postmenopausal women. *Obstet Gynecol* 1992;251:87–91.
9 Dunn T, Weaver A, Wolf D, Goddard W. Vaginal hysterectomies performed in a residency program. Can we increase the number? *J Reprod Med* 2006;51:83–86.
10 Dwyer P. Ovarian cancer and pelvic floor surgeon: the case for prophylactic bilateral salpingo-oopherectomy during POP surgery. *Int Urogynecol J* 2012;23:655–656.
11 Karp DR, Mukati M, Smith A, Suciu G, Aguilar VC, Davila GW. Predictors of successful salpingo-oopherectomy at the time of vaginal hysterectomy. *J Minim Invasive Gynecol* 2012;19:58–62.
12 Kammerer-Doak D, Magrina J, Weaver A, Lee R. Vaginal hysterectomy with and without oopherectomy: the Mayo Clinic experience. *J Pelvic Surg* 1996;2:304–306.
13 Kovac SR, Cruikshank SH. Guidelines to determine the route of oopherectomy with hysterectomy. Am J Obstet Gynecol 1996;175:1483–8.
14 Ding Z, Wable M, Rane A. Use of Ligasure bipolar diathermy system in vaginal hysterectomy. *J Obstet Gynecol* 2005;25:49–51.
15 Jansen PF, Brolmann HAH, van Kesteren PJM *et al.* Perioperative outcomes using LigaSure compared to conventional bipolar instruments in laparoscopic salpingo-oopherectomy: a randomized controlled trial. *Surg Endosc* 2012;26:2884–2891.
16 Sheth SS, Paghdiwalla KP, Hajari AR. Vaginal route: a gynaecological route for much more than hysterectomy. *Best Pract Res Clin Obstet Gynaecol* 2011;25:115–132.
17 Kovac SR. Vaginal hysterectomy. In: Rock JA, Jones HW (eds) *Te Linde's Operative Gynecology*, 10th edn. Lippincott Williams & Wilkins, Philadelphia, 2011.

CHAPTER 113

Bladder Injury During Anterior Vaginal Repair or Vaginal Hysterectomy

Pallavi Latthe[1], Suneetha Rachaneni,[2] and Mohammed Belal[3]

[1] Birmingham Women's NHS Foundation Trust, Birmingham, UK
[2] University of Birmingham, Birmingham, UK
[3] University Hospitals Birmingham NHS Foundation Trust, Birmingham, UK

Case history 1: *A 44-year-old woman with a grade 3 uterovaginal prolapse was found to have blood-stained urine following catheterization at the end of her vaginal hysterectomy and anterior repair.*

Case history 2: *A 52-year-old woman developed a bulge in the vagina 2 years following an anterior repair. She insisted on a reoperation for her anterior wall prolapse and was listed for a mesh anterior repair. A 2-cm hole was discovered in the anterior bladder wall during the dissection before mesh insertion.*

Background

Close anatomic association of genital and urinary organs predisposes the urinary tract to injury during pelvic surgery. Iatrogenic urinary tract injury results in secondary operations, prolonged catheterization, deterioration in quality of life, increased length of hospitalization, and litigation [1]. In the reports of studies involving routine cystoscopy in pelvic surgery, the overall frequency of bladder injury was 10.4 per 1000 and of ureteral injury was 6.2 per 1000. The risk of bladder injury with vaginal hysterectomy is 0.2 per 1000 [2].

Etiology

Common risk factors are previous anterior pelvic surgery (e.g., previous cesarean section or anterior vaginal wall repair), pelvic irradiation, and pelvic inflammatory disease. The limitations of transvaginal exposure, the variability in anterior vaginal wall thickness, and the proximity of the bladder base to the incision may explain the potential for bladder injury during transvaginal procedures. Bladder injuries are usually caused during dissection of the vaginal wall from the bladder. The increased incidence of bladder injuries with mesh repair is secondary to the use of trocar devices rather than the dissection of the vesicovaginal plane.

Occasionally, injuries may occur secondary to devascularization of the bladder wall or thermal injury during vaginal surgery, and may present several days after the operation.

Prevention

The best approach is to prevent lower urinary tract injury by meticulous and careful surgical technique: identifying, dissecting, and reflecting contiguous lower urinary tract structures during vaginal surgery. The role of local infiltration or hydrodissection at vaginal surgery is still debated [3], but 46% of surgeons in an international survey believed that it reduces the risk of visceral injury [4].

Use of routine intraoperative cystoscopy during major gynecologic and urogynecologic surgery might prevent the consequences of delayed recognition of lower urinary tract injuries [1]. Repair at the primary surgery is often easier and more successful. Adequate exposure, meticulous closure, and adequate duration of free drainage are essential for successful repair.

Management (see Chapter 35)

Diagnosis

Intraoperative findings can be extravasation of urine, a visible laceration, appearance of the Foley catheter in the operative area, or a sudden increase in bleeding from the wound. Intravesical instillation of methylene blue or indigo carmine through the catheter can help to diagnose bladder injury.

If ureteral injury is suspected, a cystoscopy is needed to evaluate ureteral integrity by observing for bilateral urinary jets from the ureteric orifices (Chapter 36). If there is uncertainty, it is important to seek help from a urologist. The urologist is likely to insert retrograde catheters through the ureteral orifices under fluoroscopic imaging. CT cystography may be required in cases of delayed presentation.

Treatment

If injury occurs, intraoperative repair should be carried out. This is done transvaginally in two layers using absorbable sutures (continuous non-interlocking or interrupted 2-0 or 3-0 Vicryl sutures). If the tissue is very friable, Monocryl suture causes less trauma. If the injury is in close proximity to either ureter, a ureteral stent should be placed under fluoroscopic imaging and cystoscopy guidance in order to avoid obstruction.

In case of posterior bladder injuries during dissection of scar tissues from previous cesarean section, the exposure is difficult and there is a higher risk of postoperative fistula formation. Omental interposition between bladder repair and vaginal wall may be required. Continuous bladder drainage with a large-bore Foley catheter for 7–14 days will be necessary depending on the extent of the injury. Prior to removal of the catheter, imaging such as a cystogram should be performed to confirm closure of the defect.

Gynecologic and Obstetric Surgery: Challenges and Management Options, First Edition. Edited by Arri Coomarasamy, Mahmood I. Shafi, G. Willy Davila and Kiong K. Chan.
© 2016 John Wiley & Sons, Ltd. Published 2016 by John Wiley & Sons, Ltd.

A suprapubic catheter may be necessary if there is a considerable amount of blood in the urine that could obstruct the catheter. If there is hematuria, a 22 Fr three-way catheter may be appropriate.

Persistent urinary leakage can resolve with an additional 2–4 weeks of bladder drainage. Prolonged urinary leakage after that period would indicate a vesicovaginal fistula [5].

Bladder injuries in patients undergoing mesh repair are best treated by repair of the injury in two to three layers (Case history 2). There is debate about whether these patients can have mesh inserted at the time of repair of the injury. In general, it would be prudent to avoid mesh insertion to avoid the risk of bladder mesh erosion later.

Undiagnosed injuries to the bladder that occur during surgery may become evident days after surgery as vesicovaginal fistulae. Electrocoagulation of bleeding vessels on the bladder wall during anterior repair may sometimes lead to delayed tissue necrosis and vesicovaginal fistula formation. In case of delayed presentation, transvaginal fistula closure with or without Martius graft interposition may be required. Martius graft is used for reconstruction of bladder base or urethral injuries (Figure 113.1). It is a vascularized flap taken from the labia majora with intact blood supply from the posterolateral perineal blood vessels [6]. This is best done by a surgeon with expertise in fistula surgery.

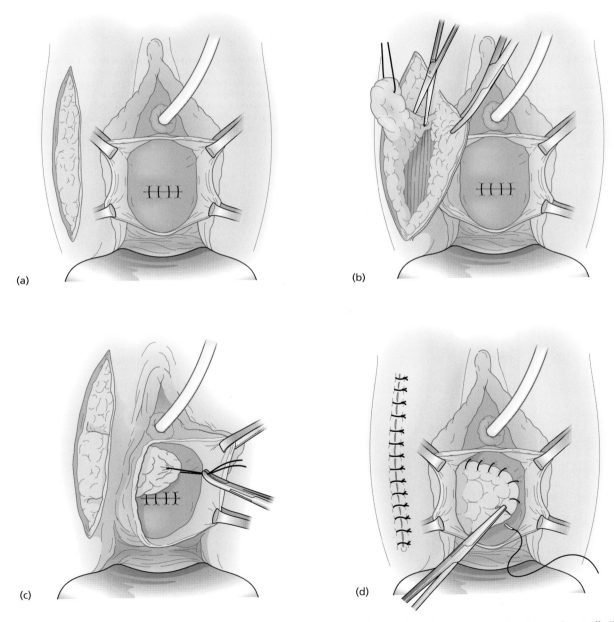

Figure 113.1 Martius fat pad graft for urethrovaginal or vesicovaginal fistula repair. (a) The lateral margin of the labia majora is incised vertically. The fat pad adjacent to the bulbocavernosus muscle is mobilized, leaving a broad pedicle attached at the inferior pole. (b, c) The fat pad is drawn through a tunnel beneath the labia minora and vaginal mucosa and sutured with delayed-absorbable sutures to the fascia of the urethra and bladder. (d) The vaginal mucosa is mobilized widely to permit closure over the pedicle without tension. The vulvar incision is closed with interrupted delayed-absorbable sutures.

KEY POINTS

Challenge: Bladder injury during anterior vaginal repair or vaginal hysterectomy.

Background
- Risk of bladder injury during anterior vaginal repair is about 0.5% but mesh insertion with trocars carries a higher risk of bladder injury.
- Only one in ten ureteral injuries and one in three bladder injuries are detected at the time of surgery without intraoperative cystoscopy.

Prevention
- Careful dissection of tissue planes, and judicious use of diathermy on bleeding vessels on the bladder surface reduce the possibility of injury.
- Use of routine intraoperative cystoscopy during major gynecologic and urogynecologic surgery can prevent the consequences from undetected lower urinary tract injuries.

Management (see Chapter 35)
- Patients with vaginal scarring from previous repair or those undergoing vaginal mesh reinforcement should be counseled about the increased risk of bladder injury.
- Transvaginal repair of vesical injury after prompt intraoperative recognition is essential for a good outcome.
- Repair is carried out in two layers with absorbable suture such Vicryl 2-0 or 3-0 (continuous non-interlocking or interrupted sutures).
- Continuous drainage with indwelling catheter for 7–14 days is required depending on the extent of bladder injury. Suprapubic catheter is not essential unless there is hematuria.
- Cystogram prior to trial without catheter should be performed.
- Vesicovaginal fistulae may be repaired transvaginally, with or without a Martius graft interposition.

References

1 Dwyer PL. Urinary tract injury: medical negligence or unavoidable complication? *Int Urogynecol J* 2010;21:903–910.
2 Härkki-Sirén P, Sjöberg J, Tiitinen A. Urinary tract injuries after hysterectomy. *Obstet Gynecol* 1998;92:113–118.
3 Ghezzi F, Cromi A, Raio L *et al*. Influence of the type of anesthesia and hydrodissection on the complication rate after tension-free vaginal tape procedure. *Eur J Obstet Gynecol Reprod Biol* 2005;118:96–100.
4 Latthe PM, Kadian S, Parsons M, Toozs-Hobson P. A survey of use of local infiltration in pelvic floor surgery. *Gynecol Surg* 2007;4:187–190.
5 Armenakas NA, Pareek G, Fracchia JA. Iatrogenic bladder perforations: longterm followup of 65 patients. *J Am Coll Surg* 2004;198:78–82.
6 Turner-Warwick R, Chapple C. The Martius labial-rotation flap support. In: *Reconstruction of the Urinary Tract and Gynaeco-Urology*, pp. 502–503. Blackwell Science Ltd, Oxford, 2002.

CHAPTER 114
Difficult Sacrocolpopexy

Orfhlaith E. O'Sullivan and Barry A. O'Reilly
Cork University Maternity Hospital, Cork, Ireland

Case history: A 50-year-old woman presented with a vault prolapse to the level of the genital hiatus. She had undergone a vaginal hysterectomy 10 years ago and the surgery was complicated by a pelvic hematoma, which required drainage under ultrasound guidance. Subsequent to the hysterectomy she was involved in a road traffic accident that left her with extensive injuries to her lower limbs, resulting in limited abduction.

Background

Up to 50% of parous women may develop pelvic organ prolapse (POP) [1]. Epidemiologic studies have shown that the lifetime risk of undergoing a single operation for prolapse or incontinence by the age of 80 is 11.1% [2]. The peak incidence of surgery is in individuals aged 60–69 years (42.1 per 10,000 women). Almost 58% of procedures are undertaken in women younger than 60 years [3]. Furthermore, reoperation was required in 29.2%, and the time intervals between repeat procedures decreased with each successive repair [2]. This highlights the importance of performing the most successful operation first.

Surgical management of vaginal vault prolapse

Surgical intervention is the mainstay for the management of POP and indeed vaginal vault prolapse (VVP). The approaches can be either vaginal or abdominal, with abdominal surgery being either open or minimally invasive (laparoscopic or robotic).

Vaginal surgery

Sacrospinous fixation (see Chapter 115)

The technique involves attaching the vault of the vagina to the sacrospinous ligament using a non-absorbable suture. A recent Cochrane review highlighted that sacrospinous fixation (SSF) was associated with higher recurrence and sexual dysfunction compared with sacrocolpopexy [1]. Risks associated with this procedure include hemorrhage, bladder injury, rectal injury, and gluteal pain. Furthermore, it is associated with a higher incidence of subsequent anterior vaginal wall prolapse because of posterior deviation of the vagina.

Iliococcygeal fixation

This involves the bilateral fixation of the vault to the iliococcygeal muscle fascia. It has a lower success rate and is more suitable for women with reduced total vaginal length.

Uterosacral suspension

This procedure is traditionally performed as an adjunct to vaginal hysterectomy to prevent further prolapse. However, it has been used in the management of vault prolapse, being performed either vaginally or abdominally. The success rates with transperitoneal approach are around 85% but with upwards of a 10% ureteric injury rate [4]. An extraperitoneal approach to reduce ureteric complications has been described by Dwyer and Fatton [5].

Vaginal mesh kits

Commercially available mesh kits have fallen out of favor following a number of high-profile court cases. A randomized controlled trial comparing mesh repair with native tissue repair found an increased incidence of surgical intervention in the mesh group at 1 year [6]. Compared with laparoscopic sacrocolpopexy, the total vaginal mesh repair is associated with a higher reoperation rate, and the objective success rate is lower [7].

Colpocleisis (see Chapter 116)

This surgery involves the obliteration of the vaginal lumen and is thus suited to frail elderly women who are no longer sexually active. It is associated with success rates of 97% [8].

Abdominal approach

Sacrocolpopexy

Abdominal sacrocolpopexy remains the gold standard for the treatment of VVP, despite the introduction of newer techniques. It is associated with success rates of 74–98%, a low recurrence rate, and reduced dyspareunia when compared with vaginal SSF [9]. It can be performed using a number of approaches including open,

Gynecologic and Obstetric Surgery: Challenges and Management Options, First Edition. Edited by Arri Coomarasamy, Mahmood I. Shafi, G. Willy Davila and Kiong K. Chan.
© 2016 John Wiley & Sons, Ltd. Published 2016 by John Wiley & Sons, Ltd.

laparoscopic, and robotic. The aim of the surgery is to suspend the vaginal vault from the anterior longitudinal ligament, which is anterior to the sacral promontory, using type 1 polypropylene mesh. Specific surgical complications include visceral injury and mesh-specific complications such as erosion.

Robot-assisted sacrocolpopexy

A typical approach for robot-assisted sacrocolpopexy follows, but the principles for open and laparoscopic approaches are the same.

- Prepare operating room for a robot-assisted sacrocolpopexy. Dock the robot and insert the ports (Figure 114.1).

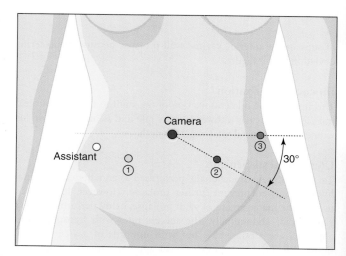

Figure 114.1 Port placement for four-arm da Vinci sacrocolpopexy. © 2013 Intuitive Surgical, Inc.

- Place the patient in a moderate Trendelenburg position.
- Use the third arm of the robot as a bowel retractor.
- Insert the rectal and vaginal probes (Figure 114.2) to aid the identification of the surgical plane.

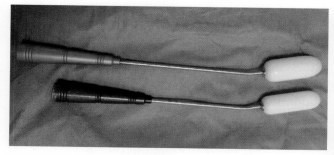

Figure 114.2 Vaginal and rectal probes.

- No bladder manipulator is available to aid with identifying the plane between the bladder and vagina. One method that can be used is to insufflate the bladder with water using a catheter. Where dissection is difficult, the surgeon must maintain a high index of suspicion for a visceral injury. An accidental cystotomy is shown in Figure 114.3.

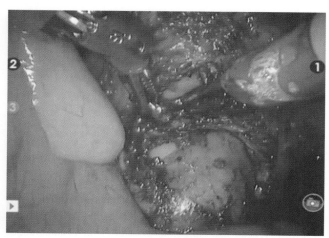

Figure 114.3 Visualization of the Foley catheter through an accidental cystotomy. © 2013 Intuitive Surgical, Inc.

- Mobilize the anterior (Figure 114.4) and posterior (Figure 114.5) vaginal walls.

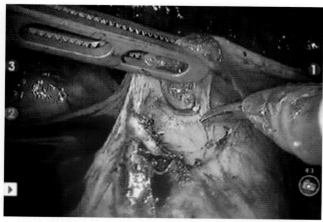

Figure 114.4 Dissection of the anterior vaginal wall. © 2013 Intuitive Surgical, Inc.

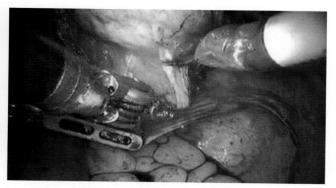

Figure 114.5 Dissection of the posterior vaginal wall. © 2013 Intuitive Surgical, Inc.

- Expose the sacral promontory, and create a track to allow the peritoneum to be closed over the mesh.
- Attach the Y-shaped polypropylene mesh from the anterior and posterior walls of the vagina to the anterior longitudinal ligament

using permanent sutures (e.g., Gore-Tex® or delayed absorbable sutures such as PDS) (Figure 114.6).
• Close the peritoneum over the graft.

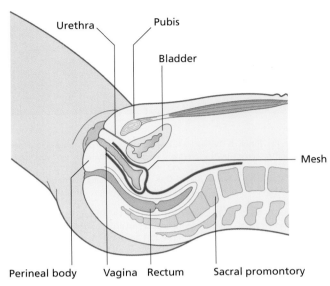

Figure 114.6 Y-shaped mesh attached from the anterior and posterior walls of the vagina to the anterior longitudinal ligament of the sacrum.

Intraoperative challenges during sacrocolpopexy

Accidental cystotomy
Management is detailed in Chapters 35 and 113, and will depend on the nature and location of the injury. A fundal cystotomy can be repaired in two layers. A posterior wall cystotomy will require on-the-table investigation to assess if the ureters are involved, before repair in two layers.

Access to the sacrum
Clear visualization of the sacral promontory and periosteum is essential for the safe and effective performance of a sacrocolpopexy. Incision of the presacral peritoneum and mobilization of the areolar connective tissue to visualize the anterior longitudinal ligament is typically straightforward, but may be challenging in repeat cases. Identification of the right ureter and colonic mesentery medially, which are the landmarks for the peritoneal incision, are important as the dissection is begun.

Dissection in rectovaginal septum
There is debate about whether the dissection off the posterior vagina needs to include dissecting the peritoneum off the posterior wall, and be followed below the levator muscle reflection to the perineum. If the peritoneum is left attached to the posterior vaginal wall, and the mesh is sutured starting cephalad to the levator reflection, there should be minimal risk of trauma to the colon or heavy bleeding. It is very important, however, to identify the superior portion of the rectovaginal attachment, by placing traction on the rectum to identify its tract carefully. This may be particularly difficult in women with previous endometriosis or cul-de-sac surgery. A rectal probe can be very useful here.

Dissection in the vesicovaginal space
This can be the most challenging part of the operation, prompting some surgeons to forgo placement of an anterior mesh arm. If a vaginal probe is placed, and the bladder partially filled (150 mL) in a retrograde fashion, the plane between vagina and bladder can be easily seen. In women with previous cesarean section or bladder surgery, the plane can be more challenging to identify or create, and intravaginal palpation or even a purposeful cystotomy may be needed for clear identification of the dissection plane. The dissection should be directed along the midline as, laterally, vascularity can be quite prominent from uterine and vaginal branches.

Bleeding from sacral periosteum
The most feared complication of a sacrocolpopexy operation is presacral hemorrhage. Although there are numerous visible vessels along the sacral promontory, including the usually obvious middle sacral artery, life-threatening bleeding can occur from periosteal perforators that cannot be seen on the surface. Fortunately, this is a rare occurrence, but the surgeon must be prepared to address this eventuality. Methodical pressure and directed cautery can be useful, but the surgeon must maintain a cool head and get help if the bleeding is brisk. Blood should be ordered for possible transfusion. With directed suction, the bleeding site can be identified and the vessel clamped with a tonsil clamp. It can then be cauterized. Placing a suture may exacerbate the bleeding. Other options include using a sterile thumbtack (if available), or coagulation of the bleeding site by applying a piece of muscle (i.e., rectus abdominis segment) over the bleeding site and cauterizing it to coagulate protein over the bleeding site.

Enterotomy or proctotomy
Proctotomy and spillage of colonic contents contraindicates placement of a synthetic mesh. Thus the procedure should be aborted once a colorectal surgeon has addressed the tear. Small bowel tears can be fixed (Chapter 37) and the abdomen copiously irrigated prior to continuing the procedure. Consultation with a colorectal surgeon is important in this scenario.

Tear into vagina
If a defect is created through the vaginal wall during the dissection, the risk of mesh erosion will increase. Thus, the defect must be carefully closed prior to continuing the procedure.

Resolution of the case

On deciding which surgery to perform for this patient, a number of issues were taken into account. In a woman with limited hip abduction, access to the vagina is difficult and so a vaginal approach was excluded. She was young at the age of 50, and if she developed a recurrence, further surgery would be even more challenging. Furthermore, there was concern that there may be adhesions from the previous hematoma after the hysterectomy, with consequent risks of bladder or bowel injuries. Following counseling, the patient elected to have a robot-assisted sacrocolpopexy.

An accidental cystotomy occurred during dissection (Figure 114.3), and this was repaired in two layers using 2-0 polyglactin 910. An indwelling catheter remained *in situ* for 7 days, following which a micturating cystourethrogram was performed confirming a completely healed bladder with no leaks.

KEY POINTS

Challenge: Difficult sacrocolpopexy.

Background
- Before performing a sacrocolpopexy, all options should be considered and management tailored to the individual patient.
- Regardless of the approach taken, sacrocolpopexy is associated with known morbidity due to the proximity to major vessels and viscera.
- Since many sacrocolpopexy procedures are not primary POP surgeries, the surgeon should be aware of the possibility of scar tissue and resultant anatomic alterations.

Prevention
- Appropriate patient positioning, bowel preparation, surgical exposure, and surgeon experience are all key factors in preventing complications.

Management
- Surgical complications do occur and where they do, one must be able to manage them appropriately.
- Bowel and bladder complications during sacrocolpopexy should be identified intraoperatively, and the surgeon should seek relevant assistance from urologist or colorectal surgeon in case of inadvertent injuries.
- Vascular injuries during sacrocolpopexy can be life-threatening, and require appropriate expertise and operative tools to be able to address this complication.

References

1 Maher C, Baessler K, Glazener CM, Adams EJ, Hagen S. Surgical management of pelvic organ prolapse in women. *Cochrane Database Syst Rev* 2013;(4):CD004014.

2 Olsen AL, Smith VJ, Bergstrom JO, Colling JC, Clark AL. Epidemiology of surgically managed pelvic organ prolapse and urinary incontinence. *Obstet Gynecol* 1997;89:501–506.

3 Brown JS, Waetjen LE, Subak LL, Thom DH, Van den Eeden S, Vittinghoff E. Pelvic organ prolapse surgery in the United States, 1997. *Am J Obstet Gynecol* 2002;186:712–716.

4 Margulies RU, Rogers MA, Morgan DM. Outcomes of transvaginal uterosacral ligament suspension: systematic review and metaanalysis. *Am J Obstet Gynecol* 2010;202:124–134.

5 Dwyer PL, Fatton B. Bilateral extraperitoneal uterosacral suspension: a new approach to correct posthysterectomy vaginal vault prolapse. *Int Urogynecol J Pelvic Floor Dysfunct* 2008;19:283–292.

6 Sokol AI, Iglesia CB, Kudish BI *et al.* One-year objective and functional outcomes of a randomized clinical trial of vaginal mesh for prolapse. *Am J Obstet Gynecol* 2012;206:86e1–9.

7 Maher CF, Feiner B, DeCuyper EM, Nichlos CJ, Hickey KV, O'Rourke P. Laparoscopic sacral colpopexy versus total vaginal mesh for vaginal vault prolapse: a randomized trial. *Am J Obstet Gynecol* 2011;204:360e1–7.

8 Cespedes RD, Winters JC, Ferguson KH. Colpocleisis for the treatment of vaginal vault prolapse. *Tech Urol* 2001;7:152–160.

9 Maher CM, Feiner B, Baessler K, Glazener CM. Surgical management of pelvic organ prolapse in women: the updated summary version Cochrane review. *Int Urogynecol J* 2011;22:1445–1457.

CHAPTER 115

Difficult Sacrospinous Fixation

Smita Rajshekhar[1] and Rohna Kearney[2]
[1] Addenbrooke's Hospital, Cambridge University Hospitals NHS Trust, Cambridge, UK
[2] St Mary's Hospital, Central Manchester University Hospitals NHS Foundation Trust, Manchester, UK

Case history: A 74-year-old woman elected to have a pelvic floor repair and sacrospinous fixation for a symptomatic large rectocele with vault descent. She had a colposuspension and total abdominal hysterectomy 20 years previously. At the time of surgery she was noted to have a severely shortened anterior vaginal wall and a large rectocele descending 3 cm outside the introitus. The vault descended to the introitus but when reduced it did not reach the sacrospinous ligament.

Background

The sacrospinous ligament (SSL), found bilaterally, is a cord-like structure in the body of the coccygeus muscle which extends in a fan shape from the ischial spine to the lateral border of the sacral bone and sacrococcygeal joint. There are important anatomic structures in close proximity to this ligament. The pudendal nerve and vessels lie directly posterior to the ischial spine. The sciatic nerve runs superior and lateral. The inferior gluteal vessels and hypogastric venous plexus are superior, and the ureter curves anteromedially at a point 1.5 cm above the ischial spine to enter the bladder.

Sacrospinous fixation is often used to treat vault prolapse in patients who are frail and in whom an abdominal approach such as a sacrocolpopexy (Chapter 114) is undesirable.

Management

Preoperative management

Preoperative management should include a thorough assessment of the patient's symptoms, an examination documenting the degree of prolapse, and a discussion of the treatment options and their associated risks. Symptom-specific questionnaires and the Pelvic Organ Prolapse Quantification (POP-Q) score are useful tools in assessment. Careful patient counseling should include a discussion about non-surgical alternatives, the choice of surgical approach (alternatives include sacrocolpopexy and colpocleisis), and the risks and complications of these techniques.

Preoperative vaginal estrogen may be helpful in women with atrophic vaginitis. Urodynamics is helpful if the woman has bothersome urinary symptoms, or the prolapse is exteriorized.

A unilateral suspension, usually the right sacrospinous ligament for the right-handed surgeon or the more accessible side, can be performed. A bilateral approach is preferred by many surgeons, as it can result in more symmetrical vaginal anatomy, but studies to date have not demonstrated a superior outcome, such as a reduced delayed cystocele recurrence rate.

Sacrospinous ligament fixation technique

Approaches to the SSL include dissecting perivesically from an incision over the anterior vaginal wall, or perirectally through a midline vertical incision on the posterior wall, or dissecting from an incision at the new apex between the enterocele sac and the vaginal wall if a four-corner suspension is to be performed [1–3]. We prefer the posterior approach.

- Infiltrate the vaginal wall with a local anesthetic agent and saline solution.
- Make a triangular or diamond-shaped incision on the perineum, as this procedure is frequently combined with a perineorrhaphy.
- Make a vertical incision in the vagina, and dissect the rectum off the vagina bilaterally.
- Perform blunt dissection to the ischial spine, usually on the right side.
- Perforate the rectal pillar, which is areolar tissue between the rectovaginal and perirectal spaces, by blunt dissection with a gauzed finger or sharp dissection by scissors.
- Identify the ischial spine and SSL by palpation. Placement of sutures through the ligament can be achieved with several techniques including using a Miya hook, a Deschamps ligature carrier, or disposable needle drivers (e.g., Capio™ needle driver, Boston Scientific Corporation) [3,4].
- Place two monofilament delayed-absorbable sutures (e.g., 0 or 1 PDS; some surgeons use non-absorbable sutures such as polypropylene) through the ligament and pass them through the new apex.
- Plicate the rectal fascia and the posterior vaginal wall closed prior to tying the SSL sutures to elevate the vault.
- Complete perineorrhaphy.

Gynecologic and Obstetric Surgery: Challenges and Management Options, First Edition. Edited by Arri Coomarasamy, Mahmood I. Shafi, G. Willy Davila and Kiong K. Chan.
© 2016 John Wiley & Sons, Ltd. Published 2016 by John Wiley & Sons, Ltd.

- Perform a rectal examination to detect any occult rectal injury.
- Place a catheter and pack, and leave therein overnight.

Challenges and complications

Selection of a new apex (resolution of the case)

There are wide variations in the anatomy of women with a vault prolapse, especially if they have undergone previous vaginal surgery. In the case history, the anterior vaginal wall was short and the vaginal vault (where the previous hysterectomy scar was) would not reach the ischial spine. A successful sacrospinous procedure can be completed in this scenario if a new location for the apex is used (Figure 115.1). In this case, a new apex was selected on the posterior wall by placing an Allis clamp on the posterior wall 9 cm from the introitus and elevating it to the ischial spine. Although a large rectocele was present, the overall vaginal length was not increased and therefore excess vagina did not need to be excised [5].

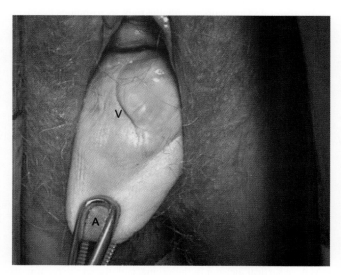

Figure 115.1 Vaginal vault eversion. The hysterectomy scar (V) can be seen anterior to the new selected apex point (A) for suspension to the sacrospinous ligament.

If the patient's apical scar had been used, the anterior wall would have been under excessive tension, and resultant stress incontinence or voiding dysfunction may have ensued. When assigning a new apex, the surgeon must consider the fact that the new apical anterior wall was in fact part of the pre-existing posterior enterocele, so it is very thin (lacking a fibromuscular layer) and could result in a future anterior enterocele. Anterior grafting may be a consideration in this scenario.

In cases such as this where the vagina is too short to reach the SSL, consideration should be given for an abdominal approach. Increasingly, sacrocolpopexy is being performed laparoscopically, with a quicker recovery and shorter length of stay than the traditional open abdominal approach.

Hemorrhage

Intraoperative hemorrhage may require application of vascular clips, packing, and subsequent embolization [6]. Bleeding can occur from vessels along the SSL, but also along the sites of posterior wall dissection, levator muscles, or rectal wall. Thus, careful methodical examination is critical when bleeding occurs during an SSL fixation.

Nerve injuries

Nerve injuries may present with pain or fecal incontinence requiring removal of the stitches. Immediate postoperative pain in the recovery room usually signifies nerve (such as pudendal) entrapment in a suspensory suture, and consideration should be given to returning to theater to replace the suture.

Rectal injury

Rectal injury can occur during dissection or placement of the sutures, and a postoperative rectal examination is an important routine step. When a patient presents with an abscess, cellulitis or sepsis following sacrospinous fixation, a rectal injury should be considered as a possible cause.

Urinary tract injuries

Bladder and ureteric injuries have been reported, more commonly with the anterior approach (Chapters 35, 36 and 113).

Obliteration of the pararectal space

This can cause difficulty in reaching the SSL, and can be found in patients with previous pelvic surgery, endometriosis, or rectal abscess. If the ischial spine and SSL cannot be easily reached and clearly dissected, consideration should be given to performing an iliococcygeal suspension, or SSL fixation on the opposite side.

Prevention

Careful patient counseling is essential prior to any prolapse procedure. This should include a discussion about non-surgical alternatives, the choice of surgical approach, and the risks and complications of these techniques. If the findings at the time of surgery differ significantly to what was expected, it may be appropriate for the surgeon to abandon the planned surgery and document the findings in favor of a more comprehensive discussion with the patient. As with any vaginal POP surgical procedure, appropriate assistance, instruments to obtain surgical exposure, lighting and suction to visualize the entire surgical field are important prerequisites.

KEY POINTS

Challenge: Difficult sacrospinous fixation.

Background
- Comprehensive anatomic knowledge is essential to the management of difficult sacrospinous fixation, due to the proximity of the ligament to important neurovascular structures.

Management
- It is important to conduct a thorough preoperative work-up, and counsel the patient about all the non-surgical and surgical options to manage VVP.

- The SSL is accessible via anterior or posterior (perirectal) routes or from the new apex of the vagina; in cases where the anterior vaginal wall has been shortened from previous surgical procedures, a new location for the vaginal vault is necessary.
- The technical steps in the procedure are:
  - Infiltrate the vaginal wall with local anesthetic and saline solution.
  - Make an incision on the perineum.
  - Make a vertical incision in the vagina and dissect the rectum off the vagina bilaterally.
  - Perform blunt dissection to the ischial spine.

- Perforate the rectal pillar by blunt dissection with a gauzed finger or by sharp dissection by scissors.
- Identify the ischial spine and SSL by palpation.
- Place sutures through the ligament with a Miya hook, Deschamps ligature carrier, or disposable devices, and pass them through the new apex.
- Prior to tying the SSL sutures, plicate the rectal fascia and the posterior vaginal wall closed.
- Complete the procedure with a perineorrhaphy.
- Perform a rectal examination to detect any occult rectal injury.
- Insert a catheter and vaginal pack and leave overnight.

- Complications of sacrospinous fixation include hemorrhage (possibly requiring vascular clips or embolization) or injury to nerves, urinary tract or rectum.
- Ongoing audit and up-to-date training with sufficient caseload can help to maintain skills and optimize efficiency.
- If surgical findings differ significantly from preoperative expectations, then it may be appropriate to abandon the planned procedure and consider other options.

References

1 Winkler HA, Tomeszko JE, Sand PK. Anterior sacrospinous vaginal vault suspension for prolapse. *Obstet Gynecol* 2000;95:612–615.
2 Goldberg RP, Tomezsko JE, Winkler HA. Anterior or posterior sacrospinous vaginal vault suspension: long-term anatomic and functional evaluation. *Obstet Gynecol* 2001;98:199–204.
3 Morley G, DeLancey JOL. Sacrospinous ligament fixation for eversion of the vagina. *Am J Obstet Gynecol* 1988;158:872–881.
4 Miyazaki FS. Miya Hook ligature carrier for sacrospinous ligament suspension. *Obstet Gynecol* 1987;70:286–288.
5 Kearney R, Delancey JOL. Selecting suspension points and excising the vagina during Michigan Four-wall sacrospinous suspension. *Obstet Gynecol* 2003;101:325–330.
6 Araco F, Gravante G, Konda D. Selective embolization of the superior vesical artery for the treatment of a severe retroperitoneal pelvic haemorrhage following Endo-Stitch sacrospinous colpopexy. *Int Urogynecol J Pelvic Floor Dysfunct* 2008:19:873–875.

CHAPTER 116

Recurrent Pelvic Organ Prolapse

Monika Vij and Robert Freeman
Plymouth Hospitals NHS Trust, Plymouth, UK

Case history: A 64-year-old woman underwent a total vaginal hysterectomy with anterior and posterior colporrhaphies 4 years ago. She now presents with sensation of a vaginal bulge which has been enlarging over the past 6 months. She states she has recently gained a significant amount of weight, and has suffered from constipation.

Background

Prolapse surgery can be classified into "primary surgery" (the first procedure required for the treatment of POP in any compartment) and "further surgery" (a global term for subsequent procedures the patient undergoes, directly or indirectly, relating to the primary surgery) [1]. Further surgery is subdivided into the following categories.

1 Primary prolapse surgery at a different site: a prolapse procedure in a new site or compartment following previous surgery (e.g., anterior repair following previous posterior repair).
2 Repeat or re-do surgery: a repeat operation for prolapse arising from the same site. Where combinations of procedures arise, such as new anterior repair plus further posterior repair, these should be reported separately as primary anterior repair and repeat posterior repair.
3 Surgery for complications: a procedure for mesh exposure or extrusion, pain, or complications such as hemorrhage.
4 Surgery for non-POP conditions: for example, subsequent surgery for stress urinary incontinence or fecal incontinence.

Incidence
Global "reoperation" rate has been reported to be 29.2% [2], but when "repeat surgery" is assessed, the rates are much lower (2.8–9.7%) [3,4,5].

Risk factors
Recurrent prolapse might result from failure related to surgical technique or because of weak connective tissue. Obesity, number of deliveries prior to surgery, and the presence of urgency or incontinence symptoms are important risk factors associated with recurrence of prolapse [6].

Management

A full assessment, including prolapse, urinary, bowel, and sexual dysfunction symptoms, is needed. The prolapse should preferably be assessed using the POP-Q system [7]. The choice of treatment will depend on the level of difficulty with symptoms, effect on quality of life, degree of prolapse, and the woman's fitness for surgery.

Conservative management
Women who do not wish to have further intervention and are asymptomatic can be managed expectantly. However, those with prolapse of grade 2 or more might be at risk of vaginal ulceration and obstructive renal, urinary, and bowel symptoms, and should be advised about prevention with vaginal pessaries or surgery. Six months of supervised pelvic floor muscle training (PFMT) has benefits in terms of anatomic and symptom improvement [8], but the efficacy of PFMT in recurrent vault prolapse is unknown.

Surgical management
The choice of operation will depend on the site of recurrence as well as associated urinary, bowel or sexual dysfunction. Surgery should be undertaken by a specialist with expertise and sufficient workload as evidenced by personal audit data.

Cystocele
Recurrences are most commonly found in the anterior compartment. The traditional anterior colporrhaphy has higher failure rates in repeat surgery compared with primary surgery [9].

The collated evidence suggests that surgical repair of recurrent anterior vaginal wall prolapse using mesh may be more efficacious than traditional surgical repair without mesh. The International Consultation on Incontinence (ICI) reported improved anatomic and subjective outcomes with non-absorbable mesh reinforcement compared with standard colporrhaphy, but with increased complication rates [10]. Both efficacy and safety vary with different types of mesh, and the data on efficacy in the long term are limited.

It is important to ensure that patients understand there is uncertainty about the long-term results and risk of complications, including sexual dysfunction and erosion into the vagina, which would require additional procedures.

Gynecologic and Obstetric Surgery: Challenges and Management Options, First Edition. Edited by Arri Coomarasamy, Mahmood I. Shafi, G. Willy Davila and Kiong K. Chan.
© 2016 John Wiley & Sons, Ltd. Published 2016 by John Wiley & Sons, Ltd.

Apical compartment or vault

There is lack of adequate evidence for the optimal surgical approach for recurrent vault prolapse. However, the approaches include the following.

Sacrospinous ligament fixation (see Chapter 115)

Repeat unilateral or bilateral sacrospinous ligament fixation (SSLF) has been reported for the management of recurrent vault prolapse [11,12]. However, such surgery can be difficult due to scarring in the pararectal space and anatomic distortion which can increase the risk of complications such as rectal injury, hemorrhage, and gluteal pain [13].

Sacrocolpopexy (see Chapter 114)

Gilleran and Zimmern [14] reported no recurrence of vault prolapse at 23 months following abdominal sacrocolpopexy for recurrent triple compartment prolapse.

McCall culdoplasty and uterosacral ligament vault suspension

These procedures and their modifications attach the vaginal vault to the origins of the uterosacral ligaments, and achieve closure of the cul-de-sac by approximating the ligaments in the midline. The ligaments are often attenuated in recurrent vault prolapse, and where the ligaments are inadequate, some surgeons advocate alternative procedures such as SSLF [15]. The rate of ureteral injury has been reported to be 1–11% [16,17].

Rectocele/posterior compartment

Posterior vaginal repair techniques include fascial plication or site-specific repair (levator plication is not recommended due to high rates of dyspareunia). There are no randomized studies for the efficacy of either procedure in recurrent rectocele. To date there is no evidence to support the use of mesh for augmentation of a posterior vaginal repair [18] in primary or recurrent rectocele [10]. The abdominal route has been used in the correction of rectocele with coexistent vault prolapse. This is a modification of sacrocolpopexy where the posterior mesh is extended down to the posterior vaginal wall [19]. However, it is unclear if this has any benefit over posterior vaginal repair.

Colpocleisis (see Chapter 117)

Colpocleisis is an effective surgical treatment for all recurrent pelvic organ prolapses in elderly women who are no longer having sexual intercourse. Advantages of this approach include shorter operative time, decreased morbidity, faster recovery, and high anatomic success rates. Colpocleisis provides high levels of patient satisfaction and improvement in quality of life without significant morbidity [20,21].

KEY POINTS

Challenge: Recurrence of vaginal prolapse after previous repair.

Background
- Prolapse surgery can be classified into "primary surgery" and "further surgery"; further surgery is subdivided into:
  - Primary prolapse surgery at different site.
  - Repeat or re-do surgery.
  - Surgery for complications (e.g., mesh exposure).
  - Surgery for non-POP conditions (e.g., for stress urinary incontinence).
- Incidence of "repeat surgery" is reported to be 3–10%.

Prevention
- Patient-related factors such as BMI, smoking, constipation, and exercise routines should be addressed with patients in order to reduce risk of recurrence.

Management
- Management of recurrent POP should be individualized.
- Surgery for recurrent POP should be performed by experienced surgeons who can address any anatomic alterations due to scar tissue from previous surgeries.
- The surgical approach will depend on the location and nature of the defect, and anticipated outcomes:
  - Cystocele: paravaginal repair, sacrocolpopexy or vaginal mesh augmentation.
  - Vault prolapse: sacrocolpopexy, sacrospinous fixation or McCall culdoplasty.
  - Rectocele: posterior colporrhaphy, sacrocolpopexy (if concomitant vault or apical prolapse) or possibly vaginal mesh augmentation.
- For elderly women who no longer wish to have intercourse: colpocleisis.

References

1 Toozs-Hobson P, Freeman R, Barber M et al. An International Urogynecological Association (IUGA)/International Continence Society (ICS) Joint Report on the terminology for reporting outcomes of surgical procedures for pelvic organ prolapse. Neurourol Urodyn 2012;31:415–421.

2 Oslen AL, Smith VJ, Bergstrom VO, Colling JC, Clark AL. Epidemiology of surgically managed pelvic organ prolapse and urinary incontinence. Obstet Gynecol 1997;89:501–506.

3 Diwadkar GB, Barber MD, Feiner B, Maher C, Jelovsek JE. Complications and reoperation rates following surgical repair for apical vaginal prolapse: a meta-analysis. Obstet Gynecol 2009;113:367–373.

4 Kapoor DS, Nemcova M, Pantazis K, Brockman P, Bombieri L, Freeman RM. Re-operation rate for traditional anterior repair: analysis of 207 cases with a median 4 year follow up. Int J Urogynecol J Pelvic Floor Dysfunct 2010;21:27–31.

5 Miedel A, Tegerstedt G, Mörlin B, Hammarström M. A 5-year prospective follow-up study of vaginal surgery for pelvic organ prolapse. Int Urogynecol J Pelvic Floor Dysfunct 2008;19:1593–1601.

6 Diez-Calzadilla NA, March-Villalba JA, Ferrandis C et al. Risk factors in the failure of surgical repair of pelvic organ prolapse. Actas Urol Esp 2011;35:448–453.

7 Bump RC, Mattiasson A, Bo K et al. The standardization of terminology of female pelvic organ prolapse and pelvic floor dysfunction. Am J Obstet Gynecol 1996;175:10–17.

8 Hagen S, Stark D. Conservative prevention and management of pelvic organ prolapse in women. Cochrane Database Syst Rev 2011;(12):CD003882.

9 Peterson TV, Karp DR, Aguilar VC, Davila GW. Primary versus recurrent prolapse surgery: differences in outcomes. Int Urogynecol J 2010;21:483–488.

10 Maher C, Baessler K, Barber M et al. Surgical management of pelvic organ prolapse. In: AbramsP, CardozoL, KhouryS, WeinA (eds) 5th International Consultation on Incontinence. Health Publication Ltd, Paris, 2013.

11 Imparato E, Asperi G, Rovertta E, Presti M. Surgical management and prevention of vaginal vault prolapse. Surg Gynecol Obstet 1992;175:233–277.

12 Lo TS, Horng SG, Huang HJ, Lee SJ, Liang CC. Repair of recurrent vaginal vault prolapse using sacrospinous ligament fixation with mesh interposition and reinforcement. Acta Obstet Gynaecol Scand 2005;84:992–995.

13 Sze EH, Karram MM. Transvaginal repair of vault prolapse: a review. Obstet Gynecol 1997;89:466–475.

14 Gilleran JP, Zimmern P. Abdominal mesh sacrocolpopexy for recurrent triple-compartment pelvic organ prolapse. BJU Int 2009;103:1090–1094.

15 Arbel R, Lavy Y. Vaginal vault prolapse: choice of operation. Best Pract Res Clin Obstet Gynaecol 2005;19:959–977.

16 Shull BL, Bachofen C, Coates KW, Kuehl TJ. A transvaginal approach to repair of apical and other associated sites of pelvic organ prolapse with uterosacral ligaments. *Am J Obstet Gynecol* 2000;183:1365–1374.

17 Silva WE, Pauls RN, Segal JL, Rooney CM, Kleeman SD, Karram MM. Uterosacral ligament vault suspension: five year outcomes. *Obstet Gynecol* 2006;108:255–263.

18 Sung VW, Rardin CR, Raker CA, Lasala CA, Myers DL. Porcine subintestinal submucosal graft augmentation for rectocele repair: a randomised controlled trial. *Obstet Gynecol* 2012;119:125–133.

19 Marinkovic SP, Stanton SL. Triple compartment prolapse: sacrocolpopexy with anterior and posterior mesh extensions. *BJOG* 2003;110:323–326.

20 Haylen BT, Freeman RM, Lee J *et al.* An International Urogynecological Association (IUGA)/International Continence Society (ICS) joint terminology and classification of the complications related to native tissue female pelvic floor surgery. *Int Urogynecol J* 2012;23:515–526.

21 Haylen BT, Freeman RM, Swift SE *et al.* An International Urogynecological Association (IUGA)/International Continence Society (ICS) joint terminology and classification of the complications related directly to the insertion of prostheses (meshes, implants, tapes) and grafts in female pelvic floor surgery. *Neurourol Urodyn* 2011;30:2–12.

CHAPTER 117

Colpocleisis

Kalaivani Ramalingam[1] and Ash Monga[2]
[1] Apollo Hospitals, Chennai, India
[2] Southampton University Hospital Trust, Southampton, UK

Case history: An 84-year-old woman presents with vaginal prolapse symptoms, having undergone an abdominal hysterectomy 40 years ago. She has occasional urgency of urine but no major urinary or bowel incontinence problems. She is not sexually active. Trials of pessaries have led to discomfort, ulceration, or falling out of the pessary. Examination shows the presence of major anterior, apical and posterior prolapse. She has multiple medical disorders.

Background

Genital prolapse occurs in 37% of women over the age of 80 years. When advanced vaginal prolapse is present, especially if it involves the apical compartment with or without the uterus *in situ*, different procedures may be appropriate depending on the patient's preferences, medical fitness, and other relevant considerations. Abdominal procedures such as sacrocolpopexy (Chapter 114) and hysteropexy (Chapter 118) are considered where sexual function is desired to be preserved or if simpler vaginal procedures have failed. Vaginal procedures include colpocleisis, site-specific repairs, sacrospinous fixation, and the use of vaginal mesh procedures. Colpocleisis is defined as surgical obliteration or closure of the lumen of the vagina [1].

A high patient satisfaction rate has been reported in most studies of colpocleisis [2]. Colpocleisis for POP has been reported to be successful in nearly 100% of patients in two recent series [3,4]. The mean duration of hospital stay is reported to be 1–5 days. Complications such as hemorrhage, ureteric injury, evisceration, and contiguous organ injury are rarely reported [4,5].

Management

Preoperative management

Preoperative evaluation should include a surgical fitness assessment for the procedure along with baseline pelvic floor function including bladder and bowel assessment. Urinary function is both difficult to assess and treat adequately in very old patients [6]. If SUI is identified preoperatively, a sling can be performed at the time of colpocleisis; bladder function is typically normalized postoperatively, although it may take longer than in younger women

[7]. Endometrial pathology (with either ultrasound or endometrial pipelle biopsy) needs to be excluded as the uterus is inaccessible for vaginal evaluation after the procedure.

Good preoperative counseling should emphasize the fact that this procedure is meant to be performed in those who have absolutely no desire to preserve their sexual function. Sexual function is not feasible after this obliterative procedure and hence there can be a small proportion of patients who may have regrets following this operation [8].

Surgical technique

The procedure can be performed under general, regional, or local anesthesia. The surgical procedure (Figure 117.1) consists of stripping the vaginal epithelium from the underlying fascia and suturing the vaginal cavity from the anterior to the posterior side to close it.

- A superficial circumscribing incision is made through the vaginal epithelium at the base of the prolapse at a level adjacent to the hymenal ring.
- The entire vaginal epithelium up to 2 cm from the urethral meatus is mobilized by sharp dissection except for 1–2 cm strips near the vault.
- The prolapse is serially reduced with absorbable sutures placed into the vaginal muscularis, beginning at the leading edge of the prolapse and continuing sequentially in interrupted pursestring fashion, or with interrupted sutures placed in an anteroposterior direction, until the prolapsed tissues are superior to the level of the levator plate.
- Colpocleisis closes the potential space into which the enterocele might protrude, so the enterocele does not need to be opened or repaired.
- Once the majority of the prolapse is reduced, the support of the vesical neck can be improved where necessary. In the caudal portion of the vagina, just above the hymenal ring, the dense connective tissue attached to the levator ani muscles and perineal membrane is closed with the lowest suture to lend firm closure of the pelvic floor.
- The procedure is completed by closing the anterior vaginal epithelium to the posterior epithelium with interrupted sutures at the level of the introitus.

Modifications described include procedures to treat SUI (e.g., tape insertion for pre-existent or occult SUI), levator plication, and perineorrhaphy [7–11].

Gynecologic and Obstetric Surgery: Challenges and Management Options, First Edition. Edited by Arri Coomarasamy, Mahmood I. Shafi, G. Willy Davila and Kiong K. Chan.
© 2016 John Wiley & Sons, Ltd. Published 2016 by John Wiley & Sons, Ltd.

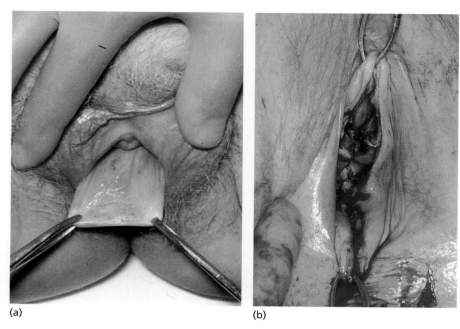

(a)   (b)

Figure 117.1 Total colpocleisis: (a) vaginal vault prolapse and (b) longitudinal incision colpocleisis with near total vaginectomy before closure.

Partial colpocleisis

This procedure is performed in women with an intact uterus and prolapse in order to allow expulsion of discharge from the uterus. Rectangular strips of vaginal epithelium of approximately equal size are removed from the anterior and posterior surfaces of the protruding vagina, leaving a canal of approximately 3 cm at each side. Care is taken not to remove vaginal epithelium from the area beneath the urethra. The anterior and posterior surfaces are approximated to each other with rows of interrupted stitches, resulting in a lateral tunnel on each side, communicating at the vault across the front of the cervix.

KEY POINTS

Challenge: Colpocleisis.

Background
- Colpocleisis is used to treat advanced POP in older women who are too frail for conventional surgery and who are absolutely no longer sexually active.
- The procedure closes the vagina and inhibits a patient from future sexual intercourse.
- It is quick, easy, effective (90–95% cure rate), and associated with low recurrence and high patient satisfaction rates.
- Postoperative pain is minimal and complications are low.
- Other procedures can be performed concomitantly for SUI and deficient perineum.

Management
- Colpocleisis can be performed using local, epidural, spinal, or general anesthesia.
- Partial colpocleisis: rectangular strips of vaginal epithelium of approximately equal size are removed from the anterior and posterior surfaces of the protruding vagina, leaving a canal of approximately 3 cm at each side (if the uterus is present).
- Complete colpocleisis: complete obliteration of the vagina is achieved.
- Care is taken not to remove vaginal epithelium from the area beneath the urethra.
- The anterior and posterior surfaces are approximated to each other with rows of interrupted stitches in the vaginal muscularis.
- The procedure is completed by closing the anterior vaginal epithelium to the posterior epithelium with interrupted sutures at the level of the introitus.
- A perineorrhaphy can be performed in cases of deficient perineum.
- A concomitant mid-urethral sling is done if the patient has demonstrable stress incontinence.

References

1 Latthe PM, Karri K, Arunkalaivanan AS. Colpocleisis revisited. *Obstetrician & Gynaecologist* 2008;10:133–138.
2 Abbasy S, Kenton K. Obliterative procedures for pelvic organ prolapse. *Clin Obstet Gynecol* 2010;53:86–98.
3 FitzGerald MP, Richter HE, Siddique S, Thompson P, Zyczynski H. Colpocleisis: a review. *Int Urogynecol J Pelvic Floor Dysfunct* 2006;17:261–271.
4 Zebede S, Smith AL, Plowright L, Hegde A, Aguilar VC, Davila GW. Obliterative LeFort colpocleisis in a large group of elderly women. *Obstet Gynecol* 2013;121:1–7.
5 Gutman RE, Bradley CS, Ye W, Markland AD, Whitehead WE, Fitzgerald MP. Effects of colpocleisis on bowel symptoms among women with severe pelvic organ prolapse. *Int Urogynecol J Pelvic Floor Dysfunct* 2010;21:461–466.
6 FitzGerald MP, Brubaker L. Colpocleisis and urinary incontinence. *Am J Obstet Gynecol* 2003;189:1241–1244.

7 Smith AL, Karp DR, Lefevre R, Aguilar VC, Davila GW. LeForte colpocleisis and stress incontinence: weighing the risk of voiding dysfunction after sling placement. *Int Urogynecol J* 2011;22:1357–1362.
8 Vij M, Bombieri L, Dua A, Freeman R. Long-term follow-up after colpocleisis: regret, bowel, and bladder function. *Int Urogynecol J* 2014;25:811–815.
9 Moore RD, Miklos JR. Colpocleisis and tension-free vaginal tape sling for severe uterine and vaginal prolapse and stress urinary incontinence under local anesthesia. *J Am Assoc Gynecol Laparosc* 2003;10:276–280.
10 Cespedes RD, Winters JC, Ferguson KH. Colpocleisis for the treatment of vaginal vault prolapse. *Tech Urol* 2001;7:152–160.
11 von Pechmann WS, Mutone M, Fyffe J, Hale DS. Total colpocleisis with high levator plication for the treatment of advanced pelvic organ prolapse. *Am J Obstet Gynecol* 2003;189:121–126.

CHAPTER 118

Uterine Suspension Procedures: Laparoscopic Hysteropexy

Natalia Price and Simon Jackson
John Radcliffe Hospital, Oxford University Hospitals NHS Trust, Oxford, UK

Case history 1: *A 36-year-old woman with two children presents with a complete procidentia, and seeks surgical remedy. She is not sure if her family is complete.*

Case history 2: *A 56-year-old woman with recurrent cystocele, uterine prolapse, and two previous anterior repairs is keen to have surgical correction.*

Background

Vaginal hysterectomy has long been the standard approach for management of uterine prolapse; however, it raises some significant questions. Vaginal hysterectomy fails to address the underlying deficiency in pelvic floor support that causes prolapse and it is therefore hardly surprising that recurrence rates are so high, with rates of up to 40% described in the literature [1,2]. It involves the removal of a healthy organ which may play a role in patients' individual and sexual identity.

In 1966, Williams [3] described a technique for transvaginal uterosacral–cervical ligament plication and reported on outcomes for 20 women undergoing this procedure, with three "failures" encountered within a 6-month follow-up period. The concept of sacrospinous hysteropexy was first described by Richardson *et al.* [4] in 1989, with unilateral fixation of the uterus to the right sacrospinous ligament. In 2001, Maher *et al.* [5] reported a small comparison study between sacrospinous hysteropexy and vaginal hysterectomy with sacrospinous vault fixation, and found no differences in objective or subjective outcomes at follow-up. The technique of posterior vaginal slingplasty [6] was first described in 2001, using mesh to create "neo-uterosacral ligaments," but mesh complication rates appear to be high.

In 1993, Addison and Timmons [7] first described a technique for resuspending the uterus to the sacrum using Mersilene® mesh. Laparoscopic abdominal surgery has, with very few exceptions, replaced laparotomy in many centers. The laparoscope confers better vision than laparotomy, allowing a magnified high-definition view. Furthermore, the long instruments allow better pelvic access, particularly behind the uterus. A number of laparoscopic uterine suspension procedures have been described using different anchoring points: the round ligaments, anterior abdominal wall, the uterosacral ligaments, and the sacral promontory.

We have developed a method of complete cervical encerclage (the Oxford hysteropexy, Figure 118.1) using a bifurcated polypropylene mesh [8]. Initial follow-up studies [8,9] show good outcomes with significant improvement in all measures of post-surgery ICIQ-VS and POP-Q scores. The Oxford technique [8] of laparoscopic hysteropexy is addressed in detail in this chapter. The aims of this treatment are as follows.

- To restore and reinforce uterine support by suspending the uterus from the sacral promontory using type 1 polypropylene mesh. Two strong attachment points are used: the cervix and the anterior longitudinal ligament overlying the sacral promontory.
- To restore vaginal length without compromising caliber.
- By restoring apical support, to reduce anterior prolapse, consistent with the importance of restoring level 1 support in cystocele repair.
- By restoring apical support, to reduce the risk of enterocele; however, low rectocele frequently requires a concurrent vaginal repair.

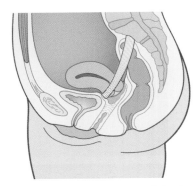

Figure 118.1 Hysteropexy: the uterus is resuspended using mesh.

The theoretical advantage is that this type of repair, by augmenting weak connective tissue with prosthetic Prolene, provides stronger apical support resulting in lower recurrence rates. It allows patients to retain their fertility and, by avoiding vaginal surgery, there is a lower potential for dyspareunia and sexual dysfunction.

Gynecologic and Obstetric Surgery: Challenges and Management Options, First Edition. Edited by Arri Coomarasamy, Mahmood I. Shafi, G. Willy Davila and Kiong K. Chan.
© 2016 John Wiley & Sons, Ltd. Published 2016 by John Wiley & Sons, Ltd.

Management

Surgical technique (Figure 118.2)

The procedure is performed under general anesthesia with the patient supine and in semi-lithotomy. A urinary catheter and uterine manipulator are inserted. A four-port laparoscopic technique is used with 10-mm umbilical, two 5-mm lateral, and a 12-mm suprapubic ports inserted. After identifying the sacral promontory the peritoneum is incised with bipolar graspers and monopolar scissors to identify a safe window of periosteum. A peritoneal relaxing incision is then used medial to the right ureter to retract it from the surgical site, and the incision is extended into the pelvis, lateral to the rectum. A flap of peritoneum is mobilized at the level of insertion of the uterosacral ligaments to facilitate re-peritonization. The vesico-uterine peritoneum is incised to reflect the bladder away, and bilateral avascular windows are created in the broad ligament.

A bifurcated polypropylene type 1 macroporous non-absorbable mesh is used, bringing the arms of the mesh through the broad ligament windows. This is transfixed to the anterior cervix using non-dissolvable non-absorbable polyester 2-0 sutures (Ethibond®). The mesh is attached to the sacral promontory under moderate tension using two to three 5-mm helical fasteners (Pro-Tack®, Covidien). The mesh is then completely re-peritonized using Monocryl® sutures. The technique has evolved over time: initially re-peritonization was not performed; however, after two patients who underwent subsequent laparoscopies were found to have bowel adhesions to the mesh, this adaptation was introduced.

Outcomes

One prospective observational study [9] has reported outcomes following laparoscopic sacrohysteropexy in 140 women. Follow-up time varied between 1 and 4 years; 89% of women felt their prolapse was "very much" or "much" better. There was significant improvement in subjective and objective scores after surgery. Approximately 4% of women experienced further apical prolapse, of whom half underwent further surgical intervention. This compares favorably with the risk of vault prolapse following vaginal hysterectomy [10]. One reason for recurrent apical prolapse was the initial mesh being left too loose and this was simply treated by mesh plication. The rate of serious complications was 4%, and comprised bowel adhesions (prior to the modified re-peritonization technique), broad ligament vascular injury, and one pulmonary embolus. Concomitant vaginal

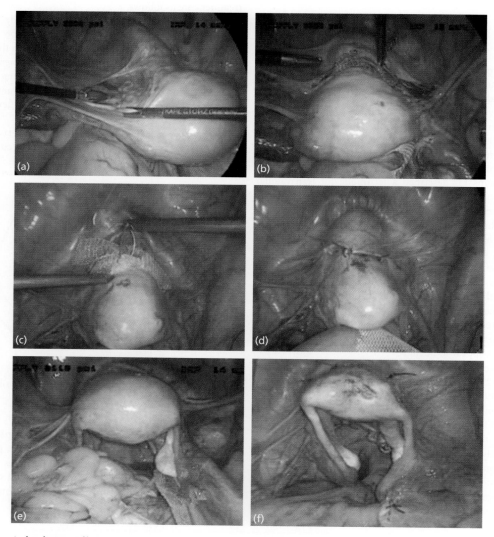

Figure 118.2 The surgical technique of laparoscopic hysteropexy: (a) opening of the left broad ligament; (b) mesh inserted through windows in the broad ligament; (c) suturing of the mesh over the anterior cervix; (d) closure of the uterovesical peritoneum; (e) peritonization of the mesh prior to fixation to the sacral promontory; (f) mesh in place and peritonization complete.

surgery was required in 91% of the patients. The majority of these were posterior repairs; although many women had anterior prolapse prior to surgery, apical support was found to correct this defect in the majority. As this is still a relatively new technique, more outcome data over a longer time frame are needed to enable comparison with more traditional approaches. The outcomes of the VUE study (a randomized multicenter trial comparing uterine preservation surgery with vaginal hysterectomy) are eagerly awaited.

Disadvantages

Vaginal hysterectomy eliminates the possibility of uterine or cervical pathology, and there are incidences of unexpected pathology being detected at pathologic examination of the removed uterus [11]. However, this benefit is less relevant with current advances in minimally invasive treatment of abnormal uterine bleeding. The cervical screening program is reducing cervical cancer incidence and endometrial cancer classically presents at an early stage with uterine bleeding. Therefore, hysterectomy to prevent future malignancy is an unnecessarily aggressive approach.

The mesh extrusion rate with an abdominal approach is considerably less, as the vaginal incision is avoided. Sacrocolpopexy mesh extrusion rates of 2–11% have been reported [12,13].

Fertility following uterine preservation surgery

Theoretically, one advantage of sacrohysteropexy is retention of reproductive potential. It may therefore be the preferred approach for younger patients who have not completed their families. However, patients must be counseled that data for pregnancy outcomes following the procedure are scarce, and that the impact of pregnancy on the surgery, and indeed of the surgery on pregnancy, are unknown. The mesh encircles the cervix, and vaginal birth is therefore not possible; in effect the mesh acts as a cervical suture. There is also concern that uterine blood flow may be compromised as the mesh potentially surrounds the uterine arteries, although it is likely that rich collateral supply will mitigate any compromise.

There have been case reports of full-term normally grown infants delivered by cesarean section after laparoscopic sacrohysteropexy [14].

NICE guidelines

The National Institute for Health and Care Excellence (NICE) has published guidance for surgeons undertaking uterine mesh suspension procedures, as summarized here [15].

- Current evidence on the safety and efficacy of mesh suspension slings for uterine prolapse repair is inadequate.
- This procedure should only be performed by surgeons specializing in pelvic organ prolapse.
- Units carrying out these procedures should have arrangements for clinical governance, consent, and audit.
- Patients should be given clear written information regarding the uncertainty about the safety and outcomes of the procedure.
- All cases should be entered onto the BSUG database.

Resolution of the cases

Case history 1

Laparoscopic hysteropexy was performed to restore the support of the uterus. Concomitant anterior and posterior repairs were also required because of the severity of vaginal prolapse. A good outcome was confirmed at initial follow-up at 8 weeks and the final follow-up at 6 months.

Case history 2

Laparoscopic hysteropexy was performed. A restoration of apical (uterine) support with laparoscopic hysteropexy reduced the cystocele completely; therefore, no vaginal surgery was required. At follow-up at 8 weeks, there were good functional and anatomic outcomes.

KEY POINTS

Challenge: Suspension of a prolapsed uterus.

Background
- The traditional approach to uterine prolapse is vaginal hysterectomy.
- Vaginal hysterectomy does not address underlying deficiencies in pelvic floor support, and recurrence of prolapse is common.

Prevention
- Numerous techniques for uterine preservation surgery have evolved and need further evaluation to enable evidence-based practice.

Management
- Laparoscopic hysteropexy aims to restore and reinforce uterine support by suspending the uterus from the sacral promontory using type 1 polypropylene mesh along the uterosacral ligament. Two strong attachment points are used: the cervix and the anterior longitudinal ligament overlying the sacral promontory.
- The short-term subjective and objective outcomes are indicating up to 90% success.
- Longer-term data are still awaited, and hence the patients have to be carefully counseled.

References

1 Symmonds R, Williams T, Lee R, Webb M. Post hysterectomy entero-cele and vaginal vault prolapse. *Am J Obstet Gynecol* 1981;140:852–859.

2 Marchionni M, Bracco GL, Checcucci V *et al.* True incidence of vaginal vault prolapse: thirteen years of experience. *J Reprod Med* 1999;44:679–684.

3 Williams BFP. Surgical treatment for uterine prolapse in young women. *Am J Obstet Gynecol* 1966;95:967–971.

4 Richardson DA, Scotti RJ, Ostergard DR. Surgical management of uterine prolapse in young women. *J Reprod Med* 1989;34:388–392.

5 Maher CF, Cary MP, Slack CJ, Murray CJ, Milligan M, Schluter P. Uterine preservation or hysterectomy at sacrospinous colpopexy for uterovaginal prolapse. *Int Urogynecol J* 2001;12:381–385.

6 Petros PE. Vault prolapse II: restoration of dynamic vaginal supports by infracoccygeal sacropexy, an axial day-case vaginal procedure. *Int Urogynecol J Pelvic Floor Dysfunct* 2001;12:296–303.

7 Addison WA, Timmons MC. Abdominal approach to vaginal eversion. *Clin Obstet Gynecol* 1993;36:995–1004.

8 Price N, Slack A, Jackson SR. Laparoscopic hysteropexy: the initial results of a uterine suspension procedure for uterovaginal prolapse. *BJOG* 2010;117:62–68.

9 Rahmanou P, White B, Price N, Jackson S. Laparoscopic hysteropexy: 1- to 4-year follow-up of women postoperatively. *Int Urogynecol J* 2014;25:131–138.

10 Prodigalidad LT, Peled Y, Stanton SL, Krissi H. Long-term results of prolapse recurrence and functional outcome after vaginal hysterectomy. *Int J Gynaecol Obstet* 2013;120:57–60.

11 Frick AC, Walters MD, Larkin KS, Barber MD. Risk of unanticipated abnormal gynecologic pathology at the time of hysterectomy for uterovaginal prolapse. *Am J Obstet Gynecol* 2010;202:507e1–4.

12 Visco AG, Weidner AC, Barber MD *et al.* Vaginal mesh erosion after abdominal sacral colpopexy. *Am J Obstet Gynecol* 2001;184:297–302.

13 Maher CM, Feiner B, Baessler K, Glazener CM. Surgical management of pelvic organ prolapse in women: the updated summary version Cochrane review. *Int Urogynecol J* 2011;22:1445–1457.

14 Lewis CM, Culligan P. Sacrohysteropexy followed by successful pregnancy and eventual reoperation for prolapse. *Int Urogynecol J* 2012;23:957–959.

15 National Institute for Health and Care Excellence. *Insertion of mesh uterine suspension sling (including sacrohysteropexy) for uterine prolapse repair.* NICE Interventional Procedure Guidance No. 282, January 2009. Available at https://www.nice.org.uk/guidance/ipg282

CHAPTER 119

Mesh Tape Exposure Following Tension-free Vaginal Tape

Helen Bolton[1] and Mark Slack[2]

[1] Hinchingbrooke Hospital, Hinchingbrooke Health Care NHS Trust, Huntingdon, UK
[2] Addenbrooke's Hospital, Cambridge University Hospitals NHS Foundation Trust, Cambridge, UK

Case history: A 48-year-old woman had a TVT for stress urinary incontinence (SUI). Postoperatively she was unable to pass any urine. She was therefore taught to perform clean intermittent self-catheterization (CISC) and discharged home. She was admitted 6 days later for examination under anesthesia (EUA) and stretching of the tape, as she was still unable to void. Her voiding function recovered fully and she no longer had symptoms of incontinence. Six months later she returned to clinic giving a history of a persistent bloody vaginal discharge and her partner was complaining of pain during intercourse. Examination revealed the tape visible in the midline of the anterior vaginal wall, confirming the diagnosis of vaginal tape exposure. This required a further surgical procedure to excise the tape.

Background

In the case history, the surgical treatment of SUI by a mid-urethral sling procedure with mesh resulted in two complications: immediate and complete urinary obstruction, followed later by vaginal mesh exposure.

The use of non-absorbable synthetic mesh in the surgical treatment of SUI is widespread. Many different meshes have been developed and their properties vary enormously (Figure 119.1). The Amid Classification of Mesh classifies synthetic mesh into four types: I, II, III, and IV [1]. The only type of mesh that should ever be used during urinary incontinence procedures or pelvic reconstructive surgery for prolapse is type I. In addition to better

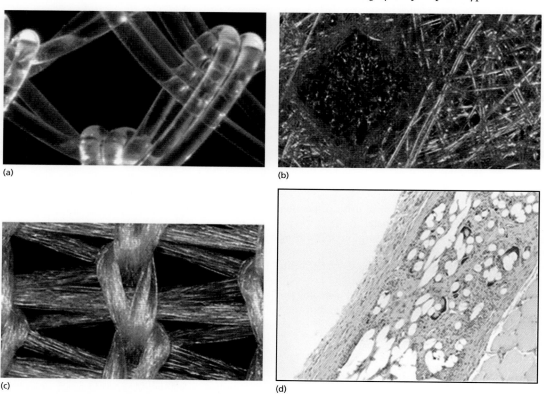

(a) (b) (c) (d)

Figure 119.1 Comparison of mesh types: (a) type I mesh (American Medical Systems); (b) type III thermally bonded mesh (ObTape); (c) type III multifilamentous mesh (Tyco); (d) type III Gore-Tex. Note that type I mesh is a monofilament mesh with large pore sizes, in contrast to the other meshes which are multifilamentous meshes with small pore sizes. In contrast to type I meshes, the others do not incorporate into the tissue and are predisposed to encapsulation and infection. From Slack *et al.*, 2012 [12] with kind permission from Springer Science and Business Media.

Gynecologic and Obstetric Surgery: Challenges and Management Options, First Edition. Edited by Arri Coomarasamy, Mahmood I. Shafi, G. Willy Davila and Kiong K. Chan.
© 2016 John Wiley & Sons, Ltd. Published 2016 by John Wiley & Sons, Ltd.

biologic incorporation rates (required for scaffolding), type I meshes are associated with significantly lower rates of mesh exposure (erosion) than other types of mesh [2]. Using an inappropriate type of mesh can result in major morbidity [2]. The surgeon is directly responsible for ensuring that the appropriate mesh is used for the procedure. Only surgeons specializing in the management of surgical treatment for female urinary incontinence and pelvic organ prolapse should be carrying out these procedures [3,4].

Postoperative voiding obstruction can complicate any surgical procedure for SUI (Chapter 106). This is usually short-lived and occurs in approximately 2–7% of cases. More permanent retention is rare [5]. However, in contrast to other incontinence surgery, the use of synthetic mesh for mid-urethral sling procedures requires expedient intervention due to the rapid biologic incorporation of the mesh into the surrounding tissue [6]. Thus early recognition and prompt treatment of obstruction are of importance in preventing secondary voiding dysfunction.

A delayed complication of TVT is mesh exposure or erosion (Chapter 107), when the mesh becomes exposed in the vagina, urethra, or bladder. In contrast to vaginal or urethral tape exposure, which is usually secondary to infection, bladder exposure is most likely the result of an unidentified bladder perforation at the time of surgery. Vaginal mesh exposure typically presents with vaginal discharge and bleeding, and the partner may complain of pain during intercourse. Symptoms associated with mesh exposure in the bladder or urethra include urinary frequency, urgency and nocturia, together with recurrent urinary tract infections, hematuria, and the development of stones.

Mesh exposure from retropubic slings is usually found along the vaginal incision line (Figure 119.2). Transobturator sling exposures typically present at either vaginal incision line or along the lateral

vaginal sulcus (Figure 119.3). Sulcus exposures may result from either inadvertent perforation during placement, or erosion over time due to very thin vaginal mucosa at the sulcus.

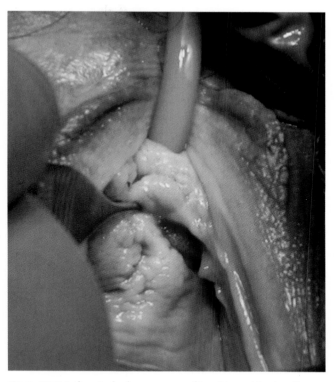

Figure 119.3 Left vaginal sulcus exposure of type I transobturator sling.

Management

Management of urinary obstruction secondary to TVT (see Chapter 106)

The woman described in the case history presented with total urinary obstruction immediately following surgery. Because of the temporal relationship between the surgery and the onset of total urinary obstruction, there is little requirement for diagnostic work-up unless the clinical presentation is atypical. The first priority is to prevent an overdistension injury to the bladder. This can be achieved either by inserting an indwelling urinary catheter or by teaching regular CISC, as in this case.

Definitive intervention for the treatment of obstruction is dictated by the degree of obstruction. Obstruction can be total or partial. Total obstruction occurs when the patient is unable to void. In partial obstruction the patient can void but is unable to empty the bladder fully, maintaining high residual volumes of urine in the bladder.

In the majority of women who experience partial obstruction following TVT, their voiding dysfunction will be transient and improve over a period of days to weeks. First-line treatment in these cases is an indwelling catheter, followed by trial without catheter (TWOC) and reassessment of voiding function a week later. In contrast, those with total obstruction, as in the Case history, rarely improve spontaneously and expedient surgical intervention is essential. Ideally, the tape can be stretched and thus retensioned within 7 days of insertion, before it becomes fixed and immobile due to the significant ingrowth of fibroblastic tissue that occurs within 1–2 weeks of the primary procedure [6]. During the procedure

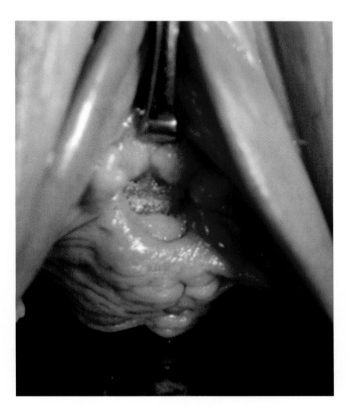

Figure 119.2 Midline exposure of type I mesh sling.

the anterior vaginal wall is reopened at the site of the original incision. The tape should be easily visualized in the midline, and an instrument such as Metzenbaum scissors or Hegar dilator is then hooked between the urethra and the sling. Gentle downward traction should be applied to loosen the tape by 1–2 cm and then the vaginal skin resutured. The patient should be allowed to void and reassessed for evidence of obstruction. Early loosening of TVT usually gives excellent results with restoration of normal voiding function, without compromising the treatment for stress incontinence. If intervention is delayed beyond 7–10 days, the ingrowth of tissue around the mesh prohibits loosening of the tape, necessitating more extensive surgical dissection and tape incision. In-the-office stretching of the tape with a Hegar dilator or another instrument in the urethra should not be performed as it has not been proven to be successful, and may increase the risk of urethral or vaginal mesh exposure.

Management of vaginal mesh exposure
Patients presenting with mesh exposure must be fully informed of their complication and referred to a surgeon experienced in treating these complications. The type of mesh used for the primary procedure must be established; non-type I meshes may require more extensive treatment.

Conservative management
Small mesh fiber exposure may respond to simple trimming in the office. In postmenopausal women, use of local estrogen may help cover any small segments of exposed mesh. If the woman (or partner) is asymptomatic from the mesh exposure, no treatment may be necessary, but regular follow-up should be instituted to ascertain lack of progression.

Surgical management
Treatment of larger segments of exposed mesh usually consists of surgical excision of the exposed mesh, as undertaken in the Case history. The procedure should begin with cystoscopy to detect any associated tape exposure in the urethra or bladder. The vaginal epithelium at the site of tape exposure is cut and the tape clearly identified. Next, the tape is undercut to 1 cm on either side of the vaginal margins, cut on both sides, and the exposed length of tape is removed. The procedure is completed by oversewing the vaginal epithelium. This process may be more challenging for transobturator slings, as the sulcus may be more difficult to expose, requiring deep Trendelenburg positioning.

Appropriate broad-spectrum antibiotics are given to treat the associated infection. Continence is typically preserved if the sling was placed more than 3–6 months before mesh exposure. If an inappropriate mesh (non-type 1) was used for the primary procedure, complete removal of the tape may be necessary, an extensive and complex procedure requiring highly specialized

surgical expertise. Type 1 mesh does not require removal of the entire sling as the sling is unlikely to be infected or be rejected.

In the UK, all cases of mesh exposure must be reported as an adverse incident to the Medicines and Healthcare products Regulatory Agency [7].

Prevention

Before any mesh-related surgical procedure, it is essential that the patient is fully informed of the potential complications of the procedure itself, including those specific to the mesh. Written information must be provided and the patient can be referred to the MHRA and FDA websites for additional information [8,9]. Consent forms should be procedure-specific and detail all the potential complications.

The expertise of the surgeon is a major factor influencing the outcome of the surgery [10]. Therefore surgeons undertaking the procedure must be fully trained and competent to carry out the procedure, and must carry out sufficient numbers of cases to maintain their competency [11]. Complex cases and those patients who develop significant complications including mesh erosion must be referred to a tertiary-level center with appropriate expertise for further management.

Obstruction can occur in any patient undergoing surgery for stress incontinence. However, patients who give a history suggestive of additional voiding abnormalities should be fully investigated (e.g., with multichannel urodynamics) prior to deciding to proceed with surgery.

At the time of surgery it is essential for the surgeon to appreciate that no tension must be placed on the tape. To prevent inadvertent tightening of a correctly positioned tape, it is recommended that Metzenbaum scissors or another instrument should be placed between the tape and urethra while the plastic sheaths are removed from the tape.

Ensuring that the integrity of the vaginal epithelium is preserved during surgery will minimize the risk of tape exposure. The vaginal skin incision should be full thickness, and hydrodissection used to separate the plane between the vaginal mucosa and urethra. Most cases of bladder tape exposure arise secondary to unrecognized bladder perforation during placement of TVT or TOT (vaginal sulcus perforation). A comprehensive cystoscopy using a 70° scope must be carried out to detect bladder perforation after the initial TVT needles are positioned. If perforation is identified, the needles must be withdrawn and repositioned, and then the bladder integrity checked again. The vagina is closed using interrupted absorbable 2-0 sutures.

Early recognition of voiding dysfunction is essential to prevent long-term complications. All postoperative patients must have at least two voids evaluated, together with ultrasound measurement of residual volumes.

KEY POINTS

Challenge: Mesh procedure-related complications.

Background
- Only type I meshes are suitable for surgical treatment of SUI or pelvic organ prolapse.
- Mesh selection is the surgeon's responsibility.

Management
- All patients should be evaluated for urinary obstruction immediately following surgery for SUI.

- Urgent action for total urinary obstruction is essential in the case of mid-urethral synthetic sling surgery.
- Mesh exposure should be treated in a specialist tertiary center with appropriate expertise.
- All significant mesh complications must be reported to the MHRA.

Prevention
- Patients must be fully informed and aware of potential risks.
- Surgeons must be appropriately trained and carry out sufficient numbers of surgical cases.
- Fastidious attention to surgical technique minimizes the risk of complications.

References

1 Amid PK. Classification of biomaterials and their related complications in abdominal wall hernia surgery. *Hernia* 1997;1:15–21.

2 Slack M. Synthetic materials for pelvic reconstructive surgery. In: CardozoL, StaskinD (eds) *Textbook of Female Urology and Urogynecology*, 2nd edn, pp. 835–844. Informa Healthcare, Abingdon, 2006.

3 Slack M, Mayne CJ. The use of mesh in gynaecological surgery. RCOG Scientific Impact Paper No. 19, April 2010. Available at https://www.rcog.org.uk/globalassets/documents/guidelines/sip_no_19.pdf

4 National Institute for Health and Care Excellence. *Surgical repair of vaginal wall prolapse using mesh*. NICE Interventional Procedure Guidance No. 267, June 2008. Available at https://www.nice.org.uk/guidance/ipg267

5 Karram MM, Segal JL, Vassallo BJ, Kleeman SD. Complications and untoward effects of the tension-free vaginal tape procedure. *Obstet Gynecol* 2003;101:929–932.

6 Shah S, Nitti VW. Diagnosis and treatment of obstruction following incontinence surgery: urethrolysis and other techniques. In: CardozoL, StaskinD (eds) *Textbook of Female Urology and Urogynecology*, 3rd edn, pp. 749–770. Informa Healthcare, London, 2010.

7 Medicines and Healthcare products Regulatory Agency. Reporting adverse incidents involving medical devices. http://www.mhra.gov.uk/Safetyinformation/Reportingsafetyproblems/Devices/index.htm

8 Medicines and Healthcare products Regulatory Agency. Vaginal mesh for pelvic organ prolapse. http://www.mhra.gov.uk/Safetyinformation/Generalsafetyinformationandadvice/Product-specificinformationandadvice/Product-specificinformationandadvice%E2%80%93M%E2%80%93T/Vaginalmeshforpelvicorganprolapse/index.htm

9 Food and Drug Administration. Surgical mesh: FDA safety communication. Available at http://www.fda.gov/MedicalDevices/Safety/AlertsandNotices/ucm142636.htm

10 Halm EA, Lee C, Chassin MR. Is volume related to outcome in health care? A systematic review and methodologic critique of the literature. *Ann Intern Med* 2002;137:511–520.

11 National Institute for Health and Care Excellence. *Urinary incontinence: the management of urinary incontinence in women*. NICE Clinical Guideline No. 171, September 2013. Available at https://www.nice.org.uk/guidance/cg171

12 Slack M, Ostergard D, Cervigni M, Deprest J. A standardized description of graft-containing meshes and recommended steps before the introduction of medical devices for prolapse surgery. Consensus of the 2nd IUGA Grafts Roundtable: optimizing safety and appropriateness of graft use in transvaginal pelvic reconstructive surgery. *Int Urogynecol J* 2012;23(Suppl 1):S15–S26.

CHAPTER 120
Vaginal Vault Evisceration

Swati Jha
Sheffield Teaching Hospitals NHS Foundation Trust, Sheffield, UK

Case history: A 42-year-old woman underwent a total laparoscopic hysterectomy for menorrhagia 3 months ago. She came back to the hospital with a 2-day history of lower abdominal pain, vaginal bleeding, and the protrusion of a mass from the vagina. Speculum examination revealed small bowel protruding into the vagina and bulging at the introitus. The bowel appeared congested but not ischemic. She had sex three days before presenting.

Background

Vaginal vault evisceration is the extrusion of intraperitoneal contents following disruption of the vaginal vault or apex. It is a rare but serious complication of a hysterectomy. It can appear immediately, or months and even years, after the initial operation. Risk factors include the triad of postmenopausal atrophy, previous vaginal surgery, and an enterocele [1]. The commonest sites of rupture are the weakest point of the vaginal vault or posterior fornix. Some studies suggest that laparoscopic hysterectomies have a higher association with vaginal evisceration than vaginal or abdominal hysterectomies [2].

In premenopausal women the commonest precipitating factors for vaginal evisceration are preceding sexual intercourse and usage of foreign objects. In postmenopausal women it can occur spontaneously, following sexual intercourse, or with activities that increase intra-abdominal pressure such as straining when passing stools and coughing.

Women with evisceration may present with abdominal pain, vaginal bleeding, discharge, and sometimes an obvious mass protruding from the vagina. If the presentation or diagnosis is delayed and the viability of intra-abdominal contents is compromised, the patient may present acutely unwell in shock and with intestinal obstruction. The most common organ to eviscerate through the vagina is the terminal ileum. Other organs that can eviscerate include the omentum, colon, fallopian tube, or appendix [3].

Management

Immediate management

Vaginal vault evisceration (Figure 120.1) is an acute gynecologic emergency. The immediate management following confirmation of the diagnosis includes stabilizing the patient, providing intravenous

fluid therapy and broad-spectrum antibiotics, wrapping the bowel or eviscerated organ with moist saline packs, and initiating surgical repair. Once stabilized, a full history is obtained and a thorough physical and pelvic examination is performed. The possibility of foreign bodies should be considered. Where bowel is protruding from the vagina, it is crucial to preserve its viability. The patient is placed in an exaggerated Trendelenburg position and attempts to replace the bowel using moist sponge sticks may be made, although this is usually not possible without anesthesia due to edema of the eviscerated contents. Arrangements should be made for surgical repair. If the patient shows signs of an acute abdomen, she should be resuscitated and immediately taken to theater for exploratory laparotomy and repair of the vaginal defect.

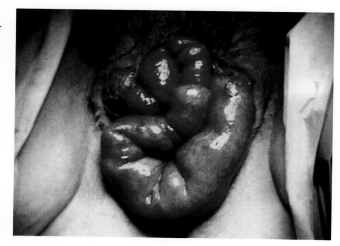

Figure 120.1 Vault evisceration with extrusion of bowel.

Surgical management

The type of approach (i.e., abdominal, vaginal, laparoscopic, combined abdominal–vaginal, or combined laparoscopic–vaginal) depends on several factors including viability of the prolapsed bowel, presence of foreign body in the peritoneal cavity, and the ability to replace the prolapsed bowels vaginally. The abdominal approach is most commonly used as it provides good exposure for inspecting the abdominal viscera, irrigation, drainage, resection of non-viable bowel, and assessment of pelvic cavity. Where the bowel appears viable and peristalsis is apparent, a vaginal approach may be used, but this can restrict the surgeon's ability to rule out concurrent trauma elsewhere in the bowel or mesentery.

Surgical treatment is a two-step process incorporating the replacement and repair of the protruding viscus, followed by closure of the vaginal defect with or without reinforcement [4]. An examination under anesthesia allows assessment of the viability of bowels or eviscerated organs and assessment of the vaginal defect. Viable bowels are reduced either abdominally or vaginally. If a section of bowel is not viable, resection and anastomosis should be carried out. The vaginal edges are excised, leaving behind fresh viable tissues and removing all necrotic areas on the vaginal cuff and supporting tissues. Most vaginal vault defects are small and easily repaired. Closure with interrupted delayed absorbable suture is preferred. Surgical help should be sought if needed. Local support and vascularity of the repair can be increased by using an omental pedicle flap (Bastiaanse procedure), bulbocavernosus muscle with labial skin interposition (Martius procedure, see Chapter 113, Figure 113.1), gracilis–myocutaneous flap (Ingelman–Sundberg procedure), gluteus maximus myocutaneous flap, or rectus muscle myocutaneous flap.

Postoperative management

Postoperative prophylactic antibiotics should be given and a pelvic drain used to minimize abscess formation. Anatomic pelvic defects should be identified and corrected to prevent future recurrence. This may be at the time of the primary surgery or as an interval procedure, and would depend on the condition of the patient, health of pelvic tissues, intestinal viability, and the experience of the operating surgeon. If major surgery is required to correct the primary defect, definitive pelvic repair is best carried out as an elective procedure at a later date. Another advantage of a two-stage procedure is that it allows a thorough reassessment after full recovery to evaluate the need for any further surgery, allows the resolution of inflammation and healing of the tissues, and minimizes the risk of postoperative infection. The advantage of simultaneous repair is that the patient does not require repeat anesthesia and surgery.

Prevention

The preventive aims are to avoid repeat vaginal operations and shortening of the vagina, and to restore pelvic support with minimal tension [4]. Enterocele formation post hysterectomy could be avoided by a concurrent McCall culdoplasty.

In view of the increased risk of vaginal vault complications after total laparoscopic hysterectomies compared with other routes of hysterectomy, the following are some recommendations to consider [2].

- A total hysterectomy should only be performed for clear indications and when a supracervical hysterectomy is not an appropriate option.

- Sharp colpotomy at the vault should be performed using a laparoscopic scalpel to minimize the use of thermal energy (which can be associated with delayed tissue damage).
- Women undergoing total laparoscopic hysterectomy should be advised to delay first intercourse postoperatively. This should be until the vagina is completely healed, usually 6 weeks after surgery, although some recommend delaying sex for up to 12 weeks after surgery.

KEY POINTS

Challenge: Vaginal vault evisceration.

Background
- This is a rare but acute and sometimes life-threatening gynecologic emergency.
- It can occur months or even years after a hysterectomy.
- Association with a total laparoscopic hysterectomy appears to be higher than with vaginal or abdominal hysterectomy.

Prevention
- Provide adequate estrogenization of the vagina preoperatively.
- Intraoperatively, avoid shortening of the vagina and tension in the repair, and address any enterocele.
- Total laparoscopic hysterectomy should be done for the appropriate indications and thermal energy minimized during a colpotomy.

Management
- Immediate management includes providing intravenous fluid therapy and broad-spectrum antibiotics, wrapping the bowel or eviscerated organ with moist saline packs, and arranging surgical repair.
- Surgical approaches to address evisceration can be abdominal, vaginal, laparoscopic, combined abdominal–vaginal, or combined laparoscopic–vaginal.
- Repair may be a one-stage or two-stage procedure and needs to be individualized:
  - One-stage procedure: incorporates the replacement and repair of the protruding viscus, as well as closure of the vaginal defect with or without reinforcement.
  - Two-stage procedure: first operation deals with replacement and repair of the viscus; a separate second operation addresses the vaginal defect.
- If a section of bowel is not viable, resection and anastomosis should be carried out (see Chapter 37).
- Repair may require a multidisciplinary approach depending on the eviscerating organs.

References

1 Croak AJ, Gebhart JB, Klingele CJ, Schroeder G, Lee RA, Podratz KC. Characteristics of patients with vaginal rupture and evisceration. *Obstet Gynecol* 2004;103:572–576.
2 Hur HC, Guido RS, Mansuria SM, Hacker MR, Sanfilippo JS, Lee TT. Incidence and patient characteristics of vaginal cuff dehiscence after different modes of hysterectomies. *J Minim Invasive Gynecol* 2007;14:311–317.
3 Ramirez PT, Klemer DP. Vaginal evisceration after hysterectomy: a literature review. *Obstet Gynecol Surv* 2002;57:462–467.
4 Gandhi P, Jha S. Vaginal vault evisceration. *Obstetrician & Gynaecologist* 2011;13: 231–237.

CHAPTER 121

Complications in Laparoscopic Pelvic Floor Surgery

Nir Haya[1] and Christopher Maher[1,2,3]

[1] Royal Brisbane and Women's Hospital, Brisbane, Queensland, Australia
[2] Wesley Hospital, Brisbane, Queensland, Australia
[3] University of Queensland, Brisbane, Queensland, Australia

Case history: *A 52-year-old woman was undergoing a laparoscopic sacrocolpopexy for vaginal vault prolapse. During the insertion of the 5-mm secondary trocar in left iliac fossa the inferior epigastric vessels were traversed.*

Background

Laparoscopic pelvic floor surgery can be complicated with port-site (Chapter 38) and other vessel bleeding (Chapter 76), injury to urinary bladder (Chapter 72), ureter (Chapter 73) or bowel (Chapter 74) during dissection and creation of retroperitoneal, rectovaginal and vesicovaginal spaces, as well as various other complications outlined in Sections 2 and 4 of this book.

Trocar site bleeding

The incidence of port-site bleeding is reported to be 0.7% [1]. Perforation of the inferior epigastric artery will produce retroperitoneal or intraperitoneal bleeding. Perforation of the superficial epigastric artery will result in intramuscular or subcutaneous bleeding. To reduce the incidence of vessel injury, the surgeon can use transillumination for locating superficial abdominal wall vessels; however, intraperitoneal

identification is required for the inferior epigastric artery (Figure 121.1). When the inferior epigastric artery is difficult to visualize, intra-abdominal landmarks can be helpful (Chapter 38). The lower ports should be placed lateral to the inferior epigastric vessels and medial to the deep circumflex vessels (Figure 121.2).

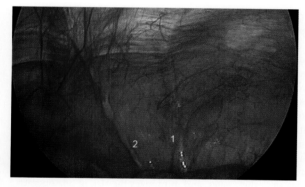

Figure 121.1 Anterior abdominal wall, with the right inferior epigastric vessels (1) lateral to the obliterated umbilical artery (2). From van der Vurst *et al.*, 2004 [2] with permission from Lippincott Williams and Wilkins.

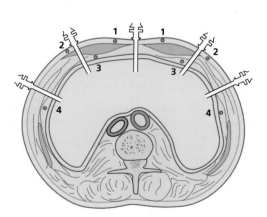

1. Superficial epigastric artery
2. Superficial circumflex iliac artery
3. Inferior epigastric artery
4. Deep circumflex iliac artery

(a)

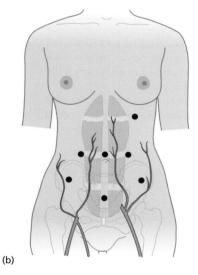

(b)

Figure 121.2 Demonstration of port placement in the transverse (a) and coronal (b) views in relation to anterior abdominal wall vasculature. Reproduced with authors' permission (© Maher/Francis).

Presacral bleeding

Presacral venous bleeding during laparoscopic sacrocolpopexy is uncommon but potentially life-threatening. The presacral fascia covers and protects the underlying plexus, which consists of venous networks both on and beneath the surface of the sacral periosteum. Inadvertent manipulation may tear the fascia and cause damage of underlying thin-walled veins, which are devoid of valves. It is well documented that conventional measures for hemostasis are ineffective in managing presacral hemorrhage [2].

Bowel injury

The incidence of bowel injuries at gynecologic laparoscopy is reported to be about 0.5% [3,4]. Approximately half of these injuries occur during entry [5–7], and the large and small bowel are equally involved [8,9]. The reported rates of intraoperative diagnosis of bowel injury vary from 43 to 61% [10,11]. A large meta-analysis of 28 studies found that thermal injury to the bowel was the most common cause of non-entry-related bowel injuries. The mortality rate from bowel injuries in gynecologic laparoscopy ranges from 2.5 to 5% [12,13], but increases to 21% in those with a delayed diagnosis of bowel injury [14].

Bladder injury

Inadvertent cystotomy has been reported in 4% of laparoscopic colposuspensions [15] and 2% of laparoscopic sacrocolpopexy, and can be identified and repaired intraoperatively without sequelae [16–18].

Ureteric injury

Ureteric injuries following pelvic floor surgery are reported in 3% of cases [19,20]. Early recognition and treatment of ureteral injuries are important to prevent morbidity.

Management

Management of trocar site bleeding

Even after using all preventive measures, experienced laparoscopic surgeons may still be faced with arterial bleeding from the inferior epigastric artery. This vessel has anastomoses with the superior epigastric artery, and therefore it is crucial to control the bleeding both cephalad and caudal to the trocar site. It is important to not remove the offending trocar, because this denotes the location of the injured artery, which may become difficult to visualize as the hematoma spreads.

If the bleeding is recognized early and the inferior epigastric artery can be identified, both ends of the transected vessel can be diathermied with bipolar forceps (Figure 121.3a). If this is unsuccessful, a size 12 Foley catheter can be passed through the 5-mm trocar, and the Foley balloon inflated with 10–15 mL of sterile water (Figure 121.3b). The trocar can then be removed over the catheter, and firm traction should be applied to tamponade the site; the catheter can be secured with an umbilical cord clamp overnight. The following morning the clamp and catheter are removed.

If this fails to secure the vessel, U-stitches can be placed into the abdominal wall under direct laparoscopic visualization; a CT-1 needle is passed through the abdominal wall into the abdomen and passed from inside the abdomen to the outside using laparoscopic

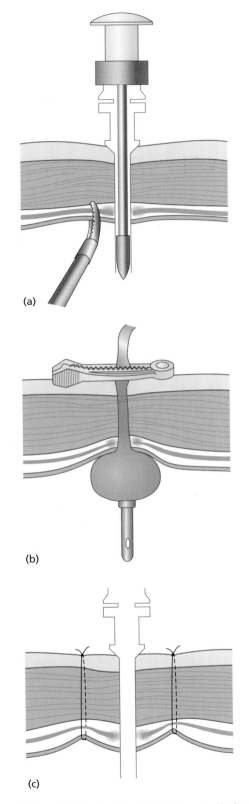

Figure 121.3 Control of inferior epigastric bleeding using diathermy (a), balloon tamponade (b), and direct suture (c). Reproduced with authors' permission (© Maher/Francis).

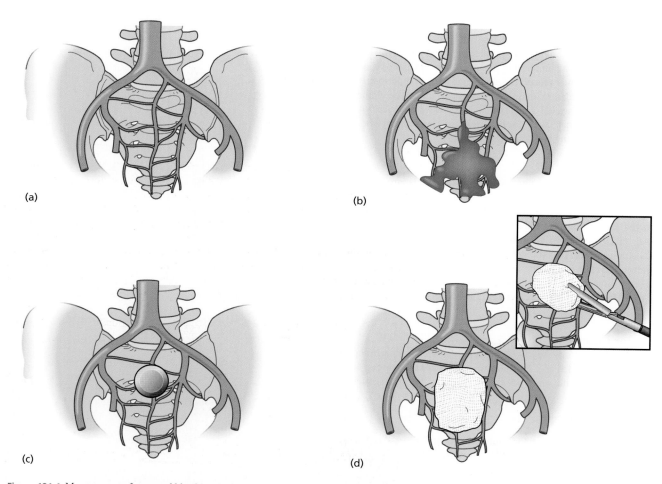

(a)

(b)

(c)

(d)

Figure 121.4 Management of presacral bleeding. Reproduced with authors' permission (© Maher/Francis).

needle holders, and tied both cephalad and caudal to the trocar (Figure 121.3c). The sutures are removed the following morning.

Management of presacral bleeding

If presacral bleeding occurs (Figure 121.4b), it is important to avoid the usual measures of coagulation and suturing because they can aggravate bleeding resulting in significant blood loss. The first step is to apply immediate direct pressure over the bleeding site using a small tampon gauze for 5 min. This may control the bleeding, but if the bleeding persists, traditionally pelvic packing and the use of sterile metallic or titanium thumbtacks are employed (Figure 121.4c). Packing has the disadvantage of reoperation for removal of the packs, with the risk of rebleeding [21]. An alternative approach is to use a hemostatic matrix agent such as FloSeal (Baxter, USA) or Surgicel Fibrillar (Ethicon, USA), followed by gauze pressure for 5 min (Figure 121.4d) [21].

Management of bowel injury (see Chapters 37, 74 and 75)

If there is a recognized Veress needle puncture injury to the bowel and there is no associated fecal spill, it is likely that the injury can be managed expectantly [5,6,22]. Trocar damage to

the bowel mandates careful inspection of the whole bowel to ensure no through-and-through injuries have occurred. Small defects of the serosal or muscularis layers may be repaired using continuous or interrupted 3-0 delayed absorbable sutures. Suture lines should be perpendicular to the long axis of the bowel to prevent stricture of the lumen. Large defects can be closed with a stapling device, or resection with re-anastomosis may be necessary. If bowel re-anastomosis cannot be performed, a temporary diverting colostomy may be required [23]. After the repair, the abdominal cavity is irrigated and broad-spectrum antibiotics are commenced.

Electrosurgical injuries are more commonly seen in bowel injuries that are diagnosed postoperatively and may result from direct application, direct or capacitive coupling or insulation failure (Chapters 70 and 71). The reported average time to diagnosis after needle or trocar injury to bowel is 1.3 days, as compared with 10.4 days for electrosurgical burns [14]. No clear guidelines exist for the management of electrosurgical bowel injuries. Surgeons should be mindful that if the area of blanching exceeds 5 mm, it is estimated the thermal damage may exceed up to 5 cm from the apparent injury and therefore resection should be considered [24].

In patients presenting postoperatively with abdominal pain or bowel symptoms, CT of the abdomen and pelvis with oral and intravenous contrast should be undertaken to assess the integrity of the bowel and urinary system.

Early consultation with a surgical colleague is recommended and damaged bowel must be repaired or resected with or without a temporary colostomy. All necrotic tissue should be removed to minimize the risk of abscess formation.

Management of bladder injury (see Chapters 35 and 72)

If bladder injury is suspected, it is important to perform a laparoscopic inspection of the bladder distended to 300 mL, and a cystoscopy. The defect can be repaired in two layers with 2-0 Vicryl or Monocryl so that the bladder is watertight at 300 mL. Cystoscopy should then be repeated to ensure there are no other unrecognized injuries and the ureters are patent.

An inadvertent cystotomy to the mobile dome of the bladder is easily repaired and the catheter can be removed after only 4–5 days [18]. However, a cystotomy close to the trigone (which happens during mobilization of the bladder from the vagina in creating the vesicovaginal space at sacrocolpopexy) is more difficult to manage as the bladder is thinner and less mobile. In this situation,

it is better to avoid introducing polypropylene mesh that can be in direct contact with the repaired cystotomy incision line, in order to minimize the risk of subsequent intravesical mesh erosion; an indwelling catheter should be left on free drainage for 7–10 days. A voiding cystogram is performed to ensure healing prior to removal of the catheter and formal trial without catheter.

Management of ureteric injury (see Chapters 36 and 73)

For intraoperative diagnosis of ureteric injury, intravenous indigo carmine or methylene blue can be administered followed by cystoscopy to look for ejection of dye from the ureteric orifices, confirming patency of the ureters. If dye is not clearly visible on cystoscopic examination following a laparoscopic pelvic floor repair, the injury is likely to be related to kinking of the ureter in the lateral retropubic space or in relation to the uterosacral/cardinal ligament sutures during sacrocolpopexy or vault suspending procedures. Lateral retropubic or vault suspending sutures should be removed one at a time until ureteric patency is demonstrated. The sutures are then placed at a safe location and ureteric patency is again confirmed. If patency is not confirmed with removal of the sutures, retrograde dye studies and intraoperative urologic consultation are required.

KEY POINTS

Challenge: Complications in laparoscopic pelvic floor surgery.

Background
- Laparoscopic pelvic floor procedures can suffer from complications, including port-site bleeding, presacral bleeding, and injury to bowel, bladder or ureters.

Prevention (of complications)
- Open entry technique and careful placement of secondary ports under vision will reduce vascular and bowel complications.
- In those with prior vertical midline incision, Palmer's point entry is advised.
- In a hostile abdomen the surgeon should re-create normal anatomy prior to commencing the surgery, and be aware that a vaginal approach to pelvic floor surgery may minimize the risk of inadvertent damage to the bladder and bowel.
- During adhesiolysis and creation of surgical spaces, traction and counter-traction with sharp dissection, while minimizing electrothermal energy use, may reduce injuries to bladder and bowel.

Management
- Early diagnosis and management of complications, preferably intraoperatively, will reduce morbidity.
- In those with persisting pain or readmission following laparoscopic pelvic floor surgery, CT of the abdomen and pelvis with oral and intravenous contrast will help delineate urinary or bowel pathology.
- Early consultation with surgical colleagues is recommended.
- The management options for port-site bleeding include:
  - Diathermy with bipolar forceps.
  - Foley balloon tamponade.
  - U-stitches.
- The management options for presacral bleeding include:
  - Direct pressure with gauze (for at least 5 min).
  - Pelvic packing.
  - Titanium thumbtacks.
  - Use of a hemostatic matrix (e.g., FloSeal or Surgicel Fibrillar).
  - Do not use diathermy or suturing because they can aggravate presacral bleeding.
- The management options for bowel, bladder and ureteric injuries are addressed in the relevant chapters.

References

1 Karthik S, Augustine AJ, Shibumon MM, Pai MV. Analysis of laparoscopic port site complications: a descriptive study. *J Minim Access Surg* 2013;9:59–64.

2 van der Vurst TJ, Bodegom ME, Rakic S. Tamponade of presacral hemorrhage with hemostatic sponges fixed to the sacrum with endoscopic helical tackers: report of two cases. *Dis Colon Rectum* 2004;47:1550–1553.

3 Quasarano RT, Kashef M, Sherman SJ, Hagglund KH. Complications of gynecologic laparoscopy. *J Am Assoc Gynecol Laparosc* 1999;6:317–321.

4 Mirhashemi R, Harlow BL, Ginsburg ES, Signorello LB, Berkowitz R, Feldman S. Predicting risk of complications with gynecologic laparoscopic surgery. *Obstet Gynecol* 1998;92:327–331.

5 Brosens I, Gordon A. Bowel injuries during gynaecological laparoscopy. A multinational survey. *Gynaecol Endosc* 2001;10:141–145.

6 Harkki Siren P, Kurki T. A nationwide analysis of laparoscopic complications. *Obstet Gynecol* 1997;89:108–112.

7 Harkki Siren P, Sjoberg J, Kurki T. Major complications of laparoscopy: a follow-up Finnish study. *Obstet Gynecol* 1999;94:94–98.

8 Chapron C, Pierre F, Harchaoui Y *et al.* Gastrointestinal injuries during gynaecological laparoscopy. *Hum Reprod* 1999;14:333–337.

9 Chapron C, Querleu D, Bruhat MA *et al.* Surgical complications of diagnostic and operative gynaecological laparoscopy: a series of 29,966 cases. *Hum Reprod* 1998;13:867–872.

10 Magrina JF. Complications of laparoscopic surgery. *Clin Obstet Gynecol* 2002;45:469–480.

11 van der Voort M, Heijnsdijk EA, Gouma DJ. Bowel injury as a complication of laparoscopy. *Br J Surg* 2004;91:1253–1258.

12 Champault G, Caracu F, Taffinder N. Serious trocar accidents in laparoscopic surgery: a French survey of 103,852 operations. *Surg Laparosc Endosc* 1996;6:367–370.

13 Hashizume M, Sugimachi K. Needle and trocar injury during laparoscopic surgery in Japan. *Surg Endosc* 1997;11:1198–1201.

14 Brosens I, Gordon A, Campo R, Gordts S. Bowel injury in gynecologic laparoscopy. *J Am Assoc Gynecol Laparosc* 2003;10:9–13.

15 Smith AR, Stanton SL. Laparoscopic colposuspension. *Br J Obstet Gynaecol* 1998;105:383–384.

16 Bruyere F, Rozenberg H, Abdelkader T. La promonto-fixation sous coelioscopie: une voie d'abord seduisante pour la cure des prolapsus. *Prog Urol* 2001;11:1320–1326.

17 Cosson M, Bogaert E, Narducci F, Querleu D, Crépin G. Promontofixation coelioscopique: resultats a court terme et complications chez 83 patientes. *J Gynecol Obstet Biol Reprod (Paris)* 2000;29:746–750.

18 Antiphon P, Elard S, Benyoussef A *et al*. Laparoscopic promontory sacral colpopexy: is the posterior, recto-vaginal, mesh mandatory? *Eur Urol* 2004;45:655–661.

19 Harris RL, Cundiff GW, Theofrastous JP, Yoon H, Bump RC, Addison WA. The value of intraoperative cystoscopy in urogynecologic and reconstructive pelvic surgery. *Am J Obstet Gynecol* 1997;177:1367–1369.

20 Jabs CF, Drutz HP. The role of intraoperative cystoscopy in prolapse and incontinence surgery. *Am J Obstet Gynecol* 2001;185:1368–1371.

21 Germanos S, Bolanis I, Saedon M, Baratsis S. Control of presacral venous bleeding during rectal surgery. *Am J Surg* 2010;200:e33–35.

22 Jansen FW, Kolkman W, Bakkum EA *et al*. Complications of laparoscopy: an inquiry about closed- versus open-entry technique. *Am J Obstet Gynecol* 2004;190:634–638.

23 Sharp HT. Prevention and management of complications from gynecologic surgery. *Obstet Gynecol Clin North Am* 2010;17:369–474.

24 Wheeless CR. Gastrointestinal injuries associated with laparoscopy. In: Phillips JM (ed.) *Endoscopy in Gynecology*, pp. 365–390. Williams & Wilkins, Baltimore, 1978.

CHAPTER 122
Robotic Urogynecology Procedures

Orfhlaith E. O'Sullivan and Barry A. O'Reilly
Cork University Maternity Hospital, Cork, Ireland

Case history: A 35-year-old woman with symptomatic prolapse was found to have uterine descent to the level of the genital hiatus. She wished to maintain her fertility. Her previous surgical history included an open appendectomy and a laparoscopic left ovarian cystectomy. Her body mass index (BMI) was raised at 35.

Background

The da Vinci® Surgical System (Intuitive Surgical, Inc., Sunnyvale, CA) gained FDA approval for gynecologic surgery in 2005 in the USA, while it has had full regulatory clearance and the CE (Conformité Européenne) mark since 1999 in Europe [1]. Since its introduction, the role of robot-assisted surgery in urogynecology has grown considerably.

Sacrocolpopexy

Sacrocolpopexy can be performed using one of three approaches: open, laparoscopic, or robot-assisted. The laparoscopic approach has been shown to have similar outcomes, with reoperation rates of approximately 6–7% and a mesh erosion rate of 3% [2]. A study comparing the three approaches found no difference in pain, length of stay, blood loss, operating time, or short-term functional outcomes [3]. Further studies have confirmed the good functional results using the robot [4], with a low complication rate and high patient satisfaction [5].

The robotic approach may assist the surgeon in dissecting over the sacral promontory [6] because of the increased range of movement of the instruments. Compared with the robot-assisted approach, a drawback of the laparoscopic approach is the technical difficulty in placing sutures and knot tying [7]. The learning curves have been shown to be higher in the laparoscopic group [8].

Hysteropexy

The aim of hysteropexy is to restore uterine anatomy where uterine preservation is required [9]. Success rates are similar for open, laparoscopic, and robot-assisted approaches, varying from 87 to 98% [10,11]. Successful pregnancies have been reported following laparoscopic hysteropexy; however, the long-term effects of pregnancy on the surgery are not fully appreciated yet [12]. Sacrohysteropexy for the treatment of prolapse is associated with

excellent subjective and objective success rates, making it a safe and feasible surgical option in the management of pelvic organ prolapse where uterine preservation is required [13].

Vesicovaginal fistula repair

The robot technology allows a complicated laparoscopic procedure to be performed safely with good results. Vesicovaginal fistulae have been treated effectively using the robot-assisted approach with minimal blood loss, short length of stay, and low recurrence rates [4].

Resolution of the case (see Chapter 118)

Given the desire to maintain fertility, a sacrohysteropexy was deemed to be the surgery of choice. The procedure was to be performed using robot assistance. The patient was counseled regarding potential complications, including the need to convert to an open procedure because of technical and surgical difficulties.

The patient was admitted to the theater complex, anesthetized, and placed in a moderate Trendelenburg position. The abdominal cavity was insufflated with CO_2 to 20 mmHg using a Veress needle, and a supra-umbilical port was placed. On inserting the camera, it was evident that there were extensive adhesions on the right side of the abdominal cavity, secondary to past appendectomy. The adhesions limited visibility and would need to be dissected to allow the procedure to continue safely. The left-sided ports (see Chapter 114, Figure 114.1) were placed under direct vision and the adhesions dissected down using laparoscopic instruments. The robot was docked, and the arms were attached. The procedure was completed using the robot-assisted approach. The technique started with identifying the sacrum and opening the overlying peritoneum. Maintaining the intra-abdominal pressure at 20 mmHg allowed the CO_2 to track between the planes, facilitating the formation of a peritoneal tunnel and dissection to the level of the anterior longitudinal ligament (Figure 122.1). A drawback of robotic surgery is the loss of haptic feedback; however, with time the surgeon develops visual haptic feedback, which overcomes the deficit.

During the procedure the third robot arm was used as a bowel retractor. Manipulation of the uterus was achieved using a uterine manipulator, which aided with acute anteversion required for suture placement. If a manipulator was unavailable or was inadequate to

Gynecologic and Obstetric Surgery: Challenges and Management Options, First Edition. Edited by Arri Coomarasamy, Mahmood I. Shafi, G. Willy Davila and Kiong K. Chan.
© 2016 John Wiley & Sons, Ltd. Published 2016 by John Wiley & Sons, Ltd.

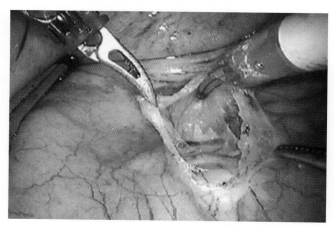

Figure 122.1 Dissection to expose the anterior longitudinal ligament.
© 2013 Intuitive Surgical, Inc.

achieve the necessary anteversion, a suture could have been placed securing the uterus to the anterior abdominal wall.

Two windows were then made through the avascular area of the broad ligament, through which the arms of the mesh were passed. They were then sutured at the uterocervical junction using a Gore-Tex suture. The long arm of the mesh was then attached to the sacrum, ensuring it was free of tension. The mesh was then covered totally with peritoneum to avoid complications such as erosion through the bowel or bladder and the formation of dense adhesions.

Challenges associated with robot-assisted surgery

The introduction of new technology brings new challenges, especially for the surgeon and the operating room team. One of the major technical issues that may occur is a robot malfunction. The incidence of device failure is reported to be 0.2–0.4% [15]. However, it does occur, highlighting the need to counsel patients and to have a contingency plan. Studies recommend conventional laparoscopic suturing skills should be maintained, thus allowing the surgery to continue [15]. All surgeons performing robotic surgery must become familiar with troubleshooting robotic technology and associated equipment. Failure to do so may add time and technical difficulty to robotic cases [16]. There is evidence that robotic failure rate decreases with increased operator and team experience [17]. Checklists have been used as an intervention to prevent these failures by promoting team-working, standardizing practice, allowing the early detection of potential errors and improving patient safety as a whole.

Patient positioning is of great importance in minimizing the adverse outcomes associated with potentially long operative times. In one study, nerve injury associated with malpositioning during urological robotic surgery had an incidence of 6.6%, with almost one-quarter persisting beyond 6 months. The injury rate was significantly affected by the operative time and the ASA group. Therefore, patients undergoing long operations should be counseled regarding the risk of nerve injury, especially if they have multiple comorbidities [18].

Robot-assisted surgery attempts to overcome some of the limitations of laparoscopic surgery while retaining the benefits of a minimally invasive approach. Specific improvements associated with robot-assisted surgery include better visualization through the use of three-dimensional magnification, availability of tools with seven degrees of freedom that mimic hand movements, along with improved ergonomics and more intuitive hand–eye coordination when controlling surgical instruments [19]. However, this has been achieved at the cost of loss of haptic and tactile feedback, as a result of the indirect manipulation of instruments by the surgeon [20]. Many surgeons using robot-assisted surgery describe attaining a new sense of visual haptic feedback, which may negate the loss of haptic feedback.

Obesity is increasing throughout the developed world. There is evidence that more complex procedures can be undertaken robotically than with traditional straight stick surgery, irrespective of body habitus.

KEY POINTS

Challenge: Robot-assisted pelvic floor surgery.

Background
- Robotic surgery can be used for sacrocolpopexy, sacrohysteropexy, and vesicovaginal fistula repair.
- Robotic surgery has a shorter learning curve than laparoscopic surgery, but is more expensive.

Prevention
- Counsel patients regarding potential complications including technical failure of the device (0.2–0.4%) and the need to convert to laparoscopic or open technique.
- Become familiar with the technology being used and be able to troubleshoot for technical problems.
- Use checklists to promote team-working, standardize practice, and identify potential errors early.
- Be cognizant of potential surgical difficulties and complications.
- Maintain laparoscopic skills, particularly the ability to suture.

References

1 Reza M, Maeso S, Blasco JA, Andradas E. Meta-analysis of observational studies on the safety and effectiveness of robotic gynaecological surgery. *Br J Surg* 2010;97:1772–1783.

2 Ganatra AM, Rozet F, Sanchez-Salas R *et al.* The current status of laparoscopic sacrocolpopexy: a review. *Eur Urol* 2009;55:1089–1103.

3 White WM, Goel RK, Swartz MA, Moore C, Rackley RR, Kaouk JH. Single-port laparoscopic abdominal sacral colpopexy: initial experience and comparative outcomes. *Urology* 2009;74:1008–1012.

4 Geller EJ, Siddiqui NY, Wu JM, Visco AG. Short-term outcomes of robotic sacrocolpopexy compared with abdominal sacrocolpopexy. *Obstet Gynecol* 2008;112:1201–1206.

5 Elliott DS, Krambeck AE, Chow GK. Long-term results of robotic assisted laparoscopic sacrocolpopexy for the treatment of high grade vaginal vault prolapse. *J Urol* 2006;176:655–659.

6 Göçmen A, Sanlikan F, Ucar MG. Robotic-assisted sacrocolpopexy/sacrocervicopexy repair of pelvic organ prolapse: initial experience. *Arch Gynecol Obstet* 2012;285:683–688.

7 Wattiez A. Laparoscopic repair of vaginal vault prolapse. *Curr Opin Obstet Gynecol* 2003;15:315–319.

8 Akl MN, Long JB, Giles DL *et al.* Robotic-assisted sacrocolpopexy: technique and learning curve. *Surg Endosc* 2009;23:2390–2394.

9 Ridgeway B, Frick AC, Walter MD. Hysteropexy. A review. *Minerva Ginecol* 2008;60:509–528.

10 Krause HG, Goh JT, Sloane K, Higgs P, Carey MP. Laparoscopic sacral suture hysteropexy for uterine prolapse. *Int Urogynecol J Pelvic Floor Dysfunct* 2006;17:378–381.

11 Price N, Slack A, Jackson SR. Laparoscopic hysteropexy: the initial results of a uterine suspension procedure for uterovaginal prolapse. *BJOG* 2010;117:62–68.

12 Busby G, Broome J. Successful pregnancy outcome following laparoscopic sacro-hysteropexy for second degree uterine prolapse. *Gynecol Surg* 2010;7: 271–273.

13 Lee T, Rosenblum N, Nitti V, Brucker BM. Uterine sparing robotic-assisted laparo-scopic sacrohysteropexy for pelvic organ prolapse: safety and feasibility. *J Endourol* 2013;27:1131–1136.

14 Sundaram BM, Kalidasan G, Hemal AK. Robotic repair of vesicovaginal fistula: case series of five patients. *Urology* 2006;67:970–973.

15 Murphy DG, Bjartell A, Ficarra V *et al*. Downsides of robot-assisted laparoscopic radical prostatectomy: limitations and complications. *Eur Urol* 2010;57:735–746.

16 Finan MA, Rocconi RP. Overcoming technical challenges with robotic surgery in gynecologic oncology. *Surg Endosc* 2010;24:1256–1260.

17 Buchs NC, Pugin F, Volonté F, Morel P. Reliability of robotic system during general surgical procedures in a university hospital. Am J Surg 2014;207:84–88.

18 Mills JT, Burris MB, Warburton DJ, Conaway MR, Schenkman NS, Krupski TL. Positioning injuries associated with robotic assisted urological surgery. *J Urol* 2013;190:580–584.

19 Coelho RF, Rocco B, Patel MB *et al*. Retropubic, laparoscopic, and robot-assisted radical prostatectomy: a critical review of outcomes reported by high-volume centers. *J Endourol* 2010;24:2003–2015.

20 Okamura AM. Haptic feedback in robot-assisted minimally invasive surgery. *Curr Opin Urol* 2009;19:102–107.

CHAPTER 123

Complications in Robotic Pelvic Floor Surgery

Amie Kawasaki

Cleveland Clinic Florida, Weston/Fort Lauderdale, Florida, USA

Case history: A 64-year-old woman with stage III vaginal vault prolapse was scheduled for a robotic sacrocolpopexy, with an anticipated operating time of 2.5 hours. The patient was positioned and draped. The trocars were placed and the robotic arms docked. During the procedure, the surgeon noticed limitations in instrument movement and the bedside assistant reported collisions between the robotic instruments externally.

Background

Robot-assisted minimally invasive surgery was widely introduced to gynecology after receiving FDA approval for gynecologic indications in 2005. Advances in three-dimensional optics, tremor filtration, and wristed instruments have led to the widespread adoption of the da Vinci Surgical System (Intuitive Surgical Inc., Sunnyvale, CA) [1]. In 2009, the American College of Obstetricians and Gynecologists published a technology assessment bulletin outlining the limited data but potential promise of the new surgical technique. The document stated that supervision by a more experienced colleague should dictate credentialing and that the foreseeable disadvantage to the robotic route was primarily the increased cost [2]. A 2012 Cochrane Review identified only two randomized controlled trials on robotic surgery for benign gynecology. One RCT was specifically designed to study laparoscopic versus robotic sacrocolpopexy for the management of pelvic organ prolapse [3]. Neither study reported a significant difference in perioperative complications when robotic cases were compared with laparoscopic operations; however, both demonstrated a significantly longer operative time among the robotic cases [3,4]. Several well-designed retrospective studies have also compared the outcomes among abdominal, laparoscopic, and robotic surgery for pelvic organ prolapse, and reported no differences [5,6]. Complications of robotic sacrocolpopexy are similar to those of laparoscopy and may include reoperation for recurrent pelvic prolapse, problems associated with patient positioning, mesh complications, and inadvertent visceral injury.

Recurrent pelvic organ prolapse

Studies comparing recurrent prolapse rates after robotic sacrocolpopexy with those after abdominal sacrocolpopexy report no differences among the surgical methods, noting composite recurrence rates of 4–8% after 1 year [7]. In addition, objective measurements of vaginal support are reported to be similar between abdominal and robotic procedures after 44 months, with composite cure rates higher for vaginal vault support than for the other vaginal compartments [8]. Recurrent pelvic prolapse is a postoperative complication that may occur after any reconstructive pelvic surgery. When comparing the robotic route to either the abdominal or laparoscopic routes, the rates of recurrence are similar.

Patient positioning

As in laparoscopic surgery, a moderate degree of Trendelenburg is utilized for robotic surgery to aid the retraction of bowel from the operative field, particularly during sacral dissection in sacrocolpopexy. Studies highlight that the operative time for robotic sacrocolpopexy is longer than for the laparoscopic route [3,9], so the patient is in this position for more time. Proper positioning is important given the length of the procedure and the importance of avoiding any movement of the patient during the procedure.

Mesh or graft complications

Mesh or graft materials are used for sacrocolpopexy regardless of the route. Similar rates of mesh erosion or infection have been described after abdominal, laparoscopic, or sacrocolpopexy routes [3,8]. Sacral diskitis is a rare but significant complication that can result from the sacral fixation of the graft in sacrocolpopexy. The proper anatomic placement of the sacral portion of the mesh is important; however, because of the decrease in tactile feedback with robotic surgery, one must be particularly conscious of the depth in which the sacral sutures are placed and avoid the improper placement of fixation sutures or devices in the L5–S1 disk space [10].

Management

The patient

Proper padding and safe positioning are important to avoid compression or hyperextension injuries of the extremities. Robot-assisted laparoscopic surgery usually requires a moderate amount of Trendelenburg in order to achieve sufficient retraction of the small bowel for visualization of the pelvis. Because of the steep angle of Trendelenburg, many anti-skid devices have been introduced. An inexpensive yet very effective method to prevent the patient shifting during surgery is to fasten egg-crate foam to the operative table, and to lay the patient directly on the disposable material. The patient's

Gynecologic and Obstetric Surgery: Challenges and Management Options, First Edition. Edited by Arri Coomarasamy, Mahmood I. Shafi, G. Willy Davila and Kiong K. Chan.
© 2016 John Wiley & Sons, Ltd. Published 2016 by John Wiley & Sons, Ltd.

upper extremities are tucked to her sides within the foam and secured using a blanket that is placed under the foam. In this manner, significant shifting is prevented, without the risk of injury from improper positioning [5]. Prior to draping, the team should confirm that all intravenous lines and ECG leads are properly functioning.

The operating room team

A singularly important safety aspect of robotic surgery is that once the patient-side cart is docked, the operating room table cannot be changed. The trocars are held at a stationary level, and therefore the patient position cannot change unless the trocars are disconnected from the robotic arms. It is recommended to perform a tilt-test once the patient is positioned. This not only confirms absence of skidding, but also gives the anesthetic team the opportunity to assess the patient's tolerance of Trendelenburg. Once this is confirmed, the robotic patient-side cart can be docked.

The ability for the surgeon to be remote from the bedside is one of the unique aspects of robotic surgery. Because of this special separation, the surgeon must rely more on the bedside assistant and scrub technician. Proper training and clear communication is necessary for safe, efficient robotic surgery. The robotic surgeon console has a built-in microphone and the Vision cart is equipped with speakers as so that the surgeon's instructions can be clearly broadcast. Communication must be two-way; therefore, the surgical team must become accustomed to verbalizing the bedside activities. For example, when the bedside assistant retrieves a needle, he or she must announce that the "needle is out" because the surgeon does not have the luxury of glancing across the table to confirm this. Finally, the bedside team should be properly familiarized with the equipment so that they may perform basic troubleshooting independently.

The procedure

The success of robotic surgery is dependent on correct trocar placement. Once the patient cart is docked, the robotic trocars rotate only along the axis of the remote center. The surgeon must anticipate the space needed for adequate range of motion of the robotic arms and instruments. The pattern for trocar placement varies with each surgery, but the basic concepts are similar (see Chapter 114, Figure 114.1). Robotic trocar sites for sacrocolpopexy should be at least 10 cm in distance from each other. The most distal portion of the robotic arm must have the space to rotate without colliding into the other robotic arms, instruments, or the patient. One may predict this obstacle by docking the robotic patient-side cart and, prior to loading any instruments, replicating the anticipated trajectory and movement of the instruments. For example, to perform a robotic sacrocolpopexy, the robotic arms must allow the instruments to point primarily to the pelvis and sacrum. Prior to loading the instruments, it is recommended to mime these actions using the robotic arms to ensure proper spacing between all the joints of the arms.

Intraoperative safety is of utmost importance regardless of the surgical approach. The surgeon must be aware of the location and operation of the instruments at all times, especially prior to activating any cautery devices. As in the laparoscopic approach, the robotic camera can offer excellent visualization of detailed anatomic structures. However, this can be at the expense of a panoramic view. One should survey the entire operative field with the camera at regular intervals and avoid "tunnel vision." Instruments should be repositioned and cautery activated only if they are directly visualized. The lack of tactile feedback may initially pose a challenge to the novice surgeon; however, this may be overcome by using visual cues to relay information regarding the texture of the tissue

in the field. In addition, the bedside assistant should be actively participating throughout the procedure and may use a laparoscopic instrument to assist in the palpation of structures.

Resolution of the case

When the surgeon felt the limitation, the robotic arms were held in this location with all instruments free from tissue and in the camera's view. The surgeon left the console to inspect the external collisions that were causing the limited range of motion. The instruments were removed under direct visualization. The robotic arms were re-configured with small movements while the trocars were supported. If larger movements were necessary, the relevant arm was undocked from the trocar to allow the positional change. Once the joints were positioned and moved freely, the instruments were introduced under direct visualization once again. The surgery was completed safely.

KEY POINTS

Challenge: Avoiding complications in robot-assisted surgery.

Background
- Several studies demonstrate that there are no significant differences in either outcomes or rates of complications when robotic sacrocolpopexy is compared with laparoscopic sacrocolpopexy.
- Complications of robotic sacrocolpopexy include reoperation for recurrent pelvic prolapse, problems associated with patient positioning, mesh complications, and inadvertent injury to surrounding organs.

Management
- Preparation, training, and a keen awareness of the technical differences are imperative for safe and efficient robotic surgery.
- As surgery often requires Trendelenburg positioning, an anti-skid device should be used. A tilt-test should be performed before docking the patient-side cart.
- As surgeon is not by the side of the patient, clear communication between the surgeon and bedside assistants is vital.
- The trocar sites should be at least 10 cm away from each other to provide enough space for the robotic arms to rotate without colliding.
- The surgeon should be fully aware of the locations of all instruments in the abdomen, particularly before using electrosurgical instruments.

References

1 Kho RM, Hilger WS, Hentz JG, Magtibay PM, Magrina JF. Robotic hysterectomy: technique and initial outcomes. *Am J Obstet Gynecol* 2007;197:113e111–114.

2 ACOG Technology Assessment in Obstetrics and Gynecology No. 6: Robot-assisted surgery. *Obstet Gynecol* 2009;114:1153–1155.

3 Paraiso MF, Jelovsek JE, Frick A, Chen CC, Barber MD. Laparoscopic compared with robotic sacrocolpopexy for vaginal prolapse: a randomized controlled trial. *Obstet Gynecol* 2011;118:1005–1013.

4 Liu H, Lu D, Wang L, Shi G, Song H, Clarke J. Robotic surgery for benign gynaecological disease. *Cochrane Database Syst Rev* 2012;(2):CD008978.

5 Geller EJ, Siddiqui NY, Wu JM, Visco AG. Short-term outcomes of robotic sacrocolpopexy compared with abdominal sacrocolpopexy. *Obstet Gynecol* 2008;112:1201–1206.

6 Robinson BL, Parnell BA, Sandbulte JT, Geller EJ, Connolly A, Matthews CA. Robotic versus vaginal urogynecologic surgery: a retrospective cohort study of perioperative complications in elderly women. *Female Pelvic Med Reconstr Surg* 2013;94:230–237.

7 Siddiqui NY, Geller EJ, Visco AG. Symptomatic and anatomic 1-year outcomes after robotic and abdominal sacrocolpopexy. *Am J Obstet Gynecol* 2012;206:435e431–435.

8 Geller EJ, Parnell BA, Dunivan GC. Robotic vs abdominal sacrocolpopexy: 44 month pelvic floor outcomes. *Urology* 2012;79:532–536.

9 Geller EJ, Lin FC, Matthews CA. Analysis of robotic performance times to improve operative efficiency. *J Minim Invasive Gynecol* 2013;20:43–48.

10 Good MM, Abele TA, Balgobin S *et al.* Preventing L5–S1 discitis associated with sacrocolpopexy. *Obstet Gynecol* 2013;121:285–290.

CHAPTER 124
Neovagina

Lynsey Hayward[1] and G. Willy Davila[2]
[1] Middlemore Hospital, Auckland, New Zealand
[2] Cleveland Clinic Florida, Weston/Fort Lauderdale, Florida, USA

Case history 1: A 17-year-old woman presents with primary amenorrhea, normal height and BMI, and normal secondary sexual characteristics. She has cyclical pain suggestive of menstruation. Examination reveals a 3-cm blind-ending vagina. She wishes to become sexually active.

Case history 2: A 45-year-old woman is referred for difficulty with resuming sexual activities after prolapse repair 16 weeks ago. On examination, she is noted to have a genital hiatus of 0.5 cm and a vaginal depth of 2.5 cm. Her tissues are atrophic.

Background

Case history 1 (see Chapter 100)

Müllerian agenesis affects 1 in 4000–10,000 females; 90% of Müllerian agenesis is associated with Mayer–Rokitansky–Kuster–Hauser (MRKH) syndrome. This is a congenital absence of the vagina, uterus, or both; the ovaries are present. Women have normal secondary sexual characteristics, normal external genitalia, normal hormone profiles, and 46XX karyotype. Up to 53% of women with MRKH syndrome also have other congenital anomalies, the commonest being renal agenesis, pelvic kidney, skeletal anomalies, and abdominal wall defects. The differential diagnosis includes androgen insensitivity syndrome (short or normal-length vagina), 17α-hydroxylase deficiency, a transverse vaginal septum (hymen present), or an imperforate hymen (no hymenal ring present).

Case history 2

Excessive trimming of vaginal epithelium at the time of pelvic organ prolapse repair can lead to a shallow and narrow vagina, making vaginal intercourse very difficult if not impossible. Contemporary surgical teaching now includes minimal vaginal skin trimming, but many surgeons may still find themselves challenged when closing the skin in a vaginal repair. This may be particularly true when the mucosa is very atrophic and tears easily during initial dissection.

Evaluation

Case history 1

A pelvic examination is needed to diagnose an imperforate hymen or a transverse vaginal septum. A rectal examination can be useful to diagnose pelvic masses. Serum gonadotropin and testosterone levels,

and karyotype analysis are essential. Ultrasound (transabdominal, translabial, or perineal) or MRI can be used to evaluate for Müllerian remnants. Investigations for renal, skeletal, and abdominal wall anomalies should be carried out with ultrasound, CT or MRI. There is a small but increased risk of hearing deficit in patients with Müllerian agenesis, so audiometry is recommended.

Case history 2

The diagnosis is usually very apparent on vaginal examination. Either an hourglass vaginal canal with an area (or multiple areas) of stricture formation, or a foreshortened vaginal canal can be identified during vaginal examination. Some strictures or vaginal apical mucosal coalescence may be easily released during examination.

Management

The diagnosis can be potentially devastating, so careful counseling is required for both the patient and the family. For women with MRKH syndrome, the presence of functional ovaries opens the possibility of a pregnancy through surrogacy. If functional endometrial tissue is present and causing pain, laparoscopic removal of Müllerian remnants is recommended (Case history 1).

For patients with postoperative vaginal scarring, most can be reassured that vaginal intercourse should be possible, but may require a great degree of motivation and/or surgery (Chapter 125).

Non-surgical management

Definitive management for vaginal agenesis should not be undertaken until the patient is of sufficient maturity to comply with treatment, including a lifelong commitment to regular vaginal dilation. Satisfactory anatomic and functional vagina can be achieved in 75–80% of women through the use of dilators. Placement of increasing sizes of vaginal dilators (Figure 124.1) using gentle pressure against the vaginal dimple will gradually result in vaginal expansion. Use of a dilator for 30 min daily over several months is usually sufficient. Dilators can be hand-held or in the form of a saddle on which the patient sits and leans into the dilator. To maintain vaginal depth and caliber, regular intercourse or ongoing use of vaginal dilators is crucial.

In the case of postoperative scarring, local estrogen (e.g., cream or pessary on two nights per week) should be used concomitantly.

Gynecologic and Obstetric Surgery: Challenges and Management Options, First Edition. Edited by Arri Coomarasamy, Mahmood I. Shafi, G. Willy Davila and Kiong K. Chan.
© 2016 John Wiley & Sons, Ltd. Published 2016 by John Wiley & Sons, Ltd.

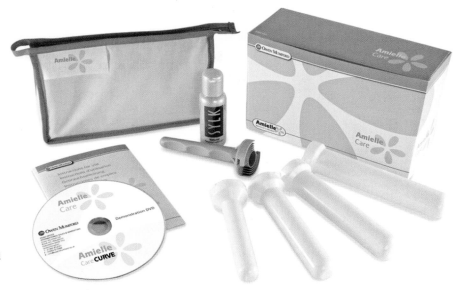

Figure 124.1 A set of plastic vaginal dilators. Amielle Care is a trademark of Owen Mumford Ltd. All rights reserved. Reproduced with permission from Owen Mumford Ltd.

If normalization of vaginal anatomy and function is not possible with these conservative measures, surgery should be considered. Various options are available.

Surgical creation of a neovagina

Surgery is the best option for women where the use of vaginal dilators has failed. The aim is to create a vagina with adequate depth, caliber, and lubrication to allow for intercourse. When anatomic success was defined as a length of 7 cm or more and functional success as coitus, all vaginoplasty techniques yielded significantly higher success rates (>90% vs. 75% after vaginal dilation), irrespective of underlying diagnosis or initial vaginal length [1]. Women must commit to either have regular intercourse or use vaginal dilators in order to maintain form and function. It is therefore essential that a patient is mature enough and willing to undertake the postoperative care required prior to performing surgery (usually around the age of 17–21 years).

Surgical management should be carried out at a center with specialist experience. Revision surgery or second procedures are associated with increased risks and poorer functional outcomes, and thus it is important to ensure the accuracy of the primary surgery.

The most commonly performed surgery is the modified Abbe–McIndoe technique. This involves dissection of the rectovesical space and insertion of a split-thickness skin graft. The graft can be obtained from the patient's lower abdominal wall or buttock, but must be prepared by removing all subcutaneous tissue and hair follicles. The graft should be of sufficient size to allow it to cover the area of desired vaginal wall surface area without tension. Once a vaginal canal tunnel is carefully created, which may require cystoscopic and rectal examination guidance, the graft is placed over a predesigned sterile mold, or a 60-mL syringe casing, and inserted into the canal. The distal skin edges are sutured to the distal vaginal skin. The patient is kept in the hospital for bed rest for 96 hours, returning to the operating room at 48–72 hours for debridement of any degenerating edges and aspiration of any subcutaneous fluid collections preventing graft incorporation. The patient is discharged with the mold sutured or held in place for up to 4 weeks, following which ongoing dilation is required to prevent graft strictures.

Alternative techniques use bowel graft, buccal mucosa, or pelvic peritoneum (Davydov procedure) for neovagina formation.

Laparoscopic procedures have increasingly replaced open abdominal techniques and have the advantage of being minimally invasive but with good reported functional outcomes. The Vecchietti technique (Chapter 100) involves the placement of a vaginal "olive" at the vaginal dimple which is attached via two sutures to an external traction device attached to the abdominal wall. The device creates upward traction and is gradually tightened to cause vaginal lengthening [2].

Postoperative care

In addition to regular intercourse or vaginal dilation, women should undergo regular vaginal examinations to assess for vaginal stenosis. Women with split-skin or bowel grafts can also develop neoplasia, ulceration, and Crohn's disease. Women should be counseled about the risk of sexually transmitted disease, but do not require Pap smears.

KEY POINTS

Challenge: Creation of a neovagina.

Background
- Congenital absence of the vagina can be secondary to genetic, hormonal, or metabolic causes.
- Acquired vaginal foreshortening or stricturing is typically due to surgical misadventure, radiation, or advanced atrophy.

Prevention
- Avoiding excessive mucosal trimming during POP surgery is important for the prevention of reduction in vaginal depth or caliber.

Management
- Conservative means of creating a vagina (with dilators) in women with Müllerian agenesis can be very successful in motivated young women.
- First surgery is the most successful surgery so referral to a specialized center of excellence is recommended.
- There are multiple surgical approaches proven to restore vaginal anatomy, but they require a patient committed to maintaining vaginal function. Options include:
  - Modified Abbe–McIndoe technique.
  - Davydov procedure.
  - Vecchietti technique.

References

1 Callens N, De Cuypere G, De Sutter P *et al*. An update on surgical and non-surgical treatments for vaginal hypoplasia. *Hum Reprod Update* 2014;20:775–801.
2 Veronikis DK, McClure GB, Nichols DH. The Vecchietti operation for constructing a neovagina: indications, instrumentation, and techniques. *Obstet Gynecol* 1997;90:301–304.

Further reading

American College of Obstetricians and Gynecologists, Committee on Adolescent Health Care. Committee opinion No. 562: Müllerian agenesis, diagnosis, management, and treatment. *Obstet Gynecol* 2013;121:1134–1137.

Edmonds DK, Rose GL, Lipton MG, Quek J. Myer Rokitansky Kuster Hauser syndrome: a review of 245 consecutive cases managed by a multi-disciplinary approach using vaginal dilators. *Fertil Steril* 2012;97:686–690.

MRKH Organization Inc., PO Box 301494, Jamaica Plain, MA 02130, USA. Center for Young Women's Health. MRKH a guide for teens. http://www.youngwomenshealth.org/mrkh/

Rock JA, Breech LL. Surgery for anomalies of the Mullerian ducts. In: Rock JA, Jones HW III (eds) *Te Linde's Operative Gynecology*, 10th edn, pp. 539–584. Lippincott Williams & Wilkins, Philadelphia, 2008.

Williams JK, Lake M, Ingram JM. The bicycle seat stool as a treatment for vaginal agenesis and stenosis. *J Obstet Gynecol Neonatal Nur* 1985;14:147–150.

CHAPTER 125

Vaginal Stricture After Pelvic Organ Prolapse Surgery

Ted M. Roth[1], G. Rodney Meeks[2], and G. Willy Davila[3]

[1] Central Maine Medical Center, Lewiston, Maine, USA
[2] University of Mississippi School of Medicine, Jackson, Mississippi, USA
[3] Cleveland Clinic Florida, Weston/Fort Lauderdale, Florida, USA

Case history: A 58-year-old woman who underwent an uneventful anterior and posterior colporrhaphy for symptomatic pelvic organ prolapse (POP) is now 6 months post operation and states that she cannot have sex due to a "blockage" and pain. She had not attempted intercourse until now. She has not been using the estrogen cream that was prescribed at her 6-week postoperative visit. On examination, an introital skin band which reduces the vaginal caliber to 1.5 cm at the level of the hymen is noted.

Background

The prevalence of dyspareunia increases after transvaginal reconstructive pelvic operations. Despite a postoperative decrease in vaginal dimensions, a causal relationship between dyspareunia and changes in vaginal dimensions has not been demonstrated [1]. Although the prevalence of iatrogenic vaginal constriction is unknown, it is likely under-reported. In 75% of the cases at one referral center the antecedent procedure involved a posterior repair [2].

Some strictures can be thin mucosal bands, while others can be thick deep connective tissue bands. Either can have the same clinical impact: difficulty and pain with sexual intercourse. This negative impact can neutralize any positive impact a woman may achieve from her POP repair. The possibility of vaginal scarring and dyspareunia should be discussed with patients in the preoperative planning and consent phase. Many surgeons go as far as considering postoperative dyspareunia as a predictable part of recovery from POP surgery, which will most commonly resolve with restoration of regular sexual intercourse.

Location

Depending on the site of the POP surgery, strictures can develop along the anterior, posterior, or lateral vaginal walls. The most common location is the posterior wall, following posterior colporrhaphy. If a levator plication or myorrhaphy is performed, the stricture tends to form at the uppermost plication suture site. Since this approach to posterior repair is not commonly used, the most common site is at the level of the introitus and hymenal ring remnants. This is typically demonstrated by insertion of the examiner's fingers and stretching of the introital skin, which demonstrates the skin fold or stricture, and reproduces the patient's reported pain. Although usually a thin skin fold, it can present as a thick band or an area of dense inelastic scar tissue. On occasion, reaction to suture material can present with granulation tissue at the site.

Apical stricture formation is less common, except when a mesh kit is used, and the fixating arms can contract and result in reduced stretchability and stricture formation (see below).

Importance of postoperative intercourse

Resumption of sexual intercourse postoperatively is crucial in reducing the possibility of stricture formation. Although discomfort and some pain may accompany the initial attempts at intercourse, patients should be warned and prepared for this eventuality. Local estrogen therapy to soften vaginal tissue, and use of local 2% lidocaine jelly prior to intercourse may be helpful. In the vast majority of cases, normal sexual function is restored within a few months. Patients who refrain from sexual activity due to discomfort may enter a vicious cycle of further discomfort from lack of sexual activity, and subsequent formation of vaginal scar tissue and stricture formation.

We routinely prescribe 2% lidocaine jelly (1–2 g) to be inserted intravaginally prior to the first few intercourse events. The jelly can be inserted with an estrogen cream applicator, and functions within about 10 min.

Prevention

Prevention of stricture formation is important, and should be on the surgeon's mind during every POP surgery.

Prepare perineal tissue

Well-estrogenized tissue allows more precise development of tissue planes during reconstructive surgery. In addition, mucosal elasticity is increased, facilitating dissection and subsequent closure. In postmenopausal women, atrophic vaginal tissues can be prepared preoperatively with local estrogen therapy (estrogen cream, tablets or ovules). Postoperative local estrogen therapy can be initiated

Gynecologic and Obstetric Surgery: Challenges and Management Options, First Edition. Edited by Arri Coomarasamy, Mahmood I. Shafi, G. Willy Davila and Kiong K. Chan.
© 2016 John Wiley & Sons, Ltd. Published 2016 by John Wiley & Sons, Ltd.

once the sutures have dissolved, and is likely to reduce stricture formation by maintaining mucosal elasticity.

Minimize vaginal mucosal trimming

When closing the vaginal epithelium at the completion of a reconstructive procedure, trimming of vaginal mucosa should be limited to a minimum: only that required to avoid formation of a mucosal tuft which the patient may sense as a recurrence of prolapse.

Avoid over-plication of soft tissue

When plicating soft fibromuscular tissue during reconstructive surgery, care must be taken to avoid reducing vaginal caliber excessively. We find it helpful to place two Allis clamps at the posterior introitus or hymenal remnants such that when approximated in the midline, a normal introital caliber results. The clamps serve to clearly identify the posterior vaginal sulci and provide the landmark needed for the surgeon to avoid over-plication. These Allis clamps are the last clamps to be removed during mucosal closure.

Manage mucosal tears rationally

Since the mucosa is rather thin, the traction/counter-traction needed to accomplish appropriate dissection can result in tears along the skin edges. These tears should be clearly identified prior to mucosal closure, such that when the mucosa is sutured closed, the original cut edges are approximated and the edges and base of the tear are not included in the suture line (Figure 125.1). If the base of a large tear is included in the suture line, a mucosal stricture may result; the larger the tear, the tighter the stricture.

Consider using vaginal dilators

When patients undergoing posterior colporrhaphy were evaluated at 3 and 6 months, there were no significant differences in *de novo* dyspareunia rates, overall postoperative sexual function scores, or global improvement scores between those using vaginal dilators during postoperative weeks 4–8 and control patients [3]. In those postmenopausal women who are not sexually active, some experts believe that the use of dilators to prevent stricture formation can

be considered postoperatively until such time that they resume intercourse. An appropriately sized dilator, and local estrogen cream, should help maintain normal vaginal caliber and elasticity.

Management

Local estrogen

As already noted, local estrogen is important for maintaining vaginal mucosal elasticity, and should be initiated, if not before now, prior to management of a vaginal stricture band [4]. Ospemifene is an effective and safe treatment for dyspareunia associated with postmenopausal vulval and vaginal atrophy [5]. An adequate trial of vaginal dilator therapy should be recommended, although some elderly women may express lack of comfort with that option (Chapter 124).

Transection and cautery of the defect base

This simple management is typically sufficient in most cases, and can be performed in an office setting. Local anesthetic is injected into the fold, followed by vertical incision until the band is relieved. Suturing can usually be avoided, and the base of the incision can be cauterized with silver nitrate to reduce bleeding. Local lidocaine jelly can be prescribed to reduce pain, and intercourse can be attempted 72 hours later.

Band transection and suturing in the operating room

This may be needed for more prominent strictures, multiple areas of stricture formation, strictures deeper within the vaginal canal, or in patients unlikely to tolerate it in the office setting. After proper positioning, the stricture bands are cut in a vertical direction and the skin edges can then be approximated in a horizontal direction (Figure 125.2) [2]. The skin edges should be closed using light sutures, such as 3-0 Vicryl, to minimize the risk of stricture recurrence. This technique can be particularly useful when vaginal lateral wall strictures are found. If limited vaginal epithelium is found (when excessive mucosal trimming has occurred, typically

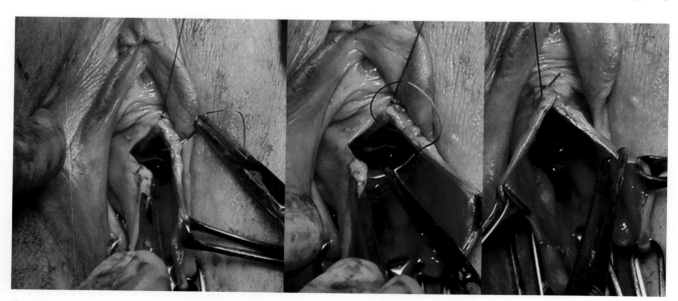

Figure 125.1 Vaginal mucosal edge tears should be clearly identified and not incorporated into closure of the original incision line.

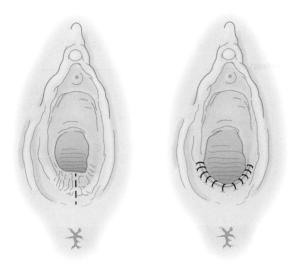

Figure 125.2 Most strictures can be addressed by simple vertical incision and horizontal closure [2].

resulting in vaginal foreshortening and markedly reduced caliber), Z-plasty can be considered [6].

Z-plasty works well for well-circumscribed constriction rings and stenotic vaginal canals. Healthy surrounding tissue is utilized to develop healthy flaps without creating further constriction or a midline scar. Z-plasty does not compromise vaginal length. Firstly, the vagina is incised, with length and angles of the "Z" typically made 2 cm long at 60° angles from one another. Increasing the angles increases the width gained. The orientation of the "Z" can be vertical or transverse, depending on the location of the stricture. Secondly, the flaps are mobilized, transposed, and sutured into place with delayed absorbable suture. Thirdly, vaginal packing and antibiotic cover are provided.

Distal strictures in women with adequate vaginal length respond well to vaginal advancement flaps. Its use is limited primarily by the surgeon's ability to mobilize adequate healthy vaginal tissue, exposure, as well as the length of the vagina (which may be compromised by the mobilization of the flap itself). To perform this procedure, firstly make a linear or curvilinear incision over the scar tissue. Secondly, create a flap of unscarred epithelium by undermining healthy tissue and excising the scar tissue. Thirdly, the epithelial flap, once adequately mobilized, is sutured without tension over the defect (usually to the perineal skin). Finally, vaginal packing for 12–24 hours helps to reduce the development of a hematoma.

If limited vaginal skin is available, relaxing incisions through the band of scar tissue can be performed. The steps involved are as follows.
- Cut all the way into the pararectal fat.
- Make multiple incisions to create adequate width, if necessary.
- Allow the incision(s) to granulate and heal by secondary intention.
- Alternatively, close the incision into the ridge perpendicularly, i.e., the incision is made vertically and closed horizontally.

Other alternatives

Abdominal wall or iliac crest full-thickness skin grafts, vulvar rotational skin flaps, and biologic grafting (SIS, buccal mucosa) can be considered in selected patients. Full-thickness grafts have

a decreased incidence of postoperative contracture as opposed to split-thickness grafts. Neovagina formation (Chapter 124) may be needed for more severe cases. The selection of a vaginal graft should be individualized and should be performed by surgeons experienced in repair of such severe strictures. Postoperative care can be quite delicate, requiring the patient to wear vaginal molds postoperatively.

When mesh is involved, mesh contraction is typically associated. One needs to remove the entire segment of hardened, firm and tender mesh, usually a band or arm located along the vaginal apex or lateral mid-vagina.

KEY POINTS

Challenge: Reduced vaginal caliber (stricture formation) following vaginal POP surgery.

Background
- Reduction in vaginal diameter is a recognized consequence of vaginal POP surgery, especially when posterior repair is performed.
- Temporary, or long-term, dyspareunia may be associated with vaginal POP surgery.

Prevention
- During POP correction, excessive mucosal trimming and/or soft-tissue plication should be avoided.
- Vaginal mucosal edge tears that occur during surgery should be clearly identified and closed separately from closure of the original suture line.
- Usage of preoperative and postoperative local estrogen may help reduce mucosal stricture formation.

Management
- Vaginal dilators and regular sexual activity, with use of local anesthetic lidocaine jelly, can help correct simple strictures.
- Most vaginal strictures can be managed by simple vertical transection and horizontal closure. Complex strictures may require referral to a specialized center.
- Z-plasty can be used for mid-vaginal and introital constrictions where the amount and depth of scar tissue is not excessive.
- Incision of the vaginal ring or ridge is useful for concentric constrictions and extensive fibrosis.
- Skin grafts may be offered when the quality of the epithelium is inadequate (e.g., patients with a history of radiation therapy, or when there is inadequate tissue for primary closure).
- Distal strictures in women with adequate vaginal length respond well to vaginal advancement flaps.

References

1 Abramov Y, Gandhi S, Botros SM et al. Do alterations in vaginal dimensions after reconstructive pelvic surgeries affect the risk for dyspareunia? *Am J Obstet Gynecol* 2005;192:1573–1577.
2 Vasallo B, Karram MM. Management of iatrogenic vaginal constriction. *Obstet Gynecol* 2003;101:512–520.
3 Antosh DD, Gutman RE, Park AJ et al. Vaginal dilators for prevention of dyspareunia after prolapse surgery: a randomized controlled trial. *Obstet Gynecol* 2013;121:1273–1280.
4 Rees M, Pérez-López FR, Ceasu I et al. EMAS clinical guide: low-dose vaginal estrogens for postmenopausal vaginal atrophy. *Maturitas* 2012;73:171–174.
5 Cui Y, Zong H, Yan H, Li N, Zhang Y. The efficacy and safety of ospemifene in treating dyspareunia associated with postmenopausal vulvar and vaginal atrophy: a systematic review and meta-analysis. *J Sex Med* 2014;11:487–497.
6 Farroha A, Hanna H. Reconstruction of symptomatic postoperative vaginal shortening using Z-plasty. *Int J Gynaecol Obstet* 2008;102:75–76.

CHAPTER 126
Urethral Diverticula and Other Periurethral Masses

Bhavin Patel and Kathleen C. Kobashi
Virginia Mason Medical Center, Seattle, Washington, USA

Case history: A 63-year-old woman presents with complaints of fullness in her anterior vagina. She has a history of incontinence (stress urinary incontinence and post-void dribbling) and recurrent urinary tract infections.

Background

Periurethral masses can be found in up to 4% of adult women [1]. They often come to the attention of the patient when they result in voiding symptoms or become a palpable mass in the anterior vaginal wall. The differential diagnosis of a periurethral mass includes urethral diverticulum, leiomyoma, Skene gland or Gartner duct abnormalities, vaginal wall cyst, urethral prolapse or caruncle, or the effects of urethral bulking agent; however, the commonest diagnosis is a urethral diverticulum, which comprises approximately 80% of periurethral masses [1].

Clinical evaluation

Physical examination
The anterior vaginal wall is carefully examined with specific attention paid to the urethral meatus and urethra. If a mass is found, its location, size, consistency, and associated symptoms should be noted. Although a periurethral mass can occur anywhere along the urethra, most are located along the ventral portion of the mid or proximal urethra. When there is clinical concern for a periurethral mass, but physical examination is inconclusive, the potential for a mass *anterior* to the urethra should be considered. Mass consistency is an important factor, as this can provide indication of a stone or malignancy within the periurethral lesion.

Once the mass has been evaluated, it is important to complete the vaginal examination by assessing for any pelvic organ prolapse, vaginal tissue atrophy, introital capacity, and for urethral hypermobility or frank stress urinary incontinence. These factors may play a role in surgical planning.

Cystoscopy
Cystoscopy can potentially identify a diverticular ostium (Figure 126.1) or anomalies of the lower urinary tract secondary to the periurethral mass. Cystoscopy can also facilitate vaginal palpation of the mass, and assessment for other causes of lower urinary tract symptoms.

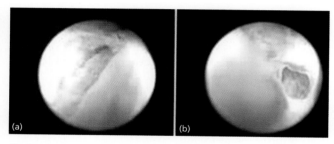

Figure 126.1 Cystourethroscopy showing orifices of a urethral diverticulum.

Urodynamics
Urodynamics are not required in patients with a periurethral mass. However, for patients with concomitant lower urinary tract symptoms or incontinence, urodynamic information can be useful in characterizing voiding symptoms and planning surgery. For example, in patients with demonstrable stress urinary incontinence, an anti-incontinence procedure at the time of periurethral mass surgery can be considered and has been shown to have good outcomes [2]. Bladder outlet obstruction can also be identified on urodynamics and may be related to the periurethral mass. A subset of patients with secondary bladder outlet obstruction may have coexistent occult stress urinary incontinence that is unmasked following repair of the periurethral mass [3].

Laboratory evaluation
Urinalysis and a urine culture should be performed. If evidence of a urinary tract infection is found, it should be treated prior to surgical management.

Imaging
The role of imaging for periurethral masses is in confirmation of the diagnosis and delineation of the anatomy of the mass and adjacent structures. Imaging can help identify multiple diverticula, which may be present in up to 50% of patients. Potential imaging modalities include voiding cystourethrography (VCUG), urethrography,

Gynecologic and Obstetric Surgery: Challenges and Management Options, First Edition. Edited by Arri Coomarasamy, Mahmood I. Shafi, G. Willy Davila and Kiong K. Chan.
© 2016 John Wiley & Sons, Ltd. Published 2016 by John Wiley & Sons, Ltd.

intravenous urography, ultrasound, and MRI. None of the imaging modalities are perfect, but each can provide useful information in the appropriate clinical setting.

- VCUG can provide excellent imaging of the bladder and urethra, particularly during and after the voiding phase. Unfortunately, not all patients are able to void in the radiology suite, and this can limit the usefulness of this test.
- Urethrography, which may include the double-balloon technique, can provide assessment of the urethra and of urethral diverticulum with a patent ostium. However, double-balloon urethrography, which involves filling of the urethra between two balloons (one at the bladder neck and the other at the meatus) can be quite uncomfortable for the patient and has therefore largely fallen out of favor.
- Intravenous urography with plain films or a CT scan may be considered in those with a vaginal mass or who are suspected to have a ureteric anomaly.
- Ultrasonography, performed transvaginally, translabially or transure-thrally, can be helpful. With ultrasound, the location and extent of the mass as well as the vascularity and internal architecture can be assessed.
- MRI has become the imaging modality of choice for many pelvic floor surgeons in evaluating a patient with a periurethral mass (Figures 126.2 and 126.3). MRI has the advantage of providing high-resolution multiplanar images of relevant anatomy and for this reason has outperformed other imaging modalities in the evaluation of a periurethral mass [4]. Despite being free from ionizing radiation, the costs of MRI and patient factors, such as claustrophobia or the presence of metallic implants, may limit its use.

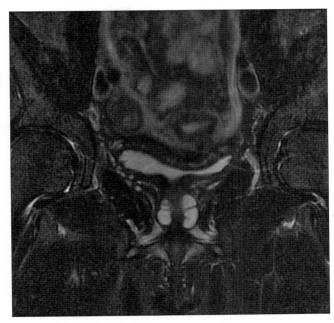

Figure 126.3 Coronal MRI showing the extent of the multilobular urethral diverticulum.

Management

Urethral diverticulum

Background

Urethral diverticula have an incidence of about 3% of adult women [1]. The cause of urethral diverticula is not clear, but the most widely accepted theory is that they form as a result of infection or inflammation of the periurethral glands. Patients with urethral diverticula typically present in the third to sixth decades of life, with a mean age of 45 years. Although the classic presentation of urethral diverticula includes the three "D"s (dysuria, dyspareunia, and post-void dribbling), patients may also be asymptomatic or have infections or other lower urinary tract symptoms. Additionally, up to 65% of patients with urethral diverticula have stress urinary incontinence [5]. Rarely, urethral diverticula can be associated with stones and malignancy, which are diagnoses to consider when imaging or examination reveals intraluminal diverticular anomalies or the patient has symptoms or signs of hematuria, induration or firmness of a periurethral mass.

Management

An experienced urologic or urogynecologic surgeon who does a reasonable number of diverticulectomies in his or her practice should undertake surgical management. The treatment options are as follows.

- In asymptomatic patients or in those with very small urethral diverticula, intervention is not indicated and observation is a reasonable option.
- Distal urethral diverticula can be managed endoscopically by using a Collins knife to incise the floor of the urethra into the diverticular cavity.

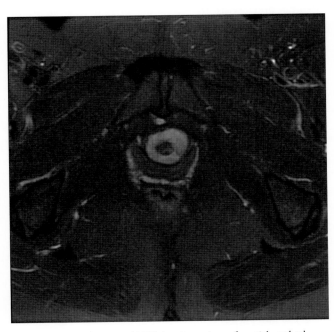

Figure 126.2 Cross-sectional MRI showing a circumferential urethral diverticulum.

- Open surgical techniques for distal diverticula include marsupialization, known as the Spence procedure, or formal diverticular excision with or without an interpositional tissue flap between the urethra and the vagina to minimize the risk of fistula formation.
- Stress urinary incontinence can be addressed with an anti-incontinence procedure [2] concomitantly, but synthetic mesh slings should never be placed at the time of diverticulectomy.

Urethral diverticulectomy surgery is performed in the operating room under general anesthesia. The procedure can take 3–4 hours, depending on the complexity. During this procedure, an inverted U-shaped incision is made in the vagina and the diverticulum carefully removed from the side of the urethra (Figure 126.4). As the diverticulum communicates with the urethra, the hole in the urethra needs to be identified and meticulously closed to prevent recurrence. Occasionally, a Martius graft is done to reinforce the repaired defect (Chapter 113).

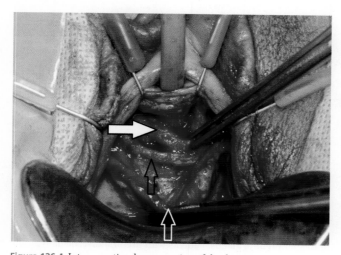

Figure 126.4 Intraoperative demonstration of the dissection involved in a urethral diverticulectomy. The hollow white arrow points to the vaginal flap, the hollow black arrow to the periurethral tissue flap, and the solid white arrow to the urethral diverticulum separated from the underlying urethra.

The bladder is drained continuously with a urethral Foley catheter (and a suprapubic catheter if necessary) for 2–3 weeks. A cystourethrogram prior to removal of catheter can be considered.

Complications that can occur with urethral diverticulectomy include wound infections, bleeding, and injury to the bladder, urethra, large blood vessels, or other organs. A urethral fistula can occasionally occur and would require another surgery.

Leiomyoma

Vaginal leiomyomas often present as smooth, round, firm but mobile masses of the anterior vaginal wall. They commonly present in the fourth and fifth decades of life and are often estrogen dependent, with regression during menopause. Direct operative excision through the vaginal wall is both diagnostic and therapeutic.

Skene gland

Skene glands are located on the anterior vaginal wall near the inferior border of the urethral meatus. Anomalies include Skene gland cysts or abscesses. Skene gland abscesses often present as exquisitely tender inflamed lesions that may express pus. They often present as masses near the inferior margin of the distal urethra in neonatal and middle-aged female patients. Differentiation from urethral diverticula can be difficult; however, unlike urethral diverticula, Skene gland anomalies do not communicate with the urethral lumen. In rare cases, Skene gland anomalies can be associated with adenocarcinoma. Treatment for symptomatic Skene gland anomalies includes needle aspiration, marsupialization, incision, and excision.

Gartner's duct

Gartner's ducts are embryologic remnants that run the length of the anterolateral vaginal wall. They can be associated with renal anomalies, such as renal agenesis, and may be drainage sites for ectopic ureters. Treatment is dependent on patient symptoms and the presence of ectopic ureteral drainage, with options including needle aspiration, marsupialization, incision, and excision with or without associated management of upper urinary tract anomalies.

Vaginal wall cyst

Vaginal wall cysts commonly present as small asymptomatic masses of the anterior vaginal wall. As they enlarge they can become symptomatic and become clinically relevant. Treatments for symptomatic vaginal wall cysts include needle aspiration, marsupialization, incision, and excision.

Urethral prolapse

Urethral prolapse is the circumferential herniation of the urethral mucosa at the urethral meatus. It can present clinically with spotting, bleeding, pain, or lower urinary tract symptoms. It commonly presents in prepubertal girls due to constipation, and in postmenopausal women due to lack of estrogen. Treatment is often with topical estrogen cream. In severe cases or cases that are refractory to estrogen, operative repair with cauterization, ligation, or circumferential excision can be considered.

Urethral caruncle

A urethral caruncle is an inflammatory lesion of the distal urethra that most commonly presents in postmenopausal women. It presents similarly to urethral prolapse, and is treated in a similar fashion.

Sterile abscess

Patients with a history of periurethral bulking agents can present for evaluation of vaginal wall masses. On imaging these masses may appear cystic or calcified. The key to diagnosis is a history of bulking agent injection. If they become symptomatic, masses related to bulking agent injections can be exposed and excised.

KEY POINTS

Challenge: Periurethral mass.

Background

- Periurethral masses are present in up to 4% of adult women.
- The differential diagnosis includes urethral diverticulum, leiomyoma, Skene gland or Gartner duct anomalies, vaginal wall cysts, urethral prolapse or caruncle, and bulking agent reaction.

Management

- Initial assessment should include a physical examination and urine microscopy and culture.

- It may be necessary to perform urodynamics and selected imaging such as a transvaginal ultrasound scan or MRI scan.
- For urethral diverticula, management options include:
  - Observation.
  - Endoscopic management: Collins knife incision.
  - Vaginal surgery: Spence procedure, or diverticular excision with or without interposition flap.
  - Cystourethroscopy should be done as part of all surgical options.

References

1 Blaivas JG, Flisser AJ, Bleustein CB, Panagopoulos G. Periurethral masses: etiology and diagnosis in a large series of women. *Obstet Gynecol* 2004;103: 842–847.

2 Faerber GJ. Urethral diverticulectomy and pubovaginal sling for simultaneous treatment of urethral diverticulum and intrinsic sphincter deficiency. *Tech Urol* 1998;4:192–197.

3 Bradely CS, Rovner ES. Urodynamically defined stress urinary incontinence and bladder outlet obstruction coexist in women. *J Urol* 2004;171:757–760.

4 Neitlich JD, Foster HE, Clickman MG, Smith RC. Detection of urethral diverticula in women: comparison of high resolution fast spin echo technique with double balloon urethrography. *J Urol* 1998;159:408–410.

5 Ganabathi K, Leach GE, Zimmern PE, Dmochowski RR. Experience with the management of urethral diverticulum in 63 women. *J Urol* 1994;152: 1445–1452.

CHAPTER 127
Vesicovaginal Fistulae

Karolynn T. Echols[1], Tamara V. Toidze[1], and Edward Stanford[2]
[1] Cooper Medical School of Rowan University, Camden, New Jersey, USA
[2] Oasis International Hospital, Beijing, China

Case history 1: *A woman with abnormal uterine bleeding secondary to uterine fibroids and a remote history of endometriosis elected to have a robotic-assisted abdominal hysterectomy with bilateral salpingo-oophorectomy. During the procedure, the surgeon encountered a difficult dissection of the vesico-uterine peritoneum off the uterus and difficulty achieving hemostasis on the left side of the vaginal cuff. Two weeks postoperatively, the patient presented with continuous leakage of urine and was found to have a vesicovaginal fistula (VVF).*

Case history 2: *A postmenopausal woman with a history of cervical cancer and radiation 10 years previously presents with continuous leakage of urine. She is found to have a pinhole vesicovaginal fistula.*

Background

In resource-limited countries, more than 90% of vesicovaginal fistulae develop from obstetric causes (obstructed labor and malpresentation, combined with poor access to obstetric care). In industrialized countries, more than 70% of fistulae are caused by direct injury to the lower urinary tract [1,2]. Other causes of urogenital fistulae include cancer or infections affecting the lower genital tract, pelvic radiation, endometriosis, foreign body (e.g., pessary), and rarely congenital defects (e.g., ectopic ureter or urethral duplication). Radiation therapy with ionizing radiation can lead to immediate fistula formation but can also lead to development of obliterative endarteritis, which can cause fistula formation months to years after treatment.

Iatrogenic urogenital fistula is a known unfortunate complication that develops in up to 0.5% of hysterectomies performed for benign causes, and in up to 10% of radical hysterectomies [3,4]. VVF is the most common of all urogenital fistulae; it is three times more common than ureterovaginal fistulae.

Prevention

The best treatment of VVF is prevention, which includes the correct approach and set-up for surgery with liberal use of retraction, light and suction, continuous bladder drainage, good surgical technique, excellent hemostasis, and avoidance of excessive electrocautery. Intraoperative cystoscopy should be used during the procedure

if necessary, and routinely performed at completion of complex cases [5].

Management

Diagnosis

Patients with VVF usually present with continuous leakage of urine. Symptoms can be painless and intermittent depending on VVF location. Most VVF will present on postoperative days 7 to 14 after an unrecognized injury, although in more severe injuries symptoms of urinary leakage can occur as soon as postoperative day 1 or after discontinuation of Foley catheter. Patients with VVF can also present with severe abdominal pain, abdominal distension, bladder spasms, and postoperative ileus. Patients can have hematuria, postoperative fever, and elevated WBCs. In cases of small fistulae, presenting signs and symptoms can be atypical, making the diagnosis more difficult. Vaginal watery discharge or drainage of a seroma during the early postoperative period can mimic VVF.

In a woman with a hysterectomy and symptoms suspicious for VVF, the most common location is in the upper third of the vagina or at the vaginal cuff. VVF may appear to be small red area(s) of granulation tissue, with no visible opening, and may be difficult to identify.

Several tests can be done to confirm or refute a VVF and these are described in the following sections.

Dye test

VVF can be identified by instilling a diluted solution of indigo carmine, methylene blue or sterile milk into the bladder through a Foley catheter (Figure 127.1). The VVF can be seen by leakage of dyed fluid into the vagina. If the test is not conclusive, a cotton tampon can be placed in the patient's vagina and then checked for dye discoloration. If no leakage is seen, the patient can be asked to cough or perform a Valsalva maneuver. If a ureterovaginal fistula is suspected, phenazopyridine can be given to the patient on the day of testing, which will turn the urine orange. A combination of phenazopyridine and indigo carmine or methylene blue dye can be used for differentiating a VVF (blue–orange discoloration) from one of ureteral origin (orange discoloration).

Gynecologic and Obstetric Surgery: Challenges and Management Options, First Edition. Edited by Arri Coomarasamy, Mahmood I. Shafi, G. Willy Davila and Kiong K. Chan.
© 2016 John Wiley & Sons, Ltd. Published 2016 by John Wiley & Sons, Ltd.

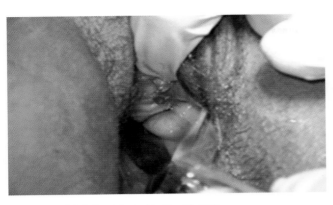

Figure 127.1 Methylene blue test to identify VVF.

Table **127.1** Classification of VVF [8–10].

Simple
VVF <2 to 3 cm
VVF proximal to vaginal cuff or supratrigonal area
No history of radiation or cancer
Normal vaginal length
First attempt at repair
Normal bladder capacity and compliance

Complicated
VVF >3 cm
VVF distant from cuff, trigonal or infratrigonal area
History of radiation
Pelvic cancer
Foreshortened vagina
Scarring
Decreased bladder capacity and compliance
Multiple fistulae
Failed previous repair

Cystourethroscopy

Cystourethroscopy can show size, site, number, and location of fistulae. It is important to determine the distance in relation to the trigone, ureteral orifices, and urethral sphincter. It is important to notice tissue characteristics surrounding the possible fistula site (i.e., level of edema, induration and scarring), which can be crucial in approach and timing of surgical repair (Figure 127.2).

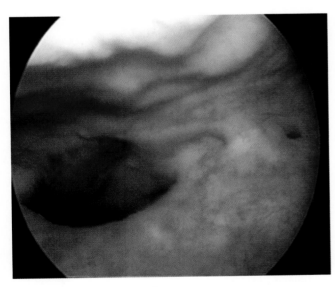

Figure 127.2 Cystoscopic view of VVF.

Imaging techniques

Imaging using intravenous pyelography (IVP) and CT can be performed. MRI with gadolinium can be more sensitive than IVP and CT [6]. Ultrasound can also be helpful in confirming diagnosis. In one study, color Doppler ultrasound with microbubble contrast agent detected fistulous tracts in 11 of 12 patients [7].

Proper classification is imperative for planning proper surgical management, and can help with the surgical approach and prognosis for cure (Table 127.1). Gynecologic fistulae are classified as simple or complicated [8].

Conservative management

VVF up to 3.5 mm in diameter may be successfully treated by electrosurgical coagulation of fistulous tract and prolonged bladder catheterization [11]. The utilization of hormones can also be beneficial for spontaneous closure, at a reported rate of almost 90% [12,13].

Timing of fistula closure is controversial and can depend on the condition of the surrounding tissue, and the cause of fistula. For example, in radiation fistulae, tissue sloughing increases in the immediate post-irradiation period; thus it is crucial to wait at least 8–12 weeks before attempting surgical repair [7]. In the case of fistula occurrence after gynecologic surgery, it is appropriate to wait 6–12 weeks to allow suture dissolution and granulation tissue ingrowth, which can increase the chances of successful repair. During the waiting period, continuous bladder drainage should be provided to allow the possible spontaneous closure of the fistula.

Abdominal, laparoscopic, or robotic repair

Abdominal repair is indicated for high fistulae (Figure 127.3e), ureterovaginal fistulae, complex fistulae, or for patients who had prior pelvic radiation.

A sagittal cystotomy is performed to provide access to the fistula, followed by sharp dissection of the base of the bladder from the anterior vaginal wall. If the fistula is in close proximity to the ureteral orifice(s), ureteral stents should be placed. After excising the entire fistulous tract, the vaginal mucosa is closed with two layers of continuous or interrupted 2-0 or 3-0 delayed absorbable suture. Cystotomy closure is then performed in two to three layers: one to approximate bladder submucosa and one to two layers to imbricate the bladder muscularis and serosa [7]. An omental or peritoneal flap can separate the bladder and vaginal layers and increase blood supply to the area to improve healing. These flaps can be particularly useful with larger fistula repairs and radiation-induced fistulae, where additional blood supply is needed.

A transvesical repair is performed extraperitoneally. Prior to the procedure, ureteral stenting should be performed. The technique is similar to that of the transvaginal flap-splitting repair except the bladder mucosa is usually closed with a running suture to achieve hemostasis.

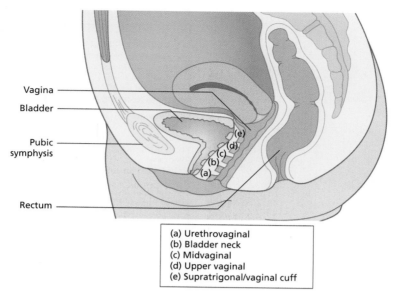

Vagina
Bladder
Pubic symphysis
Rectum

(a) Urethrovaginal
(b) Bladder neck
(c) Midvaginal
(d) Upper vaginal
(e) Supratrigonal/vaginal cuff

Figure 127.3 Anatomic fistula sites.

A transperitoneal repair is infrequent but useful in laparoscopic VVF repairs and repairs after cesarean section. A midline incision is made in the bladder and extended inferiorly around the fistula in a racquet shape to excise the tract. The vaginal defect is closed in a single layer and the bladder is then closed in two layers using 2-0 or 3-0 delayed absorbable suture.

Vaginal repair

There are two main types of VVF closure techniques for vaginal repair: the classical saucerization technique described by Sims, later modified by Latzko as a partial colpocleisis, and the commonly used dissection and layered repair or "flap-splitting" technique [14,15].

The Latzko procedure is indicated for VVF repair located at the vaginal apex. Procedure includes placement of four stay sutures around vaginal apex at least 2 cm from the margins of VVF. Tension is applied on the sutures, and the tissue around the fistula is excised in a wide circle. Hydrodissection is used to help dissect vaginal epithelium from fibromuscular layer of vagina. Multiple imbricating layers of 2-0 or 3-0 absorbable sutures are placed in transverse front-to-back interrupted fashion to bury the fistula. Usually two-layer repair is sufficient, but three or four layers might be required for repair. There can be minor shortening of vagina as a result. Retrograde filling of the bladder with indigo carmine, methylene blue, or sterile milk should be performed at the end of the procedure to test integrity of the repair.

If the VVF is more distal or larger, a Latzko procedure causes excessive shortening of the vagina. Therefore, a layered vaginal repair should be indicated. After removing the fistulous tract to expose healthy tissue, the vaginal mucosa is widely mobilized from bladder wall. The first layer of 3-0 delayed absorbable sutures is placed in the bladder submucosa to invert the mucosa into the bladder. Subsequently, a layered closure of the bladder muscularis layer and vaginal fibromuscularis layer, followed by closure of the

vaginal epithelium, is performed. A Foley catheter in the fistula tract can be used to help with the repair.

Vascular pedicles

Use of the Martius (see Chapter 113, Figure 113.1) or skin island flap modification is associated with excellent results in VVF surgery for non-obstetric fistulae. After closure of the fistula tract and before closing the vaginal epithelium, transposition of the bulbocavernosus fat pad is performed by first incising the medial aspect of the labia majora. Mobilization of the fat pad is performed, leaving its distal attachment to the blood supply (usually the external pudendal vessels). Subsequently, the pedicle is tunneled beneath the vaginal mucosa to the repaired fistula site while avoiding constriction of the distal vascular pedicle. Then, with 3-0 or 4-0 absorbable suture the pedicle is attached to the fistula site. A Penrose drain is placed in the harvested site for drainage.

Postoperative management

Continuous bladder drainage, with transurethral and/or suprapubic catheterization, is indicated to provide urine drainage until the tissues are healed. Timing of drainage varies depending on VVF complexity: 10–14 days for simple fistulae, 14–21 days for complex fistulae. The use of estrogen, steroids, or antibiotics has also been reported to be advantageous in healing after surgical repair [16]. Prior to removal of the catheter, an imaging study (i.e., cystoscopy or cystogram) should be performed to confirm an adequate repair.

Bladder capacity may be functionally decreased and patients may complain of increasing urinary urgency. The patient should be advised to monitor fluid intake and perform hourly timed voids while awake and twice nightly to prevent bladder distension. In the case of painful bladder spasms, pharmacotherapy can be used.

KEY POINTS

Challenge: Vesicovaginal fistula.

Background

- In low-income countries, 90% of fistulae are related to childbirth complications.
- In industrialized countries, more than 70% of fistulae are caused by direct injury to the lower urinary tract.
- Other causes of urogenital fistulae include cancer or infections affecting the lower genital tract, pelvic radiation, endometriosis, foreign body (e.g., pessary), and rarely congenital defects (e.g., ectopic ureter or urethral duplication).
- Iatrogenic urogenital fistula complicates up to 0.5% of hysterectomies performed for benign causes and up to 10% of radical hysterectomies.
- In prior hysterectomy, the most common location is in the upper third of the vagina or vaginal cuff.

Prevention

- The best treatment for VVF is prevention using perioperative precautions to prevent injury.

Management

- Several diagnostic tests can be used to make a diagnosis: dye test, cystourethroscopy, and imaging with IVP and CT.
- If a VVF is found, always utilize continuous bladder drainage.
- VVF up to 3.5 mm in diameter can be successfully treated by electrosurgical coagulation of fistulous tract and prolonged bladder catheterization.
- Timing of surgical treatment of fistula and success of repair depend on the condition of the surrounding tissue and cause of fistula (wait for 8–12 weeks for radiation fistulae, 6–12 weeks for gynecologic fistulae).
- An abdominal approach is indicated for high fistulae, ureterovaginal fistulae, complex fistulae or in women with prior pelvic radiation. This can be via an open, laparoscopic, or robotic approach.
- The two main types of VVF vaginal closure technique are the classical Latzko partial colpocleisis, and the commonly used dissection and layered repair or "flap-splitting" technique.
- Using the Martius or skin island flap modification has excellent results in VVF of non-obstetric etiology.
- Timing of continuous transurethral and/or suprapubic drainage varies depending on VVF complexity.
- Prior to removal of the catheter, an imaging study (i.e., cystoscopy or cystogram) should be performed to confirm an adequate repair.

References

1 Tancer ML. Observations on prevention and management of vesicovaginal fistula after total hysterectomy. *Surg Gynecol Obstet* 1992;175:501–506.

2 Hadzi-Djokic J, Pejcic TP, Acimovic M. Vesico-vaginal fistula: report of 220 cases. *Int Urol Nephrol* 2009;41:299–302.

3 Mann WJ, Arato M, Patsner B, Stone ML. Ureteral injuries in an obstetrics and gynecology training program: etiology and management. *Obstet Gynecol* 1988;72:82–85.

4 Magrina JF, Kho RM, Weaver AL, Montero RP, Magtibay PM. Robotic radical hysterectomy: comparison with laparoscopy and laparotomy. *Gynecol Oncol* 2008;109:86–91.

5 Ibeanu O, Chesson R, Echols K, Nieves M, Busangu F, Nolan T. Urinary tract injury during hysterectomy based on universal cystoscopy (phase 2): characteristics of ureteral injury. *Obstet Gynecol* 2009;113:6–10.

6 Abou-El-Ghar ME, El-Assmy AM, Refaie HF, El-Diasty TA. Radiological diagnosis of vesicouterine fistula: role of magnetic resonance imaging. *J Magn Reson Imag* 2012;36:438–442.

7 Siddighi S, Hardesty JS. *Urogynecology and Female Pelvic Reconstructive Surgery. Just the Facts*, p. 190. McGraw-Hill, New York, 2006.

8 Elkins TE, Thompson JR. Lower urinary tract fistulas. In: Walters M, Karram MM (eds) *Urogynecology and Reconstructive Pelvic Surgery*, 2nd edn, pp. 355–365. Mosby, Philadelphia, 1999.

9 Lewis G, De Bernis L (eds) *Obstetric Fistula: Guiding Principles for Clinical Management and Programme Development*. World Health Organization, Geneva, 2006.

10 Walters MD, Karram MM (eds) *Urogynecology and Reconstructive Pelvic Surgery*, 3rd edn. Mosby, Philadelphia, 2006.

11 Stovsky MD, Ignatoff JM, Blum MD, Nanninga JB, O'Conor VJ, Kursh ED. Use of electrocoagulation in the treatment of vesicovaginal fistulas. *J Urol* 1994;152:1443–1444.

12 Yokoyama M, Arisawa C, Ando M. Successful management of vesicouterine fistula by luteinizing hormone-releasing hormone analog. *Int J Urol* 2006;13:457–459.

13 Goh JT, Howat P, de Costa C. Oestrogen therapy in the management of vasicovaginal fistula. *Aust NZ Obstet Gynaecol* 2001;41:333–334.

14 Sims J. On the treatment of vesico-vaginal fistula. *Am J Med Sci* 1852;XXIII:59–82.

15 Latzko W. Postoperative vesicovaginal fistulas: genesis and therapy. *Am J Surg* 1942;58:211–218.

16 Margolis T, Mercer LJ. Vesicovaginal fistula. *Obstet Gynecol Surv* 1994;49:840–847.

CHAPTER 128

Urethrovaginal Fistulae

Sohier Elneil

University College London Hospitals NHS Foundation Trust, London, UK

Case history 1: A 23-year-old woman in her first pregnancy was admitted to her local hospital with a 2-day history of obstructed labor which necessitated an operative vaginal delivery. Three weeks later, she developed continual urinary leakage. On examination, it was determined she had both vesicovaginal and urethrovaginal fistulae.

Case history 2: A 39-year-old woman presented with a 3-month history of intermittent urinary leakage, having had a mid-urethral tape inserted 5 months previously for urinary stress incontinence. She was completely dry for the first 2 months, but noticed dampness at first and then frank urinary loss, which occurred involuntarily and usually after a micturition episode. She was examined and a small dimple was felt at the mid-urethral point. A cystoscopy revealed a small urethrovaginal fistula with tape protrusion into the urethra.

Background

Urethrovaginal fistula (UVF) is uncommon in comparison with vesicovaginal fistula (VVF, Chapter 127) and rectovaginal fistula (RVF, Chapter 129). The condition is most prevalent in the developing and emergent nations of Africa, Asia, and South America [1]. Traditionally, fistulae in the developing world occur in association with obstetric injury [2]. Many women in low-resource countries find their lives destroyed by terrible injuries because of untreated obstructed labor [3]. Access to modern obstetric care is limited for much of the world, and availability of a timely cesarean section is virtually impossible in many low-resource settings. The grinding pressure of the fetal head during obstructed labor causes ischemia to the pelvic organs, and a spectrum of injuries, including VVF, UVF and RVF, ensues.

In the developed world most urogenital fistulae arise because of direct trauma from a foreign object, malignancies, or from iatrogenic causes. Trauma can result from malignant tumors abutting on the urethra, vagina, rectum or anus, or from the complications suffered after pelvic radiotherapy. Sometimes a fistula manifests several years after radiotherapy treatment has completed. Fistulae can also arise as a consequence of urethral, abdominal, or vaginal surgery for specific conditions such as urethral diverticula (Chapter 126) or hysterectomy. A rarer cause is inappropriate placement of urethral catheters [4].

Fistulae are known to occur following standard procedures such as prolapse surgery and bladder neck injections for urinary stress incontinence [5]. More recently, mesh procedures in urogynecologic surgery have emerged as a potential cause [6].

The complications that arise after the use of mesh are usually associated with the mesh either directly infiltrating the tissues of the vagina, urethra, bladder or rectum because of inappropriate placement, or being placed in too taut, or because of an infection causing generalized necrosis of the surrounding tissue even though the mesh may have been correctly placed and at the right tension. This is a new arena for those who undertake fistula surgery [7].

Urethrovaginal fistulae, which occur between the urethral mucosa and the vaginal wall, can be pinpoint in size and not involve the continence mechanism; however, the majority vary in size between 1 and 3 cm. In those in whom the continence mechanism is preserved, there may not be any inconvenience, but in others incontinence can be a major symptom, and the repair can be complex. The degree of involvement can also be partial or full thickness, affecting the entire breadth and/or length of the urethra. Though a similar classification system to VVF (Chapter 127), using the terms "simple" and "complex," could be applied, there is a case to be made for a modification of this system as complete avulsion of the urethra also needs to be considered. The latter is commonly seen with circumferential vesicovaginal fistulae. In the end, it is the degree of scarring that determines complexity and thus prognostic outcome in almost all cases.

Management

Fistula management demands a multidisciplinary approach, often including urogynecologists, urologists, colorectal surgeons, physiotherapists, nurses, continence advisers, nutritionists, and many more supportive health workers such as social workers and occupational health therapists. Repeated repair efforts are associated with poorer prognosis, hence the importance of an effective primary management team.

Diagnosis

An accurate medical history is essential to exclude any underlying chronic medical comorbidity or urinary symptoms prior to the

Gynecologic and Obstetric Surgery: Challenges and Management Options, First Edition. Edited by Arri Coomarasamy, Mahmood I. Shafi, G. Willy Davila and Kiong K. Chan.
© 2016 John Wiley & Sons, Ltd. Published 2016 by John Wiley & Sons, Ltd.

development of the fistula. A careful examination is necessary to assess the fistula with a view to planning the repair procedure, including the possibility of ureteric reimplantation.

Classification

Classification assists appropriate management. Most classifications of fistulae are determined according to location (e.g., UVF, VVF or RVF), size, and the involvement of the sphincteric mechanism. The success of surgery is most likely to be dependent on fistula size, scarring in the operative area, involvement of the continence mechanism, and associated injuries. Thus practitioners often identify and differentiate between simple and complex, based on multiple factors (Table 128.1) [8].

Table 128.1 Classification of fistulae by complexity.

Simple
Less than 2 to 3 cm in size and near the cuff (supratrigonal), with no history of radiation or malignancy and a normal vaginal length

Complex
Greater than 3 cm in size, distant from cuff or with trigonal involvement, with a history of pelvic scarring (due to malignancy, radiation, or chronic infection) and a shortened vagina

The simple versus complex classification enables the surgeon to consider the impact on the continence mechanism. Complete avulsion of the urethra can occur in severe trauma, and is most commonly associated with a circumferential VVF. Occasionally in the case of an iatrogenic urinary fistula, it may be difficult to accurately identify and distinguish among ureterovaginal fistula, VVF, severe stress incontinence, and true sphincteric incompetence. A "three-swab test" or a double dye test, and video urodynamics can be helpful.

Routine preoperative investigations include a full blood count, renal function tests, and blood sugar levels, where indicated. Other helpful tests include IVU, ultrasonography to evaluate the upper urinary tract, and examination under anesthesia with the assistance of cystoscopy and colposcopy.

Treatment
Fistula usually develops within 3 weeks of delivery or iatrogenic intervention, and from this period onwards the condition is unlikely to respond to conservative management. Typically, surgical treatment is necessary, but the optimum surgical approaches and timings are matters of considerable debate [9].

It is at least clear that the repair procedure must adhere to universal surgical standards such as satisfactory access, light, and precautions against infection. The intervention may be carried out via any of several different routes and with an assortment of different robust techniques (including laparoscopic and even robotic surgery). In the case of a very small fistula, cauterization and laser coagulation may be sufficient to achieve the repair [10].

Most repairs are undertaken using the vaginal route, under either regional or general anesthesia. However, if a UVF occurs in tandem with another fistula, then it may be necessary to use both vaginal and abdominal routes to enable mobilization of the bladder, reimplantation of ureters, and interposition of the omentum between the vagina and bladder. Recent refinements of laparoscopic techniques, including robotics, have shown promising results, particularly in the treatment of VVF [11], which is often undertaken in tandem with UVF surgery.

Whatever the surgical approach, the constituent steps of effective management include the following.
- Excision of all the scarred tissue around the fistula, and mobilization of healthy and well-vascularized tissue (especially the pubo-cervical fascia), ensuring preservation of urethral continuity.
- Tension-free closure, using a two-layer repair technique to reform the urethra, with the use of a labial/vaginal graft if necessary to provide a good cover to the urethra (Figure 128.1).

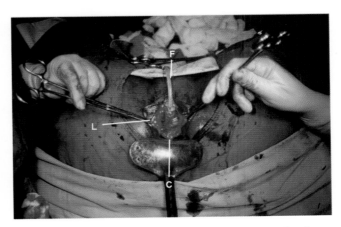

Figure 128.1 Final closure of a urethrovaginal fistula repair. C, closed pubo-cervical fascia; L, labial flaps; F, Foley catheter. © Sohier Elneil.

- Meticulous hemostasis.
- Interposition of a Martius fat graft or omentum between layers of the bladder and vagina (see Chapter 113, Figure 113.1), to provide a cushion of vascularized support to the repair site, if any tissue loss from the original trauma is greater than expected. In some cases, buccal mucosa and/or collagen implants have been used in a similar manner to restore missing tissue [12].
- Free drainage of the bladder using an indwelling urethral catheter for 14 days (in repairs not requiring ureteric cannulation) or 21 days (in repairs requiring ureteric cannulation).

Complications
Immediate postoperative complications may include secondary hemorrhage, sepsis, blocked catheters, and breakdown of the repair. More long-term complications include vaginal strictures with associated dyspareunia, hematometra, secondary amenorrhea and infertility, failure of the repair, bladder outlet obstruction, and vesical calculi.

Incontinence persists in around 10% of patients following extensive UVF surgery, not necessarily as a result of a failed repair but because the original insult or surgical procedure itself brings about a failing continence mechanism, resulting in stress incontinence. In others, where the continence mechanism is intact, problems may result from a reduced bladder capacity leading to urge incontinence. On rare occasions, different conditions may coexist, resulting in mixed incontinence. Standard treatments for these conditions can be instituted, including behavioral therapy, physiotherapy, pharmacotherapy, and continence mechanism surgery.

If the fistulous tract fails to heal without any continence mechanism failure or overactive bladder, then repeat surgery is inevitable. Otherwise, the mainstay of treatment is urinary diversion (Chapter 149), but this intervention – requiring regular access to catheters, stoma bags and medical reviews in case of further complications – presents a significant challenge in the developing world.

Prevention

Ideally, the formation of fistula may be prevented (or at least the size of the fistula reduced) following prolonged obstructed labor by maintaining an indwelling urethral catheter for 7–14 days following delivery (duration depending on the problems encountered in labor).

KEY POINTS

Challenge: Urethrovaginal fistula.

Background
- UVF is a worldwide problem but most prevalent and most difficult to manage in less developed regions.

Prevention
- The formation of fistula may be prevented (or at least the size of the fistula reduced) by maintaining an indwelling urethral catheter for a period following an obstructed delivery.

Management
- The optimum surgical approaches, routes, techniques, and timings of surgical intervention are matters of considerable debate. Most repairs are undertaken using the vaginal route, under either regional or general anesthesia.

- Principles of repair include:
  - Excision of all the scarred tissue around the fistula, and mobilization of healthy and well-vascularized tissue, ensuring preservation of urethral continuity.
  - Tension-free closure, using a two-layer repair technique to reform the urethra, with the use of a labial/vaginal graft if necessary to provide a good cover to the urethra.
  - Meticulous hemostasis.
  - Interposition of a Martius fat graft or omentum between layers of the bladder and vagina.
  - Free drainage of the bladder using an indwelling urethral catheter for 14 days (in repairs not requiring ureteric cannulation) or 21 days (in repairs requiring ureteric cannulation).
- Incontinence persists in around 10% of patients following extensive UVF surgery, for a variety of reasons involving not only the degree of surgical success but also the continence mechanism, bladder capacity, and any other associated injuries.

References

1 Lewis G, De Bernis L (eds) *Obstetric Fistula: Guiding Principles for Clinical Management and Programme Development*. World Health Organization, Geneva, 2006.

2 Kelly J. Vesico-vaginal and recto-vaginal fistulae. *J R Soc Med* 1992;85:257–258.

3 Mola G, Vangeenderhuysen C. Introduction. In: LewisG, De BernisL (eds) *Obstetric Fistula: Guiding Principles for Clinical Management and Programme Development, chapter 1*. World Health Organization, Geneva, 2006.

4 Cameron AP, Atiemo HO. Unusual presentation of an obstetrical urethro-vaginal fistula secondary to improper catheter placement. *Can Urol Assoc J* 2009;3:E21–E22.

5 Carlin BI, Klutke CG. Development of urethro-vaginal fistula following periurethral collagen injection. *J Urol* 2000;164:124.

6 Estevez JP, Colin P, Lucot JP, Collinet P, Cosson M, Boukerrou M. [Urethrovaginal fistulae resulting from sub-urethral slings for stress urinary incontinence treatment. A report of two cases and review of the literature]. *J Gynecol Obstet Biol Reprod (Paris)* 2010;39:151–155.

7 Hampel C, Naumann G, Thüroff JW, Gillitzer R. [Management of complications after sling and mesh implantations]. *Urologe A* 2009;48:496–509.

8 Elkins TE. Surgery for the obstetric vesicovaginal fistula: a review of 100 operations in 82 patients. *Am J Obstet Gynecol* 1994;170:1108–1120.

9 Meeks GR, Ghafar MA. Vesicovaginal and urethrovaginal fistulas. *Global Library of Women's Medicine*, 2012. doi: 10.3843/GLOWM.10064.

10 Dogra PN, Nabi G. Laser welding of vesicovaginal fistula. *Int Urogynecol J Pelvic Floor Dysfunct* 2001;12:69–70.

11 Wong C, Lam PN, Lucente VR. Laparoscopic transabdominal transvesical vesicovaginal fistula repair. *J Endourol* 2006;20:240–243.

12 Lowman J, Moore RD, Miklos JR. Tension-free vaginal tape sling with a porcine interposition graft in an irradiated patient with a past history of a urethrovaginal fistula and urethral mesh erosion: a case report. *J Reprod Med* 2007;52:560–562.

CHAPTER 129

Rectovaginal Fistulae

Claire Burton[1] and Simon Radley[2]
[1] Portsmouth Hospitals NHS Trust, Portsmouth, UK
[2] Birmingham Bowel Clinic, Birmingham, UK

Case history: A 34-year-old woman returns to perineal clinic 4 weeks after a forceps delivery and repair of episiotomy. She reports offensive vaginal discharge and passing of gas through the vagina. On examination there is a feculent discharge coming through a defect in the vagina, and the tissues are generally inflamed.

Background

A rectovaginal fistula is a congenital or acquired tract between the rectum (or anus) and the vagina. It may be classified according to location or the underlying cause (Table 129.1). The method of surgical repair will depend on the former, and the ultimate success of repair will be influenced by the latter, with repair of obstetric fistulae probably having the best success rate.

Table 129.1 Causes of rectovaginal fistula.

Obstetric complication	Anal sphincter injury or isolated rectal injury; missed injury; repair breakdown, often secondary to infection
Prior anorectal or vaginal surgery	Posterior repair; stapled hemorrhoidectomy; STARR (stapled transanal resection of rectum); surgery for rectal tumors (anterior resection)
Inflammatory bowel disease	Crohn's disease
Infection	Cryptoglandular abscess in anal canal rupturing through to vagina; Bartholin gland abscess; lymphogranuloma venereum; tuberculosis
Carcinoma	Invasive cervical, vaginal, rectal or anal cancer
Radiotherapy	Following pelvic irradiation (e.g., for cervical or endometrial cancer)
Congenital	
Trauma or foreign body	Retained pessary; vaginal mesh from prolapse repair

Management

The patient will usually complain of fecal or flatal incontinence through the vagina but may also complain of recurrent vaginal or urinary tract infections. Conservative management may be sufficient for small obstetric fistulae with use of analgesia and antimicrobial therapy.

Surgical repair should be undertaken by a surgeon with experience in fistula repair and often requires a multidisciplinary team approach with a colorectal surgeon, (uro)gynecologist, and specialist stoma nurse. Following surgery, there is a recognized risk of recurrence of 40% or more. Risk factors for recurrence include Crohn's disease, radiotherapy, smoking, and raised BMI [1,2].

Preoperative evaluation

This includes identification of the underlying cause of the fistula and its location together with an assessment of the continence mechanism (anal sphincter complex).

- Examination under anesthesia: the perineum, vagina and rectum are often inflamed and the patient may find examination without anesthesia very painful.
- Rigid sigmoidoscopy: to visualize the rectal mucosa, particularly if there is a possibility of inflammatory bowel disease or malignancy.
- Endoanal ultrasound and anorectal physiology: to assess sphincter anatomic integrity and function.
- Imaging such as a double-contrast CT: to demonstrate colovaginal or high rectal fistulae.
- MRI scan: to identify fistulae, secondary tracts, and associated sepsis or collections.

The timing of repair after an acute injury is debatable. There may be merit in waiting up to 12 weeks to treat infection and allow inflammation to settle. The fistula tract may decrease in size or even heal spontaneously [3]. However, the patient may find coping with pain and symptoms of leakage very distressing. Loperamide and bulking agents such as Fybogel can be used to firm stool, and may help to reduce fecal seepage through the fistula tract. A diversion procedure (e.g., ileostomy or colostomy) can be considered prior to repair, although this may not improve cure rates [1,2].

Surgical approach

High fistula

This is best treated via an abdominal approach with resection of the damaged bowel and fistula tract. The fistula is usually secondary to Crohn's disease, recent resectional surgery, radiotherapy, or cancer.

Mid or low vaginal fistula

A transrectal or transvaginal approach may be used [4]. The key to successful repair is the excision of the fistula tract, tension-free approximation, excellent hemostasis, and antibiotic cover. If there is damage to the perineal body or sphincter complex, a transperineal

Gynecologic and Obstetric Surgery: Challenges and Management Options, First Edition. Edited by Arri Coomarasamy, Mahmood I. Shafi, G. Willy Davila and Kiong K. Chan.
© 2016 John Wiley & Sons, Ltd. Published 2016 by John Wiley & Sons, Ltd.

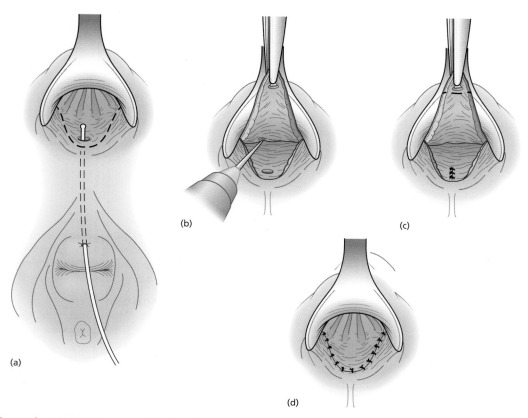

Figure 129.1 Transanal repair with advancement flap. A probe is passed down the fistula tract (a), the anal mucosa is dissected off (b), the tract is closed (c), and the flap advanced to cover the repair (d). From Hyman, 1999 [5] with permission from Elsevier.

or vaginal approach may be preferable to allow concomitant sphincteroplasty and perineorrhaphy.

Transanal repair (Figure 129.1)
Special attention must be paid to patient positioning and support; the patient should be positioned prone in a jackknife position. The fistula opening is excised and a flap developed proximally. The underlying defect in the muscular wall is closed with interrupted absorbable sutures. The flap is then advanced distally to cover the site of the defect.

Transvaginal repair
The patient should be placed in lithotomy position. The posterior vaginal wall is incised in the midline and the vaginal skin is dissected off the underlying anterior rectal wall. The fistula tract is excised and the defect is closed in layers with absorbable sutures.

Alternatively, an advancement flap can be developed. The initial incision should be horseshoe shaped including the fistula opening. The underlying defect is excised and closed before the flap is advanced distally to cover the suture line.

Prevention

Obstetric practice
Mediolateral episiotomy should be performed where indicated, rather than a midline episiotomy, as a mediolateral episiotomy is

associated with a reduced risk of rectoanal damage [6]. A thorough rectal examination is necessary after any vaginal delivery, not only to assess the integrity of the anal sphincter complex but also to check for any rectal trauma. Rectal trauma should be repaired in layers with an absorbable suture via a vaginal approach, ensuring the sutures encompass the proximal end of the defect. Colorectal surgical expertise should be sought if the surgeon is unfamiliar with the repair technique. Prophylactic antibiotics should be given to reduce the risk of infection and associated wound breakdown. Women who have experienced rectal or anal sphincter injury should be followed up in a dedicated perineal trauma clinic.

Bartholin or perineal abscess
Abscess cavities should be carefully explored to break down all loculations and check for evidence of communication with the rectum or anus. Recurrent abscesses should prompt further investigation to look for fistulae.

Posterior vaginal wall surgery
Good surgical techniques should always be employed to ensure hemostasis and avoid inadvertent damage to anus or rectum. Care should be taken to avoid perforating sutures to the rectum which may act as a tract between the rectum and vagina. A digital rectal examination should be performed at the end of any vaginal surgery involving the posterior wall to confirm rectal mucosal integrity.

KEY POINTS

Challenge: Rectovaginal fistula.

Background
- Obstetric injury is the commonest cause of rectovaginal fistula.
- Other gynecologic causes include vaginal surgery and vulval or perineal abscesses.
- Inflammatory bowel disease (i.e., Crohn's disease) is also frequently associated with RVF, but repair success rates are significantly lower.

Management
- Multidisciplinary approach with surgeons who have experience in fistula repair is essential.
- Investigations can include EUA, sigmoidoscopy, endoanal ultrasound, anorectal physiology, double-contrast CT, and MRI.

- The timing of repair should be carefully considered; it may be necessary to wait up to 12 weeks to treat infection and allow inflammation to settle.
- The repair can be via an abdominal, transrectal, or transvaginal approach. The key principles are full excision of the fistula tract and tension-free repair in multiple layers.
- A transvaginal approach to repair is preferable where there is concomitant sphincter or perineal body deficiency.

Prevention
- If an episiotomy is needed, it should be a mediolateral rather than a midline episiotomy.
- Digital rectal examination must be performed after any complex vaginal delivery or vaginal surgery.
- If a breach in rectal or anal mucosa is found and repaired, antibiotic prophylaxis should be used.

References

1 Pinto RA, Peterson TV, Shawki S, Davila GW, Wexner SD. Are there predictors of outcome following rectovaginal fistula repair? *Dis Colon Rectum* 2010;53:1240–1247

2 El-Gazzaz G, Hull TL, Mignanelli E, Hammel J, Gurland B, Zutshi M. Obstetric and cryptoglandular rectovaginal fistulas: long-term surgical outcome; quality of life; and sexual function. *J Gastrointest Surg* 2010;14:1758–1763.

3 Rahman MS, Al-Suleiman SA, El-Yahia AR, Rahman J. Surgical treatment of rectovaginal fistula of obstetric origin: a review of 15 years' experience in a teaching hospital. *J Obstet Gynaecol* 2003;23:607–610.

4 Baig MK, Zhao RH, Yuen CH et al. Simple rectovaginal fistulas. *Int J Colorectal Dis* 2000;15:323–327.

5 Hyman N. Endoanal advancement flap repair for complex anorectal fistulas. *Am J Surg* 1999;178:337–340.

6 Royal College of Obstetricians and Gynaecologists. *The Management of Third- and Fourth-degree Perineal Tears*. RCOG Green-top Guideline No. 29, June 2015. Available at https://www.rcog.org.uk/en/guidelines-research-services/guidelines/gtg29/

CHAPTER 130

Secondary Anal Sphincter Repair

Steven D. Wexner and Emanuela Silva
Cleveland Clinic Florida, Weston/Fort Lauderdale, Florida, USA

Case history: A 48-year-old woman, with a history of two vaginal births, presents with fecal urgency, soiling, and flatal incontinence. She had extension of an episiotomy to a third-degree tear with a forceps delivery 10 years ago; the tear was sutured with an end-to-end technique.

Background

It is reported that 0.5–1.0% of adults experience regular fecal incontinence that affects their quality of life [1]. The anal sphincter is the main enabling component of the intricate mechanism of fecal continence, which depends on neural integrity, rectal sensation, colonic transit, stool consistency, anorectal reflexes, pelvic floor muscles, sensory epithelium of anal mucosa, and hemorrhoidal cushions. The anal sphincter is formed by the internal anal sphincter (IAS), the external anal sphincter (EAS), and the puborectalis muscle. The latter two are innervated by the pudendal nerve, while the IAS, along with the rectum, is supplied by autonomic sympathetic and parasympathetic fibers from the pelvic and sacral roots.

Sphincter damage can potentially occur due to any anorectal or pelvic trauma. Surgical treatment of anal fissures, fistulae, tumors and, less commonly, hemorrhoids may injure the IAS, EAS, or both. Isolated or more extensive injury to the anorectal muscles may also result from trauma (impalement, rectal perforation, and damage to the soft tissue of the perineum). Nevertheless, sphincter harm secondary to obstetric trauma remains the main cause of sphincter damage.

In the United States, the prevalence of obstetric anal sphincter injury ranges from 0.5 to 7% and has been shown to be as high as 17% with midline episiotomy [2]. In addition to the physical rupture of the sphincter during vaginal delivery, prolonged labor may result in detrimental stretching of the pudendal nerve, enhancing injury. Sphincter disruption can remain latent for several years, becoming symptomatic years or even decades after the vaginal delivery.

Direct sphincter repair can be performed for isolated sphincter defects. For acute sphincter disruption, primary repair has been associated with satisfactory outcomes in 47% of patients; failure is mainly credited to its disruption [3]. Other factors such as wound infection, local hematoma, technical problems, and unacknowledged secondary defects can also contribute to poor outcomes, and require a second repair in approximately 5% [4,5]. For these patients, as well as patients in whom the rupture was unrecognized in the acute setting, or was not entirely fixed, a secondary repair may be attempted after complete resolution of infection or inflammation.

Management

People who report fecal incontinence should be offered care by healthcare professionals who have the relevant skills, training and experience and who work within an integrated continence service.

A full assessment should be carried out to discover the cause of the fecal incontinence and provide the most appropriate treatment. Detailed office evaluation includes history-taking and inviting patients to complete bowel-related quality-of-life questionnaires including the Cleveland Clinic Florida Fecal Incontinence Scale (CCF-FIS) [6]. Patients should consider appropriate changes in diet and fluid intake, establishment of a regular bowel routine, and planning of journeys so that they can use public toilets. Pelvic floor exercises should also be recommended to improve the coordination and strength of the pelvic muscles. Other treatment options to consider include biofeedback with or without electrical stimulation, stool-firming medicines such as loperamide (which are started at the lowest doses and then titrated as required), bowel retraining, percutaneous tibial nerve stimulation, sacral neuromodulation, and sphincteroplasty.

Investigations include anorectal physiology studies and endoanal ultrasonography. If endoanal ultrasound is not available, MRI, endovaginal ultrasound, and perineal ultrasound should be considered.

Overlapping sphincteroplasty

Overlapping sphincteroplasty is the most widely accepted procedure for secondary anal repair (especially with an isolated EAS lesion) because of its superior long-term functional outcomes, compared with direct apposition repair [5]. The technique evolved from the sphincter repair by direct apposition, which consisted of identification and mobilization of EAS, excision of all scar tissue, and direct suturing of the muscle ends. Modifications such as

Gynecologic and Obstetric Surgery: Challenges and Management Options, First Edition. Edited by Arri Coomarasamy, Mahmood I. Shafi, G. Willy Davila and Kiong K. Chan.
© 2016 John Wiley & Sons, Ltd. Published 2016 by John Wiley & Sons, Ltd.

preservation of the scar, overlapping of the muscle at the cut ends [7], association of levatorplasty, and plication of the IAS have since been incorporated and are associated with improved functional outcomes. With appropriate bowel preparation, this procedure is safe without need for fecal diversion.

Patient preparation

Preoperative management includes full mechanical bowel preparation. Intravenous antibiotics and subcutaneous heparin are given at the start of the procedure. The patient is placed in the prone jackknife position on a Kraske roll.

Operative technique

A 120° curvilinear incision is made anterior to the anus, approximately 0.5 cm distal and parallel to the anal verge (Figure 130.1a). The anterior portion of the sphincter muscle is identified and dissected with the index finger of the non-dominant hand inserted into the vagina (Figure 130.1b) to prevent inadvertent vaginal wall injury. Care must be taken to avoid extending the dissection through the mucosa into the anal canal or rectum, particularly where the sphincter muscle is disrupted, absent, or the rectovaginal septum is extremely thin; this may predispose to anovaginal or rectovaginal fistula formation.

EAS dissection is initiated laterally where the muscle anatomy is usually intact with a clearer plane of dissection. Specific attention should be paid to the pudendal nerve bundles as they enter the EAS bilaterally, in the posterolateral position. The intersphincteric space is dissected from lateral to medial on each side, and IAS and EAS are separated. Scar tissue connecting the two ends of the disrupted external sphincter is preserved and divided in the midline, but not excised, promoting better anchoring of the sutures. If the ends are separated, the scar is identified and preserved and the muscle mobilized.

The repair starts with imbrication of the levator muscles found just beneath the two ends of the divided scar tissue, using interrupted 2-0 polypropylene sutures. The IAS is plicated with interrupted 2-0 PDS sutures (Figure 130.1c), which are placed far enough laterally for a snug repair, and then verified by inserting the index finger into the anal canal. At this point, the ends of the EAS muscle should overlap without significant tension and are secured with interrupted 2-0 PDS mattress sutures. The scar tissue is used to provide a significant portion of the suture fixation (Figure 130.1d).

Retractors and buttock tapes are removed before tying the sutures of the overlapped ends, thereby avoiding a lax repair (Figure 130.1e). The sutures are tied snugly, but not so much as to induce muscular ischemia. The wound is closed from lateral to medial on each side using 3-0 polyglactin sutures through the skin, leaving the central-most portion of the wound open for drainage (Figure 130.1f).

Postoperative management

Postoperatively, the patient is given cefotaxime 2 g every 12 hours and metronidazole 500 mg every 6 hours for 2 days, followed by oral ciprofloxacin and metronidazole for 7 days. Ambulation is encouraged, while long periods of sitting are discouraged. The wound is not packed, so patients may need a sanitary pad to protect clothing. No constipating agents are required, and patients should be allowed to eat and drink as soon as they feel able to do so; bowel confinement is not used as there is evidence that it has no advantage over starting a regular diet [8].

Effectiveness

Short-term functional results after overlapping sphincteroplasty have been described as very good in the majority of earlier series. Success rates ranging from 71 to 86%, at a mean follow-up of 10–29 months, have been reported [2]. Unfortunately, there is a cumulative deterioration of the outcomes over the years. A systematic review on long-term outcomes, including 16 studies and 900 patients, showed that despite variable outcome measures, a clear trend toward decay of functional outcomes over time could be seen [9]. Reports of no patients remaining completely continent to liquid and solid stool at 10 years follow-up have been published [10]. Studies on whether timing of the repair, type of repair, an association with pudendal neuropathy, advanced age, postoperative wound infection, or technical factors may predict worse clinical results are still not available [11].

Resolution of the case

The patient described in the case history failed conservative treatment. She then went on to have endoanal ultrasound and manometry. She was found to have an isolated EAS lesion. After counseling about the potential benefits and limitations of each option (with particular attention to long-term results), she chose to have a sphincteroplasty. An overlapping sphincteroplasty without fecal diversion was performed, and produced good results.

KEY POINTS

Challenge: Fecal incontinence in a woman who had a previous obstetric sphincter tear.

Background
- 0.5–1.0% of adults experience regular fecal incontinence that affects their quality of life.
- The fecal continence mechanism is an intricate mechanism that comprises neural integrity, rectal sensation, colonic transit, stool consistency, anorectal reflexes, pelvic floor muscles, sensory epithelium of anal mucosa, and hemorrhoidal cushions, with the anal sphincter as the main enabling component.
- Obstetric trauma predisposes women to fecal incontinence.
- A full colorectal evaluation is required prior to any surgical intervention for fecal incontinence.

Management
- Care should be provided by a specialist team.
- Conservative management of fecal incontinence should be offered as first-line therapy, including dietary management, pelvic floor exercises, and stool-firming therapies.
- Overlapping sphincteroplasty is the procedure of choice for secondary anal sphincter repair:
  - Preoperative management includes full mechanical bowel preparation, antibiotics, and subcutaneous heparin.
  - Modifications can include preservation of the sphincter scar, levatorplasty, and plication of the IAS.
  - Postoperative management includes antibiotics, early ambulation, and timely commencement of feeding (not delayed).
- Success rates have been shown to decrease over time, making patient counseling preoperatively very important.
- Neuromodulation, as well as the use of injectable bulking agents, may offer patients with fecal incontinence additional effective therapies.

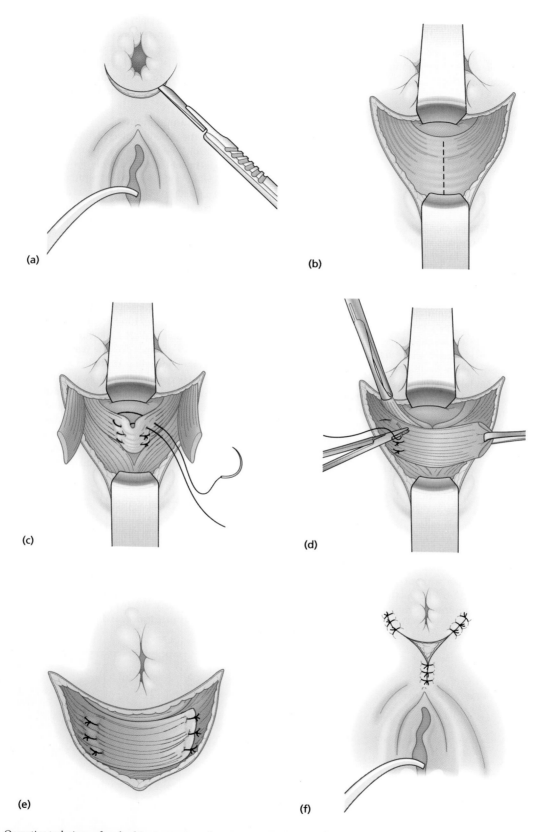

Figure 130.1 Operative technique of anal sphincter repair, with patient in prone jackknife position: (a) 120° curvilinear incision is made anterior to the anus; (b) the anterior portion of the sphincter muscle is identified and dissected; (c) the IAS is plicated with interrupted sutures; (d) the ends of the external sphincter muscle are overlapped; (e) the sutures are tied; (f) the skin wound is closed lateral to medial leaving the central-most portion open for drainage. Adapted from Cleveland Clinic Center for Medical Art & Photography © 1994–2013.

References

1 National Institute for Health and Care Excellence. *Faecal incontinence: the management of faecal incontinence in adults*. NICE Clinical Guideline No. 49, June 2007. Available at https://www.nice.org.uk/guidance/cg49

2 Fenner DE, Genberg B, Brahma P *et al.* Fecal and urinary incontinence after vaginal delivery with anal sphincter disruption in an obstetrics unit in the United States. *J Obstet Gynecol* 2003;189:1543–9.

3 Baig M, Wexner SD. Factors predictive of outcome after surgery for fecal incontinence. *Br J Surg* 2000;87:1316–1330.

4 Venkatesh KS, Ramanujam PS, Larson DM, Haywood MA. Anorectal complications of vaginal delivery. *Dis Colon Rectum* 1989;32:1039–1041.

5 Brouwer R, Duthie G. Sacral nerve neuromodulation is effective treatment for fecal incontinence in the presence of a sphincter defect, pudendal neuropathy, or previous sphincter repair. *Dis Colon Rectum* 2010;53:273–278.

6 Jorge JMN, Wexner SD. Etiology and management of fecal incontinence. *Dis Colon Rectum* 1993;36:77–97.

7 Moscovitz I, Rotholtz NA, Baig MK *et al.* Overlapping sphincteroplasty: does preservation of the scar influence immediate outcome? *Colorectal Dis* 2001;4:275–279.

8 Nessim A, Wexner SD, Agachan F *et al.* Is bowel confinement necessary after anorectal reconstructive surgery? A prospective randomized surgeon-blinded trial. *Dis Colon Rectum* 1999;42:16–23.

9 Glasgow SC, Lowry AC. Long-term outcomes of anal sphincter repair for fecal incontinence: a systematic review. *Dis Colon Rectum* 2012;55:482–490.

10 Zutshi MT, Tracey TH, Bast K, Halverson A, Na J. Ten-year outcome after anal sphincter repair for fecal incontinence. *Dis Colon Rectum* 2009;52:1089–1094.

11 Goetz LH, Lowry AC. Overlapping sphincteroplasty: is it the standard of care? *Clin Colon Rectal Surg* 2005;18:22–31.

Section 7
Gynecologic Oncology
Editors: Kavita Singh, Mahmood I. Shafi, and Kiong K. Chan

CHAPTER 131
Large Loop Excision of the Transformation Zone

Mahmood I. Shafi

Addenbrooke's Hospital, Cambridge University Hospitals NHS Foundation Trust, Cambridge, UK

Case history 1: A 35-year-old woman has been referred with severe dyskaryosis and colposcopic impression of high-grade cervical intraepithelial neoplasia (HGCIN).

Case history 2: A 28-year-old woman has been referred with mild dyskaryosis and positive high-risk human papillomavirus (HrHPV). Assessment with colposcopy and then directed biopsies have confirmed CIN2 (HGCIN).

Background

Women with high-grade cytologic abnormalities (moderate and severe dyskaryosis) and those with histologically confirmed HGCIN have cancer precursors and require treatment. The most popular method of treating CIN is with large loop excision of the transformation zone (LLETZ). This is an excisional technique which gives the benefit of further histologic assessment, exclusion of microinvasive or glandular disease, and assessment of margins of excision to ensure that preinvasive disease has been completely excised. Other treatment methods which may be used for the treatment of CIN are cold coagulation, laser ablation or cryocautery, but these techniques do not offer the facility of obtaining histologic assessment. Treatment for CIN aims at eradicating the preinvasive disease while limiting unnecessary damage to normal cervical tissue with the aim of reducing treatment-associated morbidity.

Management

LLETZ or loop electrosurgical excision procedure (LEEP) involves the use of low-voltage diathermy apparatus that is available in most surgical units. Three basic principles apply to LLETZ.
1 A competent colposcopic examination is a prelude to LLETZ.
2 The intention of LLETZ should be to remove the entire transformation zone. An adequate margin of normal epithelium should surround the dysplastic tissues and the squamocolumnar epithelium should be identifiable on histopathology.
3 LLETZ should inflict the minimal amount of damage to the specimen and to the remaining cervix.

After appropriate counseling and consent, the majority of LLETZ procedures are performed under local anesthesia where infiltration with local anesthetic and vasoconstrictor is used in the cervix just outside the transformation zone. A four quadrant or circumferential superficial infiltration is performed using a dental syringe and needle and prefilled cartridges of local anesthetic and vasoconstrictor (Citanest or Lignospan). In cases where the cervical lesion is very large or the patient is very apprehensive, LLETZ can also be performed under general anesthesia.

Treatment is ideally conducted with the whole of the transformation zone visible within one field of view with low-magnification colposcopy. The transformation zone has a variable anatomy and the loop chosen should take this into account so that adequate excision may take place (Figure 131.1). When undertaking LLETZ procedures it is important to understand the principles of desiccation and fulguration in electrosurgery. Desiccation occurs when the electrode or wire is physically touching the tissue and causes more thermal damage. With fulguration, the electrode is not in direct contact but within a millimeter or so from the tissue to be treated, causing a superficial "spray coagulation" and thereby treating a larger surface. Fulguration can be used both with the loop when excising, and with the ball when gaining hemostasis. Using a blend of cutting and coagulation for the excision, the loop is traversed across slowly so that a fulgurative cutting and coagulative effect ensues. If the loop is pushed or hurried, then desiccation occurs and there is greater thermal damage to the excised specimen.

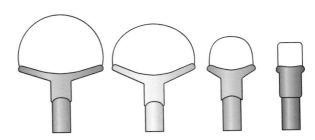

Figure 131.1 Selection of loops available for LLETZ procedure.

Gynecologic and Obstetric Surgery: Challenges and Management Options, First Edition. Edited by Arri Coomarasamy, Mahmood I. Shafi, G. Willy Davila and Kiong K. Chan.
© 2016 John Wiley & Sons, Ltd. Published 2016 by John Wiley & Sons, Ltd.

Hemostasis

Following excisional treatment, the cervical crater base is treated with ball diathermy to obtain hemostasis. A variety of techniques can be used. Using a diathermy ball in coagulative mode, the cervix can be treated quickly using either desiccation or fulguration. The rollerball makes this easier to perform as the ball rotates over the surface and fulgurates the base. With troublesome bleeding, suction, cotton tip buds or swabs are used to remove any excess blood and display bleeding points that may require coagulation. Other hemostatic techniques include the following.

- Oxycel, Surgicel or other hemostatic preparations.
- Application of ferric subsulfate (Monsel's solution or paste). The paste is prepared by aerating the solution over 48 hours, which allows a degree of evaporation to occur; the consistency of the paste can be changed by further additions of ferric subsulfate solution.
- Packing of the wound with gauze soaked in ferric subsulfate.
- Silver nitrate.

Secondary hemorrhage is usually infective in origin and settles with the use of broad-spectrum antibiotics.

Postoperative care

Following treatment, advice is given to avoid sexual intercourse and insertion of vaginal tampons for 4 weeks or until the discharge settles. Swimming should be avoided for 2 weeks. Fertility does not appear to be affected following treatment with LLETZ. Obstetric function may be compromised, with a propensity to preterm labor and preterm prelabor rupture of membranes, especially in those with deeper excisions (>1 cm depth) or those with repeated excisions. Long-term sequelae are related to the size of the loop, particularly the depth, and may be a function of the percentage of cervix removed at excision. Stenosis may occur if the depth of excision is excessive or repeat loops are performed.

The histology report should assess the excision margins as this is related to the likelihood of finding residual or recurrent disease. Both the lesion size and excision margins correlate with follow-up cytology. In those treated for HGCIN, follow-up cytology and high-risk human papillomavirus testing (HrHPV test of cure) are performed at 6 months following the treatment; if the cytology sample is negative, borderline or low grade with no HrHPV identified, then the woman can be returned to 3-yearly recall. However, in the presence of persistent HrHPV or high-grade cytology, the individual requires further colposcopic assessment. In women aged 50 years or more with endocervical or lateral margin involvement, consideration should be given to re-excision where satisfactory cytology and colposcopy cannot be guaranteed. In those with two or more margins of involvement, there is a much higher risk of residual or recurrent disease and consideration should be given to further excision. Similar consideration to further excision should be given if there is endocervical or ectocervical margin involvement in the presence of stromal involved margin (i.e., two of the three margins are involved).

Resolution of the case

In Case history 1, the colposcopy and cytology are in agreement and an option is to undertake treatment at the first visit if the woman has been appropriately informed and is agreeable to this approach.

In Case history 2, the woman had minor cytologic abnormalities, but the biopsies have confirmed HGCIN and therefore the advice is for treatment.

Prevention

Cervical precancer detection and treatment is an important aspect of preventing cervical cancer. Excisional treatments are popular for the treatment of CIN, and LLETZ is the most widely used technique. It is important that LLETZ is used appropriately in selected patients as there is a danger of overtreating minor abnormalities. Reduction of LLETZ-associated morbidity is important and is related to the amount of cervix removed with the treatment and especially depth of excision, with 1 cm being the upper limit for most situations requiring treatment of CIN.

KEY POINTS

Challenge: Large loop excision of the transformation zone.

Background
- Excisional treatments are popular for therapy of CIN.
- The basic principle is to remove the cervical abnormality with a surrounding rim of normal tissue but limit the depth of excision to around 7 mm with a maximum of 10 mm in most situations.

Management
- Selection of the patient, equipment, and loop size is very important.
- In those with plans for future pregnancy, the need to limit morbidity is even more important. Depth of excision and the amount of cervical tissue removed are important variables.
- If there is intraoperative bleeding, the options are:
  - Diathermy ball coagulation.
  - Oxycel, Surgicel or other hemostatic preparations.
  - Application of ferric subsulfate (Monsel's solution or paste).
  - Packing of the wound with gauze soaked in ferric subsulfate.
- If there is secondary bleeding, the cause is usually infective, and management will require broad-spectrum antibiotics.

Prevention
- Select and treat strategy is important for diagnosing and treating CIN. Only those patients who require treatment should be considered for LLETZ. It is important to audit treatment outcomes for women with CIN undergoing treatment.

Further reading

Luesley D, Leeson S (eds) *Colposcopy and Programme Management. Guidelines for the NHS Cervical Screening Programme*, 2nd edn. NHS Cervical Screening Programme Publication No. 20, May 2010. Available at http://www.cancerscreening.nhs.uk/cervical/publications/nhscsp20.pdf

Martin-Hirsch PPL, Parakevaidis E, Bryant A, Dickinson HO, Keep SL. Surgery for cervical intraepithelial neoplasia, *Cochrane Database Syst Rev* 2010;(6):CD001318.

Shafi MI. European quality standards for the treatment of cervical intraepithelial neoplasia (CIN). European Federation for Colposcopy. Available at http://www.e-f-c.org/pages/recommendationsguidelines/european-quality-standards-for-the-treatment-of-cervical-intraepithelial-neoplasia-cin-2007.php

Shafi MI, Nazeer S. *Colposcopy: A Practical Guide*, 2nd edn. Cambridge University Press, Cambridge, 2012.

CHAPTER 132

Knife Cone Biopsy

Najum Qureshi
Birmingham Women's NHS Foundation Trust, Birmingham, UK

Case history: A 28-year-old woman had a cervical cytology sample showing severe glandular changes. At colposcopy, villous fusion and possible glandular cuffing were noted along with dense aceto-white areas proximal to the squamocolumnar junction (SCJ). Mosaicism and coarse punctation were seen at SCJ but no vessel abnormality was noted. The colposcopic impression was suggestive of high-grade glandular and squamous lesions. A cold-knife cone (CKC) was planned for the patient under general anesthesia.

Background

Cold-knife cone (CKC) treatment has become an infrequent procedure for the treatment of cervical cytologic abnormalities with the advent of outpatient electrosurgical excisional methods (Chapter 131). However, many authorities still recommend CKC in the following situations:
- SCJ is deep in the cervical canal;
- glandular intraepithelial neoplasia is suspected;
- microinvasive disease is suspected.

Although CKC is associated with a higher morbidity compared with other modalities of treatment, it has the advantage of excision likely to be in a single piece and no risk of diathermy damage to the specimen, especially the margins.

Management

CKC is performed in the operating room under general anesthesia. Colposcopic assessment of the cervix with 5% acetic acid and Lugol's iodine stain should be performed to determine the size and location of the lesion to be excised. A gentle cleaning of the vulva, vagina, and cervix is performed. The cervix should not be scrubbed vigorously as this could traumatize the area containing the lesion.

We usually use a previously prepared combination of 2% lidocaine hydrochloride and epinephrine (1 in 80,000) via a dental syringe system to infiltrate directly into the cervix. Three ampoules are administered; one ampoule (2.2 mL) each is given at the 3 and 9 o'clock positions, and a half ampoule (1.1 mL) each at the 12 and 6 o'clock positions. Epinephrine is a vasoconstrictor and causes blanching at the injection site. The advantage of using vasoconstrictive agents such as epinephrine is that it decreases blood loss at surgery. However, as epinephrine can cause a rise in blood pressure and pulse rate, the anesthetist should be informed prior to its injection into the cervix. Although deep lateral sutures at the 3 and 9 o'clock positions have been used to occlude the descending cervical arteries to reduce primary hemorrhage, there is no evidence for such an approach.

The cervix is then repainted with Lugol's iodine to outline the lesion. To stabilize the cervix the anterior lip is grasped with a tenaculum at a site away from the anticipated line of excision. Sometimes two tenacula may be required. We prefer to use a bent Beaver® blade (Figure 132.1). The advantage of this blade over a conventional scalpel blade is that it has two sharp edges which can be used to cut in either direction, and an inward curve of the blade ensures that inadvertent injury to surrounding organs like the bladder or rectum is minimized. It is advisable to commence the cone from the 6 o'clock position and to curve upward; this prevents blood trickling down from obscuring the line of excision. As the cone is cut, it is pulled to the opposite side with a skin hook to provide visibility at the base of the incision. Every attempt should be made to remove the cone as a single piece, which should be symmetrically centered around the endocervical canal with the apex in the canal. After removal, the cone should be marked with a suture at the 12 o'clock position so that the histologist can orientate any positive margins or foci of invasive disease.

Hemostasis

There are several ways to manage the bleeding from the cone bed. If bleeding is minimal, ball diathermy could be used to achieve hemostasis and the cone bed left open to granulate. Surgicel, an absorbable hemostatic agent soaked in Monsel's solution (or paste), could also be placed in the crater. A Cochrane review has shown that vaginal packing reduces morbidity compared with elective hemostatic sutures [1]. Packs significantly reduced the amount of peroperative blood loss, the risk of dysmenorrhea, unsatisfactory colposcopy at follow-up, and cervical stenosis [2].

Meta-analysis of four trials found that the use of tranexamic acid (an antifibrinolytic drug) postoperatively was associated with a

Gynecologic and Obstetric Surgery: Challenges and Management Options, First Edition. Edited by Arri Coomarasamy, Mahmood I. Shafi, G. Willy Davila and Kiong K. Chan.
© 2016 John Wiley & Sons, Ltd. Published 2016 by John Wiley & Sons, Ltd.

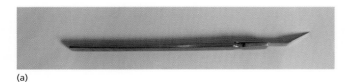

(a)

(b)

Figure 132.1 A bent Beaver blade.

statistically significant decrease in the risk of secondary hemorrhage compared with controls (RR 0.23, 95% CI 0.11–0.50) [1].

Resolution of the case

The woman needs full pre-procedure counseling about a possible threefold increased risk of preterm delivery in her subsequent pregnancies [3–5]. The background risk of preterm labor in any pregnancy is about 5%, and this could be increased up to 15% after CKC treatment.

Prevention

Other options to achieve the conization of the cervix should be considered. These can include diathermy (straight wire excision) or carbon dioxide laser. LLETZ or LEEP may be undertaken as a two-stage excision, the main traverse removing the ectocervical portion and a further traverse removing the endocervical canal. Whichever modality is used, it is important that a cone of cervix is removed for histology.

KEY POINTS

Challenge: Knife cone biopsy.

Background
- CKC has become an infrequent procedure with the advent of other excisional techniques. It may still be indicated in the following situations:
  - SCJ is deep in the cervical canal.
  - Glandular intraepithelial neoplasia is suspected.
  - Microinvasive disease is suspected.
- A larger volume of cervix is removed with CKC compared with LLETZ.
- Preterm delivery risk is increased with CKC, and patients should be counseled about the probable need for cervical cerclage (Chapter 154).

Management
- Management should be performed under general anesthesia.
- A suitable blade, such as the Beaver®, can be helpful.
- Infiltration of cervix with vasoconstrictive agents to reduce intraoperative blood loss is beneficial.
- Tranexamic acid used postoperatively may reduce risk of secondary hemorrhage.

Prevention
- CKC is associated with risk of secondary hemorrhage, cervical stenosis, and increased risk of preterm labor.
- Other less invasive options should be considered if appropriate.

References

1 Martin-Hirsch PPL, Keep SL, Bryant A. Interventions for preventing blood loss during treatment of cervical intraepithelial neoplasia. *Cochrane Database Syst Rev* 2010;(6):CD001421.

2 Gilbert L, Saunders N, Stringer R, Sharp E. Haemostasis and cold knife cone biopsy: a prospective randomised trial comparing a suture versus non-suture technique. *Obstet Gynecol* 1989;74:640–643.

3 Kyrgiou M, Koliopoulos G, Martin-Hirsch P, Prendiville W, Paraskevaidi E. Obstetric outcomes after conservative treatment for intraepithelial or early invasive cervical lesions: systematic review and meta-analysis. *Lancet* 2006;367:489–498.

4 Ørtoft G, Henriksen TB, Hansen ES, Peterson LK. After conisation of the cervix, the perinatal mortality as a result of preterm delivery increases in subsequent pregnancy. *BJOG* 2010;117:258–267.

5 Bruinsma FJ, Quin MA. The risk of preterm birth following treatment for precancerous changes in the cervix: a systematic review and meta-analysis. *BJOG* 2011;118:1031–1041.

CHAPTER 133

Staging Procedures: Examination Under Anesthesia, Cystoscopy, Sigmoidoscopy, and Biopsy Techniques

Mahmood I. Shafi

Addenbrooke's Hospital, Cambridge University Hospitals NHS Foundation Trust, Cambridge, UK

Case history 1: A 43-year-old woman has cervical cancer diagnosed at colposcopy and biopsy. She is a candidate for radical surgery and is to undergo a staging assessment.

Case history 2: A 66-year-old woman has been diagnosed with advanced cervical cancer and the plan is for her to have treatment with chemoradiotherapy.

Background

Cancers are staged surgically (e.g., ovarian), clinically (e.g., cervical), or pathologically (e.g., uterine). The most common need for undertaking an examination under anesthesia (EUA) for assessment of stage is for cervical cancer, although it can also be helpful in certain cases of vaginal or vulval cancer. The stage of the cervical cancer (Figure 133.1) is decided by clinical examination, although additional information can be obtained from other investigations that would assist in devising a treatment plan.

Management

EUA for staging of cervical cancer is best performed with sedation or general anesthesia so that full information is obtained to guide subsequent treatment. The examination is also best performed in the presence of appropriate personnel such as the surgical and clinical oncologists, to decide on stage and appropriate further treatment plans. Usually there will have been confirmation of the diagnosis by a suitably sized biopsy but if this has not previously been done, then this should be performed as part of the EUA assessment. Other tests should already have been performed including chest X-ray and an MRI scan of the abdomen and pelvis.

The EUA is performed by a bimanual vaginal and a combined rectovaginal examination, following visual assessment of the disease state. During the visual inspection, the site and size of the tumor is documented and if appropriate measured using a tape measure or other measuring device. The vaginal fornices are visualized and felt during the digital examination. This determines the size of the cervical tumor; because there is complete relaxation,

the parametrium and uterosacral ligaments are assessed, as this may not have been feasible in the conscious patient due to discomfort. If nodularity and shortening of the uterosacral ligament are noted, then this likely represents tumor involvement. If there is no cancer-free space between the tumor and the pelvic sidewall, then a higher stage is assigned. There is much debate about the accuracy of clinical assessment compared with MRI, with the latter having better predictability when assessed against histologic findings.

The role of cystoscopy and sigmoidoscopy is debated. These form part of the tests used for staging cervical cancers. MRI will usually confirm the cervical tumor and its site and size. If the tumor is small and there is a clear rim of normal cervix surrounding the tumor, it is highly unlikely that cystoscopy or sigmoidoscopy will give any additional information. However, if the tumor is more advanced or affecting the cervix in an asymmetric manner (e.g., anterior or posterior lip), then cystoscopy and/or sigmoidoscopy may prove helpful.

Cystoscopy

Cystoscopy is usually undertaken with a rigid cystoscope as the female urethra is relatively straight. The cystoscope is introduced with the obturator *in situ*. The obturator is then replaced by a telescope, usually with a 70° lens. The bladder is visualized by angling the surgeon's end of the cystoscope away from the side of interest. A conical motion is undertaken, with the tip or pivot point being the urethra. Video camera is used to better visualize and magnify areas of interest to allow easier viewing of the ureteric orifices. It is important not to overinflate the bladder with distension fluid. Any area of abnormality should be biopsied through the cystoscope to confirm or refute involvement with the tumor (Figure 133.2). Bullous edema within the bladder may be seen but this may not signify a higher stage of cervical cancer. Following biopsy of the bladder, the area may need to be cauterized for hemostasis. When taking the biopsy, the ureteral orifice should be avoided if at all possible. If ureteral orifice damage is unavoidable because of the location of the suspicious lesion, then a ureteral stent should be placed. Following cystoscopy and biopsy, patients are informed that minor hematuria or dysuria is normal.

Gynecologic and Obstetric Surgery: Challenges and Management Options, First Edition. Edited by Arri Coomarasamy, Mahmood I. Shafi, G. Willy Davila and Kiong K. Chan.
© 2016 John Wiley & Sons, Ltd. Published 2016 by John Wiley & Sons, Ltd.

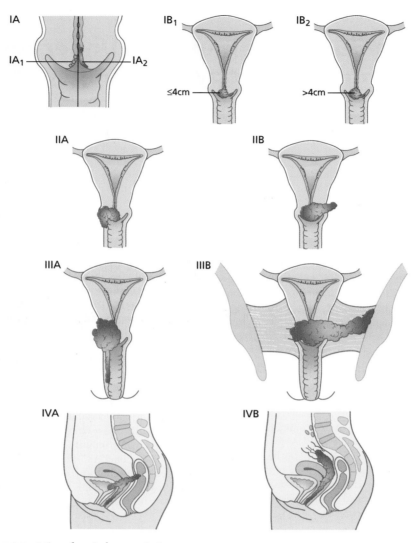

Figure 133.1 Diagrammatic representation of cervical cancer staging.

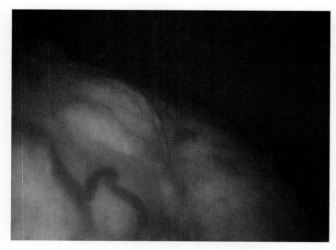

Figure 133.2 Cervical cancer pushing into the bladder at cystoscopy.

Sigmoidoscopy

Rigid sigmoidoscopy is used if there is suspected rectal involvement, usually from posterior spread of cervical cancer. Absolute contraindications to sigmoidoscopy are suspected bowel perforation or anal stenosis. Prior to the sigmoidoscopy, digital examination should always be performed to assess the general anatomy, any palpable lesions, and contents of the rectum. After generous lubrication up to 4 cm into the anus, the sigmoidoscope is introduced in the direction of the patient's umbilicus. The obturator of the sigmoidoscope is then removed and the eyepiece is sealed with the glass window. The sigmoidoscope is advanced under direct vision using the bellows to gently insufflate air into the rectum intermittently to expand the rectum as the sigmoidoscope advances carefully to the middle of the expanded segment. Beyond 4 cm from the anus, the rectum angulates posteriorly over the puborectalis sling towards the sacral hollow and the direction of the sigmoidoscope should change from pointing anteriorly to posteriorly. The insufflate–advance steps are repeated as the sigmoidoscope is moved along, and any abnormalities are noted. Around the 12-cm level, the sacral promontory produces a sharp angulation of the rectum anteriorly and the sigmoidoscope direction is likewise changed so that it points anterosuperiorly. The usual distance of examination is 15–20 cm and any further examination would need a flexible scope. As the sigmoidoscope is withdrawn, small circular motions allow complete examination and may reveal lesions missed during insertion of the sigmoidoscope.

Cervical biopsies

If a tissue diagnosis has not already been made, then appropriate biopsies will need to be undertaken during the EUA and staging procedure. Depending on the lesion, these can be taken as punch biopsies using biopsy forceps (Figure 133.3A) but these will need to be of sufficient depth to confirm the invasive process. Alternative techniques involve using a small LLETZ (Figure 133.3B) which can be used especially if bleeding is anticipated. The base of the biopsies can be fulgurated for hemostatic control, or a hemostatic agent such as Surgicel, silver nitrate, or Monsel's solution or paste can be applied (Chapter 131). If the lesion to be biopsied is deep, then a Trucut-type procedure is appropriate (Figure 133.3C). These are conducted with care so that the appropriate tissue is biopsied without risking normal structures. The Trucut can be advanced several times if necessary and the biopsy material checked to ascertain if sufficient amount has been obtained for histologic assessment.

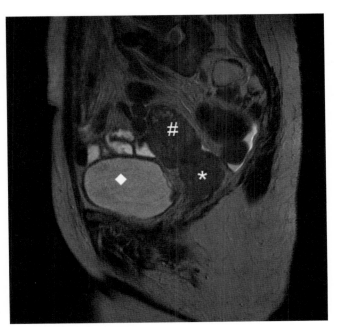

Figure 133.4 MRI of bulky cervical cancer. *, cervix; #, uterus; ◊, urinary bladder.

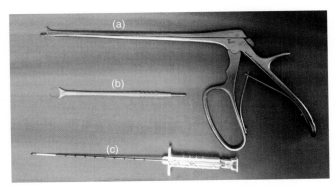

Figure 133.3 Biopsies can be taken using (a) biopsy forceps Tischler type, (b) small loop biopsy, and (c) Trucut.

Prevention

Staging procedures are still important despite much information being available from other diagnostic techniques such as MRI (Figure 133.4). As staging of cervical cancer is clinical, this can be undertaken during the EUA and by having a multidisciplinary approach. Accurate representation of the findings on a proforma is useful for future reference. Biopsy to confirm or refute disease can also be undertaken as necessary with the appropriate technique.

KEY POINTS

Challenge: Staging procedures for gynecologic cancer.

Background
- Staging of certain gynecologic cancers such as cervix is clinical.
- Important pretreatment information can be obtained from EUA and selective use of cystoscopy, sigmoidoscopy, and appropriate biopsies.

Management
- Multidisciplinary assessment should be undertaken so that the appropriate treatment stratagem can be adopted.
- Assessment of the size, site, and mobility of the tumor is important.
- Cystoscopy and sigmoidoscopy should be undertaken systematically.

Prevention
- Information from other diagnostics may aid the clinician but it is important to undertake the EUA without prejudice so that a complete picture can be developed for better management.
- Biopsies, especially if bleeding is anticipated, can be deferred to the EUA procedure as the clinician has more techniques available should bleeding be a problem.
- Other imaging modalities such as MRI and PET-CT may provide additional information.

Further reading

Kyrgiou M, Shafi MI. Invasive cancer of the cervix. *Obstet Gynaecol Reprod Med* 2010;20:147–154.
Shafi MI, Earl H, Tan LT (eds) *Gynaecological Oncology.* Cambridge University Press, Cambridge, 2009.

CHAPTER 134
Radicality of Surgery for Cervical Cancer

Mahmood I. Shafi
Addenbrooke's Hospital, Cambridge University Hospitals NHS Foundation Trust, Cambridge, UK

Case history 1: A 38-year-old woman with stage IB1 adenosquamous cancer of the cervix measuring 2 cm in maximal diameter has been advised to have radical surgery.

Case history 2: A 48-year-old woman with stage IIA squamous cell cancer of the cervix, maximal diameter 3 cm but with extension to involve 1 cm of upper vagina, has elected to have radical surgery as opposed to treatment with chemoradiation.

Background

Surgery for cancers follows the principles of en bloc resection of the tumor and its draining lymph nodes with an emphasis on achieving clear surgical margins. The exact choice of treatment will take into account key prognostic features, including extent of disease, nodal status (on MRI or CT scans), and lymphovascular space invasion (LVSI), as well as fertility wishes and long-term impact on quality of life. For cervical cancers of stages IA, IB and IIA, surgery should generally be considered the first-line approach as it is associated with better long-term quality of life than radiotherapy. The earliest results described for radical surgery for cervical cancer were by Ernst Wertheim in 1906, and involved removing the cervix with a good safety margin that included the uterus superiorly, a cuff of vagina inferiorly and around the cervix, uterovesical fascia anteriorly, uterosacral ligaments posteriorly, and the lateral cervical ligaments and parametrial tissues laterally. Various radical procedures have been described with differing degrees of radicality. The balance is between the curative effect of surgery and adverse effects, such as bladder dysfunction [1].

For women who wish to preserve fertility and have stage IA2 or small (<2 cm) IB1 squamous cell cervical cancers, radical trachelectomy (Chapter 136) and laparoscopic lymphadenectomy (Chapter 135) may be an acceptable option.

Management

Both women in the case histories can undergo curative radical surgery. Various classifications for radicality of surgery for cervical cancer have been published. The 1974 classification in popular use (Table 134.1) relates only to open surgery, and since then advances have led to the procedures being undertaken laparoscopically or with robot assistance.

Table 134.1 Piver–Rutledge classification of hysterectomy for cervical cancer (1974).

Type	Description
1	Extrafascial hysterectomy: removal of all cervical tissue
2	Modified radical hysterectomy: removal of medial 50% of cardinal and uterosacral ligaments; uterine vessels divided medial to ureter
3	Equivalent to the classical Wertheim–Meigs operation: wide radical resection of the parametrium and paravaginal tissues; ureter dissected completely to bladder entry; uterosacral ligaments divided at their origin from the sacrum; cardinal ligaments divided at pelvic sidewall
4	Ureter separated from pubovesical ligament; superior vesical artery ligated and upper two-thirds of vagina excised
5	More radical procedure with possible bowel, bladder, or ureteric dissection

Source: Piver *et al.*, 1974 [2].

In Case history 1, a type 2 radical hysterectomy would suffice with curative intent. In Case history 2, a type 3 radical hysterectomy would be appropriate to get good surgical margins, which is generally accepted to be 5 mm for cervical cancer. The removal of ovaries is individualized after discussion with the woman, taking into consideration her wishes, loss of hormonal function, and the possible need for adjuvant treatment (chemotherapy and/or radiotherapy).

The application of the above system to laparoscopic or vaginal approaches is inappropriate. A new classification has been developed that is anatomically based and is applicable to all surgical approaches (Table 134.2) [3]. The curative effect of surgery correlates with the anatomic extent of resection and there is a balance between benefit and risk associated with the degree of radicality. Some of the adverse effects, such as bladder dysfunction, are correlated with the anatomic extent of resection and nerve preservation.

Classifications regarding radicality are not descriptions of technique but do encompass the basis upon which curative surgery is undertaken. The lymph node dissection is classified separately from the primary tumor surgery. The extent of vaginal surgery is a modifiable component of this classification in cases of vaginal extension of disease (as in Case history 2) or in those with other associated pathology (e.g., vaginal intraepithelial neoplasia).

The extent of lymph node dissection corresponds anatomically to the arteries in the region, which are the most stable landmarks in this area. The removal of lymph nodes is not curative and extent is dependent on tumor characteristics. Sentinel lymph node dissection is an option in cervical cancer and may limit the extent of surgery and adverse effects. In those with enlarged

Gynecologic and Obstetric Surgery: Challenges and Management Options, First Edition. Edited by Arri Coomarasamy, Mahmood I. Shafi, G. Willy Davila and Kiong K. Chan.
© 2016 John Wiley & Sons, Ltd. Published 2016 by John Wiley & Sons, Ltd.

Table 134.2 Querleu–Morrow classification of radical hysterectomy (2008). This classification can be applied to fertility-sparing surgery and can be adapted to open, vaginal, laparoscopic, or robotic surgery.

Type	Description
Type A	*Minimum resection of paracervix*: this is an extrafascial hysterectomy. The paracervix is transected medial to the ureter but lateral to the cervix. The uterosacral and vesicouterine ligaments are not transected at a distance from the uterus. Vaginal resection is generally at a minimum, routinely less than 10 mm, without removal of the vaginal part of the paracervix (paracolpos)
Type B	*Transection of the paracervix at the ureter*: partial resection of the uterosacral and vesicouterine ligaments, ureter is unroofed and rolled laterally, permitting transection of the paracervix at the level of the ureteral tunnel. At least 10 mm of the vagina from the cervix or tumor is resected
Type C	*Transection of paracervix at junction with internal iliac vasculature system*: transection of the uterosacral ligament at the rectum and vesicouterine ligament at the bladder. The ureter is mobilized completely. Between 15 and 20 mm of vagina from the tumor or cervix and the corresponding paracolpos is resected routinely, depending on vaginal and paracervical extent
Type D	*Laterally extended resection*: rare operations feature additional ultra-radical procedures. The most radical corresponds to the laterally extended endopelvic resection (LEER) procedure

Lymph node dissection

Level 1	External and internal iliac nodes
Level 2	Common iliac (including presacral) nodes
Level 3	Aortic inframesenteric nodes
Level 4	Aortic infrarenal nodes

Source: Querleu & Morrow, 2008 [3] with permission from Elsevier.

lymph nodes (>2 cm), these should be removed as a debulking type procedure. In both case histories described here, a level 2 systematic dissection would be adequate unless there was other information available on MRI or intraoperatively to suggest enlarged or suspicious lymph nodes.

Prevention

Cervical cancer is staged clinically and a decision is made with regard to treatment by surgery or chemoradiotherapy depending on stage and tumor size. Additional information can be ascertained using MRI, which is highly accurate in evaluating tumor volume, parametrial invasion, and the assessment of pelvic and abdominal lymphadenopathy. Using all this information, and after discussion within a multidisciplinary team, appropriate management can

be recommended. As a general principle, it is good to avoid multimodality treatment with surgery and chemoradiotherapy. If the likelihood is high that chemoradiotherapy will be needed, then surgery will increase morbidity while having no discernible effect on cure rates.

KEY POINTS

Challenge: Radicality of surgery for cervical cancer.

Background
- Radical surgery for cancer is a balance between the curative intent and adverse effects of surgery.
- The basic principle is to achieve tumor clearance with an adequate clear surgical margin of at least 5 mm.
- Surgery is generally considered the first-line approach for cervical cancers of stages IA, IB and IIA.

Management
- Classifications of radicality of surgery are not descriptions of the surgery, but allow broad classifications of the approaches. The commonly used Piver–Rutledge classification is suitable for open approaches. The newer Querleu–Morrow classification is anatomically based and suitable for all surgical approaches.
- Radical surgery is tailored according to disease status, intentions of surgery, and the wishes of the woman.
- Extrafascial hysterectomy (in which the ureters are not dissected out from their beds) may be appropriate for small cervical tumors (<2 cm in diameter).
- A modified radical hysterectomy (in which the lateral cervical and uterosacral ligaments are only partially excised) may be appropriate for many early cervical cancers.
- A classical radical hysterectomy (in which the lateral cervical ligaments are excised at the pelvic sidewall and the uterosacral ligaments from their origin at the sacrum) may be necessary with larger cancers.

Prevention
- Adequate clinical staging and additional information from MRI will inform the decision for treatment and the radicality of any surgery.

References

1 Ahmed A, Tan LT, Shafi MI. Cervical and vaginal cancer. In: Shafi MI, Earl H, Tan LT (eds) *Gynaecological Oncology*, pp. 147–161. Cambridge University Press, Cambridge, 2009.

2 Piver MS, Rutledge F, Smith JP. Five classes of extended hysterectomy for women with cervical cancer. *Obstet Gynecol* 1974;44:265–272.

3 Querleu D, Morrow CP. Classification of radical hysterectomy. *Lancet Oncol* 2008;9:297–303.

CHAPTER 135

Pelvic and Para-aortic Lymphadenectomy in Gynecologic Cancers

Kavita Singh and Rami Fares

City Hospital, Sandwell and West Birmingham Hospitals NHS Trust, Birmingham, UK

Case history: A 62-year-old woman was diagnosed to have uterine serous carcinoma on endometrial biopsy; MRI revealed deep myometrial invasion of endometrial tumor, and bilateral enlarged external iliac nodes. She underwent total hysterectomy, bilateral salpingo-oophorectomy, systematic pelvic lymphadenectomy, para-aortic node sampling, and omental biopsy. Histology revealed metastatic involvement of right external iliac node (stage IIIC1). She was referred for adjuvant chemotherapy and radiotherapy.

Background

Pelvic and para-aortic lymphadenectomy is a common surgical procedure in gynecologic oncology. It can have both diagnostic and therapeutic roles. It facilitates staging, provides information about prognosis, and influences the type of adjuvant treatment given to the patient.

Lymphadenectomy may be necessary to achieve optimal debulking in ovarian cancers, as well as staging of endometrial cancer. While lymphadenectomy is not part of the staging for cervical cancer, it can provide prognostic information.

Lymphadenectomy can be either selective or systematic. In selective lymphadenectomy, representative sampling of only a few lymph nodes is performed, whereas in systematic or complete lymphadenectomy all the lymph nodes in the affected field are removed. Systematic is preferred over selective lymphadenectomy as it increases the detection of metastases in lymph nodes, thus avoiding understaging of patients.

Surgical routes for lymphadenectomy

Pelvic and para-aortic lymphadenectomy can be performed via a laparotomy or laparoscopy. Laparotomy is usually through a vertical midline incision. Laparoscopy can be through either a transperitoneal or retroperitoneal approach. Benefits of laparoscopy include superior surgical magnification, lower morbidity, better recovery, shorter hospital stay, better esthetic outcome, and reduced incidence of wound infection and incisional hernia, especially in obese patients. Laparoscopy may also be associated with better sealing of lymphatic channels,

and thus a potentially lower risk of postoperative lymphatic complications such as lymphedema and lymphocyst formation. However, laparoscopy does have a steep learning curve and requires a coordinated team approach with adequate provision for laparoscopy equipment and instruments. Introduction of ultrasonic devices for dissection, coagulation and sealing has immensely influenced laparoscopic surgery.

Respiratory and cardiac compromise and inadequate access may limit the success of laparoscopic lymphadenectomy, and necessitate conversion to open surgery. Women who have had previous abdominal surgery and have intense scarring may not be suitable for a laparoscopic approach. Women with cervical and endometrial cancers are increasingly having their surgery and lymphadenectomy laparoscopically; however, lymphadenectomy in ovarian cancer is still performed mostly through a laparotomy to achieve a thorough cytoreduction.

Robotic surgery is also being used in gynecologic oncology, but its use is limited by high cost and lack of availability.

Surgical anatomy of pelvic lymph nodes

Anatomic boundaries for pelvic lymphadenectomy include common iliac bifurcation superiorly, deep circumflex vein inferiorly, genitofemoral nerve on the iliopsoas muscle laterally, and obliterated umbilical artery medially. There are four main groups of lymph nodes in the pelvis: external iliac, internal iliac, obturator, and presacral (Figure 135.1) [1].

Surgical anatomy of para-aortic lymph nodes

Para-aortic lymph nodes include pre-aortic, paracaval, left lateral para-aortic, and retro-aortic groups (Figure 135.2). Para-aortic lymphadenectomy can be classified anatomically into the following.

1 Inframesenteric (low para-aortic): dissection extends below the origin of the inferior mesenteric artery, which usually lies at the level of L3, about two finger breadths above the aortic bifurcation.

2 Infrarenal (high para-aortic): dissection extends superiorly to the crossing of the left renal vein over the aorta.

Gynecologic and Obstetric Surgery: Challenges and Management Options, First Edition. Edited by Arri Coomarasamy, Mahmood I. Shafi, G. Willy Davila and Kiong K. Chan.
© 2016 John Wiley & Sons, Ltd. Published 2016 by John Wiley & Sons, Ltd.

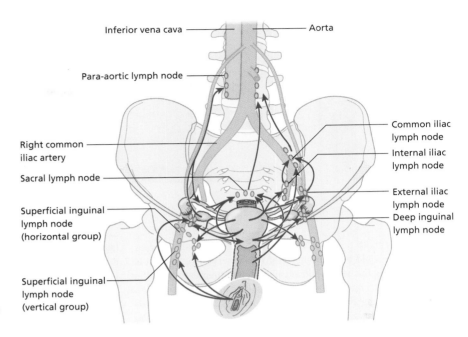

Figure 135.1 Lymphatic drainage of the female genitalia.

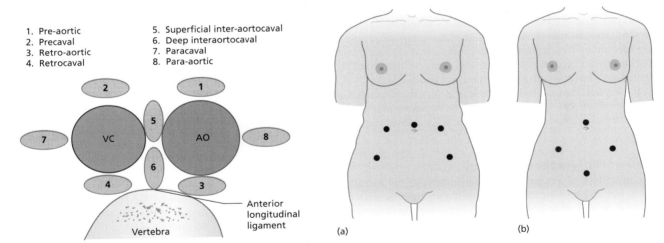

1. Pre-aortic
2. Precaval
3. Retro-aortic
4. Retrocaval
5. Superficial inter-aortocaval
6. Deep interaortocaval
7. Paracaval
8. Para-aortic

Figure 135.2 Para-aortic lymph node regions.

Figure 135.3 Ports distribution in (a) fan shape and (b) diamond shape.

Management

Pelvic lymphadenectomy

The patient is positioned in a dorsal lithotomy position with hands tucked to the sides of the pelvis. Laparoscopy is performed by open or closed technique; a 12-mm primary trocar is inserted at the umbilicus, and a 0° or 30° telescope is introduced, followed by side ports, which are inserted under vision. The ports are placed in a fan- or diamond-shaped distribution according to the patient's habitus and the surgeon's preference (Figure 135.3). For open surgical route a conventional extended vertical midline incision from the symphysis pubis up to midway between the umbilicus and xiphisternal junction is performed.

A thorough exploration of the abdomen and the retroperitoneum is carried out. The round ligament is identified, cut and secured, followed by opening of the broad ligament which is incised in a cephalad direction lateral and parallel to the infundibulopelvic ligament. The obliterated umbilical artery is identified and retracted medially to access the paravesical space, which is situated between the bladder medially and the lateral pelvic wall [2].

The subsequent step is gaining access to the obturator fossa, which is bounded by the external iliac vein superiorly, the internal iliac artery and the paravesical space medially, obturator nerve inferiorly, and the obturator internus muscle laterally (Figure 135.4). Lymphoareolar tissue is harvested along the dissection planes. Special care should be taken to avoid injury to the obturator vessels

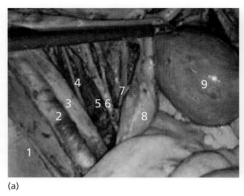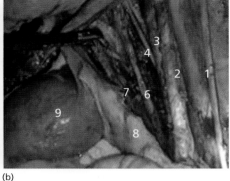

1 Ileo-psoas with overlying genitofemoral nerve
2 External iliac artery
3 External iliac vein
4 Obturator nerve
5 Obturator fossa
6 Internal iliac artery
7 Ureter
8 Adnexa
9 Uterus

(a)   (b)

Figure 135.4 (a) Left and (b) right pelvic sidewalls.

which are normally posterior to the nerve; however, an aberrant obturator vein could be found anterior to the nerve. The harvest is carried out along the nerves and vessels down to their entry into the obturator foramen and up to the common iliac bifurcation.

The fascia along the psoas muscle is incised laterally so as to avoid injury to the genitofemoral nerve, which is found over the muscle lateral to the external iliac vessels and sometimes overlying them. The lymph nodes are dissected from the lateral, front, and medial aspects of the iliac vessels down to the deep circumflex iliac vein, which is the inferior boundary of dissection. Then the vessels are retracted medially and the psoas laterally to remove the lateral lymph nodes. The lymph nodes medial to the internal iliac vessels are harvested, with attention paid to bleeding that can result from cutting uterine, vaginal, and superior vesical vessels. They should be ligated or coagulated with a bipolar or ultrasonic device.

If the lymphadenectomy is extended to include the common iliac nodes, then attention should be focused on the ureter which could be injured as it crosses the common iliac bifurcation at the pelvic brim.

Para-aortic lymphadenectomy

The procedure is commenced by mobilization of the ascending colon through opening of the peritoneum at the right paracolic gutter along the white line of Toldt up to the hepatic flexure, with attention to the ureter, right kidney and the duodenum that may need to be mobilized medially by incising the peritoneal attachment

lateral to the C-shaped curve of the duodenum (Kocherization of the duodenum). In addition, the peritoneum along the small intestinal mesentery needs to be incised from the ileocecal junction, passing through the sacral promontory up to the duodenojejunal junction. Sometimes the descending colon may need to be mobilized in a similar manner [3].

The right ureter is then lateralized and the paracaval lymph nodes medial to it and the lymph nodes along the right ovarian vessels are dissected, with special attention to the lumbar vessels that can cause troublesome bleeding. The inter-aortocaval lymph nodes are dissected.

Dissection of the left para-aortic lymph nodes is more challenging as the left ureter is closely related to the sigmoid mesocolon and the inferior mesenteric artery. The inferior mesenteric artery arises from the anterolateral aspect of the aorta at the level of L3, and can be easily injured. The lymphoareolar tissue along the left ovarian vessels should be traced and excised up to its insertion in the left renal vein.

Complications of lymphadenectomy

Lymphedema, lymphocyst, and chylous ascites are known to occur after extensive pelvic and para-aortic lymphadenectomy. Injury can occur to major vessels (including iliac vessels, inferior mesenteric vessels, aorta, and IVC), ureters, and nerves (obturator, genitofemoral, and sympathetic chain). Meticulous and systematic surgical approach is necessary to minimize the risk of complications.

KEY POINTS

Challenge: Pelvic and para-aortic lymphadenectomy in gynecologic cancers.

Background
- Lymphadenectomy has a diagnostic and a therapeutic role. It facilitates staging, gives information about prognosis, and determines the type of adjuvant treatment.
- Lymphadenectomy may be necessary to achieve optimal debulking in ovarian cancer.
- Lymphadenectomy can be either selective or systematic.
- Good understanding of surgical anatomy and adequate experience are crucial for successful lymphadenectomy.
- Para-aortic lymphadenectomy is not accepted as standard practice in the treatment of cervical and endometrial cancers.

Management
- Systematic complete lymphadenectomy is preferred over selective lymphadenectomy for accurate staging of cancer.

- Laparoscopy is a safe and effective technique for performing a thorough lymphadenectomy.
- Lymphadenectomy should be carried out in a systematic manner, paying particular attention to tissue planes, anatomic variations, and hemostasis.
- Pelvic lymphadenectomy can involve the removal of external iliac, internal iliac, obturator, and presacral nodes.
- Para-aortic lymphadenectomy can involve the removal of pre-aortic, precaval, para-aortic, paracaval, and retro-aortic nodes. It can be inframesenteric (low para-aortic) or infrarenal (high para-aortic).

Prevention
- Most of the lymphatic complications after surgery subside with conservative treatment.
- An open entry should be considered in patients with respiratory or cardiac conditions as these may limit the success of a laparoscopic approach.

References

1 Cibula D, Abu-Rustum NR. Pelvic lymphadenectomy in cervical cancer: surgical anatomy and proposal for a new classification system. *Gynecol Oncol* 2010;116:33–37.

2 Benedetti Panici P, Basile S, Angioli R. Pelvic and aortic lymphadenectomy in cervical cancer. The standardization of the surgical procedure and its clinical impact. *Gynecol Oncol* 2009;113:284–290.

3 Ercoli A, Fanfani F, D'Asta M *et al*. Role of different approaches to the abdominal retroperitoneum for lymphadenectomy in patients with gynaecologic cancers. *Eur J Surg Oncol* 2013;39:94–99.

CHAPTER 136
Trachelectomy for Treatment of Cervical Cancer

Kavita Singh and Janos Balega

City Hospital, Sandwell and West Birmingham Hospitals NHS Trust, Birmingham, UK

Case history: A 26-year-old nulliparous woman presented with severely dyskaryotic cervical cytology, and underwent a loop biopsy which diagnosed a superficial stage IB1 squamous cell carcinoma measuring 7 mm wide, 8 mm across, and 2.5 mm deep with associated CIN 3 reaching endocervical excision margins. On clinical examination she had a short infravaginal cervix. MRI of abdomen and pelvis excluded any obvious pelvic and para-aortic lymphadenopathy, and found no visible tumor.

Background

Surgical treatment of cervical cancer is advocated for early-stage disease (stages IA1, IA2 and IB1); type of surgery is tailored according to the tumor profile. Surgical options vary from simple cone biopsy, trachelectomy, simple hysterectomy to radical hysterectomy. Factors that influence the choice of surgical treatment include stage, histologic type, size of tumor, depth of tumor invasion, presence or absence of lymphovascular invasion, and future fertility desires of the patient.

Trachelectomy is a fertility-preserving operation aimed at preserving the uterus in a woman who wants a future pregnancy (Figure 136.1). There are different types of trachelectomy and different surgical approaches to the procedure. Trachelectomy could be simple or radical; simple trachelectomy involves supravaginal amputation of cervix, whereas radical trachelectomy involves removal of cervix with the parametrium and vaginal cuff.

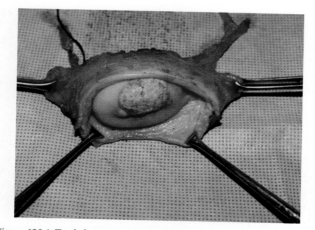

Figure 136.1 Trachelectomy specimen with cervical cancer.

In the UK, the peak incidence of cervical cancer is in women aged 35–39 years [1]. As there is a progressive increase in maternal age at first childbirth, it is not uncommon to find women with cervical cancer who have not yet started or completed their fertility goals. Daniel Dargent first published a series of radical vaginal trachelectomy (RVT) cases in 1994 [2,3]. This operation has subsequently been performed in other centers with similar survival outcomes to the traditional approach of radical Wertheim hysterectomy. The shortfalls of this operation are the need for stringent case selection, and the lack of long-term follow-up data on cancer recurrence, impact on fertility, and subsequent pregnancies.

Management

Patient selection

MRI is needed to ensure that there will be a sufficient length of residual cervix to allow adequate preservation of functional cervical length following surgical excision. The cervical tumor should be less than 2 cm in size. Adverse rare histologic types like neuroendocrine tumor or clear cell carcinoma of cervix are not suitable for trachelectomy. Adenocarcinoma is not regarded as a contraindication to trachelectomy. Pelvic lymphatic metastasis should have been excluded, usually by histologic assessment after lymphadenectomy.

In the case history, the patient is young and nulliparous with future fertility desires; as per FIGO classification, she has a stage IB1 cervical cancer but regarded as small volume superficial as it has less than 3 mm depth of invasion and tumor volume less than 500 mm³ ($8 \times 7 \times 2.5 = 140$ mm³). She is negative for lymphadenopathy on MRI. It would be reasonable to consider trachelectomy for this patient.

Surgical technique

Simple trachelectomy is performed through a vaginal approach. Radical trachelectomy has been performed most commonly via a vaginal approach, although abdominal and laparoscopic approaches are now being favored in view of the radicality of excision of parametrium. Laparoscopic radical trachelectomy is an accepted surgical route that is now being performed with robotics to improve precision and ease of dissection. Fertility outcome after abdominal and laparoscopic radical trachelectomy has not been published as

Gynecologic and Obstetric Surgery: Challenges and Management Options, First Edition. Edited by Arri Coomarasamy, Mahmood I. Shafi, G. Willy Davila and Kiong K. Chan.
© 2016 John Wiley & Sons, Ltd. Published 2016 by John Wiley & Sons, Ltd.

sufficient numbers of cases have not been performed worldwide via these routes.

Radical vaginal trachelectomy is performed in two steps. Firstly, a laparoscopic lymphadenectomy (Chapter 135) is carried out to assess the pelvic lymph nodes. Secondly, a radical resection of cervix along with a vaginal cuff and the paracervical tissue is performed. It is feasible to perform both procedures on the same day if there is a reliable frozen-section facility available; if not, laparoscopic lymphadenectomy can precede the radical trachelectomy by a few days.

For radical trachelectomy, the patient is placed in dorsal lithotomy position and the cervix is exposed. A circumferential incision is made on the upper vagina to create a 2-cm vaginal cuff, which is folded over the cervix and held with Chrobak clamps for downward traction. The vesicovaginal and paravesical spaces are dissected anteriorly and pouch of Douglas opened posteriorly. The ureter is palpated in the bladder pillar and is reflected upward and medially. The bladder pillars are divided inferiorly, further releasing the bladder and ureters superiorly. The lateral cardinal ligaments are identified, and with a right angle clamp a window is created just beneath the uterine vessels to identify the upper limit of the cardinal ligament and clamps are applied on the cardinal ligament, which is divided just below the ureter. The cervicovaginal vessels are ligated. The uterosacral ligaments and proximal parametrium are resected posteriorly. A size 6 Hegar dilator is placed within the cervical canal and cervix is horizontally excised below the isthmus. The trachelectomy specimen, where feasible, should be sent for frozen section to ensure the margins are tumor-free. Endocervical surgical margins and vaginal cuff should be tumor-free by 1 cm. Satisfactory hemostasis is achieved on the raw surface of the cervix with diathermy or interrupted Vicryl sutures. The vagina is sutured in a circular fashion around the cervix with interrupted sutures and a new vagino-isthmic junction is created.

Two additional procedures to consider are cervical cerclage to prevent cervical incompetence in the future, and placement of an intrauterine catheter for up to 3 weeks to prevent cervical stenosis. Both these procedures may interfere with function of the residual cervix. Cervical incompetence can be dealt with as an interval procedure or cerclage during pregnancy. Cervical stenosis can be treated by cervical dilatation if it develops. If cervical cerclage is carried out, Ethilon® suture or Mersilene® tape can be used with the knot tied and buried at the 6 o'clock position.

This operation originally described by the vaginal route can also be performed by abdominal [4] and laparoscopic [5] routes. The abdominal approach is suitable if the cervix is flushed with the vault or the vagina is constricted with narrow subpubic arch. The abdominal radical trachelectomy is the technique of choice in centers with limited experience in vaginal radical surgery, and in certain specific indications, such as pediatric patients, distorted vaginal anatomy, bulky exophytic tumor, or cervical cancer in the first half of pregnancy [6].

Outcomes

The important primary outcome measures of cancer treatment are survival, recurrence, and morbidity. Reported morbidities of RVT are bladder and ureteral injury, bladder dysfunction, hematoma, and vulval and upper thigh edema [7]. The average recurrence rate was 4.1% with a mortality rate of 2.5%. Common sites of recurrence are parametrium, para-aortic nodes, and pelvic sidewall. Central recurrences are attributable to either persistent disease in uterus or persistent high-risk HPV infection [8].

Risk factors for recurrence are high-grade tumor, close excision margins, deep stromal invasion, and presence of LVSI and lymph node metastasis. Additional treatment (e.g., completion of radical hysterectomy) is offered if margins of clearance are less than 1 cm, and chemoradiation is considered if more than one risk factor exists. Following trachelectomy all cases should be followed up at a cancer center. All patients are encouraged to avoid pregnancy for the first 6 months to ensure adequate healing and no persistence or recurrence of disease.

KEY POINTS

Challenge: Trachelectomy for treatment of cervical cancer.

Background
- Trachelectomy is an accepted surgical option for treatment of early-stage cervical cancer in women of childbearing age with future fertility wishes.
- Trachelectomy can be simple (removal of cervix) or radical (removal of cervix, parametrium and vaginal cuff).

Management
- Careful counseling is required for women with cervical cancer wishing to retain fertility.
- Trachelectomy is reserved for early-stage cervical cancer in the absence of adverse histologic markers like LVSI, deep stromal invasion, or histologic types such as neuroendocrine and clear cell carcinoma.
- Simple trachelectomy is a suitable option for cervical cancer with superficial invasion <3 mm and low volume <500 mm³.
- Radical trachelectomy is a recognized surgical treatment option for stage IB1 cervical cancer.
- Laparoscopic approach is now favored over the vaginal route for radical trachelectomy.
- Cervical cerclage can be performed at the time of trachelectomy, or as an interval procedure, or during pregnancy.
- Regular follow-up at a cancer center is recommended.

References

1 Bosch FX, Lorincz A, Muñoz N, Meijer CJ, Shah KV. The causal relation between human papillomavirus and cervical cancer. *J Clin Pathol* 2002;55:244–265.
2 Dargent D, Burn JL, Roy M, Remi I. Pregnancies following radical trachelectomy-for invasive cevical cancer. *Gynecol Oncol* 1994;52:105 (Abstract 14).
3 Dursun P, Leblanc E, Nogueira MC. Radical vaginal trachelectomy (Dargent's operation): a critical review of the literature. *Eur J Surg Oncol* 2007;33:933–941.
4 Cibula D, Ungar L, Svarovsky J, Zivny J, Freitag P. [Abdominal radical trachelectomy: technique and experience.] *Ceska Gynekol* 2005;70:117–122.
5 Cibula D, Ungar L, Palfalvi L, Bino B, Kuzel D. Laparoscopic abdominal radical trachelectomy. *Gynecol Oncol* 2005;97:707–709.
6 Cibula D, Slama J, Fischerova D. Update on abdominal radical trachelectomy. *Gynecol Oncol* 2008;111(2 Suppl):S111–S115.
7 Plante M, Renaud MC, Roy M. Radical vaginal trachelectomy: a fertility-preserving option for young women with early stage cervical cancer. *Gynecol Oncol* 2005;99(3 Suppl 1):S143–S146.
8 Morice P, Dargent D, Haie-Meder C, Duvillard P, Castaigne D. First case of a centropelvic recurrence after radical trachelectomy: literature review and implications for the preoperative selection of patients. *Gynecol Oncol* 2004;92:1002–1005.
Further reading

Further reading

Shepherd JH, Milliken DA. Conservative surgery for carcinoma of the cervix. *Clin Oncol (R Coll Radiol)* 2008;20:395–400.
Singh N, Titmuss E, Chin AJ *et al.* A review of post-trachelectomy isthmic and vaginal smear cytology. *Cytopathology* 2004;15:97–103.

CHAPTER 137

Laparoscopic Radical Surgery for Cervical Cancer

Mohamed Mehasseb

Glasgow Royal Infirmary, Glasgow, Scotland, UK

Case history 1: A 35-year-old woman with screen-detected stage IB1 cervical squamous cell carcinoma is undergoing laparoscopic radical hysterectomy and bilateral pelvic lymphadenectomy. The surgeon starts with the pelvic sidewall preparation, only to find the right obturator group of lymph nodes to be enlarged. The hysterectomy has not been done yet.

Case history 2: A 45-year-old woman presented with a clinical stage IB1 cervical adenocarcinoma. She has a BMI of 40 and had two cesarean section deliveries. Intraoperatively, the bladder is morbidly adherent to the uterus, and an inadvertent cystotomy occurs during a particularly difficult dissection.

Background

Since its initial description in 1990, the feasibility, safety, and oncologic efficacy of total laparoscopic radical hysterectomy for cervical cancer have been confirmed. Performed properly, this minimally invasive approach has minimal impact on the patient's quality of life, with reduced perioperative morbidity and faster recovery time.

Laparoscopic radical hysterectomy (LRH) is offered to women with early-stage cervical cancer. In general, LRH is contraindicated where the cervical tumor is larger than 4 cm, or where there is evidence of metastatic nodal involvement or peritoneal spread. The procedure should be performed by surgeons with specific training in advanced laparoscopic and oncologic surgery [1].

Although obesity is not an absolute contraindication, it may increase rates of complications and conversion to laparotomy. LRH in obese women is more difficult, lasts longer, and is associated with greater blood loss. Obese women present a particular anesthetic challenge, with difficult ventilation resulting from prolonged periods in the steep Trendelenburg position. Relative contraindications to LRH include the presence of multiple medical comorbidities and a history of multiple prior laparotomies [2].

Management

Preparation

Mechanical bowel preparation and the use of heparin can be considered on the day before the surgery. On the day of the surgery, the woman's legs are placed in the Lloyd-Davies position, with the arms tucked at the sides. A sandbag or gel bag may be placed under the buttocks to tilt the pelvis. This helps to keep the bowel out of the pelvis and reduces the degree of Trendelenburg tilt required. A 12-mm trocar is placed at the level of the umbilicus. Two additional 5-mm trocars are then placed in the right and left lower quadrants. An additional 12-mm trocar is inserted in the midline in the suprapubic area. Alternatively, two additional 5-mm trocars could be inserted higher up above the lower-quadrant trocars. The table is then placed in a steep Trendelenburg position.

Surgical technique

The pelvis and abdomen are thoroughly explored to rule out peritoneal disease. The retroperitoneal spaces on the pelvic sidewalls are then entered by division of the round ligaments. The ureters are identified and the iliac vessels are also exposed. The lymph-bearing tissue along the pelvis is then evaluated for obvious metastatic disease. The pararectal and paravesical spaces are developed, followed by identification and transection of the uterine vessels at their point of origin from the internal iliac vessels. The bladder is then mobilized from the anterior vagina, allowing for adequate resection of a 2-cm vaginal cuff. The parametrial tissue is dissected and brought over the ureters, which are dissected to the point of their insertion into the bladder bilaterally. The rectovaginal space is exposed and developed. The uterosacral ligaments are then transected. The cervix and uterus are now free of all their vascular and suspensory attachments and can be removed. The vaginal vault is sutured laparoscopically.

Management of lymph nodes

Metastatic disease in clinically positive or enlarged pelvic lymph nodes cannot be cured by surgery alone, and women with this condition will require postoperative radiation. If the diseased lymph nodes had been discovered preoperatively, such patients would not have been offered primary surgery. Although modern surgical and radiotherapy techniques have minimized risks, complications may be more common when both surgery and radiation are used, compared with a single modality of treatment.

The ideal management of enlarged suspicious lymph nodes found at the time of radical surgery is controversial. The first option available to the surgeon is to send the suspicious lymph nodes for frozen-section histologic assessment and abandon the procedure

Gynecologic and Obstetric Surgery: Challenges and Management Options, First Edition. Edited by Arri Coomarasamy, Mahmood I. Shafi, G. Willy Davila and Kiong K. Chan.
© 2016 John Wiley & Sons, Ltd. Published 2016 by John Wiley & Sons, Ltd.

should these prove positive for malignant metastases. However, the unavailability of the frozen-section technique, and its sensitivity and specificity for assessment of lymph node metastases do not make it a universal option.

The second alternative is to complete the pelvic lymphadenectomy and obtain a formal histologic assessment, planning the radical hysterectomy as a second-stage procedure if the lymph nodes are negative. This approach allows for ultra-sectioning of the lymph nodes, with higher sensitivity and specificity for detecting lymphatic metastases. Nevertheless, a second anesthesia and operative procedure are not without morbidity. Inevitably, some degree of scarring and adhesions will develop on the pelvic sidewall, making the second procedure challenging.

The last option is to fully complete the lymphadenectomy and radical hysterectomy, with adjuvant radiotherapy offered should the lymph nodes be positive on final histology examination. Some studies suggest an improved outcome when enlarged malignant pelvic nodes are removed, whenever possible.

There is disagreement among gynecologic oncologists regarding the order of procedures during radical surgery for cervical cancer. Some surgeons prefer performing the lymph node dissection first, allowing modification of the radicality of the lateral dissection or even aborting the procedure completely depending on the results of the lymphadenectomy. Other gynecologic oncologists prefer to perform the radical hysterectomy first, as it is the most difficult part of the operation, especially the dissection of the distal ureters.

Complications of laparoscopic radical hysterectomy

The intraoperative complications of LRH combine those associated with laparoscopic and radical gynecologic surgery (Table 137.1).

The commonest complication is postoperative bladder dysfunction, resulting from injury to the sensory and motor nerve supply to the detrusor muscle. Most women with bladder dysfunction quickly recover to near normal function; however, some occasionally need long periods of indwelling catheter bladder drainage, or intermittent self-catheterization. Limiting the extent and radicality of surgery, especially in women with early lesions, can minimize this morbidity. Identification and preservation of the hypogastric nerves also help to minimize bowel and bladder dysfunction. One of the advantages of laparoscopic surgery is that the hypogastric nerves are usually easy to identify.

Intraoperative bladder injury is more common with LRH compared with open surgery (6% vs. 2%), with higher rates of vesicovaginal fistula formation. However, both approaches carry the same risks of intra-operative ureteric or bowel injuries [3]. Faced with a viscus injury during laparoscopic surgery, the operator has the choice of repairing it laparoscopically or converting to an open procedure (Sections 2 and 4).

Patients may also experience neuropathy (genitofemoral or obturator) following extensive lymphadenectomy. Most neurologic injuries are transient and resolve with minimal intervention [4].

Prevention

The preoperative evaluation of women with cervical cancer should include confirmation of the histologic diagnosis and accurate staging. If there is evidence of lymphatic, systemic, or intraperitoneal spread, then the patient can be spared unnecessary surgery. Nevertheless, the FIGO staging for cervical cancer only includes the use of widely available imaging modalities, in addition to EUA. This clinical staging using only simple permitted radiologic assessment remains relatively inaccurate and variable. Assessment of tumor size, patency of the ureters, and lymphatic and parametrial involvement are all more accurately assessed by advanced radiologic techniques, with pelvic MRI gaining popularity and gradually replacing clinical staging in many centers. Positron emission tomography (PET-CT) remains the most accurate means of detecting malignant pelvic lymph nodes. However, PET-CT is not universally available.

KEY POINTS

Challenge: Laparoscopic radical hysterectomy.

Background
- LRH should be performed by surgeons with specific training in advanced laparoscopic and oncologic surgery.
- Obesity and previous abdominal or pelvic surgery may increase rates of complications and conversion to laparotomy.
- The intraoperative complications of LRH combine those associated with laparoscopic and radical gynecologic surgery.

Management
- The ideal management of enlarged suspicious lymph nodes found at the time of radical surgery is controversial. Intraoperative frozen-section histologic assessment, a two-stage procedure, or completion of the full primary procedure are all acceptable options.
- The ideal order of procedures during radical surgery for cervical cancer (hysterectomy or lymphadenectomy first) is debated.
- Faced with a viscus injury during laparoscopic surgery, the operator has the choice of repairing it laparoscopically, or converting to an open procedure.

Prevention
- The preoperative evaluation of women with cervical cancer should include confirmation of the histologic diagnosis and accurate staging using pelvic MRI and PET-CT. If there is evidence of lymphatic, systemic, or intraperitoneal spread, then the patient can be spared unnecessary surgery.
- Patients should be counseled appropriately regarding the risks of complications and conversion to laparotomy.

References

1 Canis M, Mage G, Wattiez A, Pouly JL, Manhes H, Bruhat MA. [Does endoscopic surgery have a role in radical surgery of cancer of the cervix uteri?] *J Gynecol Obstetrique Biol Reprod (Paris)* 1990;19:921.
2 Pomel C, Atallah D, Le Bouedec G *et al.* Laparoscopic radical hysterectomy for invasive cervical cancer: 8-year experience of a pilot study. *Gynecol Oncol* 2003;91:534–539.
3 Hwang JH. Urologic complication in laparoscopic radical hysterectomy: meta-analysis of 20 studies. *Eur J Cancer* 2012;48:3177–3185.
4 Xu H, Chen Y, Li Y, Zhang Q, Wang D, Liang Z. Complications of laparoscopic radical hysterectomy and lymphadenectomy for invasive cervical cancer: experience based on 317 procedures. *Surg Endosc* 2007;21:960–964.

Table 137.1 Complications of radical hysterectomy.

Severe bladder atony	4%
Vesicovaginal fistula	1%
Ureterovaginal fistula	2%
Thrombophlebitis	2%
Pulmonary embolus	1%
Bowel complications	1%
Lymphocyst requiring drainage	3%

CHAPTER 138
Groin and Retroperitoneal Lymphocele

David M. Luesley
City Hospital, Sandwell and West Birmingham Hospitals NHS Trust, Birmingham, UK

Case history: A 65-year-old woman with a triple incision radical vulvectomy and groin node dissection for a clitoral cancer developed a swelling in the left groin extending to the mons pubis, 4 weeks after the operation. Clinical examination confirmed a lymphocyst.

Background

A lymphocyst or lymphocele is an abnormal collection of lymph that usually occurs following a surgical intervention that either damages or transects regional lymphatics. The condition was first described by Mori [1] in 1955 as part of a large series of patients who had undergone radical hysterectomy. The term "lymphocyst" was replaced by "lymphocele" in the 1970s.

A lymphocele contains lymphatic fluid in a space that does not have a distinct epithelial lining. Classically, it follows procedures that result in excessive collection of lymph (lymphadenectomies). Lymphatics, unlike blood vessels, do not have the advantage of containing platelets or high concentrations of clotting factors; furthermore, lymphatic vessels lack smooth muscle in their walls, so once transected they continue to leak fluid.

Lymphoceles have been reported after many types of surgery and in most anatomic sites of high-density lymphatics. In gynecology, they are most associated with inguinofemoral, pelvic, and para-aortic lymphadenectomies.

Management

Inguinofemoral lymphocele occurs after dissection of the inguinofemoral lymph nodes, which is mostly performed as part of the management of vulval cancer. Diabetes and the amount of lymphatic drainage on the last day of drainage are predictors for the occurrence of short-term complications. In turn, young age and the development of a lymphocele are the main predictors of long-term lymphedema.

Presentation and evaluation

Lymphoceles present as a fluctuant swelling in the groin (Figure 138.1) and can be quite large. They typically present within 4 weeks of surgery, and most are asymptomatic. It seems logical to assume that as soon as natural drainage, or leakage, is interrupted by either healing of the skin or removal of suction drains, the lymphatic fluid will continue to accumulate, expanding the artificial space created by the surgery.

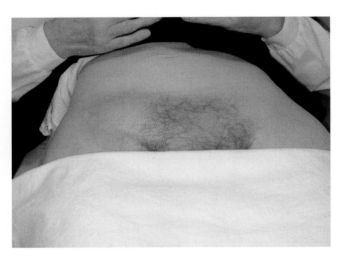

Figure 138.1 Right-sided lymphocele 6 months after surgery.

If symptoms are present, they reflect the discomfort of a swelling or occasionally pain and tenderness. From the patient's perspective, they raise the possibility of recurrent disease. While this is possible, a lymphocele is usually clinically quite distinct, being soft and fluctuant, and occasionally they transilluminate. It is also very unusual to see cancer recurrence in the groin so soon after surgery. If the groin swelling is tender, erythematous, and warm to the touch, then infection and associated cellulitis need to be considered. If there is any doubt about the diagnosis, ultrasound examination is usually diagnostic and will confirm the presence of a simple unilocular structure in the groin. Occasionally internal septations may be identified [2]. Ultrasonography is probably essential if percutaneous drainage is to be considered.

Management of groin lymphoceles

Once groin lymphoceles have formed, concerns arise about whether or not intervention is necessary. Some practitioners consider percutaneous drainage is justified regardless of symptoms, as there is a relationship between lymphocele formation and chronic lymphedema. The counter-argument is that while the relationship between the two is quite clear, it is possible that a lymphocele does not cause lymphedema, but they are both caused by the same process (lymphatic transection). Furthermore, percutaneous aspiration is an invasive procedure that breaches the integrity of a closed and sterile space and thus risks introducing infection. As yet, there are no data indicating that drainage offers any advantage over observation, and as drainage has a potential risk, drainage should only be employed when there is evidence of established infection or the patient is severely symptomatic. In this situation, it should be managed in a similar fashion to an abscess. Sclerosing agents have also been used on an ad hoc basis; bleomycin and doxycycline have both been reported as useful sclerosants in this situation [3,4].

Some centers have used a technique of opening the lymphocele and applying a vacuum-assisted closure (VAC) technique, and this can yield a slow but clinically excellent outcome, but data are limited at present.

Management of retroperitoneal lymphoceles

Retroperitoneal lymphoceles are usually the result of either pelvic lymphadenectomy or para-aortic lymphadenectomy, performed as part of a radical surgical approach to cervical, endometrial, and ovarian cancer. One prospective observational study using three-dimensional ultrasound scans at 2 and 6 weeks and 3, 6, 9 and 12 months after pelvic lymphadenectomy confirmed lymphoceles in 44% of patients, with 80% of them being diagnosed within 2 weeks of surgery. Four lymphoceles were detected by physical examination before the ultrasound diagnosis [2]. The occurrence of lymphoceles was unrelated to the diagnosis, surgery performed, operating surgeon, blood loss, or the number of lymph nodes removed. Importantly, there was no relationship with concurrent symptoms, including pain over the abdomen, pelvis, thigh, legs or back, lymphedema, fever, or symptoms of cystitis. In this well-documented series of 108 patients, only one required intervention because of infection.

Although symptoms appear to be uncommon, much effort has been directed at treatment. Some of this enthusiasm undoubtedly results from lymphocele management in other scenarios (particularly renal transplant patients). However, extrapolation of the problems of lymphocele from other scenarios might not be appropriate. Percutaneous drainage, laparotomy and fenestration, and more recently laparoscopic fenestration, have all been used with variable to good outcomes. Most recently a laparoscopic approach has been recommended, but these data are uncontrolled and insufficient to guide practice [5].

Prevention

There have been several approaches to attempt to prevent lymphocele formation in the groin and retroperitoneally; these have included measures to minimize lymph leakage by sparing the saphenous vein, transposing sartorius, and lymphatic ligation. Selective lymphadenectomy or sentinel lymph node biopsy is associated with a lower risk of lymphocele formation but is not suitable for more advanced or multifocal cancers [6]. Prolonged suction drainage remains the most frequent strategy used to minimize the risk of lymphocele and there are anecdotal reports of the use of collagen-based coagulation factors and fibrin glue.

None of the approaches has been associated with consistent success. Minimizing lymphatic damage can only go so far because the removal of lymph nodes must, by definition, transect major lymphatic trunks. Encouraging fibrosis in the wound is also logical, although it is only likely to be successful if fibrosis precedes

the accumulation of lymph. Prolonged suction drainage is also associated with its own problems. As patients begin to mobilize, it becomes increasingly difficult to maintain a closed drainage system and leakage around the drain is a common occurrence. Finally, prolonged drainage represents an infection risk, which probably poses a greater threat to the patient than lymphocele formation.

Attempts at prevention of retroperitoneal lymphoceles follow those employed in the groin. There is a published Cochrane Review [7] comparing drainage with no drainage for the prevention of lymphocyst formation, concluding that there did not appear to be any benefit associated with drainage. A pilot study using a collagen patch coated with human coagulation factors suggested a moderate reduction in lymphocyst formation [8].

KEY POINTS

Challenge: Groin and retroperitoneal lymphocele.

Background
- Inguinofemoral lymphoceles occur in 20–50% of cases after groin lymphadenectomy.

Management
- Percutaneous aspiration is discouraged because of the possibility of producing infection, except in severely symptomatic patients.
- Groin lymphocysts may be treated with sclerosing agents (e.g., bleomycin and doxycycline).
- Retroperitoneal lymphocysts can be treated with peritoneal fenestrations.

Prevention
- Groin lymphocysts may be prevented by the use of sentinel lymph node biopsies to allow selective lymphadenectomy. Other strategies, but with limited evidence, include:
  - Prolonged suction drainage of the surgical site.
  - Use of collagen-based coagulation factors and fibrin glue.

References

1 Mori N. Clinical and experimental studies on the so-called lymphocyst which develops after radical hysterectomy in cancer of the uterine cervix. *J Jpn Obstet Gynecol Soc* 1955;2:178–203.
2 Tam KF, Lam KW, Chan KK, Ngan HY. Natural history of pelvic lymphocysts as observed by ultrasonography after bilateral pelvic lymphadenectomy. *Ultrasound Obstet Gynecol* 2008;32:87–90.
3 Elsandabesee D, Sharma B, Preston J, Ostrowski J, Nieto J. Sclerotherapy with bleomycin for recurrent massive inguinal lymphoceles following partial vulvectomy and bilateral lymphadenectomy. Case report and literature review. *Gynecol Oncol* 2004;92:716–718.
4 Folk JJ, Musa AG. Management of persistent lymphocele by sclerotherapy with doxycycline. *Eur J Obstet Gynecol Reprod Biol* 1995;60:191–193.
5 Radosa MP, Diebolder H, Camara O, Mothes A, Anschuetz J, Runnebaum IB. Laparoscopic lymphocele fenestration in gynaecological cancer patients after retroperitoneal lymph node dissection as a first line treatment option. *BJOG* 2013;120:628–636.
6 Van der Zee AG, Oonk MH, De Hullu JA *et al.* Sentinel node dissection is safe in the treatment of early-stage vulvar cancer. *J Clin Oncol* 2008;26:884–889.
7 Charoenkwan K, Kietpeerakool C. Retroperitoneal drainage versus no drainage after pelvic lymphadenectomy for the prevention of lymphocyst formation in patients with gynaecological malignancies. *Cochrane Database Syst Rev* 2010;(1):CD007387.
8 Tinelli A, Giorda G, Manca C *et al.* Prevention of lymphocele in female pelvic lymphadenectomy by a collagen patch coated with the human coagulation factors: a pilot study. *J Surg Oncol* 2012;105:835–840.

CHAPTER 139

Laparotomy for a Pelvic Mass of Uncertain Nature

Mahmood I. Shafi

Addenbrooke's Hospital, Cambridge University Hospitals NHS Foundation Trust, Cambridge, UK

Case history 1: *A 32-year-old nulliparous woman has a lower abdominal/pelvic mass and a laparotomy is planned.*

Case history 2: *A 68-year-old woman with abdominal distension and a mass in the lower abdomen/pelvis is having a laparotomy planned.*

Background

Laparotomy is a common surgical procedure, usually undertaken when a diagnosis is strongly supported by the clinical scenario and findings on imaging. In some patients, the diagnosis can be unclear despite using all these modalities. In these women, laparotomy becomes the final arbiter in their diagnosis and management. The age of the patient and fertility intentions become important in planning surgery as there is always a desire to retain normal tissue, but without compromising outcome for the individual.

Management

Women requiring laparotomy will usually have a strong indication with a provisional diagnosis. The information from clinical history, examination, and investigations should be reviewed and a surgical approach agreed with the patient.

Age is an important predictor of likely findings at surgery. In the case histories, even if they have similar biochemical and imaging findings, the 32 year old is more likely to have benign pathology and the 68 year old is more likely to have a malignant process. A formal assessment of the risk of malignancy is important, and a key tool for this purpose is the risk of malignancy index (RMI) [1]. The formula for calculating the RMI score is given in Table 139.1, and a protocol for triaging women using RMI is given in Table 139.2. The RMI system is currently the most widely used model, but there is emerging evidence that the IOTA (International Ovarian Tumor Analysis) system based on specific ultrasound parameters offers increased accuracy [1].

Table 139.1 Calculation of RMI score.

Feature	RMI score
Ultrasound features:	0, none
Multilocular cyst	1, one abnormality
Solid areas	3, two or more abnormalities
Bilateral lesions	
Ascites	
Intra-abdominal metastases	
Premenopausal	1
Postmenopausal	3
CA125	units/mL

RMI score = ultrasound score × menopausal score × CA125 level (units/mL).

Table 139.2 An example of a protocol for triaging women using the RMI.

Risk grade	RMI	Women (%)	Risk of ovarian cancer (%)
Low	<25	40	<3
Moderate	25–250	30	20
High	>250	30	75

From this it is clear that in the two cases described, even if they have similar CA125 results and imaging, the RMI is significantly different based on the score for menopausal status. If there is concern about the mass, then additional tests for CEA, AFP, HCG, and LDH are important, especially in the case of the 32 year old who is at a higher risk of germ cell tumors.

Imaging using ultrasound, CT or MRI provides vital additional information. Ultrasound is good for initial assessment of a mass of unknown origin. CT is good at assessing abdomen and nodal status. If a differential diagnosis for a pelvic mass is needed, then MRI is usually superior in differentiating uterine pathology from ovarian pathology. Other investigations that may be needed include bowel studies (e.g., sigmoidoscopy or colonoscopy) and cystoscopy. In situations where there is uncertainty about the tissue origin of a complex pelvic mass, the use of different panels of immunohistochemistry markers on biopsy specimens or ascitic cytology can be informative. For example, a combination of cytokeratin, CA125, and CEA markers may help differentiate a gastrointestinal tumor from a female genital tract cancer.

With the use of these tests, it is unusual not to have a working diagnosis prior to the laparotomy. Multidisciplinary discussions can be helpful in deciding on further management options and appropriate documentation. However, the final arbiter is the operative assessment and the patient may need careful counseling (especially in younger women, for whom fertility issues are likely to be important). As a general rule, in these individuals it is appropriate to undertake fertility-conserving surgery with the attendant risk that if malignancy is confirmed, further surgery may be necessary. This is preferred to a radical surgical approach without fertility preservation when the diagnosis is uncertain.

Technique

Most laparotomies are conducted in the supine flat position. However, if there is any suggestion of possible bowel pathology, then access may be important and the legs should be positioned to allow movement and perineal access. A lower midline incision is usually preferred as it gives the advantage of being able to be extended if needed depending on the intraoperative findings. At surgery, once the peritoneal cavity is entered, ascites or peritoneal washings for cytology are taken before undertaking a formal assessment of the extent of disease. The pelvic and abdominal contents are then carefully examined and any abnormalities are noted, preferably on a proforma so that there is complete capture of data. Depending on the findings and discussions prior to surgery, appropriate excisions and biopsies are performed. In some situations, ready recourse to frozen sampling for histology can be important and the necessary arrangements should be made available and ideally histopathology departments prewarned of this possibility.

Prevention

Laparotomy for pelvic masses that are uncertain in nature should be rare given the range of investigations available. Despite these, it can be difficult in some cases to be sure of what the operative findings will be and what the definitive management should be. As a general principle, if fertility is an issue, then the most conservative surgery appropriate to the situation is undertaken, with the proviso that further surgery may be necessary. Frozen-section histologic assessment intraoperatively may prove helpful in selected cases.

KEY POINTS

Challenge: Laparotomy for a pelvic mass of uncertain nature.

Background
- Clinical situation, age, and other variables should be used to assess cases of pelvic mass.
- Use of RMI allows risk stratification for ovarian cancers. IOTA classification is also useful for assessing the risk of malignancy.
- In certain situations, despite appropriate diagnostic procedures, the precise nature of the condition is uncertain until the time of laparotomy.

Management
- Multidisciplinary working is important to guide management.
- Counseling and documentation of possible outcomes are important.
- A lower midline incision is usually the preferred approach.
- As soon as the peritoneal cavity is opened, ascites or peritoneal washings should be taken for cytologic examination.
- In those with fertility issues, conservative surgery is appropriate with the knowledge that further surgery may become necessary.
- Cystoscopy and sigmoidoscopy may be appropriate for some patients.
- A systematic assessment of the pelvis and abdomen should be carried out to allow planning of further management.

Prevention
- With appropriate diagnostics, laparotomy for a mass of uncertain nature should be a decreasing common scenario.
- Multidisciplinary discussions are helpful in garnering all opinions.

Reference

1 Royal College of Obstetricians and Gynaecologists. *Management of Suspected Ovarian Masses in Premenopausal Women*. RCOG Green-top Guideline No. 62, December 2011. Available at https://www.rcog.org.uk/en/guidelines-research-services/guidelines/gtg62/

Further reading

Mazhar SB, Shafi MI. Principles of surgical technique. *Obstet Gynaecol Reprod Med* 2012;22:215–222.

National Institute for Health and Care Excellence. *Ovarian cancer: the recognition and management of ovarian cancer*. NICE Clinical Guideline No. 122, April 2011. Available at https://www.nice.org.uk/guidance/cg122

Shafi MI, Earl H, Tan LT (eds) *Gynaecological Oncology*. Cambridge University Press, Cambridge, 2009.

CHAPTER 140

Gynecologic Cancer Extending to the Bowel

Kiong K. Chan

City Hospital, Sandwell and West Birmingham Hospitals NHS Trust, Birmingham, UK

Case history: A 42-year-old woman presented with abdominal distension and a mass arising from the pelvis. Clinical examination revealed ascites, an omental "cake," and a mass in the lower abdomen. CA125 was 780 kU/L, but CEA was normal. A CT scan of the abdomen and pelvis revealed the possibility of sigmoid colon involvement. The chest X-ray was clear. There was no family history of cancer.

Background

Advanced gynecologic cancers can involve adjacent organs, including the bladder and the bowel. Epithelial ovarian cancer is the first cancer in which surgical debulking of tumor has been shown to be of survival benefit. The greatest benefit is gained in those patients in whom it has been possible to remove all macroscopic disease, especially if this can be achieved before starting chemotherapy.

Management

Patient preparation

The patient was seen and examined by a gynecologic oncologist and then counseled jointly with a gynecologic oncology clinical nurse specialist. The patient's details, including her imaging, were presented and discussed at a gynecologic oncology multidisciplinary team meeting. The imaging suggested that it would be possible to obtain total macroscopic clearance of tumor, so it was agreed that the patient should be recommended a laparotomy with a view to primary debulking surgery if the operative findings showed that complete debulking was achievable. The patient was counseled regarding the possibility of bowel surgery, including the formation of a stoma. Written consent was obtained and arrangements were made for admission for surgery and for preoperative bowel preparation to be carried out at home. Admission on the day of surgery was arranged. Intravenous fluid infusion was instituted soon after admission in order to minimize dehydration brought on by a combination of starvation and bowel preparation.

Surgical technique

The patient was given a general anesthetic and an epidural. Her legs were placed in adjustable Lloyd-Davies supports. This allowed easy access to the anus which would be required for the use of an anastomosis gun. The vagina and perineum were prepared with aqueous povidone iodine and the whole of the abdomen prepared with alcoholic Hibitane up to and including the lower thorax.

A 10-cm midline incision was made below the umbilicus to allow an early assessment of the spread of the tumor. A 25-cm diameter left ovarian tumor was found attached to the sigmoid colon and the left pelvic sidewall. Particular attention was paid to the small bowel serosa and mesentery since extensive involvement of these would mean that complete macroscopic removal of tumor would not be achieved. These were not involved, so the diaphragm and liver were palpated to confirm that it was possible to perform total macroscopic clearance. The incision was then extended upwards and downwards. The ascites was removed by suction and a thorough assessment was carried out. The omentum was extensively involved, forming an omental "cake." This was mobilized from the transverse colon to allow a careful assessment of the lesser sac since metastatic disease here is often not resectable and would mean that total macroscopic clearance of tumor would not be feasible. No disease was found in the lesser sac. There was disease greater than 2 cm in diameter involving the omentum, the sigmoid colon, the pelvic peritoneum, the pouch of Douglas, the peritoneum overlying the bladder, the uterus, and the tubes and right ovary.

Following mobilization of the splenic flexure, a total omentectomy was performed (Chapter 141). The pelvic peritoneum was incised at the level of the pelvic brim and an extraperitoneal approach was used to identify the ovarian pedicles and the ureters. Both round ligaments were divided and ligated with 2-0 Vicryl sutures. Both ovarian pedicles were picked up with Babcock forceps. After the ureters were mobilized away, the pedicles were divided between slightly curved Zeppelin clamps. The proximal ends were doubly ligated first with a 2-0 Vicryl tie and then with a 2-0 Vicryl suture. The pelvic peritoneum was further dissected, which included lifting it off the dome of the bladder as the bladder wall itself was not involved. It was obvious that the involvement of the sigmoid colon and the pouch of Douglas would require an anterior resection of the upper rectum and a sigmoid colectomy. In essence what was required was a modified posterior exenteration. Consequently, the sigmoid colon and the descending colon were mobilized up to and including the splenic flexure. The sigmoid colon mesenteric vessels and the sigmoid mesentery were divided up to the sigmoid serosa. The sigmoid colon was divided with an 80-mm GIA stapling gun. The posterior part of the pelvic peritoneum was then mobilized to expose the superior rectal artery and vein. As the primary was ovarian rather than rectal, a "high tie" for the inferior mesenteric vessels was not necessary (although it is as well to remember that the nearer a vessel approaches the organ it supplies, the more likely it is to branch). The inferior mesenteric vein and artery were clamped and divided individually. They were doubly ligated with 2-0 Vicryl ties. The rectum was mobilized away from the sacrum, taking care to remain in the total mesorectal excision (TME) plane to avoid injuring any of the sacral vessels. The pelvic tumor was further mobilized by dividing the uterine vessels between slightly curved Zeppelin clamps and ligating them with 2-0 Vicryl sutures. Care was taken to "skeletonize" these vessels so that no pelvic peritoneum was included in the clamps, thereby performing an extraperitoneal hysterectomy. The cardinal ligaments were clamped with straight Zeppelin clamps, divided and ligated with 2-0 Vicryl sutures. The anterior vaginal wall was picked up and incised between two Littlewoods forceps. The vaginal angles were clamped with slightly curved Zeppelin clamps and transfixed with 2-0 Vicryl sutures. The posterior vaginal wall was incised and the rectovaginal space was dissected and the uterus left attached to the rectosigmoid. The rectum was mobilized using a combination of diathermy and Roberts artery forceps to clamp lateral vascular pedicles, containing branches of the middle rectal arteries. When the wall of the upper rectum was clearly defined by dissection, the rectum was divided just below the reflection of the peritoneum from the anterior rectal wall. This was achieved with a TA60 stapler. The rectum was cut free with a scalpel, allowing the whole specimen to be removed.

The vagina was closed with 2-0 Vicryl. A figure-of-eight suture was inserted medial to each of the vaginal angles to ligate the vaginal vessels. The rest of the vagina was closed with a continuous locking 2-0 Vicryl suture. The descending and transverse colon were mobilized to ensure that the proximal end of resected bowel would reach the rectal stump without tension. A curved Doyen soft bowel clamp was applied to the descending colon about 10 cm from its cut end. The stapled end was cut off just proximal to the staples. Adequate dilation of the distal end of descending colon was performed using sizers to prevent constriction at the anastomosis site. The proximal end of the colon was sutured with a continuous 2-0 Prolene suture on a round-bodied needle. Care was taken to see that it was running freely. The anvil of a CEEA31 anastomotic stapling gun was inserted into the colon and the suture tied firmly around its stem (Figure 140.1). The cut ends of the suture were left long (approximately 15 cm) and its free ends held by a pair of small Dunhill artery forceps. The legs were raised to allow access to the anus. A washout of the anal canal produced very little fecal material. The anal sphincter was stretched gently digitally. The CEEA31 stapling gun was inserted into the anal canal with the spike retracted (Figure 140.1). The gun was guided to the staple line. The spike was ejected out so that it perforated the staple line. It was removed with a pair of forceps and the stem of the anvil inserted in its place, care being taken to avoid any rotation of the bowel. The two parts of the bowel were approximated by winding the top part down until the marker was within the green zone of the gun. The safety catch was released and the gun was fired. This resulted in the Prolene suture being cut free. The gun was unwound for two full rotations to allow the anvil to tilt. It was then rotated 90° one way and then 90° the other way to ensure that it was no longer attached to any part of the bowel. The gun was then withdrawn and the "doughnuts" removed for inspection. They were seen to be intact. The pelvis was filled with water and care taken to ensure that no air was trapped. Air was insufflated into the rectum using a short disposable sigmoidoscope.

No air leakage was seen so the sigmoidoscope was withdrawn and the Doyen soft bowel clamp removed. The colon had been adequately mobilized and there was no tension on the anastomosis.

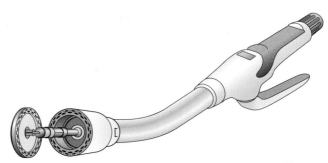

Figure 140.1 Circular stapling gun. Adapted from Covidien EEA™.

The rest of the abdomen was checked for metastases. A few small metastases were found on the peritoneum of the right paracolic gutter. These were excised with a small margin of normal peritoneum. No other metastases were found so excision of macroscopic tumor was complete. The pelvis was washed out with 2 L of water. A 12 FG Robinson drain was placed in the pelvis behind the bowel anastomosis. A thorough check was made to ensure good hemostasis. The abdomen was closed with continuous 1-Ethilon sutures starting at each end of the incision using a mass closure technique. The skin was closed with staples.

The patient's recovery was uneventful. Her Robinson drain was removed 4 days postoperatively. Her histology showed a serous carcinoma of the ovary so she was started on chemotherapy with a combination of carboplatin and paclitaxel in her fourth postoperative week.

Prevention

Gynecologic oncologists not proficient in bowel surgery must involve colorectal surgeons in these operations. Colorectal surgeons should certainly be involved in all complex cases such as those patients who have had radiation, previous bowel surgery, previous inflammatory bowel disease, and cases requiring multiple bowel anastomoses. If a colorectal on-table opinion is needed due to unexpected bowel involvement, it may become necessary to reposition the patient if initial laparotomy was conducted in a supine flat position. If at all possible, colorectal and stoma opinion should be obtained prior to planned involvement at surgery.

KEY POINTS

Challenge: Gynecologic cancer extending to the bowel.

Background
- Epithelial ovarian cancer is the first cancer in which surgical debulking of tumor has been shown to be of survival benefit.
- The greatest benefit is gained in those patients in whom it has been possible to remove all macroscopic disease, especially if this can be achieved before starting chemotherapy.

Management

- To remove all macroscopic disease, a surgeon must be prepared to remove bowel and other organs such as the spleen or parts of the diaphragm.
- Whenever possible bowel continuity should be restored, but this may not be possible either because of technical difficulties or due to the absence of someone with the necessary expertise. Under such circumstances, if the removal of a segment of large bowel will result in the complete clearance of macroscopic disease, then that resection should be carried out and a colostomy formed. If possible, bowel continuity can be restored when postoperative chemotherapy has been completed.
- It is important to ensure that chemotherapy is started (or restarted in those patients treated with neoadjuvant chemotherapy) as soon as the patient has made sufficient recovery from the surgery. However, there is a general agreement that a 3-week delay is required in those patients who have had bowel anastomoses.

Prevention

- It is important to involve colorectal surgeons if one is inexperienced in bowel surgery and in all complex cases with previous bowel pathology, irradiation or surgery, or requiring multiple anastomoses.

Further reading

Barlin JN, Jelinic P, Olvera N et al. Validated gene targets associated with curatively treated advanced serous ovarian carcinoma. *Gynecol Oncol* 2013;128:512–517.

Bristow RE, Tomacruz RS, Armstrong DK, Trimble EL, Montz FJ. Survival effect of maximal cytoreduction surgery for advanced ovarian carcinoma during the platinum era: a meta-analysis. *J Clin Oncol* 2002;20:1248–1259.

Chi DS, Musa F, Dao F et al. An analysis of patients with bulky advanced stage ovarian, tubal and peritoneal cancer treated with primary debulking surgery (PDS) during an identical time period as the randomised EORTC-NCIC trial of PDS vs neoadjuvant chemotherapy (NACT). *Gynecol Oncol* 2012;124:10–14.

Rose PG, Brady MF. EORTC 55971: Does it apply to all patients with advanced state ovarian cancer? *Gynecol Oncol* 2011;120:300–301.

Vergote I, Tropé CG, Amant F et al. Neoadjuvant chemotherapy or primary surgery in Stage IIIC or IV ovarian cancer. I Vergote et al. N Engl J Med 2010;363:943–953.

CHAPTER 141

Omental Procedures: Supracolic Omentectomy, Infracolic Omentectomy, Omental Biopsy

Kiong K. Chan

City Hospital, Sandwell and West Birmingham Hospitals NHS Trust, Birmingham, UK

Case history 1: *A 42-year-old woman presented with abdominal distension. CA125 was 458 kU/L. A CT scan revealed ascites, a 25-cm pelvic mass, and involvement of the omentum. The liver and chest were clear so the multidisciplinary team decided that primary debulking surgery should be carried out.*

Case history 2: *A 57-year-old woman was found to have an asymptomatic mass in the left upper quadrant of the abdomen on a CT scan performed for an unrelated reason. Two and a half years previously, she had surgery and adjuvant chemotherapy and radiotherapy for a leiomyosarcoma of the vagina. Imaging-guided needle biopsy suggested a gastrointestinal stromal tumor (GIST), so a laparotomy was carried out.*

Background

The omentum is a common site for metastases from a large variety of cancers. The commonest causes of omental metastases are ovarian cancer and primary peritoneal or tubal cancer, through transperitoneal or transcoelomic spread. Advanced endometrial and bowel cancers also spread to the omentum. Omentum can also be affected by distant cancers such as breast cancer.

Although the lesser omentum can be affected, it is usually the greater omentum that contains the metastases, which often coalesce to form an omental "cake." The term "omentectomy" is generally taken to imply removal of the greater omentum (Figure 141.1). Omentectomy is subdivided into infracolic, supracolic, and total. Infracolic omentectomy is the removal of the greater omentum below the transverse colon. Supracolic omentectomy includes the part of the greater omentum between the transverse colon and the greater curvature of the stomach. Total omentectomy includes removal of the omentum which extends to the hilum of the spleen in addition to the parts removed by supracolic omentectomy.

The prognosis of patients with advanced epithelial ovarian cancer is dependent on the completeness of surgical debulking. Although no randomized study has been undertaken to demonstrate the value of debulking surgery, there is no doubt that residual disease status is the single most important prognostic factor in advanced ovarian cancer. This is the reason why total omentectomy is important in the surgical management of advanced ovarian cancer.

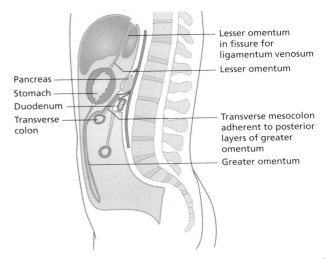

Figure 141.1 Sagittal section through the abdomen illustrating anatomy of omentum.

Management

Omentectomy is most often carried out in patients with epithelial ovarian cancers. A total omentectomy should be performed if there is obvious involvement of the omentum. Infracolic omentectomy should be confined to the removal of normal-looking omentum for staging purposes. Under such circumstances, a large omental biopsy would also suffice. There is no agreement among gynecologic oncologists regarding the size of an adequate biopsy [1]. Omentectomy is also required as part of the staging of uterine papillary serous carcinoma of the endometrium.

Resolution of the cases

In both patients a midline abdominal incision was made. A Gray retractor was used to hold the wound apart. In Case history 1, the ascitic fluid was sent for cytology. The liver and diaphragm

Gynecologic and Obstetric Surgery: Challenges and Management Options, First Edition. Edited by Arri Coomarasamy, Mahmood I. Shafi, G. Willy Davila and Kiong K. Chan.
© 2016 John Wiley & Sons, Ltd. Published 2016 by John Wiley & Sons, Ltd.

were normal. The gastrointestinal tract was normal. There was an omental "cake" measuring 23 × 5 × 2.5 cm. There were multiple metastases on the paracolic peritoneum. There was a 25-cm diameter right ovarian tumor with metastases on the left ovary, the uterine serosa, and the pelvic peritoneum including the pouch of Douglas and the uterovesical fold of peritoneum. The ovarian tumor and its metastases were removed in the manner described in Chapter 140. In Case history 2, the uterus, tubes and ovaries were absent because of her previous surgery. The liver and diaphragm were normal. The only abnormality was a tumor measuring 10 cm in diameter involving the left half of the greater omentum. There were no enlarged retroperitoneal lymph nodes. Omentectomy was carried out in both cases.

The anterior two leaves of the greater omentum were dissected off the transverse colon giving access to the lesser sac. No involvement of the stomach or pancreas was found. The splenic flexure of the transverse colon was mobilized to avoid traction on the spleen. The omentum was mobilized from the hepatic flexure. It was then excised from the greater curve of the stomach inside the gastro-epiploic arcade of vessels using a combination of diathermy and Autosuture clips for the small vessels running between the arcade and the greater curve of the stomach. The short gastric arteries at the cardia of the stomach were divided between Roberts forceps and ligated with 2-0 Vicryl mounted ties. The omentum was carefully mobilized from the splenic hilum to complete the total omentectomy. A careful check was made to ensure complete hemostasis. In this area, any bleeding is likely to continue and have serious consequences as tamponade does not occur. For the patient in Case history 2, histology showed the tumor to be a recurrence of the leiomyosarcoma (illustrating that the histology from a needle biopsy can be wrong); the patient was treated with further chemotherapy.

Omentectomy may result in a paralytic ileus, particularly if the operation is prolonged and there has been significant disturbance of the bowel (e.g., resection or extensive adhesiolysis). In such cases, it is wise to request the anesthetist to insert a nasogastric tube at the time of the operation. This can be guided to an optimal position by the surgeon and saves the patient an unpleasant experience of swallowing a nasogastric tube postoperatively. The ileus will resolve with time provided a careful watch is kept regarding fluid and electrolyte balance. Potassium supplements are important and must be given routinely unless a contraindication exists.

Although ileus is the more common complication, bowel obstruction can occur. This diagnosis must be considered if postoperative vomiting fails to settle.

KEY POINTS

Challenge: Omental procedures.

Background
- The omentum is a site for metastases of ovarian cancer, peritoneal or tubal cancer, advanced endometrial or bowel cancer, and uncommonly distant cancers such as breast cancer.
- Omentectomy can be infracolic, supracolic, or total.

Management
- A total omentectomy should be performed if there is obvious involvement of the omentum.
- Infracolic omentectomy should be confined to the removal of normal-looking omentum for staging purposes; a large omental biopsy can be an alternative approach.

- The omentum is intimately related to the transverse colon, the stomach and the spleen, all of which can be easily injured if care is not taken during the dissection. In particular, traction on the spleen can tear its capsule, resulting in an unnecessary splenectomy. This is why the splenic flexure of the transverse colon must be mobilized when performing a supracolic or total omentectomy.
- Meticulous hemostasis is important as any bleeding from the omental vessels may continue due to the absence of tamponade effect.
- Omentectomy may result in paralytic ileus particularly if the operation is prolonged or if there has been significant disturbance of the bowel; in such situations, a nasogastric tube can be inserted at the time of the operation.
- If the patient shows worsening gastrointestinal symptoms, bowel obstruction should be considered; if this does not settle with conservative management, it may require surgical correction.

Further reading

Gehrig PA, Van Le L, Fowler WC Jr. The role of omentectomy during the surgical staging of uterine serous carcinoma. *Int J Gynecol Cancer* 2003;13:212–215.

Hagiwara A, Sawai K, Sakakura C et al. Complete omentectomy and extensive lymphadenectomy with gastrectomy improves the survival of gastric cancer patients with metstases in the adjacent peritoneum. *Hepatogastroenterology* 1998;45:1922–1929.

Usubütün A, Ozseker HS, Himmetoglu C, Balci S, Ayhan A. Omentectomy for gynecologic cancer: how much sampling is adequate for microscopic examination? *Arch Pathol Lab Med* 2007;131:1578–1581.

CHAPTER 142
Diaphragmatic Surgery in Advanced Ovarian Cancer

Ariella Jakobson-Setton[1] and Kavita Singh[2]
[1] Sheba Medical Center and Tel Aviv University, Tel Hashomer, Israel
[2] City Hospital, Sandwell and West Birmingham Hospitals NHS Trust, Birmingham, UK

Case history: A 65-year-old woman presented with a history of abdominal discomfort and bloatedness. CA125 was 4521 kU/L. CT scan suggested advanced ovarian cancer. Laparoscopic biopsies were performed confirming high-grade serous ovarian cancer. Neoadjuvant chemotherapy (NACT) was commenced and a favorable response was noted after three cycles of NACT, so the patient underwent delayed debulking surgery that involved hysterectomy, bilateral salpingo-oophorectomy, total omentectomy, and right diaphragmatic stripping. Complete debulking was achieved, followed by administration of further chemotherapy.

Background

Ovarian carcinoma is usually diagnosed at an advanced stage. Cytoreductive surgery and platinum/taxane-based chemotherapy are considered the standard of care [1,2]. Cytoreduction can be complete (with no residual macroscopic disease), optimal (<1 cm diameter residual disease left), or suboptimal (>1 cm gross residual disease left). Complete resection of all macroscopic disease has been shown to be the single most important independent prognostic factor affecting outcome in advanced ovarian cancer (AOC) [1].

Diaphragm involvement is common with AOC, and the right hemidiaphragm is more commonly and extensively involved compared with the left hemidiaphragm; this may be due to the clockwise flow of intraperitoneal fluid, which is indirectly linked to peristalsis of the bowel and the diagonal attachment of the small bowel mesentery.

Diaphragm involvement can be superficial or infiltrative which can extend to the pleural surface. In infiltrative diaphragm lesions, full-thickness diaphragm resection is required, whereas superficial lesions require diaphragm stripping or excision of surface peritoneum. It is noted that 40% of patients with AOC have bulky disease on the diaphragm, and require liver mobilization, diaphragm peritonectomy and/or resection to achieve complete cytoreduction. Splenectomy and distal pancreatectomy may be required in some cases to complete cytoreduction of diaphragmatic disease [3]. Inability to achieve cytoreduction for diaphragmatic disease has been reported as the leading cause for suboptimal cytoreduction.

Hepatophrenic anatomy

The diaphragm is a dome-shaped musculofibrous septum that separates the thoracic from the abdominal cavity. It is attached to the spine, ribs and sternum and contains two parts: a peripheral muscular part and the central aponeurosis. The muscular part is separated into the sternal, costal, and lumbar parts. The sternal part is made up of two muscular slips from the back of the xiphoid process. The costal portion is attached to the inner surfaces of the cartilages and the lower ribs, and continuous with the transversus abdominis muscle. The lumbar portion, called the musculotendinous crura, comes from the lumbar vertebrae and attaches on both sides of the aorta. The diaphragm has openings for the esophagus, phrenic nerve, aorta, and inferior vena cava (IVC) (Figure 142.1).

The liver is attached to the diaphragm and the abdominal wall by ligaments and loose connective tissue (Figure 142.2). The falciform ligament attaches the liver to the abdominal wall anteriorly, and superiorly continues into the right and left coronary ligaments which connect the liver to the diaphragm, and posteriorly to form the right and left triangular ligaments. These fix the liver to the diaphragm and to the right renal Gerota's fascia. These ligaments need to be dissected in order to mobilize the liver and expose the diaphragm. The blood vessels in this area comprise the superior hepatic veins, which leave the liver cranially and empty into the IVC, and the inferior phrenic arteries that arise from the aorta or celiac trunk and divide into a medial and a lateral branch. One needs to be aware of the anatomic variations so as to avoid any surgical complications [4].

Management

Tumor volume and distribution in the diaphragm will dictate the type of surgical procedure required. It may be superficial and localized or widespread and infiltrative.

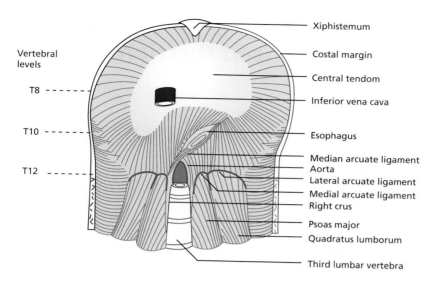

Figure 142.1 Anatomy of the diaphragm. *Source*: Faiz O, Blackburn S, Moffat D. *Anatomy at a Glance*, 3rd edn. Wiley-Blackwell, Oxford, 2011, http://www.ataglanceseries.com/anatomy/thorax-4-3-flashcards.asp, with permission from John Wiley & Sons, Ltd.

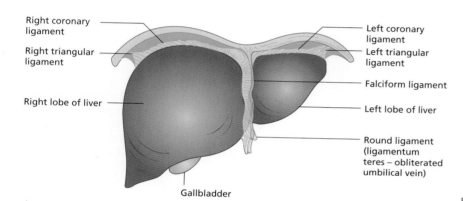

Figure 142.2 Ligaments of liver.

Types of diaphragm surgery in ovarian cancer cytoreductive surgery

Superficial coagulation of nodules

This is performed when there are only a few superficial nodules. Ablative techniques using any of the electrosurgical instruments, such as monopolar, bipolar, ultrasonic, argon beam coagulator, or laser systems, may be used. Usually only a partial liver mobilization is required for these procedures.

Diaphragmatic peritoneal stripping

This involves dissection and resection of the peritoneum from the diaphragm muscle, and is performed in cases of more extensive but superficial disease. Partial or full liver mobilization will be required according to the extent of disease.

Full-thickness diaphragm resection

The resection can include the muscle, or central tendon and the overlying peritoneum and pleura. This procedure is required when no dissection plane can be found, and for deep lesions that penetrate through the peritoneal layer into the muscle, the tendon or to the

pleural surface. The defects are then sutured using a monofilament suture like Prolene or PDS. This procedure has the potential risk of injuring the lung, vessels of the central tendon, and the phrenic nerves.

Surgical technique

The patient is positioned in dorsal lithotomy with a jelly bag underneath the chest to facilitate the exposure of the diaphragm. An extended midline incision is used, reaching the sternum on the right side, just above the xiphoid, which is sacrificed if necessary. Self-retaining retractors are used for retraction and elevation of the abdominal wall and costal margins upwards and laterally, thus ensuring an optimal view into the subphrenic space.

The falciform ligament is first divided from its peritoneal attachments and ligamentum teres is then divided in its membranous part. The anterior and posterior coronary ligaments are divided, followed by the triangular ligaments, leading to exposure of the bare area of the liver where the IVC and right hepatic vein are in proximity.

To undertake diaphragmatic stripping, an incision is made through the anterior peritoneum of the diaphragm, near the costal margin, and then a plane between the peritoneum and the muscular diaphragm is developed, while placing traction on the peritoneal edge. The peritoneum usually strips easily from the diaphragm except over the central tendon, where the attachment of the peritoneum to the central tendon is much stronger. The dissection will continue up to the coronary and right triangular ligaments, exposing the bare area, where extra care should be taken to avoid injury to the vessels.

Mobilization and rotation of the liver can cause a transient bradycardia and hypotension, and occasionally light bleeding from small branches of the inferior phrenic artery and vein, which will require coagulation. The retroperitoneal dissection on the left side is usually less extensive due to the lower frequency and volume of left-sided diaphragm involvement.

After completing the stripping procedure, the integrity of the diaphragm should be checked by covering the dissection area with saline; as the anesthetist inflates the lungs, with the patient in the Trendelenburg position, a check is made for any air bubbles in the fluid. If a hole in the diaphragm is identified, it is repaired with late absorbable or non-absorbable sutures, over a suction catheter inserted to the chest cavity, which will be pulled out with the tying of the last knot. The air leak test will be repeated.

Complications

Potential complications attributable to diaphragmatic surgery are rare (<5%) except for pleural effusion. An important intraoperative complication is injury of blood vessels, namely phrenic vessels, IVC, and (accessory) hepatic veins. The vessels are injured mainly due to liver mobilization, and can be treated by vascular sutures. Liver capsule laceration occurs during liver mobilization, and can be treated by pressure, suture, coagulation, or hemostatic patch.

Opening of the pericardium has been described rarely during left-sided diaphragmatic surgery, but can be sutured. Lung laceration can rarely occur in full-thickness diaphragmatic resection. The treatment would include placement of chest tube, hemostatic patch, sutures, or coagulation.

A number of late complications are associated with diaphragm surgery. Pleural effusions are common (37–59%) irrespective of the kind of surgical procedure performed. Larger diaphragm resections or complete liver mobilization are associated with higher risk of pleural effusion. This can be treated by thoracocentesis or insertion of chest tube. Pneumothorax can occur in 4–5% of patients, and can be treated by thoracic drainage. Hemothorax and subdiaphragm hematomas can also be treated by insertion of a chest drain.

Pleural empyema or other pulmonary infection (2%) and subdiaphragm abscesses will need appropriate management. Other late complications include hemidiaphragm paralysis (diaphragmatic elevation due to phrenic nerve injury), flattening of the diaphragm, incisional diaphragmatic hernia, and pulmonary embolism (5%).

Insertion of a chest drain is not mandatory but is at the discretion of the surgeon; it can be used as a prophylactic procedure intraoperatively, especially in patients with larger pleural openings or extensive resections.

Prevention

After extensive debulking surgery with diaphragm resection, patients are best managed in a high-dependency unit. Chest radiography should be performed postoperatively. If any significant pleural effusion or pneumothorax is detected, it is best managed with chest drainage. Active chest physiotherapy to prevent atelectasis and vigilance for consolidation and chest infection are advised.

KEY POINTS

Challenge: Diaphragmatic surgery in advanced ovarian cancer.

Background
- Diaphragmatic surgery is feasible and should be a part of the skill-set of any surgeon performing surgical cytoreduction for patients with advanced ovarian cancer.
- Maximal cytoreduction improves patient outcomes in ovarian cancer.

Management
- Diaphragmatic surgery requires detailed understanding of hepatophrenic anatomy.
- Diaphragmatic surgery involves techniques of liver mobilization and cytoreductive surgery, which can include:
  - Superficial coagulation of nodules: this is performed when there are only a few superficial nodules.
  - Diaphragmatic peritoneal stripping: this involves dissection and removal of the peritoneum from the diaphragm muscle, and is performed in cases of more extensive but superficial disease.
  - Full-thickness diaphragm resection: The resection can include the muscle, or central tendon and the overlying peritoneum and pleura. This procedure is required for deep lesions.
- Potential intraoperative complications include injury to blood vessels, liver capsule laceration, lung laceration, and opening of pericardium. The surgeon should have the ability to manage these complications.
- The procedure may be associated with postoperative morbidities such as pleural effusions and infection, which require careful vigilance and active postoperative management.

Prevention
- Patients are best managed in a high-dependency unit.
- Chest radiography should be performed postoperatively.
- Postoperative chest physiotherapy is advised.

References

1 Bristow RE, Tomacruz RS, Armstrong DK, Trimble EL, Montz FJ. Survival effect of maximal cytoreductive surgery for advanced ovarian carcinoma during the platinum era: a meta-analysis. *J Clin Oncol* 2002;20:1248–1259.

2 Chi DS, Eisenhauer EL, Lang J *et al.* What is the optimal goal of primary cytoreductive surgery for bulky stage IIIC epithelial ovarian carcinoma (EOC)? *Gynecol Oncol* 2006;103:559–564.

3 Kehoe SM, Eisenhauer EL, Chi DS. Upper abdominal surgical procedures: liver mobilization and diaphragm peritonectomy/resection, splenectomy, and distal pancreatectomy. *Gynecol Oncol* 2008;111:S51–S55.

4 Eisenhauer EL, Chi DS. Liver mobilization and diaphragm peritonectomy/resection. *Gynecol Oncol* 2007;104:25–28.

CHAPTER 143

Fine-needle Aspiration Biopsy of Superficial Groin Lymph Node

Moji Balogun

Birmingham Women's NHS Foundation Trust, Birmingham, UK

Case history: A 72-year-old patient presented with a vulval tumor and enlarged nodes in both inguinal regions on MRI scan. She was known to have diabetes, with bilateral leg ulcers. There was uncertainty about whether the adenopathy was a result of the leg ulcers or due to infiltration by the vulval tumor. This differentiation would have significant implications for her management and it was therefore decided to sample the groin nodes using the technique of ultrasound-guided fine-needle aspiration cytology (US-FNAC).

Background

Lymphatic spread is one of the three main ways of tumor dissemination; others are direct spread to local or adjacent structures and hematogenous spread. Nodal metastases are an adverse prognostic factor in many cancers and are a part of the FIGO staging criteria in a number of gynecologic cancers including endometrial and vulval cancers [1].

Superficial inguinal nodes drain lymph from the gluteal region and lower anterior abdominal wall, external genitalia, lower anal canal and perianal region, and from the uterine lymphatics via the round ligament [2]. This drainage area reflects the extent of probable primaries for lymph node involvement, hence the need for further evaluation for more accurate localization. In gynecology, vulval and endometrial cancers are particularly implicated.

Traditionally, lymph node evaluation has been based on size, as infiltrated nodes are often enlarged, but it is recognized that for many primary tumors, up to 20% of normal-sized local nodes contain small tumor deposits [3–5]. Conversely, more than one-third of enlarged nodes will be reactive, only showing inflammatory changes [4,6].

Identification of nodal metastases helps to plan definitive treatment. Clinical assessment of inguinal nodes by palpation is inadequate; in reviews of vulval cancer patients with clinically normal nodes nearly one-quarter have metastases, whereas in those with clinically involved nodes up to 40% are negative at histology [7,8].

Inguinal node dissection in vulval cancer patients is associated with both short- and long-term morbidity. There are reports that up to half of all patients who have undergone inguinofemoral

lymphadenectomy suffer postoperative debilitating complications such as wound infection, wound breakdown, and lymphedema [9].

A review has evaluated the accuracy of various diagnostic tests in the assessment of groin nodal status in squamous cell vulval cancer [10]. It suggested that non-invasive tests were less accurate than invasive tests in predicting groin node status. In practice, the choice of technique used in nodal assessment is usually based on local availability of the technique and expertise. The primary tumor also has a bearing on this selection.

High-resolution ultrasound may be used for inguinal node assessment in patients with vulval cancer or a peripheral melanoma. Cross-sectional imaging methods such as CT and MRI are also used to assess nodal status and for the diagnosis of metastases, based on criteria such as size and enhancement or signal characteristics. Ultrasound morphologic assessment with or without fine-needle aspiration and cytology has also been used to aid identification of involved nodes.

Functional imaging techniques such as 2-[^{18}F]fluoro-2-deoxy-d-glucose positron emission tomography (FDG-PET) can be used to detect metabolic changes in metastatic nodes, while sentinel lymph node (SLN) detection using blue dye and technetium-99m nanocolloid is also widely used (Chapter 145).

Management

US-FNAC is often performed as an outpatient procedure. An initial ultrasound scan of the groin is performed using a high-frequency linear transducer (7–14 MHz). The nodes are assessed using the recognized criteria of increased size (short axis diameter >15 mm), altered shape (round or irregular rather than ovoid), loss of the fatty hilum, and perinodal irregularity (Figure 143.1). The presence of necrosis or abnormal blood flow pattern is also suspicious.

Local anesthesia with 1% lidocaine to the skin and subcutaneous tissues is sometimes used; it is especially useful when more than one node is to be sampled. A 21 or 25 gauge needle is then introduced into the selected node(s) under ultrasound guidance. Two methods of specimen collection may be used.

Gynecologic and Obstetric Surgery: Challenges and Management Options, First Edition. Edited by Arri Coomarasamy, Mahmood I. Shafi, G. Willy Davila and Kiong K. Chan.
© 2016 John Wiley & Sons, Ltd. Published 2016 by John Wiley & Sons, Ltd.

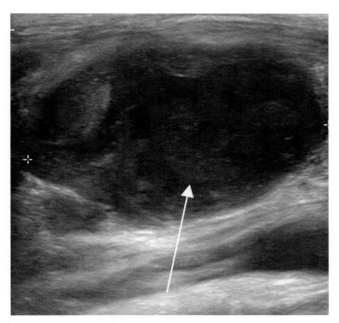

Figure 143.1 Enlarged node with an irregular outline, loss of the normal ovoid shape and fatty hilum. A heterogeneous echogenicity with irregular hypoechoic areas (arrow) suggests infiltration and necrosis.

- Non-aspiration capillary-action technique: the needle is vigorously manipulated in a to-and-fro motion through the lymph node until a small amount of cellular material is seen in the needle well.
- Suction aspiration technique: a 10-mL syringe is applied to the hub of the needle and a similar to-and-fro manipulation is performed with minimal suction (1–2 mL) to aspirate a cellular specimen.

The method used, either non-aspiration or suction aspiration, is operator-dependent [11]. An abnormal node with the needle in position within the node during a guided aspiration is shown in Figure 143.2.

After each biopsy pass, the needle is withdrawn and the sample smeared onto a glass slide and fixed in alcohol. Multiple passes may be made into the same node to increase the detection rate for a cellular specimen. The specimen is then analyzed by a cytopathologist. A cytology technician may be present at the time of the procedure to facilitate specimen preparation and initial assessment to ascertain adequacy.

Patients are warned about the possibility of bleeding from the site and discomfort, which may be alleviated by using standard pain relief. This is more likely to occur (though still uncommon) in patients who have had multiple passes.

KEY POINTS

Challenge: Ultrasound guided fine-needle aspiration.

Background
- Groin adenopathy is a common occurrence in inflammatory conditions of the lower limbs, perineal and perianal regions, as well as the vulval regions.
- Neoplastic conditions in this area can also give rise to adenopathy.

Management
- Various techniques of lymph node assessment have shown varying accuracy and user acceptability.
- The options for assessing lymph nodes include ultrasound, CT, MRI, FDG-PET, SLN biopsy, and US-FNAC.
- US-FNAC has the added advantage of assessing both morphology and enabling cytologic analysis.
- US-FNAC is often performed as an outpatient procedure with the following steps:
  - An ultrasound scan of the groin is performed and the nodes are assessed using recognized criteria.
  - Local anesthesia with 1% lidocaine to the skin and subcutaneous tissues is sometimes used; it is especially useful when more than one node is to be sampled.
  - A 21 or 25 gauge needle is then introduced into selected node(s) under ultrasound guidance, and specimens are collected via the non-aspiration capillary-action technique or the suction aspiration technique.
  - After each biopsy pass, the needle is withdrawn and the sample smeared onto a glass slide and fixed in alcohol, for analysis by a cytopathologist. Multiple passes may be made into the same node to increase the detection rate for a cellular specimen.
  - Patients (especially those who have had multiple passes) should be warned of a low risk of bleeding or discomfort, which may be alleviated by using standard pain relief.

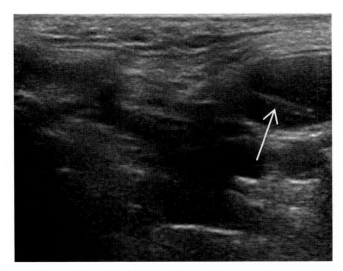

Figure 143.2 Hypoechoic node with a needle within the node at fine-needle aspiration (arrow).

References

1 Pecorelli S. Revised FIGO staging for carcinoma of the vulva, cervix, and endometrium. *Int J Gynaecol Obstet* 2009;105:103–104.
2 Warwick R, Williams PL (eds) The lymphatic drainage of the lower limbs. In: *Gray's Anatomy*, 36th edn, p. 791. Churchill Livingstone, London, 1980.
3 Gross BH, Glazer GM, Orringer MB, Spizarny DL, Flint A. Bronchogenic carcinoma metastatic to normal-sized lymph nodes: frequency and significance. *Radiology* 1988;166:71–74.
4 Kayser K, Bach S, Bülzebruck H, Vogt-Moykopf I, Probst G. Site, size and tumour involvement of resected extrapulmonary lymph nodes in lung cancer. *J Surg Oncol* 1990;43:45–49.
5 Staples CA, Müller NL, Miller RR, Evans KG, Nelems B. Mediastinal nodes in bronchogenic carcinoma: comparison between CT and mediastinoscopy. *Radiology* 1988;167:367–372.
6 McLoud TC, Bourgouin PM, Greenberg RW *et al.* Bronchogenic carcinoma: analysis of staging in the mediastinum with CT by correlative lymph node mapping and sampling. *Radiology* 1992;182:319–323.

7 Sedlis A, Homesley H, Bundy B. Positive groin lymph nodes in superficial squamous vulvar cancer. *Am J Obstet Gynecol* 1987;156:1159–1164.

8 Homesley H, Bundy B, Sedlis A. Prognostic factors for groin node metastasis in squamous cell carcinoma of the vulva. *Gynecol Oncol* 1993;49:279–283.

9 Gaarenstroom KN, Kenter CG, Trimbos JB *et al*. Post operative complications after vulvectomy and inguinofemoral lymphadenectomy using separate groin incisions. *Int J Gynecol Cancer* 2003;13:522–527.

10 Selman TJ, Luesley DM, Acheson N, Khan KS, Mann CH. A systematic review of the accuracy of diagnostic tests for inguinal lymph node status in vulvar cancer. *Gynecol Oncol* 2009;99:206–214.

11 Titton RL, Gervais DA, Boland GW, Maher MM, Mueller PR. Sonography and sonographically guided fine-needle aspiration biopsy of the thyroid gland: indications and techniques, pearls and pitfalls. *Am J Roentgenol* 2003;181:267–271.

CHAPTER 144
Vulval Surgery: Wide Local Excision and Vulvectomy

Mahmood I. Shafi
Addenbrooke's Hospital, Cambridge University Hospitals NHS Foundation Trust, Cambridge, UK

Case history 1: A 45-year-old woman has a 1.5 × 1 cm suspected vulval cancer on the left labium majus; there is no previous history of vulval problems.

Case history 2: A 78-year-old woman has a 5 × 3 cm fungating anterior vulval cancer which has been bleeding; she has a previous history of vulval lichen sclerosus.

Background

Vulval cancers are relatively rare. Predisposing factors include vulval intraepithelial neoplasia and lichen sclerosus. The majority of vulval tumors are squamous cell (~90%), with the remainder being adenocarcinoma, Bartholin's gland tumor, basal cell carcinoma, or melanoma. Most will present with symptoms and a visible lesion (~90%).

Staging of vulval cancers is surgicopathologic. Management consists of surgery for the primary tumor, and surgery for locoregional lymph nodes, with or without adjuvant treatment with radiotherapy and/or chemotherapy. Surgery has increasingly become more conservative given the psychosexual sequelae associated with surgery on the vulva. This has been achieved without compromising survival outcomes.

Management

Vulval cancer is managed within gynecologic cancer centers by multidisciplinary teams.

Assessment

Diagnosis and documentation of the lesion (site and size) are important, and ideally photographs should be taken. The relationship of the tumor to central structures (urethra, base of bladder, perineal body, and anus) should be noted. Palpation may give information about infiltration deep to the pubic or ischial bones. Groin nodes should be palpated and any enlarged ones noted. If necessary, examination can be undertaken under general anesthesia.

Radical treatment of vulval tumors should not be undertaken without biopsy confirmation of malignancy. This should be performed by including the transformation point between normal and malignant tissue. This should be adequate to give diagnosis, depth of invasion, and assessment of lymphovascular space invasion. A staging MRI is useful prior to planning surgery.

Surgical management

The surgical approach for vulval cancers has become individualized depending on tumor characteristics and comorbidities (the patients are often elderly). Vulvoscopy may aid in assessment of the area but is not necessary in all cases.

Surgery aims to remove the primary tumor with at least 1 cm resection margin (in the fixed specimen, equating to approximately 1.5 cm fresh tissue margin). For early-stage cancers (Case history 1) with depth of tumor less than 1 mm, groin dissection is not necessary as the risk of lymph node metastasis is negligible. If the tumor is more advanced, then either sentinel node biopsy (Chapter 145) or groin node dissection (Chapter 146) is required.

Resolution of the cases

Case history 1

A wide local excision of the tumor will likely suffice. At the time of operation, it is advised that the surgical margin is delineated with indelible marker pen using a ruler. This should be a 1.5-cm margin around any abnormal skin identified. Depth of excision is also important so as not to jeopardize deep excision margins. Diathermy, or clamp and tie techniques are utilized to remove the tumor. The surgical specimen can be pinned to a board with a marker suture so as to make orientation easier for the pathologist.

Case history 2

Careful assessment is necessary to decide on extent of surgery. This anterior tumor may involve or be close to the urethra or urethral opening. There may additionally be atypical skin surrounding the malignancy as there is a history of lichen sclerosus. If primary closure is likely to be an issue, then preoperative planning should be undertaken in conjunction with a plastic surgeon. Excising the large tumor with a 1.5-cm margin will result in a defect of 8 × 6 cm. Flaps or other reconstructive techniques may become necessary to achieve primary closure of the defect (Chapter 147). If the terminal urethra has to be sacrificed to obtain good surgical margins, then

---

Gynecologic and Obstetric Surgery: Challenges and Management Options, First Edition. Edited by Arri Coomarasamy, Mahmood I. Shafi, G. Willy Davila and Kiong K. Chan.

this should be undertaken. The female urethra is approximately 4 cm in length. Depending on the length of the remaining urethra, there may be postoperative urinary issues (e.g., incontinence). This is especially the case if less than 2 cm urethral length remains after surgery. Delineation of the planned excision and flap is vital in these procedures and again should be considered carefully given the anatomic site of the tumor and the patient characteristics and comorbidities, especially those that may impact on vascular supply to the surgical site. Drainage of the surgical site may be necessary and is decided upon intraoperatively.

Postoperative management

Postoperative nursing care is of vital importance. An air mattress can be useful and nursing in the supine position can minimize the risk of dependent edema. Keeping the area clean with irrigation and drying with cold air hairdryer may be necessary.

Despite these measures, many of the surgical wounds break down. If this happens, then an appropriate dressing should be applied. If possible, a VAC dressing (negative pressure wound therapy) may be beneficial as it speeds up the healing process and aids healing by secondary intention (Chapter 47).

Prevention

Management of vulval cancer is conducted by a multidisciplinary team. Appropriate assessment and investigations will indicate the optimal treatment pathway. Surgery is the primary treatment modality. Excision with an adequate margin is required but in some circumstances a palliative procedure may be appropriate. Surgery should be as conservative as possible while not compromising clinical outcome.

KEY POINTS

Challenge: Vulval surgery: wide local excision and vulvectomy.

Background
- Surgery is the primary modality of treatment for vulval cancer.
- Site and size of the lesion are important.
- Many women will have comorbidities that may impact on radicality of the surgery.
- Radical treatment should not be undertaken without prior confirmation of malignancy.

Management
- Multidisciplinary assessment and management should be undertaken in a gynecologic cancer center so that an individualized treatment plan can be made.
- Surgery should be to excise the tumor with an adequate margin of 1 cm in the fixed specimen (approximately 1.5 cm margin in the fresh specimen).
- The management of groin and pelvic lymph nodes is an important aspect of treatment of vulval cancer.
- Depending on the defect following excision of the tumor, reconstructive surgery may involve the need for flaps or other plastic surgical approaches.

Prevention
- With careful planning, good outcomes can be achieved.
- Psychosexual support is important as the surgery can be disfiguring in nature.

Further reading

Royal College of Obstetricians and Gynaecologists. *Management of Vulval Cancer.* RCOG Press, London, 2006. Available at https://www.rcog.org.uk/globalassets/ documents/guidelines/wprvulvalcancerfull2006.pdf

Shafi MI, Earl H, Tan LT (eds) *Gynaecological Oncology.* Cambridge University Press, Cambridge, 2009.

CHAPTER 145

Sentinel Node Biopsy in Gynecologic Cancer

Kavita Singh
City Hospital, Sandwell and West Birmingham Hospitals NHS Trust, Birmingham, UK

Case history: *A 65-year-old woman presented with a 2 × 2 cm indurated ulcer on the left labium majus, with no palpable inguinofemoral lymphadenopathy. Biopsy from the edge of the ulcer confirmed a moderately differentiated squamous cell carcinoma with 5 mm depth of invasion. She underwent a wide local excision and sentinel node biopsy. Histology confirmed completely excised vulval cancer with 1-cm margin of clearance and negative sentinel node from the left groin. She made an uncomplicated postoperative recovery and is on regular follow-up.*

Background

The sentinel lymph node (SLN) is defined as any lymph node that receives a direct drainage from the tumor site and is the first node to be involved with metastasis, and is therefore regarded as the "gatekeeper of the nodal basin" (Figure 145.1). SLNs are identified by a procedure called lymphatic mapping. We use both the radioactive tracer (immunoscintigraphy) and blue dye test for detecting the sentinel node so as to improve the detection rate and reduce false-negative rates. SLN detection has become an accepted clinical practice in the management of breast cancer and melanoma in the UK since 2004. In the case of gynecologic cancers, the greatest progress has been made in patients with vulval cancer [1].

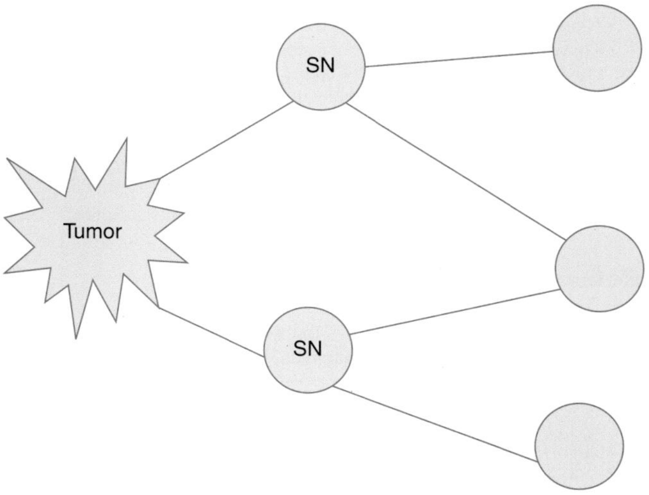

Figure 145.1 Sentinel lymph nodes (SN): "gatekeepers of the nodal basin."

SLN biopsy (SLNB) identifies metastatic nodal spread accurately and offsets the need for a systematic lymphadenectomy. This reduces the morbidity of a systematic lymphadenectomy, such as lymphedema and wound breakdown, without compromising safety. Secondly, SLNB improves identification of metastatic nodal involvement in unusual locations such as the presacral area in cervical cancer, which can otherwise be missed. Thirdly, ultra-staging and frozen sections used for analyzing the SLN improve the detection rate of metastasis and ability to detect macrometastasis, micrometastasis, and isolated tumor cells (ITCs) in the harvested node. Ultra-staging is an exhaustive procedure; it is thus not practical for systematic lymphadenectomy but feasible for one or two nodes harvested as sentinel nodes. Macrometastases are defined as tumor deposits larger than 2.0 mm; micrometastases are defined as deposits between 0.2 and 2.0 mm; and ITCs are defined as deposits no larger than 0.2 mm, including the presence of single non-cohesive cytokeratin-positive tumor cells.

Presence of micrometastases in SLN in patients with early-stage cervical cancer is associated with a significant reduction in overall survival, equivalent to patients with macrometastases. No prognostic significance has been found for ITCs. These data highlight the importance of SLNB and pathologic ultra-staging in the management of cervical cancer [2]. Sensitivity of SLNB is higher than current imaging technologies such as PET, CT or MRI.

Management

The management includes preoperative lymphoscintigraphy, which involves an injection of 1 mL of ^{99m}Tc (~0.4 mCi) sulfur colloid in four equal parts circumferentially in the four quadrants of the tumor, and CT lymphoscintigraphy is performed 2–4 hours prior to the surgery.

After induction of anesthesia, prepping and draping, a total of 4 mL of blue dye (isosulfan blue mixed 1:1 with normal saline) is injected in exactly the same manner as the radiocolloid. The diluted dye is used in an attempt to decrease the possibility of severe anaphylactic reactions, which increase in incidence when greater than 4 mL of undiluted dye is injected.

A gamma probe is used to localize the sentinel nodes. For vulval cancer a hand-held device is used and for cervical and endometrial

Gynecologic and Obstetric Surgery: Challenges and Management Options, First Edition. Edited by Arri Coomarasamy, Mahmood I. Shafi, G. Willy Davila and Kiong K. Chan.

cancers a laparoscopic gamma probe is used to allow for laparoscopic retrieval of SLNs. The gamma probe identifies hotspots, which are further confirmed by visual inspection for localization of the SLN with the aid of the blue dye test.

Gamma counts are recorded, including *in situ*, extracorporeal, and residual bed counts. A node is considered "hot" only if it contains at least 10 times the residual bed radioactivity. For an SLN to be considered completely removed, the residual count is required to be the same as background in the region. SLNs are labeled by location as well as radioactivity and dye status (i.e., blue only, blue and hot, hot only). All SLNs are harvested and submitted for frozen section or routine histology. When routine sectioning is found to be negative, then micro-staging is performed (including 100-μm slices and cytokeratin immunohistochemical staining) to detect micrometastasis.

SLN detection in vulval cancer

For vulval cancer, the most important prognostic factor is the presence or absence of metastasis in the inguinofemoral lymph nodes [3]. Levenback *et al.* [1] introduced the SLNB procedure for vulval cancer in 1994 and since then it has been validated in multiple studies [4]. With approximately 25–35% of patients initially presenting with occult lymph node metastases, SLNB spares patients an unnecessary inguinofemoral lymphadenectomy, and its associated morbidity, in 65–75% of patients. Almost 400 cases have been reported of SLNB followed by inguinofemoral lymphadenectomy in case series; in this combined experience, the sensitivity of the SLNB is 97.6% and the false-negative rate is 2.4% [5]. With 2-year follow-up on more than 200 patients, the groin relapse rate in patients with unifocal disease was 2.3%. These data suggest that when performed by a skilled multidisciplinary team, the groin relapse rate for SLNB only is similar to the groin relapse rate of inguinofemoral lymphadenectomy as currently performed.

Selection criteria for SLNB in vulval cancer include small-size vulval cancers (<4 cm), clinically negative groin nodes, no infiltration to adjacent organs, and unifocal cancer.

The safety of SLN detection is questionable in the following situations: central tumors and unilateral SLN identified, scar tissue of previous vulval surgery, Bartholin's gland cancer, and detection of SLN in patients with increased BMI.

SLN detection in cervical cancer

In early-stage cervical cancer SLN detection is feasible and aims to reduce morbidity of systematic pelvic lymphadenectomy. As the tumor is visible on the cervix it is easy to inject both the radiocolloid and the blue dye. It is feasible to retrieve the lymph nodes laparoscopically. Role of SLNB is limited to early stages of cervical cancer (IA2 and IIB1). In cervical cancer, sentinel nodes should be harvested from each hemipelvis. If a unilateral sentinel node is identified, complete lymphadenectomy should be performed, and all bulky nodes should be removed.

Advantages of SLN detection in cervical cancer

SLNB improves detection rate of nodes in unusual areas such as presacral, common iliac, and para-aortic regions in 10% of cases, which would otherwise have not been explored with routine pelvic lymphadenectomy in a conventional approach. SLNB may allow tailoring of surgery in small-volume cervical cancer; if SLN is negative for metastatic disease, then it may be safe to favor a simple hysterectomy rather than radical hysterectomy in cervical cancer of more than 2 cm size. If SLN is positive on frozen section, then radical hysterectomy can be abandoned as these patients are treated better

with chemoradiotherapy. This helps to reduce post-radical surgery radiotherapy complications. Finally, it may be possible to extend radical surgery for cervical cancer cases with early parametrial infiltration in the absence of metastatic SLN involvement.

Difficulties with SLN detection in cervical cancer

The cervix has a circumferential lymphatic drainage, and so more than one SLN may be identified. It is sometimes technically difficult to identify the parametrial nodes if the gamma probe cannot be angulated to receive adequate signals, and if there is interference with the signals in the parametrium due to the close proximity of the primary tumor bed. A multicenter (AGO Study Group) validation study of SLN detection in cervical cancer reported the safety of this procedure for cervical cancers of less than 2 cm, with a sensitivity of 91%, a negative predictive value of 99%, and a false-negative rate of 2% [6]. However, every institution needs to validate their SLN detection rate and adopt this practice with careful scrutiny of the technique and expertise.

SLN detection in endometrial cancer

The role of SLNB in endometrial cancer is less well established. Different techniques have been used for injection of the radiocolloid and the blue dye, but they have not been adequately validated. Different routes of injection have been used, such as cervical, fundal, and endometrial injection via hysteroscopy. However, early-stage endometrial cancer has a low incidence of lymphatic spread, and thus the utility of SLNB needs further evaluation in this population.

KEY POINTS

Challenge: Sentinel node biopsy in gynecologic cancer.

Background
- SLN is the "gatekeeper of the nodal basin" and the first node to be involved in metastasis.
- Achieving an acceptably low false-negative rate is crucial before SLN detection can be considered as an alternative to the current treatment standards.

Management
- Careful selection of patients for SLNB and technical expertise are vital.
- Sentinel node detection requires immunoscintigraphy and blue dye test for surgical localization of these nodes.
- Sentinel nodes for vulval cancer are removed from the groin, while for cervical and endometrial cancers SLN can be laparoscopically retrieved.
- There is a learning curve required for skill acquisition, with rigorous monitoring of surgical performance and outcomes; SLNB should be offered as a centralized service within a cancer center.

References

1 Levenback C, Burke TW, Gershenson DM, Morris M, Malpica A, Ross MI. Intra-operative lymphatic mapping for vulvar cancer. *Obstet Gynecol* 1994;84:163–167.

2 Cibula D, Abu-Rustum NR, Dusek L *et al.* Prognostic significance of low volume sentinel lymph node disease in early-stage cervical cancer. *Gynecol Oncol* 2012;124:496–501.

3 Burger MP, Hollema H, Emanuels AG, Krans M, Pras E, Bouma J. The importance of the groin node status for the survival of T1 and T2 vulval carcinoma patients. *Gynecol Oncol* 1995;57:327–334.

4 Hassanzade M, Attaran M, Treglia G, Yousefi Z, Sadeghi R. Lymphatic mapping and sentinel node biopsy in squamous cell carcinoma of the vulva: systematic review and meta-analysis of the literature. *Gynecol Oncol* 2013;130:237–245.

5 Van der Zee AG, Oonk MH, De Hullu JA *et al.* Sentinel node dissection is safe in the treatment of early-stage vulvar cancer. *J Clin Oncol* 2008;26:884–889.

6 Altgassen C, Hertel H, Brandstädt A, Köhler C, Dürst M, Schneider A. Multi-center validation study of the sentinel lymph node concept in cervical cancer: AGO Study Group. *J Clin Oncol* 2008;26:2943–2951.

CHAPTER 146
Groin Lymphadenectomy

Ketan Gajjar

Addenbrooke's Hospital, Cambridge University Hospitals NHS Foundation Trust, Cambridge, UK

Case history 1: A 43-year-old woman with a 2-cm vulval lump near the fourchette underwent excision biopsy, which showed a squamous cell carcinoma. Clinical examination and MRI did not show lymphadenopathy.

Case history 2: A 76-year-old woman with vulval itching and soreness was diagnosed with squamous cell carcinoma of vulva on wedge biopsy of a unifocal lesion. The depth of invasion was larger than 1 mm. On examination, a tumor of 2 × 2 cm was seen on the left labium minor. Clinical and MRI assessment of groin region did not show enlarged groin nodes.

Background

The inguinal and femoral nodes are the sites of regional spread from vulval cancer, and appropriate groin lymphadenectomy is the single most important factor in reducing mortality from this cancer. Overall risk of lymph node spread is dependent on the type, size, and location of the vulval tumor. Up to the 1990s, radical vulvectomy en bloc with bilateral inguinofemoral lymphadenectomy ("butterfly" resection) was the standard therapy for vulval cancer. However, severe morbidity and psychosexual impairment led to a change in surgical approach. Increasingly, the management of groin nodes in vulval cancer is carried out through separate incisions (triple incision technique). Groin lymphadenectomy is individualized to meet the patient's need. Lower limb lymphedema occurs in 85% of patients following inguinal lymphadenectomy. Increasingly, sentinel node biopsy is used in carefully selected patients to reduce unnecessary lymphadenectomy and associated surgical morbidity.

Management

FIGO stage IA squamous cell carcinoma does not require groin lymphadenectomy due to the low risk (<1%) of metastasis [1]. All patients with FIGO stage IB or stage II lesions or with a vulval lesion with more than 1 mm stromal invasion should undergo groin lymphadenectomy in addition to vulval surgery. Bilateral groin lymphadenectomy should be performed for midline and large lateral tumors. The incidence of positive contralateral groin nodes in patients with smaller-size lateral FIGO stage IB tumors is less than 1%, so unilateral groin lymphadenectomy is appropriate for such lesions [1].

Following correct initial surgery, groin recurrence is rare and should be managed on an individual basis. Operable groin recurrences that occur after prolonged remission can be considered for surgery followed by postoperative radiotherapy or chemoradiotherapy, rather than radiotherapy alone.

Verrucous carcinoma and basal cell carcinoma do not metastasize to lymph nodes. Adenoid cystic carcinoma of Bartholin's gland is a slow-growing tumor and also does not require lymphadenectomy. Inguinal lymphadenectomy has no place in the management of sarcoma or malignant melanoma of the vulva since it confers no survival benefit.

Assessment

Overall, 30% of patients with vulval cancer are diagnosed with metastatic disease to the inguinal or pelvic lymph nodes. Independent risk factors for inguinal lymph node metastases include clinical lymph node status, tumor grade, lymphovascular space invasion, depth of invasion, and age. Therefore, it is desirable to determine the status of the groin nodes prior to planning the overall treatment [2]. Clinical examination can identify grossly enlarged superficial groin nodes but remains an unreliable method, especially for deep-seated nodes or in obese patients. Such groin nodes should be assessed with a groin ultrasound scan or more commonly with MRI scan. MRI is of particular value in the case of ulcerated or fixed nodes for identifying deeper infiltration to muscle or femoral vessels. Groin ultrasound can be used for ultrasound-guided fine-needle aspiration cytology (FNAC). Other radiologic imaging modalities include CT, functional MRI, and PET-CT. These studies are helpful in detecting metastases in pelvic as well as inguinal lymph nodes. However, false-negative rates with current imaging methods are too high to reliably avoid groin lymphadenectomy or SLNB.

Planning of surgery

When treating vulval cancers, both superficial and deep nodes are to be removed, because selective superficial inguinal lymphadenectomy constitutes undertreatment with a risk of nodal recurrence in 5% of patients before central recurrence,

Gynecologic and Obstetric Surgery: Challenges and Management Options, First Edition. Edited by Arri Coomarasamy, Mahmood I. Shafi, G. Willy Davila and Kiong K. Chan.
© 2016 John Wiley & Sons, Ltd. Published 2016 by John Wiley & Sons, Ltd.

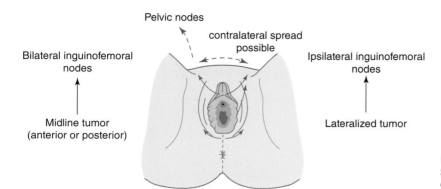

Figure 146.1 Lymphatic drainage of the vulva. *Source*: Shafi *et al.*, 2009 [3]. Reproduced with permission from Cambridge University Press.

and the mortality rate in these patients is high (92%). Groin lymphadenectomy should be performed through separate groin incisions as the incidence of skin bridge recurrence in early-stage cancers is low. The traditional butterfly incision extending into the groin region has limited indications in modern gynecologic oncology and should be reserved for tumors localized near skin bridges between the vulva and groins. In lateral tumors (>2 cm from midline), only an ipsilateral groin node dissection needs to be performed initially (Figure 146.1) [3]. Contralateral groin lymphadenectomy may be required if ipsilateral nodes are positive for metastasis [2]. In case of lateral lesions, most lymphatics flow through the superficial inguinal nodes, deep inguinal nodes, and the node of Cloquet to the pelvic lymph node chains. Deep inguinal nodes are positive approximately 3% of the time when superficial inguinal node findings are negative (Figure 146.2) [4].

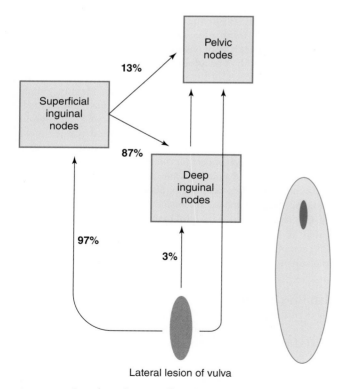

Figure 146.2 Lymphatic drainage of lateral lesions. Source: Iversen & Aas, 1983 [4]. Reproduced with permission from Cambridge University Press.

Surgical technique

For groin lymphadenectomy, an incision is made along a line drawn between the anterior superior iliac spine and the pubic tubercle, about 1 cm above and parallel to the groin crease. The incision is carried through the subcutaneous tissue to the superficial Camper's fascia, which is then incised. The subcutaneous tissue between this superficial fascia and skin should be preserved to avoid skin necrosis. The tissue below the superficial fascia down to fascia lata is removed, with the upper limit of dissection being 2 cm above the inguinal ligament to include all the inguinal nodes. The dissection is then carried on downward over the femoral triangle and around the femoral vessels. After splitting the fascia lata, the fatty tissue medial to the femoral vessels within the opening of the fossa ovalis is resected to perform femoral lymphadenectomy. The long saphenous vein can be preserved or tied off at the apex of femoral triangle. Preservation of the long saphenous vein may reduce both groin wound and subsequent lower limb problems [2]. The fascia lata lateral to the femoral vessels can be preserved. Cloquet's node should be checked for by retraction of the inguinal ligament, and removed if detected. At the conclusion adequate hemostasis should be confirmed and a suction drain is placed in the groin. The wound should be closed in two layers. Skin closure with an absorbable subcuticular suture followed by adhesive glue is a good technique.

Survival rates

The 5-year survival rates with lymph node metastasis are given in Table 146.1. The prognostic impact of the number of lymph nodes removed is unclear. Certain authors recommend at least six nodes per groin to assure complete dissection, but variations in anatomy and other factors make node counting an unreliable measure of surgical quality.

Table 146.1 Lymph node status and 5-year survival rates in vulval cancer.

Groin node status (all stages)	5-year survival rate (%)
Positive	52.4
Negative	91.3
Positive pelvic nodes	11

Source: Royal College of Obstetricians and Gynaecologists, 2006 [2].

Complications

The risk factors for the development of early and late complications include age, diabetes, en bloc surgery, and higher drain production on the last day the drain was *in situ* [5]. Complications of groin lymphadenectomy are summarized in Table 146.2.

Table 146.2 Morbidity from groin lymphadenectomy.

Short-term morbidities (up to 6 weeks after surgery)
Wound infection (Chapter 47) and breakdown
Wound necrosis and necrotizing fasciitis (Chapter 50)
Hemorrhage including femoral blowout
Femoral nerve injury leading to anesthesia of anterior thigh and paralysis of quadriceps femoris
Groin lymphocyst (collection of lymph in groin) (Chapter 138)
Pulmonary embolism/deep vein thrombosis
Pressure sores

Long-term morbidities
Chronic leg edema
Recurrent groin lymphocysts (Chapter 138)
Femoral hernia
Recurrent leg lymphangitis (Chapter 57)
Chronic and recurrent skin infections (Chapter 47)
Reduced mobility

Resolution of the cases

Case history 1

The patient underwent definitive treatment with wide local excision of the primary lesion site and bilateral groin lymphadenectomy. She was deemed not suitable for sentinel node detection as previous excision biopsy affects the reliability of the sentinel node detection with local injection of radioactive and patent blue dye. The patient suffered from recurrent lymphocyst requiring drainage. She required referral to lymphedema services for chronic leg lymphedema.

Case history 2

The patient received wide local excision for primary vulval tumor, which was approaching the midline. The groins were managed with a sentinel node detection approach using ^{99m}Tc radioactive sulfur colloid and patent blue dye. The sentinel nodes were detected bilaterally by radioactivity and blue dye, and removed. The histology of nodes was negative and excision margins of primary tumor were adequate. The patient had wound breakdown on the left groin wound which required VAC dressing (Chapter 47) and wound care over 4–6 weeks.

Prevention

Sentinel node detection and biopsy appear to be the way forward for reducing the need for full groin lymphadenectomy in selected cases (Chapter 145). The need for groin lymphadenectomy should be tailored to the individual patient after discussion within a multidisciplinary team and should take into consideration the

cancer type, the disease stage, long-term morbidity and its effect on the patient's quality of life, and the patient's wishes. Detecting vulval lesions at early stages may negate the need for groin lymphadenectomy and related debilitating sequelae. Efforts are ongoing to develop HPV vaccines that prevent premalignant and malignant lesions of the vulva. Further research is needed in the prevention and optimal management of lymphedema and lymphocyst.

KEY POINTS

Challenge: Groin lymphadenectomy.

Background
- The presence of metastasis in the inguinal lymph nodes is one of the most important prognostic factors in women with squamous cell cancer of the vulva.
- Recurrence in the groin carries a very high mortality risk; therefore appropriate groin treatment is the single most important factor in reducing mortality from early vulval cancer.
- Short-term complications of groin lymphadenectomy include wound infection and breakdown, wound necrosis and necrotizing fasciitis, hemorrhage, femoral nerve injury, groin lymphocyst, pulmonary embolism, and pressure sores.
- Long-term complications of groin lymphadenectomy include chronic leg edema, recurrent groin lymphocysts, femoral hernia, recurrent leg lymphangitis, chronic and recurrent skin infections, and reduced mobility.

Management
- In managing groin nodes for vulval cancer, MRI scan should be performed prior to surgery, and should include pelvic lymph nodes.
- In patients presenting with enlarged, fixed and/or ulcerated groin lymph nodes, biopsy or fine-needle aspiration should be considered prior to initial treatment with radiation or chemoradiation.
- The Bassett–Way operation, which emphasized en bloc resection of the vulva and both groins, has been replaced by radical wide excision and selective groin lymphadenectomy through separate groin incisions.
- Sentinel node biopsy is an option in patients with a squamous cell carcinoma of the vulva with >1 mm of invasion, a tumor <4 cm in diameter, and no obvious metastatic disease on physical examination or imaging studies (Chapter 145).

Prevention
- Detecting vulval cancers in early stages can reduce the need for lymphadenectomy and related sequelae.

References

1 Hacker NF, Eifel PJ, Van der Velden J. Cancer of the vulva. *Int J Gynaecol Obstet* 2012;119(Suppl 2):S90–S96.
2 Royal College of Obstetricians and Gynaecologists. *Management of Vulval Cancer.* RCOG Press, London, 2006. Available at https://www.rcog.org.uk/globalassets/documents/guidelines/wprvulvalcancerfull2006.pdf
3 Shafi MI, Earl HM, Tan LT (eds) *Gynaecological Oncology.* Cambridge University Press, Cambridge, 2009.
4 Iversen T, Aas M. Lymph drainage from the vulva. *Gynecol Oncol* 1983;16:179–189.
5 Hinten F, Van den Einden LCG, Hendriks JCM *et al.* Risk factors for short- and long-term complications after groin surgery in vulvar cancer. *Br J Cancer* 2011;105:1279–1287.

Plastic Surgical Techniques in Vulval or Perineal Procedures

Mahmood I. Shafi

Addenbrooke's Hospital, Cambridge University Hospitals NHS Foundation Trust, Cambridge, UK

Case history 1: A woman undergoes excision of a vulval tumor of 4 × 2 cm diameter with necessary surgical margins. There is difficulty in closing the defect without tension.

Case history 2: A perineal lesion with intraepithelial disease is excised, but the area proves difficult to close as a primary procedure.

Background

Following excision of vulval and perineal lesions, ideally primary closure of the defect is undertaken. In some patients, especially if a good surgical margin is required for cancer surgery (deemed to be 10–15 mm), then the defect becomes large and primary closure may not be possible. In such patients the surgical defect may be closed using plastic surgical techniques. This requires planning and adoption of certain principles [1,2].

Management

In those women with vulval and perineal lesions that are excised, especially with a good surgical margin, and in those with limited remnant skin, it becomes inappropriate to attempt primary closure under tension. These closures are at high risk of wound breakdown. If the surgical site cannot be primarily closed, then consideration of healing by secondary intention or with a flap is appropriate. Secondary intention healing is often prolonged and risks infection at the surgical site.

The use of skin flaps allows the surgical site (recipient skin) to be closed by transferring tissue from the donor site while maintaining its blood supply. These flaps vary in shape and form and range from simple advancement of skin to composites of different types of tissue (Box 147.1). The flap is transferred with its own blood supply intact. Flaps may be classified as random, where the blood supply is not derived from a recognized or named artery (many cutaneous skin flaps fall into this category) or axial, where the blood supply comes from a recognized (named) artery or group of arteries (most muscle flaps have an axial blood supply). Grafts, as opposed to flaps, are transferred without a blood supply from the source, and rely entirely on blood supply from the recipient site. Flaps can be moved in two directions, either advancement in a straight line or rotation into the recipient site. Some flaps can have elements of advancement and rotation [3].

> ## BOX 147.1 CLASSIFICATION OF FLAPS
>
> - Blood supply: random, where there is no named blood vessel; or axial, where there is a named blood vessel.
> - Tissue transferred: flaps may be composed of one type or several types of tissue (e.g., fasciocutaneous or musculocutaneous).
> - Location of donor site: flaps may be transferred from adjacent areas (local flap) or transferred from a non-contiguous site (distant flap). A distant flap may be pedicled or free, the latter requiring microsurgical anastomosis.

Within gynecology, the principle is to try to use the most similar tissue to that which has been excised. Rotational flaps afford good cosmetic results and can be undertaken by using basic surgical principles. This allows mobilization and rotation of large areas of tissue with a wide vascular base for reconstruction.

V-Y flap

Local pivotal flaps such as V-Y or rotational flaps are usually employed in the vulval and perineal areas. For smaller areas, a V-Y advancement flap (Figure 147.1) is simple and ideal. To close the primary surgical defect, a V-shaped incision is employed by cutting down to the dermis, thereby preserving the blood supply to this island of skin. The skin is then mobilized to cover the defect and the donor site is closed as a "Y" shape.

Rotational flap

A rotational flap may also be considered to close a triangular defect. However, in clinical practice, defects are typically round or oval. Imagining the oval or circular defect within a triangle is useful for planning the flap. The circular cut is typically three to four times the width of the defect. The flap is undermined within the fat and the leading edge is rotated beyond the defect to ensure closure. A tacking suture can be used to assess whether closure without undue tension is possible. Once the optimal location is decided, the flap can be sutured in place, initially with deeper sutures and then closure of the skin. In Figure 147.2, C is the pivotal point and A is rotated to B to obtain closure.

Gynecologic and Obstetric Surgery: Challenges and Management Options, First Edition. Edited by Arri Coomarasamy, Mahmood I. Shafi, G. Willy Davila and Kiong K. Chan.
© 2016 John Wiley & Sons, Ltd. Published 2016 by John Wiley & Sons, Ltd.

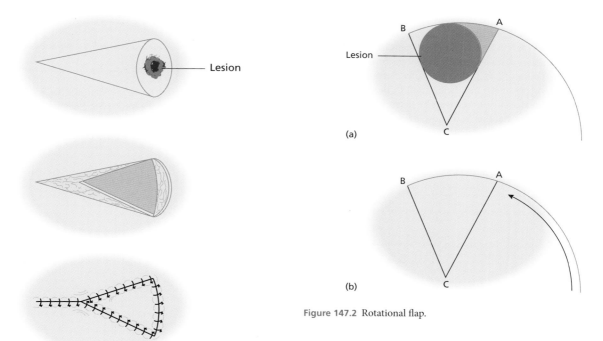

Figure 147.2 Rotational flap.

Figure 147.1 V-Y flap.

Rhombic transposition flap

In larger defects, such as in Case history 1 with a vulval tumor requiring excision with surgical margin, other flap techniques may be necessary. The defect created by excising vulval tumors is often rhomboid in shape. Use of the rhombic transposition flap (Figure 147.3) gives good results and can be varied according to anatomic findings at the time of surgery [4]. In the diagram, ABCD is the surgical defect following excision of the lesion. The length of DE is equivalent to that of AB. The line EF is parallel and of similar length to CD. By rotation, the primary defect can be closed as well as the donor site by adequate undermining and planning. Care must be taken to anchor the flap with deeper sutures before closing the skin edges.

Prevention

Planning of any surgical procedure is vital, especially where skin lesions are being excised. Vulval procedures are associated with psychological sequelae and altered physical appearance. These can be mitigated with counseling and surgical techniques to minimize any distortion of surface anatomy.

By using plastic surgical techniques, most lesions in the vulval or perineal area can be excised and closed either primarily or using flap procedures. Women who smoke or are diabetic (especially insulin dependent) have higher complications associated with this type of surgery because of compromised skin vascularization. It is important not to compromise with regard to surgical cure with good excision margins of tumors. Flaps should be as simple as possible to obtain closure with least tension. Working in conjunction

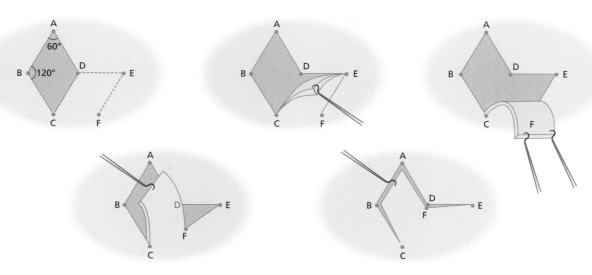

Figure 147.3 Rhombic transposition flap.

with plastic or reconstructive surgeons is ideal for increasing the likelihood of a favorable outcome.

Considerations to take into account are lesion diameters, anatomy affected, scar orientation with respect to relaxed tension lines, arc of skin rotation, and the vector of maximal tension after closure of all surgical incisions. Blood supply to the skin being used in the flap procedure is of vital importance and care needs to be taken in preserving the deep perforators, with attention to closure of dead space as well as meticulous hemostasis. By adhering to these principles, a good clinical and cosmetic outcome can be achieved in the vast majority of patients.

KEY POINTS

Challenge: Plastic surgical techniques in vulval or perineal procedures.

Background
- Excisional procedures on skin may leave defects that are difficult to close without tension.

Management
- Be thoughtful: consider all options from simple to complex prior to any flap surgery.
- Know and understand the anatomy, blood supply, comorbidities, and quality of tissue available.
- Be flexible and have a back-up plan available.
- For flap surgery, working with plastic or reconstructive surgeons is ideal. Some options include:
  - V-Y flaps for small defects.
  - Rotational flaps.
  - Rhombic transposition flaps for larger defects.

Prevention
- By adhering to good surgical principles, most surgical skin defects may be closed with an appropriate flap.

References

1 Mathes SJ, Hentz VR (eds) *Plastic Surgery*, 2nd edn. WB Saunders, Philadelphia, 2005.
2 Mardini S, Wei FC (eds) *Flaps and Reconstructive Surgery*. Saunders Elsevier, Philadelphia, 2009.
3 Rohrer TE, Cook JL, Nguyen TH, Mellette JR Jr (eds) *Flaps and Grafts in Dermatologic Surgery*. WB Saunders Elsevier, Philadelphia, 2007.
4 Townend J. A template for the planning of rhombic skin flaps. *Plast Reconstr Surg* 2008;92:968–971.

CHAPTER 148
Vaginectomy

Janos Balega and Kavita Singh
City Hospital, Sandwell and West Birmingham Hospitals NHS Trust, Birmingham, UK

Case history 1: *A 28-year-old nulliparous patient has been diagnosed with FIGO stage IB1 grade 1 squamous cell carcinoma of the cervix. She is desperate to preserve fertility. Colposcopy assessment revealed Schiller-test positive areas of VAIN3 on the upper third of the anterior and posterior vaginal fornix.*

Case history 2: *A 55-year-old patient who received total laparoscopic simple hysterectomy for CIN3 2 years previously was found to have moderately dyskaryotic cells on follow-up smears. Colposcopy showed acetowhite coarse mosaic occupying the vaginal vault.*

Background

Surgical removal of the vagina, called vaginectomy or colpectomy, is rarely performed as a stand-alone operation, and is usually performed as part of a more extensive procedure such as radical hysterectomy, radical vulvectomy, or exenteration. It is usually performed for primary or recurrent malignant or premalignant lesions either arising from the vagina itself or extending or metastasizing from the cervix, uterus, rectum, bladder, or vulva. Primary vaginal cancers are rare, and only 16–27% of all vaginal cancers arise from the vagina [1].

Simple vaginectomy consists of the removal of vaginal mucosa and the underlying muscularis layer, while during radical vaginectomy the paravaginal connective tissue is also resected. Partial vaginectomy is the removal of a smaller part of vagina, while the removal of the full length of the vagina is called a total vaginectomy. Small premalignant lesions such as VAIN (vaginal intraepithelial neoplasia) are usually removed through the vaginal route as a simple partial vaginectomy; frankly invasive lesions usually require radical vaginectomy.

Management

Diagnostic work-up
The most important initial investigation is an examination under anesthesia, which provides great details of the extent of the disease and resectability by excluding fixation to the underlying bony structures. Colposcopy with multiple mapping biopsies from the lesion to establish the histologic diagnosis is mandatory. Cystoscopy and rectosigmoidoscopy to exclude bladder or rectal involvement are also performed.

The purpose of diagnostic imaging is twofold: firstly, the extent of local spread can be precisely assessed by pelvic MRI, and secondly an abdominal and chest CT scan or PET-CT scan can exclude distant metastasis prior to the surgical intervention.

Preparation for surgery
As the rectum is very close to the vagina, preoperative bowel preparation is considered useful. Although there is no clear evidence, a low-residue diet with light laxatives for a few days prior to the operation followed by a phosphate enema on the morning of the procedure yields an empty rectum and greatly facilitates the dissection and also the repair of bowel complications.

Preoperative psychosexual counseling is important. Depending on the extent of the vaginal lesion, patients can lose all or a significant proportion of the vagina. Although neovagina formation at the same time as vaginectomy or later is an option, changes in sexual life, both at physical and psychological levels, can occur.

Technique: vaginal simple vaginectomy
The patient is placed in lithotomy position and a Foley catheter is inserted into the bladder. The extent of the lesion is visualized with colposcopy using acetic acid and Lugol's iodine (Schiller's test). These tests will indicate the site and extent of resection. If a focal lesion is identified, infiltration of the submucosal space with saline will help with the dissection. Incision is made below the level of the lesion and careful dissection is carried out around the lesion in a similar fashion to an anterior repair. Careful hemostasis is achieved, with due attention paid to the underlying organs such as the rectum and the bladder.

Technique: abdominal or laparoscopic vaginectomy after hysterectomy
The patient is placed in the modified lithotomy (Lloyd-Davies) position with a jelly bag under the sacrum if the operation is performed laparoscopically. A Foley catheter is placed into the bladder. The extent of the lesion is visualized with colposcopy using acetic acid and Lugol's iodine (Schiller's test). These tests will indicate the lowest level of resection.

Gynecologic and Obstetric Surgery: Challenges and Management Options, First Edition. Edited by Arri Coomarasamy, Mahmood I. Shafi, G. Willy Davila and Kiong K. Chan.
© 2016 John Wiley & Sons, Ltd. Published 2016 by John Wiley & Sons, Ltd.

A swab on a sponge-holder is placed into the vagina to stretch the vault. This will facilitate the dissection. Adhesions around the vault are released and the bladder is sharply dissected off the vaginal vault. If total or subtotal vaginectomy is performed, complete ureterolysis with releasing of the ureteric tunnels (lateralization of the ureters) is necessary to avoid ureteric injuries near the trigone of the bladder.

Transection of the paravaginal tissues by straight clamps near or far from the vagina is then performed, according to the oncologic need (simple or radical vaginectomy). One has to ascertain by performing a vaginal speculum examination that the lesion has been completely removed before the vagina is transected. The final step is the closure of vagina or the creation of a neovagina (Chapter 124).

Risks and risk-reduction strategies

- During vaginal approach, the risk of visceral injury can be reduced by adequate infiltration of submucosal tissues prior to incision and by careful dissection.
- If vaginal vault resection is performed post hysterectomy, small bowel loops can be attached to the vaginal vault. The risk of bowel injury is more likely if the colpectomy is performed vaginally; an abdominal approach can significantly reduce such risk.
- Injury to bladder, ureters, and bowel loops is the most common surgical complication due to adhesions and fibrosis. Meticulous dissection can help to prevent such injuries.
- Fistula formation is a rare but potential complication due to impaired blood supply.
- Scarring, narrowing, or shortening of the vagina resulting in sexual dysfunction can be prevented by creating a neovagina at the time of the operation (Chapters 124 and 125) [2].

Resolution of the case

In Case history 1, a laparoscopic radical trachelectomy (resection of the cervix) with upper vaginectomy and pelvic lymphadenectomy can be undertaken. In Case history 2, a vaginal simple colpectomy can be performed.

KEY POINTS

Challenge: Vaginectomy.

Background
- Vaginectomy is mostly required for recurrent malignant lesion or premalignant lesion of the vagina and rarely for primary vaginal cancers.

Management
- A simple vaginectomy consists of the removal of vaginal mucosa and the underlying muscularis layer, whereas during a radical vaginectomy the paravaginal connective tissue is also resected.
- Vaginectomy can be partial when only part of the vagina is removed, or total where the whole length of vagina is removed which is usually associated with total pelvic exenteration.
- Vaginectomy can be performed vaginally, laparoscopically, or via laparotomy.

Prevention
- Vaginectomy is associated with both surgical and psychological morbidity and requires careful case selection, preoperative work-up, and counseling.

References

1 Choi YJ, Hur SY, Park JS, Lee KH. Laparoscopic upper vaginectomy for post-hysterectomy high risk vaginal intraepithelial neoplasia and superficially invasive vaginal carcinoma. *World J Surg Oncol* 2013;11:126.
2 Hendren SK, Swallow CJ, Smith A, Lipa JE. Complications and sexual function after vaginectomy for anorectal tumors. *Dis Colon Rectum* 2007;50:810–816.

CHAPTER 149
Urinary Diversion

John Parkin

City Hospital, Sandwell and Birmingham Hospitals NHS Trust, Birmingham, UK

Case history: A 49-year-old woman, treated 10 years previously with chemoradiotherapy for a stage IIIA cervical carcinoma, presented with recurrent disease involving the cervix and proximal vagina. Following EUA and staging scans which confirmed localized disease, a total pelvic exenteration was proposed. Understanding that this would involve removal of her bladder, the patient asked what the options were regarding urinary reconstruction.

Background

There are two fundamental principles to major pelvic cancer surgery: firstly oncologic integrity, and secondly acceptable functional recovery. With regard to function, none of the currently available reconstructive procedures following removal of the bladder are able to exactly reproduce the "normal" bladder conditions of inert urinary storage together with sensations and innervation related to storage and voiding. However, there are situations when bladder excision is unavoidable in order to completely remove a tumor with adequate margins. In such situations, urinary reconstruction can be achieved in one of three ways: creation of a bladder substitute that empties via the native urethra (orthotopic neobladder) [1]; developing an intra-abdominal reservoir that can be emptied by a catheter (continent urinary diversion) [2]; or diverting the urine directly into a stoma, usually via an interposing section of small bowel (ileal conduit) [3].

Management

There are benefits for both quality of life and self-image from a well-functioning neobladder that avoids any form of stoma; however, this must be balanced against any additional surgical risk, and anatomic and metabolic considerations. If surgery necessitates a complete vaginectomy or excision of the levator ani muscles, or the patient has had a significant radiotherapy dose to the pelvic floor, it is unlikely that an orthotopic (i.e., utilizing the native urethra) reconstruction would be feasible due to lack of sphincter function. In these circumstances the second-best option from the functional point of view may be a continent diversion, although the simplest approach, with the lowest rate of complications, is an ileal

conduit. Since the more complex procedure of reservoir formation usually requires de-tabularization of the selected bowel segment, followed by long anastomotic suture lines, radical radiotherapy increases the risk of anastomotic leakage in the early postoperative period. There is also some evidence that previous radiotherapy may increase the risk of delayed anastomotic complications such as stenosis.

Complications of urinary diversion procedures

The complications of urinary diversion are listed in Table 149.1. Absolute contraindications for urinary reservoir (i.e., either neobladder or continent diversion) include severe renal or hepatic impairment, inflammatory bowel disease, radiation-affected bowel segments, and an inability to self-catheterize [4].

Table 149.1 Complications of urinary diversion surgery.

Early complications
Paralytic ileus
Bowel obstruction
Anastomotic leak

Late complications
Metabolic complications
Anastomotic stricture
Stomal stenosis
Diarrhea
Urinary tract infections
Vitamin B_{12} deficiency
Stone formation

All urinary diversion procedures involving the bowel have a risk of subsequent metabolic abnormalities (usually a hyperchloremic metabolic acidosis) due to absorption of ammonia and chlorine from the urine. However, the risk of these metabolic abnormalities varies depending on how much bowel and which segment is used, as well as whether the urine is stored in a reservoir. An ileal conduit is not designed to be a storage reservoir, but simply a channel to the abdominal wall with a wider lumen than the ureters, and hence reduces the risk of obstruction due to stenosis and the skin. It also uses the shortest length of bowel, and is therefore the least likely of the surgical options to produce significant metabolic

Gynecologic and Obstetric Surgery: Challenges and Management Options, First Edition. Edited by Arri Coomarasamy, Mahmood I. Shafi, G. Willy Davila and Kiong K. Chan.
© 2016 John Wiley & Sons, Ltd. Published 2016 by John Wiley & Sons, Ltd.

disturbances (although metabolic disturbances still occur in up to 10% of patients) and is therefore the safest option in this regard, particularly in patients with underlying renal or hepatic dysfunction. The rate of metabolic acidosis following continent urinary diversion or orthotopic neobladder varies and has been reported to be between 29 and 45% [5–8]. The specific type of reconstruction chosen will have some impact on this, as different segments can be used as well as slightly varying lengths of bowel (e.g., ileal or ileocolic) [9].

There are several reasons for diarrhea to develop following this type of surgery. Firstly, there may be a critical reduction in the length of bowel due to either the longer lengths used for ileal pouches or previous bowel resections. Secondly, there may be a pre-existing functional deficiency despite adequate bowel length because of previous radiotherapy or concurrent inflammatory bowel disease. Thirdly, there may be reduced bile salt and fat absorption caused by dysfunction of the terminal ileum, which may be due to ileal resection as part of the reconstructive procedure or bacterial colonization caused by loss of the ileocecal valve (such as with an ileocolic or ileocecal pouch). Again, the risk of diarrhea is least with an ileal conduit since this utilizes the shortest length of ileum and maintains the integrity of the ileocecal valve.

Operative technique for ileal conduit

On initial laparotomy the bowel is inspected to ensure there would be an adequate segment of distal ileum to use as an ileal conduit. During the exenteration the ureters are handled carefully and as much surrounding tissue preserved as feasible. The ureteric lengths are kept as long as is oncologically possible.

Once the exenteration is complete, the left ureter is brought across the retroperitoneal structures to lie alongside the right ureter (Figure 149.1) [10]. This is easier when a total exenteration is performed as the left colon will have already been fully mobilized. When surgery is limited to an anterior exenteration, a window is formed retroperitoneally over the aorta and IVC through which the left ureter can be redirected (Figure 149.1b). Care must be taken during this maneuver to keep the ureter in the correct alignment and avoid rotation.

We favor a Wallace uretero-ileal anastomosis, although other approaches have been described including Bricker and Le Duc (Figure 149.2) [11–13]. The ureters are shortened appropriately so that the distal ends lie adjacent to each other and the ends are spatulated. The ureters can be oriented such that they are either side by side or head to tail, and a continuous 4-0 Vicryl suture is used to anastomose one edge of each ureter to the other and a Bard urinary diversion catheter inserted in each ureter with the aid of a guidewire. The catheters (stents) are anchored to the ureteric anastomosis with a 3-0 Vicryl Rapide suture.

The distal ileum is used for the conduit. The last 15 cm of terminal ileum is preserved for its specialist metabolic function. Proximal to this, an appropriate 15–20 cm loop of ileum is identified, with a mesenteric length allowing reach to both the ureters on the posterior abdominal wall, and the stoma site which is usually placed in the right iliac fossa. In the more obese patient a longer length of bowel may be required. The small bowel mesentery is incised, ligating the vessels, the bowel divided and the conduit irrigated with a Betadine and saline mixture. Ileal continuity is re-established with either a sutured or stapled anastomosis. The ureteric stents are brought through the conduit and the uretero-ileal anastomosis is

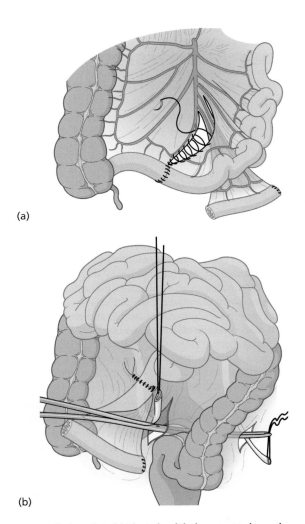

(a)

(b)

Figure 149.1 Ileal conduit. (a) The isolated ileal segment to be used as a conduit is lying below the digestive anastomosis, and the mesentery window of the ileo-ileal anastomosis is sutured. (b) Isolation of the ureters. Transposition of the left ureter to the right side of the pelvis through a tunnel prepared at the base of the sigmoid mesentery in front of the common iliac vessels. *Source*: Adapted from Colombo & Naspro, 2010 [10]. Reproduced with permission from Elsevier.

completed with a continuous 3-0 Vicryl suture running along each remaining edge of the ureters.

The stoma is formed as marked preoperatively, anchoring the bowel conduit to the rectus sheath with three or four 2-0 Vicryl sutures and folding back the end of the conduit to produce a spout.

Resolution of the case

The various issues were discussed in detail with the patient and her partner. She also had a session with the stoma team for additional counseling. In view of a degree of renal impairment, previous high-dose radiotherapy, and need for bowel resection with or without a permanent colostomy, she opted for an ileal conduit urinary diversion.

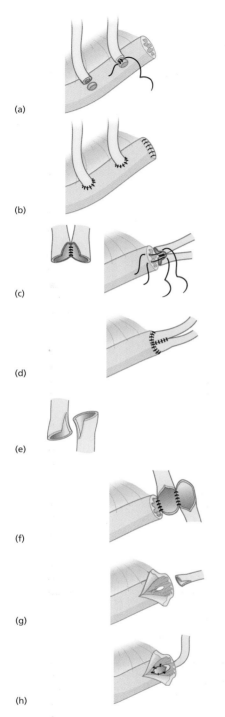

(a)

(b)

(c)

(d)

(e)

(f)

(g)

(h)

Figure 149.2 Ileo-ureteral anastomosis. (a, b) The original Nesbit technique adopted by Bricker: the proximal end of the conduit is left closed, and the ureteral ends are spatulated and anastomosed directly and separately along the antimesenteric side of the conduit. (c–f) Wallace variants: the ends of the ureters are widely spatulated and (c, d) conjoined together "head to head" (Wallace I) or (e, f) oriented in the opposite, "head to tail" direction (Wallace II), and then directly anastomosed to the proximal end of the ileal segment. (g, h) Le Duc antirefluxing anastomosis technique: the ends of ureters are spatulated, laid down on the ileal tracks, and secured to mucosal margins. *Source*: Adapted from Colombo & Naspro, 2010 [10]. Reproduced with permission from Elsevier.

KEY POINTS

Challenge: Urinary diversion.

Background
- There are three options when considering urinary reconstruction following bladder removal as part of pelvic exenteration:
  - Ileal conduit.
  - Continent urinary diversion (catheterizable reservoir).
  - Orthotopic neobladder.
- Although all these techniques share specific risks related to anastomotic leaks and stenosis, long-term acid–base metabolism and altered bowel function, these are limited with an ileal conduit.

Management
- Counseling the patient requires a full and frank discussion regarding the risks and implications of urinary reconstruction.
- Although the option of complex reconstruction may appear desirable at first glance, due to previous interventions and comorbidities many patients may not be considered suitable.

Operative technique for ileal conduit
- Ensure adequate segment of ileum is present to use as a conduit.
- Dissect and bring the left ureter across the retroperitoneal structures to lie alongside the right ureter.
- Shorten the ureters appropriately and spatulate the ends.
- Prepare a 15–20 cm loop of ileum as a conduit.
- Anastomose ureteral ends to the ileal conduit using Bricker, Wallace, or Le Duc techniques.
- Form the stoma (usually in the right iliac fossa).

References

1 Studer UE, Burkhard FC, Schumacher M *et al.* Twenty years experience with an ileal orthotopic low pressure bladder substitute: lessons to be learned. *J Urol* 2006;176:161–66.
2 Bissada NK, Abdallah MM, Aaronson I, Hammouda HM. Continent cutaneous urinary diversion in children: experience with Charleston pouch 1. *J Uol* 2007;177:307–311.
3 Urology BOP. Urinary diversion. Available at http://urobop.co.nz/urology-patient-information/procedure-information/urinary-diversion/
4 Kaufman MR, Cookson MS. Complications of orthotopic neobladder. In: TanejaSS (ed.) *Complications of Urologic Surgery: Prevention and Management*, 4th edn, pp. 559–570. Saunders Elsevier, Philadelphia, 2010.
5 Kamidono S, Oda Y, Ogawa T. Clinical study of urinary diversion. II. Review of 41 ileocolic conduit cases, their complications and long term (6–9 years) follow-up. *Nishinihon J Urol* 1985;47:415–420.
6 Hall MC, Koch MO, McDougal WS. Metabolic consequences of urinary diversion through intestinal segments. *Urol Clin North Am* 1991;18:725–735.
7 McDougal WS. Metabolic complications of urinary intestinal diversion. *J Urol* 1992;147:1199–1208.
8 Gerharz EW, Turner WH, Kälble T, Woodhouse CRJ. Metabolic and functional consequences of urinary reconstruction with bowel. *BJU Int* 2003;91:143–149.
9 Rink M, Kluth L Eichelberg E, Fisch M, Dahlem R. Continent catheterizable pouches for urinary diversion. *Eur Urol* 2010;Suppl 9:754–762.
10 Colombo R, Naspro R. Ileal conduit as the standard for urinary diversion after radical cystectomy for bladder cancer. *Eur Urol* 2010;Suppl 9:736–744.
11 Wallace DM. Uretero-ileostomy. *Br J Urol* 1970;42:529–534.
12 Bricker EM. Bladdder substitution after pelvic evisceration. *Surg Clin North Am* 1950;30:1511–1513.
13 Le Duc A, Camey M, Teillac P. An original antireflux ureteroileal implantation technique: long term follow-up. *J Urol* 1987;137:1156–1158.

CHAPTER 150
Pelvic Exenteration

Kavita Singh

City Hospital, Sandwell and West Birmingham Hospitals NHS Trust, Birmingham, UK

Case history: A 42-year-old patient treated with chemoradiotherapy for stage IB2 cervical cancer 2 years previously has now presented with thickening at the posterior vaginal vault suggestive of recurrence.

Background

Pelvic exenteration is an extensive surgical procedure undertaken for recurrent localized gynecologic cancers. Sometimes it is required as the primary treatment for an extensive gynecologic cancer confined to the pelvis. It is possible to achieve over 50% overall 5-year survival rate in recurrent gynecologic cancers with exenterative surgery [1–4]. However, it is associated with high morbidity (30–50%) and mortality (8–10%), and is therefore usually offered when other modalities of treatment like radiotherapy and chemotherapy are no longer suitable options.

Pelvic exenteration was first described by Brunschwig [5] in 1948, when it was performed for palliation of symptoms. The operation later evolved into a potentially curative intervention for patients with central recurrences. Over time, the indications for exenteration have extended to pelvic sidewall recurrences whenever resection with clear margins is achievable [6]. Recurrent cervical cancer is the most common indication for pelvic exenteration.

Effective preoperative assessment by expert teams working in cancer centers is paramount to ensure patients are appropriately identified for exenteration, and outcomes are optimized. Informed consent and extensive counseling are essential elements of management to ensure patients are fully aware of the potential risks associated with this surgery.

Pelvic exenteration involves radical excision of the uterus in conjunction with the adjacent viscera from the urologic or rectal compartments. It is referred to as anterior exenteration when the bladder is removed, and as posterior exenteration when the rectum is removed (Figure 150.1). When surgical excision extends to all the three compartments (bladder, uterus and rectum), it is referred to as total pelvic exenteration.

Management

The extent of exenterative surgery is tailored to tumor profile and is aimed to achieve clear excision margins. Exenteration involving total colpectomy (removal of vagina) extends below the levator

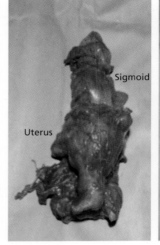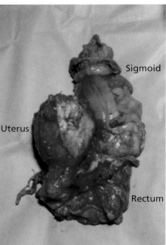

Figure 150.1 Supra-levator posterior exenteration.

ani muscle and is referred to as infra-levator or trans-levator exenteration. It is associated with complete excision of the anal canal and the perineal body. In cases where the lower third of the vagina is not involved, an attempt to conserve the lower vagina, perineal body, and anal canal is appropriate. This is referred to as supra-levator pelvic exenteration as it does not include the excision of levator ani muscles.

Pelvic exenteration is associated with diversion procedures for urine (Chapter 149) and feces (Chapter 37). Rectal excision is usually associated with a colostomy except where it is feasible to perform low anorectal anastomosis. However, many patients may have had prior radiation, and in such patients low anorectal anastomosis is associated with high anastomotic leaks and therefore a colostomy is favored.

Case selection for pelvic exenteration

Careful case selection is essential. After having excluded non-surgical options (chemotherapy and radiotherapy), exenterations should only be offered to well-motivated patients who understand the surgical morbidity and consequences of the procedure on their

---

Gynecologic and Obstetric Surgery: Challenges and Management Options, First Edition. Edited by Arri Coomarasamy, Mahmood I. Shafi, G. Willy Davila and Kiong K. Chan.
© 2016 John Wiley & Sons, Ltd. Published 2016 by John Wiley & Sons, Ltd.

CHAPTER 151

Gynecologic Cancer and Concurrent Pregnancy

Nirmala Rai Talapadi[1] and Sudha Sundar[2]

[1] College of Medical and Dental Sciences, University of Birmingham, Birmingham, UK
[2] City Hospital, Sandwell and West Birmingham Hospitals NHS Trust, Birmingham, UK

Case history 1: *A 32-year-old woman in her first pregnancy presents at 20 weeks of gestation with post-coital bleeding. On speculum examination an irregular growth measuring less than 2 cm is noted on the anterior lip of the cervix.*

Case history 2: *A 26-year-old woman at 18 weeks of gestation presented with worsening abdominal pain, associated with nausea and vomiting. Ultrasound of the abdomen showed a complex 10-cm mass with solid components and septae, and free fluid in the pelvis. Left ovary was not visualized. Lactate dehydrogenase (LDH) and CA125 were raised, but other tumor markers were normal.*

Background

Gynecologic cancers in pregnancy are uncommon, although women occasionally present with cervical or ovarian cancer in pregnancy [1]. Management requires a multidisciplinary approach and needs to consider gestational age, stage of cancer, tumor biology, maternal wishes, impact on the fetus, future fertility, and ethics. The decision to undertake surgery is complex and must aim to optimize both maternal outcome and fetal well-being.

The first peak age of cervical cancer is 30–34 years. The reported incidence of cervical cancer in pregnancy varies from 1 to 12 per 10,000 pregnancies [2]. Cervical cancer in pregnancy can be detected incidentally on speculum examination, or in patients presenting with increased discharge or vaginal bleeding. Pregnancy-associated changes can make it difficult to diagnose early lesions but a low threshold of suspicion should be maintained especially in the presence of recurrent bleeding; colposcopic examination by an experienced colposcopist should be considered if the cervix looks abnormal. Cancer may also be diagnosed during colposcopy follow-up. Approximately 70% of cervical cancers diagnosed during pregnancy are detected at stage I.

Incidence of adnexal mass in pregnancy is 2–4%; only 6% of all operated adnexal masses in pregnancy are cancerous [3]. Incidence of ovarian cancer is 1 in 100,000 to 1 in 10,000 pregnancies. The commonest tumors are germ cell tumors, followed by borderline ovarian tumors and epithelial cancers. Over 90% of ovarian tumors in pregnancy present in stage I. Most ovarian cancers present as adnexal masses, either acutely or incidentally detected on ultrasound during planned obstetric scans. Ultrasound is useful for differentiating morphology and determining the malignant potential [4].

Management

Management of suspected cervical cancer

In Case history 1, a loop or wedge biopsy is required to confirm cancer, as punch biopsy is insufficient to exclude invasion. Biopsy is preferably performed in the operating room by an experienced doctor as the risk of hemorrhage is up to 25% [5]. The pathologist must have full information including the pregnancy status. The interpretation of histology in pregnancy is challenging as decidual changes may mimic invasive changes.

Clinical staging is undertaken once cancer is confirmed. MRI does not use ionizing radiation and is safe in pregnancy; it aids clinical management [6] by providing information on the size and the location of the tumor, as well as the extent of spread to parametrium and lymph nodes. Management is multidisciplinary and should be individualized; it is guided by the stage of cancer, gestational age, and the patient's wishes. Prognosis is influenced by the stage of cancer, nodal status, and histologic subtype. For instance, small cell subtype is aggressive, and a radical hysterectomy is often recommended. However, treatment during pregnancy should generally consider preserving fetal viability whenever feasible without compromising maternal prognosis.

The patient in Case history 1 has a stage IB1 cancer; the management options will include termination of pregnancy and radical hysterectomy if prolongation of pregnancy or fertility preservation is not desired. If continuation of pregnancy is desired, she could be offered lymphadenectomy; if lymph nodes are negative, it may be reasonable to offer planned delay of treatment until delivery, with careful observation [7]. European guidelines recommend trachelectomy (abdominal or vaginal) or neoadjuvant chemotherapy (NACT) followed by large cone biopsy or trachelectomy [8]. The risks of bleeding, fetal loss with trachelectomy, and exposure to chemotherapy with NACT should be discussed with the patient. With conservative management, treatment is delayed until fetal viability (28 weeks, ideally 32–35 weeks) and steroids are given to improve lung maturity.

Lymphadenectomy can be performed by either laparotomy (retroperitoneal approach preferred) or laparoscopy, which reduces uterine handling and irritation. Laparoscopic approach is feasible up to 22 weeks of gestation [9] by experienced and skilled surgeons (Chapter 25). Open technique (Hasson entry) is preferred during laparoscopy to reduce the risk of uterine damage.

Gynecologic and Obstetric Surgery: Challenges and Management Options, First Edition. Edited by Arri Coomarasamy, Mahmood I. Shafi, G. Willy Davila and Kiong K. Chan.
© 2016 John Wiley & Sons, Ltd. Published 2016 by John Wiley & Sons, Ltd.

The survival statistics in patients with planned (intentional or patient refusal) delays (4–40 weeks, averaging 16 weeks) in treatment, especially up to stage IB1 with negative nodes, are good [2]. However, if lymph nodes are positive, guidelines recommend immediate standard treatment (i.e., radical hysterectomy).

Except in stage IA1 cancers with negative margins, cesarean section is the preferred mode of delivery, as metastases in episiotomy wounds have been reported. Vaginal delivery can be considered if the cervix is cleared of the tumor.

Management of suspected ovarian cancer

In Case history 2, the decision for surgery is based on clinical presentation (acute abdomen or suspicion of malignancy) and radiologic appearance (complex mass). Tumor markers are unreliable in pregnancy. MRI may help select patients for surgical procedures and frozen section, if available, is useful. In this patient, a midline laparotomy is indicated. Surgery confirmed a solid torted right ovary. The other ovary, the peritoneal cavity, and the upper abdomen were normal. Peritoneal washings were taken, and unilateral salpingo-oophorectomy was performed.

Frozen section was suggestive of dysgerminoma (the commonest tumor associated with pregnancy), and therefore infracolic omentectomy and removal of enlarged lymph nodes were undertaken. Biopsy of contralateral ovary is indicated only if affected; in the absence of advanced disease, no further treatment is required, and follow-up can be arranged with imaging.

If frozen section is unavailable, it would be reasonable to await histology, and further surgery can often be postponed until after delivery. Dysgerminomas are very sensitive to chemotherapy and surgical treatment is limited to staging laparotomy and unilateral salpingo-oophorectomy. Adjuvant chemotherapy is indicated only for advanced dysgerminomas. Staging laparotomy is performed ideally between 18 and 20 weeks, when there is reduced risk of miscarriage as corpus luteal dependency is minimal. If staging laparotomy is not done at the time of primary surgery for a torted ovary, then secondary surgery for staging may be necessary; the timing of staging surgery will be influenced by the gestational age. If the primary surgery is before 20 weeks, secondary surgery for staging can be considered between 18 and 20 weeks if the mother wishes to continue the pregnancy. If the primary surgery is in the late second trimester or third trimester, it may be reasonable to wait until after delivery before considering further surgery. In selected cases, a laparoscopic procedure could be undertaken by experienced surgeons. Avoidance of spillage is important to prevent upstaging of the cancer.

Before and after surgery the fetus should be monitored appropriately by either ultrasound or CTG depending on the gestational age. After surgery, the variability on CTG may be reduced because of the effects of anesthesia. The mother is operated and nursed in a lateral position to prevent caval compression. There is an increased risk of preterm delivery following surgery but there is no evidence to support prophylactic tocolysis. However, if uterine contractions develop, a tocolytic drug can be used.

Cesarean section is also preferred in women with ovarian cancers, as vaginal delivery may lead to cyst rupture or obstructed labor, but care has to be individualized. There are no reported cases of the fetus being affected either in cervical or ovarian cancer; however, the placenta should be examined for metastases.

KEY POINTS

Challenge: Gynecologic cancer and concurrent pregnancy.

Background
- Gynecologic cancers are uncommon in pregnancy, and therefore there is limited experience and expertise.
  - Incidence of cervical cancer is 1–12 per 10,000 pregnancies.
  - Incidence of ovarian cancer is 1 in 100,000 to 1 in 10,000 pregnancies.
  - In pregnancy, 70% of cervical cancers and 90% of ovarian cancers present in stage I.
- Management often poses a therapeutic challenge and ethical dilemma of balancing the interests of the mother and the fetus.

Management
- Management should be in a cancer center by a multidisciplinary team.
- Management depends on the stage of the tumor, histologic type, gestational age, and maternal wishes.
- The current trend is toward close monitoring and planned delay of surgery to try to achieve good outcomes for the mother while preserving fetal well-being.
- Surgery should be carried out with the patient in left lateral position to avoid caval compression.
- Viability of the fetus should be confirmed before and after the surgery with ultrasound or CTG.
- Steroids should be administered to improve fetal lung maturity if the fetus is being delivered early.

Management of suspected cervical cancer
- A loop or wedge biopsy is needed to confirm cancer; punch biopsy is often insufficient.
- If cervical cancer is confirmed, clinical staging and MRI are needed.
- For early-stage cancers, one option is termination of pregnancy and radical hysterectomy if prolongation of pregnancy or fertility preservation is not required.
- If pregnancy continuation is desired, the patient could be offered lymphadenectomy; if nodes are negative, surgery can be delayed until after delivery (after 28 weeks of gestation); if nodes are positive, immediate treatment of cervical cancer should be recommended.
- Role of trachelectomy and neoadjuvant chemotherapy should be considered.

Management of suspected ovarian cancer
- Tumor markers are unhelpful; imaging with ultrasound and MRI can be helpful in understanding the nature of an adnexal mass.
- Midline laparotomy is indicated; peritoneal washings should be taken, and the pelvis and abdomen should be thoroughly evaluated.
- Frozen section of the removed ovarian mass can be useful in guiding the extent of surgery. If frozen section is unavailable, it may be reasonable to await histology of the removed ovary, and perform definitive surgery after delivery.
- Role of staging laparotomy during pregnancy and adjuvant chemotherapy should be considered.

References

1 Latimer J. Gynaecological malignancies in pregnancy. *Curr Opin Obstet Gynecol* 2007;19:140–144.
2 Morice P, Uzan C, Gouy S, Verschraegen C, Haie-Meder C. Gynaecological cancers in pregnancy. *Lancet* 2012;379:558–569.
3 Giuntoli RL II, Vang RS, Bristow RE. Evaluation and management of adnexal masses during pregnancy. *Clin Obstet Gynecol* 2006;49:492–505.
4 Bromley B, Benacerraf B. Adnexal masses during pregnancy: accuracy of sonographic diagnosis and outcome. *J Ultrasound Med* 1997;16:447–452.
5 Robinson WR, Webb S, Tirpack J, Degefu S, O'Quinn AG. Management of cervical intraepithelial neoplasia during pregnancy with LOOP excision. *Gynecol Oncol* 1997;64:153–155.

6 Nicklas AH, Baker ME. Imaging strategies in the pregnant cancer patient. *Semin Oncol* 2000;27:623–632.

7 Morice P, Narducci F, Mathevet P, Marret H, Darai E, Querleu D. French recommendations on the management of invasive cervical cancer during pregnancy. *Int J Gynecol Cancer* 2009;19:1638–1641.

8 Pentheroudakis G, Orecchia R, Hoekstra HJ, Pavlidis N. Cancer, fertility and pregnancy: ESMO Clinical Practice Guidelines for diagnosis, treatment and follow-up. *Ann Oncol* 2010;21(Suppl 5):v266–v273.

9 Yumi H. Guidelines for diagnosis, treatment, and use of laparoscopy for surgical problems during pregnancy. *Surg Endosc* 2008;22:849–861.

Section 8
Obstetric Surgery
Editors: Pallavi Latthe, Kiong K. Chan and Arri Coomarasamy

CHAPTER 152

Ovarian Cyst Identified at Cesarean Section

Kiong K. Chan[1] and Ioannis Gallos[2]
[1] City Hospital, Sandwell and West Birmingham Hospitals NHS Trust, Birmingham, UK
[2] University of Birmingham, Birmingham, UK

Case history: A 34-year-old woman with a term pregnancy had a cesarean section for fetal distress. The baby was delivered uneventfully. Exploration of the pelvis following closure of the uterine incision revealed a right ovarian cyst measuring 8 cm in diameter. A gynecologist was summoned to the operating room.

Background

Ovarian cysts are usually diagnosed antenatally, permitting a plan of management to be devised before delivery. Incidental ovarian cysts at the time of cesarean section are detected in approximately 1 in 200 women undergoing the operation. These cysts are usually benign, but there are no large prevalence studies to accurately estimate the risk of malignancy. In a series of 43 adnexal masses incidentally diagnosed and excised during cesarean section, the histopathologic diagnoses were mature cystic teratoma (35%), mucinous cystadenoma (16%), serous cyst or cystadenoma (14.0%), endometrioma (12%), luteoma (7%), paraovarian cyst (5%), corpus luteum cyst (2%), fibroma (2%), inclusion cyst (2%), serous-mucinous cyst (2%), and borderline serous cystadenoma (2%) [1,2]. Despite such reassuring data, the obstetrician should not be lulled into a false sense of security as the possibility of an ovarian cancer exists [3].

There is no consensus regarding the management of ovarian cysts in pregnancy. An RCOG guideline for premenopausal women with ovarian cysts recommends surgical removal of ovarian cysts that are symptomatic, large (>7 cm in diameter), enlarging on serial scanning, or that appear complex sonographically, especially if the RMI is raised [4,5]. However, this guideline was not developed to advise on the management of an incidental finding of an ovarian cyst during a cesarean section.

Management

The RCOG Consent Advice No. 7 states that additional procedures during a cesarean section should not be carried out without further discussion with the woman [6]. This includes procedures which may be appropriate but not essential at the time, such as ovarian cystectomy or oophorectomy.

Women under general anesthesia

Cystectomy or oophorectomy for an incidentally identified cyst should not be performed in a woman under general anesthesia, in the absence of prior informed consent. If the ovarian cyst appears suspicious for cancer, a gynecologic oncologist can be summoned to the operating room for an opinion. Peritoneal washings should be taken for cytology, and biopsies of cyst wall or visible peritoneal lesions can be considered on the grounds that these procedures may be diagnostic and carry minimal risks. At the end of the surgery, when the woman is conscious, she should be informed of the findings, and consent should be sought before sending any specimen to the laboratory for examination.

Women under regional anesthesia

A woman undergoing regional anesthesia can be sensitively counseled about the findings at the time of surgery, and her consent can be sought for further management. If the woman does not wish to have an additional procedure or finds it difficult to make a decision at that time, the consent criteria are not satisfied and a cystectomy or oophorectomy should not be performed; the woman can be given more time to make a decision about definitive management after the procedure. If she agrees to further management at the time, then the gynecologist must decide whether to perform a cystectomy or oophorectomy. If the cyst appears to be benign, a cystectomy is preferred, but should be done without spillage of cyst contents (see below). If it appears to be malignant, an oophorectomy (without or without more extensive surgery) is appropriate, but this should be done by a gynecologic oncologist. In general the aim of ovarian cancer surgery is total macroscopic clearance; however, this may not be possible or appropriate at the time of cesarean section, and an interval staging laparotomy after histology confirms an ovarian cancer can be more appropriate. At the time of surgery further investigations such as tumor markers and imaging are both inappropriate and impractical.

Avoiding spillage during cystectomy

A large cyst containing few or no solid elements can be removed without spillage by aspirating its contents via a bowel bag fused to its capsule. The technique is straightforward. A bonding glue such as Dermabond is applied to a 5-cm area of the cyst capsule, taking care not to allow the glue to spread to any other structures. The bag

Gynecologic and Obstetric Surgery: Challenges and Management Options, First Edition. Edited by Arri Coomarasamy, Mahmood I. Shafi, G. Willy Davila and Kiong K. Chan.
© 2016 John Wiley & Sons, Ltd. Published 2016 by John Wiley & Sons, Ltd.

is applied to that part of the cyst wall and firmly kept in place with a swab to ensure a good bond between capsule and bag. A small incision is made in the middle of the bonded area and the sucker inserted to empty the cyst. The bowel bag prevents any spillage. When the cyst is empty, the bag is tied around the sucker and its tubing. Gloves are changed to further minimize the possibility of contamination, before proceeding with cystectomy. If the technique described is unavailable, it may be possible to exteriorize the ovary (particularly since the pedicles are long in pregnancy), surround the pedicle with packs or swabs on the abdominal surface, and then carry out the cystectomy.

Resolution of the case

The woman was under regional anesthesia and the gynecologist counseled her for further management of the cyst, and offered removal at the time. He explained the benefits and risks, and advised that if she preferred this could be done at a later stage. The woman consented to further management and the gynecologic oncologist was asked for an opinion.

The cyst was well encapsulated with no external excrescences. In view of this the gynecologic oncologist decided to perform an ovarian cystectomy after carrying out peritoneal washings with normal saline.

The right ovary was mobile and could be lifted out of the abdomen despite its size and the confines of a Pfannenstiel incision. A cystectomy was carried out using standard techniques. The remnant capsule was closed with 2-0 Vicryl to minimize adhesions. A careful exploration of the abdominal cavity and its contents was carried out to look for metastases or suspicious areas. Special attention was paid to the omentum, the undersurface of the diaphragm, the retroperitoneal lymph nodes, the gastrointestinal tract, and the peritoneal surfaces.

The abdominal cavity was washed out with warm water as this reveals bleeding points easily and in theory would cause lysis of any shed cells. The abdomen was closed in layers. Histologic examination revealed the cyst to be a benign cystic teratoma.

KEY POINTS

Challenge: Ovarian cyst at cesarean section.

Background
- Incidental ovarian cysts are detected at the time of the cesarean section in approximately 1 in 200 women undergoing the procedure.
- Most cysts are benign, but there are anecdotal reports of malignancies.

Management
- Additional non-emergency procedures during a cesarean section should not be carried out without the consent of the woman.

Under general anesthesia
If an ovarian cyst with features suggestive of malignancy is identified:
- Seek an on-the-table review by an oncology specialist.

- Take peritoneal washings for cytology.
- Consider biopsies of cyst wall or visible peritoneal lesions.
- Inform the patient of the findings when she is conscious, and seek her permission to send any specimens for laboratory investigations.
- Plan definitive management in consultation with a gynecologic oncologist.

Under regional anesthesia
- Inform and seek consent for further management.
- If the cyst appears to be benign, consider performing a cystectomy, but without spillage of cyst contents.
- If the cyst has features suggestive of malignancy, take peritoneal washings, and consider performing an oophorectomy with or without additional surgery. The procedure should be performed by an oncology specialist. Once histology is available, interval staging laparotomy can be planned as appropriate.

References

1 Hobeika EM, Usta IM, Ghazeeri GS, Mehio G, Nassar AH. Histopathology of adnexal masses incidentally diagnosed during cesarean delivery. *Eur J Obstet Gynecol Reprod Biol* 2008;140:124–125.
2 Royal College of Obstetricians and Gynaecologists. Ovarian mass at caesarean section (query bank). Available at https://www.rcog.org.uk/en/guidelines-research-services/guidelines/ovarian-mass-at-caesarean-section—query-bank/ (accessed 15 October 2014).
3 Li X, Yang X. Ovarian malignancies incidentally diagnosed during cesarean section: analysis of 13 cases. *Am J Med Sci* 2011;341:181–184.
4 Royal College of Obstetricians and Gynaecologists. *Ovarian Cysts in Postmenopausal Women.* RCOG Green-top Guideline No. 34, October 2003, reviewed 2010. Available at https://www.rcog.org.uk/en/guidelines-research-services/guidelines/gtg34/
5 Royal College of Obstetricians and Gynaecologists. *Management of Suspected Ovarian Masses in Premenopausal Women.* RCOG Green-top Guideline No. 62, December 2011. Available at https://www.rcog.org.uk/en/guidelines-research-services/guidelines/gtg62/
6 Royal College of Obstetricians and Gynaecologists. Caesarean section. RCOG Consent Advice No. 7, October 2009. Available at https://www.rcog.org.uk/globalassets/documents/guidelines/consent-advice/ca7-15072010.pdf (accessed 15 October 2014).

CHAPTER 153

Laparoscopy in Pregnancy

Kevin J.E. Stepp and Anjana Nair
Carolinas Healthcare System, Charlotte, North Carolina, USA

Case history: *A 36-year-old woman presented with acute lower abdominal pain and nausea at 12 weeks of gestation. An ultrasound showed a 7-cm, complex, probably torted, cystic adnexal mass, along with a viable intrauterine pregnancy.*

Background

Pregnancy is no longer considered a contraindication for laparoscopic surgery. However, there are specific risks associated with laparoscopy during pregnancy (Chapter 25).

Adnexal masses are relatively common during pregnancy. While most of these are corpus luteal cysts that will resolve prior to the second trimester, other types of masses may persist and predispose the patient to complications later in pregnancy. Adnexal masses greater than 5 cm and persisting beyond 14–16 weeks of gestation may expose the patient to higher risks of complications such as torsion, rupture, or hemorrhage, potentially also necessitating higher-risk emergency intervention [1].

Appendicitis, reported in 0.05–0.1% of pregnant women, is the most common non-gynecologic surgical condition requiring a laparoscopy [2], followed by cholecystitis. Concern for appendicitis should prompt surgical evaluation regardless of gestational age because fetal mortality is increased with perforated appendix [2,3]. Laparoscopy may also be carried out in pregnancy for adrenalectomy and nephrectomy.

The advantages of laparoscopy may be particularly important during pregnancy. Smaller incisions offer lower risks of wound complications (infections, dehiscence and hernias), lower postoperative pain, and less fetal depression from narcotics. Minimal bowel manipulation allows for early return of bowel function. Pregnancy is a hypercoagulable state due to several changes in the coagulation cascade and increased venous stasis. Early ambulation after minimally invasive surgery helps to decrease the risk of venous thromboembolism.

Physiologic concerns of laparoscopy and pregnancy (Chapter 25)

Metabolic and mechanical changes associated with advancing gestation lead to significant changes in maternal pulmonary function. As gestation progresses, the diaphragm is elevated and functional residual capacity and residual lung volume are decreased. However, blood volume, heart rate, cardiac output,

minute ventilation, and oxygen consumption are increased. Carbon dioxide production is also increased and a compensatory mild respiratory alkalosis is seen. General endotracheal anesthesia is considered safe in pregnancy. Most of the anesthetic drugs, muscle relaxants and morphine-like drugs used in general anesthesia are not teratogenic or toxic to the fetus.

Pregnant patients are at risk of aspiration but this can be reduced with a nasogastric or orogastric tube. Gastric drainage will also decrease the risk of visceral injury during left upper quadrant trocar placement. The physical effects of pneumoperitoneum decrease excursion of the diaphragm, reduce the compliance of the thoracic cavity, and further reduce residual lung volume and functional residual capacity. Increased intra-abdominal pressure may also reduce maternal venous return, cardiac output, and uterine blood flow, causing maternal hypotension. Trendelenburg position will accentuate these changes by increasing intrathoracic pressure. Importantly, general anesthesia combined with pneumoperitoneum and the reverse-Trendelenburg position can reduce cardiac output by as much as 50% secondary to pooling of blood in the lower extremities.

Fetal concerns with laparoscopy

Carbon dioxide readily diffuses into the maternal circulation and between the maternal–fetal circulations. In theory, the excess CO_2 absorption from prolonged pneumoperitoneum may cause adverse effects. The resulting maternal acidosis can cause decreased removal of fetal CO_2 and potential fetal acidosis, but no long-term adverse effects have been identified [4]. Non-invasive continuous monitoring of end-tidal CO_2 ($ETCO_2$) with waveform capnography is recommended. Controlled hyperventilation will eliminate the excess CO_2 and maintain $ETCO_2$ at less than 35 mmHg [5]. Close monitoring with $ETCO_2$ and ensuring adequate maternal oxygenation is the best way to ensure adequate fetal oxygenation and prevent fetal acidosis. There is little or no role for routine invasive monitoring of maternal arterial blood gases unless there is significantly prolonged ventilation [6].

Management (Chapters 25 and 78)

Timing of intervention

The optimal time for surgery in pregnancy is considered to be the second trimester. The background risk of spontaneous miscarriage is lower in the second trimester (5.6%) compared with the first

Gynecologic and Obstetric Surgery: Challenges and Management Options, First Edition. Edited by Arri Coomarasamy, Mahmood I. Shafi, G. Willy Davila and Kiong K. Chan.
© 2016 John Wiley & Sons, Ltd. Published 2016 by John Wiley & Sons, Ltd.

457

trimester (12–15%) [7]. Since organogenesis is complete by 12 weeks, the risk of teratogenesis is low beyond the first trimester. Surgery in the third trimester may require manipulation of the gravid uterus to provide adequate exposure, possibly predisposing the patient to uterine irritability and preterm labor.

Patient positioning

The patient should be positioned in lateral tilt to displace the gravid uterus off the inferior vena cava and aorta. In the supine position, the gravid uterus (even in the second trimester) can compress the inferior vena cava and reduce venous return to the heart, thereby affecting the cardiac output of the pregnant patient. If reverse-Trendelenburg position is needed, it should be done gradually to minimize the hemodynamic effects.

Entry techniques

The primary entry site should be carefully chosen after considering the height of the uterine fundus, the planned procedure, and the patient's tilt. We recommend making the primary entry high enough above the uterine fundus to provide adequate visualization (see Chapter 25, Figure 25.1). Potential locations to be used in the second trimester include the base of the umbilicus, supraumbilical, subxiphoid midline, or left upper quadrant (Palmer's point) sites. Options of primary entry include the Veress needle technique, optical trocars, or open entry (e.g., Hasson technique). The open entry method may be the safest to avoid injury to the gravid uterus. The gravid uterus may move the small bowel out of the pelvis, thus potentially increasing the risk of bowel injury with Veress needle or trocar. Secondary trocars should only be inserted under direct visualization.

Intraoperative recommendations

Studies have reported intra-abdominal pressures up to 15 mmHg for laparoscopies in pregnancy without increasing adverse maternal or fetal effects. However, the maximum pressure may be decreased to 8–12 mmHg after initial entry provided that visualization is not compromised. In an euvolemic pregnant patient, the raised intra-abdominal pressure should not lead to reductions in blood flow to mother or fetus [8,9].

If electrosurgery is used, there may be a risk from potential fetal exposure to carbon monoxide from surgical smoke. Ultrasonic devices may be preferred because they generate less smoke. Any intra-abdominal smoke from electrocautery devices should be immediately evacuated.

The risks of preterm labor and pregnancy loss are increased by emergency procedures and third-trimester surgeries, either as a result of the surgical procedure per se or the condition that necessitated the surgical intervention. Although there are no definitive data, the risk of premature labor may be higher if the uterus or cervix is manipulated; such manipulation should therefore be minimized. Tocolytics may be considered if there are signs of uterine irritability or preterm labor.

The safety of hemostatic agents has not been established and these should be avoided in pregnancy if possible. Gasless laparoscopy has been considered for use in pregnant patients. In this technique, mechanical abdominal wall elevators are utilized to provide visualization. No pneumoperitoneum is used. Visualization is often limited and the technique is not commonly employed. Data are still inadequate and further research is necessary prior to use of this approach in pregnancy.

Fetal monitoring

Fetal heart rate should be documented preoperatively and postoperatively in all patients. Routine intraoperative fetal monitoring is not recommended and is not practical. In cases involving a viable fetus, a cardiotocograph may be considered preoperatively, and if non-reassuring may be a contraindication to proceeding with surgery until the woman and the fetus are better resuscitated.

Postoperative management

Paracetamol or non-steroidal anti-inflammatory drugs (NSAIDs) may be used in the second trimester. NSAIDs are not recommended beyond the second trimester because of concerns about premature closure of the ductus arteriosus. In some cases narcotic pain medication may be needed.

KEY POINTS

Challenge: Pregnant patient requiring laparoscopy.

Background
- In a life-threatening situation, surgical management may be necessary regardless of the trimester of pregnancy, as maternal well-being should be prioritized over fetal well-being.
- In non-emergency situations, it is ideal to wait until 6 weeks postpartum. If surgery is indicated during pregnancy, it is best performed electively in the second trimester.
- Studies to date have not shown any long-term adverse effects on the mother or the fetus from laparoscopic surgery during pregnancy.

Management
- No intrauterine manipulator or any cervical instrumentation should be used.
- The patient should be placed in lateral tilt in the late second trimester and beyond.
- Entry by open technique is generally preferred, although entry by Veress needle or optical trocar may be used in certain circumstances.
- Primary trocar should be high above the uterine fundus.
- Pneumoperitoneum should be kept as low as possible to permit adequate visualization and no greater than 15 mmHg.
- Any intra-abdominal smoke from electrocautery devices should be evacuated.
- Maternal $ETCO_2$ should be maintained at 35 mmHg or lower if possible.
- Fetal heart rate should be checked preoperatively and postoperatively.
- Appropriate thromboprophylaxis, early ambulation, hydration, and analgesia should be considered.

References

1 Nezhat FR, Tazuke S, Nezhat CH, Seidman DS, Phillips DR, Nezhat CR. Laparoscopy during pregnancy: a literature review. *J Soc Laparoendosc Surg* 1997;1:17–27.

2 Babaknia A, Parsa H, Woodruff JD. Appendicitis during pregnancy. *Obstet Gynecol* 1977;50:40–44.

3 McComb P, Laimon H. Appendicitis complicating pregnancy. *Can J Surg* 1980;23:92–94.

4 Hunter JG, Swanstrom L, Thornberg K. Carbon dioxide pneumoperitoneum induces fetal acidosis in a pregnant ewe model. *Surg Endosc* 1995;9:272–279.

5 Nezhat C, Nicoll LM. Laparosocpic management of pelvic pathology during pregnancy. *Expert Rev Obstet Gynecol* 2009;4:53–60.

6 Bhavani-Shankar K, Steinbrook RA, Brooks DC, Datta S. Arterial to end-tidal carbon dioxide pressure difference during laparoscopic surgery in pregnancy. *Anesthesiology* 2000;93:370–373.

7 Novak E, Lambrou C. Ovarian tumors in pregnancy: an ovarian tumor registry review. *Obstet Gynecol* 1975;46:401–406.

8 Lanzafame RJ. Laparoscopic cholecystectomy during pregnancy. *Surgery* 1995;118:627–631.

9 Rizzo AG. Laparosocpic surgery in pregnancy: long-term follow up. *J Laparoendosc Adv Surg Tech* 2003;13:11–15.

CHAPTER 154
Cervical Cerclage

Ayesha Mahmud and Yousri Afifi
Birmingham Women's NHS Foundation Trust, Birmingham, UK

Case history *A 24-year-old woman with a history of three recurrent mid-trimester miscarriages presents at 11 weeks of gestation. The last pregnancy loss was after a failed vaginal cervical suture.*

Background

Cervical cerclage was first performed in 1902 in women with a history of mid-trimester miscarriages suggestive of cervical incompetence. Shirodkar and then McDonald made this procedure common in obstetrics [1]. The efficacy of cerclage remains uncertain [2]. There is a lack of agreement about the optimal procedure, suture, technique, and timing of insertion. Available evidence suggests that cerclage is associated with significant decreases in preterm birth outcomes, as well as improvements in composite neonatal morbidity and mortality, and may be considered in high-risk women [3]. However, it should be noted that cervical cerclage itself is associated with risks such as maternal pyrexia, cervical laceration or trauma, bladder damage, membrane rupture, and bleeding during insertion [3].

Criteria for offering cervical cerclage
Various criteria have been suggested by the Royal College of Obstetricians and Gynaecologists (RCOG, UK) to provide guidance on the indications for cervical cerclage (Table 154.1) [3]. Cervical cerclage can be considered in other circumstances; in complex cases, senior clinical input and a multidisciplinary team approach are advisable.

Table 154.1 Criteria for offering cervical cerclage.

Cerclage category	Criteria for offering cerclage
History-indicated cerclage	Women with history of three or more previous preterm births and/or second-trimester losses
Ultrasound-indicated cerclage	Women with history of one or more spontaneous mid-trimester losses or preterm births, with ultrasound surveillance indicating a cervical length of ≤25 mm before 24 weeks of gestation
Rescue cerclage	Individualized decision, taking into account gestation and cervical dilatation

Approaches for cervical cerclage
The options have evolved over the years. The approach for cervical cerclage can be transvaginal or transabdominal; with the latter, it can be an open or laparoscopic procedure (Figure 154.1). A transabdominal cerclage is usually inserted in cases following a failed vaginal cerclage or in cases where extensive cervical surgery has shortened the cervix significantly [3]. Transabdominal cerclage carries a greater risk of complications in comparison with the transvaginal approach, and necessitates a planned cesarean section at term.

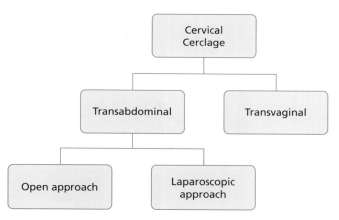

Figure 154.1 Types of cervical cerclage.

Management

The patient should be counseled fully about potential benefits and risks and the uncertainty in the evidence. In a pregnant woman, it is important to confirm fetal viability prior to insertion of cerclage; transabdominal cerclage can generally be inserted at up to 12 weeks of gestation.

Transvaginal cervical cerclage
The choice of technique for transvaginal cervical cerclage is usually operator-dependant. Shirodkar and McDonald techniques have been commonly used (Figure 154.2). McDonald cerclage is a pursestring suture placed at the cervico-vaginal junction, without

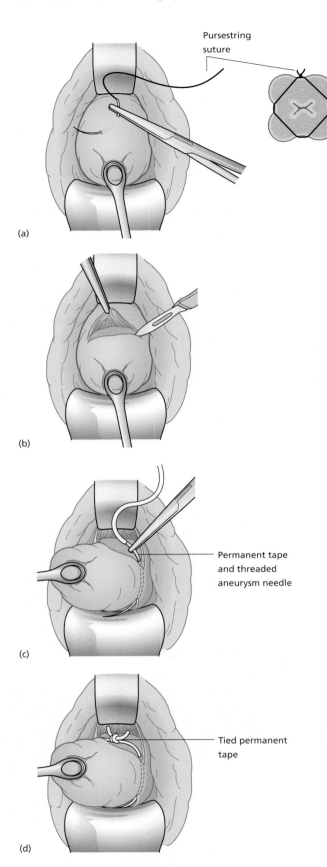

Pursestring suture

(a)

(b)

Permanent tape and threaded aneurysm needle

(c)

Tied permanent tape

(d)

Figure 154.2 Transvaginal cervical cerclage: (a) McDonald cerclage and (b–d) Shirodkar cerclage.

bladder mobilization. Shirodkar procedure is a high vaginal cervical cerclage; a transvaginal pursestring suture is placed following bladder mobilization, to allow insertion above the level of the cardinal ligaments. It may require regional anesthesia for removal at 37 weeks, given that the technique often involves suture burial [4].

Surgical technique for transvaginal cerclage [5]

The procedure may be done under regional anesthesia. With the patient in lithotomy position, the vulva and vagina are cleaned using surgical soap solution. With an assistant's help, the vaginal walls are retracted, including the bladder anteriorly, with right-angled retractors. A weighted speculum can be used to retract the posterior vaginal wall.

The anterior and posterior lip of the cervix are gently grasped using a grasping sponge forceps. The cervico-vaginal fold is identified while retracting the bladder anteriorly and the posterior fornix posteriorly. The distance from the external os to the cervico-vesical fold should be at least 2 cm; if it is less than 2 cm, another type of cerclage is indicated.

A pursestring suture is driven through the cervix using a 5-mm Mersilene (multifilament) tape or No. 1 Prolene or nylon suture (monofilament) on a round-bodied needle (Figure 154.2). The suture should be placed at the level of the internal os, and exit at the 5 and 7 o'clock positions. Once the tape insertion is complete, the bladder should be emptied with a catheter to ensure the presence of clear urine. The needles can then be cut off, and the tape or suture ends tied in three separate knots. A small gap between each knot is necessary to allow easy identification and removal.

Transabdominal cerclage

There is no evidence to support a laparoscopic approach over laparotomy for the insertion of abdominal cerclage [3]. Therefore the choice of approach is dependent on the clinical needs, surgeon's expertise, and patient's choice. Open approach involves the placement of a cerclage at the cervical isthmus, positioned in the avascular space above the cardinal and uterosacral ligaments following a laparotomy [6]. There are various approaches for laparoscopic insertion of abdominal cerclage, reflecting the lack of evidence and consensus on the choice of material and techniques.

Surgical technique for laparoscopic transabdominal cerclage

In non-pregnant patients, a standard laparoscopic entry technique with four ports is used. Open umbilical entry or Palmer's point entry is the first choice for pregnant patients, but the site of primary trocar will depend on the size of the uterus (Chapter 25) and previous surgical history (Chapter 27).

Vaginal manipulation of the uterus facilitates the operation, and is therefore recommended in non-pregnant patients. However, during pregnancy, vaginal manipulation of the uterus should be avoided, and instead an atraumatic retractor such as a liver retractor can be used for uterine manipulation (Figure 154.3).

The first step is to open the vesico-uterine peritoneal space and reflect down the vesico-uterine peritoneum. In a pregnant uterus this area may be more vascular in comparison with a non-pregnant uterus. Filling the bladder with saline can be used during pregnancy for easy outlining of bladder.

The operator then needs to identify the uterine vessel complex (Figure 154.4), the uterosacral ligaments and the ureters. An Endoclose needle is subsequently inserted through the space

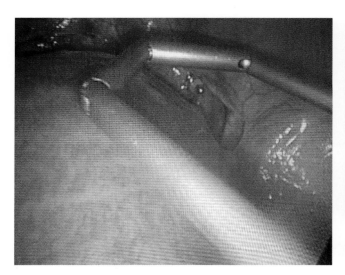

Figure 154.3 Liver retractor.

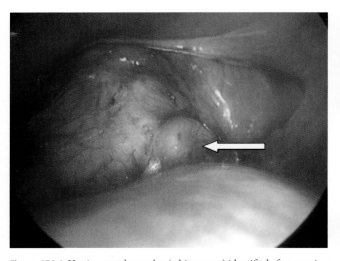

Figure 154.4 Uterine vessel complex (white arrow) identified after opening the vesico-uterine peritoneal space.

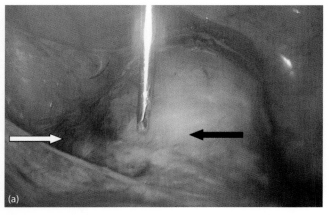

(a)

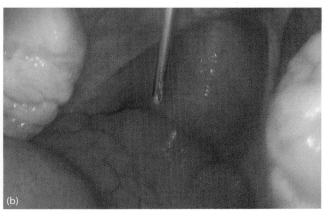

(b)

Figure 154.5 (a) Endoclose needle about to be inserted in the space between the uterine vessel complex (white arrow) and cervix (black arrow) on the left side. (b) Endoclose needle now visible in the pouch of Douglas after it has traversed the side of the cervix on the left.

between the uterine vessel complex and the cervix at the level of the internal os (Figure 154.5). The chosen suture (e.g., 5-mm Mersilene, Prolene or nylon) is introduced into the pouch of Douglas via one of the laparoscopic ports, and the suture is picked up and pulled through the cervix to the anterior cervical surface with the aid of the Endoclose needle. The Endoclose needle is then introduced through the other side of the cervix, and the procedure is repeated. The suture can now be tied using an intracorporeal square knot (Figure 154.6).

Postoperative care

The choice of operative technique dictates postoperative care. There is no need for routine tocolytic drugs. Timing of removal of cerclage in the transvaginal group should be set at 37 weeks of gestation to avoid cervical lacerations or trauma in the event of labor. In the transabdominal group a planned cesarean section at term is recommended [3].

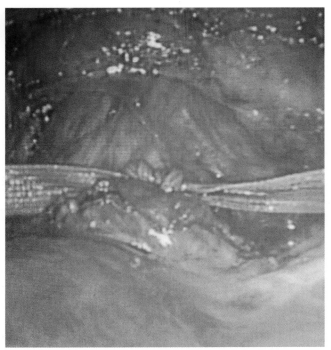

Figure 154.6 Position of Mersilene tape knot.

KEY POINTS

Challenge: Cervical cerclage.

Background
- Cerclage may be indicated in women with a history of multiple mid-trimester miscarriages or preterm births, women with a short cervix (≤25 mm) on ultrasound scan, or as a rescue therapy in women with cervical dilation.
- The choice between transvaginal or transabdominal cerclage depends on prior obstetric history, and patient and clinician preferences.

Management
- Perform a comprehensive preoperative clinical assessment, and ultrasound scan to assess cervical length.
- If the patient is pregnant, check fetal viability before and after the procedure.
- Perform McDonald or Shirodkar suture if vaginal cerclage is appropriate. The cervical length should be at least 2 cm for a vaginal cerclage.
- Women with a history of trachelectomy or a typical history of cervical insufficiency in whom prior vaginal cerclage has been unsuccessful should be considered for abdominal cerclage.
- After transabdominal cerclage, the mode of delivery should be cesarean section. After transvaginal cerclage, if there is no contraindication to vaginal birth, the suture should be removed at 37 weeks.

References

1 Fox N, Chervenak F. Cervical cerclage: a review of the evidence. *Obstet Gynecol Surv* 2008;63:58–65.
2 MRC/RCOG Working Party on Cervical Cerclage. Final report of the Medical Research Council/Royal College of Obstetricians and Gynaecologists multicentre randomised trial of cervical cerclage. *Br J Obstet Gynaecol* 1993;100:516–523.
3 Royal College of Obstetricians and Gynaecologists. *Cervical Cerclage*. RCOG Green-top Guideline No. 60, May 2011. Available at https://www.rcog.org.uk/en/guidelines-research-services/guidelines/gtg60/
4 Abbott D, To M, Shennan A. Cervical cerclage: a review of current evidence. *Aust NZ J Obstet Gynaecol* 2012;52:220–223.
5 Karl K, Katz M. Surgical technique: a stepwise approach to cervical cerclage. *OBG Managment* 2012;24(6). Available at http://www.obgmanagement.com/home/article/a-stepwise-approach-to-cervical-cerclage/2e7b822ade39843ac1394ef6d393df56.html
6 Benson RC, Durfee RB. Transabdominal cervico-uterine cerclage during pregnancy for the treatment of cervical incompetency. *Obstet Gynecol* 1965;25:145–155.

CHAPTER 155

Cesarean Section in a Woman with Fibroids

Andrew Prentice

Addenbrooke's Hospital, Cambridge University Hospitals NHS Foundation Trust, Cambridge, UK

Case history: A women with a fibroid uterus presents at term with non-engagement of the presenting part. Clinical examination indicates that there is a fibroid below the presenting part, preventing it from entering the pelvis. Vaginal delivery will not be possible and delivery by cesarean section is required.

Background

Uterine fibroids are common benign tumors; the incidence of fibroids in women of reproductive age is 25–40%. Fibroids have been reported to have an effect on pregnancy and be affected by pregnancy. However, fibroids do not always enlarge during pregnancy as commonly believed. In a longitudinal study undertaken through the course of pregnancy, 78% of fibroids remained unchanged during pregnancy, and of those that increased in size none increased by more than 25% [1]. Nevertheless, fibroids may change during pregnancy and undergo red degeneration, giving rise to pain, in approximately 10% of cases [2].

Fibroids have been reported to have a significant impact on pregnancy outcomes and increase the risk of miscarriage, bleeding in early pregnancy, preterm labor, placental abruption, malpresentation, dystocia, cesarean section, postpartum hemorrhage, and puerperal hysterectomy [3].

Management

Surgical delivery by cesarean section will be required for obstruction of the pelvic inlet or outlet leading to dystocia, non-engagement of the presenting part, or malpresentation. The type of incision and surgical technique depend on the size and site of the fibroids. Women need to be counseled about the possible need for midline incision with or without a classical uterine incision, especially when anterior lower segment fibroids are present. If a classical incision on the uterus is chosen, the patient should be informed of the implications for future pregnancy. For women with fibroids having cesarean section, there is an increased risk of cesarean hysterectomy (3.3%, compared with the baseline risk of 0.2%) and blood transfusion.

Preoperative management

It is important to accurately map the location and size of the fibroids, along with the presentation of the fetus, using ultrasound or, uncommonly, other forms of imaging such as MRI. The preoperative hemoglobin should be checked, and blood should be cross-matched. A prospective plan for the management of severe hemorrhage should be made, with consideration for interventional radiologic involvement if facilities for uterine artery embolization are available.

Intraoperative management

The skin incision should allow good access to the anterior aspect of the uterus, and this may require a midline incision. A final decision on the incision can be made by examining the patient once she has been positioned on the operating table.

Once the abdomen is open, an assessment can be made to decide which uterine incision should be used. If the fibroid is in the fundus or high in the uterus, the presenting part can descend normally, and the lower segment is usually normally formed; a standard lower segment incision can be used in this situation. If the fibroid is in posterior cervix or low in the uterus posteriorly, the presenting part is likely to be high, and the lower segment poorly formed; a transverse incision in the upper part of the lower segment can often be used in this situation. Challenges exist when the fibroids are in the anterior uterus. If the fibroid is arising low in the cervix there may still be a lower segment through which the uterine cavity may be opened, but it is more likely that a classical incision in the upper segment may be required.

The greatest difficulty is encountered when multiple fibroids are present in the anterior uterus, limiting access to normal myometrium. Wherever possible a linear incision should be made in normal myometrium sufficiently distant from the fibroids to allow closure. When fibroids prevent access to the uterine cavity through normal myometrium, myomectomy may be required to allow the safe delivery of the fetus. Occasionally, myomectomy may also be required to facilitate the closure of the uterine incision. However, myomectomy should generally be avoided because of the risk of severe hemorrhage, and consequent hysterectomy. Myomectomy has been reported in a number of small series as being a safe procedure with no increased morbidity, but these reports [4,5] have not changed the consensus view [3].

Before the uterine incision is made, the fetal position should also be confirmed. Where there is a malpresentation and delivery has to be achieved by breech extraction, care should be taken that a fetal leg is brought out through the wound first rather than a fetal arm.

Gynecologic and Obstetric Surgery: Challenges and Management Options, First Edition. Edited by Arri Coomarasamy, Mahmood I. Shafi, G. Willy Davila and Kiong K. Chan.
© 2016 John Wiley & Sons, Ltd. Published 2016 by John Wiley & Sons, Ltd.

When the cesarean section is complicated by hemorrhage, this should be managed in the conventional manner (Chapters 40 and 158). When bleeding is due to uterine atony the position of the fibroids may complicate the insertion of brace sutures, such as the B-Lynch suture [6]. An alternative approach is to insert compression sutures in other locations avoiding individual fibroids, as illustrated in Figure 155.1 [7].

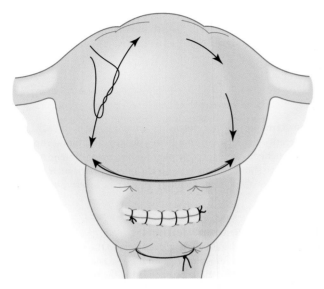

Figure 155.1 Compression sutures in a uterus complicated with fibroids. *Source*: Ouahba *et al.*, 2007 [7]. Reproduced with permission from John Wiley & Sons, Ltd.

Traditional textbooks of gynecologic surgery have suggested that an elective hysterectomy may be considered as definitive management of multiple fibroids at the time of cesarean section [8]. However, this approach cannot be considered ideal in modern practice. Nevertheless, the woman should be counseled fully about the possibility of needing an emergency hysterectomy should there be uncontrollable bleeding after delivery of the baby.

Postpartum management

Women will require detailed debrief of the intraoperative findings, the surgery performed, and implications to recovery and future childbirth. The information should also be communicated to the general practitioner. If the woman suffers from menorrhagia or pressure symptoms in the postpartum period, referral to a gynecologist is appropriate. If further pregnancy is desired, an elective myomectomy might be considered before future conception.

KEY POINTS

Challenge: Cesarean section in a woman with fibroids.

Background
- Fibroids are commonly occurring tumors in women of reproductive age.
- Fibroids can undergo red degeneration in pregnancy.
- Fibroids can be associated with increased risks of miscarriage, bleeding in early pregnancy, preterm labor, placental abruption, malpresentation, dystocia, cesarean section, postpartum hemorrhage, and peripartum hysterectomy.

Management
- Hemoglobin should be checked and blood should be cross-matched.
- Informed consent should include a discussion of the possibility of hysterectomy.
- Careful consideration should be given to the choice of both the abdominal and uterine incisions; midline incision on the skin with or without classical uterine incision might be essential to allow good access if the fibroid is in the anterior lower uterine segment.
- Uterine incisions should avoid fibroids whenever possible.
- Myomectomy may be performed to allow access for delivery or to facilitate closure of the uterine incision, but is generally considered inadvisable.
- Alternative site uterine compression sutures may prove a useful alternative to the usual B-Lynch compression suture.
- If further pregnancy is desired, an elective myomectomy might be considered before future conception.

References

1 Aharoni A, Reiter A, Golan D, Paltiely Y, Sharf M. Patterns of growth of uterine leiomyomas during pregnancy. A prospective longitudinal study. *Br J Obstet Gynaecol* 1988;95:510–513.
2 Katz VL, Dotters DJ, Droegemeuller W. Complications of uterine leiomyomas in pregnancy. *Obstet Gynecol* 1989;73:593–596.
3 Lee HJ, Norwitz ER, Shaw J Contemporary management of fibroids in pregnancy. *Rev Obstet Gynecol* 2010;3:20–27.
4 Mu YL, Wang S, Hao J, Shi M, Yelian FD, Wang XT. Successful pregnancies with uterine leiomyomas and myomectomy at the time of caesarean section. *Postgrad Med J* 2011;87:601–604.
5 Brown D, Fletcher HM, Myrie MO, Reid M. Caesarean myomectomy: a safe procedure. A retrospective case controlled study. *J Obstet Gynaecol* 1999;19:139–141.
6 B-Lynch C, Coker A, Lawal AH, Abu J, Cowen MJ. The B-Lynch surgical technique for the control of massive postpartum haemorrhage: an alternative to hysterectomy? Five cases reported. *Br J Obstet Gynaecol* 1997;104:372–375.
7 Ouahba J, Piketty M, Huel C *et al*. Uterine compression sutures for postpartum bleeding with uterine atony. *BJOG* 2007;114:619–622.
8 Monaghan JM. Myomectomy and management of fibroids in pregnancy. In: *Bonney's Gynaecological Surgery*, 9th edn. Baillière Tindall, London, 1986.

CHAPTER 156

Cesarean Section at the Limits of Viability

Catherine Aiken[1] and Jeremy Brockelsby[2]

[1] University of Cambridge, Cambridge, UK

[2] Rosie Maternity Hospital, Cambridge, UK

Case history 1: *A woman presented at 24 weeks and 3 days of gestation with severe ongoing antepartum hemorrhage. Appropriate resuscitative measures were instituted, and an emergency cesarean section was commenced.*

Case history 2*: A woman presented with severe pre-eclampsia at 24 weeks and 6 days of gestation. She was stabilized with antihypertensive drugs and magnesium sulfate. However, her renal function continued to deteriorate rapidly, and a cesarean section was undertaken.*

Background

Cesarean section at the limits of fetal viability is a complicated surgical challenge, where morbidity to the mother and the fetus should be carefully considered. Such cesarean sections may be required for maternal reasons, as given in the two case histories, or may be undertaken for fetal reasons. Whether cesarean section at the limits of viability is advisable for fetal reasons is debatable, but the technical issues remain similar nonetheless.

The operative difficulties for extreme preterm cesarean section include considerations of the optimal surgical approach, the uterine incision, and management of peripartum fetal and maternal morbidity. The surgeon needs to anticipate a poorly developed lower uterine segment, increased likelihood of fetal malpresentation, difficulty in avoiding an anterior placenta, increased risk of intraoperative hemorrhage, and the possible need for a hysterectomy if there is uncontrollable bleeding.

The extremely preterm baby is at high risk of birth trauma, even in the context of a cesarean section. Possible injuries include fractures, nerve damage, and intracranial hemorrhage. Babies with extensive ecchymosis from delivery have increased rates of mortality and cerebral hemorrhage [1].

An upper segment (classical) cesarean section may be needed in about 10% of babies born at 27–28 weeks, with consequent impact on future pregnancies.

Management

Preoperative management

Multidisciplinary team involvement in the preoperative planning is mandated; this should include an obstetrician, a neonatologist, a midwife, and an anesthetist. It is good practice for the neonatologist to counsel the woman directly about the risks of neonatal morbidity and mortality. Steroids should be administered for fetal lung maturation whenever possible, as long as there is no contraindication. Pre-delivery magnesium sulfate treatment should be considered for newborn neuroprotection. Blood tests including full blood count and group and cross-match are necessary. The patient should be counseled about the risks for the mother and baby, and a neonatal team should be arranged to attend the delivery. If time allows, preoperative sonography is useful for determining fetal lie and placental site.

Optimization of surgical approach

The procedure should be performed by an experienced senior obstetrician. The choice of the abdominal incision is a critical factor in allowing appropriate access to the uterus. A generous (larger than usual) transverse incision on the skin can allow adequate access. Entry into the abdominal cavity is best achieved by a modified Joel-Cohen incision [2], which is placed approximately 3 cm above the usual level of a Pfannenstiel incision. When compared with a Pfannenstiel incision, a Joel-Cohen incision is associated with less blood loss, fever, pain, and analgesic requirements, as well as shorter duration of surgery [3].

The use of retractors will enhance surgical access. The use of ring retractors (Figure 156.1) may be particularly valuable in women with high BMI, and may help reduce birth trauma and infection.

The use of a midline vertical abdominal incision will not directly reduce birth trauma; however, it may allow better access to the surgical site in some women (Chapter 26). A midline incision has the advantage of allowing the easy placement of vertical (classical) uterine incision or modifications of surgical technique (Figure 156.2) as appropriate. In emergency situations, delivery may be achieved more rapidly via a vertical incision, but this is not associated with improved neonatal outcomes; unfamiliarity with the approach makes it less suitable for many obstetricians [4].

Method of uterine incision

The decision on which uterine incision is most appropriate should be taken intraoperatively based on the evaluation of the uterus. Even at the limits of viability there may still be a well-formed lower segment, which allows the option of a transverse incision.

A transverse lower segment uterine incision (Figure 156.2a) is preferred because the lower uterine segment is less vascular than

---

Gynecologic and Obstetric Surgery: Challenges and Management Options, First Edition. Edited by Arri Coomarasamy, Mahmood I. Shafi, G. Willy Davila and Kiong K. Chan.
© 2016 John Wiley & Sons, Ltd. Published 2016 by John Wiley & Sons, Ltd.

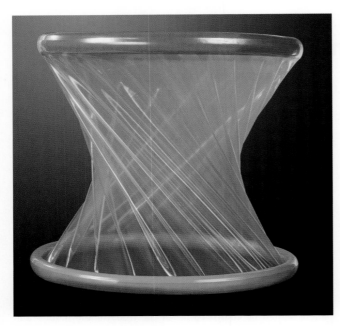

Figure 156.1 Alexis O retractor for cesarean section. Reproduced with permission from Applied Medical.

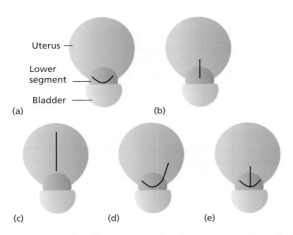

Figure 156.2 Possible uterine incisions for cesarean section at the limits of viability: (a) low transverse; (b) low vertical; (c) classical; (d) J incision; (e) inverted T.

the body of the uterus, and the incision is easier to repair. This leads to a reduction in operative complications, especially hemorrhage, and also a reduction in morbidity. Lower segment incisions are also associated with a lower incidence of uterine dehiscence or rupture in subsequent pregnancies [5]. Occasionally, after a transverse lower segment incision has been made, the incision needs to be extended to facilitate the delivery, particularly if the fetus is in transverse lie or if the after-coming head is trapped. In this situation, the incision may be extended vertically, in the midline, into the upper segment of the uterus forming an inverted T-shaped incision (Figure 156.2e). Alternatively, the incision may be extended vertically from the end of the transverse incision to form a J-shaped incision (Figure 156.2d).

In extremely early gestations, the lower uterine segment may be poorly formed; a vertical (classical) incision (Figure 156.2c) may then be necessary, especially when the baby is in a transverse lie.

Hemorrhage is potentially more severe with a classical incision, and the placenta will often occupy the anterior uterine upper segment [4]. In order to minimize potential blood loss from the fetus, the placenta must be avoided if at all possible, and separated rather than cut. If a vertical incision is contemplated, some surgeons advocate the use of a midline stay suture above the bladder to help prevent downward extension of the incision.

Although recent evidence suggests the development of a bladder flap confers no advantage in term cesarean sections, it is likely to be required at the limits of viability for access to the lower segment area.

With classical or any upper segment incision, a three-layer closure is the usual method of repair.

Minimizing fetal injury

Several techniques have been described to minimize fetal injury. Delivery of the fetus while preserving the amniotic membranes is believed to reduce trauma at the time of delivery. The "splint technique," whereby the operator's hand is inserted into the cavity to cup the fetal head, and the fetal trunk rests against the forearm, has been advocated by some [6]. For the malpresenting fetus, internal or external podalic version may be needed to facilitate delivery.

Delivery into a plastic bag to reduce the risk of hypothermia [7] and direct transfer to waiting neonatologists is recommended. Delayed cord clamping and cord milking are associated with improved hemodynamic stability, a decreased blood transfusion requirement, and a lower incidence of intraventricular hemorrhage in preterm babies [8].

Prevention

The conditions that prompt cesarean section at the limits of viability are often such that preoperative planning time is curtailed, but where possible all necessary preparations should be made. These include a senior obstetrician, availability of blood products and cell salvage facility, and the presence of an experienced neonatal team in the operating room.

Complications for future pregnancies from a classical incision include a scar rupture rate of approximately 5% [9], some of which will be pre-labor. Cesarean section is recommended for future deliveries, although vaginal birth may be considered for low vertical incisions. The risk of subsequent placenta praevia or accreta following a vertical uterine incision is unknown.

KEY POINTS

Challenge: Cesarean section at the limits of fetal viability.

Background
- Cesarean section may be undertaken at the limits of fetal viability for maternal reasons, or occasionally for fetal reasons.
- The extremely preterm infant is at high risk of birth trauma.
- Challenges include a poorly developed lower uterine segment, increased likelihood of fetal malpresentation, difficulty in avoiding an anterior placenta, increased risk of intraoperative hemorrhage, and the possible need for a hysterectomy.
- There is a 5% scar rupture rate in future pregnancies in women with a history of classical uterine incision.
- The procedure should be performed by an experienced obstetrician.

Management

- The decision for delivery should ideally be made by a multidisciplinary team, and with full counseling of the woman or couple.
- Pre-delivery steroids and magnesium sulfate should be considered for fetal lung maturation and newborn neuroprotection, respectively.
- Full blood count, cross-match of blood, and cell salvage equipment (if available) should be arranged.

Skin incision

- Adequate exposure can be obtained via a transverse or vertical skin incision; however, a larger than usual incision is advisable.
- A modified Joel-Cohen incision may be preferable to a standard Pfannenstiel incision.
- The use of ring retractors can enhance surgical access.

Method of uterine incision

- If the lower segment is found to be adequately formed, a lower segment transverse incision is preferred.
- Having performed a lower segment transverse incision, if it is found to be inadequate, it can be extended with an inverted-T or J-shaped incision.
- If lower segment is not formed, a vertical (classical) incision may be necessary.
- Upper segment incisions should be closed in three layers.

Minimizing fetal morbidity

- Delivering the baby in the amniotic sac may reduce fetal injury.
- The "splint technique" may help to minimize fetal injury.
- Delivery into a plastic bag and direct transfer to waiting neonatologists is recommended.
- Delayed cord clamping and cord milking may be of benefit.

References

1 Arad I, Braunstein R, Ergaz Z, Peleg O. Bruising at birth: antenatal associations and neonatal outcome of extremely low birth weight infants. *Neonatology* 2007;92:258–263.

2 Wallin G, Fall O. Modified Joel-Cohen technique for caesarean delivery. *Br J Obstet Gynaecol* 1999;106:221–226.

3 Mathai M, Hofmeyr GJ, Mathai NE. Abdominal surgical incisions for caesarean section. *Cochrane Database Syst Rev* 2013;(5):CD004453.

4 Wylie BJ, Gilbert S, Landon MB *et al.* Comparison of transverse and vertical skin incision for emergency cesarean delivery. *Obstet Gynecol* 2010;115:1134–1140.

5 National Institute for Health and Care Excellence. *Caesarean Section*, 2nd edn. RCOG Press, London, 2011. Available at http://www.nice.org.uk/guidance/cg132/documents/caesarean-section-update-full-guideline2 (accessed 21 September 2014).

6 Druzin ML. Atraumatic delivery in cases of malpresentation of the very low birth weight fetus at cesarean section: the splint technique. *Am J Obstet Gynecol* 1986;154:941–942.

7 Jin Z, Wang X, Xu Q, Wang P, Ai W. Cesarean section en caul and asphyxia in preterm infants. *Acta Obstet Gynecol Scand* 2013;92:338–341.

8 Raju TN. Timing of umbilical cord clamping after birth for optimizing placental transfusion. *Curr Opin Pediatr* 2013;25:180–187.

9 Halperin ME, Moore DC, Hannah WJ. Classical versus low-segment transverse incision for preterm caesarean section: maternal complications and outcome of subsequent pregnancies. *Br J Obstet Gynaecol* 1988;95:990–996.

CHAPTER 157

Difficult Delivery of the Fetal Head During Cesarean Section

Parveen Abedin

Birmingham Women's NHS Foundation Trust, Birmingham, UK

Case history: *A 34-year-old nulliparous woman at term made slow progress to full dilatation in labor. After an hour of pushing, she had an unsuccessful trial of ventouse in theater. A cesarean section was initiated, but the clinician could not deliver the head as it was wedged deep in the pelvis. A senior obstetrician was immediately summoned to operating room.*

Background

Cesarean sections at full dilatation, often after a prolonged second stage of labor, are associated with fetal and maternal trauma. As a result of the fetal head being deeply engaged and wedged in the pelvis, disengagement can be difficult. The surgeon carrying out a cesarean section with a deeply engaged head can find it extremely difficult to insert the hand between the lower pole of the fetal head and the pelvis in order to lift the head out of the pelvis to effect delivery of the baby. The fact that the lower uterine segment is thinned out with a blurring of the anatomic landmarks complicates the situation further, and can result in a very low uterine incision extending into the vagina; such injuries can also cause broad ligament tears resulting in hemorrhage, and potentially injury to the ureters.

Management

Several techniques can be used to help with the delivery of a deeply engaged head at cesarean section. These include the "push" method, the "pull" methods (reverse breech extraction and Patwardhan technique), and more recently the Fetal Pillow®. The choice of method will depend on the surgeon's experience and preference, although the available evidence favors the "pull" methods.

"Push" method

This involves an assistant pushing the fetal head upwards via the vaginal route after abducting the maternal legs [1]. At the same time, the surgeon should apply steady upward pressure via the uterine incision on the fetal shoulders [2]. These procedures should be carried out when the uterus is in the relaxation phase; alternatively, tocolytics such as terbutaline can be considered to induce uterine relaxation.

It has been suggested that the surgeon can deliver the head with one hand in the uterus and the other hand in the vagina to push up the head [3]. This approach may be useful when good assistance is unavailable.

With the push method, considerable force is needed to push the fetal head up to the level of the uterine incision, resulting in potential skull fractures and damage to the head. Extensive lacerations often occur, including extensions into the vagina or the broad ligament.

Reverse breech extraction method

After making the uterine incision, the surgeon should grasp one or both fetal feet at the uterine fundus and bring them out with steady traction via the uterine incision [4]. Once the legs are brought out, the buttocks follow; the fetal head now ascends to the level of the lower segment, and the baby is extracted as a breech.

Patwardhan technique

The incision over the lower uterine segment is made high at the level of the anterior shoulder, which is then delivered along with the anterior arm by hooking a finger in the elbow if needed [5]. The posterior shoulder is now rotated forward and delivered. The trunk, breech, and lower limbs are successively delivered by traction aided by fundal pressure by the assistant. The head is now disengaged and lifted out of the pelvis.

Fetal Pillow®

The Fetal Pillow® is a soft silicone balloon that inflates in only one direction (Figure 157.1). It occupies minimal space in the pelvis when inserted. It is placed on the anococcygeal ligament, thus preventing any downward movement, and elevates the fetal head by 3–4 cm when inflated.

Insertion is carried out just before performing a cesarean section; the device is positioned like a posterior ventouse cup. The patient's legs are then placed flat before inflation is carried out using 180 mL of saline. The time taken for this maneuver is approximately 30 seconds.

A recent randomized controlled trial of 240 patients showed a reduction in uterine extensions, blood loss and transfusions, uterine incision to delivery interval, and length of hospital stay with the use of the Fetal Pillow [6].

Gynecologic and Obstetric Surgery: Challenges and Management Options, First Edition. Edited by Arri Coomarasamy, Mahmood I. Shafi, G. Willy Davila and Kiong K. Chan.
© 2016 John Wiley & Sons, Ltd. Published 2016 by John Wiley & Sons, Ltd.

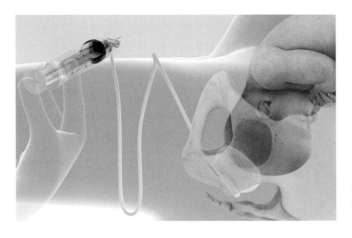

Figure 157.1 Fetal Pillow® in use.
Source: Safe Obstetric Systems. Reproduced with permission.

Evidence

Both the "push" and the "pull" methods have been compared in several studies [4,7–11], although only one study was a randomized trial [11]. In this study, 108 women undergoing cesarean section for obstructed labor at term were assigned randomly to either the "push" or the "pull" methods of delivery as already detailed. Patients in the "push" group had significantly greater blood loss, extension of the uterine incision, and postpartum endometritis, as well as fetal morbidity. These findings are similar to the findings from the other studies. In one of the retrospective studies [4], extension of the

uterine incision occurred in 22.8% when the baby was delivered as cephalic compared with 2.2% when delivered as breech. Although there are no large-scale randomized controlled trials, the available evidence suggests less maternal and fetal morbidity with the "pull" methods.

A survey conducted among UK trainees [12] revealed that 80% faced difficulties when delivering a deeply engaged head. Only 42% of trainees were confident of doing a "pull" method of delivery, and 80% agreed that supervised training was necessary to improve their confidence.

KEY POINTS

Challenge: Cesarean section delivery of a deeply engaged fetal head.

Background
- A deeply engaged head at cesarean section poses risk of significant morbidity for mother and baby.
- Maternal risks include tear extensions to vagina, broad ligament, cervix, and bladder, leading to increased blood loss and transfusions.

Management
- It is important to wait until the uterus is relaxed before attempting to deliver the head; alternatively, a tocolytic (e.g., terbutaline) can be given to induce uterine relaxation.
- The options for delivery are as follows:
  - "Push" method: involves an assistant pushing up the head via the vaginal route, while the obstetrician applies steady upward pressure on the fetal shoulders via the uterine incision.

- Reverse breech extraction method: involves the obstetrician grasping one or both fetal feet and delivering the baby as a breech.
- Patwardhan technique: involves making a lower segment uterine incision high at the level of the fetal anterior shoulder, which is then delivered along with the anterior arm, followed by rotation and delivery of the posterior arm, and then the trunk, breech and lower limbs, and finally the fetal head.
- Fetal Pillow®: involves inflating a purpose-made balloon placed under the fetal head to elevate the head before a cesarean section delivery.
- Available evidence suggests that "pull" methods (reverse breech extraction or Patwardhan technique) may be superior to the "push" method.

References

1 Blickstein L. Difficult delivery of the impacted fetal head during caesarean section: intraoperative disengagement dystocia. *J Perinat Med* 2004;32:465–469.
2 Landesman R, Graber EA. Abdominovaginal delivery: modification of the caesarian section operation to facilitate delivery of the impacted head. *Am J Obstet Gynecol* 1984;148:707–710.
3 Lippert TH. Abdominovaginal delivery in case of impacted head in caesarian section operation. *Am J Obstet Gynecol* 1985;151:703.
4 Chopra S, Bagga R, Keepanasseril A, Jain V, Kalra J, Suri V. Disengagement of the deeply engaged fetal head during caesarean section in advanced labour: conventional method versus breech extraction. *Acta Obstet Gynecol Scand* 2009;88:1163–1166.
5 Patwardhan BB, Motashaw ND. Caesarian section. *J Obstet Gynecol India* 1957;8:1–15.
6 Seal S, Tibriwal R, Kanrar P, De A, Mukherjee J. Elevating fetal head prior to performing a cesarean section at full dilation using fetal pillow: a prospective randomised trial. BJOG 2015 suppl EP10.131.

7 Bastani P, Pourabolghasem S, Abbasalizadeh F, Motvalli L. Comparison of neonatal and maternal outcomes associated with head-pushing and head-pulling methods for impacted fetal head extraction during caesarean delivery. *Int J Gynaecol Obstet* 2012;118:1–3.
8 Mukhopadhyay P, Naskar T, Dalui R, Hazra S, Bhattacharya D. Evaluation of Patwardhan technique: a four year study in a rural teaching hospital. *J Obstet Gynecol India* 2005;55:244–246.
9 Ziyauddin F, Hakim S, Khan T. Delivery of the deeply engaged head during caesarean section in advanced labour: a comparative study of head pushing versus reverse breech extraction. *Curr Pediatr Res* 2013;17:41–43.
10 Veisi F, Zangeneh M, Malekkhosravi S, Rezavand N. Comparison of "push" and "pull" methods for impacted fetal head extraction during caesarean delivery. *Int J Gynaecol Obstet* 2012;118:4–6.
11 Fasubaa OB, Ezechi OC, Orji EO et al. Delivery of the impacted head of the fetus at caesarean section after prolonged obstructed labour: a randomised comparative study of two methods. *J Obstet Gynecol* 2002;22:375–378.
12 Sethuram R, Jamjute P, Kevelighan E. Delivery of the deeply engaged head: a lacuna in training. *J Obstet Gynecol* 2010;30:545–549.

CHAPTER 158

Surgical Management of Massive Obstetric Hemorrhage from the Uterus, Cervix, or Vagina

Phil Steer

Faculty of Medicine, Imperial College London, London, UK

Case history: *A 37-year-old woman in her first pregnancy agreed to induction of labor at 7 days past her due date. She had a prolonged first and second stage followed by a forceps delivery of a baby weighing 4.1 kg. By 10 min after the birth, measured blood loss per vaginam had already reached 1000 mL and the bleeding showed no sign of abating.*

Background

Primary postpartum hemorrhage (PPH) is most commonly due to uterine atony; other causes include vaginal or cervical tears, retained placental tissues, coagulation defects, uterine rupture, and uterine inversion (Chapter 162). It is customary to define PPH as the loss of more than 500 mL of blood, but detailed studies have shown that this level of blood loss is common in childbirth. Estimation of blood loss is notoriously difficult and often underestimated. Therefore continued monitoring of vital signs such as a pulse rate and blood pressure are essential, and a dedicated member of staff should be assigned to this task. Ideally, this person will be an obstetric anesthetist.

Management

Most hospitals have a PPH protocol that is initiated when the estimated blood loss is excessive. The initial steps would be as in any emergency: call for help; assess airway, breathing and circulation; lie the patient flat; commence oxygen administration; ensure venous access along with blood withdrawals for hemoglobin, group and cross-match and coagulation; and start fluid resuscitation. The management will then focus on assessing the cause of bleeding, and instituting timely management with uterotonic drugs and surgery. The focus of this chapter is on the surgical management of PPH; however, aggressive medical management with uterotonic drugs, blood, and blood products (Chapter 40) is a core aspect of management, and all obstetricians should have the necessary competency to provide timely and effective management.

Repairing trauma to the vagina or cervix

The obstetrician should perform a detailed assessment to ascertain the source of bleeding. It may be coming from a tear in the vagina or cervix, or it may be coming from an atonic uterus. Proper assessment requires the woman to be in the lithotomy position, with a good spotlight for inspection. At least two Sims speculae will be necessary to enable inspection of the vagina, and it is often helpful to have a third, held by an assistant, to allow three-point traction, giving better visibility. If the blood loss is due to a tear in the vagina, then local pressure will usually slow it down sufficiently to allow proper visualization. Once identified, the tear should be sutured using an absorbable suture such as Dexon or Vicryl, starting at the upper apex. A simple continuous suture is usually appropriate because it provides longitudinal as well as lateral compression. If the tear is very deep, then it may be necessary to use two layers of sutures, one for the deeper tissues and one for the vaginal skin. If the tear extends up into the fornix, and is anterolateral, then a potential danger is including the ureter if a suture is placed too deeply. In such an event, it may be necessary to perform a laparotomy in case the tear has extended into the broad ligament, causing a hematoma that can be difficult to diagnose in any other way. This will require a second surgeon so that the repair can be visualized from both below and above. If the tear is posterior, then care must be taken not to include the wall of the rectum in the suture. This should be checked by rectal examinations at intervals during the repair. If the tear is anterior, it is advisable to place an indwelling Foley catheter so that the urethra can be clearly identified and one can avoid including it in any sutures.

If the cause of the bleeding is a tear in the cervix, then it should also be repaired by suturing. In order to check the cervix, a useful way is to place a sponge-holder at the 12 o'clock position and another at the 2 o'clock position; the intervening tissue can then be inspected. If a tear is not found, then the 12 o'clock sponge-holder can be removed and placed at the 4 o'clock position, and the intervening cervix inspected, and so on until the cervix has been inspected over its full circumference. If a tear is found, it can be repaired with a single continuous suture, using Dexon or Vicryl.

Surgical management of uterine bleeding

Uterotonic drugs should be administered without delay, but if the bleeding continues, plans for surgical management should be made. Surgical options include intrauterine balloon tamponade, uterine artery embolization, uterine compression sutures, ligation

---

of uterine or internal iliac arteries, aortic compression, and hysterectomy. An important interim measure is the application of bimanual compression (Figure 158.1). This is achieved by placing a fist in the vagina, and using the other hand per abdomen to compress the body of the uterus against the fist. The uterus can also be massaged with the abdominal hand as this will stimulate uterine activity at least temporarily, often producing a marked reduction in the bleeding for up to a minute or so until uterus naturally relaxes again. This can provide important time to resuscitate a mother if she is already showing signs of volume decompensation. It is also a useful way to assess whether it is uterine atony that is responsible for the hemorrhage.

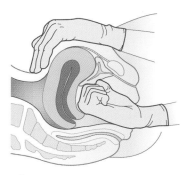

Figure 158.1 Bimanual compression.

Although medical management with uterotonic drugs is not addressed in this surgical book, one caveat regarding the use of uterotonic drugs should be noted: some clinicians advocate giving prostaglandin F2α (Hemabate) directly into the uterus through the abdomen using a long needle, but this risks intravenous injection which can result in acute maternal collapse.

Intrauterine balloons

The insertion and inflation of an intrauterine balloon should be considered if medical therapy is not effective. Inflation must be done with normal saline and not air, because rupture of a balloon containing air could give rise to an air embolism. The use of a Rusch urologic hydrostatic balloon is common, although there is now a device specific for use in uterine atony called the Bakri tamponade balloon catheter. This has the advantage of a central lumen with an opening above the balloon, allowing drainage of any blood within the uterus above the balloon, and revealing any ongoing bleeding which could otherwise be missed. However, if such specialized balloons are not available, then a tamponade balloon can be constructed with a condom tied to a Foley catheter.

A study of pressures and volumes in the normal postpartum uterus showed that up to 1.5 L of fluid could be infused before the maximum intrauterine pressure of 50–60 mmHg was reached [1]; the authors of this study commented that the existing restriction of balloon inflation to 500 mL may limit the usefulness of balloon tamponade and that sometimes greater volumes are needed. They also suggested that the mode of action might not be a direct compression effect on the uterus, but lateral wall pressure in the pelvis reducing uterine artery blood flow.

The usual recommendation is that the balloon be kept inflated for 24 hours and that removal should be accomplished by reducing the intra-balloon volume by 50–100 mL every 2 hours or so. However, deflating the balloon completely after 24 hours and removing it is a common practice. There is currently no agreed policy regarding antibiotic prophylaxis.

EDITOR'S NOTE ON A NEW UTERINE TAMPONADE DEVICE: AMMALIFE MITTEN

Arri Coomarasamy

There are uncertainties about the most effective way to use a tamponade balloon. The three key challenges include (i) the correct placement of the balloon, (ii) achieving the correct intrauterine volume and pressure, and (iii) retention of the balloon in the correct place during and after inflation. A new device in development (Ammalife Mitten, Figures 158.2 and 158.3) may overcome all three challenges, but rigorous clinical studies are needed to evaluate its effects. In a partially contracted uterus with a smaller uterine cavity, the "two finger" technique can be used to inflate the balloon with a smaller volume of fluid (Figure 158.4).

Balloon tamponade can also be used to arrest bleeding from multiple vaginal sites where suturing has not proved to be effective [2]. Ammalife Mitten is particularly suited for this purpose as the "sleeve" can be packed with gauze or sponge to provide vaginal tamponade (Figure 158.3e). This device also eliminates the risk of any retained swabs as all swabs are contained within the "sleeve" and removed automatically when the device is removed (Figure 158.5).

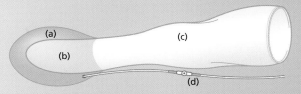

Figure 158.2 The Ammalife Mitten has an inflatable balloon (a), which is mounted on a "mitten" (b); the mitten is continuous with a long "sleeve" (c). A fluid channel (d) runs along the sleeve to enter the inflatable balloon. *Source*: Image courtesy of Ammalife: www.ammalife.org.

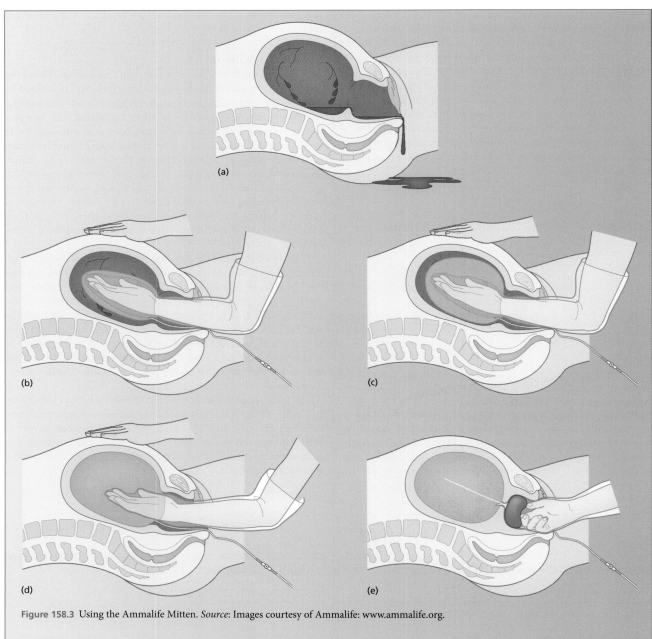

Figure 158.3 Using the Ammalife Mitten. *Source*: Images courtesy of Ammalife: www.ammalife.org.

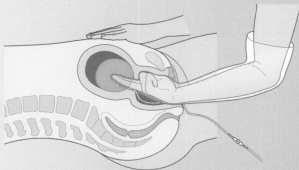

Figure 158.4 Using the Ammalife Mitten in a partially contracted uterus using the "two finger" technique. *Source*: Image courtesy of Ammalife: www.ammalife.org.

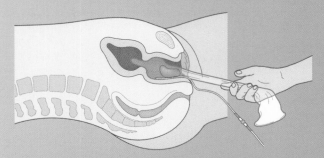

Figure 158.5 Removal of the Ammalife Mitten. Swabs in the "sleeve" are automatically removed, eliminating the risk of retained swabs in the vagina.
Source: Image courtesy of Ammalife: www.ammalife.org.

quality of life. The indications for pelvic exenterative surgery include the following.

- Cervical cancer: recurrent disease confined to the pelvis, and not extending to the pelvic bones; persistent residual disease following chemoradiation; stage III or IV cancer, often with palliative intent.
- Endometrial cancer: recurrent disease confined centrally to the vaginal vault.
- Vulval or vaginal cancer: primary or recurrent disease of the vulva or vagina involving adjacent pelvic organs.
- Ovarian cancer: rarely used in ovarian cancer; pelvic exenterative surgery may be performed if recurrent disease is confined to the pelvis.

Contraindications for exenteration

Leg pain, lymphedema, and hydronephrosis were regarded as the classic triad of doom and were contraindications for exenterative procedures as they signified nerve involvement, lymphatic involvement, or lateral pelvic sidewall extension, respectively. However, with the practice of lateral pelvic sidewall excision of tumor (Hockel's LEER procedure), unilateral hydronephrosis is not regarded as an absolute contraindication. The following clinical situations are regarded as contraindications for exenteration:

- multifocal or extrapelvic presence of recurrence;
- pelvic or para-aortic nodes found positive for metastasis at frozen section performed at the start of the exenteration;
- lesion larger than 5 cm, where it will be difficult to achieve clear surgical excision margins;
- tumor extending to the lateral pelvic sidewall in close proximity to sacrosciatic notch where possible nerve involvement or infiltration is suspected.

Preoperative preparations

After a potential patient for exenteration has been identified, her case should be discussed formally with the team who will be involved in her subsequent care, and this will include: gynecologic oncologist, colorectal oncologist, urologic oncologist, clinical psychologist, clinical nurse specialists (in gynecologic oncology, colorectal surgery and urology), psychosexual nurse counselor, and nutrition team.

Detailed preoperative assessment requires a thorough evaluation by the gynecologic oncologist followed by appropriate imaging of the disease with CT and/or PET. If the patient is suitable for exenteration, then a careful psychological review needs to take place so that she fully understands the procedure, its associated risks, outcomes, sometimes protracted recovery, and alteration in body image. The clinical nurse specialists in each team need to be involved from the start. Full anesthetic assessment including liaison with an intensive care anesthetist regarding the immediate postoperative care is essential.

Surgical procedure

Adequate staffing of the surgical and anesthetic teams is mandatory as two surgical scrub teams are required for a combined abdominal and vaginal approach. Frozen section facility should be set up to exclude any possible extrapelvic metastatic disease. As these are prolonged operations, careful monitoring and adequate hydration of the patient is essential. An epidural is usually inserted for postoperative analgesia. Vertical midline incision is performed followed by thorough intra-abdominal exploration and taking of samples from pelvic and para-aortic nodes for frozen section analysis.

The success of exenteration depends on obtaining a histologic clearance. Depending on the excision margins, one may obtain total microscopic clearance (referred to as R0), margins with macroscopic clearance but microscopic involvement (referred to as R1), or margins with macroscopic and microscopic involvement (referred to as R2). Compared with R0, R1 has a poorer prognosis and R2 has the least favorable prognosis.

A careful assessment is undertaken of the disease distribution and plans are made for the extent of surgery. An exenteration is performed with curative intent if it is feasible to obtain complete microscopic clearance of tumor (R0), or with palliative intent when the aim is to improve the patient's symptoms and the surgical excision margins are not free of tumor (R2). The latter is performed usually in cases with malignant fistulae or impending bowel obstruction.

Postoperative management

Postoperative management should include adequate hydration, thromboprophylaxis, nutrition supplementation (enteral or parenteral feeding), chest physiotherapy, early mobilization, wound care, and stoma care. The support of a clinical psychologist is crucial in the perioperative period.

Vigilance for complications is necessary. Potential complications include chest, urinary tract, pelvic and wound infections; hematoma; perineal discharge; perineal hernia, chronic perineal discomfort or pain; thrombosis and embolism; anastomotic leakage; stoma complications; ileal conduit complications (pyelonephritis, stone formation, ureteral stricture, urostomy stricture, and renal failure); fistulae; and depression.

Resolution of the case

An MRI scan was arranged to investigate the thickening in the posterior vaginal fornix; it confirmed a 2 × 2 cm lesion suggestive of cancer recurrence, with no obvious nodal involvement or hydronephrosis, indicating probable unifocal recurrence with no extension to pelvic sidewall. The patient underwent an examination under anesthesia and a vault biopsy, which confirmed recurrence of her squamous cell carcinoma of the cervix. As she was young with no other medical comorbidities and had previously been treated with chemoradiotherapy, a total pelvic exenteration was recommended. She was informed about the proposed surgical procedure, its effect on her body image, double stomas, and associated morbidity and mortality. She was assessed by a clinical psychologist and after she was deemed fit to tolerate this extensive surgical procedure both psychologically and physically, she underwent PET-CT to ensure there was no extrapelvic recurrence. She underwent a total pelvic exenteration with ileal conduit and a colostomy. She was managed in the high-dependency unit for 24 hours and carefully monitored on the ward; she made an uncomplicated postoperative recovery. Her histology revealed recurrent cervical cancer with clear excision margins.

Quality of life after exenterative surgery

Although patients report lingering gastrointestinal symptoms and some decline in physical function after exenterative surgery, most adjust well, returning to almost baseline functioning within a year. Providers can counsel patients that many, though not all, symptoms in the first 3 months following exenteration are likely to improve as they adapt to their changed health status [7].

KEY POINTS

Challenge: Pelvic exenteration.

Background
- Exenterations may be offered for central pelvic recurrences when other treatment options are not suitable.
- Exenterations are associated with more than 50% overall 5-year survival rates, but 30–50% risk of morbidity and 8–10% mortality.
- Pelvic exenterations can be anterior, posterior, or total.

Management
- Exenterative surgery requires multidisciplinary management of the patient.
- Psychological assessment and support is important.
- Intraoperative frozen section analysis is useful to provide guidance on the need and extent of exenterative surgery.
- The aim of surgery should be to remove all macroscopic and microscopic lesions.
- Exenteration often requires urinary diversion (Chapter 149) and colostomy (Chapter 37).
- Postoperative management should include adequate hydration, thromboprophylaxis, enteral or parenteral nutrition, chest physiotherapy, early mobilization, wound care, and stoma care.

References

1 Lopez MJ, Petros JG, Augustinos P. Development and evolution of pelvic exenteration: historical notes. *Semin Surg Oncol* 1999;17:147–151.
2 Khoury-Collado F, Einstein MH, Bochner BH *et al*. Pelvic exenteration with curative intent for recurrent uterine malignancies. *Gynecol Oncol* 2012;124: 42–47.
3 Berek JS, Howe C, Lagasse LD, Hacker NF. Pelvic exenteration for recurrent gynecologic malignancy: survival and morbidity analysis of the 45-year experience at UCLA. *Gynecol Oncol* 2005;99:153–159.
4 Andikyan V, Khoury-Collado F, Gerst SR *et al*. Anterior pelvic exenteration with total vaginectomy for recurrent or persistent genitourinary malignancies: review of surgical technique, complications, and outcome. *Gynecol Oncol* 2012;126 :346–350.
5 Brunschwig A. Complete excision of pelvic viscera for advanced carcinoma: a one-stage abdominoperineal operation with end colostomy and bilateral ureteral implantation into the colon above the colostomy. *Cancer* 1948;1:177–183.
6 Höckel M. Laterally extended endopelvic resection (LEER): principles and practice. *Gynecol Oncol* 2008;111(2 Suppl):S13–S17.
7 Rezk YA, Hurley KE, Carter J *et al*. A prospective study of quality of life in patients undergoing pelvic exenteration: interim results. *Gynecol Oncol* 2013;128: 191–197.

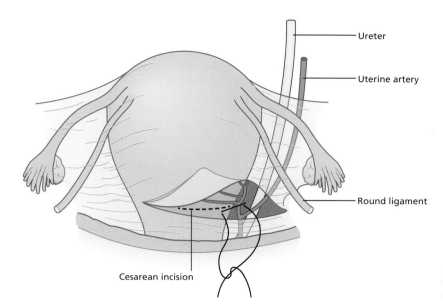

Ureter

Uterine artery

Round ligament

Cesarean incision

Figure 158.6 Uterine artery ligation. *Source*: Adapted from O'Leary, 1995 [3]. Reproduced with permission from the *Journal of Reproductive Medicine*.

Uterine compression sutures

The details of this technique are discussed in Chapter 159.

Uterine artery ligation

Both uterine arteries can be ligated without any risk of devitalizing the uterus, and will often reduce uterine bleeding, especially if this is due to extension of the lower segment incision at cesarean section. Indeed, it is possible that often the uterine artery is ligated inadvertently when such extensions are sutured. It is important to open the broad ligament to visualize the uterine artery before it is ligated, so that one can be sure of avoiding ligation of the ureter (Figure 158.6) [3].

Internal iliac ligation

Internal iliac ligation is a specialist procedure that should only be performed by an experienced surgeon, ideally a vascular surgeon or a gynecologic oncologist. The main dangers are accidentally ligating the external iliac artery and thereby devitalizing the leg, or damaging the internal iliac vein, which lies just behind the artery. If this is torn, it can cause torrential bleeding, and it is very difficult to repair without seriously compromising venous drainage of the pelvis.

Aortic compression

If there is ongoing pelvic hemorrhage that cannot readily be controlled, then the obstetrician should consider temporarily compressing the aorta over the sacral promontory. This can provide good control of hemorrhage until a vascular surgeon arrives. The aorta can be clamped at this point for up to 4 hours before serious tissue damage occurs in the lower limbs, and this approach is often used in vascular repair procedures. Pressure can be applied with the hand, or a suitable atraumatic instrument which has been designed for the purpose.

Cesarean hysterectomy

If it is clear that the above procedures have been unsuccessful and the uterus continues to bleed, a hysterectomy is needed. This is done by addressing the two main pedicles, the ovarian and the uterine artery pedicles. The safest approach is to perform a subtotal hysterectomy first, because if the cervix itself is not bleeding, a subtotal hysterectomy is a simpler and safer alternative to a total

hysterectomy. Even if the cervix is bleeding, once the uterus has been removed, access and visibility are greatly improved, and it may be possible to stop the cervical bleeding with appropriate stitches. The purpose of the procedure is to arrest bleeding, so the procedure should be stopped when the bleeding is controlled. Attempting to complete a total hysterectomy by removing the cervix can sometimes restart the bleeding; removal of the cervix should therefore be reserved for when there is substantial cervical bleeding.

If there is continuous oozing from the pelvic sidewalls without a specific bleeding point being identified, one can consider inserting a Logothetopulos pack (Figure 158.7) [4,5]. This consists of a large sterile plastic bag (which may, for example, have been used as packaging for sterile equipment) packed with sterile gauze and tied at the neck using plastic tubing (e.g., from a sterile intravenous infusion giving set). The tubing is passed through the pelvis and through the vagina, and over the end of the operating table with a weight attached (e.g., a 1-L bag of saline), which applies traction, pulling the pack into the pelvis and applying tamponade to the pelvic sidewalls.

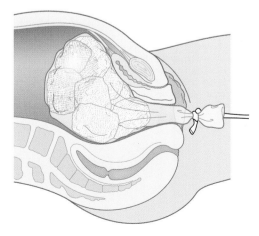

Figure 158.7 Logothetopulos pack [4,5].

Prevention

The birth attendants should be prepared to deal with PPH when it occurs. Such preparation will include having a range of uterotonic drugs, sufficiently senior staff with experience of dealing with PPH, a plan of management that can be promptly implemented, and surgical facilities available should they be needed.

It is wise to avoid iatrogenic factors that can lead to PPH, in particular prolonged infusion of oxytocin at high dosage for augmentation of labor; this is likely to lead to downregulation of the oxytocin receptors, and in such situations the risk of a serious PPH is increased. Prolonged labor in general is an important risk factor, as is a known large baby.

For many years an important prophylactic procedure in otherwise normal labors and deliveries has been the active management of the third stage of labor. This has traditionally included the routine use of uterotonic drugs, early clamping and cutting of the cord, and controlled cord traction [6]. However, recent evidence suggests that early cord clamping maybe disadvantageous for the baby because it limits blood transfusion to the baby from the placenta as the uterus contracts with the placenta still *in situ* [7,8]. Controlled cord traction should therefore be delayed by a few minutes, usually until pulsations stop in the cord.

There are many randomized controlled trials showing that the routine use of oxytocic drugs following delivery of the baby (usually administered either intramuscularly following the delivery of the anterior shoulder, or intravenously following delivery of the baby) reduces PPH rates by approximately 40%. Currently, the most commonly advocated regimen is Syntocinon 10 units i.m. following vaginal birth, or 5 units i.v. over approximately 5 min at cesarean section. An alternative is the uterotonic drug carbetocin, a long-acting Syntocinon analog; there is a heat-stable version of this drug that does not require refrigerated storage, and thus may have an important role in low-income countries.

KEY POINTS

Challenge: Surgical management of postpartum hemorrhage.

Background
- Primary PPH can be caused by uterine atony, vaginal or cervical tears, retained placental tissues, coagulation defects, uterine rupture, and uterine inversion.
- Someone in the delivery team must be nominated to monitor blood loss (this is commonly the anesthetist).

Management
- An emergency PPH protocol should be followed. This should include call for help, assess ABC, give oxygen, give uterotonic drugs, withdraw bloods (for hemoglobin, clotting and cross-match), resuscitate with fluids and blood, and assess and manage cause(s) of bleeding.
- Primary suturing of vaginal or cervical tears:
  - Single or double layer continuous suturing with an absorbable suture is generally appropriate to repair cervical or vaginal tears.
  - If the tear extends to deeper tissues, care should be taken to avoid including ureter, bladder or bowel in the stitches.
- Bimanual compression and uterine massage can produce important temporary reductions in blood loss, which improves visualization and buys time for definitive management.

- Surgical management options include:
  - Insertion and inflation of an intrauterine balloon.
  - Uterine artery embolization.
  - Laparotomy and insertion of uterine compression sutures.
  - Uterine artery ligation.
  - Internal iliac ligation.
  - Aortic compression.
  - Hysterectomy.
- Uterine artery ligation can be a useful and relatively safe maneuver. However, internal iliac ligation should only be done by an expert.
- Aortic compression can be a useful temporary measure to reduce blood loss while expert assistance is obtained.
- A Logothetopulos pack can be used to control diffuse pelvic bleeding following cesarean hysterectomy.

Prevention
- Birth attendants should be competent at recognizing and managing PPH.
- Prolonged use of high-dose oxytocin infusion for labor augmentation should be avoided.
- Prophylactic uterotonic drugs should be routinely recommended as part of management of third stage of labor.

References

1 Belfort MA, Dildy GA, Garrido J, White GL. Intraluminal pressure in a uterine tamponade balloon is curvilinearly related to the volume of fluid infused. *Am J Perinatol* 2011;28:659–666.

2 Tattersall M, Braithwaite W. Balloon tamponade for vaginal lacerations causing severe postpartum haemorrhage. *BJOG* 2007;114:647–648.

3 O'Leary JA. Uterine artery ligation in the control of postcesarean hemorrhage. *J Reprod Med* 1995;40:189–193.

4 Robie GF, Morgan MA, Payne GG Jr, Wasemiller-Smith L. Logothetopulos pack for the management of uncontrollable postpartum hemorrhage. *Am J Perinatol* 1990;7:327–328.

5 Hallak M, Dildy GA III, Hurley TJ, Moise KJ Jr. Transvaginal pressure pack for life-threatening pelvic hemorrhage secondary to placenta accreta. *Obstet Gynecol* 1991;78:938–940.

6 Royal College of Obstetricians and Gynaecologists. RCOG statement on NICE Clinical Guideline No. 55. Intrapartum care: care of healthy women and their babies during childbirth, September 2007. Available at https://www.rcog.org.uk/en/news/rcog-statement-on-nice-clinical-guideline-55-intrapartum-care–care-of-healthy-women-and-their-babies-during-childbirth/. Original NICE guidance available at http://www.nice.org.uk/guidance/CG55

7 Duley L, Batey N. Optimal timing of umbilical cord clamping for term and preterm babies. *Early Hum Dev* 2013;89:905–908.

8 Diaz-Castro J, Florido J, Kajarabille N *et al.* The timing of cord clamping and oxidative stress in term newborns. *Pediatrics* 2014;134:257–264.

CHAPTER 159
Surgical Management of Placenta Praevia

Vibha Giri and Mohan Kumar

Good Hope Hospital, Heart of England NHS Foundation Trust, Sutton Coldfield, West Midlands, UK

Case history: *A woman presented at 35 weeks of gestation with antepartum hemorrhage, with an estimated blood loss of approximately 500 mL. A scan at 32 weeks had identified a major placenta praevia. She has had few mild bleeding episodes in this pregnancy and has already received steroids.*

Background

Placenta praevia occurs when the placenta is implanted either partly or completely into the lower uterine segment. It is an important cause of antepartum hemorrhage and is subclassified as major when the placenta covers the internal cervical os, or minor when the leading edge is not covering the cervical os.

The incidence of placenta praevia has increased in the last two decades and seems to be associated with pregnancy at an older age, termination of pregnancy, and increasing cesarean section rate [1]. Maternal deaths from hemorrhage are rare in the developed world. In the developing countries, with widespread pre-existing anemia, transport difficulties, and limited medical facilities, placenta praevia continues to be a cause of many maternal deaths [2].

Management

Timing of delivery

The timing of delivery depends on maternal and fetal conditions. Elective delivery by cesarean section is recommended at or after 38 weeks of gestation for asymptomatic women with major placenta praevia [3]. However, about 40% of women with major placenta praevia deliver before 38 weeks of gestation. Emergency delivery by cesarean section is indicated in women with vaginal bleeding with fetal heart rate abnormalities, life-threatening maternal hemorrhage, and onset of labor with major praevia [4]. If there is recurrent bleeding, particularly after 34 weeks of gestation, delivery may be considered.

Mode of delivery

There is general consensus that a trial of labor is appropriate if the placenta is more than 20 mm from the internal os, confirmed on a scan at 32–36 weeks of gestation, and if there are no other contraindications to vaginal birth [3,5]. After a diagnosis of low-lying placenta at the mid-trimester scan, a placental localization scan, preferably via the transvaginal route, is recommended at 36 weeks of gestation for minor praevia and at 32 weeks of gestation for major praevia.

For major praevia or placenta less than 20 mm from internal os, a cesarean section is indicated to minimize risk of hemorrhage. There is a place for transvaginal ultrasound scan if fetal head is engaged prior to the planned cesarean section to recheck placental location and distance from the internal cervical os.

Preoperative preparations

Cesarean section should be carried out by senior clinicians in a hospital with blood bank and facilities for high-dependency care. The choice of anesthetic technique must be made by the anesthetist; there is insufficient evidence to support one technique over the others [3,6–8]. At least 2–4 units of packed red cells should be available for delivery [4]. In cases of massive blood loss or suspicion of coexisting abruption, fibrinogen level, Kleihauer test, and prothrombin time should be checked. Cell salvage may be considered, especially in women who refuse donor blood [9,10].

Incision

Cesarean section is usually performed through a transverse or Pfannenstiel skin incision. The surgeon should aim to avoid disrupting the placenta when entering the uterus. Careful ultrasound mapping of the placental site before surgery may assist the surgeon in planning the direction of uterine incision [3,4].

In the case of anterior placenta, a transverse incision is made in the lower uterine segment. The placenta will be met underneath the uterine incision; the baby may be delivered by the obstetrician passing a hand around the margins of the placenta. Occasionally, the placenta is incised if it is not possible to avoid it. If the placenta is cut, the baby should be delivered immediately, and immediate cord clamping is essential to prevent fetal exsanguination.

If the placenta is in anterolateral location, a low vertical incision can be made in the lower uterine segment on the opposite side from the placenta. If the placenta wraps around the cervix from anterior to posterior lower uterine segment, a transverse or vertical incision may be possible above it, although it may lead to extension into upper uterine segment [11,12].

Gynecologic and Obstetric Surgery: Challenges and Management Options, First Edition. Edited by Arri Coomarasamy, Mahmood I. Shafi, G. Willy Davila and Kiong K. Chan.
© 2016 John Wiley & Sons, Ltd. Published 2016 by John Wiley & Sons, Ltd.

Management of hemorrhage

After placental delivery, severe bleeding may occur from the placental bed. It is important to always anticipate massive obstetric hemorrhage in a woman with placenta praevia. Hemostasis may be achieved by one or more of the following.

- Oversewing of the placental bed.
- Circular interrupted ligation around the lower uterine segment both above and below the transverse incision [13].
- Tamponade with an intrauterine balloon (Chapter 158).
- Uterine compression stitches:
  ○ B-Lynch brace suture: has been successfully used with no apparent complications [14].
  ○ Cho's square and Hayman's modification of B-Lynch suture: morbidity and fertility data are limited.
  ○ Parallel vertical compression stitches: a small study has provided reassuring evidence [15].
- Subendometrial vasopressin (4 units in 20 mL of saline) injections into the placental bed [16].
- Bilateral uterine or internal iliac artery ligation (Chapter 158), or uterine artery embolization through interventional radiology.
- Cesarean hysterectomy: performed as a last resort but should not be delayed in cases of life-threatening hemorrhage (Chapter 158).

B-Lynch compression suture [14]

The patient is placed in Lloyd-Davies position for access to the vagina to assess the control of bleeding. The bladder has to be adequately dissected off the lower uterine segment. The uterine cavity is evacuated, examined, and swabbed out. A round-bodied needle

with Monocryl No. 1 suture is used to puncture 3 cm below the left inferior edge of the uterine incision and 3 cm from the lateral border (Figure 159.1). The suture is passed through the uterine cavity to emerge at the upper incision margin 3 cm above and approximately 4 cm from the lateral border (because the uterus widens from below upward). The suture now visible is passed anteriorly, around the fundus and the posterior wall, to enter the uterine cavity at a low level (Figure 159.1b). The suture is pulled under moderate tension assisted by manual compression. The suture is fed through posteriorly and vertically over the fundus to lie anteriorly and vertically compressing the fundus on the right side, in a similar fashion to the left side. The two lengths of the suture are pulled tightly assisted by bimanual compression to minimize trauma, and a secure knot is placed. The lower uterine incision is then closed in one or two layers in the usual way.

Parallel vertical compression sutures [15]

Cesarean section with a Pfannenstiel incision is performed in the usual way. After the placenta is removed, the bladder is reflected downward so as to adequately expose the underlying lower uterine segment. The bladder is retained behind a retractor to keep it away from the uterus.

A No. 1 Monocryl on a round-bodied needle is used to place a stitch through the anterior wall of the lower uterine segment and the posterior wall of the lower segment (Figure 159.2). The needle does not penetrate the entire thickness of the posterior wall (Figure 159.2a). The exact entry and exit sites of the needle can be positioned in the lower segment as needed near the site of active bleeding so as to achieve effective compression of the bleeding vessels. Another suture

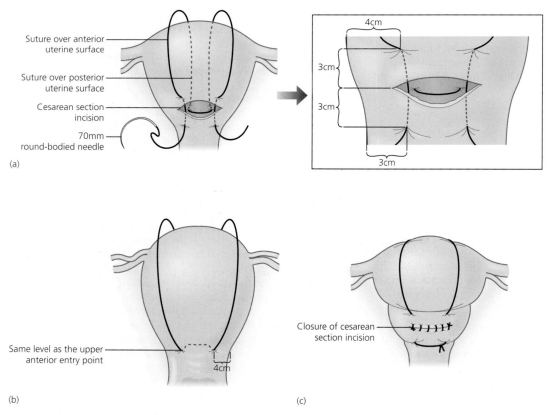

Figure 159.1 Application of the B-Lynch procedure: (a) Anterior view. (b) Posterior view. (c) Anterior view after completion of the procedure. *Source*: Adapted from Keith & B-Lynch, 2005 [17] © B-Lynch 2005.

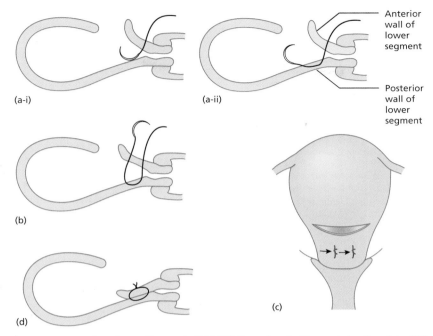

Figure 159.2 Parallel vertical compression stitches. *Source*: Hwu *et al.*, 2005 [15]. Reproduced with permission from John Wiley & Sons, Ltd.

is used in the same manner on the other side. The two vertical sutures are thus parallel to each other (Figure 159.2c).

After placing the sutures, the knots are tied as tightly as possible to compress the lower segment of the uterine cavity by opposing the anterior and posterior walls (Figure 159.2d).The uterine incision is then closed in the usual fashion.

Resolution of the case

After cross-matching 4 units of blood preoperatively, an emergency cesarean section was carried out. Hemostasis was achieved by hemostatic square sutures placed in the placental bed and an intrauterine tamponade balloon.

KEY POINTS

Challenge: Surgical management of placenta praevia.

Background
- Placenta praevia occurs when the placenta is implanted either partly or completely in the lower uterine segment.
- The incidence of placenta praevia has increased in the last two decades and seems to be associated with pregnancy at an older age, termination of pregnancy, and cesarean section.

Management
- Timing of delivery depends on maternal and fetal status.
- Elective delivery by cesarean section is recommended at or after 38 weeks of gestation for asymptomatic women with major placenta praevia or placenta <20 mm from internal cervical os.
- Careful ultrasound mapping of placental site before surgery may assist the surgeon to plan the direction of uterine incision and avoid disrupting the placenta when entering the uterus.

- After placental delivery at cesarean section, hemostasis may be achieved by one or more of the following:
  - Oversewing of the placental bed.
  - Circular interrupted ligation around the lower uterine segment both above and below the transverse incision.
  - Tamponade with an intrauterine balloon.
  - Uterine compression stitches: B-Lynch brace suture or parallel vertical compression stitches.
  - Subendometrial vasopressin (4 units in 20 mL of saline) injections into the placental bed.
  - Bilateral uterine or internal iliac artery ligation, or uterine artery embolization through interventional radiology.
  - Cesarean hysterectomy.
- Hysterectomy is performed as a last resort, but should not be delayed in cases of life-threatening hemorrhage.

References

1 Miller DA, Chollet JA, Goodwin TM. Clinical risk factors for placenta praevia–placenta accreta. *Am J Obstet Gynecol* 1997;177:210–214.
2 Neilson JP. Interventions for suspected placenta praevia. *Cochrane Database Syst Rev* 2003;(2):CD001998.
3 Royal College of Obstetricians and Gynaecologists. *Placenta Praevia, Placenta Praevia Accreta and Vasa Praevia: Diagnosis and Management*. RCOG Green-top Guideline No. 27, January 2011. Available at https://www.rcog.org.uk/en/guide-lines-research-services/guidelines/gtg27/
4 Lockwood CJ, Russo-Stieglitz K. Clinical features, diagnosis, and course of placenta previa. *UpToDate*, May 5, 2014. http://www.uptodate.com/contents/clinical-features-diagnosis-and-course-of-placenta-previa#H2532737269
5 Bhide A, Prefumo F, Moore J, Hollis B, Thilaganathan B. Placental edge to internal os distance in the late third trimester and mode of delivery in placenta praevia. *BJOG* 2003;110:860–864.

6   Bonner SM, Haynes SR, Ryall D. The anaesthetic management of caesarean section for placenta praevia: a questionnaire survey. *Anaesthesia* 1995;50:992–994.

7   Parekh N, Husaini SW, Russell IF. Ceasarean section for placenta praevia: a retrospective study of anaesthetic management. *Br J Anaesth* 2000;84:725–730.

8   Peel WJ. A survey of the anaesthetic management of patients presenting for caesarean section with high risk obstetric conditions. *Int J Obstet Anesth* 1996;5:219–220.

9   Yamada T, Mori H, Ueki M. Autologous blood transfusion in patients with placenta previa. *Acta Obstet Gynecol Scand* 2005;84:255–259.

10 Watanabe N, Suzuki T, Ogawa K, Kubo T, Sago H. Five-year study assessing the feasibility and safety of autologous blood transfusion in pregnant Japanese women. *Obstet Gynaecol Res* 2011;37:1773–1777.

11 Kayem G, Davy C, Goffinet F, Thomas C, Clément D, Cabrol D. Conservative versus extirpative management in cases of placenta accreta. *Obstet Gynecol* 2004;104:531–536.

12 Kotsuji F, Nishijima K, Kurokawa T *et al*. Transverse uterine fundal incision for placenta praevia with accreta, involving the entire anterior uterine wall: a case series. *BJOG* 2013;120:1144–1149.

13 Joy S. Placenta previa: treatment and management. *Medscape*, updated March 23, 2015. Available at http://emedicine.medscape.com/article/262063-treatment

14 B-Lynch C, Coker A, Lawal AH, Abu J, Cowen MJ. The B-Lynch surgical technique for the control of massive postpartum haemorrhage: an alternative to hysterectomy? Five cases reported. *BJOG* 1997;104:372–375.

15 Hwu YM, Chen CP, Chen HS, Su TH. Parallel vertical compression sutures: a technique to control bleeding from placenta praevia or accreta during caesarean section. *BJOG* 2005;112:1420–1423.

16 Kato S, Tanabe A, Kanki K *et al*. Local injection of vasopressin reduces the blood loss during cesarean section in placenta previa. *J Obstet Gynaecol Res* 2014;40:1249–1256.

17 Keith LG, B-Lynch C. Surgical management of intractable pelvic hemorrhage. Available at http://www.cblynch.co.uk/surgical-management-of-intractable-pelvic-hemorrhage/ (accessed October 2014).

CHAPTER 160

Surgical Management of Placenta Accreta

Vibha Giri and Mohan Kumar

Good Hope Hospital, Heart of England NHS Foundation Trust, Sutton Coldfield, West Midlands, UK

Case history: A 28-year-old woman with two previous cesarean sections was found to have an anterior low-lying placenta on a mid-trimester scan. A follow-up scan at 32 weeks showed features suggestive of placenta accreta.

Background

Placenta accreta occurs in approximately 1 in 2500 pregnancies (Figure 160.1). Placenta accreta can be classified as follows.
- Placenta accreta vera: villi are attached directly to the myometrium, but do not invade it (75–80%).
- Placenta increta: villi invade the myometrium (17%).
- Placenta percreta: villi invade beyond the whole myometrium, and possibly into other organs such as the bladder (5%).

The incidence of placenta accreta has increased and seems to parallel the rising cesarean section rate [1]. Three-quarters of placenta accreta are associated with placenta praevia (Chapter 159). The risk of accreta in women with placenta praevia increases from 24% with one previous cesarean section to 67% with three or more cesarean sections [2]. Other predisposing factors for placenta praevia include advanced maternal age, high parity, any condition resulting in myometrial damage such as previous myomectomy, intrauterine adhesions, submucous leiomyoma, endometrial ablation, and uterine artery embolization [3–5].

Management

Placenta accreta is a potentially life-threatening condition that requires a multidisciplinary approach to management.

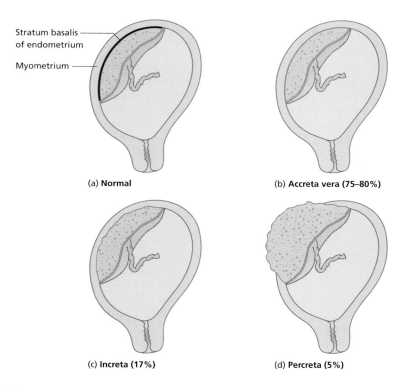

Figure 160.1 (a–d) Classification of placenta accreta.
Source: http://en.wikipedia.org/wiki/Placenta_accreta

Gynecologic and Obstetric Surgery: Challenges and Management Options, First Edition. Edited by Arri Coomarasamy, Mahmood I. Shafi, G. Willy Davila and Kiong K. Chan.
© 2016 John Wiley & Sons, Ltd. Published 2016 by John Wiley & Sons, Ltd.

Diagnosis

Women who have had a previous cesarean section and now have a placenta praevia or an anterior placenta underlying an old cesarean section scar should be evaluated for placenta accreta, and managed as if they have placenta accreta [6]. Diagnosis is usually established by ultrasonography. The use of three-dimensional power Doppler and color Doppler can further help to improve the diagnosis [6–8].

If placenta percreta is suspected, in addition to ultrasonography, MRI and cystoscopy may be indicated to evaluate the extent of the placental invasion. Gross hematuria is rare even when the bladder is invaded [9].

Preoperative planning

The optimum gestation for scheduled delivery is controversial. For asymptomatic women, elective delivery by cesarean section at 36–37 weeks of gestation is generally recommended [6].

The multidisciplinary team may include an obstetrician, pelvic surgeon or gynecologic oncologist, anesthetist, intensivist, neonatologist, urologist, hematologist, and interventional radiologist [1,6,10]. Current recommendations for blood replacement in trauma situations support transfusion of packed red blood cells and fresh frozen plasma (FFP) in a 1:1 ratio, and these should be made available in the operating room [1]. Where available, cell salvage should be considered, particularly if the woman refuses donor blood.

Pneumatic compression stockings should be placed preoperatively, and continued until the patient is fully ambulatory. Prophylactic antibiotics should be given, particularly if the surgery is prolonged or if estimated blood loss exceeds 2 L. For patients with suspected percreta, preoperative cystoscopy with placement of ureteric stents may help prevent inadvertent urinary tract injury [11].

The risk of hysterectomy should be discussed with the patient.

Incision

The choice of skin and uterine incisions will depend on the location of the placenta. It is useful to perform ultrasound mapping of the placental site before surgery [1,6]. A classical (vertical) uterine incision, often transfundal, may be necessary to avoid the placenta and allow delivery of the baby. Planned attempt at manual removal of the placenta should be avoided [1]. A high transverse incision above the upper border of the placenta has also been suggested by some authors [12].

Uterine conservation

A decision will need to be made on whether manual placental removal in pieces is a reasonable option, or a hysterectomy is indicated. The removal of placenta in pieces may be possible if placental bed invasion is minimal; however, any adherent pieces of placenta will need to be left behind, and any bleeding should be controlled. The majority of patients in whom uterine conservation is attempted will need additional treatment for control of hemorrhage, including arterial embolization, arterial ligation, and balloon tamponade [13].

Leaving the placenta *in situ* in the uterus, with or without the addition of methotrexate treatment, has been reported as an option. However, this approach can be associated with severe vaginal bleeding (53%), sepsis (6%), secondary hysterectomy (19%), and maternal mortality [14]. If a patient opts to have this approach, she should be counseled about these risks.

Delivery with hysterectomy

The recommended management of placenta accreta is generally a planned cesarean hysterectomy with the placenta left *in situ*. After delivery of the baby, the cord is cut close to the placenta, the uterine incision is sewn circumferentially or using a whip stitch, and a hysterectomy is performed [1]. This approach may not be considered first line for women who have a strong desire for future fertility; conservative management may be tried in these cases.

Focal accreta

Separated placenta needs to be delivered, and hemorrhage should be controlled in the usual way. Adherent portions should be left attached. It may be possible to remove a small wedge of uterine tissue with adherent placenta, followed by repair of the defect.

Fundal or posterior accreta

Uterine conservation may be a reasonable option for a posterior or fundal accreta since bleeding after placenta removal may be more readily controlled with interventional radiology or balloon tamponade in these areas. The option of hysterectomy is still available if bleeding cannot be controlled.

Placenta percreta with bladder invasion

Preoperative cystoscopy with ureteric stenting should be considered if bladder invasion is suspected. Treatment usually involves partial cystectomy with repair of the bladder [15,16]. A urologist should be involved in the management of these cases. Anterior bladder cystotomy is recommended for defining dissection planes; it also helps in assessing the degree of bladder involvement and determining whether posterior wall resection is required [17,18].

Follow-up of women who have uterus-conserving surgery

Women should be warned of the risks of bleeding and infection. Prophylactic antibiotics are recommended. Neither methotrexate nor arterial embolization reduces the risks and neither is recommended routinely [6]. Follow-up of women with weekly HCG and ultrasound serial scans to check placental resolution is recommended.

Prevention

As placenta accreta is mostly a consequence of the rising cesarean section rate, proactive measures to reduce the number of cesarean sections will help to reduce both placenta praevia and placenta accreta. Avoidance of vigorous uterine curettage and measures to prevent formation of intrauterine adhesions can help to reduce the incidence of placenta accreta. All patients with previous cesarean section and placenta praevia should be assessed for ultrasonographic evidence of placenta accreta.

KEY POINTS

Challenge: Management of placenta accreta.

Background
- Placenta accreta is a life-threatening obstetric condition.
- Three-quarters of cases of placenta accreta are associated with placenta praevia.

Management

Diagnosis
- Diagnosis is usually established by ultrasonography.
- MRI is considered useful when scan findings are ambiguous.
- A cystoscopy may be needed if bladder involvement is suspected.

Preoperative planning
- Multidisciplinary involvement is recommended.
- Packed red blood cells and thawed FFP should be made available in the operating room.
- Ultrasound mapping of the placental site before surgery helps to plot the extent of placenta and plan both skin and uterine incisions.

Surgical approach
- A classical or vertical uterine incision (often transfundal) may be necessary to avoid the placenta and allow delivery of the baby.
- If considering cesarean hysterectomy, then placenta should be left *in situ*.
- If uterine conservation is to be attempted, the options are:
  - Removal of placenta in pieces (suitable only in women with superficial accreta), followed by hemostatic procedures (e.g., oversewing of placental bed, uterine artery embolization, and uterine balloon tamponade).
  - Leaving placenta *in situ* in the uterus, with or without the addition of methotrexate treatment.
- The recommended management of placenta accreta is generally a planned cesarean hysterectomy.
- If there is bladder involvement, the patient may require partial cystectomy with repair of the bladder.
- Women who have uterus-conserving surgery should receive prophylactic antibiotics, and weekly HCG and serial ultrasound scans to check on placental resolution.

Prevention
- Attempts should be made to reduce the cesarean section rate.
- All patients with previous cesarean section and placenta praevia should be assessed for ultrasonographic evidence of placenta accreta.

References

1 American College of Obstetricians and Gynecologists. ACOG Committee opinion No. 529, July 2012. Placenta accreta. *Obstet Gynecol* 2012;120:207.

2 Clark SL, Koonings PP, Phelan JP, Read JA, Cotton DB, Miller FC. Placenta previa/accreta and prior cesarean section. *Obstet Gynecol* 1985;66:89-92.

3 Al-Serehi A, Mhoyan A, Brown M, Benirschke K, Hull A, Pretorius DH. Placenta accreta: an association with fibroids and Asherman syndrome. *J Ultrasound Med* 2008;27:1623–1628.

4 Hamar BD, Wolff EF, Kodaman PH, Marcovici I. Premature rupture of membranes, placenta increta, and hysterectomy in a pregnancy following endometrial ablation. *J Perinatol* 2006;26:135–137.

5 Pron G, Mocarski E, Bennett J, Vilos G, Common A, Vanderburgh L. Pregnancy after uterine artery embolization for leiomyomata: the Ontario multicenter trial. *Obstet Gynecol* 2005;105:67–76.

6 Royal College of Obstetricians and Gynaecologists. *Placenta Praevia, Placenta Praevia Accreta and Vasa Praevia: Diagnosis and Management*. RCOG Green-top Guideline No. 27, January 2011. Available at https://www.rcog.org.uk/en/guidelines-research-services/guidelines/gtg27/

7 Comstock CH. Antenatal diagnosis of placenta accreta: a review. *Ultrasound Obstet Gynecol* 2005;26:89–96.

8 Warshak CR, Eskander R, Hull AD *et al*. Accuracy of ultrasonography and magnetic resonance imaging in the diagnosis of placenta accreta. *Obstet Gynecol* 2006;108:573–581.

9 Takai N, Eto M, Sato F, Mimata H, Miyakawa I. Placenta percreta invading the urinary bladder. *Arch Gynecol Obstet* 2005;271:274–275.

10 Eller AG, Bennett MA, Sharshiner M *et al*. Maternal morbidity in cases of placenta accreta managed by a multidisciplinary care team compared with standard obstetric care. *Obstet Gynecol* 2011;117:331–337.

11 Tam Tam KB, Dozier J, Martin JN Jr. Approaches to reduce urinary tract injury during management of placenta accreta, increta and percreta: a systematic review. *J Matern Fetal Neonatal Med* 2012;25:329–334.

12 Chandraharan E, Rao S, Belli AM, Arulkumaran S. The Triple-P procedure as a conservative surgical alternative to peripartum hysterectomy for placenta percreta. *Int J Gynaecol Obstet* 2012;117:191–194.

13 Bretelle F, Courbiere B, Mazouni C *et al*. Management of placenta accreta: morbidity and outcome. *Eur J Obstet Gynecol Reprod Biol* 2007;133:34–39.

14 Steins Bisschop CN, Schaap TP, Vogelvang TE, Scholten PC. Invasive placentation and uterus preserving treatment modalities: a systematic review. *Arch Gynecol Obstet* 2011;284:491–502.

15 Washecka R, Behling A. Urologic complications of placenta percreta invading the urinary bladder: a case report and review of literature. *Hawaii Med J* 2002;61:66–69.

16 Matsubara S. Ureteral catheter is useful to prevent ureteral injuries not only for gynaecologic surgery but also for caesarean hysterectomy for placenta previa accreta: the obstetrician's opinion. *Urologica* 2014;81:187–188.

17 Abbas F, Talati J, Wasti S, Akram S, Ghaffar S, Qureshi R. Placenta percreta with bladder invasion as a cause of life threatening hemorrhage. *J Urol* 2000;164:1270–1274

18 Bakri YN, Sundin T. Cystotomy for placenta previa percreta with bladder invasion. *Urology* 1992;40:580.

CHAPTER 161

Surgical Management Options for Shoulder Dystocia: Zavanelli Maneuver, Abdominal Rescue, Symphysiotomy, and Cleidotomy

Syeda Batool Mazhar and Asia Nazir
Pakistan Institute of Medical Sciences, Islamabad, Pakistan

Case history: *A woman had a prolonged second stage of labor, necessitating an outlet forceps delivery. The fetal head was delivered with ease; however, the shoulders did not deliver over the next 2 min despite suprapubic pressure and McRoberts maneuver.*

Background

Shoulder dystocia occurs when either the anterior or, less commonly, the posterior fetal shoulder is impacted on the maternal symphysis or sacral promontory, respectively. Shoulder dystocia complicates 0.6–1.4% of vaginal deliveries [1]. There can be significant perinatal morbidity and mortality associated with the condition, even when it is managed appropriately. Brachial plexus injury (BPI) is one of the most important fetal complications of shoulder dystocia, complicating 2.3–16% of such deliveries. Most cases of BPI resolve without permanent disability, with fewer than 10% resulting in permanent neurologic dysfunction. Maternal morbidity is increased, particularly the incidence of postpartum hemorrhage (11%), and third and fourth-degree perineal tears (3.8%) [1].

The risk factors for shoulder dystocia are maternal BMI greater than 30 kg/m², previous shoulder dystocia, macrosomia above 4.5 kg, diabetes mellitus, induction of labor, oxytocin augmentation, prolonged first or second stage of labor, and assisted vaginal delivery [1,2].

Management

Details of first-line and second-line management maneuvers can be found in standard obstetric textbooks and clinical guidelines [1,2], and are not addressed in this surgical textbook. In this chapter, we focus on third-line surgical approaches. However, two useful mnemonics for the management approach to shoulder dystocia are worth recounting here: MAPS (M, McRoberts maneuver; A, anterior shoulder delivery; P, posterior shoulder delivery; S, salvage maneuvers) [3], and HELPERR (H, call for help; E, evaluate for episiotomy; L, legs (McRoberts maneuver); P, suprapubic pressure; E, enter (rotational maneuvers); R, remove the posterior arm; R, roll the patient to her hands and knees) [4].

If first-line and second-line maneuvers are unsuccessful, the following third-line procedures are considered as a last resort: Zavanelli maneuver, abdominal rescue, symphysiotomy, and clavicular fracture. Less frequently, Shute parallel forceps [5] for fetal shoulder rotation, use of a shoulder horn [6], and posterior axillary sling traction [7] have been used.

Cephalic replacement (Zavanelli maneuver)

The patient is prepared for a cesarean section delivery, and a tocolytic drug (e.g., terbutaline) is administered to facilitate the maneuver. The head is replaced with constant and firm pressure on the occiput with the palm of one hand, while depressing the posterior vaginal wall with the other hand [8]. If the head has rotated to the side, it must first be rotated to occiput-anterior or occiput-posterior position, followed by flexion of the head, and slow replacement into the vagina. The head is pushed to the level of zero station. A Foley catheter is inserted, and a cesarean section is carried out. A cesarean section at full cervical dilation poses several challenges, and the operator needs to be prepared to tackle these (Chapter 157).

Continuous fetal surveillance is necessary during the procedure of cephalic replacement; often there is an episode of bradycardia for 2–4 min, but the CTG normally recovers soon after the fetal head has been replaced in the vagina [8]. Sepsis is the most common postpartum complication after cephalic replacement, and therefore antibiotics should be prescribed. Uterine rupture is the most serious complication, with a reported incidence of 5%, often requiring emergency hysterectomy.

Abdominal rescue

If the Zavanelli maneuver fails, one option is to proceed with a lower segment uterine incision to allow manual rotation of the anterior shoulder into an oblique diameter, permitting descent of the shoulders. Through the uterine incision, the fetal shoulder is pushed below the symphysis pubis, followed by a vaginal delivery. Failure of abdominal rescue after an unsuccessful Zavanelli maneuver has been corrected by breech extraction through the hysterotomy [9].

Symphysiotomy

The cartilage joining the pubic bones can be surgically divided to increase the size of the pelvic outlet to help with the delivery of an obstructed fetus (cephalopelvic disproportion) or as a third-line management approach to shoulder dystocia [10]. The procedure may have a particular role in low-resource countries where access to cesarean operations can be limited. A WHO commentary noted

Gynecologic and Obstetric Surgery: Challenges and Management Options, First Edition. Edited by Arri Coomarasamy, Mahmood I. Shafi, G. Willy Davila and Kiong K. Chan.
© 2016 John Wiley & Sons, Ltd. Published 2016 by John Wiley & Sons, Ltd.

that symphysiotomy is controversial, but could be a life-saving intervention [11].

To perform a symphysiotomy, an indwelling catheter is first inserted. The patient's thighs are abducted to 80° and steadied by two assistants. Local anesthesia is infiltrated into the skin over the symphysis pubis and into the joint. The index and middle fingers of the left hand are inserted into the vagina and placed against the posterior aspect of the symphysis; the urethra (with the indwelling catheter inside it) is now pushed to the side with the index finger, and the middle finger is used to monitor the forthcoming action of the scalpel (Figure 161.1). A 2-cm vertical skin incision is made over the mons pubis; the scalpel is held vertical and advanced further down to incise the fibrocartilaginous symphysis joint. A 2–3 cm symphyseal separation is achieved [12]. The patient is catheterized for 5 days, immobilized for 3 days, allowed to sit on the fourth day, and can have a walk on the fifth day. Full ambulation and pelvic stability is achieved soon afterwards, but the patient is advised against undue physical activity for 3 months.

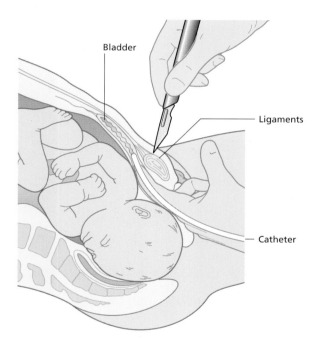

Figure 161.1 Symphysiotomy technique.

The complications of this procedure include hemorrhage, retropubic hematoma (mostly self-limiting), and soft-tissue trauma to bladder and urethra.

Cleidotomy

Cleidotomy is the deliberate fracture of the fetal clavicle to reduce the fetal bisacromial diameter [1,2]. The safest site is the mid-portion of the clavicle; by applying upward digital pressure the risk of subclavicular vascular injury can be reduced. Fractures of the clavicle usually heal rapidly without permanent sequelae.

Prevention

Risk assessment for the prediction of shoulder dystocia is not accurate enough to allow prevention in the majority of cases. However, elective cesarean section can be considered for high-risk women, for example women with fetuses with an estimated weight greater than 5 kg, or women with diabetes and a large fetus.

Practical training using mannequins has been associated with improvements in the management in simulation and in clinical practice.

KEY POINTS

Challenge: Third-line surgical options for shoulder dystocia.

Background
- If first-line and second-line maneuvers for shoulder dystocia are unsuccessful, the following third-line procedures can be considered as a last resort:
  - Cephalic replacement (Zavanelli maneuver).
  - Abdominal rescue.
  - Symphysiotomy.
  - Clavicular fracture (cleidotomy).

Surgical (third-line) management
Cephalic replacement (Zavanelli maneuver)
- Prepare for cesarean section.
- Administer a tocolytic drug.
- Rotate the head to occiput-anterior or occiput-posterior position, flex the head, and slowly push it into the vagina, to reach zero station.
- Insert a Foley catheter into the bladder.
- Perform a cesarean section.

Abdominal rescue
- Open the abdomen and perform a lower segment transverse uterine incision.
- Dislodge the anterior shoulder from the pubic symphysis, and manually rotate it to an oblique diameter to permit descent into the pelvis.
- Carry out a vaginal delivery.

Symphysiotomy
- Insert an indwelling catheter.
- Abduct patient's thighs to 80° and stabilize them.
- Infiltrate the skin over the symphysis pubis and the joint with local anesthetic drugs.
- Place index and middle fingers in the vagina and push the urethra (with the catheter inside it) to the side.
- Make a 2-cm skin incision over the symphyseal joint, and extend the incision into the joint with a vertically held knife.
- Keep the patient catheterized for 5 days, and immobilized for 3 days.

Cleidotomy
- Apply upward digital pressure in the mid-portion of the clavicle.

Prevention
- Consider elective cesarean section in high-risk women.
- Ensure the obstetric team has regular practical training in managing emergencies, including shoulder dystocia.

References

1 American College of Obstetricians and Gynecologists. ACOG Practice Bulletin 40. Shoulder dystocia. *Obstet Gynecol* 2002;100:1045–1050.

2 Royal College of Obstetricians and Gynaecologists. *Shoulder Dystocia*. RCOG Green-top Guideline No. 42, 2nd edn, March 2012. https://www.rcog.org.uk/en/guidelines-research-services/guidelines/gtg42/

3 Cluver CA, Hofmeyr GJ. Shoulder dystocia: an update and review of new technique. *S Afr J Obstet Gynaecol* 2009;15:90–93.

4 Baxley EG, Gobbo RW. Shoulder dystocia. *Am Fam Physician* 2004;69:1707–1714.

5 Shute WB. Management of shoulder dystocia with the Shute/parallel dystocia forceps. *Am J Obstet Gynecol* 1962;84:936–939.

6 Chavis WM. A new instrument for the management of shoulder dystocia. *Int J Gynecol Obstet 1978–1979*;16:331–332.

7 Hoffmyer GJ, Cluver CA. Posterior axilla sling traction for intractable shoulder dystocia. *BJOG* 2009;116:1818–1820.

8 O'Leary JA (ed.) *Shoulder Dystocia and Birth Injury: Prevention and Treatment.* Humana Press, Totowa, NJ, 2009.

9 O'Shaughnessy MJ. Hysterotomy facilitation of the vaginal delivery of the posterior arm in a case of severe shoulder dystocia. *Obstet Gynecol* 1998;92:693–695.

10 Gebbie DAM. Symphysiotomy. *Clin Obstet Gynaecol* 1982;9:663–683.

11 Tukur J. Symphysiotomy for feto-pelvic disproportion (last revised 1 October 2011). *The WHO Reproductive Health Library.* World Health Organization, Geneva.

12 Bergstrom S, Hojer B, Liljestrand J, Tunell R. Appendix III: Symphysiotomy. Appendix IV: Cesarean section under local anesthesia. In: *Perinatal Health Care with Limited Resources*, pp. 164–177. Macmillan Education, London, 1994.

CHAPTER 162
Uterine Inversion

Phil Steer

Faculty of Medicine, Imperial College London, London, UK

Case history: *A multiparous woman has a quick labor and delivery, with the first stage of labor lasting only 3 hours, and the baby delivering precipitately with only three pushes. There is a sudden gush of bleeding per vaginam and she collapses, and becomes pale and sweaty with a pulse rate of 160 bpm. The placenta appears at the vaginal introitus but attempts to deliver it are unsuccessful and the woman's condition continues to deteriorate.*

Background

Inversion of the uterus is rare [1]. Because of its rarity, many obstetricians and midwives may never manage a case in their career. However, it is a serious obstetric emergency that requires prompt and effective management to ensure good outcomes.

Pulling on the umbilical cord excessively before separation of the placenta is believed to contribute to this condition. Predisposing factors include multiparity, a broad uterine shape (including bicornuate), a fundal placenta, short umbilical cord, retained or adherent placenta, and precipitate labor [1].

It can cause severe postpartum hemorrhage (94% of women), sudden cardiovascular collapse or shock (39% of women), infection, and severe abdominal pain [2,3].

Management

The first steps of management are similar to other obstetric emergencies: calling for help, securing airway, breathing and circulation (ABC), and proceeding to treat the condition. The patient should be resuscitated by placing at least two large-bore intravenous cannulas and infusing crystalloid or colloid fluid. Blood should be withdrawn for full blood count, clotting and cross-match.

There are two non-surgical methods for replacing the uterus: manual replacement and hydrostatic methods. If these fail then surgery can be considered.

Non-surgical methods
The uterus and the attached placenta should ideally be replaced as soon as possible, before the lower segment and cervix start to contract, trapping the body of the uterus in the inverted position. Attempts to remove the placenta should not be made until the uterus is replaced, because this is only likely to increase bleeding

and waste time, although in some cases it detaches spontaneously. Immediate replacement is possible in 43–88% of women [3].

The manual replacement technique involves placing the whole hand in the vagina, and lifting the uterus while holding the fundus in the palm, and keeping the tips of the fingers at the uterocervical junction [1,4].

The hydrostatic method was first described by O'Sullivan [4] in 1945, and consists of filling the vagina with up to 3 L of warm normal saline (the fluid is infused using an intravenous giving set, and the hand of the accoucheur is used to block the introitus and prevent the fluid leaking out). This expands the cervix and the hydrostatic pressure of the infused fluid pushes the uterus back into the usual position. A useful modification of the original technique consists of using a Silastic vacuum extractor to produce a seal at the vaginal introitus (Figure 162.1), preventing the infused normal saline from leaking out [5]. This is more efficient than using the operator's hand to seal the introitus. Sometimes it is necessary to give a uterine relaxant drug such as magnesium sulfate, nitroglycerine, or a β-adrenergic agonist such as terbutaline. Occasionally, general anesthesia will be needed, in which case uterine relaxant anesthetics such as halothane can be

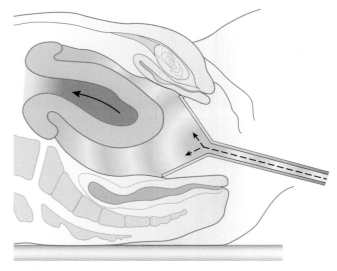

Figure 162.1 Use of the Silastic vacuum extractor to facilitate the O'Sullivan hydrostatic uterine replacement technique.

Gynecologic and Obstetric Surgery: Challenges and Management Options, First Edition. Edited by Arri Coomarasamy, Mahmood I. Shafi, G. Willy Davila and Kiong K. Chan.
© 2016 John Wiley & Sons, Ltd. Published 2016 by John Wiley & Sons, Ltd.

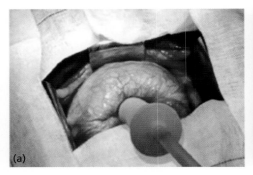
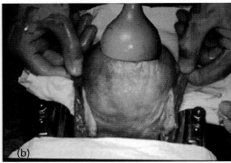

Figure 162.2 (a) An obstetric ventouse applied to the inverted uterine fundus. (b) Reduction of the inverted uterus after traction with the ventouse. *Source:* Antonelli *et al.*, 2006 [6]. Reproduced with permission from John Wiley & Sons, Ltd.

used, although it is best if possible to avoid uterine relaxants as these are likely to increase blood loss.

Surgical methods

If vaginal maneuvers are not successful, then it is necessary to consider an operative technique. Standard surgical methods include surgical exposure of the inversion site and upward traction of the inverted uterine fundus. This can be done together with a longitudinal incision to the cervical ring posteriorly to facilitate uterine replacement. In 2006, Antonelli and colleagues [6] described the use of the ventouse, not per vaginam but at laparotomy. The ventouse is inserted through the inversion and then suction is applied, allowing traction on the fundus to pull the uterus back into position (Figure 162.2). It has even been suggested that correction of the inversion can be done laparoscopically by pushing the fundus of the uterus from below and applying counter-pressure using a laparoscopic instrument to prevent undue stretching of the parauterine ligaments (Figure 162.3) [7].

Prevention

Uncontrolled traction on the umbilical cord should be avoided, particularly in parous women. Early recognition of uterine inversion is important as (i) non-surgical replacement is more likely to work soon after the inversion, before the cervix has contracted, and (ii) the sooner the inversion is reversed, the quicker the control of postpartum hemorrhage. Women who have had uterine inversion should be given broad-spectrum antibiotics to prevent endometritis and pelvic infection. As soon as uterine inversion is corrected, uterotonic drugs should be commenced to prevent recurrence of uterine inversion.

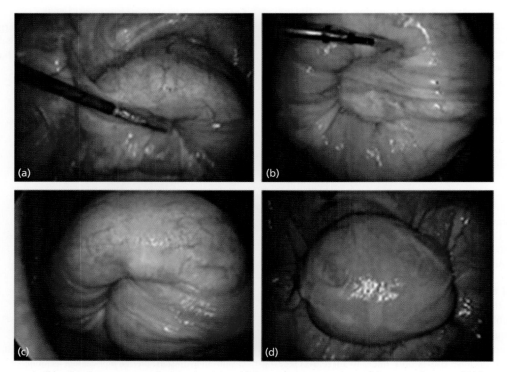

Figure 162.3 Laparoscopically assisted management of uterine inversion. (a) Laparoscopic appearance of the inverted uterus; (b) a laparoscopic forceps being used to provide counter-pressure on the inverted uterus; (c) partial reduction is achieved, with further reduction completed using a 10-mm blunt-tipped Teflon rod to press down on the inverted uterus; (d) complete reduction is achieved. Source: Vijayaraghavan & Sujatha, 2006 [7]. Reproduced with permission from John Wiley & Sons, Ltd.

KEY POINTS

Challenge: Management of uterine inversion.

Background
- Uterine inversion is a rare but serious complication.
- Risk factors include excessive cord traction, multiparity, broad uterine shape, fundal placenta, short umbilical cord, retained or adherent placenta, and precipitate labor.

Management
- First steps of management include calling for help, assessing and managing ABC, providing fluid resuscitation, and arranging blood count, clotting and cross-match.
- Uterine inversion is best managed by immediate replacement if possible. Reposition the uterus (with the placenta still attached) by slowly and steadily pushing upward.
- If this fails then a general anesthetic is usually required. The uterus may then be returned by placing a fist on the fundus and gradually pushing it back manually into the pelvis through the cervix.

- The next step is use of the O'Sullivan hydrostatic technique, and a vacuum extractor can be used to improve the vaginal seal.
- If vaginal approaches are not successful, it will be necessary to resort to a laparotomy or laparoscopy, permitting a combined transabdominal and transvaginal reduction of the inversion. A longitudinal incision to the cervical ring posteriorly may be necessary to facilitate uterine replacement.
- Uterine relaxants or general anesthesia may relax the cervix, aiding uterine replacement.

Prevention
- Uncontrolled cord traction should be avoided.
- Early recognition of inversion is important to minimize morbidity.
- Women with uterine inversion should be given prophylactic antibiotics to prevent endometritis.
- As soon as the uterine inversion is corrected, uterotonic drugs should be commenced to prevent recurrence of inversion.

References

1 Calder A. Emergencies in operative obstetrics. *Best Pract Res Clin Obstet Gynaecol* 2000;14:43–55.

2 Beringer RM, Patteril M. Puerperal uterine inversion and shock. *Br J Anaesth* 2004;92:439–441.

3 Mehra U, Ostapowicz F. Acute puerperal inversion of the uterus in a primipara. *Obstet Gynecol* 1976;47:30S–32S.

4 O'Sullivan JV. Acute inversion of the uterus. *BMJ* 1945;2:282–283.

5 Ogueh O, Ayida G. Acute uterine inversion: a new technique of hydrostatic replacement. *Br J Obstet Gynaecol* 1997;104:951–952.

6 Antonelli E, Irion O, Tolck P, Morales M. Subacute uterine inversion: description of a novel replacement technique using the obstetric ventouse. *BJOG* 2006;113:846–847.

7 Vijayaraghavan R, Sujatha Y. Acute postpartum uterine inversion with haemorrhagic shock: laparoscopic reduction: a new method of management? *BJOG* 2006;113:1100–1102.

CHAPTER 163

Episiotomy and Second-degree Tear

Khaled M.K. Ismail and Sara S. Webb

Birmingham Women's NHS Foundation Trust, Birmingham, UK

Case history: A nulliparous woman, with meconium-stained liquor, has been pushing for 90 min. The vertex is advancing well with good maternal pushing. The fetal heart rate is now demonstrating late, prolonged decelerations.

Background

Perineal injuries during childbirth are common and most occur at the vaginal orifice as the baby's head delivers. Perineal tears related to childbirth are classified according to the anatomic structures involved: first degree (skin only), second degree (perineal muscles and skin), third degree (injury to the anal sphincter complex), and fourth degree (injury to the perineum, anal sphincter complex, and rectal epithelium).

An episiotomy is a deliberate surgical incision through the perineum and perineal body, performed during the last part of the second stage of labor or delivery, in order to enlarge the vaginal orifice and facilitate birth [1,2]. Episiotomy has become one of the most commonly performed surgical procedures worldwide, with mediolateral and midline incisions being the most common types chosen. By enlarging the vaginal opening, an episiotomy enables more room to allow easier forceps application or procedures to be undertaken during fetal shoulder dystocia. There is a growing body of evidence suggesting that the angle of the episiotomy affects the risk of obstetric anal sphincter injury. Moreover, the type of episiotomy performed may also impact on the extent of perineal trauma, with midline episiotomies associated with a higher risk of obstetric anal sphincter injuries (OASIS) [3,4].

Evidence shows that a continuous non-locking suturing technique using absorbable suture for repair of episiotomy and second-degree tears is associated with less pain in the immediate postpartum period, less need for suture removal, and less analgesia requirement compared with the traditional methods of using interrupted sutures. The majority of sutured perineal tears will heal quickly by primary intention [5,6].

Management

The options for the woman in the case history are either to perform an episiotomy to enlarge the vaginal orifice and expedite delivery of the fetus or, alternatively, if the vertex is advancing well and delivery is imminent, to allow spontaneous delivery with the possibility of a second-degree perineal tear.

Perform an episiotomy

If the woman has no analgesia, or does not have adequate perineal analgesia from an existing regional anesthesia, infiltration of the perineum with local anesthetic agents should be performed before an episiotomy is made.

Mediolateral episiotomy

Mediolateral episiotomy is an incision that begins at the midline and is directed laterally, at an angle of at least 60° from the midline at crowning [7] (Figure 163.1). This is the type of episiotomy most frequently used in Europe and evidence suggests that mediolateral episiotomy is associated with a reduced risk of OASIS.

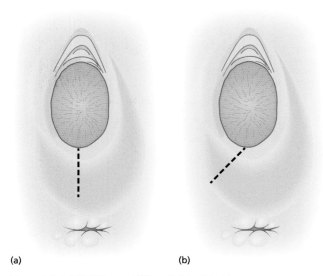

(a)   (b)

Figure 163.1 (a) Midline and (b) mediolateral incisions.

Midline (median, medial) episiotomy

Midline episiotomy starts at the posterior fourchette and proceeds along the midline through the central tendon of the perineal body. This

Gynecologic and Obstetric Surgery: Challenges and Management Options, First Edition. Edited by Arri Coomarasamy, Mahmood I. Shafi, G. Willy Davila and Kiong K. Chan.
© 2016 John Wiley & Sons, Ltd. Published 2016 by John Wiley & Sons, Ltd.

incision should only extend to half the length of the perineum (Figure 163.1). The midline episiotomy is commonly used in both the USA and Canada. Midline episiotomy is associated with a significant risk of extending to the anal sphincter complex and is therefore not advisable.

Repair techniques for episiotomy and second-degree tear

Evidence suggests that a three-layer continuous non-locking technique using an absorbable suture (such as 2-0 Vicryl Rapide) is the optimal approach. After completing the suturing of the vaginal wall and the muscle layer with continuous suturing, skin surface is closed with a continuous suture. The continuous non-locking suturing technique transfers tension across the whole suture area and avoids the over-tightening of traditional interrupted or locked sutures, which can cause tissue edema and increased pain. Absorbable suture material is associated with less short-term pain, reduction in the use of analgesia, and less dehiscence.

Complications of episiotomy

Possible complications of an episiotomy include bleeding, extended tears past the incision into anal sphincter, perineal pain, dyspareunia, infection, perineal hematoma, wound dehiscence, and formation of rectovaginal fistula. Patients should therefore be advised to report symptoms or signs suggestive of complications, including bleeding or pain at the episiotomy site, foul-smelling vaginal discharge, fever, or a perineal swelling. Perineal, vaginal and rectal examinations should be performed if a complication is suspected.

Wound dehiscence

Risk factors for wound breakdown include infection, extended tears, hematoma, smoking, and poor repair technique. Management of wound dehiscence varies worldwide. In the UK, the standard practice is to manage these expectantly. However, healing by secondary intention can result in extensive scar tissue that can lead to ongoing problems such as dyspareunia. In some countries, an early repair of dehiscence may be more usual practice [8]. With re-repair, the first step is the full debridement of the wound and the removal of all suture fragments. A thorough vaginal and rectal examination is then carried out to look for any hematomas and rectal sphincter or mucosal damage. A repair can then be performed using a standard technique. The patient should be started on antibiotics, low-residue diet, and a stool-softening drug.

Rectovaginal fistula

Although uncommon, rectovaginal fistula can be caused by either unrecognized tears in the rectovaginal septum or from breakdown of a hematoma. Risk factors include obesity, malnutrition, connective tissue disorders, inflammatory bowel disease, and past radiation therapy. Management of rectovaginal fistula is addressed in Chapter 129.

KEY POINTS

Challenge: Episiotomy and second-degree tear.

Background
- Perineal trauma can be first degree (skin only), second degree (perineal muscles and skin), third degree (injury to the anal sphincter complex), and fourth degree (injury to the perineum, anal sphincter complex, and rectal epithelium).
- If the vertex is advancing well and delivery is imminent, an episiotomy may not be required.
- The decision on whether to perform an episiotomy at delivery depends on whether the vaginal orifice needs widening to allow intervention and facilitate an easier or expedited delivery.

Management
- If an episiotomy is necessary, evidence suggests a mediolateral episiotomy reduces the risk of an obstetric anal sphincter injury.
- Both episiotomy and second-degree tears should be sutured with a three-layer continuous non-locking technique using an absorbable suture such as 2-0 Vicryl Rapide.
- Postoperatively, vigilance is required for possible complications including bleeding, infection, perineal hematoma, wound dehiscence, and rectovaginal fistula formation.
- When episiotomy dehiscence occurs, the management may be expectant or re-repair of the wound.

References

1 Carroli G, Mignini L. Episiotomy for vaginal birth. *Cochrane Database Syst Rev* 2009;(1):CD000081.

2 Fernando R, Williams AA, Adams EJ. *The Management of Third- and Fourth-degree Perineal Tears*. RCOG Green-top Guideline No. 29, 3rd edn, June 2015. Available at https://www.rcog.org.uk/en/guidelines-research-services/guidelines/gtg29/

3 Kalis V, Laine K, de Leeuw J, Ismail K, Tincello D. Classification of episiotomy: towards a standardisation of terminology. *BJOG* 2012;119:1284–1285.

4 Hartmann K, Viswanathan M, Palmieri R, Gartlehner G, Thorp J, Lohr KN. Outcomes of routine episiotomy: a systematic review. *JAMA* 2005;293:2141–2148.

5 Kettle C, Dowswell T, Ismail KMK. Continuous and interrupted suturing techniques for repair of episiotomy or second-degree tears. *Cochrane Database Syst Rev* 2012;(11):CD000947.

6 Dudley L, Kettle C, Ismail K. Prevalence, pathophysiology and current management of dehisced perineal wounds following childbirth. *Br J Midwifery* 2013;21:160–171.

7. Royal College of Obstetricians and Gynaecologists. The Management of Third- and Fourth-Degree Perineal Tears. Green-top Guideline No. 29. June 2015.

8 Graves CR. Obstetric problems. In: RockJA, JonesHW (eds) *Te Linde's Operative Gynecology*, 10th edn. Lippincott Williams & Wilkins, Philadephia, 2008.

CHAPTER 164
Obstetric Anal Sphincter Tear

Natalie P. Nunes[1], Helen Stevenson[2] and Matthew Parsons[2]
[1] West Middlesex University Hospital, London, UK
[2] Birmingham Women's NHS Foundation Trust, Birmingham, UK

Case history: Following a long second stage exacerbated by a persistent occipito-posterior position, a woman needed an instrumental delivery. She had a forceps delivery with an episiotomy. On examination of her perineum after delivery, it was noted that she had sustained an extensive perineal tear.

Background

The risk of third- and fourth-degree tears is approximately 1% of all vaginal births. Anal sphincter damage that is not identified and correctly repaired could lead to long-term physical and psychosexual complications.

Different degrees of perineal tears were defined in Chapter 163. A third-degree tear, involving the anal sphincter, can be subcategorized as follows.

- 3A: Tear involving less than 50% of the thickness of the external anal sphincter.
- 3B: Tear involving more than 50% of the thickness of the external anal sphincter.
- 3C: Tear involving both the external and internal anal sphincter.

A fourth-degree tear is characterized by involvement of the rectal mucosa.

Obstetric risk factors for third- and fourth-degree tears include occipito-posterior position, birthweight over 4 kg, prolonged second stage, instrumental delivery, shoulder dystocia, midline episiotomy (Chapter 163), and primiparity.

Management

Written consent should be obtained for examination under anesthesia and perineal repair. Repair of an anal sphincter injury should be performed in an operating room with good lighting and appropriate instruments, rather than in a labor room where the lighting and the provision of instruments are likely to be suboptimal. Regional or general anesthesia is recommended as it allows the anal sphincter to relax, which facilitates adequate exposure and visualization of the muscle ends. Anal sphincter repair should always be undertaken by (or under the supervision of) a properly trained clinician.

Surgical technique

The first step is to repair the rectal or anal mucosa with an interrupted absorbable 2-0 or 3-0 braided suture such as polyglactin (Vicryl) with the knot in the lumen. The second step is to repair the internal anal sphincter (IAS) with interrupted absorbable sutures such as 3-0 PDS (absorbed by 180 days) or 2-0 Vicryl (absorbed by 60–90 days). The third step is to repair the external anal sphincter (EAS) with an end-to-end technique (bringing the two cut edges together; Figure 164.1) or an overlap technique (overlapping the cut edges; Figure 164.2). A monofilament suture such as polydioxanone (PDS) or Vicryl interrupted sutures can be used. Figure of eight sutures should be avoided during the repair of obstetric anal sphincter injuries (OASIS), to preclude any hemostatic effect causing tissue ischemia [1]. The final step is to suture the vaginal and perineal skin tears.

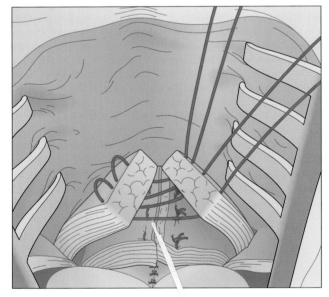

Figure 164.1 End-to-end technique for repairing external anal sphincter.

A Cochrane review comparing end-to-end and overlapping techniques found no differences in perineal pain, dyspareunia, or flatal incontinence at 12 months [2]. However statistically significant

Gynecologic and Obstetric Surgery: Challenges and Management Options, First Edition. Edited by Arri Coomarasamy, Mahmood I. Shafi, G. Willy Davila and Kiong K. Chan.
© 2016 John Wiley & Sons, Ltd. Published 2016 by John Wiley & Sons, Ltd.

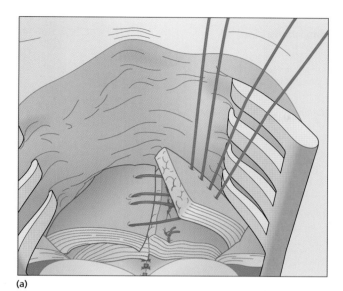

(a)

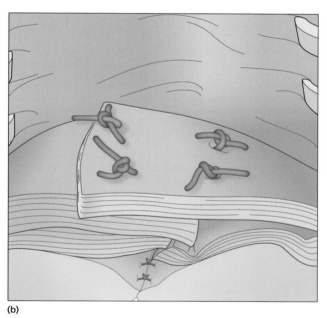

(b)

Figure 164.2 Overlap technique for repairing external anal sphincter.

reductions in the incidence of fecal urgency and anal incontinence symptoms were noted in the overlap group [2]. Studies of longer-term follow-up are small and few, but found no difference in flatal or fecal incontinence between the two techniques at 36 months.

Postoperative care

Regular analgesia is essential to reduce pain associated with walking, sitting, passing urine, and opening of bowels [3]. Ice packs or cool gel packs also improve pain relief [4]. A broad-spectrum intravenous antibiotic such as a second-generation cephalosporin or co-amoxiclav is recommended, followed by a 1-week oral course of antibiotics to reduce wound complications such as breakdown or purulent discharge [5].

Laxatives are associated with earlier and less painful bowel motion and earlier discharge, but there is no evidence of a difference in other symptoms [6]. Pelvic floor exercises are recommended for all postpartum women.

Follow-up is recommended in a dedicated clinic with a specialist team to assess recovery and make a plan for future pregnancies. Recovery assessment can be done via symptom evaluation, endoanal ultrasound (EAU), transperineal ultrasound (TPU), and endoanal manometry. Women who have a normal scan at follow-up are known to have the same incontinence rates as the normal controls [7].

Guidance for next pregnancy

If there are no residual symptoms and no EAU evidence of a defect, then a woman can be advised to have a vaginal delivery. If the woman had significant symptoms which have now resolved, or EAU evidence of a defect, then she may consider a cesarean section to avoid the risk of recurrence of the symptoms. If a woman has significant current symptoms, and is planning to have a secondary repair, then she may consider proceeding with a vaginal delivery and having a secondary repair on completing her family.

Resolution of the case

The patient should now be thoroughly and systematically examined to establish the extent of the tear. An adequately trained individual should perform the examination. It should include a rectal examination to determine any injury to the anal sphincter and rectum. Any injury can then be appropriately repaired.

Prevention

A range of preventive measures have been tried, with varying degrees of evidence to support their use.
• Ventouse rather than forceps as an instrument of choice for delivery.
• Perineal massage from 34 weeks onwards until delivery to reduce the risk of second-degree but not third-degree tears.
• Using warm compression on the perineum at delivery to reduce the risk of third-degree perineal tear [8].
• Using a "hands-on" technique for the delivery rather than a "hands-off" technique.

It is good practice to perform a vaginal and rectal examination after every vaginal delivery to avoid missing a third-degree or button-hole tear. If detected, a tear should be sutured by an experienced obstetrician with adequate lighting and analgesia in place.

There is no evidence for using a prophylactic episiotomy. If an episiotomy is required, then a mediolateral one should be performed; this is in fact a horizontal cut when the fetal head is distending the perineum. A prospective study showed a 50% reduction in relative risk of sustaining a third-degree tear for every 6° away from the perineal midline during an episiotomy cut [9].

KEY POINTS

Challenge: Obstetric anal sphincter tear.

Background
- The risk of third- and fourth-degree tears is approximately 1% of all vaginal births.
- Obstetric risk factors include occipito-posterior position, birthweight over 4 kg, prolonged second stage, instrumental delivery, shoulder dystocia, midline episiotomy, and primiparity.
- At the time of delivery, recognition and categorization of the tear and expert repair are vital to reduce short- and long-term symptoms.

Management
- The degree of the tear must be assessed in an operating room under good lighting and analgesia.
- The appropriate type of repair must be done to ensure all layers are opposed:
  - Repair the rectal or anal mucosa with an interrupted absorbable 2-0 or 3-0 braided suture, with the knot in the lumen.
  - Repair the IAS with interrupted absorbable sutures.
  - Repair the EAS with an end-to-end technique (bringing the two cut edges together) or an overlap technique (overlapping the cut edges).
  - Suture the vaginal and perineal skin tears.

Postoperative care
- Regular analgesia.
- Use of ice packs or cool gel packs.
- Antibiotics for a week.
- Consider use of laxatives.
- Follow-up in a dedicated clinic.

Guidance for the next pregnancy
- If there are no residual symptoms and no EAU evidence of a defect, then a woman can consider a vaginal delivery.
- If the woman had significant symptoms which have now resolved, or EAU evidence of a defect, then she may consider a cesarean section.
- If a woman has significant current symptoms, and is planning to have a secondary repair, then she may consider proceeding with a vaginal delivery (and having a secondary repair on completing her family).

Prevention
- Strategies aimed at prevention include ventouse delivery (in preference to forceps delivery), warm perineal compressions at delivery, correctly angled mediolateral episiotomy (when an episiotomy is required), and a "hands-on" or "hands-poised" technique.
- After every vaginal delivery, it is good practice to perform a vaginal and rectal examination.

References

1 Royal College of Obstetricians and Gynaecologists. The Management of Third- and Fourth-Degree Perineal Tears. Green-top Guideline No. 29. June 2015.
2 Fernando R, Sultan AH, Kettle C, Thakar R. Methods of repair for obstetric anal sphincter injury. *Cochrane Database Syst Rev* 2013;(12):CD002866.
3 Dodd JM, Hedayati H, Pearce E, Hotham N, Crowther CA. Rectal analgesia for the relief of perineal pain after childbirth: a randomised controlled trial of diclofenac suppositories. *BJOG* 2004;111:1059–1064.
4 East CE, Begg L, Henshall NE, Marchant PR, Wallace K. Local cooling for relieving pain from perineal trauma sustained during childbirth. *Cochrane Database Syst Rev* 2012;(5):CD006304.
5 Kettle C, Dowswell T, Ismail KMK. Absorbable suture materials for primary repair of episiotomy and second degree tears. *Cochrane Database Syst Rev* 2010;(6):CD000006.
6 Mahony R, Behan M, O'Herlihy C, O'Connell PR. Randomized, clinical trial of bowel confinement vs. laxative use after primary repair of a third-degree obstetric anal sphincter tear. *Dis Colon Rectum* 2004;47:12–17.
7 Valsky DV, Messing B, Petkova R et al. Postpartum evaluation of the anal sphincter by transperineal three-dimensional ultrasound in primiparous women after vaginal delivery and following surgical repair of third-degree tears by the overlapping technique. *Ultrasound Obstet Gynecol* 2007;29:195–204.
8 Aasheim V, Nilsen AB, Lukasse M, Reinar LM. Trauma. *Cochrane Database Syst Rev* 2011;(12):CD006672.
9 Eogan M, Daly L, O'Connell PR, O'Herlihy C. Does the angle of episiotomy affect the incidence of anal sphincter injury? *BJOG* 2006;113:190–194.

CHAPTER 165

Pregnancy and Female Genital Mutilation

Naomi Low-Beer and Gubby Ayida
Chelsea and Westminster Hospital NHS Foundation Trust, London, UK

Case history: A 19-year-old black woman of Somali origin presented with painful reg contractions at term in her first pregnancy. The pregnancy had been uncomplicated, except for two urinary tract infections. The midwife was about to perform a vaginal examination but called for help as she was unable to interpret the findings on genital inspection. A senior midwife confirmed female genital mutilation (FGM). A thick band of scar tissue obscured the urethra and introitus, and a vaginal examination was deemed to be difficult.

Background

It is estimated by the World Health Organization that 130 million women worldwide have undergone genital mutilation and that some 2 million women undergo some form of genital mutilation annually. FGM is a traditional cultural practice in 29 African countries and in some parts of Asia and the Middle East. FGM type III (infibulation) is found almost exclusively in Africa, and has a particularly high prevalence in northeastern Africa (Somalia, Sudan, Ethiopia, Eritrea, Djibouti). Age at FGM varies among countries, but it is almost always carried out on girls under the age of 15 years. It can have severe health consequences in the short and long term [1].

FGM is prohibited by law in England, Scotland and Wales, whether it is committed against a UK national or permanent UK resident in the UK or abroad. FGM is an abuse of human rights and is also a child protection issue.

Classification

FGM is defined as all procedures involving partial or total removal of the external female genitalia or other injury to the female genital organs, whether for cultural or other non-therapeutic reasons [2]. The WHO classifies FGM into four types [3].

  I Clitoridectomy: partial or total removal of the clitoris and/or the prepuce.
 II Excision: partial or total removal of the clitoris and the labia minora, with or without excision of the labia majora.
III Infibulation: narrowing of the vaginal orifice with creation of a covering seal by cutting and appositioning the labia minora and/or the labia majora, with or without excision of the clitoris.

IV Other: all other harmful procedures to the female genitalia for non-medical purposes (e.g., pricking, incising, scraping and cauterizing).

FGM type III (infibulation) leaves a bridge of scar tissue almost closing the vagina, except for a small hole (often the size of a matchstick head) for the passage of urine and menstrual blood. Re-infibulation is the resuturing of FGM type III to reclose the vagina again after childbirth, and is illegal in the UK.

De-infibulation (the surgical procedure to open up the vagina) is generally required for all women with type III FGM and some women with type II FGM.

Management

Obstetric care for a pregnant woman with FGM should ensure that (i) a plan of care is developed, documented, and clearly communicated; (ii) psychological support is provided; (iii) the risk of maternal morbidity is minimized; and (iv) the newborn infant's welfare is safeguarded. Healthcare workers should actively demonstrate knowledge and respect, and use terminology that is appropriate with the woman and her family to avoid causing unnecessary upset [4,5].

For women with severe type III FGM, where adequate vaginal assessment during labor is unlikely to be possible, antenatal de-infibulation, ideally in the second trimester, is recommended (Figure 165.1). For other women requiring de-infibulation, the woman's preferred choice of timing should be discussed, agreed, and documented. Antenatal de-infibulation has the advantage of being an elective procedure without the added stresses of labor, with a greater likelihood that an appropriately trained midwife or obstetrician can be present to perform or supervise the procedure. Antenatal de-infibulation is usually performed in the second trimester, but can be done at any time during pregnancy. De-infibulation at the time of delivery (also known as anterior episiotomy) is preferred by some women because this may be usual practice in their country of origin.

Surgical technique

The patient should have adequate pain relief (e.g., epidural or local anesthesia). The infibulation scar should be generously infiltrated with local anesthetic drug in and around the midline. In lithotomy

---

Gynecologic and Obstetric Surgery: Challenges and Management Options, First Edition. Edited by Arri Coomarasamy, Mahmood I. Shafi, G. Willy Davila and Kiong K. Chan.
© 2016 John Wiley & Sons, Ltd. Published 2016 by John Wiley & Sons, Ltd.

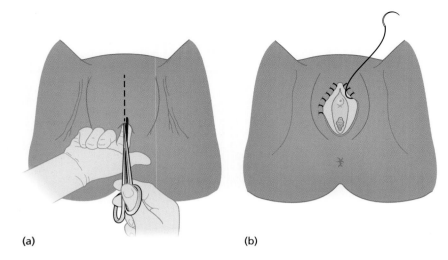

(a) (b)

Figure 165.1 (a, b) Technique of de-infibulation. *Source:* Clark N. (Leeds Teaching Hospital Trust). Female Genital Mutilation (FGM) Clinical Guidelines, 2007. Reproduced with permission.

position, an attempt should be made to identify the urethra and catheterize the bladder, although this may not be possible until the tissue bridge over the vulva has been incised. Forceps or a finger placed behind the scar during infiltration and incision will protect the underlying urethra and reduce the risk of injury (Figure 165.1a). An incision is then made along the midline with a knife blade, cutting diathermy or scissors up to the point where the urethral meatus is visualized, but not so far as to risk injury to the buried clitoris or clitoral stump. It is important to keep the incision strictly on the midline.

The cut edges are then oversewn separately with fine absorbable suture material such as polyglactin 910 (Vicryl Rapide) with subcuticular or interrupted stitch (Figure 165.1b). Prophylactic antibiotic therapy is often administered by many practitioners. The woman should be advised not to have sexual intercourse for 2 weeks after the procedure, and told to expect changes in urination (a steady stream, as opposed to dribbling), menstruation, and sexual intercourse.

Intrapartum care

Intrapartum de-infibulation is appropriate for many women with FGM [2]. De-infibulation should be carried out in the first stage of labor, before the cervix is fully dilated and the fetal head is low. Genital mutilation is not an absolute indication for cesarean birth unless the woman has such an extreme form of mutilation with anatomic distortion that makes de-infibulation impossible. Decisions about delivery must take into account the psychological needs of the woman.

Postpartum care

A review by a specialist FGM midwife should be arranged to give information about FGM, including its long-term consequences, complications, and the law (the UK FGM Act 2003 makes it a criminal act to carry out FGM on a child born in the UK). Appropriate measures should be taken to safeguard the welfare of a newborn girl [5]. A postnatal follow-up appointment should be offered to all women who have had intrapartum de-infibulation to check for the presence of adhesions or re-fusion of the incised scar.

KEY POINTS

Challenge: Female genital mutilation and pregnancy.

Background
- 130 million women worldwide live with FGM.
- WHO classifies FGM into four types:
  - I: Clitoridectomy.
  - II: Excision: partial or total removal of the clitoris and the labia.
  - III: Infibulation: narrowing of the vaginal orifice with creation of a covering seal by cutting and appositioning the labia.
  - IV: Other: all other harmful procedures to the female genitalia.
- FGM type III (infibulation) leaves a bridge of scar tissue almost closing the vagina, except for a small hole for passage of urine and menstrual blood.
- De-infibulation (the surgical procedure to open up the vagina) is generally required for all women with type III FGM and some women with type II FGM.

Management
- De-infibulation can be performed before conception, antenatally (usually in the second trimester), or intrapartum (during the first stage of labor).
- Some women with extreme forms of mutilation with anatomic distortions may benefit from a cesarean section.
- Surgical technique for de-infibulation:
  - Provide adequate anesthesia.
  - Attempt to identify the urethra and catheterize the bladder, although this may not be possible.
  - Pass a forceps or a finger behind the scar tissue bridge, and incise along the midline; incise up to a point where urethral meatus is visible, and not further up.
  - Oversew the cut edges with continuous or interrupted sutures to secure hemostasis.
  - After suturing of the cut edges, use paraffin gauze dressing to reduce the risk of re-fusion of the incised scar.
- Postoperative care: ask the woman to avoid intercourse for 2 weeks while the tissues heal, and prescribe antibiotics.
- Child safeguarding guidance must be followed; all girls born to women with FGM are considered at risk.

References

1 Banks E, Meirik O, Farley T, Akande O, Bathija H, Ali M. Female genital mutilation and obstetric outcome: WHO collaborative prospective study in six African countries. *Lancet* 2006;367:1835–1841.

2 Royal College of Obstetricians and Gynaecologists. *Female Genital Mutilation and its Management*. RCOG Green-top Guideline No. 53, 2nd edn, July 2015. Available at https://www.rcog.org.uk/en/guidelines-research-services/guidelines/gtg53/

3 World Health Organization. Eliminating female genital mutilation. An interagency statement. Available at http://www.who.int/reproductivehealth/publications/fgm/9789241596442/en/

4 HM Government. *Multi-agency Practice Guidelines: Female Genital Mutilation.* Available at https://www.gov.uk/government/uploads/system/uploads/attachment_data/file/288819/Multi-Agency_Practice_Guidelines_-_Female_Genital_Mutilation.pdf

5 RCM, RCN, RCOG, Equality Now, UNITE. *Tackling FGM in the UK: Intercollegiate Recommendations for Identifying, Recording and Reporting.* Royal College of Midwives, London, 2013.

CHAPTER 166

Destructive Operations on a Dead Fetus

Hany Abdel-Aleem

Faculty of Medicine, Assiut University, Assiut, Egypt

Case history: A 38-year-old woman who did not receive any antenatal care was admitted in labor. History suggested a term pregnancy; this was confirmed with an ultrasound scan, but sadly fetal heart activity was absent. An ultrasound examination by another sonographer confirmed intrauterine death with a large hydrocephalic head. A decision needed to be taken about the mode of delivery.

Background

Destructive operations on the fetus are rarely done in modern obstetrics. These procedures have, as their objective, the diminution of the bulk of the fetus in order to permit its passage through the birth canal. Such procedures are only performed on a fetus with a lethal abnormality or on a fetus which is already dead. These operations include craniotomy (perforation of the cranium), decapitation (severing the head of the dead fetus from its trunk followed by extraction of trunk and head in case of neglected shoulder presentation), cleidotomy (division of one or both clavicles, in case of arrested shoulders), and evisceration (removal of the abdominal and/or thoracic contents with the object of diminishing the bulk of the fetus so that it can be extracted vaginally). Other than the special case of drainage of the hydrocephalic fetal head (craniocentesis), these procedures appear to have no place in modern obstetric practice in high-income countries [1]. However, they have a place in settings where women present with obstructed labor and intrauterine fetal death, and emergency cesarean section is not feasible or is deemed to be unsafe. A destructive operation will leave a woman with an intact uterus, which is far less likely to rupture in a future pregnancy, and this will be of particular advantage for women in low-income countries where access to expert medical care and cesarean operation may be limited or indeed unavailable. An obstetrician's queasiness is not a legitimate reason to avoid a destructive operation; an obstetrician must not lose sight of the fact that a fetal craniotomy avoids a uterine scar, and may thus prevent a future uterine rupture and save a woman's life. The incidence of fetal destructive operations varies between 0.2 and 1.6% of deliveries from reports originating in Nigeria, Ghana, and India [2,3].

Management

A woman whose fetus is being considered for a destructive operation may be very ill, and require aggressive resuscitation. A thorough evaluation of the patient is needed, including vital signs for hemodynamic stability and examination for exclusion of a ruptured uterus. Ultrasound confirmation of intrauterine death should be performed by two competent practitioners.

Craniocentesis

Craniocentesis refers to the drainage of cerebrospinal fluid (CSF) from a hydrocephalic fetal head. Under ultrasound guidance, the CSF can be drained abdominally using a large-bore spinal needle which is passed through the abdominal wall, uterine wall, and hydrocephalic skull (Figure 166.1) [4]. If the fetal presentation is cephalic, and the vagina is dilated, it may be possible to perform the drainage vaginally by inserting a large-bore needle through the fontanelle or suture line, after steadying the fetal head with a tenaculum.

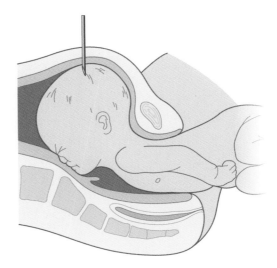

Figure 166.1 Transabdominal craniocentesis. *Source:* Hanretty, 2003 [4]. Reproduced with permission from Elsevier.

Craniotomy

Craniotomy is the most commonly performed destructive operation; the usual indication for craniotomy is a neglected labor resulting in fetal death and fetal head impaction in the pelvis. If the fetal head is mobile or palpable more than three-fifths in the abdomen, or the cervix is less than 7 cm dilated, craniotomy is difficult and dangerous, and a cesarean section should be recommended [5].

Craniotomy should be performed in an operating room, with facilities for a laparotomy if necessary. General anesthesia is administered, the woman is placed in lithotomy position, and the bladder is emptied. The fetal head is stabilized with abdominal pressure by one assistant, while another assistant exposes the fetal head with two Sims specula.

An X-shaped incision is made on the fetal scalp, right down to the level of the bone. This incision creates four flaps, which are peeled off the skull. The skull is palpated for a suture line or fontanelle, and a closed pair of strong pointed scissors or Simpson's perforator is inserted between the bones. For a face presentation, the insertion point can be through the fetal hard palate or orbit. The instrument is advanced to the center of the skull and the blades are opened and closed a few times, while turning around the instrument. The contents of the skull will flow from the hole, and any remaining tissue can be removed, resulting in the collapse of the skull. The frontal and parietal bones, and any loose pieces of bone, are removed as they can cause vaginal tears. Three or four strong tissue-grasping forceps (e.g., vulsellum forceps) are now attached to the fetal scalp and the remains of the skull (Figure 166.2a).

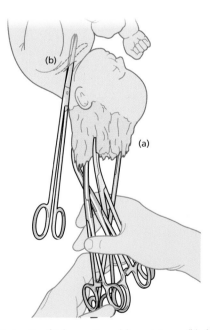

Figure 166.2 Destructive fetal operations: (a) craniotomy; (b) cleidotomy. *Source:* King *et al.,* 1990 [6]. Reproduced with permission from Oxford University Press.

When the woman has a contraction, all the tissue-grasping forceps are held together, and pulled with a twisting motion. It is important to protect the vagina with the operator's fingers to avoid the risk of vaginal injury from any bony fragments of the fetal skull. The fetal head should deliver and the body will follow. If there is difficulty in delivering the shoulders, turning the anterior shoulder by 90° may help; if not, a cleidotomy can be performed (Figure 166.2b). When performing a cleidotomy, it is important to ensure that it is the clavicle that is fractured or incised, and not the scapula.

After delivery of the fetus, the placenta can be manually removed. The operator should then check the uterine cavity to ensure there is no evidence of rupture, tears, or retained tissues.

Postoperative care

If the uterus is not contracted, uterotonic drugs should be administered, and steps should be taken for managing postpartum hemorrhage (Chapters 40 and 158). An indwelling bladder catheter should be left *in situ* for 2 weeks in the case of obstructed labor; this will minimize the risk of fistula formation. Antibiotics should be prescribed according to local guidelines.

KEY POINTS

Challenge: Destructive operations on a dead fetus.

Background
- Destructive operations on a dead fetus are rarely done in modern obstetrics, except the drainage of the hydrocephalic fetal head (craniocentesis).
- Craniotomy still has a place in settings where women present with obstructed labor and fetal death, and emergency cesarean section is not feasible or safe.
- A destructive operation has the advantage of not leaving a uterine scar, which has a clear benefit for future pregnancies.

Destructive operations
- Craniotomy: perforation of the cranium, and delivery of the fetus in cases of obstructed labor.
- Decapitation: severing the head of the dead fetus from its trunk followed by extraction of the trunk and the head in cases of neglected shoulder presentation.
- Cleidotomy: division of one or both clavicles, in cases of arrested shoulders.
- Evisceration: removal of the abdominal and/or thoracic contents with the objective of diminishing the bulk of the fetus to aid vaginal delivery.

Management
- Stabilize the woman with aggressive resuscitation.
- Weigh up the options carefully in consultation with the woman or couple, and only proceed with a destructive operation if the net benefit outweighs potential harm, the patient consents to the operation, and the necessary preconditions for a destructive operation are met.
- The following preconditions need to be met for a destructive craniotomy:
  - Fetus is dead.
  - No evidence of uterine rupture.
  - Fetal head is impacted in the pelvis, with the head low and immobile in the pelvis.
  - Cervix is at least 7 cm dilated.

Craniotomy technique
- Steady the fetal head with abdominal pressure, and expose the fetal head with two Sims specula in the vagina.
- Make an X-shaped incision on the fetal scalp and peel off the skin from the skull.
- Identify the skull suture line or fontanelle, and insert a closed pair of strong pointed scissors or Simpson's perforator.
- Open and close the instrument in the center of the skull, while turning the instrument around. This allows the contents of the skull to flow out or be extracted, resulting in the collapse of the skull.

- Grasp the edges of the fetal skull with three or four strong tissue-grasping forceps, and deliver the fetus by putting traction on the forceps when the uterus contracts. Guard the vaginal tissue with one hand during the delivery.
- If delivery of the shoulders proves to be difficult, perform cleidotomy.
- Remove placenta manually, and check uterine cavity to ensure there is no rupture.

Postoperative care
- Administer uterotonic drugs and antibiotics.
- Catheterize for 14 days to minimize the risk of fistula formation from prolonged obstructed labor.

References

1 Baskett TF, Calder AA, Arulkumaran S. Symphysiotomy. In: *Munro Kerr's Operative Obstetrics*, 11th edn, pp. 315–320. Saunders Elsevier, Philadelphia, 2007.
2 Harrison K. Approaches to reducing maternal and perinatal mortality in Africa. In: Philpot RH (ed.) *Maternal Services in the Developing World: What the Community Needs*, pp. 52–69. RCOG Press, London, 1980.
3 Amo-Mensah S, Elkins TE, Ghosh TS, Greenway F, Waite V. Obstetric destructive procedures. *Int J Gynaecol Obstet* 1996;54:167–168.
4 Hanretty KP. *Obstetrics Illustrated*, 6th edn, p. 319. Churchill Livingstone, London, 2003.
5 Maharaj D, Moodley J. Symphysiotomy and fetal destructive operations. *Best Pract Res Clin Obstet Gynaecol* 2002;16:117–131.
6 King M, Bewes PC, Cairns J, Thornton J (eds) *Primary Surgery, Vol. 1. Non-Trauma.* Oxford University Press, Oxford, 1990.

CHAPTER 167

Development of a Basic Obstetric Theater Facility in a Low-resource Setting

Zahida Qureshi[1] and Alfred Murage[2]

[1] University of Nairobi, Nairobi, Kenya
[2] Aga Khan University Hospital, Nairobi, Kenya

Case history: *A young woman arrived at the local health center after being in labor for 24 hours at home. A diagnosis of cephalopelvic disproportion was made, necessitating an emergency cesarean section. However, the health center had no capacity to perform cesarean sections and therefore she was referred to a higher-level facility 2 hours away. Unfortunately the obstetric theater was non-functional at this higher-level facility.*

Background

In any given population or community, 15% of pregnant women can be expected to develop complications during pregnancy or delivery, and will require emergency obstetric care [1]. Emergency preparedness should include establishing a functional operating theater (OT) to deal with complications and avert maternal and neonatal morbidity and mortality [2]. The resource constraints in low-income countries provide a continuing challenge for realizing a sustained reduction in perinatal and maternal deaths. Whereas developed countries have at least 15 OTs per 100,000 people, resource-constrained countries have fewer than two OTs per 100,000 people, with more than half of these OTs not having basic functionalities such as facilities to monitor oxygen saturation during anesthesia [3]. Establishing and maintaining a functional emergency obstetric (basic and comprehensive) healthcare system requires careful planning to achieve optimal balance in availability, accessibility, quality, and cost-effectiveness of services. Technical competence must also be available in an integrated healthcare service delivery system.

The World Health Organization (WHO), UNICEF, and the UN Population Fund (UNFPA) recommend a minimum acceptable level of EmOC (emergency obstetric care) services stating: "For every 500,000 population, there should be at least four basic and one comprehensive Emergency Obstetric Care (EmOC) facilities" [1]. A comprehensive EmOC facility should be able to offer cesarean sections and blood transfusion in addition to the functions of a basic facility, namely administration of parenteral antibiotics, oxytocic drugs, and anticonvulsants; manual removal of placenta (MROP); removal of retained products of conception; neonatal resuscitation; and assisted vaginal delivery. These functions need to be performed on a regular basis for a health institution to qualify as either a basic or comprehensive EmOC facility.

The basic obstetric OT

Establishing and maintaining a well-functioning obstetric OT is expensive. The local community administration should be involved at the outset, ensuring allocation of funds and commitment to continued maintenance of the facility. The feasibility of an effective referral system, with availability of transport and communication channels from the catchment area to the hospital with the OT should be planned from the outset [4].

The OT must be adequately equipped to handle common obstetric problems that include the following.
- Cesarean sections.
- Uterine evacuations and MROP.
- Perineal repairs.
- EUA for hemorrhage and other conditions.
- Laparotomy.
- Immediate neonatal care.

Physical infrastructure

The obstetric OT should be housed within a building that fulfills structural safety standards. The architectural plan (Figure 167.1) should take into account the following considerations:
- be on the same floor as the maternity unit or have a ramp from the maternity area to theater if not on same floor;
- running water and adequate reservoirs;
- power supply compatible with solar (preferably) or generator back-up system to provide overhead or portable lighting and extra power points;
- impermeable washable walls and floors;
- extra rooms including staff changing area, anesthesia induction room, scrubbing and recovery area.

A total area of 372 m^2 (or about 4000 square feet) provides ample space.

Gynecologic and Obstetric Surgery: Challenges and Management Options, First Edition. Edited by Arri Coomarasamy, Mahmood I. Shafi, G. Willy Davila and Kiong K. Chan.
© 2016 John Wiley & Sons, Ltd. Published 2016 by John Wiley & Sons, Ltd.

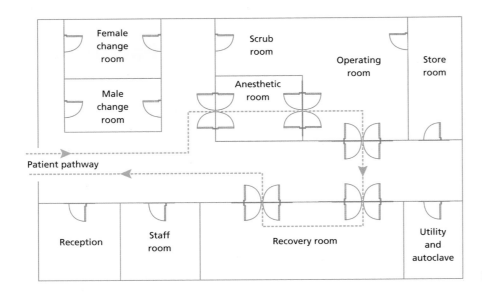

Figure 167.1 Sample obstetric theater layout.

Design of the OT

The OT is divided into four zones requiring varying levels of cleanliness.

Zone 1 Protective area: reception, waiting room, trolley bay, changing rooms.

Zone 2 Clean area: preoperative and recovery areas, staff lounges, store room.

Zone 3 Sterile area: operating room, scrub area, anesthesia room, set-up room.

Zone 4 Disposal area: dirty utility room, disposal corridor.

Basic surgical equipment and supplies

As a minimum, the equipment should include:

- OT table (this can be locally assembled to minimum specifications);
- patient trolleys and wheelchairs;
- overhead lighting;
- cesarean section surgical trays (these are adaptable to perform laparotomies);
- perineal repair trays;
- manual vacuum aspiration (MVA) kits;
- reusable drapes and gowns;
- consumables (e.g., catheters, sutures, gloves, waste disposal bags).

Drugs such as uterotonics, anesthetics, analgesics, antibiotics and fluids should be available. Supplies such as scrubs, OT shoes, caps and masks are essential items. Small inexpensive autoclaves that require minimal maintenance are the sterilizing equipment of choice.

Anesthetic equipment

Preference should be for regional anesthesia, but the capability for general anesthesia for selected cases should be in place [5].

- Basic anesthetic machine:
  - Airway maintenance equipment.
  - Airways, endotracheal tubes, bag and mask equipment, laryngoscopes.
- Oxygen cylinders with monitoring gauges.
- Spinal and epidural catheters.

Neonatal equipment

- Locally assembled Resuscitaire® with heat source.
- Neonatal bag and mask equipment, oropharyngeal suckers, endotracheal tube.
- Reusable linen.
- Makeshift neonatal transfer cots.

Staffing

Obstetric OT staffing should be dictated by competencies required to perform emergency obstetric procedures. Consultant-level obstetricians and anesthetists are usually unavailable and not necessarily appropriate in small facilities in low-resource countries. Task-shifting to non-physician clinicians and midwives is common in these settings, but appropriate training, competency assessment, and lifelong professional development are important. A typical arrangement can involve a non-physician clinician performing the cesarean section assisted by a midwife, with another non-physician clinician acting as the anesthetist [6]. An additional midwife can be responsible for neonatal resuscitation, with a nursing assistant slotting in as the runner nurse. The staff should be available around the clock or within, at most, 30 min of the facility.

A buddy system with a referral center can be established. An obstetrician-led specialist team can make planned visits aimed at up-scaling competencies through CME or jointly operating with the local team. Technical staff tasked with routine maintenance of equipment should also be easily available.

Autoclave room

Each EmOC facility should have a designated area or separate autoclave room, with a person trained in autoclaving. The following items should be in place:

- functioning autoclave machine with temperature and pressure gauges;
- supply of indicator papers;
- reliable and safe electric connections or supply of kerosene oil or gas;
- table with marked areas, indicating space for non-sterilized and sterilized areas;
- manual for packaging for different procedures.

Quality measures

Systems for quality improvement and monitoring should be in place. The operating room should gather information on procedures done and their indications, complication rates, maternal and neonatal outcomes, morbidity and mortality reviews, and infection rates. The information gathered should be used for continuous quality improvement.

KEY POINTS

Challenge: Development of an obstetric operating theater in a low-income country.

Background
- For a population of 500,000, there should be at least four basic and one comprehensive EmOC facilities:
  - Basic EmOC should provide administration of parenteral antibiotics, oxytocic drugs, and anticonvulsants; MROP; removal of retained products of conception; neonatal resuscitation; and assisted vaginal delivery.
  - Comprehensive EmOC should provide all of the above, plus cesarean section and blood transfusion.

Management
- A comprehensive EmOC can only be achieved if there is an integrated healthcare system in place.

- Continued maintenance of the facility should be considered from the outset of developing a new facility.
- When setting up an OT facility, the following should be considered:
  - Financing of the facility.
  - Referral pathways and systems.
  - Access to the facility.
  - Physical infrastructure.
  - Provision of drugs, surgical equipment and supplies.
  - Anesthetic equipment.
  - Neonatal equipment.
  - Staffing.
  - Arrangements for maintenance of equipment and facility.
  - Systems for continuous quality improvement.
- Monitoring and evaluation must be integral components of an obstetric OT, with defined analyses of outcomes and consequent remedial measures to maintain quality of service provision.

References

1 UNICEF, WHO, UNFPA. *Guidelines for Monitoring the Availability and Use of Obstetric Services*, 2nd edn. UNICEF, New York, 1997. Available at http://www.childinfo.org/files/maternal_mortality_finalgui.pdf
2 Hofmeyr GJ, Haws RA, Bergström S *et al*. Obstetric care in low-resource settings: what, who, and how to overcome challenges to scale up. *Int J Gynaecol Obstet* 2009;107(Suppl 1):S21–S45.
3 Lawn JE, Lee AC, Kinney M, Bateman M, Paul V, Darmstadt GL. Reducing intrapartum-related deaths and disability: can the health system deliver? *Int J Gynaecol Obstet* 2009;107(Suppl 1):S123–S142.
4 World Health Organization. *Surgical Care at the District Hospital*. WHO, Geneva, 2003. Available at http://www.who.int/surgery/publications/en/SCDH.pdf
5 Dobson MB. *Anaesthesia at the District Hospital*, 2nd edn. WHO, Geneva, 2000.
6 Block FE Jr, Helfman S (eds) *Operating Room Design Manual*. American Society of Anesthesiologists, 2010–2011. Available at https://www.asahq.org/resources/resources-from-asa-committees/operating-room-design-manual

Section 9
Miscellaneous
Editors: Mahmood I. Shafi and Arri Coomarasamy

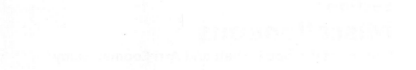

CHAPTER 168

Enhanced Recovery

Manjeet Shehmar

Birmingham Women's NHS Foundation Trust, Birmingham, UK

Case history: A 49-year-old woman has a hysterectomy for heavy menstrual bleeding due to large fibroids. She has hypertension controlled with an ACE inhibitor. She has a midline laparotomy at around 2 pm on an all-day theater list and the surgery is uncomplicated.

Background

Interventions aimed at reducing the postoperative recovery time have the potential for huge benefits to individual patients, the health service, society, and the economy. There is evidence that a formal "fast-track" or enhanced recovery (ER) program for surgery improves recovery and reduces hospital stay. ER is now a recognized model of care for the elective surgery pathway. The aim is to reduce the physiological and psychological stress responses during surgery to minimize organ dysfunction and aid faster recovery. The pathway was first described in 1990 [1] in a Danish model for colorectal surgery patients taking into account the decision for surgery, surgical work-up, anesthesia, postoperative care, and advice for the recovery period [2]. In the UK, the ESTReP (Enhanced Surgical Treatment and Recovery Programme) [3] transformed the way in which colorectal surgery is delivered. The program combined known clinical predictors of recovery (such as early feeding after surgery, not using nasogastric tubes or surgical drains) with positive psychological factors such as patient education and health promotion. ESTReP led to a reduction in the average hospital stay from 9–10 days per patient to 6 days. The program was shown to be cost-efficient, and gained support from the Department of Health. Further programs with a variety of components of the ER pathway have been compared in two meta-analyses [4,5]. One review found significant reductions in length of hospital stay (weighted mean difference –2.5 days, 95% CI –3.2 to –1.9) and complication rates (RR 0.5, 95% CI 0.4–0.6) in the ER group if at least four individual elements of the pathway were implemented [4]. The other review also found a significant reduction in hospital stay without an increase in readmission rates or mortality [5]. A Cochrane review of ER in gynecologic cancer [6] concluded that there were no RCTs in ER for this population, and so the Enhanced Recovery Partnership Programme [7] was set up as a partnership with the Department of Health, the National Cancer Action Team, NHS Improvement, and the NHS Institute of Innovation and Improvement in 2009–2011. This initiative included studies in gynecology, urology, and musculoskeletal surgery.

Management

The four fundamental aspects of an ER program are patient education, aggressive pain management, early nutrition, and early mobilization.

Preoperative management

In order to optimize recovery, a plan is formalized using a multidisciplinary approach involving the anesthetist and ward staff. The patient is counseled by the surgeon and preoperative staff about positive measures to help her to recover and is given information about surgery and recovery. This plan includes recovery in the immediate postoperative period in an enhanced recovery unit with specialist trained nursing care to optimize pain control, posture, breathing, early feeding, and mobilization. The patient is asked to fast for 6 hours prior to surgery, but to drink clear fluids until 2 hours before surgery. A clear carbohydrate drink should be administered orally the night before surgery and 3 hours prior to induction of anesthesia. This will reduce dehydration and starvation effects on recovery. The patient's comorbidities should be well managed (e.g., blood pressure control for the patient in the case history) and the importance of healthy eating and regular exercise should be stressed.

Care on admission

Venous thromboembolism scoring is carried out and appropriate prophylaxis is given. The patient is again seen by the surgical and anesthetic team and the importance of faster return to normality is advocated in order to reduce patient anxiety and empower the patient to aid her own recovery. Pre-anesthetic medications are not recommended.

Intraoperative management

A World Health Organization (WHO) checklist is completed so that the whole operating room team is aware of the plan and potential risks. The patient should receive prophylactic antibiotics, Flowtron®, and a regional TAP block for analgesia. It is important to keep the patient warm during the operation, and use warmed-up fluids. Attention is paid to hemostasis and no drain is used. A WHO debrief is conducted with a plan for care in recovery.

Gynecologic and Obstetric Surgery: Challenges and Management Options, First Edition. Edited by Arri Coomarasamy, Mahmood I. Shafi, G. Willy Davila and Kiong K. Chan.
© 2016 John Wiley & Sons, Ltd. Published 2016 by John Wiley & Sons, Ltd.

Immediate postoperative management

The post-surgical ward round includes the anesthetist, surgeon, and the nurse responsible for the patient. A plan is documented for the next 24 hours that involves the use of oxygen, optimal positioning, early feeding, optimizing pain control, and observations using an early warning chart. The medical and nursing team should review progress during the evening.

Hospital recovery

Opiate analgesia is discontinued on day 1 after the operation and replaced with simple analgesia and NSAIDs. However, it is important to treat pain aggressively and pre-emptively to reduce stress responses. It is sometimes possible to use a low-dose epidural without compromising mobility.

The patient is mobilized and the urinary catheter is removed when she is able to walk to the toilet. Once her saturations are adequate, the oxygen is discontinued. She is taught how to breathe and mobilize effectively. If the patient has not opened her bowels by the second day after the surgery, she can be examined and, if appropriate, glycerin suppositories can be prescribed to aid her bowels; she should also be encouraged to drink plenty of clear fluids. When the patient fulfills the discharge criteria, she can be discharged home with advice about recovery on a DVD and contact numbers for ER nurses. A structured and comprehensive discharge summary to the GP includes the ER plan with contact information for advice and support.

Prevention

It is important that any ER program is evaluated to ensure patient safety, positive experience, and pathway efficiency. This will include collection of morbidity and patient satisfaction data. ER programs are complex and multi-modal, resulting in difficulties in studying whole programs for effectiveness. Future research in ER needs well-designed collaborative trials involving surgeons, anesthetists, nurses, and physiotherapists in order to establish which parts of the programs are effective.

The preoperative ER pathway is vital for performing a thorough risk assessment, managing risks, and providing information and psychological preparation to the patient. The discharge plan is based on criteria such as mobilization, control of pain by oral analgesia, being able to eat and drink, and passing flatus. It is recommended that patients be given information regarding practical advice to aid recovery and expected time to return of normal function. It is important to maximize recovery at every point of the surgical journey, and examples of approaches are given in Table 168.1.

Table 168.1 Example of enhanced recovery pathway.

	Principle	Examples
Preoperative	Provide patient information	Provide clear information
		Control comorbidities
	Reduce medical morbidity	Stop smoking
		Lose weight
Intraoperative	Reduce physiological stress	Provide goal-directed fluid replacement
		Aim to use regional anesthesia
		Aim to use minimally invasive approach
		Avoid drains
Postoperative	Reduce opioid analgesia	Switch to non-opioid analgesia
	Reduce ileus	Encourage early oral feeding
	Reduce physiological stress	Mobilize
	Provide long-term recovery advice	Provide VTE prophylaxis until early mobilization
		Provide advice for returning to normal activities

KEY POINTS

Challenge: Enhanced recovery.

Background
- Enhanced recovery asks the question "Why is this postoperative patient in hospital today?"
- The four cornerstones of ER are patient education, aggressive pain management, early nutrition, and early mobilization.

Management
- ER programs involve optimizing the preoperative, intraoperative, and postoperative surgical phases by:
  - Patient information and support.
  - Reducing comorbidities.
  - Allowing food up to 6 hours before surgery.
- Allowing clear fluids up to 2 hours before surgery.
- Using preoperative carbohydrate loading.
- Using regional anesthesia.
- Providing goal-directed intraoperative fluid therapy.
- Employing minimal access approaches.
- Keeping the patient warm.
- Avoiding drain and nasogastric tube use.
- Optimizing pain control (and switching to non-opioid drugs as soon as possible).
- Encouraging early feeding.
- Encouraging early and structured mobilization.
- Providing clear advice on returning to normal activities.
- It is important to provide thromboprophylaxis and prophylactic antibiotics according to local or national policy.
- Audit of an ER program is essential to ensure safety, positive patient experience, and efficiency.

References

1 Kehlet H. Multimodal approach to control postoperative pathophysiology and rehabilitation. *Br J Anaesth* 1997;78:606–617.
2 Kehlet H, Slim K. The future of fast-track surgery. *Br J Surg* 2012;99:1025–1026.
3 Windsor AL. Improving surgical outcomes, reducing length of stay. http://www.reducinglengthofstay.org.uk/doc/healthdirectoroct07.pdf
4 Varadhan KK, Neal KR, Dejong CH, Fearon KC, Ljungqvist O, Lobo DN. The enhanced recovery after surgery (ERAS) pathway for patients undergoing major elective open colorectal surgery: a meta-analysis of randomized controlled trials. *Clin Nutr* 2010;29:434–440.
5 Gouvas N, Tan E, Windsor A, Xynos E, Tekkis PP. Fast-track vs standard care in colorectal surgery: a meta-analysis update. *Int J Colorectal Dis* 2009;24:1119–1131.
6 Lu D, Wang X, Shi G. Perioperative enhanced recovery programmes for gynaecological cancer patients. *Cochrane Database Syst Rev* 2012;(12):CD008239.
7 National Health Service. Enhanced recovery. http://www.nhsiq.nhs.uk/improvement-programmes/acute-care/enhanced-recovery.aspx (accessed 9 January 2014).

CHAPTER 169
Major Surgery in a Jehovah's Witness Patient

Martyn Underwood and William Parry-Smith
Shrewsbury and Telford Hospitals NHS Trust, Telford, Shropshire, UK

Case history 1: *A Jehovah's Witness is 37^{+4} weeks pregnant and attends in spontaneous labor. She has a raised BMI of 40. The presentation of the fetus has been confirmed as breech and the mother has opted for a cesarean section. Her most recent hemoglobin is 10.9 g/dL.*

Case history 2: *A 54-year-old Jehovah's Witness presents with a history of postmenopausal bleeding. An ultrasound suggested a thickened endometrium at 14 mm with a bulky uterus. An endometrial biopsy histology reports an endometrioid adenocarcinoma and she has opted to have an abdominal hysterectomy and bilateral salpingo-oophorectomy.*

Background

There are over 1.2 million Jehovah's Witnesses in the USA and 136,000 in the UK [1] with established congregations gathering on a regular basis worldwide.

A Jehovah's Witness will consider all routine care and surgical interventions apart from the use of the following: transfusions of whole blood or the four primary components of blood: red blood cells, white blood cells, platelets, and plasma (FFP). However some Jehovah's Witnesses may make a choice to accept or decline (i) intraoperative or postoperative blood cell salvage or (ii) blood fractions (e.g., albumin, clotting factors and immunoglobulins). This can lead to challenges in the management of obstetric and operative hemorrhages. There have been several case reports of patients dying after declining a blood transfusion. A recent review of maternal deaths and serious obstetric morbidity found that

> women who are Jehovah's Witnesses are at a six times increased risk for maternal death, at a 130 times increased risk for maternal death because of major obstetric hemorrhage and at a 3.1 times increased risk for serious maternal morbidity because of obstetric hemorrhage, compared with the general Dutch population [2].

Management

Obstetric patients (Case history 1)

Preoperative management

It is imperative to complete an advanced directive prior to contemplating surgery on a patient who declines blood products. This establishes the boundaries and all staff involved in the patient's care are clearly informed of what the patient will and will not accept should the need arise for the transfusion of blood products.

Even in a situation where the patient's life is at risk by declining a transfusion, the patient's wishes and beliefs must be respected.

Preoperative management is essential when undertaking surgery in patients who will decline blood products. Optimizing the patient's hemoglobin count before surgery if possible will leave a greater reserve should the patient go on to bleed. This can be done by optimizing iron, folate, and vitamin B$_{12}$ stores if the patient is deficient in any of these. The use of recombinant human erythropoietin (EPO), which does not cross the placenta, is reportedly safely used in pregnancy and enhances the hemoglobin response [3].

Optimizing the patient's health prior to surgery can lead to less challenging surgery and a reduction in the rate of complications that require a blood transfusion; for example, losing weight may benefit an obese patient's general health and make the surgery easier.

Uterine artery catheter balloons can be considered in those with known placental anomalies such as placenta praevia, as this may aid reduction in blood loss during surgery [4]. A senior surgeon who feels competent and comfortable to operate in these situations should perform the surgery. Close liaison with the patient, their family and elders can help overcome many potential problems.

Intraoperative management

Requesting senior support at an early stage from a consultant obstetrician and anesthetist is advised by both the Royal College of Obstetricians and Gynaecologists (RCOG) and the Association of Anaesthetists [5]. The obstetrician should re-confirm with the patient which blood products she will and will not accept, and confirm that the advanced directive is complete.

By aiming to keep blood loss to a minimum during surgery, the need for transfusion can be significantly reduced. This can be achieved by operating at a lower blood pressure threshold once the fetus has been delivered, the use of diathermy and diligent suturing of any bleeding points, along with the use of topical hemostatic agents. The operating surgeon should have a low threshold for calling senior assistance from a fellow consultant if bleeding becomes excessive.

Some Jehovah's Witnesses will allow the use of cell salvage, whereby the patient's own blood is aspirated from the surgical field and filtered prior to being stored or transfused directly back to the patient. It is important to clearly establish with the patient if storage of her own blood is an option or if the continuous loop method is acceptable.

A large systematic review established that there is increased blood loss associated with general anesthesia compared with

Gynecologic and Obstetric Surgery: Challenges and Management Options, First Edition. Edited by Arri Coomarasamy, Mahmood I. Shafi, G. Willy Davila and Kiong K. Chan.
© 2016 John Wiley & Sons, Ltd. Published 2016 by John Wiley & Sons, Ltd.

neuraxial anesthesia [6]. However, the rate of blood transfusion was not altered. Nevertheless, it would seem logical to keep blood loss to a minimum and if a spinal anesthetic or epidural is feasible, it should be preferred.

After delivery of the fetus, prophylactic use of a Syntocinon infusion will aid uterine contractility, and has been shown to reduce the need for other uterotonic agents [7]. Local guidelines for the management of major obstetric hemorrhage should be followed if there is excessive blood loss.

Prior to closure of the abdomen, it is important to ensure the patient's blood pressure is adequate to suggest good perfusion of the pelvic organs, as hypotensive patients may go on to bleed postoperatively when the blood pressure normalizes.

A low threshold for radiologic intervention should be considered in those with an ongoing bleed. An early recourse to hysterectomy should also be considered if there is significant ongoing bleeding. Tamponading the uterus can be considered using either a B-Lynch suture or an intrauterine tamponade balloon (Chapter 158). The use of recombinant factor VIIa (NovoSeven) has been demonstrated to stop (64%) or decrease (32%) [8] bleeding in these cases and significantly reduce the need for blood products.

The use of drains should be considered as these may act as an early warning sign of intra-abdominal bleeding. However, they can cause patient discomfort and reduce mobility following the surgery.

Postoperative management

Close observation of the patient following the surgery is necessary. Syntocinon infusion should be considered for several hours. Active management of anemia with early commencement of iron supplementation is indicated.

Gynecologic patients (Case history 2)

Preoperative management

The management is the same as for obstetric patients, although in this situation there is often more time to plan for the surgery and optimize the patient's condition.

Intraoperative management

Good surgical technique is important to minimize blood loss at every step of an operation. There are numerous topical hemostatic agents available and their early use should be considered, particularly when dealing with larger areas of generalized ooze or when operating close to important structures or difficult to reach places. An experienced assistant can aid the speed and safety of the surgery and reduce the risk of bleeding.

Maintaining a low blood pressure during the surgery may help reduce the loss of blood during the procedure, but the blood pressure has to be normalized prior to closing to identify any potential bleeding points. If there is an increased amount of blood loss, then consideration should be given to occluding pelvic vessels either radiologically or with the help of vascular surgeons.

If bleeding is still difficult to control, tight abdominal packing may allow time for clotting products such as FFP, cryoprecipitate, and platelets (if the patient has agreed to these prior to surgery) or agents such as tranexamic acid, vitamin K, and NovoSeven to be given. The use of cell salvage in surgery for cancer is controversial and needs to be discussed on an individualized basis taking into consideration risks and benefits.

Postoperative management

In discussion with a hematologist, it may be advisable to commence oral or intravenous iron supplements in combination with erythropoiesis-stimulating agents (ESAs) in life-threatening anaemia [3]. Hyperbaric oxygen therapy may be considered [3] if facilities are available in extreme cases. The collection of blood using pediatric tubes and microsampling can help reduce the amount of circulating blood that is removed for important hematologic tests [3].

KEY POINTS

Challenge: Major surgery in a Jehovah's Witness patient.

Background
- Jehovah's Witness patients differ in their permission to allow blood or blood products in any planned surgery.

Management
Preoperative management
- Complete advanced directive.
- Optimize Hb, iron, vitamin B_{12}, and folate if indicated.
- For severe anemia consider use of recombinant human EPO.
- Liaise with interventional radiology.
- Request senior support or attendance.
- Operate in a center which has appropriate facilities (e.g., HDU and interventional radiology).

Intraoperative management
- Consider cell salvage (continuous or storage depending on the patient's wishes).
- Consider hypotensive surgery.
- Use meticulous surgical techniques and topical hemostatic agents to minimize blood loss.
- Liaise closely with a hematologist regarding alternatives to blood products such as factor VIIa.
- Liaise with the family and elders in cases of ongoing bleed.
- Consider hyperbaric oxygen in specialist centers for those with life-threatening anemia.

Postoperative care
- Be vigilant for blood loss.
- Treat anemia aggressively.

References

1 Historical Watchtower Publisher and Memorial Data. Complete publisher report. http://www.jwfacts.com/watchtower/statistics-historical-data.php (accessed 6 April 2014).

2 Van Wolfswinkel M, Zwart J, Schutte J, Duvekot JJ, Pel M, Van Roosmalen J. Maternal mortality and serious maternal morbidity in Jehovah's witnesses in the Netherlands. *BJOG* 2009;116:1103–1110.

3 Sienas L, Wong T, Collins R, Smith J. Contemporary uses of erythropoietin in pregnancy: a literature review. *Obstet Gynecol Surv* 2013;68:594–602.

4 Royal College of Obstetricians and Gynaecologists. *Placenta Praevia, Placenta Praevia Accreta and Vasa Praevia: Diagnosis and Management.* RCOG Green-top Guideline No. 27, January 2011. Available at https://www.rcog.org.uk/en/guidelines-research-services/guidelines/gtg27/

5 Association of Anaesthetists of Great Britain and Ireland. *Management of Anaesthesia for Jehovah's Witnesses,* 2nd edn. AAGBI, London, 2005.

6 Heesen M, Hofmann T, Klöhr S et al. Is general anaesthesia for caesarean section associated with postpartum haemorrhage? Systematic review and meta-analysis. *Acta Anaesthesiol Scand* 2013;57:1092–1102.

7 Sheehan SR, Montgomery AA, Carey M et al. Oxytocin bolus versus oxytocin bolus and infusion for control of blood loss at elective caesarean section: double blind, placebo controlled, randomized trial. *BMJ* 2011;343:d4661.

8 Kobayashi T, Nakabayashi M, Yoshioka A, Maeda M, Ikenoue T. Recombinant activated factor VII (rFVIIa/NovoSeven®) in the management of severe postpartum haemorrhage: initial report of a multicentre case series in Japan. *Int J Hematol* 2012;95:57–63.

CHAPTER 170

Termination of Pregnancy at Advanced Gestation

Rohan Chodankar[1] and Janesh Gupta[2]
[1] Frimley Health NHS Foundation Trust, Frimley, Surrey, UK
[2] Birmingham Women's NHS Foundation Trust, Birmingham, UK

Case history: A 25-year-old woman with two previous pregnancies with good outcomes seeks an abortion at 19 weeks of gestation.

Background

Women may request or need a termination of pregnancy at an advanced gestation, when the risks are greater than at a lower gestation. The Abortion Act 1967, as amended by the Human Fertilisation and Embryology Act 1990, governs abortion in England, Scotland and Wales (Great Britain).

Treatment for abortion (medical and surgical) must be carried out in an NHS hospital or approved independent sector facility. Surgical terminations at advanced gestations should be carried out by practitioners with appropriate training and experience.

Management

Pre-abortion management

Pre-abortion counseling and support should be provided to women who need it. However, women who are certain of their decision to have an abortion should not be subjected to compulsory counseling. It is important to provide evidence-based information with regard to the method of abortion best suited to the gestation, risks of complications, and clinical implications; however, women should be supported in their choice of a particular method.

Pre-abortion assessment should include Rh typing in order that anti-D prophylaxis can be instituted as appropriate. Ultrasound scanning prior to an abortion is dictated by clinical need, for example suspicion of an ectopic pregnancy, discrepancy in dates and period of gestation, and very obese patients. It is important to perform screening for *Chlamydia trachomatis* and consider risk assessment and screening for other sexually transmitted infections (HIV, syphilis, and gonorrhea). If screening is not performed, prophylactic antibiotic therapy is indicated.

Inducing fetal death before medical abortion may have beneficial emotional, ethical, and legal consequences. The RCOG recommends feticide for abortions over 21 weeks and 6 days of gestation, except in the case of lethal fetal abnormality, and that feticide should always be performed by an appropriately trained practitioner using aseptic conditions and with continuous ultrasound guidance. Drugs such as intracardiac KCl, intra-amniotic or intrathoracic injection of digoxin, and umbilical venous or intracardiac injection of 1% lidocaine can be used to induce feticide. In the case history described, with a gestational age of 19 weeks, feticide would not be necessary.

Medical termination of pregnancy

The following regimen is recommended for medical abortion between 13 and 24 weeks of gestation: mifepristone 200 mg orally, followed 36–48 hours later by misoprostol 800 μg vaginally, then misoprostol 400 μg orally or vaginally, 3-hourly, to a maximum of four further doses. If abortion does not occur, mifepristone can be repeated 3 hours after the last dose of misoprostol and 12 hours later misoprostol may be recommenced.

Surgical evacuation of the uterus is not required routinely following medical abortion between 13 and 24 weeks of gestation. It should only be undertaken if there is clinical evidence that the abortion is incomplete.

Surgical termination of pregnancy

Cervical preparation followed by dilatation and evacuation under ultrasound guidance (to reduce the risk of uterine perforations and retained tissues) is appropriate for pregnancies above 14 weeks of gestation.

Cervical preparation should be considered in all cases as it is associated with a reduction in risk of cervical lacerations, uterine perforations, and time taken to perform an abortion procedure when compared with mechanical cervical dilatation. After 14 weeks of gestation, overnight use of osmotic dilators provides superior dilatation to medical methods; however, misoprostol is an acceptable alternative up to 18 weeks of gestation. Misoprostol 400 μg is administered vaginally 3 hours prior to surgery, or sublingually 2–3 hours prior to surgery. Vaginal misoprostol can be administered either by the woman herself or by a clinician.

Women and clinicians in the UK are relatively unfamiliar with abortion under local anesthesia, although its use is increasing. The majority of abortions in the second trimester will be performed under general anesthesia, although there is increasing evidence that

Gynecologic and Obstetric Surgery: Challenges and Management Options, First Edition. Edited by Arri Coomarasamy, Mahmood I. Shafi, G. Willy Davila and Kiong K. Chan.
© 2016 John Wiley & Sons, Ltd. Published 2016 by John Wiley & Sons, Ltd.

induced abortions may be safely undertaken using local anesthesia or conscious sedation. Typical regimens include an intravenous opioid (such as fentanyl) plus an intravenous sedative (such as midazolam or propofol).

Vacuum aspiration is appropriate up to 14 weeks of gestation, although it may be done up to 16 weeks with the use of specialized instrumentation, namely using a large-bore cannula and tubing or completion of the abortion (to remove larger fetal parts) using a forceps.

It is important not to perform routine sharp curettage after vacuum aspiration as it linked to increased bleeding, pain, and intrauterine adhesions possibly resulting in Asherman's syndrome.

Post-abortion care

Anti-D IgG should be given to non-sensitized RhD-negative women within 72 hours of medical or surgical abortion. The recommended dose is 250 IU for gestations below 20 weeks, and 500 IU for gestations of 20 weeks and above. For gestations of 20 weeks and above, the amount of fetomaternal hemorrhage should be assessed using either the traditional Kleihauer acid elution test or the more accurate flow cytometry. If the test indicates a fetomaternal hemorrhage of over 4 mL, additional anti-D IgG should be administered.

Initiation of contraception immediately following induced abortion has several advantages. Options include copper IUD, levonorgestrel intrauterine system (LNG-IUS), and implants (e.g., Nexplanon). NICE recommends that a copper IUD or LNG-IUS can be inserted immediately after a first- or second-trimester abortion or at any time thereafter. Sterilization can be safely performed at the time of induced abortion, although the risk of regret should be considered.

Routine histopathology assessment and gestational trophoblastic neoplasia screening are not recommended. Fetal tissue must be treated with dignity and respect. Any personal wishes that are expressed should be met wherever possible. In general, abortion service providers arrange for fetal material from late medical and surgical abortions to be incinerated. Some have a contract with local crematoria or burial authorities.

KEY POINTS

Challenge: Termination of pregnancy at late gestations.

Background
- Termination at late gestations may be performed through a medical or surgical approach.
- Women should be counseled about potential risks, including uterine perforation, hemorrhage, pelvic infection, and persistent pregnancy tissues.

Management
- A policy of universal STI screening or antibiotic prophylaxis is recommended regardless of the method of abortion used.
- The RCOG recommends feticide for abortions over 21 weeks and 6 days of gestation, except in the case of lethal fetal abnormality.
- Medical abortions are performed using a combination of mifepristone and misoprostol.
- Surgical abortions are performed using manual or electric vacuum aspiration, and dilatation and evacuation with prior cervical preparation:
  - Cervical preparation can be achieved by administering misoprostol 400 µg vaginally 3 hours before surgery.
  - Large-bore cannula should be used for evacuation of the uterus.
  - In advanced gestations, it may be necessary to remove large fetal parts using forceps.
  - Performing surgical termination under ultrasound guidance will reduce the risks of perforation and persistent tissues.
- Rh typing should be undertaken prior to an abortion and all non-sensitized RhD-negative women should receive anti-D IgG within 72 hours of medical or surgical abortion.
- A plan for post-abortion contraception should ideally be agreed upon prior to the abortion.

Further reading

National Institute for Health and Care Excellence. *Long-acting reversible contraception.* NICE Clinical Guideline No. 30, October 2005. Available at https://www.nice.org.uk/guidance/cg30/resources/cg30-longacting-reversible-contraception-full-guideline2

Royal College of Obstetricians and Gynaecologists. *The Care of Women Requesting Induced Abortion.* RCOG Evidence-based Clinical Guideline No. 7, November 2011. Available at https://www.rcog.org.uk/en/guidelines-research-services/guidelines/the-care-of-women-requesting-induced-abortion/

CHAPTER 171

Cervical Fibroids: Techniques for Myomectomy and Hysterectomy

Deborah R. Karp

School of Medicine, Emory University, Atlanta, Georgia, USA

Case history: *A 45-year-old woman with an enlarging fibroid has elected to undergo a hysterectomy. Because of the increasing size of the mass, preoperative imaging is performed. This imaging reveals the fibroid to be originating from the cervix.*

Background

Fibroids originating from the cervix are thought to account for 0.6% of all fibroids [1]. Cervical fibroids can be extracervical (subserosal) or intracervical. Unlike uterine fibroids, which are located within the peritoneal cavity, cervical fibroids are most commonly retroperitoneal. They may be classified according to their anatomic location; anterior, posterior, lateral, or deep-rooted/vaginal. In rare circumstances they may be found prolapsing into the vagina and are then considered submucosal or polypoidal. Unlike fibroids originating in the uterine body, cervical fibroids are most often solitary tumors. They may grow rapidly, and because of their retroperitoneal location, may often reach massive sizes before symptoms manifest [2].

Symptoms of cervical fibroids include pressure effects on surrounding pelvic organs such as the bladder, urethra, and rectum. Symptoms can include urinary retention or frequency, constipation with tenesmus, back pain, or dyspareunia. Cervical fibroids may also cause menstrual bleeding problems and dysmenorrhea. Reproductive sequelae of cervical fibroids include infertility with anatomic blockage of the endocervical canal or uterine cavity, recurrent pregnancy loss, and obstruction of labor with dystocia leading to high rates of cesarean delivery, cesarean hysterectomy, postpartum hemorrhage, and blood transfusion [3].

Preoperative examination of women with cervical fibroids will reveal a fixed mass with little or no mobility. The mass may often bulge into the vaginal fornix and distort normal vaginal anatomy making the cervix difficult to identify (Figure 171.1). In cases of intracervical and submucosal cervical fibroids, the cervical os is often dilated. Preoperative imaging to aid diagnosis and surgical planning includes transvaginal ultrasound and pelvic MRI. In cases of large cervical fibroids, acoustic shadowing may limit the ability of sonography to determine the fibroid location with accuracy. Pelvic MRI is considered the most accurate imaging modality for determining the origin and location of fibroids. Cervical fibroids

are easily identified on pelvic MRI because their epicenter will be below the internal os of the cervix on T2-weighted sagittal imaging [4].

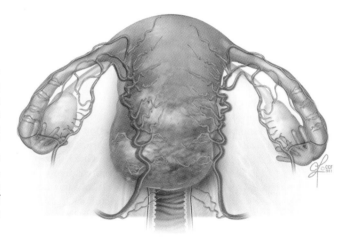

Figure 171.1 Anterior cervical fibroid. *Source*: Colombo & Naspro, 2010 [5]. Reproduced with permission from John Wiley & Sons, Ltd.

Management

Angiographic embolization of the uterine artery for cervical fibroids yields poor results, with incomplete necrosis of the fibroids in 8 of 10 patients (80%) in one series [4]. This is largely thought to be due to the fine plexus of collateral vessels supplying the cervix, which may not even be visualized on standard angiography and are thus not amenable to embolization. Collateral arterial supply is vast and often aberrant, incorporating the cervico-vaginal or descending branch of the uterine artery and branches of the ovarian, vaginal, and middle hemorrhoidal arteries. Reported complications with attempts at embolization of these fibroids include vaginal expulsion of fibroid material and necrosis of the vagina.

Surgery for cervical fibroids should only be undertaken in appropriately equipped settings, by expert pelvic surgeons who are skilled in radical dissection of the pelvis, as there are challenges from the large size, retroperitoneal location, and close proximity of

Gynecologic and Obstetric Surgery: Challenges and Management Options, First Edition. Edited by Arri Coomarasamy, Mahmood I. Shafi, G. Willy Davila and Kiong K. Chan.
© 2016 John Wiley & Sons, Ltd. Published 2016 by John Wiley & Sons, Ltd.

the cervical fibroid to important pelvic structures and vasculature. Impaction and distortion of normal pelvic anatomy increases the risk of operative complications such as urinary tract injury, inadvertent enterotomy, and massive intraoperative hemorrhage. Cervical fibroids are typically fixed in place even after peritoneal flaps and deep attachments are freed. In rare circumstances, vaginal fibroids have been discovered postoperatively and are thought to be due to either incomplete excision of cervical fibroids or possibly inadvertent expulsion of cervical fibroid cells into the adjacent spaces [6].

Fertility-sparing surgery

Vaginal myomectomy (Chapter 96)
In cases of a prolapsing submucosal or polypoidal cervical fibroid, a vaginal myomectomy can be considered. Care should be taken as these fibroids can grow large enough to completely fill the vaginal vault, limiting safe and easy access from a vaginal approach. Vaginal myomectomy is an ideal approach for small prolapsing fibroids on a stalk. In these cases where a stalk or sessile attachment is identified, infiltration of the fibroid with dilute vasopressin aided with careful blunt and sharp dissection should be used to remove the fibroid and its attachment from the cervix [7]. Blindly twisting out the fibroid without a thorough understanding of its origin and attachment may cause damage to the myometrium and hemorrhage.

Abdominal myomectomy
Abdominal myomectomy, performed either by a laparoscopic or open route, should be the fertility preservation procedure of choice for cervical fibroids that are intracervical or deep-rooted within the cervix. Preoperative administration of GnRH analog or ulipristal acetate can reduce fibroid size and improve preoperative hemoglobin level, especially where women are already anemic.

Intraoperatively, injection of a vasoconstrictor such as vasopressin (e.g., 20 units diluted in 100 mL saline) between the fibroids and the serosa is useful in temporarily reducing blood flow, enhancing visualization during surgery, and minimizing hemorrhage. Bilateral uterine artery ligation where they originate as a branch of the internal iliac artery should be considered at the onset of surgery. The origin of the uterine artery is located by placing gentle traction along the obliterated umbilical ligament on the lower anterior surface of the peritoneum, which will place the anterior division of the internal iliac artery under tension. This is easily visualized from a laparoscopic viewpoint. In cases where the fibroid is completely filling the pelvic cavity, access to the retroperitoneal space may not be possible. In such cases the use of angiographic interventional procedures should be contemplated. Temporary placement of CT-guided endovascular balloons may be used to occlude the internal iliac arteries during the critical portions of the procedure in order to reduce hemorrhage [8].

After securing the major blood supply, the cervical fibroid is injected with 20–30 mL of dilute vasopressin. A transverse incision is made along the prominent portion of the cervical fibroid at the proximal junction of the fibroid and the uterine body, taking care to prevent injury to nearby organs such as the bladder (anterior fibroid), rectum (posterior fibroid), and ureters (lateral or deep-rooted fibroid). If possible, the fibroid is then completely enucleated with the use of a myoma screw placed to provide traction. Because of their large size, there may be a lack of space for application of traction and counter-traction. If the fibroid cannot be

enucleated completely due to limited working space in the pelvis, *in situ* morcellation can be performed [9].

The approach for removing subserosal cervical fibroids should be as follows.
- *Anterior*: the vesico-uterine peritoneum is incised in a standard transverse fashion and the bladder separated from the anterior surface of the fibroid prior to enucleation or morcellation.
- *Posterior*: in cases of posterior subserosal cervical fibroids, the fibroid will be found anterior to the rectum. A transverse incision is made at the anterior-most aspect of the fibroid in order to expose the fibroid capsule. After ensuring the rectum, both ureters, and uterine arteries are adequately separated, the fibroid is enucleated or morcellated.
- *Lateral*: the fibroid will be found extending into the broad ligament. An incision is made within the peritoneum overlying the broad portion of the fibroid and the capsule is identified. Morcellation or enucleation proceeds after identification and separation of the ureter and ligation of the uterine vessels.
- *Deep infiltrating*: for such fibroids located within the cervix and with their main portion protruding into the vagina, it may be necessary to have a vaginal assistant push cephalad on the fibroid to bring it adequately into the pelvis. Once the fibroid is pushed in a cephalad manner, it will be accessible within the pelvis, and the fibroid may be approached in a similar manner to subserosal fibroids.

In all cases, the base of the capsule should be coagulated to reduce bleeding and the cervix is then closed in multiple layers; consideration should be given to placing a drain within the cul-de-sac as there is likely to be serous oozing from the bed of the tumor that may lead to a pelvic collection and postoperative febrile illness.

Hysterectomy
The transvaginal approach for hysterectomy, unless laparoscopically assisted, is considered to be largely inaccessible [8]. Cervical fibroids obliterate the vaginal fornices making an anterior or posterior colpotomy difficult, and ligation of the uterine arteries prior to fibroid removal impossible from a vaginal approach.

After access to the peritoneal cavity is obtained, a complete retroperitoneal dissection is performed in order to facilitate safe dissection of the anterior, lateral, and posterior aspects of the fibroid from the bladder, ureter, and rectum, respectively. When undertaking a hysterectomy, ligation of arterial blood supply, careful ureterolysis, and maximal debulking of the cervical fibroid are advisable in order to maintain adequate hemostasis, protect the genitourinary tract, and correct anatomic distortions of the uterine cervix prior to proceeding with hysterectomy. If debulking is not undertaken, then a modified radical abdominal or laparoscopic hysterectomy can be undertaken.

The hysterectomy procedure should be undertaken as follows.
- After gaining access to the pelvis through either a laparoscopic or abdominal approach, secure the utero-ovarian vessels and open up and divide the broad and round ligaments.
- Open up the rectovaginal space by incising the posterior peritoneum overlying the posterior vaginal wall and dissecting the posterior vagina from the perirectal fascia. This will mobilize the rectum in a posterior manner.
- The vesicovaginal space is then entered to dissect the bladder in an anterior and caudad fashion off the pubocervical fascia. This will facilitate mobilization of the bladder off the cervical fibroid.

- The paravesical and pararectal spaces are developed and a ureterolysis is performed beginning at the pelvic brim and proceeding in a cephalad to caudad direction up to the insertion into the bladder trigone. Ligation of the uterine arteries is then performed at their origin from the anterior branch of the internal iliac artery.
- A transverse incision along the most proximal and widest portion of the cervical fibroid is made in order to expose the capsule. In cases of large intracervical fibroids, the walls of the cervix will be severely attenuated.

- Enucleate the mass if possible. It may be helpful to have a vaginal assistant push the mass firmly in a cephalad direction. In cases of isthmic cervical fibroids, the cervico-vaginal junction may be obscured. Placement of the surgeon's fingers in the vagina may help delineate the vaginal fornices from the mass in order to prevent inadvertent vaginectomy.
- Once the mass is removed, the hysterectomy may be completed in a standard fashion.

KEY POINTS

Challenge: Myomectomy or hysterectomy for cervical fibroids.

Background
- Cervical leiomyomas are rare, accounting for approximately 0.6% of all fibroids.
- They are classified as extracervical (subserosal) or intracervical.
  - They may be located in an anterior, posterior, lateral, or deep-rooted/vaginal position.
  - Rarely, they may be found prolapsing into the vagina and are then classified as submucosal or polypoidal.
  - Unlike uterine fibroids, which are located within the peritoneal cavity, cervical fibroids are more commonly retroperitoneal.
- Cervical fibroids can grow rapidly and often reach massive sizes before symptoms manifest.

Management
- Pelvic MRI is the most accurate imaging modality for the mapping and characterization of cervical fibroids.

- Preoperative administration of GnRH agonists or ulipristal acetate may be given to shrink the fibroid and cease heavy menstrual loss, thereby helping to correct pre-existing anemia.
- The injection of dilute vasopressin will help minimize bleeding by inducing vasoconstriction (Chapter 95).
- In cases where the cervical fibroid is thought to completely fill the retroperitoneal space within the abdomen and pelvis, thereby severely limiting access for surgical ligation of the uterine arteries, preoperative angiographic evaluation and intervention may be warranted.
- Surgical mobilization of the vesicovaginal, rectovaginal, paravesical, and pararectal spaces will help to mobilize the bladder, ureters, and rectum out of the immediate operative field.
- In cases of fertility preservation, a myomectomy may be offered. If enucleation of the fibroid is not possible, then morcellation of the fibroid from its capsule while still attached to uterus should be considered.

References

1 Tiltman AJ. Leiomyomas of the uterine cervix: a study of frequency. *Int J Gynecol Pathol* 1998;17:231–234.
2 Lewers AHN. On fibroids of the cervix uteri. *BMJ* 1901;2(2115):63–66.
3 Tian J, Hu W. Cervical leiomyomas in pregnancy: report of 17 cases. *Aust NZ J Obstet Gynaecol* 2012;52:258–261.
4 Kim MD, Lee M, Jung DC *et al.* Limited efficacy of uterine artery embolisation for cervical leiomyomas. *J Vasc Interv Radiol* 2012;23:236–240.
5 Colombo R, Naspro R. Ileal conduit as the standard for urinary diversion after radical cystectomy for bladder cancer. *Eur Urol* 2010;Suppl 9:736–744.
6 Yanamandra SR, Redman CWE, Coomarasamy A, Varma R. Leiomyoma appearing in the vaginal vault following hysterectomy. *J Obstet Gynaecol* 2007;27:91–92.
7 Garg R. Two uncommon presentation of cervical fibroids. *People's Journal of Scientific Research* 2012;5(2):36–38.
8 Takeda A, Koyama K, Imoto S, Mori M, Nakano T, Nakamura H. Temporary endovascular balloon occlusion of the bilateral internal iliac arteries to control hemorrhage during laparoscopic-assisted vaginal hysterectomy for cervical myoma. *Eur J Obstet Gynecol Reprod Biol* 2011;158:319–324.
9 Chang WC, Chen SY, Huang SC, Chang DY, Chou LY, Sheu BC. Strategy of cervical myomectomy under laparoscopy. *Fertil Steril* 2010;94:2710–2715.

CHAPTER 172

Hysterectomy for Broad Ligament Fibroids

Kiong K. Chan

City Hospital, Sandwell and West Birmingham Hospitals NHS Trust, Birmingham, UK

Case history: *A 47-year-old parous woman presents with heavy menstrual bleeding. Abdominal examination reveals an irregular firm 22-week mass arising from the pelvis. Bimanual palpation of the mass suggests that it is of uterine origin and that much of the mass extends to the right side of the pelvis from the level of the isthmus. An ultrasound scan confirms the presence of fibroids and a subsequent MRI scan shows no suspicious features but demonstrates several fibroids extending subserosally toward the right pelvic sidewall. After consultation with her gynecologist, the patient decides to have a total abdominal hysterectomy and bilateral salpingo-oophorectomy. At laparotomy three fibroids measuring 5, 4 and 2 cm are seen extending from the uterus into the broad ligament toward the pelvic sidewall.*

Background

Hysterectomy for an enlarged fibroid uterus can be challenging mainly because surgical access is limited. Enlarged fibroid uteri often have an enhanced blood supply, which increases the risks of intraoperative bleeding, and anatomy can become distorted, increasing the potential for inadvertent damage to surrounding pelvic structures such as the bladder, ureter, and major pelvic blood vessels. These risks are further increased when fibroids originate near the uterine blood supply in the vicinity of the cervix and uterine isthmus and extend subserosally into the broad ligament.

Management

Pretreatment for 3–6 months with a GnRH analog or ulipristal acetate should be considered to reduce the fibroid volume, facilitating surgical access.

The patient should be admitted and prepared for a laparotomy under general anesthesia with or without an epidural to aid postoperative pain relief. Laparoscopic surgery would be difficult because of restricted access down the side of the uterus, compromising safe dissection and control of uterine blood vessels. A midline abdominal incision provides the best access.

A thorough exploration of the abdominal cavity and its contents should be made. Sarcomatous change within fibroids is rare but as preoperative imaging is non-discriminatory, it is prudent to inspect the diaphragm, liver, omentum, retroperitoneal lymph nodes, and the gastrointestinal tract in light of the woman's age and the large uterine mass. Surgeons should orientate themselves within the pelvis as the uterine and related pelvic anatomy is likely to be distorted.

Operative technique

The round ligaments on each side should be picked up with atraumatic (e.g., Babcock) or traumatic (e.g., Kocher) forceps and divided between vascular (e.g., Roberts) clamps and the cut ends should be ligated with an appropriate suture (e.g., 2-0 Vicryl). The pelvic sidewall peritoneum should then be divided parallel to the ovarian pedicle, a maneuver which can help to mobilize the uterus. The ovarian pedicle should then be elevated using atraumatic Babcock forceps and the right ureter identified visually. A small opening can then be created in the posterior leaf of the broad ligament between the Babcock forceps and the ureter, and the ovarian pedicle safely divided between two slightly curved heavy vascular (e.g., Zeppelin) clamps. By applying the distal clamp first, the surgeon should be able to lift the pedicle slightly and reveal the peritoneal window, facilitating application of the proximal clamp. The pedicle is then ligated using an absorbable suture; our preferred technique is to do this with an initial 2-0 Vicryl tie followed by a 2-0 Vicryl suture on a round-bodied needle placed distal to the tie.

In the presence of broad ligament fibroids, ureteric damage is more likely and so it is now important to trace the ureter to where it is crossed by the uterine artery. This requires extraperitoneal dissection within the broad ligament, which is facilitated by division of the posterior leaf. This maneuver then allows the uterus to be mobilized further, elevating the broad ligament fibroids out of the pelvis. It is more common for broad ligament fibroids to be found superior to the uterine vessels; isthmic or cervical fibroids would be situated below the uterine vessels, thus requiring more extensive dissection. Once the ureter has been displaced downward and laterally and the broad ligament fibroids mobilized upward, the uterine vessels can be safely divided between two slightly curved vascular Zeppelin clamps and the uterine pedicle can be ligated. The round ligament and ovarian pedicle on the other side are divided and secured in the same manner as previously described. The bladder should be dissected away from the cervix and displaced downward to expose the vagina. Often a degree of bladder dissection is required to help expose the uterine pedicles prior to their division.

Gynecologic and Obstetric Surgery: Challenges and Management Options, First Edition. Edited by Arri Coomarasamy, Mahmood I. Shafi, G. Willy Davila and Kiong K. Chan.
© 2016 John Wiley & Sons, Ltd. Published 2016 by John Wiley & Sons, Ltd.

The anterior wall of the vagina should then be picked up with two Littlewood forceps. Entry into the vagina is then made between the two Littlewood forceps using a scalpel. The vaginal angles are then clamped with two slightly curved vascular Zeppelin forceps. These clamps are applied so that one jaw is located inside the vagina and the other external to ensure that they are holding the entire thickness of the vaginal wall. A scalpel or scissors is then used to cut along the length of the clamps to separate the cervix from the vagina. Hemostasis is secured by ligating the vaginal angles and placing either continuous or figure-of-eight sutures to close the vaginal vault.

The pelvis should then be inspected to ensure good hemostasis and the abdomen closed; our preferred method is a mass closure using a strong, delayed absorbable suture such as No. 1 Ethilon (747) or PDS. The skin is then closed with a continuous or interrupted suture or staples.

KEY POINTS

Challenge: Hysterectomy for broad ligament fibroids.

Background
- Hysterectomy for an enlarged fibroid uterus can be challenging mainly because surgical access is limited.
- The risks of intraoperative bleeding and inadvertent damage to surrounding pelvic structures (e.g., bladder, ureter, and major pelvic blood vessels) are increased when fibroids originate near the uterine blood supply in the vicinity of the cervix and uterine isthmus and extend subserosally into the broad ligament.

Management
- MRI scans are useful for distinguishing ovarian from uterine masses and for mapping the fibroids.

- Large fibroids may be treated with GnRH analogs or ulipristal acetate to shrink uterine size.
- Broad ligament fibroids are not a contraindication for laparoscopic surgery but they need to be small enough to allow adequate access laterally for ureteric dissection.
- Adequate access through a midline laparotomy incision is necessary.
- Experience in dissecting retroperitoneally within the broad ligament to identify and separate the ureter and uterine vessels is essential.
- Broad ligament fibroids have an intimate relationship with the ureter. Consequently, it is important to trace the ureter along its course if injury is to be avoided.
- Although myomectomy is useful in operations on cervical fibroids, it is less so in the case of broad ligament fibroids except when they are impacted because of their size.

Further reading

Brown RSD, Marley JL, Cassoni AM. Pseudo-Meigs' syndrome due to broad ligament leiomyoma: a mimic of metastatic ovarian carcinoma. *Clin Oncol* 1998;10:198–201.

Bulun SE. Uterine fibroids. *N Engl J Med* 2013;369:1344–1355.

Ferrari MM, Berlanda N, Mezzopane R, Ragusa G, Cavallo M, Pardi G. Identifying the indications for laparoscopically assisted vaginal hysterectomy: a prospective comparison with abdominal hysterectomy in patients with symptomatic uterine fibroids. *BJOG* 2000;107:620–625.

Gowri V, Sudheendra R, Oumachigui A, Sankaran V. Giant broad ligament leiomyoma. *Int J Gynaecol Obstet* 1992;37:207–210.

Liapis A, Bakas P, Giannapoulos V, Creatsas G. Ureteral injuries during gynecological surgery. *Int Urogynecol J* 2001;12:391–394.

Liebsohn S, d'Ablaing G, Mishell D Jr, Schlaerth J. Leiomyosarcoma in a series of hysterectomies performed for presumed uterine leiomyomas. *Am J Obstet Gynecol* 1990;162:968–976.

CHAPTER 173

Hysterectomy for a Double Uterus

Kiong K. Chan

City Hospital, Sandwell and West Birmingham Hospitals NHS Trust, Birmingham, UK

Case history: A 49-year-old woman with heavy menstrual bleeding resistant to systemic medical treatment was diagnosed with a uterus didelphys and an incomplete vaginal septum. On examination, the uterus was found to be mobile and of normal size. She was listed for a total abdominal hysterectomy with bilateral salpingo-oophorectomy. An MRI scan confirmed the presence of a double uterus including cervices and an upper longitudinal vaginal septum. No renal anomalies were detected.

Background

A double uterus (uterus didelphys) is a congenital uterine malformation resulting from the failure of the paramesonephric (Müllerian) ducts to fuse during embryologic development (Chapter 100). This can result in a double uterus with two uterine horns, two cervices and, frequently, a vaginal septum. This congenital anomaly is less commonly encountered than arcuate, septated, or bicornuate uteri [1]. It is important to diagnose the condition because it has obstetric and gynecologic implications that include difficulties in conception, miscarriage, preterm delivery, and intrauterine growth restriction [2]. Furthermore, duplication of the cervix necessitates taking two cervical smears from each cervix.

In general gynecologic practice, failure of systemic medical treatments would indicate a need to consider more effective conservative interventions such as levonorgestrel-releasing intrauterine system or second-generation endometrial ablation. If these fail, hysterectomy is an option.

Management

Preoperative investigations

Renal anomalies are present in 10% of women with double uteri. MRI is now accepted as the best form of imaging for classifying the uterine abnormality and for excluding renal anomalies [3,4]. It is important to review the actual images as well as the report since reports may be incorrect even in the best radiologic departments. It is important to be aware of such anomalies as renal agenesis [5] and duplicated ureters to help plan the surgical approach and anesthetic management.

Surgical route and incision

All routes for performing a hysterectomy should be considered [6]. The technique described here relates to open hysterectomy but the principles of safe delineation of anatomy apply to all routes of surgery.

After sterile cleaning with a disinfectant such as aqueous Betadine, a Foley catheter should be inserted into the bladder using a no-touch technique. A careful assessment of the size and mobility of the double uterus should be made on bimanual palpation by the operating surgeon; this key task should not simply be delegated to an assistant. A lack of mobility may suggest the presence of adhesions from either pelvic inflammatory disease or endometriosis, indicating that a vertical incision may be more appropriate. The choice of incision and the need for a vertical incision should have been discussed with the patient preoperatively. When in doubt the vertical incision is the wiser choice as it is better to place safety before cosmesis.

Operative technique

Following a Pfannenstiel or vertical incision, the layers of the anterior abdominal wall are traversed and the peritoneal cavity is opened. The contents of the abdominal cavity are examined, the bowels are packed, and a self-retaining retractor is inserted. The surgeon should then examine and become familiar with the pelvic anatomy, especially the shape and axis of the double uterus, the location of the duplicated cervices, and their relationships to the pelvic sidewall.

Total abdominal hysterectomy can then be performed in a number of ways utilizing variations in surgical technique, favored sutures, and choice of equipment. The following surgical description is my preferred approach and highlights the principles of safe systematic surgery, especially germane to this case where abnormal pelvic anatomy is present.

- The round ligaments are picked up with atraumatic Babcock forceps before clamping with Roberts artery forceps prior to dividing them with dissecting scissors and ligating the pedicles with absorbable 2-0 Vicryl ties.
- The uterovesical fold of peritoneum is then divided to dissect the bladder downward, exposing the anterior wall of the vagina. The two cervices are often found adherent to each other, giving the impression of a broad single cervix.

Gynecologic and Obstetric Surgery: Challenges and Management Options, First Edition. Edited by Arri Coomarasamy, Mahmood I. Shafi, G. Willy Davila and Kiong K. Chan.
© 2016 John Wiley & Sons, Ltd. Published 2016 by John Wiley & Sons, Ltd.

- It is important to identify the ureters and their proximity to the cervices to avoid inadvertent injury. This is achieved by incising the peritoneum of the broad ligament parallel to the ovarian pedicle on each side, facilitating extraperitoneal dissection and identification of the ureters. The surgeon should be vigilant for the presence of a double ureter because this renal tract anomaly may be missed on imaging.
- The ovarian pedicle is then picked up using Babcock tissue forceps to visualize the ureter on that side. A peritoneal window is then made in the posterior leaf of the broad ligament just below the Babcock tissue forceps and above the ureter. This isolates the infundibulopelvic pedicle, which is then clamped with two slightly curved Zeppelin vascular forceps, and divided. The pedicle is ligated proximally with 2-0 Vicryl and a second, more distal transfixing suture, thereby avoiding bleeding when the needle is passed through the pedicle.
- The posterior leaf of the broad ligament is then divided and the pouch of Douglas is opened to ensure that the rectum is not adherent to the posterior part of the cervices.

- The uterosacral ligaments are then divided close to the uteri to minimize the risk of ureteric damage, which are kept under direct vision.
- The uterine vessels are then "skeletonized" to allow precise placement of a slightly curved Zeppelin vascular forceps. Back-bleeding from the uterus is prevented using Roberts or Spencer Wells artery forceps. The uterine pedicles are then sutured with 2-0 Vicryl.
- The cardinal ligaments are then clamped with straight Zeppelin forceps and divided with a scalpel flush to the clamps to minimize bleeding and the pedicles sutured with 2-0 Vicryl.
- The vagina is then picked up and divided between two Littlewoods tissue forceps and the vaginal angles clamped with curved Zeppelin forceps. Cholecystectomy forceps are used to clamp the posterior vaginal wall and the double uterus is then detached and removed.
- The vaginal angles are secured with 2-0 Vicryl sutures and the vagina closed in continuous fashion with the same suture.
- The anterior abdominal wall is closed in layers using continuous sutures: 2-0 Vicryl to the parietal peritoneum, No. 1 PDS to the rectus sheath, and subcuticular 4-0 Prolene to close the skin.

KEY POINTS

Challenge: Hysterectomy for a double uterus.

Background
- A double uterus (uterus didelphys) is a congenital uterine malformation resulting in two uterine horns, two cervices, and often a vaginal septum.
- This congenital anomaly is less commonly encountered than arcuate, septated, or bicornuate uteri, and has an estimated prevalence of 1 in 3000 women [1].
- Coexisting renal tract anomalies are found in 10% of women with double uteri.
- Hysterectomy is more complex in the presence of congenital genital and renal tract abnormalities, and the risk of complications is higher.

Prevention
- It is important to perform appropriate imaging before a hysterectomy in order to minimize the risk of injury to the urinary tract.
- MRI is the best form of imaging in the investigation of uterine anomalies and can detect associated pelvic and urinary tract anomalies. It is also able

to demonstrate clearly the presence or absence of a plane between the uteri and the bladder or rectum.
- Alternatives to hysterectomy should be considered for benign disease.

Management
- A careful and systematic approach to hysterectomy, regardless of the route chosen, is mandatory.
- The surgeon should appreciate the possibility of ureteric abnormalities and the operative challenges of abnormal uterine anatomy, especially the increased size often associated with duplicated cervices.
- Identification of the ureter by extraperitoneal dissection minimizes the risk of inadvertent injury.
- Abdominal hysterectomy has traditionally been used over vaginal hysterectomy because access and visualization of the pelvic sidewall is facilitated. However, most double uteri can now be removed without a laparotomy using laparoscopic surgical techniques by an appropriately experienced surgeon.

References

1 Grimbizis GF, Camus M, Tarlatzis BC, Bontis JN, Devroey P. Clinical implications of uterine malformations and hysteroscopic treatment results. *Hum Reprod Update* 2001;7:161–174.
2 Heinonen PK, Saarikoski S, Pystynen P. Reproductive performance of women with uterine anomalies: an evaluation of 182 cases. *Acta Obstet Gynecol Scand* 1982;61:157–162.
3 Saleem SN. MR imaging diagnosis of uterovaginal anomalies: current state of the art. *Radiographics* 2003;23:e13.

4 Takagi H, Matsunami K, Noda K, Furui T, Imai I. Magnetic resonance imaging in the evaluating of the double uterus and associated urinary tract anomalies: a report of five cases. *J Obstet Gynaecol* 2003;23:525–527.
5 Zurawin RK, Dietrich JE, Heend MJ, Edwards CL. Didelphic uterus and obstructed hemivagina with renal agenesis: a case report and review of the literature. *J Pediatr Adolesc Gynecol* 2004;7:137–141.
6 Lee CL, Wang CJ, Swei LD, Yen CF, Soong YK. Laparoscopic hemi-hysterectomy in treatment of didelphic uterus with hypoplastic cervix and obstructed hemivagina. *Hum Reprod* 1999;14:1741–1743.

CHAPTER 174
Cervical Stump Excision

Kiong K. Chan

City Hospital, Sandwell and West Birmingham Hospitals NHS Trust, Birmingham, UK

Case history: A 44-year-old woman with fibroids was treated with an abdominal subtotal hysterectomy and bilateral salpingo-oophorectomy through a Pfannenstiel incision. Unfortunately, her histology revealed a stage IA endometrioid endometrial carcinoma. Her BMI was 20.

Background

The patient was referred to a gynecologic oncologist who explained that it would be prudent to remove the cervical stump even though it was a well-differentiated tumor and may well have been completely excised, particularly as there was endometrium at the excision margin. There was no cervical descent and the vagina was of normal size. The recent surgery would have made the presence of adhesions more likely. Consequently, the abdominal approach was deemed safer than the vaginal route. The patient was advised to have laparoscopic surgery with the option of converting to open surgery should extensive adhesions be encountered.

If cervical descent had been present, then the vaginal route for removing the cervical stump would have been preferable because it is associated with a lower morbidity and a shorter hospital stay. However, the abdominal route is generally safer in those patients who require removal of the cervical stump following recent surgery or in those who have a history suggestive of bowel or bladder adhesions to the stump. If possible a laparoscopic approach is desirable but not always possible and the patient should be made aware of this during the consenting process.

Management

Preoperative preparation

The patient was admitted on the day of surgery and prepared for a laparotomy. She was given general anesthesia and placed in lithotomy position using movable Lloyd-Davies poles. A gel-filled bag was placed under her buttocks to tilt the pelvis and help keep the bowel away from the pelvic organs. The vagina and perineum were prepared by painting with aqueous Betadine. The bladder was catheterized with a Foley catheter attached to a continuous drainage bag. An examination under anesthesia was performed. This revealed a normal mobile cervix. A swab on a sponge-holder was placed in the vagina to allow the cervical stump to be elevated in the

pelvis. Meanwhile the skin of the whole of the anterior abdominal wall was sterilized with an alcoholic preparation of Hibitane. This was allowed to dry by evaporation to ensure effective sterilization of the area. The legs were lowered and the abdomen draped as for a laparotomy.

Laparoscopic entry

In view of the patient's recent hysterectomy undertaken via a Pfannenstiel incision, an open entry using the Hasson technique was used in preference to insufflation using a Veress needle. This technique was chosen to minimize the risk of major vascular injury, which is increased with closed entry in slim patients [1]. It was also felt that because of the increased likelihood of adhesions from her previous abdominal surgery, the open approach could aid identification of inadvertent bowel injury. A small vertical incision was made at the umbilicus. The rectus sheath was grasped with two Roberts (or Kocher) forceps and divided between them. A 0 PDS suture was inserted to hold the sheath on each side. A J-shaped needle was used to allow ease of access. The peritoneum was then grasped with two Roberts forceps and divided. Two further 0 PDS sutures were inserted to encompass the sheath and peritoneum on each side. The Hasson cannula was inserted, followed by a 10-mm telescope. Once it was confirmed that entry into the peritoneal cavity had been made, the gas tubing was connected and insufflation of carbon dioxide gas to a pressure of 20 mmHg was achieved. Under direct vision, three 5-mm trocars and cannulas were inserted, two on the left and one on the right side of the abdomen. Following insertion of the side ports the insufflation pressure was reduced to 15 mmHg.

Conversion to laparotomy

There were small bowel adhesions to the anterior abdominal wall scar. The sigmoid colon was attached by some of its appendices epiploicae to the inferior part of the scar. The bladder was found to be densely adherent to the cervical stump. In view of these findings it was considered unsafe by the surgeon to continue with laparoscopic surgery. Consequently, the decision was made to convert to open laparotomy (Chapter 89). While the threshold at which a decision to convert to a laparotomy is made will vary from surgeon to surgeon and among centers according to experience and available infrastructure, it should be considered part of standard surgical practice (and not "failed" surgery).

Gynecologic and Obstetric Surgery: Challenges and Management Options, First Edition. Edited by Arri Coomarasamy, Mahmood I. Shafi, G. Willy Davila and Kiong K. Chan.
© 2016 John Wiley & Sons, Ltd. Published 2016 by John Wiley & Sons, Ltd.

Laparotomy

A vertical midline incision was made extending to 3 cm above the umbilicus. A midline incision was considered preferable to reopening the Pfannenstiel incision because access was important for the safe dissection of adhesions. The small and large bowel adhesions were divided mainly with careful sharp dissection. Both ureters were identified using an extraperitoneal approach. This approach is important after previous pelvic surgery because the pelvic peritoneum is often opaque, which makes transperitoneal identification of the ureters difficult. The ureters were then traced down to either side of the cervical stump and displaced laterally to ensure their safety. The densely adherent bladder was dissected free with sharp dissection because blunt dissection of an adherent bladder is more likely to produce bladder injury. The plane of dissection between the bladder and cervix can often be found if the uterine vessels are skeletonized anteriorly and the dissection of that plane extended medially.

The cardinal ligament on each side of the pelvis was then clamped with straight Zeppelin clamps and divided. Each was secured with a 2-0 Vicryl suture on a round-bodied needle (9136). The vagina was picked up and divided between two Littlewood clamps. A slightly curved Zeppelin clamp was used to hold each vaginal angle. The cervix was then divided with a knife. The vaginal angles were then secured with 2-0 Vicryl sutures and the vault was then sutured. I use a lateral and a medial suture to close the angles on each side of the vault in the belief that when the continuous suture for vault closure is anchored to the medial suture it is less likely to endanger the hemostasis of the vaginal angles.

To ensure complete hemostasis a check was carried out for residual bleeding after pelvic lavage with 1 L of warm water. Water is preferred to normal saline as blood mixes with it less readily and bleeding points are more easily identified. The abdomen was closed with No. 1 Ethilon (747) using a mass closure technique. The skin was closed with staples.

Histologic examination did not reveal any pathology so no further treatment was required.

Prevention

Reassurance from cervical screening and the unproven belief of reduced sexual dysfunction has encouraged some gynecologists to revive the old operation of subtotal or supracervical hysterectomy as opposed to performing a total hysterectomy. However, subsequent excision of the cervical stump may become necessary for ongoing symptoms or for premalignant or malignant pathology as highlighted in this case [2,3]. The patient and surgeon should consider this possibility, especially because the morbidity of subsequently removing a cervical stump is higher than that of a total hysterectomy. Furthermore, should a carcinoma develop in the cervical stump it can be extremely difficult to treat particularly if it is not operable, as it is difficult to safely or adequately irradiate the cervical stump.

There is no strong evidence that a subtotal hysterectomy is associated with reduced risks of long-term complications such as genital prolapse or sexual dysfunction, compared with a total hysterectomy [4–6]. The available evidence from randomized trials would point to the surgical morbidity being the same. In addition to the uncommon but serious threat of the development of cervical neoplasia, patients with subtotal hysterectomy may continue to experience some vaginal bleeding (up to 25% in one series) and vaginal discharge.

The subtotal operation should be avoided in women with previous cervical intraepithelial neoplasia or ongoing cervical smear abnormalities, endometrial hyperplasia, and probably in the presence of significant fibroids because of the possible existence of leiomyosarcoma. In addition, women with endometriosis or menstrual pain may be more likely to have continuing problems after subtotal hysterectomy.

Advocates of subtotal hysterectomy argue that it is technically simpler and quicker to perform, either as an open or laparoscopic procedure, compared with total hysterectomy. Indeed, prior pelvic infection and endometriosis may result in adhesions of the bladder or rectum to the cervix, making total hysterectomy hazardous. Nevertheless, a total hysterectomy is feasible and safe in the vast majority of cases for a proficient surgeon with the appropriate surgical experience and expertise. An easier operation for the surgeon is not always in the patient's interest.

KEY POINTS

Challenge: Cervical stump excision.

Background
- Excision of the cervical stump may become necessary for ongoing symptoms or for premalignant or malignant pathology after a subtotal or supracervical hysterectomy.
- Excision of the cervical stump can be surgically challenging; the patient and surgeon should consider this possibility, especially because the morbidity of subsequently removing a cervical stump is higher than that of a total hysterectomy.

Prevention
- There is no strong evidence that a subtotal hysterectomy is associated with less risk of long-term complications (e.g., genital prolapse and sexual dysfunction) compared with total hysterectomy.
- The subtotal operation should be avoided in women with previous or ongoing cervical intraepithelial neoplasia or endometrial hyperplasia.
- A total hysterectomy is feasible and safe in the vast majority of cases for a proficient surgeon with the appropriate surgical experience and expertise.

Management
- The cervical stump can be removed using a laparoscopic or open approach. However, in the presence of cervical prolapse, a vaginal route is preferable.
- A systematic approach to surgery is necessary and the choice of surgical route should provide enough access to identify and dissect free the ureters and uterine blood vessels to minimize complications.

References

1 Altun H, Banli O, Kavlakoglu B, Kücükkayikci B, Kelesoglu C, Erez N. Comparison between direct trocar and Veress needle insertion in laparoscopic cholecystectomy. *J Laparoendosc Adv Surg Tech* 2007;17:709–712.
2 van der Stege JG, van Beek JJ. Problems related to the cervical stump at follow-up in laparoscopic supracervical hysterectomy. *J Soc Laparoendosc Surg* 1999;3:5–7.
3 Hilger WS, Pizarro AR, Magrina JF. Removal of the retained cervical stump. *Am J Obstet Gynecol* 2005;193:2117–2121.
4 Lieng M, Qvigstad E, Istre O, Langebrekke A, Ballard K. Long-term outcome following laparoscopic supracervical hysterectomy. *BJOG* 2008;115:1605–1610.
5 Gimbel H, Zobbe V, Andersen BM et al. Randomised controlled trial of total compared with subtotal hysterectomy with one-year follow up results. *BJOG* 2003;110:1088–1098.
6 Thakar R, Ayers S, Clarkson P, Stanton S, Manyonda I. Outcomes after total versus subtotal abdominal hysterectomy. *N Engl J Med* 2002;347:1318–1325.

CHAPTER 175

Surgery for Ovarian Remnant

Kiong K. Chan[1] and Arri Coomarasamy[2]

[1] City Hospital, Sandwell and West Birmingham Hospitals NHS Trust, Birmingham, UK
[2] College of Medical and Dental Sciences, University of Birmingham, Birmingham, UK

Case history: *A 38-year-old woman had total abdomino hysterectomy and bilateral salpingo-oophorectomy for endometriosis. Seven months after the procedure she presented with persisting lower abdominal pain and abdominal distension. Clinical examination was not helpful as the patient was obese. The patient was reassured without any investigations. At follow-up, an ultrasound scan showed a complex left adnexal mass. Serum FSH, LH, and estradiol showed that the patient was premenopausal. CA125 was 113 kU/L. CT scan of the abdomen and pelvis showed a complex pelvic mass measuring 6.3 × 3.3 × 3 cm on the left. The patient was on estrogen replacement therapy.*

Background

Ovarian remnant syndrome (ORS) occurs when fragments of ovarian tissue are unintentionally left behind after an oophorectomy (Figure 175.1). The remnant ovarian tissue can result in pelvic pain and an adnexal mass. Risk factors for ORS include endometriosis, pelvic adhesions, multiple pelvic surgery, and anatomic distortions [1]. Most women who have ORS are premenopausal, as in the case history [2,3]. The syndrome is reported to appear after a mean period of 4 years (range 5 months to 12 years) following oophorectomy [4].

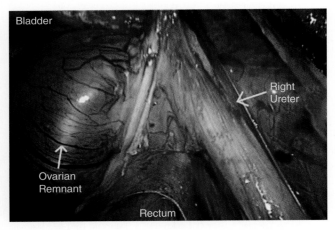

Figure 175.1 Ovarian remnant adherent to the dissected right ureter.
Source: Nezhat *et al.*, 2000 [3]. Reproduced with permission from Elsevier.

Management

Diagnosis

The first step is to review previous operation records to identify any operative difficulties and histology reports to assess the possibility of a partial resection of an ovary.

Clinical history

Most patients (84%) present with constant chronic pelvic pain, while a smaller proportion have cyclic pelvic pain (9%) and dyspareunia (26%) [1]. Other symptoms include cyclic vaginal bleeding, dysuria, and pain on defecation.

Hormonal assays

As most women with ORS are premenopausal, the functional status of any remaining ovarian tissue can be assessed with measurement of estradiol and follicle-stimulating hormone (FSH). If the woman is not taking estrogen replacement therapy, a hormone assay can be performed without delay; for patients on oral estrogen replacement therapy (as in the case history), the replacement should be stopped for 2 weeks and then the hormone assays can be performed, avoiding confounding by any exogenous hormones. In women with ORS, premenopausal levels of estrogen (>35 pg/mL) and FSH (<30 IU/L) can be expected. However, reproductive hormone levels in the postmenopausal reference range should not always be interpreted as absence of ORS because false-negative results are possible.

An ovarian stimulation test (clomiphene 100 mg for 10 days) followed by an ultrasound scan can be useful in locating the ovarian remnant [5]. Such an approach may also aid identification of the ovarian remnant at surgery. However, false-negative results are again possible with a clomiphene challenge test. A GnRH analog suppression test can aid diagnosis of ORS when pain without an obvious adnexal mass is the main presenting complaint; pain is likely to improve if the diagnosis is ORS.

Imaging

Ultrasound, MRI, and CT can all be useful in diagnosing ORS. The size, nature (simple or complex), and location of any adnexal mass should be noted.

Gynecologic and Obstetric Surgery: Challenges and Management Options, First Edition. Edited by Arri Coomarasamy, Mahmood I. Shafi, G. Willy Davila and Kiong K. Chan.
© 2016 John Wiley & Sons, Ltd. Published 2016 by John Wiley & Sons, Ltd.

Treatment

The mainstay of treatment is surgery, particularly in postmenopausal women in whom there is an age-related increase in the risk of cancer. In some premenopausal women medical treatment may have a role.

Medical treatment

Premenopausal women with ORS can be treated with oral contraceptive pill, progestins, or GnRH agonists. However, treatment failures appear to be high in the published data [1].

Surgery

Surgical removal of ovarian remnants can be achieved via laparoscopy, laparotomy, or robotic surgery [6]. Regardless of the operative approach, the key steps are similar, and the principles of surgical management are as follows [1].

- Involvement of general surgeons and urologists is prudent if appropriate and consideration should be given to preoperative bowel preparation.
- Cystoscopy and ureteral stenting can help identify the ureters, and may reduce the risk of injury depending on findings at imaging (e.g., MRI).
- The pelvic peritoneum is incised parallel to the ovarian vessels to enter the retroperitoneum. The ovarian vessels are isolated and ligated high to ensure no ovarian remnant is missed along the ovarian vessels. The ureter is mobilized off the pelvic sidewall peritoneum, from pelvic brim down to the level of the bladder. In most patients, the ovarian remnant can now be removed with a good margin from the pelvic sidewall. Some authors recommend stripping and excising the entire pelvic sidewall peritoneum as the ovarian remnant can be situated anywhere on the pelvic sidewall [1].

Resolution of the case

The patient was advised to undergo a laparotomy. Cystoscopy was performed to insert ureteric stents at the start of the operation. A midline incision was performed. The right ovary was found to be densely adherent to the pelvic sidewall. Using an extraperitoneal approach, the right ureter was identified and dissected away from the ovary. The ovarian pedicle was identified, clamped, divided, and ligated. The ureteric stents were removed at the end of the operation. Her postoperative recovery was uneventful and her symptoms vanished. Histology confirmed the pressure of endometriosis in the ovarian remnant.

Prevention

The problem of ORS could be avoided in the first place by identifying the ovarian pedicles properly and dividing them. This is best done by identifying the ureters using an extraperitoneal approach. The ovarian pedicles are always anterior to the ureters. In cases where extensive fibrosis is expected, such as endometriosis or previous extensive surgery, it is wise to insert ureteric stents so that the ureters can be identified by palpation as well as visually.

The risk of ORS is thought to be increased with blunt dissection of ovarian adhesions, as fragments of ovarian tissue may be left behind [1]. Sharp dissection of ovarian adhesions may therefore reduce the risk of ORS.

KEY POINTS

Challenge: Surgery for ovarian remnant.

Background
- Occurs when fragments of ovarian tissue are unintentionally left behind after an oophorectomy.
- Risk factors include endometriosis, pelvic adhesions, multiple pelvic surgery, and anatomic distortions.

Management
Diagnosis
- Previous operation notes and histopathology reports should be reviewed.
- Hormonal assays should be performed to measure estradiol and FSH levels indicating the degree of any residual ovarian activity.
- An ovarian stimulation test with clomiphene (100 mg for 10 days) can be considered.
- In the presence of a pelvic mass, CA125 and other tumor markers should be taken to assess risk of malignancy.
- Imaging with ultrasound, CT, or MRI is useful for identifying, locating, and assessing the nature of a pelvic mass.

Treatment
- Medical management may be appropriate in premenopausal age women. However, there is high risk of treatment failure.
- The key principles of surgical management are:
  - Adopt a laparoscopic or laparotomic approach.
  - Involve general surgeons and urologists as appropriate.
  - Consider preoperative bowel preparation.
  - Cystoscopy and ureteral stenting may be necessary.
  - Incise the pelvic sidewall peritoneum to enter the retroperitoneum and then dissect the paravesical and pararectal spaces.
  - Isolate and ligate the ovarian vessels high in the pelvis to avoid leaving any further ovarian remnant.
  - Mobilize the ureter from the pelvic brim along its course to the bladder.
  - Remove the ovarian remnant and consider stripping the entire pelvic sidewall peritoneum.

Prevention
- Identify and ligate ovarian pedicles properly.
- Use sharp rather than blunt dissection of ovarian adhesions.

References

1 Magtibay PM, Magrina JF. Ovarian remnant syndrome. *Clin Obstet Gynecol* 2006;49:526–534.
2 Magtibay PM, Nyholm JL, Hernandez JL, Podratz KC. Ovarian remnant syndrome. *Am J Obstet Gynecol* 2005;193:2062–2066.
3 Nezhat CH, Seidman DS, Nezhat FR, Mirmalek SA, Nezhat CR. Ovarian remnant syndrome after laparoscopic oophorectomy. *Fertil Steril* 2000;74:1024–1028.
4 Fat BC, Terzibachian JJ, Bertrand V *et al.* [Ovarian remnant syndrome: diagnostic difficulties and management.] *Gynecol Obstet Fertil* 2009;37:488–494.
5 Kaminski PF, Sorosky JI, Mandell MJ, Broadstreet RP, Zaino RJ. Clomiphene citrate stimulation as an adjunct in locating ovarian tissue in ovarian remnant syndrome. *Obstet Gynecol* 1990;76:924–926.
6 Zapardiel I, Zanagnolo V, Kho R, Magrina J, Magtibay P. Ovarian remnant syndrome: comparison of laparotomy, laparoscopy and robotic surgery. *Acta Obstet Gynecol Scand* 2012;91:965–969.

CHAPTER 176

Surgery for Missing Intrauterine Contraceptive Device

Toh Lick Tan
KK Women's and Children's Hospital, Singapore

Case history 1: A woman attended for replacement of her copper intrauterine device (Cu-IUD). The Cu-IUD thread was seen in the vagina but attempts to remove the device caused immense pain, and the removal had to be abandoned. A transvaginal pelvic ultrasound showed a Cu-IUD sited within the lower uterine cavity.

Case history 2: A woman using levonorgestrel intrauterine system (LNG-IUS) found herself to be pregnant, although the thread from the device was not seen on speculum examination. A transvaginal pelvic ultrasound found a viable early intrauterine pregnancy with the LNG-IUS in the pouch of Douglas. Following counseling on the risks of retaining or removing the LNG-IUS, she opted to continue with the pregnancy with the LNG-IUS in situ. Abdominal X-ray after an uncomplicated term vaginal delivery confirmed that the LNG-IUS was in the pelvis.

Background

A missing IUD is associated with device expulsion or uterine perforation. The risk of expulsion of IUD is common at around 1 in 20 [1]. This usually occurs within 3 months of insertion. In contrast, the risk of uterine perforation associated with IUD is uncommon at up to 2 per 1000 insertions [1]. However, apart from a loss of contraceptive effect, misplaced IUD secondary to perforation can lead to pelvic adhesions, visceral damage, infection, and abscess formation. Furthermore, the device can also translocate into various abdominal structures including the omentum, ovary, rectosigmoid colon, small bowel, and bladder. Active localization of the missing device is therefore important.

There is no significant difference in perforation rates or expulsion rates with different Cu-IUD, or between Cu-IUD and LNG-IUS [1]. However, with a perforated LNG-IUS, there is the added complication of systemic absorption of levonorgestrel, which can be 10 times higher than when the device is *in utero* [2]. Despite this, concerns about congenital anomalies, clitoral hypertrophy, or other urinary tract anomalies in female infants in pregnancies complicated by the presence of LNG-IUS have yet to be substantiated [3,4].

Management

When the thread of the IUD is not visualized on speculum examination, a transvaginal pelvic ultrasound is required to localize the device. Both two-dimensional and three-dimensional ultrasound may be used, although IUDs are significantly more conspicuous on three-dimensional ultrasound, particularly in the case of LNG-IUS [5]. The accuracy of ultrasound in localizing the device in the endocervical canal or uterine cavity is unknown and should only be attempted after a pregnancy is excluded. Advice on emergency contraception and alternative contraception such as condoms should be discussed.

If the IUD cannot be retrieved in an outpatient setting, surgery is indicated. The type of surgery required to retrieve the missing IUD depends on the location of the device and the anticipated complexity of the retrieval. In most cases, these are performed as elective day surgery under general anesthesia, although sedation and local anesthesia can be used in non-incisional approaches. Intraoperative broad-spectrum antibiotic cover is recommended, and this should be continued if any abscess or visceral perforation is found.

If the woman has completed her family and sterilization is indicated, the clinician should discuss potential concurrent hysteroscopic or laparoscopic sterilization during IUD retrieval.

The surgical options are summarized in Figure 176.1 and detailed in the following sections. However, if the woman is pregnant, intervention should generally be delayed. In such instances, the IUD is best sought at delivery or termination; if not found, abdominal X-ray is indicated to determine if the device is extrauterine.

Hysteroscopy

The majority of missing IUDs are found within the uterine cavity [6]. Hysteroscopic removal may be indicated as outpatient removal of IUD can be complicated by missing or short threads, inadequate analgesia, an embedded IUD, or mechanical obstruction such as fibroids. Occasionally, the IUD thread may have eroded through the cervix making it unfeasible to remove the IUD in an outpatient setting. This was the situation in Case history 1 (Figure 176.2). Hysteroscopic removal may also be indicated during an evacuation of the uterus in a miscarriage or termination of pregnancy.

Gynecologic and Obstetric Surgery: Challenges and Management Options, First Edition. Edited by Arri Coomarasamy, Mahmood I. Shafi, G. Willy Davila and Kiong K. Chan.
© 2016 John Wiley & Sons, Ltd. Published 2016 by John Wiley & Sons, Ltd.

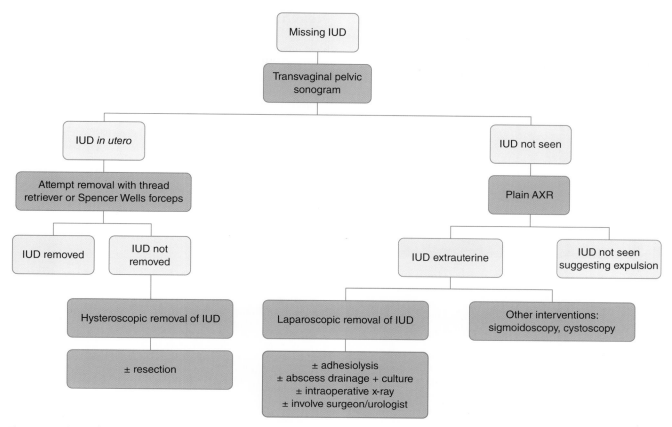

Figure 176.1 Surgical options for missing intrauterine contraception device outside pregnancy.

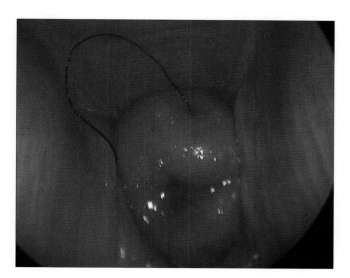

Figure 176.2 Intrauterine contraceptive device thread eroded through the cervix.

During hysteroscopy, the entire IUD must be visualized within the uterine cavity before removal is attempted. If there is any suggestion of a perforated IUD, laparoscopy is indicated to exclude bowel or bladder involvement. Removal of the IUD is usually achieved with a Spencer Wells forceps directed to the stem of the IUD. Hysteroscopic resection may be required if the IUD is embedded.

A check hysteroscopy is recommended following retrieval to confirm that no remnant has been left behind and good hemostasis has been achieved, and to exclude visceral damage.

Laparoscopy

This should ideally be performed by experienced laparoscopic gynecologists who are able to deal with the coexisting morbidity of a perforated IUD.

During laparoscopy, the IUD is frequently found to be adherent to viscera and therefore adhesiolysis and hemostatic control are usually required, as was the situation in Case history 2 (Figure 176.3). If the IUD is found to have translocated in part into the bowel or bladder, it is good practice to involve surgical or urologic colleagues to perform a sigmoidoscopy or cystoscopy, respectively. A multidisciplinary approach should be considered in laparoscopic retrieval of IUD [7]. Any pelvic abscess associated with the perforated IUD should be drained and cultured, followed by a thorough pelvic wash with normal saline.

Occasionally, the IUD is not easily seen at laparoscopy if it is located beyond loops of bowel or high in the abdominal cavity, or has translocated into the bowel lumen or bladder. Intraoperative X-ray may therefore be required to locate the IUD and to minimize unnecessary visceral trauma in attempting to find the IUD.

Laparotomy

Laparotomy may be indicated in complex cases where the procedure cannot be completed safely laparoscopically.

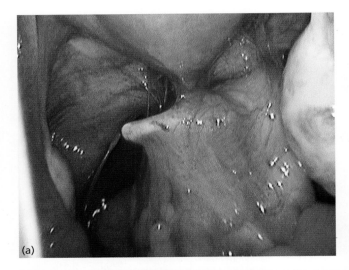

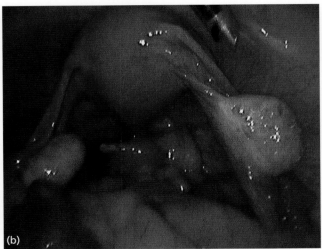

Figure 176.3 (a, b) Perforated intrauterine contraceptive device embedded in the rectal serosa.

Combined hysteroscopy and laparoscopy (with or without cystoscopy)

When consenting patients for hysteroscopic removal of IUD, it is good practice to obtain consent for laparoscopy and cystoscopy so that these may be performed if necessary.

During hysteroscopy, if the entire IUD is not visualized within the uterine cavity or there is any suggestion of a perforation, laparoscopy to exclude bowel or bladder involvement should be performed. If there is no involvement of other viscera, the IUD may be removed with a Spencer Wells forceps and hemostasis confirmed in the combined procedure.

Consent for combined laparoscopy and hysteroscopy is also indicated when the IUD is *in utero* with a concurrent ectopic pregnancy.

Other interventions

Ultrasound or preoperative CT may localize the IUD in the bowel or bladder. These cases should be referred to a colorectal surgeon or urologist for retrieval by sigmoidoscopy or cystoscopy as appropriate.

Prevention

Most uterine perforations associated with IUD occur during insertion. An acutely flexed uterus or previous cesarean section may predispose the woman to this complication. Insertion of IUD under ultrasound guidance may help prevent this complication.

Previous uterine perforation is not a contraindication for IUD and is not established as a risk factor for uterine perforation. The Faculty of Sexual and Reproductive Healthcare (UK) suggests that repeat attempts to insert an IUD should be made at intervals of at least 6 weeks [1].

The IUD thread should be cut at about 2 cm from the external cervical os. A short IUD thread may be associated with "lost thread" and can be uncomfortable for the sexual partner.

KEY POINTS

Challenge: Surgery for missing intrauterine contraceptive device.

Background
- Most surgical retrieval of IUD involves *in utero* IUD with a "lost thread."
- Uterine perforation associated with IUD is uncommon. However, it can lead to pelvic adhesions, visceral damage, infection, and abscess formation.
- Perforated IUD can translocate into various abdominal structures. Laparoscopic retrieval may involve a multidisciplinary team.
- The IUD should be localized by ultrasound prior to surgery. If the IUD is not seen *in utero*, a plain abdominal X-ray is required to confirm an extrauterine IUD.

Prevention
- In cases with acutely flexed uterus or previous cesarean section, ultrasound-guided insertion may be helpful.
- The IUD thread should be cut at about 2 cm from the external cervical os.

Management
- If the IUD is found in the uterus on transvaginal ultrasound, removal can be attempted with thread retriever or Spencer Wells forceps. If this is not possible, hysteroscopic removal may be needed.
- If the IUD is not seen in the uterus on ultrasound, a plain abdominal X-ray should be performed. If IUD is found in the pelvis or abdomen, laparoscopic removal may be possible. Intraoperative X-ray may be needed to locate the IUD.
- Patients should be counseled about (and consent obtained for) conversion to laparotomy, adhesiolysis, cystoscopy, and sigmoidoscopy.
- Antibiotic prophylaxis is often needed.
- Consider multidisciplinary team approach, particularly the involvement of bowel surgeons or urologists.

References

1 Faculty of Sexual and Reproductive Healthcare Clinical Effectiveness Unit. Intrauterine contraception, November 2007. http://www.fsrh.org/pdfs/CEUGuidanceIntrauterineContraceptionNov07.pdf (accessed 31 December 2011).

2 Zhou L, Harrison-Woolrych M, Coulter DM. Use of the New Zealand Intensive Medicines Monitoring Programme to study the levonorgestrel releasing intrauterine device (Mirena). *Pharmacoepidemiol Drug Saf* 2003;12:371–377.

3 Hopkins MR, Agudelo-Suarez P, El-Nashar SA, Creedon DJ, Rose CH, Famuyide AO. Term pregnancy with intraperitoneal levonorgestrel intrauterine system: a case report and review of the literature. *Contraception* 2009;79:323–327.

4 Zhang L, Chen J, Wang Y, Ren F, Yu W, Cheng L. Pregnancy outcome after levonorgestrel-only emergency contraception failure: a prospective cohort study. *Hum Reprod* 2009;24:1605–1611.

5 Moschos E, Twickler DM. Does the type of intrauterine device affect conspicuity on 2D and 3D ultrasound? *AJR Am J Roentgenol* 2011;196:1439–1443.

6 Turok DK, Gurtcheff SE, Gibson K, Handley E, Simonsen S, Murphy PA. Operative management of intrauterine device complications: a case series report. *Contraception* 2010;82:354–357.

7 Cook J, Martin A, Warren O, Tan TL. Term pregnancy with LNG-IUS embedded in the rectal mucosa. *J Obstet Gynaecol* 2011;31:546.

CHAPTER 177

Management of Imperforate Hymen, Transverse and other Vaginal Septa

Jane MacDougall

Addenbrooke's Hospital, Cambridge University Hospitals NHS Foundation Trust, Cambridge, UK

Case history: A 16-year-old girl was referred with a history of cyclical pelvic pain, and a palpable pelvic mass. She was diagnosed with primary amenorrhea and a hematocolpos secondary to an imperforate hymen. She was added to an emergency gynecology list for incision of the hymen. A pregnancy test was negative and an ultrasound confirmed a hematocolpos.

Background

The hematocolpos identified in the case history may be due to an imperforate hymen (Figure 177.1). However, it is vital to exclude a transverse vaginal septum as the surgical management is different (Figure 177.2). Other causes of a hematocolpos include vaginal or cervical agenesis and other complex Müllerian anomalies. It is important to seek the opinion of a clinician with expertise in pediatric and adolescent gynecology with complex cases.

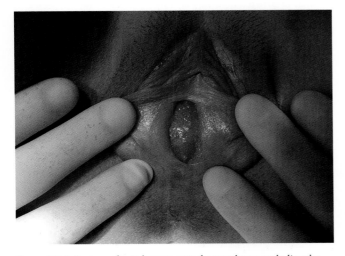

Figure 177.1 An imperforate hymen: note the membrane occluding the vagina is at the level of the hymenal ring and is bluish, translucent and bulging. Source: Ecran *et al.*, 2011 [13]. Reproduced with permission.

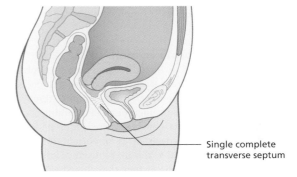

Single complete transverse septum

Figure 177.2 Schematic diagram of a transverse vaginal septum.

Classification and embryology

There have been several attempts at classifying Müllerian anomalies. The American Society of Reproductive Medicine (previously the American Fertility Society) classification (Chapter 100), which is based on the degree of failure of normal development, is probably the most useful [1].

Transverse vaginal septa are thought to arise as a result of failure in either the fusion or canalization of the urogenital sinus and Müllerian ducts. Their position varies from low (15–20%), to middle (30–40%) to high (46%) and they can vary in thickness from a few millimeters to several centimeters [2,3]. Occasionally there are two separate septa. They may be further complicated by hematometra, bilateral hematosalpinges, pelvic endometriosis, and pressure symptoms, causing urinary retention and constipation.

Examination and investigations

It is important to exclude pregnancy. Puberty should be staged from both the history (onset of pubarche and thelarche) and examination (Tanner staging). The appearance of the introitus is the key to making the right diagnosis. If the membrane occluding the vagina is at the level of the hymenal ring and is bluish, translucent and bulging, then this suggests an imperforate hymen. However, if the tissue is pink and flat, then the diagnosis is likely to be a transverse vaginal septum.

Gynecologic and Obstetric Surgery: Challenges and Management Options, First Edition. Edited by Arri Coomarasamy, Mahmood I. Shafi, G. Willy Davila and Kiong K. Chan.
© 2016 John Wiley & Sons, Ltd. Published 2016 by John Wiley & Sons, Ltd.

An MRI scan should be organized in all patients where a transverse vaginal septum is suspected from the clinical appearances, or if there is any doubt about the diagnosis [4]. This will help to define the site and thickness of the septum, confirm the presence of a cervix, and identify the amount of vagina above and below the septum. The renal tracts should also be imaged as associated anomalies occur [5,6].

Symptoms can be controlled by downregulation with a GnRH analog with or without HRT (or alternatively with the oral contraceptive pill taken continuously) while the diagnosis is confirmed. Patients with thick, middle or upper transverse septa should be referred to a tertiary center. With inadequate initial surgery the vagina will restenose and subsequent surgery is very difficult; outcomes can be poor.

Management

Surgery for an imperforate hymen
If there is a clear diagnosis of an intact hymen, surgery involves incision of the hymen. Different authors have recommended variations in technique from simple incision to complete removal [3,7]. Many advise a cruciate or radial incision with trimming of the tissue back to the level of the hymenal ring. There is little evidence to support any particular approach. It is important to avoid instrumenting the vagina or uterus as this may introduce infection. Patients and their parents should be warned that altered old blood will continue to drain for some days. Patients should not use tampons until their next normal menses, again to avoid infection.

Surgery for a transverse vaginal septum
Surgical management involves the removal of the whole septum and re-anastomosis of the upper and lower vaginal mucosa by a surgeon who is familiar with the necessary technique. If the septum is thought to be thin and low, then an EUA can be performed. It is helpful to insert a needle attached to a syringe into the septum under antibiotic cover; if brown fluid is obtained within 0.5 cm, then excision of the septum should be straightforward. If the septum is thick this will involve mobilization of the vaginal walls in order to reattach the upper to the lower vagina [2,3]. A combined abdominoperineal approach may be necessary [2]. Occasionally the distance to be bridged is too great and an interposition skin or intestinal graft is required. Some authors recommend preoperative dilation of the transverse septum to decrease its thickness [8]. It is often easier if there is a hematocolpos present as this will have stretched the upper vagina and there will therefore be more vaginal tissue available for the re-anastomosis. Care must be taken to avoid damage to the urethra or rectum. For the more complex repairs some authors recommend leaving a large catheter or mold in the vagina to prevent stricture formation [9]. A balloon catheter has also been used with serial dilation over a transvaginally inserted guidewire to create an outflow tract without surgery [10]. Some authors have recommended the use of vaginal dilators postoperatively to maintain patency and avoid stricture, although the appropriateness of this approach is contentious given the young age at which these patients often present.

There are few studies that have assessed long-term outcomes. These patients are at risk of developing endometriosis, menstrual irregularity, dyspareunia, and infertility [5,6,11]. Patients with middle or high transverse vaginal septa are less likely to conceive than patients with low septa or imperforate hymen [12].

It is important to address a patient's psychological, sexual, and reproductive needs both preoperatively and postoperatively.

Other vaginal septa
Cyclical pain and a unilateral hematocolpos in a patient who has been menstruating may be due to another type of vaginal septum, an obstructed hemivagina. In this case there is uterine duplication with vaginal septation; blood collects behind the lateral septum and at EUA there is a patent vagina with a cervix and a paravaginal mass. The kidney on the obstructed side is often absent (uterus didelphys with obstructed hemivagina and ipsilateral renal agenesis).

Unobstructive longitudinal vaginal septa are often asymptomatic and will not cause hematocolpos. They may present with difficulties in inserting tampons or dyspareunia [2] or when a cervical smear is first attempted. Longitudinal vaginal septa are often associated with other duplications of the internal genitalia (uterine didelphys, bicornuate uterus, and uterine septum) and are secondary to fusion abnormalities of the two Müllerian ducts.

In an obstructed hemivagina, surgery involves the excision of a window in the vaginal septum. The septal wall is then excised to create a single vagina. It is usually difficult to assess the optimum amount of tissue to resect at the initial surgery, so a two-stage procedure may be necessary. Surgical excision of a longitudinal septum is relatively straightforward, although the vagina is very vascular and care must be taken with hemostasis and to avoid causing a defect or vaginal stricture.

KEY POINTS

Challenge: Management of imperforate hymen, transverse and other vaginal septa.

Background
- Primary amenorrhea and cyclical abdominal pain with normal pubertal development and a hematocolpos may be due to:
  - Imperforate hymen.
  - Transverse vaginal septum.
  - Other Müllerian duct anomalies (rare).

Management
- It is vital to make the correct diagnosis as the surgical management is different.
- An imperforate hymen is characterized by a bulging bluish translucent membrane and can be managed surgically with a cruciate or radial incision.

- A transverse vaginal septum is characterized by flat pink tissue.
- Preoperative work-up for transverse vaginal septa includes:
  - MRI will clarify the diagnosis, the position, and thickness of the septum.
  - Downregulation with GnRH analog with or without HRT can control symptoms and allow time to make the diagnosis and plan treatment.
- The type of surgery depends on the nature of the transverse vaginal septum:
  - Surgery for low, thin, transverse septa involves removal of the whole septum by an experienced surgeon.
  - Patients with thick, middle, or upper transverse vaginal septa should be referred to a tertiary center.
- The patient's psychological, sexual, and reproductive needs should be addressed by a multidisciplinary team both preoperatively and postoperatively.

References

1 American Fertility Society. The American Fertility Society classification of adnexal adhesions, distal tubal occlusion, tubal occlusion secondary to tubal ligation, tubal pregnancies, mullerian abnormalities and intrauterine adhesions. *Fertil Steril* 1988;49:1944–1955.

2 MacDougall J, Creighton S. Surgical correction of vaginal and other anomalies. In: Balen AH, Creighton SM, Davies MC, MacDougall J, Stanhope R (eds) *Paediatric and Adolescent Gynaecology. A Multidisciplinary Approach*, pp. 120–130. Cambridge University Press, Cambridge, 2004.

3 Edmonds DK, Rose GL. Outflow tract disorders of the female genital tract. *Obstetrician & Gynaecologist* 2013;15:11–17.

4 Minto CL, Hollings N, Hall-Craggs M, Creighton S. Magnetic resonance imaging in the assessment of complex Mullerian anomalies. *Br J Obstet Gynaecol* 2001;108:791–797.

5 Joki-Erkkila MM, Heinonen PK. Presenting and long-term implications and fecundity in females with obstructing vaginal malformations. *J Pediatr Adolesc Gynecol* 2003;16:307–312.

6 Nazir Z, Rizvi RM, Qureshi RN, Khan ZS, Khan Z. Congenital vaginal obstructions: varied presentation and outcome. *Pediatr Surg Int* 2006;22:749–753.

7 Basaran M, Usal D, Aydemir C. Hymen sparing surgery for imperforate hymen: case reports and review of literature. *J Pediatr Adolesc Gynecol* 2009;22:e61–e64.

8 Hurst BS, Rock JA. Preoperative dilatation to facilitate repair of the high transverse vaginal septum. *Fertil Steril* 1992;57:1351–1353.

9 Van Bijsterveldt C, Willemsen W. Treatment of patients with a congenital transverse vaginal septum or a partial aplasia of the vagina. The vaginal pull through versus the pushthrough technique. *J Pediatr Adolesc Gynecol* 2009;22:157–161.

10 Kansagra AP, Miller CB, Roberts AC. A novel image-guided balloon vaginoplasty method to treat obstructive vaginal anomalies. *J Vasc Interv Radiol* 2011;22:691–694.

11 Deligeoroglou E, Iavazzo C, Sofoudis C, Kalampokas T, Creatsas G. Management of hematocolpos in adolescents with transverse vaginal septum. *Arch Gynecol Obstet* 2012;285:1083–1087.

12 Rock JA, Zacur HA, Dlugi AM, Jones HW Jr, Te Linde RW. Pregnancy success following surgical correction of imperforate hymen and complete transverse vaginal septum. *Obstet Gynecol* 1982;59:448–451.

13 Ecran CM, Karasahin KE, Alanbay I, Ulubay M, Baser, I. Imperforate hymen causing hematocolpos and acute urinary retention in an adolescent girl. *Taiwanese J Obstet Gynecol* 2011:50;118–120.

CHAPTER 178

Benign Lesions in the Groin and Vulva

Jennifer Byrom

Birmingham Women's NHS Foundation Trust, Birmingham, UK

Case history: A 56-year-old woman presents as an emergency with a painful lesion in the vulva. She explains that for 6 months she has had an itchy lump which has now become painful. She describes having had a vulval swelling operated on 10 years previously under general anesthesia. She is keen to avoid general anesthesia.

Background

Benign conditions affecting the vulva and groin include dermatoses, infections, neoplasms, and non-neoplastic cysts or lesions (Box 178.1). The requirements for accurate diagnosis and appropriate management are a thorough history, clinical examination, and relevant microbiology and histology specimens.

Management

Preparation

For examining the vulva, taking biopsies and performing minor operations, a colposcopy couch has advantages; however, this is not always necessary or possible. Adequate exposure with good lighting at the foot of a bed is the minimum requirement.

The area for biopsy or treatment should be prepared with a mild antiseptic solution (e.g., 0.05% chlorhexidine gluconate). The area is then infiltrated with 1–3 mL of local anesthetic such as 1% lidocaine via a dental syringe or 25-gauge needle. Anesthetics containing epinephrine prolong the anesthetic effect and promote vasoconstriction. Hemostasis can be achieved with silver nitrate, ferric subsulfate (Monsel's solution), or with interrupted absorbable sutures (e.g., 4-0 Vicryl Rapide).

Biopsy technique

An adequate biopsy of the vulval skin can usually be obtained with a Keyes punch, available in diameters ranging from 2 to 5 mm. As well as taking diagnostic biopsies, the Keyes punch can often be used to remove small lesions. When performing a diagnostic biopsy, the site selected should be representative of the abnormality; however, inflamed, ulcerated or necrotic areas should be avoided as they often yield minimal useful tissue for analysis. The cutting edge of the Keyes punch is applied perpendicular to the skin surface and rotated to the end of the metal "blade" to ensure a full skin thickness specimen. The area can then be excised with a scalpel blade.

BOX 178.1 CONDITIONS AFFECTING THE VULVA

Non-infectious dermatoses
Contact dermatitis
Lichen sclerosus
Lichen planus
Lichen simplex
Zoon's vulvitis
Psoriasis
Seborrheic dermatitis
Pemphigus/pemphigoid
Erythema multiforme
Hailey–Hailey disease
Crohn's disease
Urticaria
Behçet's disease

Neoplasms
Seborrheic keratosis
Vulval intraepithelial neoplasia
Extramammary Paget's disease
Squamous cell carcinoma
Basal cell carcinoma
Melanoma
Adenocarcinoma
Lentigo
Moles
Angiomyxoma
Lipoma

Non-neoplastic cysts or swellings
Epidermal inclusion cysts
Skin tags
Fibroepithelial polyps
Hemangioma
Pyogenic granuloma
Epidermoid cyst
Endometriosis
Paraurethral cysts
Bartholin's cysts
Vestibular gland cysts
Abscesses

Gynecologic and Obstetric Surgery: Challenges and Management Options, First Edition. Edited by Arri Coomarasamy, Mahmood I. Shafi, G. Willy Davila and Kiong K. Chan.
© 2016 John Wiley & Sons, Ltd. Published 2016 by John Wiley & Sons, Ltd.

Larger lesions can be removed under local anesthetic using an elliptical incision around the lesion and closed with an absorbable suture. If larger excisional biopsies or multiple biopsies are required, then general anesthesia may be more appropriate depending on the woman's general medical health.

Cysts and abscesses

Vulval and groin cysts are generally asymptomatic but can cause extreme acute pain due to enlargement or infection. The most commonly affected area is within the Bartholin's glands, which are located posteriorly at the base of the labia minora and drain through 2.5-cm ducts that exit into the vestibule at approximately the 4 and 8 o'clock positions. The glands are usually the size of a pea and are not palpable unless the duct becomes blocked or in the presence of infection. Appropriate swabs should be performed as up to 20% of Bartholin's gland abscesses are associated with *Neisseria gonorrhoeae* [1]. However, more recent reports suggest much lower incidences of gonorrhea [2], with most cases with positive cultures being caused by opportunistic organisms (coliforms being the most commonly detected).

Bartholin's abscesses rarely resolve with antibiotic therapy alone and hence usually require drainage. Marsupialization is the conventional surgical management approach [3]. Whether adjuvant antibiotic therapy is necessary following surgical treatment of Bartholin's abscess is controversial and the optimal initial therapy is not known. In cases of gonorrhea or *Chlamydia* appropriate antibiotic therapy should be administered. However, as most other infections are polymicrobial, a broad-spectrum drug such as co-amoxiclav may be the most suitable empirical treatment until cultures become available.

The ducts of the Skene glands, which drain on either side of the urethra, can also become blocked resulting in cyst formation or infection necessitating drainage.

Surgical techniques

The aim of treatment is to preserve the gland and its function, and can usually be performed under local anesthesia, reserving general anesthesia for larger cysts and abscesses. Although lancing an abscess or cyst will provide immediate relief, many clinicians discourage the approach of simple incision and drainage as recurrence rates are high. Furthermore, incision and drainage may make later Word catheter placement or marsupialization difficult. However, a systematic review of the management of Bartholin's cysts and abscesses failed to identify the best treatment approach [4].

Cyst removal

Removal of a Bartholin's cyst is associated with hemorrhage and scarring and does not preserve the function of the gland, hence it should be reserved for recurrent cysts or for postmenopausal women in whom a carcinoma, though rare, may be detected.

Under general anesthesia, the cyst is elevated by gentle pressure from within the vagina. An incision is made over the cyst at the medial aspect of the labia minora longitudinally. The skin edges can be grasped with delicate clamps and the cyst mobilized by blunt and sharp dissection. The lower pole should be detached first, after performing a rectal examination to gauge proximity of the cyst

wall to the rectum. After mobilizing the lower pole, dissection can continue to the upper pole. The wound should be closed in layers with absorbable sutures [5].

Complications include damage to adjacent organs, severe hemorrhage, hematoma formation, infection, and recurrence. If hemostasis is difficult to achieve, the placement of a small drain may minimize postoperative hematoma formation.

Ablation

After incising the cyst or abscess there are several techniques for destroying the cyst base [4]. Reported techniques include the application of silver nitrate, alcohol instillation, and use of the carbon dioxide (CO_2) laser. In one study the use of silver nitrate was compared with marsupialization in the outpatient setting; both approaches were found to be equally effective with similar recurrence rates [6]. A study evaluating CO_2 laser vaporization showed that it was well tolerated under local anesthetic, with cure rates of over 85% [7].

Marsupialization

After appropriate anesthesia, a 1–2 cm incision is made in a longitudinal direction at the region of the gland opening over the cyst or abscess. The contents can then drain. Any loculations should be broken down digitally. The wall of the cyst is then sutured to the vestibular skin with interrupted sutures. A small wick soaked in saline or proflavine can be inserted and allowed to fall out. The opening shrinks over the following few weeks [5].

Recurrences tend to occur if the incision was too small, the cyst wall was not sutured properly to the skin, or loculations were not drained. Recurrence rates of 0–15% have been reported [1,4].

Fistulization

This is a technique whereby a new epithelialized outflow tract for an obstructed Bartholin's duct is created. This can be achieved by a small Foley catheter, Jacobi ring, or Word catheter (Figure 178.1). The Word catheter is a safe and simple outpatient alternative to marsupialization [4].

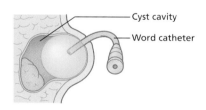

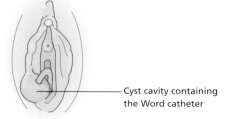

Figure 178.1 Word catheter being used to treat a Bartholin's cyst or abscess. Adapted from Mol *et al.*, 2011 [8].

The technique for placement of a Word catheter involves making a 5-mm stab incision through the vestibular mucosa. This incision should be within the introitus external to the hymenal ring in the area of the duct orifice. Any loculations should be broken down. The bulb of the Word catheter is inserted and inflated up to 3 mL with sterile saline to hold it in place; a suture may also be placed around the catheter. The short free end of the catheter is then placed in the vagina. The catheter is left *in situ* for

4–6 weeks. Recurrence rates are reported as 4–17%. Premature loss of the device is the most commonly reported complication. A multicenter randomized controlled trial (the Woman study) comparing recurrence rates and acceptability between traditional surgical marsupialization under general anesthesia and placement of a Word catheter in the outpatient setting has just finished recruiting. The results from this study will help inform best practice.

KEY POINTS

Challenge: Benign lesions in the groin and vulva.

Background
- Benign conditions affecting the vulva and groin include dermatoses, infections, neoplasms, and non-neoplastic cysts or lesions.
- There are several techniques that can be used for taking vulval biopsies and for managing vulval cysts or abscesses.
- Most procedures can be performed with local anesthesia.

Management
- Adequate exposure with good lighting is the minimum requirement for examination.
- Any biopsy area should be prepared with a mild antiseptic solution (e.g., 0.05% chlorhexidine gluconate).
- A biopsy area can be infiltrated with 1–3 mL of local anesthetic with or without epinephrine.
- A biopsy can be obtained with Keyes punch or scalpel.
- Hemostasis can be achieved with silver nitrate, Monsel's solution, or absorbable sutures.
- Cysts and abscesses can be managed by a number of techniques which include:
  - Marsupialization.
  - Cyst removal.
  - Ablation.
  - Fistulization with a Word catheter.

References

1 Cheetham DR. Bartholin's cyst: marsupialization or aspiration? *Am J Obstet Gynecol* 1985;152:569–570.
2 Bhide A, Nama V, Patel S, Kalu E. Microbiology of cysts/abscesses of Bartholin's gland: review of empirical antibiotic therapy against microbial culture. *J Obstet Gynaecol* 2010;30:701–703.
3 Kaufman RH, Faro S (eds) *Benign Diseases of the Vulva and Vagina*, 4th edn, pp. 168–248. Mosby, St Louis, MO, 1994.
4 Wechter MA, Wu JM, Marzano D, Haefner H. Management of Bartholin duct cysts and abscesses. *Obstet Gynecol Surv* 2009;64:395–404.
5 Raz S. *Atlas of Transvaginal Surgery*, 2nd edn, pp. 303–304. WB Saunders, Philadelphia, 2002.
6 Mungan Q, Uğur M, Yalçin H, Alan S, Sayilgan A. Treatment of Bartholin's cyst and abscess: excision versus silver nitrate insertion. *Eur J Obstet Gynecol Reprod Biol* 1995;63:61–63.
7 Figueiredo AC, Duarte PE, Gomes TP, Borrego JM, Marques CA. Bartholin's gland cysts: management with carbon-dioxide laser vaporization. *Rev Bras Ginecol Obstet* 2012;34:550–554.
8 Mol BWJ, Roovers JP, Morssink LP, Reesink-Peters N, Kroese JA, Kop PAL. Management of Bartholin gland cyst and abscess: marsupialization or Word catheter. *Protocol Version* 3, 23 March 2011 (unpublished).

CHAPTER 179

Cystic Structure in the Upper Vagina

Ted M. Roth[1] and G. Rodney Meeks[2]

[1] Central Maine Medical Center, Lewiston, Maine, USA
[2] University of Mississippi School of Medicine, Jackson, Mississippi, USA

Case history: A 54-year-old woman was noted to have a vaginal bulge during a routine cervical screen. A cystic structure was noted along the anterior vaginal wall and was initially thought to be a urethral diverticulum. The patient did admit to some mild feelings of vaginal pressure, but did not complain of urgency, frequency, incontinence, or obstructive voiding symptoms. She denied recurrent urinary tract infections. The mass measured 3 × 3 cm. The urethral meatus itself was unremarkable. Cystoscopy showed normally located ureteral orifices. An MRI was obtained which was consistent with a Gartner's duct cyst (GDC). Marsupialization of the cyst drained clear fluid and the resultant cavity was smooth with a blind end.

Background

The urogenital system develops from intermediate mesoderm and forms the urogenital ridge and mesonephric ducts between 3 and 8 weeks of gestation. Distal portions of the mesonephric ducts and attached ureteric buds become incorporated into the posterior wall of the primitive bladder to become the ureters, trigone, and bladder neck. The paramesonephric ducts develop lateral to the mesonephric ducts and form the fallopian tubes and uterus. Distal mesonephric ducts in the female are typically absorbed. GDCs arise from vestigial remnants of the mesonephric ducts. The cysts are classically located along the anterolateral vaginal wall, as the duct extends from the mesosalpinx between layers of the broad ligament to the cervix. While most GDCs are limited to the vaginal walls, larger cysts may reach the ischiorectal fossa. In contrast, Bartholin cysts are usually located in the posterolateral wall of the inferior third of the vagina.

There is an association between GDCs and abnormalities of the metanephric urinary system, with cases of ectopic ureter, unilateral renal agenesis and hypoplasia reported [1–3]. There are case reports of GDCs associated with congenital vesicovaginal fistula and adult urethrovaginal fistula [4].

Management

Assessment

Patient history should include onset and duration of symptoms including pain, voiding dysfunction, dyspareunia, association with menses, and urogynecologic surgical history. A history of urgency, frequency, and recurrent urinary tract infections should alert the surgeon to the possible presence of a urethral diverticulum (Chapter 126) in the differential diagnosis. Continuous urinary incontinence may represent an ectopic ureterocele. Physical examination should assess the lesion in terms of location, consistency, tenderness, mobility, and the possibility of pelvic organ prolapse. A GDC is retrovesical and bulges into the bladder wall. The cyst does not communicate with the bladder, bladder neck, or urethra, and does not change in shape and size with alterations in intravesical pressure, so pressure applied to the cyst will not lead to leakage of urine or extrusion of purulent material from the urethral meatus.

Differential diagnoses includes urethral diverticulum, Skene's gland cyst or abscess, vaginal wall cyst, leiomyoma, ectopic ureterocele, and obstructed hemivagina often associated with uterine didelphys. When GDCs are large enough, they may also be mistaken for cystoceles.

Imaging may be required to help further characterize the lesion. MRI is particularly useful in the diagnosis of vaginal cysts and urethral diverticulum. GDCs have been observed in 1–2% of female pelvic MRI scans [5]. A GDC exhibits low signal intensity on T1-weighted images and high signal intensity on T2 images as simple cysts. However, when intracystic contents are present (e.g., protein, mucin, or blood), GDCs have intermediate to high signal intensity on T1-weighted images. Neither the cyst nor its wall enhances with intravenous contrast. Ultrasonographic depiction of GDCs is also described [6] and allows for evaluation of the upper tracts.

In cases where the patient complains of urinary incontinence, urodynamics, cystourethroscopy, and voiding cystourethrography may also be appropriate to help confirm the cause of the urinary incontinence and assess for the presence of ureteral ectopy, ureteral reflux, and urethrovaginal fistula. MRI can be used in lieu of voiding cystourethrography.

Surgical technique

Under general anesthesia, we typically approach a GDC via a superficial sagittal incision along the vaginal sidewall. Epithelial flaps are developed and the cyst is skeletonized and removed. Small vascular pedicles are uncommonly encountered. At times, opening and decompressing the cyst, especially larger ones, may facilitate visualizing the surrounding anatomy. In this way, portions of the cyst wall can be peeled from the surrounding fibromuscular tissue. We obliterate the dead space with

Gynecologic and Obstetric Surgery: Challenges and Management Options, First Edition. Edited by Arri Coomarasamy, Mahmood I. Shafi, G. Willy Davila and Kiong K. Chan.
© 2016 John Wiley & Sons, Ltd. Published 2016 by John Wiley & Sons, Ltd.

sutures reapproximating the surrounding fibromuscular tissue and close the vaginal epithelium separately. Depending on the size of the cyst bed, a drain may be left in place.

Marsupialization may also be performed in the same way as for symptomatic Bartholin's cysts. Cyst aspiration and sclerosis with 5% tetracycline injection has been reported [7]. There are no long-term follow-up data or grade A studies.

Recurrence rates are not reported in the literature. If a GDC is associated with an ectopic ureter, then further surgical intervention may be warranted including ureteral reimplantation, fistula repair, or removal of a dysplastic kidney.

Prevention

Steps should be taken to minimize the chances of discovering unexpected pathology during surgical management of GDC. While there is no standard of care for preoperative imaging of vaginal cysts, a pelvic MRI may be a useful diagnostic modality to help with surgical planning and is the gold standard for excluding paraurethral pathology. It is also helpful for patient counseling.

KEY POINTS

Challenge: Cystic structure in the vagina (Gartner's duct cyst).

Background
- GDCs arise from vestigial remnants of the mesonephric ducts.
- The cysts are classically located along the anterolateral vaginal wall, as the duct extends from the mesosalpinx between layers of the broad ligament to the cervix.

Management
- Patient history should include onset and duration of symptoms including pain, voiding dysfunction, urgency, recurrent UTIs, dyspareunia, association with menses, and urogynecologic surgical history.

- Physical examination should assess the lesion in terms of location, consistency, tenderness, mobility, and the possibility of pelvic organ prolapse.
- MRI is recommended for GDCs and suspected urethral diverticulum.
- Symptomatic GDCs may be treated by cyst excision, marsupialization, or sclerosis.
- If the GDC is associated with upper tract anomalies, more extensive surgery may be warranted.

Prevention
- Minimize chances of discovering unexpected pathology or associated upper tract anomalies.
- Consider MRI prior to surgical intervention and to help with patient counseling.

References

1 Gotoh T, Koyonagi T. Clinicopathological and embryological considerations of single ectopic ureters in Gartner's duct cyst: a unique subtype of single vaginal ectopia. *J Urol* 1987;137:969–972.
2 Currarino G. Single vaginal ectopic ureter and Gartner's duct cyst with ipsilateral renal hypoplasia and dysplasia (or agenesis). *J Urol* 1982;128:988–993.
3 Sheih C, Hung C, Wei C, Lin C. Cystic dilatations within the pelvis in patients with ipsilateral renal agenesis or dysplasia. *J Urol* 1990;144:324–327.

4 Dwyer PL, Rosamilia A. Congenital urogenital anomalies that are associated with the persistence of Gartner's duct: a review. *Am J Obstet Gynecol* 2006;195:354–359.
5 Eilber KS, Raz S. Benign cystic lesions of the vagina: a literature review. *J Urol* 2003;170:717–722.
6 Sherer DM, Abulafia O. Transvaginal ultrasonographic depiction of a Gartner duct cyst. *J Ultrasound Med* 2001;20:1253–1255.
7 Abd-Rabbo MS, Atta MA. Aspiration and tetracycline schlerotherapy: a novel method for management of vaginal and vulval Gartner cysts. *Int J Gynaecol Obstet* 1991;35:235–237.

CHAPTER 180
Adnexal Masses in Infants and Children

Rachel J. Miller and Kris Ann P. Schultz
Children's Hospitals and Clinics of Minnesota, Minneapolis, Minnesota, USA

Case history: A 2-year-old child presents with precocious puberty and a protruberant abdomen. Laboratory studies show normal α-fetoprotein (AFP) and bHCG but elevated inhibin A and B. Unilateral salpingo-oophorectomy is performed with appropriate intraoperative staging including peritoneal fluid cytology. Pathology shows a juvenile granulosa cell tumor.

Background

Clinical presentation and evaluation in infants

Adnexal masses in neonates are usually first discovered on antenatal sonography. They may also present as an abdominal mass. Neonatal cysts are usually physiologic, reflecting the influence of maternal hormones. They may be simple or have a complex appearance if there is hemorrhage or torsion.

Antenatally diagnosed ovarian cysts should be followed with an early postnatal ultrasound prior to hospital discharge. The imaging quality will be superior to antenatal imaging. The initial evaluation should include a careful history and physical examination with attention to any prenatal or family history of congenital genitourinary anomalies or maternal health problems such as thyroid disease.

Clinical presentation and evaluation in children

Children with adnexal masses may present with pain from torsion, rupture, infarction or hemorrhage, or with non-specific symptoms such as abdominal swelling, distension, urinary frequency or retention, a palpable mass, or as an incidental finding detected on imaging for a separate condition [1]. Systemic signs including fever and poor weight gain or rarely respiratory distress due to increased intra-abdominal pressure may be present. However, most malignancies present with an asymptomatic mass. Ovarian stromal tumors may present with hormonal symptoms including precocious puberty, or signs of virilization including voice changes, acne, hirsutism, or cliteromegaly.

The initial evaluation should include a careful history and physical examination with attention to any personal or family history of neoplastic or dysplastic conditions, congenital genitourinary anomalies, and the presence of endocrine manifestations such as precocious puberty, virilization or thyroid nodules [2–6].

When an adnexal mass is suspected based on clinical findings, a pelvic ultrasound is usually the first imaging modality used. Advantages of ultrasound over other imaging modalities include the lack of exposure to radiation and avoidance of the need for sedation. The addition of Doppler is not helpful in determining the presence or absence of torsion [7].

CT may provide additional details for patients with a particularly large or heterogeneous mass, but is not necessary in all cases. When imaging in addition to ultrasound is deemed necessary, MRI may provide additional detail without the concern for radiation exposure raised by CT, but this option may be limited in young children by the potential need for sedation. When MRI is used for evaluation of a suspected ovarian tumor, the radiologist should be notified of the clinical concern so that the appropriate imaging protocol may be used.

Germ cell tumors are the most common ovarian neoplasms in children. Therefore, when a mass suspicious for neoplasm is seen, tumor markers including AFP, bHCG and LDH should be drawn. When signs of hormone production such as precocious puberty or virilization or other clinical findings associated with an ovarian stromal tumor are present, additional tumor markers comprising inhibin A and B, testosterone, and CA125 should also be evaluated. Although most classically elevated in germ cell tumors, ovarian stromal tumors may also be associated with elevated AFP, especially Sertoli–Leydig cell tumors with retiform differentiation. If imaging shows concern for a malignant neoplasm, CA125 and measurement of serum calcium may also be helpful as elevated serum calcium may provide an important clue to the presence of small cell carcinoma of the hypercalcemic type, a rare but aggressive epithelial malignancy requiring specific intraoperative and postoperative management.

Differential diagnosis

The differential diagnosis of adnexal masses in childhood includes both non-neoplastic and neoplastic conditions. Pelvic non-neoplastic masses in infancy and childhood include simple follicular cysts, complex functional cysts, and congenital malformations including hydrocolpos.

Physiologic cysts are uncommon during childhood prior to puberty because of low gonadotropin stimulation of the ovaries. Follicular cysts remain the most common cause of simple cysts. Follicular cysts may be seen in McCune–Albright syndrome, characterized by precocious puberty, lytic bone lesions, and

Gynecologic and Obstetric Surgery: Challenges and Management Options, First Edition. Edited by Arri Coomarasamy, Mahmood I. Shafi, G. Willy Davila and Kiong K. Chan.
© 2016 John Wiley & Sons, Ltd. Published 2016 by John Wiley & Sons, Ltd.

café-au-lait spots [8]. Other ovarian cysts can occur in response to central precocious puberty.

An asymptomatic ovarian cystic mass that has few internal echoes consistent with hemorrhage and no calcifications or septations is usually benign. Suspected torsion is likely to result from a benign tumor, as the presentation is rare with malignant neoplasms [9–11]. Ovarian malignancies comprise 1% of childhood cancers [12].

Management

Management in infants
Small simple and complex cysts measuring less than 4–5 cm can be followed with serial ultrasound imaging. Interventions such as aspiration or surgery should be considered for cysts that are symptomatic, more than 4–5 cm in size, enlarging, or persisting for greater than 6 months [13]. Congenital vaginal anomalies resulting in hydrocolpos can be confused for an adnexal cyst. This condition can be expectantly managed until puberty.

Management in children
Simple cysts may be expectantly managed with serial ultrasound scans as the majority will spontaneously resolve. Cystectomy may be undertaken for large persistent benign cysts as they are more likely to represent a serous or mucinous cystadenoma and place the adnexa at risk for torsion.

Surgical approach via laparotomy and robotic or standard laparoscopy will vary based on surgical experience and preferences. Clinical factors to take into account when selecting the type of surgery include the age and size of the patient relative to mass. Intraoperative management must consider the likelihood of malignancy and the potential impact on future reproductive function and fertility.

When severe pain is present, torsion should be suspected and urgent surgical intervention undertaken to preserve ovarian function. Detorsion is the initial procedure of choice [14]. A follow-up ultrasound can be performed to further assess a potential underlying neoplasm and interval procedure undertaken as necessary. Ovarian cystectomy is the preferred approach for managing non-malignant neoplasms; however, in the setting of significant edema, tissue planes may be compromised and hence the benefits of an interval procedure [15].

If clinical and radiographic findings are suggestive of a benign mature teratoma, ovarian-sparing surgery such as cystectomy should be considered. However, if the clinical findings are suggestive of a germ cell tumor with malignant potential (age <10 years, tumor >10 cm, and elevation of tumor markers), then appropriate staging per Children's Oncology Group guidelines should be performed [16,17]. Referral to a subspecialist with surgical experience in pediatric ovarian cancers is indicated. For most patients with germ cell tumors, a fertility-sparing approach is reasonable and preferred. Adequate staging includes collection of ascitic fluid or peritoneal washings for cytologic examination. Adequate staging also includes palpation of pelvic viscera and pelvic and retroperitoneal lymph nodes and inspection of the contralateral ovary with biopsy of any suspicious findings. If peritoneal studding is seen, these nodules should be biopsied. Presence of multiple peritoneal implants containing mature neuroepithelial components is deemed gliomatosis peritonei, a finding which is considered benign and does not change staging. The tumor capsule should not be violated or aspirated as this will result in upstaging.

If clinical and laboratory findings are suggestive of an ovarian stromal tumor, FIGO fertility-sparing staging procedures are necessary and should include unilateral salpingo-oophorectomy, but not hysterectomy [18]. Care to avoid intraoperative rupture is necessary. If rupture occurs, it is important to clearly denote whether the rupture occurred preoperatively or intraoperatively, because rupture may indicate the need for adjuvant therapy.

KEY POINTS

Challenge: Adnexal mass in an infant or child.

Background
- Adnexal masses in infants and children may present with abdominal fullness, palpable mass, or abdominal pain. Hormonal symptoms may be present.
- Physicians should be alert to the possibility of non-neoplastic or neoplastic conditions.
- Malignant adnexal neoplasms are rare in childhood.

Evaluation
- Careful clinical history, family history, and physical examination are integral to the diagnosis.
- Judicious use of imaging studies may provide clues to the underlying diagnosis.
- Tumor markers should be drawn preoperatively when a neoplastic lesion is suspected.

Management
- Operative approaches that spare fertility and future hormone production are preferred in infants and children.
- If preoperative evaluation suggests malignancy, appropriate staging is required.

References

1 Schultz KA, Sencer SF, Messinger Y, Neglia JP, Steiner ME. Pediatric ovarian tumours: a review of 67 cases. *Pediatr Blood Cancer* 2005;44:167–173.
2 Young RH. Sex cord-stromal tumours of the ovary and testis: their similarities and differences with consideration of selected problems. *Mod Pathol* 2005;18(Suppl 2):S81–S98.
3 Velasco-Oses A, Alonso-Alvaro A, Blanco-Pozo A, Nogales FF Jr. Ollier's disease associated with ovarian juvenile granulosa cell tumour. *Cancer* 1988;62:222–225.
4 Schultz KA, Pacheco MC, Yang J *et al.* Ovarian sex cord-stromal tumours, pleuropulmonary blastoma and DICER1 mutations: a report from the International Pleuropulmonary Blastoma Registry. *Gynecol Oncol* 2011;122:246–250.
5 Rio Frio T, Bahubeshi A, Kanellopoulou C *et al.* DICER1 mutations in familial multinodular goiter with and without ovarian Sertoli–Leydig cell tumours. *JAMA* 2011;305:68–77.

6 Heravi-Moussavi A, Anglesio MS, Cheng SW *et al.* Recurrent somatic DICER1 mutations in nonepithelial ovarian cancers. *N Engl J Med* 2012;366:234–242.
7 Linam LE, Darolia R, Naffaa LN *et al.* US findings of adnexal torsion in children and adolescents: size really does matter. *Pediatr Radiol* 2007;37:1013–1019.
8 Pienkowski C, Baunin C, Gayrard M, Lemasson F, Vaysse P, Tauber M. Ovarian cysts in prepubertal girls. *Pediatr Adolesc Gynecol* 2004;7:66–76.
9 Guthrie BD, Adler MD, Powell EC. Incidence and trends of pediatric ovarian torsion hospitalizations in the United States, 2000–2006. *Pediatrics* 2010;125:532–538.
10 Savic D, Stankovic ZB, Djukic M, Mikovic Z, Djuricic S. Torsion of malignant ovarian tumours in childhood and adolescence. *J Pediatr Endocrinol Metab* 2008;21:1073–1078.
11 Oltmann SC, Fischer A, Barber R, Huang R, Hicks B, Garcia N. Pediatric ovarian malignancy presenting as ovarian torsion: incidence and relevance. *J Pediatr Surg* 2010;45:135–139.

12 Breen JL, Maxson WS. Ovarian tumours in children and adolescents. *Clin Obstet Gynecol* 1977;20:607–623.

13 Ben-Ami I, Kogan A, Fuchs N *et al*. Long-term follow-up of children with ovarian cysts diagnosed prenatally. *Prenat Diagn* 2010;30:342–347.

14 Oltmann SC, Fischer A, Barber R, Huang R, Hicks B, Garcia N. Cannot exclude torsion: a 15-year review. *J Pediatr Surg* 2009;44:1212–1216; discussion 1217.

15 Oelsner G, Cohen SB, Soriano D, Admon D, Mashiach S, Carp H. Minimal surgery for the twisted ischaemic adnexa can preserve ovarian function. *Hum Reprod* 2003;18:2599–2602.

16 Oltmann SC, Garcia NM, Barber R, Hicks B, Fischer AC. Pediatric ovarian malignancies: how efficacious are current staging practices? *J Pediatr Surg* 2010;45:1096–1102.

17 Billmire D, Vinocur C, Rescorla F *et al*. Outcome and staging evaluation in malignant germ cell tumours of the ovary in children and adolescents: an intergroup study. *J Pediatr Surg* 2004;39:424–429.

18 FIGO Committee on Gynecologic Oncology. Current FIGO staging for cancer of the vagina, fallopian tube, ovary, and gestational trophoblastic neoplasia. *Int J Gynaecol Obstet* 2009;105:3–4.

CHAPTER 181

Nerve Injuries Associated with Gynecologic and Obstetric Surgery

Djavid Alleemudder

Salisbury NHS Foundation Trust, Salisbury, UK

Case history: A 45-year-old woman had an abdominal hysterectomy for menorrhagia due to a large multifibroid uterus. She presented postoperatively with weakness of hip flexion, adduction, and knee extension. There was also loss of the knee jerk reflex, and paresthesia over the anterior and medial thigh as well as the medial aspect of the calf. Electromyographic studies confirmed neuropraxia of the femoral nerve, likely due to nerve compression from self-retaining retractors used intraoperatively.

Background

The incidence of neuropathy following gynecologic surgery is between 1.1 and 1.9% [1]. Patient malpositioning, improper incision sites, and self-retaining retractors are major contributors to the origins of intraoperative gynecologic nerve injury. Prognosis is good for the majority of cases, with minimal or no intervention necessary for resolution of the neurologic impairment. However, a minority will sustain long-term complications necessitating prolonged treatment or even restorative surgery.

Three types of nerve injury can occur (Table 181.1). *Neuropraxia* is the result of external nerve compression, leading to disruption

Table 181.1 Pathophysiology of nerve injury.

Type of injury	Pathophysiology	Prognosis
Neuropraxia	External nerve compression	Recovery within weeks to months
Axonotmesis	Severe nerve compression with axon damage	Recovery takes longer, usually several months
Neurotmesis	Nerve transection with damage to Schwann cells	Poor prognosis without restorative surgery

of conduction across a small portion of the axon. *Axonotmesis* is caused by profound nerve compression or traction. Damage occurs to the axon only, with preservation of the supporting Schwann cells. Regeneration is possible because supporting Schwann cells remain intact. *Neurotmesis* is the most severe form of nerve injury and results from complete nerve transection or ligation, where both the axon and Schwann cells are disrupted and regeneration is impossible without restorative surgery.

The nerves most commonly injured during gynecologic surgery originate from the lumbosacral (L1–S3, Figure 181.1) and brachial (C5–T1, Figure 181.2) plexuses. A summary of the function of each nerve, the mechanism of intraoperative nerve injury, and clinical presentation if neuropathy occurs is provided in Tables 181.2 and 181.3.

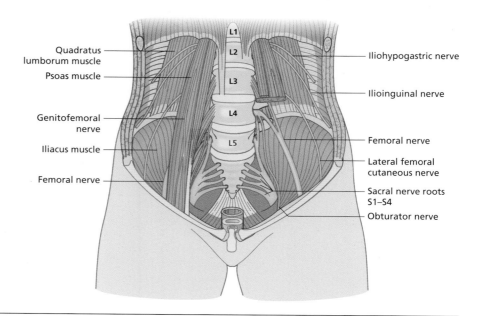

Quadratus lumborum muscle

Psoas muscle

Genitofemoral nerve

Iliacus muscle

Femoral nerve

Iliohypogastric nerve

Ilioinguinal nerve

Femoral nerve

Lateral femoral cutaneous nerve

Sacral nerve roots S1–S4

Obturator nerve

Figure 181.1 Lumbosacral plexus.

Gynecologic and Obstetric Surgery: Challenges and Management Options, First Edition. Edited by Arri Coomarasamy, Mahmood I. Shafi, G. Willy Davila and Kiong K. Chan.
© 2016 John Wiley & Sons, Ltd. Published 2016 by John Wiley & Sons, Ltd.

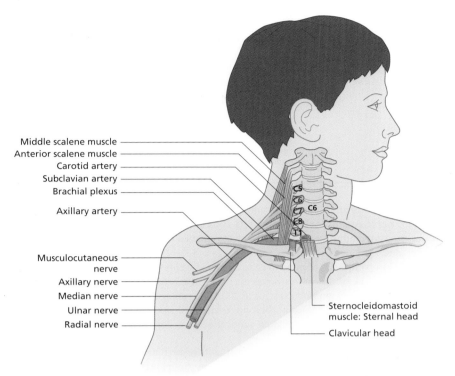

Figure 181.2 Brachial plexus.

Table 181.2 Lumbosacral plexus: summary of common nerve injuries.

Nerve	Origin	Sensory function	Motor function	Clinical presentation	Method of injury
Femoral	L2–L4	Anterior/medial thigh, medial aspect calf	Hip flexion/adduction Knee extension	Unable to climb stairs	Compression from deep or laterally placed retractors. Stretch injuries from improper lithotomy positioning
Obturator	L2–L4	Upper medial thigh	Thigh adduction	Minor ambulatory problems	Transection during retroperitoneal surgery, excision of endometriosis, and paravaginal defect repairs. Trocar insertion through obturator foramen and insertion of TOT tapes

Sciatic
  Common peroneal
  Tibial
	L4–S3	Below knee except medial foot
		  Lateral calf, dorsum foot
		  Toes, plantar surface foot
			Hip extension/knee flexion
			  Dorsiflexion/eversion foot
			  Plantar flexion/inversion foot
				Sciatica
				  Foot drop
				  Cavus deformity foot
					Stretch injuries from hyperflexion of thighs in improper lithotomy positions

Iliohypogastric	T12–L1	Mons, lateral labia, upper inner thigh	None	Sharp, burning pain radiating from incision site to mons, labia, or thigh	Suture entrapment at lateral borders of low transverse or Pfannenstiel incisions
Ilioinguinal	T12–L1	Groin, symphysis	None	Sharp, burning pain to groin, symphysis	Suture entrapment at lateral borders of low transverse or Pfannenstiel incisions
Pudendal	S2–S3	Perineum	None	Perineal pain	Entrapment during sacrospinous ligament fixation
Lateral cutaneous	L2–L3	Anterior/posterolateral thigh	None	Pain/paresthesia anterior/posterolateral thigh: meralgia paresthetica	Compression from deep or laterally placed retractors. Stretch injuries from improper lithotomy positioning
Genitofemoral	L1–L2	Labia, femoral triangle	None	Pain/paresthesia labia, femoral triangle	Transection during pelvic sidewall surgery and removal of the external iliac nodes

Management

The majority of neuropathies will resolve spontaneously with minimal intervention. Sensory neuropathies typically resolve within 5 days, whereas motor deficits may take up to 10 weeks to recover. Occasionally neuropathies persist beyond 1 year.

Neuropathic complaints are sometimes dismissed in the setting of residual anesthesia, incision pain, and postoperative analgesia, especially during the acute postoperative period. The opinion of a neurologist should be sought once a neuropathy has been identified. Detailed neurologic examination and electromyography (EMG) are key to diagnosing a neurologic deficit. EMG is useful in

Table 181.3 Brachial plexus: summary of common nerve injuries.

Nerve	Origin	Sensory function	Motor function	Clinical presentation	Method of injury
Ulnar	C8–T1	Medial 1½ fingers	Small muscles of hand	Claw hand	Compression injury from pressure placed on medial aspect of elbow during arm board positioning
Radial	C5–T1	Dorsal tips of lateral 3½ fingers	Wrist and finger extension	Wrist drop Unable to extend fingers	Compression injury from pressure on humerus during arm positioning
Erb's palsy	C5–C6	None	Abduction of shoulder, flexion of elbow, supination	Waiters tip	Stretch injury from arm boards extending beyond 90° from the long axis of the operating table or when the arm unknowingly falls from the arm board
Klumpke's palsy	C8–T1	Medial arm/forearm/hand and medial 2 fingers	Intrinsic muscles of hand	Claw hand	Stretch injury if shoulder brace positioned too laterally

identifying and localizing acute nerve injury by measuring sensory and motor nerve conduction velocity. EMG is usually performed 3–4 weeks postoperatively, as denervation of the afflicted muscle is often delayed.

Painful neuropathies can respond to pharmacologic agents known to be effective in the treatment of neurogenic pain, such as tricyclic antidepressants and γ-aminobutyric acid (GABA) antagonists. Painful neuropathies rarely persist beyond 6 months; however, if they do, local nerve blockade or even surgical nerve excision or decompression can be considered.

Motor impairment from retraction or stretch-related nerve injuries can be managed by physiotherapy, so as to maintain flexibility and range of movement. Active use of the muscles afflicted is generally recommended, although splinting may be protective against further injury.

Nerve lesions that do not heal are often the result of complete nerve transection. These nerves may be amenable to specialist repair using microsurgical techniques such as tension-free end-to-end anastomosis. The aim is to regain alignment of the epineurial sheath and neural fascicles.

Prevention

A thorough understanding of the anatomy of the lumbosacral and brachial nerve plexuses is necessary to minimize the risk of nerve injury during gynecologic operations. It is also important to preoperatively identify patients who are more prone to neurologic complications. Studies have shown that patients who have a thin body habitus, ill-developed abdominal wall muscles, or a narrow pelvis are more at risk of retractor blade-associated nerve injury [2–5]. Patients are at further risk if the operating time exceeds 4 hours.

A large number of iatrogenic lumbosacral nerve injuries during gynecologic surgery can be attributed to the incorrect positioning of self-retaining retractor blades. The gold standard of correct positioning is for the self-retractor blades to cradle the rectus muscle without compressing the psoas muscle underneath.

When positioning the retractors, the surgeon must check visually and by direct palpation that the psoas muscle is not entrapped between the blades and the pelvic sidewall. Furthermore, the shallowest retractor blade sufficient to provide adequate exposure should be chosen, as it has been suggested that the degree of nerve injury is proportional to blade length [6]. Rolled-up laparotomy pads may be used to cushion the retractor blades against the pelvic sidewall as a precaution. Retractor blade position should be monitored intermittently during the operation and readjusted accordingly.

I recommend undoing the retractors and repositioning at regular intervals to relieve blade pressure against the pelvic sidewall if a lengthy operation is being undertaken. As hand-held retractors will only exert intermittent as opposed to continual pressure on retracted tissue, they should be selected over self-retaining ones wherever possible [2].

Particular attention must be paid to the correct preoperative positioning of the patient in lithotomy stirrups. The proper lithotomy position dictates that the hip and knee are only moderately flexed. At the hip, there should be minimal abduction and external rotation. The stirrups or boots should be at equal height. Excessive movement around the hip joint results in stretch and/or compression of the sciatic and femoral nerves.

Common peroneal nerve injury is avoided when there is padding in place between the lateral fibular heads and the stirrup, thus preventing nerve compression against a hard surface. As with abdominal surgery, the length of operative time during lithotomy has been cited as a significant risk factor for increasing the risk of nerve injury, especially if operating time exceeds 2 hours [7].

A surgeon should avoid extending the incision beyond the lateral margins of the rectus muscles, where the ilioinguinal and iliohypogastric nerves lie. If wide margins are necessary, upward curving incisions should be made to avoid the path of the underlying nerves.

Shoulder braces, if used during steep Trendelenburg, should be positioned over the acromio-clavicular joint, thus preventing brachial plexus injury. During surgery, the upper arm must be pronated and padding should be adequately draped over the posteromedial elbow to prevent ulnar nerve compression against the operating table.

KEY POINTS

Challenge: Nerve injuries in obstetric and gynecologic surgery.

Background
- Nerve injuries are a common complication of gynecologic surgery, occurring in 1.1–1.9% of cases.

- Patient malpositioning, incorrect placement of self-retaining retractors, hematoma formation, and direct nerve entrapment or transection are the primary mechanisms for perioperative nerve injury.
- Nerves most commonly injured during surgery include the femoral, ilioinguinal, pudendal, obturator, lateral cutaneous, iliohypogastric, and genitofemoral nerves.

Management
- The majority of neuropathies resolve with conservative management and physiotherapy.
- Patients with significant neurologic deficit should be seen by a neurologist and have detailed neurologic examination, as well as EMG studies as appropriate.
- SSRIs, tricyclic antidepressants, and GABA antagonists are of significant benefit in managing painful neuropathies.
- Transected nerves may require specialist surgical repair.

Prevention
- Correct positioning of self-retaining retractor blades is important. The retractor blades should be regularly loosened and repositioned in long operations.
- The retractor blades should be cushioned in slim patients; it is ideal practice to cushion the blades in all patients.
- Correct positioning and padding of the patient in lithotomy stirrups will reduce the risk of nerve injuries.
- In prolonged laparoscopic surgery, it is important to regularly reposition the legs.
- Abdominal incisions should aim to avoid injury to ilioinguinal and iliohypogastric nerves that lie beyond the lateral margins of the rectus muscles.

References

1 Bohrer JC, Walters MD, Park A, Polston D, Barber MD. Pelvic nerve injury following gynecologic surgery: a prospective cohort study. *Am J Obstet Gynecol* 2009;201:531e1–7.
2 Goldman JA, Feldberg D, Dicker D, Samuel N, Dekel A. Femoral neuropathy subsequent to abdominal hysterectomy. A comparative study. *Eur J Obstet Gynecol Reprod Biol* 1985;20:385–392.
3 Kenrick MM. Femoral nerve injuries following pelvic surgery. *South Med J* 1963;56:152–156.
4 Rosenblum J, Schwartz GA, Bendler E. Femoral neuropathy: a neurological complication of hysterectomy. *JAMA* 1966;195:409–414.
5 Vosburgh LF, Finn WF. Femoral nerve impairment subsequent to hysterectomy. *Am J Obstet Gynecol* 1961;82:931–937.
6 Georgy FM. Femoral neuropathy following abdominal hysterectomy. *Am J Obstet Gynecol* 1975;123:819–822.
7 Warner MA, Martin JT, Schroeder DR, Offord KP, Chute CG. Lower-extremity motor neuropathy associated with surgery performed on patients in a lithotomy position. *Anesthesiology* 1994;81:6–12.

CHAPTER 182
Consent Challenges

William Parry-Smith and Martyn Underwood
Shrewsbury and Telford Hospitals NHS Trust, Telford, Shropshire, UK

Case history 1: A 35-year-old patient has a diagnosis of deep transverse arrest at 8 cm dilatation with a pathologic CTG. The recommendation of the obstetrician is that a cesarean section is performed to reduce harm to both the mother and the baby. The risks and benefit of cesarean section are discussed with the patient, who refuses to consent to the cesarean section.

Case history 2: A 25-year-old patient with learning difficulties attends the gynecology department accompanied by her mother. The patient's mother requests that her daughter is sterilized as she is concerned that if her daughter became pregnant she would be unable to care for the baby.

Background

Consent in the field of obstetrics and gynecology can be a challenge from a variety of situations as illustrated in the case histories. The law varies from country to country, and even within one country, for example the devolved nations of the UK. As a general rule for avoiding consent pitfalls, it is important to work in partnership with patients and respect their decisions about their care, to exercise clinical judgment, and to ensure patients have capacity to make a decision about their care [1]. If in doubt, it is advisable to seek senior support, and the advice of the hospital legal department and defense union; if safe and practical, it is prudent to delay surgery while the appropriate advice is obtained.

Management

The Mental Capacity Act (MCA) 2005 (UK) sets out a framework intended to empower and protect people who may lack capacity, and has the aim of ensuring any decisions made in the circumstances where the patient may lack capacity are in their best interests [2]. The safeguarding and protection of the vulnerable is at the heart of the legislation, and it is not intended to complicate or hinder the consent process. The decision and assessment of capacity rest on whether the patient can understand the information relevant to the decision, retain that information, use that information as part of a process of making a decision, and communicate the decision.

The principles of the MCA [2] include the following.
- A person must be assumed to have capacity unless it is established that the person lacks capacity.
- A person is not to be treated as unable to make a decision unless all practicable steps to help the individual to do so have been taken.
- A person is not to be treated as unable to make a decision merely because he or she makes an unwise decision.
- An act done, or decision made, under this Act for or on behalf of a person who lacks capacity must be done, or made, in his or her best interests.
- Before the act is done, or the decision is made, regard must be had to whether the purpose for which it is needed can be as effectively achieved in a way that is less restrictive of the person's rights and freedom of action.

If it is judged that the patient lacks capacity, then the advice in Box 182.1 should be followed. The General Medical Council (GMC, UK) has published detailed and clear guidance relating to consent and the documentation of consent [1]. The guidance suggests that the written documentation of consent should be used when a complex treatment with significant risks is involved, when significant consequences for the patient are at stake, and in situations such as research participation. In emergency situations, such as those encountered on a labor ward, oral consent with documentation in the medical notes is satisfactory instead of a signed consent form. However, if feasible and if the situation allows, a signed consent form should be sought. In situations where the patient is in significant pain or distress, oral consent with a record in the medical notes of their oral consent is permissible [1].

BOX 182.1 PATIENT LACKING CAPACITY: ADVICE

- Act in the person's best interest
- Involve family, friends, and carers in decision-making; if they are not available consider an independent mental capacity advocate (IMCA)
- Always seek advice from experienced colleagues and the hospital legal service

In the event of dispute
- Involve an advocate who is independent of all the parties involved
- Get a second opinion
- Hold a formal or informal case conference
- Go to mediation
- An application could be made to the Court of Protection for a ruling

Source: adapted from Office of the Public Guardian [3].

It is advisable to re-confirm consent prior to proceeding with treatment, especially in the situation where consent has been taken in the clinic prior to surgery. The majority of hospital consent forms are designed in such a way that confirmation of consent on the day of surgery can be readily documented.

Children and young people pose a particular challenge in terms of consent, and must always be involved in discussions about their care. The basic principles of acting in the best interests of the patient, fostering a collaborative approach between the child, parents or guardian, combined with clear communication, holds true. Given the complexity of consent involving children and young people, the use of senior colleagues and legal advice is encouraged if required. As a rule, parents are likely to be the best judges of what is in their child's best interest and should make decisions in this regard, until such a time as the child or young person has capacity to take over this role [4]. The mental capacity of children and young people is assessed in the same way as that of adults; 16 year olds are presumed to have capacity but if younger than 16 they may have capacity depending on maturity and understanding. A 15-year-old child may have the capacity to consent to any procedure, from a vaccination to a laparotomy; however, the decision-making process and complexity of the latter situation requires greater maturity. If a child lacks capacity, the consent of a parent or guardian is required. In the situation where there is dispute between parents or their decision is not in the best interest of their child in the opinion of the medical team caring for the child, legal advice and a court ruling may be required. It is the duty of a doctor to act in the best interest of their patient and this duty may on occasion be in conflict with the wishes of a parent or guardian.

The provision of contraception to a young person less than 16 years of age has been much discussed in the literature. In effect the right of a young person to access medical services, not just relating to contraception, provided they have capacity, has been confirmed by case law. The implications for child protection in cases where underage sexual activity occurs need to be balanced with the rights and wishes of a young person; however, it is worth noting that sexual activity under the age of 13 years should trigger a child protection referral [5].

Resolution of the cases

Case history 1

A detailed assessment of the patient's mental capacity must be made and it would be wise to check with her family and the birth partner if her behavior and thought processes were usual for her. The risks and consequences of not agreeing to a cesarean section must be discussed, including uterine rupture and maternal and fetal death, or disability or lifelong impairment. The involvement of a second senior clinician and consultation with the hospital's legal team is advisable.

If after detailed discussion and having ensured that the patient has capacity and is acting voluntarily and not under duress, consent is not given for cesarean section, then the patient must be supported in her decision and afforded all necessary ongoing care and treatment as required.

Case history 2

Assessing the capacity of the patient is the key issue. If the patient's learning difficulties are mild and it is deemed that capacity is not impaired, then one could proceed to sterilization at the patient's request, and not the mother's request. However, if the patient does not have capacity and the mother requests sterilization, based on the judgment of Mr Justice Cobb in the Court of Protection in 2013 and his recommendations, an application for a decision by the Court of Protection should be made [6]. The key to understanding how best to act in this case is the argument set out in the MCA that any treatment should be as least restrictive as possible. In the case of sterilization, there are arguably less permanent and as effective options available, which would achieve the same objective and be more aligned to the principle of acting in the patient's best interests.

KEY POINTS

Challenge: Consent challenges.

Background
- Consent in surgery, and particularly obstetrics and gynecology, can be complex.
- A person must be assumed to have capacity unless it is established that the person lacks capacity.
- A person is not to be treated as unable to make a decision merely because he or she makes an unwise decision.

Management
- Act in the person's best interest.
- Involve family, friends, and carers in decision-making; if they are not available, consider an independent mental capacity advocate (IMCA).
- Always seek advice from experienced colleagues and the hospital legal service.

In the event of dispute
- Involve an advocate who is independent of all the parties involved.
- Get a second opinion.
- Hold a formal or informal case conference.
- Go to mediation.
- An application could be made to the Court of Protection for a ruling.

References

1 General Medical Council. *Consent: patients and doctors making decisions together.* Available at http://www.gmc-uk.org/guidance/ethical_guidance/consent_guidance_index.asp

2 Mental Capacity Act 2005 c. 9. http://www.legislation.gov.uk/ukpga/2005/9

3 Office of the Public Guardian. *Making decisions: a guide for people who work in health and social care.* https://www.gov.uk/government/uploads/system/uploads/attachment_data/file/348440/OPG603-Health-care-workers-MCA-decisions.pdf

4 General Medical Council. *0–18 years: guidance for all doctors.* Available at http://www.gmc-uk.org/guidance/ethical_guidance/children_guidance_index.asp

5 NSPCC. Gillick competency and Fraser guidelines. NSPCC factsheet, March 2014. http://www.nspcc.org.uk/Inform/research/briefings/gillick_wda101615.html (accessed 5 April 2014).

6 A Local Authority v K [2013] EWHC 242 (COP) (15 February 2013).

CHAPTER 183
Dealing with Complaints

Mahmood I. Shafi

Addenbrooke's Hospital, Cambridge University Hospitals NHS Foundation Trust, Cambridge, UK

Case history 1: A 55-year-old woman attending the gynecology clinic complained to the Patient Advice and Liaison Service that the doctor seeing her had been rude and dismissive during the consultation and did not show any respect.

Case history 2: A 90-year-old woman's daughter wrote a letter after her mother was operated on, to complain that her care on the ward had been substandard, the ward was dirty, and she was discharged home too early.

Background

Complaints in healthcare can arise from a variety of different issues. They can be initiated immediately or a considerable time after the event. The issues often revolve around one of the following.

- The patient is not happy with the environment (ward, clinic or another clinical area).
- The patient feels that the staff have been disrespectful.
- The patient has had transport or parking problems causing inconvenience (a common complaint in the UK).
- The patient feels that outcome from medical encounter was not satisfactory.
- The patient does not understand her management or has received conflicting information.

Patients are encouraged to raise any concerns immediately to staff, but if this does not happen, then the Patient Advisory and Liaison Service (PALS) is available; PALS aims to improve patient satisfaction and to reduce any confusion or anxiety about any issues raised. Most complainants have a genuine desire to try to improve the system so that others do not encounter similar experiences.

Management

A complaint can occasionally be expected but often occurs without notice. Patients are encouraged to take any concerns to PALS within the NHS as PALS can act quickly to deal with the situation before it becomes more serious.

In the case histories, a letter has been received by PALS, and there is a legal requirement to investigate and respond in a timely manner, usually taken as 25 working days. In exceptional or complex circumstances, there can be a mutually agreed extension.

Complaints should generally be relevant to the preceding 12 months of the event. The arrangements for dealing with a complaint comprise the following.

- Complaints are dealt with efficiently.
- Complaints are properly investigated.
- Complainants are treated with respect and courtesy.
- Complainants receive, so far as is reasonably practical, the assistance to enable them to understand the procedure in relation to complaints, or advice on where they may obtain such assistance.
- Complainants receive a timely and appropriate response.
- Complainants are told the outcome of the investigation of their complaint.
- Action is taken if necessary in the light of the outcome of a complaint.

The relevant healthcare providers should be advised of the complaint and a written report of the event should be obtained. During the response, all issues or questions should be addressed and the medical and nursing notes should always be used to construct the response.

In Case history 1, while a report from the doctor concerned is relevant, it may be beneficial to obtain additional reports from the nursing staff who may have been present during the consultation. It is important to find out if any issues were raised at the time and, if so, how were they addressed. Outcomes of the investigations should be used as a reflective exercise to improve future behavior.

In Case history 2, there are issues of perceived substandard care (medical and nursing), the environment (cleanliness), and early hospital discharge while the patient did not feel able to cope. All of these are equally important matters and reports should be sought from the relevant staff. If there has been substandard care, this should be acknowledged and an apology given. Necessary lessons should be learnt and disseminated. Managing the patient's expectations regarding hospital discharge should occur from the time of initial consultation, with uniform advice given in relation to expected length of stay. It is important to take into account home circumstances in planning discharge. Social services may need to be involved as well as the family to make sure that appropriate support is in place for the patient's discharge from hospital.

Very rarely, if there is failure to come to a satisfactory conclusion with a complaint, the patient has recourse to involve the Health Service Ombudsman, which will act as a neutral party in any dispute.

Gynecologic and Obstetric Surgery: Challenges and Management Options, First Edition. Edited by Arri Coomarasamy, Mahmood I. Shafi, G. Willy Davila and Kiong K. Chan.
© 2016 John Wiley & Sons, Ltd. Published 2016 by John Wiley & Sons, Ltd.

Prevention

Complaints (and "thank you" letters) provide feedback regarding a service. This can be relevant to the individual or the organization. Complaints must be used to improve the quality of services and outcomes for patients. The vast majority of patients are satisfied with the explanation and, if appropriate, an apology.

Meeting the expectations of patients and their relatives is an important aspect of healthcare provision. When there is a real or perceived failure to provide adequate professional care in a clean safe environment, complaints can arise. Patients should be encouraged to voice these contemporaneously as they can then be addressed immediately for an improved outcome. If this is not possible or the patient does not feel empowered, then a well-developed PALS system can help patients understand the issues, and many complaints can be appropriately dealt with in an informal manner. Organizations need a "learning culture" in that senior individuals within the healthcare system need to take a personal interest and disseminate learning to the rest of the organization. This should reduce the recurrence of issues raised and improve clinical outcomes.

KEY POINTS

Challenge: Dealing with complaints.

Background
- Patients have certain statutory rights within the NHS.
- Complaints can arise from a variety of issues either directly or indirectly related to patient care.

Management
- Many complaints can be managed informally with the right approach.

- There is a statutory response mechanism.
- Once a complaint is received, a comprehensive response to the relevant issues needs to be provided in a timely manner.
- A senior individual within the organization needs to take responsibility for managing or overseeing all complaints.

Prevention
- Having a learning and open environment to complaints can be beneficial in reducing complaints.
- Good medical, nursing and associated care should be striven for in all caregiving institutions.

Further reading

http://www.nhs.uk/Service-Search/Patient-advice-and-liaison-services-(PALS)/Location/363

http://www.nhs.uk/chq/Pages/1082.aspx?CategoryID=68

Bennett L, MacDougall J. Responding to complaints. *Obstet Gynaecol Reprod Med* 2008;18:23–24.

CHAPTER 184

Dealing with Litigation

Rebekah Ley and Mahmood I. Shafi
Cambridge University Hospitals NHS Foundation Trust, Cambridge, UK

Case history: A 58-year-old woman attended for an elective hysterectomy. She suffered a bladder injury which was not recognized during the operation. Diagnosis of the injury was made 7 days after the operation, and was successfully repaired via a laparoscopic approach. Her hospital stay was prolonged and complicated by a bladder infection.

Background

Investigations and treatment for gynecologic problems are among the most common of medical procedures, as most women will need some form of gynecologic care during their lives. Claims in respect of gynecologic care can be due to an action by a doctor that causes a gynecologic injury or a failure to recognize or treat a gynecologic complication or injury.

Common claims include postoperative complications, infection, failed sterilization operations and wrongful birth, unnecessary or failed procedures, cancer misdiagnosis, misinterpretation of test result(s), and failure to warn.

Management

A clinical negligence claim is a demand for financial compensation for alleged harm caused by substandard clinical care. While the common reasons for claims in gynecology are listed above, it is also important to note that many claims arise out of poor communication.

It is important to remember that if the claim relates to care and treatment that a clinician provided on a private basis, he or she must immediately inform the body providing professional indemnity. If the claim relates to care and treatment provided as part of NHS duties, it is likely that the clinician will be informed about any claim via the hospital department that deals with claims.

In order to bring a successful claim, the patient has to prove on the balance of probabilities that the treatment she received was such that no reasonable practitioner would have delivered that care (known as *breach of duty*), and that the breach of duty or negligence caused or contributed to the patient's suffering or poor outcome (known as *causation*).

The *clinical negligence pre-action protocol* aims to resolve claims without the need to go to court. The protocol represents an opportunity to resolve matters swiftly and efficiently, so avoiding the stress, time and costs associated with formal court proceedings, where it is appropriate and possible to do so. The time limits under the protocol are short and require close cooperation from clinicians to maximize the chance of resolution.

If a lawyer or patient requests copies of the patient's medical records and has the appropriate consent, the request must be acknowledged within 14 days and copies of the records must be supplied within 40 days. If the patient wishes to bring a claim, she must send the doctor a *Letter of Claim* setting out her version of events, the alleged injury, and the compensation sought. The doctor's representatives then have 4 months to send the patient a *Letter of Response*. If a clinician is asked to respond to the allegations set out in a Letter of Claim, he or she needs to respond and include the following: (i) what was done, (ii) why it was done, setting out the reasoning, and (iii) what the medical records contain to support the clinician's version of events.

A Letter of Response may make admissions (i.e., agree with some of the alleged points of negligence). If a Letter of Response denies liability (i.e., there was no negligent care) and a claimant still wishes to claim compensation, then they have to issue *proceedings*. Less than 2% of claims go to court for a trial. Even when formal legal proceedings are issued, most claims are either discontinued, or settled by mediation or negotiation before trial. It is very unlikely that attendance at court to give evidence will be required. However, in some cases claims do progress to formal proceedings and trial.

The first stage of court proceedings is that a summons is prepared and issued in a court (followed by it being served). The basic time limit for issuing proceedings is 3 years from the date of injury, or the date the patient knew she had been caused an injury. However, this can be longer in certain circumstances: if the patient was a child, then time does not start to run until the child reaches the age of 18; if the injured party was mentally ill; if there was an interval before the patient realized, or could be expected to know about the injury. For example, a child who was brain damaged during birth could bring a claim as an adult. What this means in practice is that there could be many years between the incident and the claim.

Gynecologic and Obstetric Surgery: Challenges and Management Options, First Edition. Edited by Arri Coomarasamy, Mahmood I. Shafi, G. Willy Davila and Kiong K. Chan.
© 2016 John Wiley & Sons, Ltd. Published 2016 by John Wiley & Sons, Ltd.

Once court proceedings are issued the claimant has 4 months to serve the claim form, which means sending it to the defendant's hospital. It must be acknowledged within 14 days. In the unlikely event that a clinician receives court papers directly, he or she must alert the person who deals with claims immediately and this person can then acknowledge the claim form.

Prevention

After a clinical incident it is important for a patient to know what has gone wrong and why. An open explanation is important to restore trust and reduce the frustration and anger a patient will feel if he or she thinks they are being ignored; this can often be a catalyst for litigation.

In any clinical situation the clinician should undertake the following.

- Write legible and detailed notes. The medical records are essential evidential documents which can help demonstrate that the standards of care were appropriate. This is especially important as claims can be brought several years after the events. After a long time interval the clinician may only have the records to reconstruct details of what happened.
- Consider what colleagues would do in a similar situation. Clinical judgment is always important. However, if a doctor departs from guidelines or policy without clear and documented reasons for doing so, he or she will be left in the uncomfortable position of having to demonstrate this course of action was reasonable.
- Recognize and work within the limits of his or her competence and seek advice as appropriate. If advice is sought from a colleague about care and treatment, it is important to document this.

KEY POINTS

Challenge: Dealing with litigation.

Background
- A clinical negligence claim is a demand for financial compensation from a patient.
- In gynecology, claims might typically relate to an action by a doctor that causes a gynecologic injury or a failure to recognize or treat a gynecologic complication or injury.
- In order to bring a successful claim, the patient has to prove *breach of duty*, and *causation*.

Management
- Good communication is paramount.

- When responding to the allegations set out in a *Letter of Claim*, the *Letter of Response* must set out (i) what was done, (ii) why it was done, and (iii) what the medical records contain to support (i) and (ii).
- If a Letter of Response denies liability and the claimant still wishes to seek compensation, then formal proceedings may be issued, but it may yet be possible to resolve the claim by mediation or negotiation before trial.

Prevention
- Medical notes must always be written with sufficient detail to clearly show the treatment provided and reasons.
- It is important to work within the limitations of individual competence.
- If something goes wrong, then the patient must be given a prompt and open explanation of what happened.

Further reading

Medical Defence Union. http://www.themdu.com/
NHS Litigation Authority. http://www.nhsla.com/Pages/Home.aspx

Index

Page numbers in *italics* denote figures, those in **bold** denote tables.

Gynecologic and Obstetric Surgery: Challenges and Management Options, First Edition. Edited by Arri Coomarasamy, Mahmood I. Shafi, G. Willy Davila and Kiong K. Chan.
© 2016 John Wiley & Sons, Ltd. Published 2016 by John Wiley & Sons, Ltd.